Graber and Wilbur's

FAMILY MEDICINE
EXAMINATION
& BOARD REVIEW

Graber and Wilbur's
FAMILY MEDICINE EXAMINATION & BOARD REVIEW

FIFTH EDITION

Editors

Mark A. Graber, MD, MSHCE, FACEP
Clinical Professor
Departments of Family Medicine and Emergency Medicine
Roy J. and Lucille A. Carver College of Medicine
University of Iowa
Iowa City, Iowa

Brigit E. Ray, MD, MME
Clinical Assistant Professor
Department of Family Medicine
Roy J. and Lucille A. Carver College of Medicine
University of Iowa
Iowa City, Iowa

Jason K. Wilbur, MD, FAAFP
Clinical Professor
Department of Family Medicine
Roy J. and Lucille A. Carver College of Medicine
University of Iowa
Iowa City, Iowa

McGraw Hill

New York/Chicago/San Francisco/Athens/London/Madrid/Mexico City/
New Delhi/Milan/Singapore/Sydney/Toronto

Graber and Wilbur's Family Medicine Examination & Board Review, Fifth Edition

1 2 3 4 5 6 7 8 9 LWI 25 24 23 22 21 20

ISBN 978-1-260-44107-9
MHID 1-260-44107-5

Notice

Medicine is an ever-changing science. As new research and clinical experience broaden our knowledge, changes in treatment and drug therapy are required. The authors and the publisher of this work have checked with sources believed to be reliable in their efforts to provide information that is complete and generally in accord with the standards accepted at the time of publication. However, in view of the possibility of human error or changes in medical sciences, neither the authors nor the publisher nor any other party who has been involved in the preparation or publication of this work warrants that the information contained herein is in every respect accurate or complete, and they disclaim all responsibility for any errors or omissions or for the results obtained from use of the information contained in this work. Readers are encouraged to confirm the information contained herein with other sources. For example and in particular, readers are advised to check the product information sheet included in the package of each drug they plan to administer to be certain that the information contained in this work is accurate and that changes have not been made in the recommended dose or in the contraindications for administration. This recommendation is of particular importance in connection with new or infrequently used drugs.

This book was set in Minion Pro Regular by MPS Limited.
The editors were Kay Conerly and Kim J. Davis.
The production supervisor was Catherine H. Saggese.
Project management was provided by Ishan Chaudhary, MPS Limited.

This book is printed on acid-free paper.

Library of Congress Cataloging-in-Publication Data

Names: Graber, Mark A. (Mark Alan), editor. | Ray, Brigit E., editor. |
    Wilbur, Jason K., editor.
Title: Graber and Wilbur's family medicine examination & board review /
    editors, Mark A. Graber, Brigit E. Ray, Jason K. Wilbur.
Other titles: Family practice examination and board review. | Family
    medicine examination & board review
Description: Fifth edition. | New York : McGraw Hill Education, [2020] |
    Includes bibliographical references and index. | Summary: "In addition
    to its use as a board review book for family medicine, this publication
    can be employed as a general review for primary care physicians,
    physician assistants, and nurse practitioners"– Provided by publisher.
Identifiers: LCCN 2019043442 (print) | LCCN 2019043443 (ebook) | ISBN
    9781260441079 (paperback) | ISBN 9781260441086 (ebook)
Subjects: MESH: Family Practice | Examination Question
Classification: LCC R834.5 (print) | LCC R834.5 (ebook) | NLM WB 18.2 |
    DDC 610.76–dc23
LC record available at https://lccn.loc.gov/2019043442
LC ebook record available at https://lccn.loc.gov/2019043443

McGraw-Hill books are available at special quantity discounts to use as premiums and sales promotions, or for use in corporate training programs. To contact a representative, please visit the Contact Us pages at www.mhprofessional.com.

*To the people who make Family Medicine happen. **Jogjakarta**: Dr. Mora Claramita, Dr. Adi Heru Husodo, Dr. Wahyudi Istiono, and Dr. Fitriana Murriya. **Moscow**: Professor Dr. Gregorii Efimovich Roitberg, Dr. Olga Sharkun, Dr. Irina Slastnikova, Dr. Janna Dorosh, and Professor Timothy O'Connor. **Haiphong**: Dr. Hùng Nguyễn Văn, Dr. Linh Nguyễn, and Dr. Nguyễn Thuý Hiếu.*
—MAG

To my parents, Bill and Bonnie Ray, for always loving, supporting, and encouraging me to follow my dreams to become a family physician. To all of my Family Medicine and education mentors including: Drs. George Bergus, Rick Dobyns, Jason Wilbur, Bob Tallitsch, Jeff Pettit, and Marcy Rosenbaum. Your guidance and support along this journey have shaped me into the family physician educator I have become!
—BER

To my many mentors in Family Medicine, including Drs. John Ely, Mark Graber, Paul James, Gerald Jogerst, and Barcey Levy; and to Dr. Kate Thoma and all the Family Medicine program directors and faculty members who work tirelessly (and mostly thanklessly) to develop the next generation of excellent family doctors. Keep teaching; keep leading!
—JKW

Contents

Contributors

Emad Abou-Arab, MD, CME
Clinical Assistant Professor
Department of Family Medicine
Roy J. and Lucille A. Carver College of Medicine
University of Iowa
Iowa City, Iowa
10. Endocrinology

Daniel M. Anderson, DO
Senior Associate Consultant
Department of Neurology
Mayo Clinic Health System Franciscan Healthcare
La Crosse, Wisconsin
18. Neurology

A. Ben Appenheimer, MD
Clinical Assistant Professor
Department of Internal Medicine
Division of Infectious Diseases
Roy J. and Lucille A. Carver College of Medicine
University of Iowa
Iowa City, Iowa
8. Infectious Diseases
9. HIV/AIDS

Stacey Appenheimer, MD
Clinical Assistant Professor
Department of Family Medicine
Roy J. and Lucille A. Carver College of Medicine
University of Iowa
Iowa City, Iowa
14. Adolescent Medicine

Olivia E. Bailey, MD
Clinical Associate Professor
Department of Emergency Medicine
Roy J. and Lucille A. Carver College of Medicine
University of Iowa
Iowa City, Iowa
1. Emergency Medicine

Maresi Berry-Stoelzle, MD
Department of Family Medicine
Roy J. and Lucille A. Carver College of Medicine
University of Iowa
Iowa City, Iowa
6. Hematology and Oncology

Guru V. Bhoojhawon, MBBS, MD, FAAP
Clinical Associate Professor
Department of Pediatrics
Roy J. and Lucille A. Carver College of Medicine
University of Iowa
Iowa City, Iowa
13. Pediatrics

Nicholas R. Butler, MD, MBA
Clinical Associate Professor
Department of Family Medicine
Roy J. and Lucille A. Carver College of Medicine
University of Iowa
Iowa City, Iowa
21. Care of the Older Patient

Rachel R. Butler, MD
Clinical Assistant Professor
Department of Internal Medicine
Division of Pulmonary, Critical Care, and Occupational
   Medicine
Roy J. and Lucille A. Carver College of Medicine
University of Iowa
Iowa City, IA
3. Pulmonology

Meghan Connett, MD
Clinical Assistant Professor
Department of Family Medicine
Roy J. and Lucille A. Carver College of Medicine
University of Iowa
Iowa City, Iowa
15. Obstetrics and Women's Health

Dustin Z. DeYoung, MD
Psychiatrist
Behavioral Health Associates
University of California, Los Angeles
Los Angeles, California

Austin R. Fox, MD
Department of Ophthalmology and Visual Sciences
University of Iowa
Iowa City, Iowa
19. Ophthalmology

Mark A. Graber, MD, MSHCE, FACEP
Clinical Professor
Departments of Family Medicine and Emergency Medicine
Roy J. and Lucille A. Carver College of Medicine
University of Iowa
Iowa City, Iowa
1. Emergency Medicine
2. Cardiology
7. Gastroenterology
12. Orthopedics and Sports Medicine
26. Ethics
28. Evidence-Based Medicine
30. Final Examination

Erin Hayward, MD
Clinical Assistant Professor
Department of Family Medicine
University of Iowa
Iowa City, Iowa
22. Care of the Surgical Patient

Priyanka Iyer, MD, MPH
Clinical Associate Professor
Department of Internal Medicine
Division of Immunology
University of Iowa Clinics and Hospitals
Iowa City, Iowa
11. Rheumatology

Monika Jindal, MD
Instructor, University of Colorado School of Medicine
Department of Psychiatry
Department of Family Medicine
Denver Health Medical Center
Denver, Colorado
23. Psychiatry

Nicholas H. Kluesner, MD, FACEP
Associate Medical Director
Department of Emergency Medicine
UnityPoint Health – Des Moines
Des Moines, Iowa
26. Ethics

Jason Kruse, DO
Department of Internal Medicine
Broadlawns Medical Center
Des Moines, Iowa
7. Gastroenterology

Bharat Kumar, MD, MME, FACP, RhMSUS
Department of Internal Medicine and Division of
    Immunology
Department of Internal Medicine
Roy J. and Lucille A. Carver College of Medicine
University of Iowa
Iowa City, Iowa
11. Rheumatology

Aaron R. Kunz, DO, MA, MME
Clinical Assistant Professor
Department of Family Medicine
Roy J. and Lucille A. Carver College of Medicine
University of Iowa
Iowa City, Iowa
16. Men's Health

Victoria Linares, MD
CAQ Geriatric Medicine
Clinical Assistant Professor
Department of Primary Care
Loyola University Medical Center
Maywood, IL
21. Care of the Older Patient

Britt L. Marcussen, MD
CAQ Sports Medicine
Clinical Associate Professor
Department of Family Medicine
Roy J. and Lucille A. Carver College of Medicine
University of Iowa
Iowa City, Iowa
12. Orthopedics and Sports Medicine

Denise A. Martinez, MD
Clinical Associate Professor
Associate Dean for Diversity, Equity, and Inclusion
Department of Family Medicine
Roy J. and Lucille A. Carver College of Medicine
University of Iowa
Iowa City, Iowa
29. Patient-Centered Care

Patrick J. McCarthy, MD, MME
Assistant Professor
Section of Hospital Medicine, Department of Pediatrics
Medical College of Wisconsin/Children's Hospital of
    Wisconsin
Milwaukee, Wisconsin
13. Pediatrics

Sarah L. Miller, MD, FACEP, FAAP
Clinical Associate Professor
Department of Emergency Medicine
Roy J. and Lucille A. Carver College of Medicine
University of Iowa
Iowa City, Iowa
1. Emergency Medicine

Megan H. Noe, MD, MPH, MSCE
Instructor
Department of Dermatology
Brigham & Women's Hospital
Harvard Medical School
Boston, Massachusetts
17. Dermatology

Scott R. Owen, MD
Assistant Professor
Director of Facial Plastic and Reconstructive Surgery
Department of Otolaryngology, Head and Neck Surgery
University of Iowa
Iowa City, Iowa
20. Otolaryngology

Juan R. Pagan-Ferrer, MD, DABIM, Ger, HPM
Clinical Assistant Professor
Department of Internal Medicine
Roy J. and Lucille A. Carver College of Medicine
University of Iowa
Iowa City, Iowa
27. End-of-Life Care

Sanjeev Patil
Assistant Professor
Department of Rheumatology and Immunology
University of Vermont Medical Center
Burlington, VT

Brigit E. Ray, MD, MME
Clinical Assistant Professor
Department of Family Medicine
Roy J. and Lucille A. Carver College of Medicine
University of Iowa
Iowa City, Iowa
15. Obstetrics and Women's Health
22. Care of the Surgical Patient
30. Final Examination

Wendy W. Shen, MD, PhD
Clinical Associate Professor
Department of Family Medicine
Roy J. and Lucille A. Carver College of Medicine
University of Iowa
Iowa City, Iowa
4. Allergy and Immunology

Tameem A. Shoukih, MD
Clinical Assistant Professor
Departments of Emergency Medicine and Pediatrics
Roy J. and Lucille A. Carver College of Medicine
University of Iowa
Iowa City, Iowa
12. Orthopedics and Sports Medicine

Kelly Skelly, MD
Clinical Associate Professor
Department of Family Medicine
Roy J. and Lucille A. Carver College of Medicine
University of Iowa
Iowa City, Iowa
14. Adolescent Medicine

C. Blake Sullivan, MD
Resident Physician
Otolaryngology – Head and Neck Surgery
University of Iowa
Iowa City, Iowa
20. Otolaryngology

Melissa L. Swee, MD, MME
Clinical Assistant Professor
Department of Internal Medicine
Division of Nephrology
Roy J. and Lucille A. Carver College of Medicine
University of Iowa
Iowa City, Iowa
5. Nephrology

Teri Thomsen, MD
Clinical Associate Professor
Department of Neurology
Roy J. and Lucille A. Carver College of Medicine
University of Iowa
Iowa City, Iowa
18. Neurology

Alka Walter, MBBS, MS
Clinical Assistant Professor
Department of Family Medicine
Roy J. and Lucille A. Carver College of Medicine
University of Iowa
Iowa City, Iowa
22. Care of the Surgical Patient

Karolyn A. Wanat, MD, FAAD
Associate Professor
Department of Dermatology
Medical College of Wisconsin
Milwaukee, Wisconsin
17. Dermatology

Jason K. Wilbur, MD, FAAFP
Clinical Professor
Department of Family Medicine
Roy J. and Lucille A. Carver College of Medicine
University of Iowa
Iowa City, Iowa
2. Cardiology
6. Hematology and Oncology
16. Men's Health
24. Nutrition and Herbal Medicine
30. Final Examination

Qiang Zhang, MD
Movement Disorder Fellow
Department of Neurology and Iowa Neuroscience Institute
Physician Scientist Training Program
Clinical NeuroScientist Training Program
Roy J. and Lucille A. Carver College of Medicine
University of Iowa
Iowa City, Iowa
18. Neurology

Preface

Welcome to the fifth edition of *Graber & Wilbur's Family Medicine Examination & Board Review* book. We hope that you are as excited to be here as we are. The whole book has been meticulously updated to not only serve you well as a study guide, but also to provide you with cutting edge, up-to-date, information pertinent to your practice. For those of you who love your e-readers and tablets, there is a portable, electronic version of the book. You can also now find us on "AccessMedicine."

What is new? We have added a succinct guide to the recommended health maintenances for children and adults, perfect for a quick review. We estimate that 30% of the material has been changed since our last edition: think of hepatitis C diagnosis and treatment, new cholesterol and blood pressure guidelines, new heart failure guidelines (and drugs), the ever-changing anticoagulation guidelines, etc.

What has not changed? Our essential style remains the same. The book is divided into 29 chapters based on body system and elements of patient care, followed by the "Final Examination" (Chapter 30). The thousands of questions in the book are woven into cases, which we hope you will find interesting, practical, and relevant. To test your acquisition of knowledge, each case ends with the learning objectives. To break the monotony of slogging through a study guide, you will find "Quick Quizzes" and "Helpful Tips" peppered throughout each chapter.

A dozen years ago when we wrote the first edition, we made the decision to use the second-person voice in order to engage the reader better and to give the book a conversational appeal. We have tried to keep the book from being boring. Yes, we are aware that this is a study aid. But why must studying be an exercise in tedium and endurance? It should be enjoyable, applicable to real life and provide a surprise every now and again. You will find (sometimes feeble) attempts at humor throughout the book. We have noticed that an occasional reader does not appreciate our sense of humor. As Abraham Lincoln famously never said, "You can please some of the people all of the time, and then again, some people just won't think you're funny."

We have been impressed with the level of engagement of our readers. Over the years, we have received scores of e-mails from readers who have thanked us, corrected us, and sometimes chided us. No matter the intent of the message, the tone is almost universally positive—readers are invested in the book and want to offer helpful suggestions. Likewise, the comments posted online (not usually the place one goes for affirmation) have been mostly approving, constructive, and enthusiastic.

The first edition was published amid a less-than-friendly environment, with declining interest in print media and several well-known board review books already on the market. Because our book carried a different tone, readers slowly gravitated to it, and its market share grew by word-of-mouth. Engaged and supportive readers play a huge role!

In preparation for work on the fifth edition, we saved all of your e-mails and scoured the Internet for reader comments and reviews. We read and considered all that we could find—which amounted to several hundred readers' ideas. So, you, the reader, have helped shape this book. Keep those e-mails coming!

With all of the board review books out there, why should you choose our text? **There are two crucial differences between this book and other board review books on the market.** First, we have written this book not only to help you pass the boards but also to broaden your knowledge of family medicine. The majority of questions contain a detailed explanation not only of why an answer is right but also why the other answers are wrong. In the rapidly changing world of medical knowledge, we have endeavored to provide you with the most relevant and up-to-date evidence. When the current evidence is controversial and we are not certain what the American Board of Family Medicine (ABFM) will do with it, we acknowledge the uncertainty and try to help you navigate the current evidence.

We have tried to make this book as broad and as comprehensive as possible. In addition to its use as a board review book for family medicine, it can be employed as a general review for primary care physicians, physician assistants, and nurse practitioners. Students and residents studying for Step 3 of the licensing examination should find the book helpful as well. However, no board review book can possibly cover the entire scope of family medicine. Use these questions as a guide: what areas are your strengths and what do you need to study further? Each answer of the "Final Examination" is referenced in the book so you can go back and review any topic that you might have missed.

In this book, the use of eponymous medical terms such as Crohn disease and Wilson disease reflects the current American Medical Association recommendations for these and similar terms where the possessive form is dropped. In addition, there is a general trend toward using fewer eponyms, such as Wegener, which has been dropped completely. We have made note of both new and old terms when we have deemed the old term more recognizable.

We enjoyed writing this book and we hope that you enjoy using it. If you have suggestions or complaints (okay, maybe all of our jokes aren't politically correct or even funny), do not hesitate to write us at mark-graber@uiowa.edu, jason-wilbur@uiowa.edu, or brigit-ray@uiowa.edu. We take your comments seriously as we endeavor to make studying for the board examination more effective and more fun.

We acknowledge and thank all our chapter authors who have brought their expertise to bear on this project. We also want to thank the good people at McGraw-Hill who have edited the book to keep errors to a minimum and created a handsome and readable layout.

Mark would like to thank you, the reader, for buying this book. Thanks also to his family: Hetty, Rachel, and Abe (as always). But not to the dogs, Nietzsche and "Vash the Stampede." They need to learn to stay either in or out of the house. No more of this back and forth. Music that has kept Mark awake: "Hellborg, Lane, and Sipe" (check out "Time is the Enemy" and "Personae" [yes, it is spelled with an "e"]), Stephane Wrembel (Barbes-Brooklyn is Mark's favorite but you can't go wrong), and the Kinks. Finally, thanks to his bicycle for keeping Mark sane … although some would argue this point.

Jason thanks his loving and supportive family. After some initial threats, Deb has granted her patience and understanding to the project, and Jason simply owes her dinner every night … for a year. Jason thanks his boys, Ken and Ted, who offer a great distraction from work (like learning to drive—yikes!) and find it entertaining that their dad is some form of an author. Finally, as with every edition, Jason must acknowledge that the book would never get finished without large amounts of coffee; so, he thanks everyone involved in the worldwide production of coffee, from the pickers on the Central American fincas to the local baristas. He's really hoping that we all do something about climate change to at least save the coffee-growing regions of the world.

Brigit thanks her husband, Austin, for being so patient when she has been cranky and sleep deprived. She is so proud of her husband's hard work and dedication in the completion of his research, residency, and fellowship. He has been an inspiration and her greatest sidekick, friend, and love, and she can't wait to start this new chapter in their life together; by FINALLY living in the same location! She would like to acknowledge the "Academy" (no really, she's not joking) as she has spent many hours on her couch with the movies and the AAFP editing this book and completing her CME questions. Lastly, she would like to thank the open roads, blue skies, and sunshine for always providing her with much needed "run therapy" and happiness.

Also, the AAFP markets a comprehensive board review self-study course, which will set you back over $1,000 if you are a member and more if you are not. Indeed, it covers everything you need to know for the examination. But so does this book! So, the choice is yours, but we doubt that you will need both our book and the AAFP board examination self-study package.

What about texts and primary sources? Well, while we would admire your perseverance in slogging through whole texts preparing for the examination, we do not recommend attempting to read cover-to-cover texts like Robert Rakel's *Textbook of Family Medicine* or reference material like *UpToDate*. Don't get us wrong. We like these sources and recommend them to you as references as you are studying, but you should not rely on them as your sole study material. Likewise, using primary sources, like medical journals, is impractical as a study foundation but useful to expand your knowledge when you don't understand something.

As far as board review courses: to each his or her own. If you are considering attending a course, the AAFP offers comprehensive courses multiple times per year in locations all across the country. For-profit entities provide additional options. If you learn best in a live lecture setting, these courses may be a good option for you, but you need not attend a course to get all that information (c'mon—you've got this book!).

There are some important basic things you need to know about the examination. As of the writing of this book, the examination is composed of 4 sections, each consisting of 80 multiple choice questions and 100 minutes in length. Sections 1, 3 and 4 have questions from a wide variety of family medicine topics. Section 2 consists of 40 questions from a chosen module and 40 questions pertaining to the general breadth of family medicine. It is best to choose modules with which you are more familiar. For example, if you practice primarily in an emergency department, you may want to choose Emergent/Urgent Care or Hospital Medicine rather than Maternity Care (unless you're looking for the additional challenge). We highly recommend to check out the ABFM website (https://www.theabfm.org/continue-certification/cognitive-expertise/one-day-fmc-exam) for exam information as this may change.

The examination consists entirely of four-item multiple-choice questions. You are not penalized for guessing. An unanswered question will always be wrong; whereas, a guessed question has a 25% chance of being right. If you have no idea, go ahead and guess. As a corollary to that rule, never exit the examination without first completing all the items. You cannot return to answer unmarked items.

Read every stem and option carefully. Although we doubt that the ABFM writes "trick questions," they do use catch words/phrases, such as "except," "most likely," "first step," and "least likely." If you are not attending to the catch phrase, you are likely to answer the question wrong.

In the past, the ABFM recommended relying on evidence in place up to 2 years before the examination rather than the most recent medical evidence. Now, the ABFM recommends examinees rely on the most up-to-date evidence available. So, when you are looking at a question and thinking, "Well, the answer last year might have been 'A' but now the evidence points to 'B'." Choose "B."

Successful test-takers do not use grand strategies to outsmart the question writers; instead they tend to employ a few simple rules when answering multiple-choice questions. These simple rules that follow amount to guidelines that cannot be blindly applied to the entire test, but are often true. No secret to many of you, perhaps, but here they are:

- Go with your first thoughtful choice unless you have a solid reason to change it (e.g., you misread the question).
- Look for catch words in the answers, such as "always" and "never." These will often be incorrect.
- Avoid answers with unfamiliar terms (e.g., obscure disease names or rarely performed procedures). These are often incorrect.
- The most detailed answer is often the correct answer.
- If two answers are similar, they are probably both wrong.
- Stick with family medicine principles (e.g., answers with "more history" or "shared decision making" are more likely to be correct).
- If you don't know, guess and move on. Do not waste time deliberating on a single question.

Finally, we part offering advice that we know busy doctors seldom follow: get plenty of rest. Seriously! Be prepared for the examination day by getting a good night's sleep. Don't stop taking care of your health prior to the examination, and that includes rest. Eat a good breakfast, bring a snack for your breaks, and plan to take yourself out for a nice lunch (but skip the martini—you've got an examination to finish). Just like a mountain climber, wear layers. Some of those test-taking centers are freezing; some are boiling. Stay positive, take a deep breath and keep moving through it. You will pass this thing! Good luck.

A Few Words on Studying and Taking the Board Examination

Throughout the book, you will find that we give advice on what we think is likely to be on the examination. That's what you're paying for, right? However, the fourth edition marked the first time that we offered advice on studying for and taking the examination. We thought it worthwhile to keep this section for the fifth edition. **We recommend you read this section prior to diving into the rest of the book**.

While we acknowledge that some people are simply better test takers than others, there is good evidence to show that anyone can improve his or her scores. In fact, examination scores are directly proportional to time spent studying for the examination (although this association grows weaker for those who have high scores already). The point is, you don't have to be a genius who got a 36 on the ACT in order to rock the ABFM Certification/Recertification Examination. But you may need to put in the work.

Your first step in studying for the examination—after purchasing this book, of course—should be to develop a study plan. Plotting out time and dedicating that time to uninterrupted study is important. How much time do you have before the examination? How many hours per week can you devote to studying? When are you most productive in your studying—morning or night? What are the chances of a worldwide failure of coffee crops? Will a new *Star Wars* movie open before the examination? Thinking through these questions, get a calendar, mark the examination date, and plot out days and times that you will devote to studying. If you have taken the examination before and it didn't turn out so well, you may need to change your daily work schedule for 2 to 3 months before the examination to accommodate studying 10 to 15 hours per week. We endorse neither "cramming" for the examination nor "adding on" studying to an already full schedule. To get the most out of studying, you need to approach it like a daily devotion.

In order to maximize your return on your studying and to focus on deficiencies, try taking a pre-test. The best pre-test is the ABFM In-Training Examination (ITE) — keep reading for more on this. You can use your results on the pre-test to see what areas are your weakest. Studying weak areas is less fun but will net higher yield results than studying areas of relative strength. If your practice is narrow in scope (e.g., a hospitalist),

you probably already have a sense of areas of strength and ⟨ ness. Make sure you address your weak areas with rela more time on them.

Next, know what is on the examination. The percent examination content devoted to various systems is post the ABFM website, and we recommend you review it. Th systems tested are usually cardiovascular, respiratory, and culoskeletal systems. If you are weak in any of these are certain to focus your studying on them.

Now, what material should you use when studying? So our readers have been overly kind, suggesting in their re that this book is the only study tool needed for the board e nation. While we would like to believe it, we cannot endor point of view.

To get a flavor for the questions on the examinatio best strategy is to go to the source. The ABFM posts i for the last 3 years on its website (www.theabfm.org). A is required, which board-certified family physicians sho have. **The ITEs are perhaps the best source for assessin knowledge—we strongly recommend you use them.** Alt we do not recommend relying on the ITEs as your only st (obviously; we're trying to sell books here!), you can us as a way to measure your progress as you study. The cr are available as well, so you can learn what the ABFM you should know. The ABFM also has extensive informat what you should expect when you sit for the certifying/r fying examination, including a tutorial that simulates the ination. If you are an anxious test-taker, be certain to ch the tutorial. While the ABFM has several useful tools, be that the Self-Assessment Modules are **not** representative types of questions you will find on the certifying/recer examination; however, the more recent Continuous Kno Self-Assessment activity, where the diplomate answers 2 tions per quarter, is a closer representation.

Another great source for questions is the American Ac of Family Physicians (AAFP) website. If you are a men AAFP, you can access questions for free. They are categori body system and can be done in chunks of ten at a time 0.25 CME credits. This question bank offers another op nity to test your knowledge and determine where you r focus your studying.

Emergency Medicine

Olivia E. Bailey, Sarah L. Miller, and Mark A. Graber

> ▶ **CASE 1.1**

You get a call from a panicked mother because her 4-year-old drank a bottle of children's Tylenol. She found the empty bottle in her child's bed after a nap, and her child had been in bed for 90 minutes. She thinks there were about 3 ounces of liquid left in the bottle. She is about 35 minutes from the hospital. She states her child weighs 15 kg.

Question 1.1.1 Your advice to her is:
A) Induce vomiting to reduce acetaminophen absorption
B) Have the child eat to slow absorption and proceed directly to the hospital
C) Proceed to the hospital
D) Breathe deeply and calm down; the amount of acetaminophen this child could have ingested is harmless

Answer 1.1.1 **The correct answer is "C."** Proceed to the hospital. "A" is incorrect for a couple of reasons. After 90 minutes, it is not likely that there is significant medication left in the stomach and induced vomiting can lead to aspiration (this is true of liquids *and* pills). "B" is incorrect because you do not want to delay definitive treatment. "D" is incorrect as this patient may have ingested up to 3 oz (90 mL) of 160 mg/5 mL solution (total dose of 2880 mg or 192 mg/kg).

> **HELPFUL TIP:**
> Acetaminophen is the most common agent involved in pediatric ED visits for over-the-counter medication exposures. Reasons for these high exposure rates include the medication's reputation as "safe," its ubiquity in medicine cabinets, errors in dosing, as well as co-administration of medications that also contain acetaminophen.

The patient arrives in your emergency department (ED). She is alert with stable vital signs. The mother states she now

believes the ingestion occurred about 50 minutes ago as her child told her she found the bottle in the bathroom when she woke up from her nap. You contemplate gastrointestinal (GI) decontamination.

Question 1.1.2 Which of the following statements is true about gastric lavage?
A) Except in extraordinary circumstances it should only be done in the first hour after an overdose
B) Patients who have had gastric lavage have higher incidence of pulmonary aspiration than patients who have not
C) Patients who undergo gastric lavage have a higher incidence of esophageal perforation
D) It can push pill fragments beyond the pylorus
E) All of the above are true

Answer 1.1.2 **The correct answer is "E."** All of the options are true. Generally, the efficacy of gastric lavage is limited. Outcome data do not support the use of gastric lavage after the first hour. In a particularly severe overdose or in an overdose that is likely to delay gastric emptying (e.g., tricyclic antidepressants), you might want to consider lavage, but such circumstances are unusual. Gastric lavage increases the risk of aspiration, esophageal perforation, and can push pill fragments beyond the pylorus.

Question 1.1.3 After careful consideration, you decided not to lavage. She is now 90 minutes after the ingestion. Her physical exam is normal other than some dried sticky liquid on her face, shirt, and hands that smells like cherry flavoring. The next best step to take in this patient is to:
A) Check blood acetaminophen levels and refer for hemodialysis if markedly elevated
B) Administer 5 g/kg of charcoal with sorbitol
C) Start treatment with *N*-acetylcysteine (NAC)
D) Prophylactically treat this patient for seizures using phenytoin
E) Observe and measure acetaminophen level at 4 hours after ingestion

Answer 1.1.3 The correct answer is "E." Giving charcoal is likely helpful only *within the first hour after ingestion*, and even this remains controversial. "A" is incorrect because hemodialysis is not indicated for acetaminophen (APAP) overdose and measuring levels at 90 minutes will not allow appropriate risk stratification for this child. "C" and "D" are incorrect because seizure prophylaxis is not indicated in this patient, and although NAC could be initiated for a known dose of >150 mg/kg, this child clearly had spilled medication on her skin and clothing. In order to determine the risk of APAP-induced hepatotoxicity and treatment via the Rumack–Matthew nomogram, a 4-hour APAP level is necessary.

HELPFUL TIP:
Although frequently given, single dose activated charcoal has limited or no *effect on outcomes of poisonings*. It reduces absorption by about 30% if given within 1 hour of ingestion and likely has no benefit after 1 hour. It can also cause vomiting with aspiration. For this reason, it has fallen out of favor (we don't remember the last time we used it in our ED). We are not sure what the correct answer on the test will be.

HELPFUL TIP:
Do NOT give activated charcoal to patients with an altered mental status or who are otherwise unable to protect their airway. To prevent aspiration, do not give charcoal to a patient likely to have a seizure (such as with tricyclic overdose).

Question 1.1.4 *Assuming you are using charcoal,* **for which of these overdoses is charcoal NOT indicated?**
A) Acetaminophen
B) Aspirin
C) Iron
D) Digoxin
E) Opiates

Answer 1.1.4 The correct answer is "C." Charcoal will not bind iron. Charcoal will also not bind **C**austics/corrosives, **H**eavy metals, **A**lcohols, **R**apid-onset cyanide, **C**hlorine (or iodine), **O**ther insoluble tablets, **A**liphatics (hydrocarbons), or **L**axatives (**mnemonic: CHARCOAL**). Some of you may have answered "A." Theoretically, charcoal could interfere with the action of *N*-acetylcysteine, the antidote for acetaminophen ingestion by absorbing it. However, this is more of a theoretical concern than an actual one. First, the drugs should be used at different times. Charcoal should be given immediately, while *N*-acetylcysteine is given only after 4-hour levels are available. Second, the doses of *N*-acetylcysteine recommended are quite high, and you can give a higher dose if you will be using it with charcoal. Finally, intravenous (IV) *N*-acetylcysteine is available and is obviously not affected by charcoal. "B," "D," and "E" are all incorrect. While we do have antidotes for digoxin and opiates (Digibind, naloxone), charcoal may still be indicated to reduce absorption within the first hour.

▶ **Objectives: Did you learn to …**
- Manage a patient with an acute ingestion?
- Describe the appropriate use of gastric lavage and charcoal administration?
- Identify situations where charcoal may not be indicated?

 QUICK QUIZ: BIOTERRORISM AND THE ATTACK OF GODZILLA

Oh, no. Godzilla is attacking Tokyo. And this time it is with weapons of mass destruction. Which of the following properly describes the isolation requirements of a patient with pulmonary anthrax?
A) No isolation necessary. The patient may be in the same room with an uninfected patient
B) Respiratory isolation only
C) Respiratory and contact isolation
D) Negative pressure room (such as with tuberculosis) + contact isolation

The correct answer is "A." Pulmonary anthrax is NOT transmitted person to person. Contact isolation is indicated in those with cutaneous anthrax and GI anthrax (where diarrhea may be infectious).

Godzilla is not done yet… Which of the following drugs should be used as prophylaxis against inhaled anthrax, should exposure to aerosolized spores be documented?
A) A first-generation cephalosporin
B) Trimethoprim/sulfamethoxazole
C) Ciprofloxacin
D) A third-generation cephalosporin

The correct answer is "C." Fluoroquinolones are the drugs of choice when treating those exposed to anthrax. Doxycycline may also be used. Cephalosporins and TMP/SMX are not active against anthrax.

Godzilla, frustrated by his failed anthrax attack, is now spreading smallpox. Which of the following is NOT true about smallpox?
A) Isolation is best done at home if possible
B) The patient is infectious until he or she becomes afebrile
C) All lesions are generally in the same stage of evolution, unlike what is seen in varicella
D) Smallpox immunization causes an encephalitis in 1:300,000 of which 25% of cases are fatal

The correct answer is "B." The patient is infectious until all lesions crust over. Infectivity has nothing to do with the presence or absence of fever. "A" is true. Isolation is best done at home since this will limit spread (as those in the household have likely already been exposed). "C" is also true; all lesions are in a similar state of evolution. Finally, "D" is true and is the reason we do not currently immunize against smallpox—well, that and the fact we eradicated it in the wild (Way to go, humans!).

▶ CASE 1.2

A 22-year-old female presents to the ED with an overdose. She has a history of depression, and there were empty bottles found at her bedside. The bottles had contained clonazepam and nortriptyline. The patient is unconscious with diminished breathing and is unable to protect her airway.

Question 1.2.1 The BEST next step is to:
A) Intubate the patient
B) Begin gastric lavage and administer charcoal
C) Administer flumazenil, a benzodiazepine antagonist, to awaken her and improve her respirations
D) Administer bicarbonate
E) Administer lipid emulsion

Answer 1.2.1 The correct answer is "A." This patient should be intubated. Remember in any emergency situation that the ABCs (airway, breathing, and circulation) are the priority. "B" is incorrect because, as noted earlier, patients who undergo gastric lavage have a higher incidence of pulmonary aspiration—an even greater concern in the obtunded patient. In fact, airway protection is MANDATORY before undertaking lavage. "C" is incorrect. Flumazenil *will* reverse the benzodiazepine. However, we know from experience that seizures in patients who have had flumazenil are particularly difficult to control. This would be particularly problematic in a patient with a mixed overdose, such as with a tricyclic, where seizures are common. Thus, it is recommended that flumazenil be used only as a reversal agent after procedural sedation in patients who are not on chronic benzodiazepines. "E" is incorrect. Lipid emulsion refers to the liquid fatty acids given as part of total parenteral nutrition and theoretically can be used to bind fat-soluble drugs in the blood. Case series support consideration of lipid emulsion for calcium channel blocker, beta-blocker, and tricyclic antidepressant overdoses, as well as other fat-soluble drugs but only in cases of refractory cardiac arrest or cardiovascular collapse—and certainly not before the airway has been secured. Keep reading for a discussion of answer "D."

You notice that the patient begins to have an abnormal tracing on the cardiac monitor, so you order an ECG.

Question 1.2.2 Which of the following findings would you expect to find in a tricyclic overdose?
A) Normal QRS complex
B) Second- and third-degree heart block
C) Widened QRS complex
D) Sinus tachycardia
E) Any of the above

Answer 1.2.2 The correct answer is "E." All of the above findings can be seen with a tricyclic overdose. In fact, the most common presenting rhythm is a narrow-complex sinus tachycardia. As toxicity progresses, you can see a prolonged PR interval, a widened QRS complex, and a prolonged QT interval. A QRS >100 ms is predictive of seizures and QRS >160 ms is highly predictive of ventricular arrhythmia in patients with a tricyclic antidepressant overdose. Heart blocks (second- and third-degree) herald a poor outcome and may be seen late in the course. Asystole is not a primary rhythm in tricyclic overdose and tends to reflect the end stage of another arrhythmia.

YIKES!! The patient becomes unresponsive and you look at the monitor. You obtain an ECG which shows the following (Fig. 1-1).

Question 1.2.3 What is the patient's rhythm?
A) Monomorphic ventricular tachycardia
B) Sinus tachycardia with a bundle branch block
C) Paroxysmal supraventricular tachycardia
D) Torsades de pointes
E) Third degree heart block

Answer 1.2.3 The correct answer is "D." This is torsades de pointes which is a subtype of polymorphic ventricular tachycardia. In French, it literally means "twisting of the points," but in every language it means "bad news." Torsades de pointes can be recognized by the varying amplitude of the complex in a somewhat regular pattern. "A" is incorrect because the complexes are not monomorphic. "B" is incorrect for two reasons. First, there are no P waves visible. Second, sinus tachycardia should not have varied amplitude. "C" is incorrect because, again, there are no P waves and the complexes are polymorphic. "E" is incorrect because there are no P waves.

Question 1.2.4 This patient needs treatment post haste. After taking care of the ABCs, what is the ONE BEST drug for the treatment of this arrhythmia in a patient with a tricyclic overdose?
A) Esmolol
B) Lidocaine
C) Sodium bicarbonate
D) Procainamide
E) Amiodarone

Answer 1.2.4 The correct answer is "C." The treatment of choice for arrhythmias in patients with a tricyclic overdose is sodium bicarbonate. Raising the pH and administering sodium seem to "prime" the sodium channels in the heart, reversing the toxicity of the tricyclic. Procainamide ("D") and quinidine should not be used because they act in similar fashion to tricyclics and may worsen the problem. Lidocaine ("B") can be used as can amiodarone ("E"), but they are not the best choices. Beta-blockers such as esmolol ("A") can worsen hypotension and should be avoided.

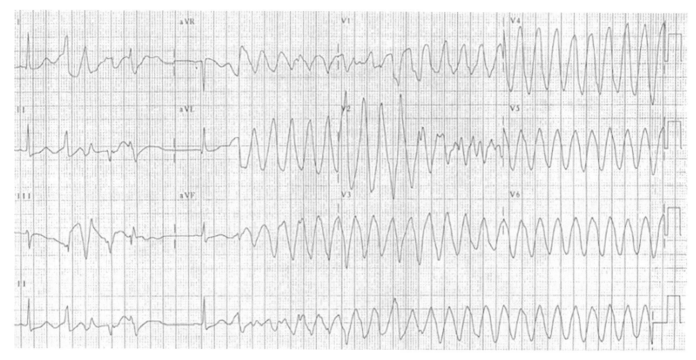

FIGURE 1-1.   ECG for patient in question 1.2.3.

This is not your patient's lucky day. She begins to seize after the administration of the bicarbonate.

Question 1.2.5 The treatment of choice for this seizing patient is:
A) Lorazepam (Ativan)
B) Repeat the bolus of sodium bicarbonate and start a bicarbonate drip
C) Phenytoin (Dilantin)
D) Fosphenytoin (Cerebryx)
E) None of the above

Answer 1.2.5 **The correct answer is "A."** Benzodiazepines are the treatments of choice in tricyclic-induced seizures. While most seizures are self-limited, it is important to control seizures because the resultant acidosis can worsen tricyclic toxicity (beyond the fact that prolonged seizures can cause CNS injury). "B" is incorrect. This patient is already alkalinized, and although sodium bicarbonate is the preferred therapy for tricyclic-induced cardiovascular toxicity, sodium bicarbonate is not particularly effective in tricyclic-induced seizures. "C," phenytoin, can be used, but benzodiazepines and phenobarbital should be administered first if possible. In addition to not working well as an antiepileptic drug in tricyclic overdose, phenytoin is also a class Ib antiarrhythmic, which may further prolong the QRS and worsen the cardiac toxicity of the tricyclic. "D" is incorrect for two reasons. First, since fosphenytoin is metabolized to phenytoin, the concern about efficacy applies. Second, fosphenytoin is a prodrug and requires adequate circulation and renal and hepatic function to be converted into active drug. If our patient becomes hypotensive with poor liver and renal perfusion, adequate drug levels might not be achieved. Finally, both phenytoin and fosphenytoin can cause hypotension—not what you need in this unstable patient.

You correct the arrhythmia and stop the seizures, and she is admitted to the intensive care unit.

HELPFUL TIP:
A patient who is *entirely* asymptomatic 6 hours after a tricyclic overdose is unlikely to have any serious consequences from the ingestion. They can be "medically cleared" at that point for admission to a psychiatric unit. Note that "symptomatic" may just be tachycardia or mild confusion. We mean the *entirely* asymptomatic patient.

▶ Objectives: Did you learn to ...
• Understand the importance of the ABCs in an unstable patient?
• Describe the role of flumazenil in toxicologic emergencies?
• Manage a tricyclic overdose?
• Recognize ECG findings in a tricyclic overdose?
• Recognize torsades de pointes and its treatment in the context of a tricyclic overdose?

 QUICK QUIZ: DESIGNER AND CLUB DRUGS

An 18-year-old male presents after a party. He is having alternating episodes of combative behavior interspersed with episodes of coma. He becomes almost apneic during the episodes of coma. He has alternating bradycardia (while in coma) and

TABLE 1-1   TOXIDROMES

Drug Class	Examples	Signs and Symptoms
Anticholinergic	Tricyclics, diphenhydramine, scopolamine, loco weed (jimson weed), some mushrooms, etc.	Tachycardia, flushing, dilated pupils, low-grade temperature, and confusion. **Mnemonic:** Dry as a bone, red as a beet, mad as a hatter, blind as a bat
Opiates	Morphine, heroin, codeine, oxycodone, etc.	Pinpoint pupils, hypotension, hypopnea, coma, hypothermia
Cholinergic	Organophosphate or carbamate pesticides, some mushrooms	Lacrimation, salivation, muscle weakness, diarrhea, vomiting, miosis. **Mnemonic:** SLUDGE BBB (salivation, lacrimation, urination, diarrhea, GI upset, emesis … Bradycardia, bronchorrhea, bronchospasm)
Sympathomimetic	Cocaine, ecstasy, methamphetamine	Tachycardia, hypertension, elevated temperature, dilated pupils (mydriasis)
Gamma-hydroxybutyrate (GHB)	GHB, liquid ecstasy, etc.	Alternating coma with agitation, hypopnea while comatose, bradycardia while comatose, and myoclonus

tachycardia when awake. The patient is also having myoclonic seizures. His serum alcohol level is zero, and his pupils are miotic.

The most likely drug causing this is:
A) Ecstasy (MDMA)
B) GHB (gamma-hydroxybutyrate aka "liquid ecstasy")
C) Methamphetamine
D) LSD (lysergic acid diethylamine aka "acid")
E) Oxycodone

The correct answer is "B." The episodic coma and bradycardia interspersed with episodes of extreme agitation are almost pathognomonic of GHB overdose. GHB intoxication also causes pinpoint pupils. "A" is incorrect because MDMA causes an amphetamine-like reaction with agitation, hypertension, hyperthermia, tachycardia, etc. "C" is incorrect for the same reason. "D" is incorrect because LSD rarely (if ever) causes coma. "E" is incorrect because patients with opioid overdoses are generally somnolent or comatose without interspersed episodes of agitation, although opioids *may* also cause miosis (be aware that not all narcotic overdoses are associated with pinpoint pupils). GHB is odorless and has slight salty taste. Besides being a street drug, GHB is available by prescription as "sodium oxybate" for narcolepsy (Xyrem). It has become a drug of choice for "date rape" since it cannot be detected in the urine. The toxicity tends to be self-limited and can be treated with intubation if needed along with tincture of time. The half-life is only 27 minutes.

 QUICK QUIZ: TOXIDROMES

A patient presents to the hospital with a diphenhydramine overdose.

Which of the following signs and symptoms are you likely to find in this patient?
A) Bradycardia, dilated pupils, flushing, and increased bowel sounds
B) Bradycardia, pinpoint pupils, flushing, and decreased bowel sounds
C) Tachycardia, dilated pupils, diaphoresis, and increased bowel sounds
D) Tachycardia, dilated pupils, flushing, and decreased bowel sounds
E) Tachycardia, pinpoint pupils, flushing, and increased bowel sounds

The correct answer is "D." This patient has an anticholinergic toxidrome. Toxidromes are symptom complexes associated with a particular overdose that should be immediately recognized by the clinician. Common toxidromes are listed in Table 1-1.

▶ CASE 1.3

A patient presents to your office with neck pain after a motor vehicle accident. He was restrained and the airbag deployed. He notes that he had some lateral neck pain at the scene. He continues to have lateral neck pain.

Question 1.3.1 **Which of the following IS NOT a criterion for clearing the cervical spine clinically?**
A) Absence of all neck pain
B) Normal mental status including no drugs or alcohol
C) Absence of a distracting injury (such as an ankle fracture)
D) Absence of paralysis or another "hard" sign that could be caused by a neck injury
E) Absence of retrograde amnesia

Answer 1.3.1 **The correct answer is "A."** Patients can have lateral neck pain and still have their cervical spines cleared clinically. However, no one will fault you for obtaining radiographs in patients with lateral muscular (e.g., trapezius) neck pain. Patients with central neck pain (e.g., over the spinous processes) DO need imaging (radiographs ± CT) to clear their cervical spine. All of the other criteria are required in order to clinically clear the cervical spine (Table 1-2). These criteria have been validated in both adult and adolescent patients.

TABLE 1-2 CLEARING THE CERVICAL SPINE CLINICALLY

No central neck pain on questioning or palpation

No distracting, painful injury (e.g., bone fracture)

No symptoms or signs referable to the neck (paralysis, stinger-type injury, etc.)

Normal mental status including no drugs or alcohol. This includes any retrograde amnesia, etc.

HELPFUL TIP:
CT has pretty much replaced plain x-rays in the evaluation of the bones of the neck. If you are doing plain films, the most common cause of missed fractures is an inadequate series of radiographs. An adequate series of radiographs for the cervical spine includes an AP film, a lateral film including the top of T-1, and an odontoid film. Flexion–extension views add little and should be avoided.

The patient's daughter, aged 4 years, was in the same motor vehicle accident and also had her cervical spine cleared by radiograph. However, you get a call from the ED 48 hours after the initial accident that she is paralyzed from just above the nipple line down (never a good thing—you quickly make a mental note to make sure your malpractice insurance premiums are paid up). You review the initial radiographs with the radiologist, which are negative as is a CT of the cervical spine bones done after the onset of the paralysis.

Question 1.3.2 The most likely cause of this patient's paralysis is:
A) Missed transection of the thoracic cord
B) Conversion reaction from the psychological trauma of the accident
C) Subarachnoid hemorrhage
D) SCIWORA syndrome
E) Guillain–Barre syndrome

Answer 1.3.2 The correct answer is "D." This likely represents SCIWORA syndrome (**s**pinal **c**ord **i**njury **w**ithout **r**adiologic **a**bnormality). SCIWORA has become a bit of a misnomer in the age of MRI, as up to two-thirds of children with this diagnosis will have abnormal MRI findings. This entity occurs from stretching of the cord secondary to flexion/extension-type movement in an accident. Patients with SCIWORA syndrome may be paralyzed at the time of initial presentation (in the event of cord transection) or may have a delayed presentation up to 72 hours after the injury. "A" is incorrect because a cord transection would present with paralysis immediately at the time of injury. "B" is incorrect because this child is 4 years old, and conversion reaction is unlikely in children. In addition, conversion reaction *is always* a diagnosis of exclusion. "C" and "E" are incorrect because this is neither the presentation of a subarachnoid hemorrhage (headache, stiff neck, perhaps focal neurologic symptoms) nor of Guillain–Barre

syndrome (progressive numbness and weakness from autoimmune myelitis).

Question 1.3.3 The next step in the management of this patient is:
A) Avoid hypotension and hypoxia to prevent secondary insult to the cord
B) Fluid restriction and diuretics to reduce cord edema
C) Mannitol to reduce cord edema
D) Neurosurgical intervention to decompress the cord
E) Lollipop and a gift card for "service recovery"

Answer 1.3.3 The correct answer is "A." Patients with a cord injury should be monitored closely to avoid hypotension and hypoxia, both of which will further damage the already compromised spinal cord. Neither diuretics ("B") nor mannitol ("C") will be useful in this situation. "D" is incorrect because the process of SCIWORA involves stretching of the cord (and subsequent dysfunction) rather than cord compression such as would be seen with a bony injury. "E" might be the right choice if you are taking this test as a "patient experience expert" instead of a doctor; but doctors should choose "A."

HELPFUL TIP:
Don't use steroids for spinal cord injuries. It doesn't work. There are also secondary complications from the steroids, including hyperglycemia, myopathy, and infections (e.g., pneumonia).

Question 1.3.4 The father is, understandably, irate that his child is now paralyzed. You can tell him that the natural history of SCIWORA syndrome in THIS CHILD is likely to be the following:
A) Continued paralysis with the necessity of long-term, permanent adaptation to the injury
B) Progression of the injury over the next week to include further paralysis in an ascending fashion
C) Resolution of paralysis and sensory symptoms over the next several months
D) Resolution of all symptoms except sensory symptoms over the next several months
E) Large lawsuit payout on the way. Do not pass go; do not collect $200; go directly to a malpractice attorney

Answer 1.3.4 The correct answer is "C." Generally, patients with SCIWORA syndrome regain their strength and sensory abilities over time. **However, this depends on when they present with symptoms!** Patients who present with paralysis right after the accident may have complete cord transection and thus will not regain function. For this reason, it is important to obtain an MRI on all patients with SCIWORA syndrome (and any trauma-induced paralysis for that matter). Patients with significant spinal cord findings on MRI are more likely to have persistent deficits.

▶ **Objectives: Did you learn to …**
- Clinically "clear" the cervical spine and decide when to order cervical spine radiographs?
- Understand the physiology, natural history, and management of SCIWORA syndrome?

▶ CASE 1.4

A patient with an extensive history of alcohol use presents to the ED after drinking a bottle of automobile winter gas treatment (Rothschild Vintage, 1954). He is intoxicated, has a headache, and describes a "misty" vision, "like a snowstorm" (if you live in southern Florida or Hawaii, call one of us in Iowa for a description). He is tachycardic and tachypneic. You start an IV and administer saline. You obtain a blood gas, which shows a mild metabolic acidosis.

Question 1.4.1 **A metabolic acidosis is consistent with all of the following ingestions EXCEPT:**
A) Ethylene glycol
B) Methanol
C) Ethanol (e.g., vodka, gin)
D) Petroleum distillates (e.g., non-alcohol-containing gasoline products)

Answer 1.4.1 **The correct answer is "D."** Ethylene glycol, methanol, and ethanol can all cause a metabolic acidosis. Hydrocarbons (e.g., gasoline products) do not cause a metabolic acidosis. The main manifestation of hydrocarbon toxicity is secondary to the inhalation and aspiration of the hydrocarbon and the resulting pneumonitis.

This patient's electrolytes are as follows: sodium 135 mEq/L, bicarbonate 12 mEq/L, chloride 108 mEq/L, BUN 12 mg/dL, Cr. 1 mg/dL.

Question 1.4.2 **This patient's anion gap is:**
A) 13
B) 15
C) 23
D) Unable to calculate the anion gap with the information provided

Answer 1.4.2 **The correct answer is "B."** By convention, the anion gap is calculated without using a major cation, potassium. Thus, the anion gap is calculated as follows:

$$sodium - (chloride + bicarbonate)$$

In this patient, the anion gap = 135 − (108 + 12) = 15.

The normal anion gap is typically considered to be 12 or less. However, since albumin is the major unmeasured anion in the serum, the anion gap should be adjusted for hypoalbuminemia. Every 1 g decrease in albumin will decrease the anion gap by about 3. Therefore, you should subtract (3 × [normal albumin − actual albumin]) to get the "real" anion gap. The normal albumin is considered to be 4. So, let us say we calculate an anion gap of 16 but the albumin is 2. In this case, the corrected anion gap will be (16 − [3 × (4 − 2)] = 16 − 6), or 10.

HELPFUL TIP:
In methanol ingestions, the severity of acid–base disturbance is generally a better predictor of outcome than serum methanol levels.

Question 1.4.3 **All of the following are causes of an anion gap acidosis EXCEPT:**
A) Lactic acidosis
B) Diabetic ketoacidosis
C) Renal tubular acidosis
D) Uremia
E) Ingestions such as methanol

Answer 1.4.3 **The correct answer is "C."** See Table 1-3 for more on causes of anion gap acidosis.

TABLE 1-3 CAUSES OF ACIDOSIS

Causes of an **elevated** anion gap acidosis	Lactic acidosis Diabetic ketoacidosis Ingestions such as ethanol, methanol, etc. Uremia Alcoholic ketoacidosis
Causes of a **normal** anion gap acidosis	GI bicarbonate loss (e.g., chronic diarrhea) Renal tubular acidosis (types I, II, and IV) Interstitial renal disease Ureterosigmoid loop Acetazolamide and other ingestions Small bowel drainage

Question 1.4.4 Which of the following findings IS NOT frequently seen in patients with methanol ingestion?
A) Hypopnea
B) Optic disk abnormalities
C) Abdominal pain and vomiting
D) Basal ganglia hemorrhage
E) Meningeal signs, such as nuchal rigidity

Answer 1.4.4 The correct answer is "A." Hypopnea is not commonly seen in methanol poisoning until the patient is close to death. In fact, the reverse is true. Tachypnea is a frequent finding in methanol overdose. This makes sense. The patient is trying to compensate for a metabolic acidosis by blowing off CO_2. Optic disk abnormalities, abdominal pain and vomiting, basal ganglia hemorrhage, and meningeal signs are all seen as part of methanol toxicity. It is thought that many of these signs and symptoms are secondary to central nervous system (CNS) hemorrhage.

You can test for ethanol at your hospital but do not have a test for methanol on a stat basis and want to be sure that this patient is not just saying he has a methanol ingestion in order to obtain alcohol (a treatment for methanol ingestion—break out the single malt scotch!).

Question 1.4.5 What test is most likely to help you determine if the patient has methanol ingestion?
A) Complete blood cell count (CBC)
B) BUN/creatinine
C) Liver enzymes
D) Measured serum osmolality
E) Amylase and lipase

Answer 1.4.5 The correct answer is "D." With a measured serum osmolality, you can calculate the osmolar gap. To do so, subtract the total *measured* serum osmoles from the osmoles known to be due to ethanol (each 100 mg/dL of ethanol accounts for approximately 22 osmoles). If there is an elevated osmolar gap, it is evidence of a circulating, unmeasured osmole. A normal osmolar gap is usually about 6 mOsm/L or less. Any osmolar gap over 10 mOsm/L suggests a concurrent ingestion with the alcohol (such as in our case, methanol).

In this case, for example:

$$\text{Measured serum osmolality} = 368$$

$$\text{Blood alcohol} = 200 \text{ mg/dL or about } 44 \text{ osmoles}$$

$$\text{Calculated osmolality} = 2(\text{Na}) + \text{BUN}/2.8 + \text{glucose}/18$$
$$= 280 + 6 + 8 = 294$$

$$\text{So, osmolar gap} = 368 - (294 + 44) = 30$$

This means that there are 30 unmeasured osmoles that could, in the clinical context of the case, represent methanol. Thus, we know that the patient did not simply overindulge on ethanol (methanol, such as "gas dry," *will* make one intensely drunk ... but has obvious downsides).

You decide that there is sufficient evidence that this patient has ingested methanol to institute treatment.

Question 1.4.6 Appropriate treatment(s) for this patient include:
A) Fomepizole (4-MP)
B) Acetylsalicylic acid
C) Ethanol
D) A and C
E) All of the above

Answer 1.4.6 The correct answer is "D." Both fomepizole (4-MP) and ethanol are used for methanol ingestion. The idea is to slow down the metabolism of the methanol. The toxicity of methanol is caused by formic acid, which is a by-product of methanol metabolism. Ethanol is metabolized by alcohol dehydrogenase, the same enzyme that breaks down methanol. Thus, methanol metabolism is competitively inhibited by ethanol. The same holds true for fomepizole, which is a competitive inhibitor of alcohol dehydrogenase. Fomepizole and ethanol can both be used for ethylene glycol ingestion as well. "B" is incorrect. Acetylsalicylic acid (ASA), or aspirin, has no role in methanol ingestion, and would likely worsen any gastritis or hemorrhaging.

HELPFUL TIP:
Hemodialysis should be available for any patient who has ingested methanol. Indications for hemodialysis include methanol level >50 mg/dL, severe and resistant acidosis, and renal failure.

▶ **Objectives: Did you learn to ...**
- Recognize manifestations of alcohol ingestion?
- Identify causes of metabolic acidosis with elevated and normal anion gaps?
- Use the osmolar gap to narrow down the differential diagnosis of metabolic acidosis?

 QUICK QUIZ: BETA-BLOCKER OVERDOSE

Which of the following has been shown to be useful in beta-blocker overdose when conventional, adrenergic vasopressors are ineffective?
A) Calcium chloride
B) Glucagon
C) Milrinone
D) High-dose insulin
E) All of the above

The correct answer is "E." In beta-blocker overdoses, the following findings may be observed: bradycardia, AV block, hypotension, bronchospasm, nausea, emesis, and *hypoglycemia*. This is very similar to the presentation of a calcium channel blocker overdose, but calcium channel blocker overdose often lacks bronchospasm and patients are *hyperglycemic* as insulin release from the islet cells is calcium dependent. When a beta-blocker overdose has been identified, the usual treatments are employed (e.g., IV fluids, vasopressors, airway protection). If conventional vasopressors have failed, glucagon in a dose of 3 to 5 mg IV bolus and a drip at 1 to 5 mg/hr may be effective in treating beta-blocker overdose. It is generally preferred over atropine in this situation. Milrinone and other phosphodiesterase inhibitors may also be used but are considered third-line agent. Likewise, calcium is considered a third-line agent in beta-blocker overdose. Calcium chloride may potentiate the action of glucagon. There is also a growing body of literature supporting use of high-dose insulin (while maintaining *euglycemia*) for beta-blocker, calcium channel blocker, or combination overdoses. The insulin is started at 0.5 U/kg/hr and titrated to as high as 10 U/kg/hr, titrated by hemodynamic improvement (*Clin Toxicol (Phila)*. 2011;49(4):277–283). Dextrose infusion may be required to maintain euglycemia. Does it seem counterintuitive to give glucagon and insulin? Both appear to mitigate the deleterious effects of beta-blockers on cardiac myocyte metabolism, although the mechanism is not completely understood. Both can be given (usually in sequence with the glucagon first) to the same patient for beta-blocker overdose. **Remember to maintain euglycemia if using insulin for beta-blocker or calcium channel blocker overdose.**

 QUICK QUIZ: TOXICOLOGY 1

Which of the following can be used to increase the metabolism of alcohol in an intoxicated patient?
A) IV fluids
B) Charcoal
C) Forced diuresis
D) GABA antagonists such as flumazenil
E) None of the above

The correct answer is "E." Drunk patients, no matter how much they annoy you, will just have to sleep it off. The rate of alcohol metabolism is fixed with zero-order kinetics at lower doses (fixed metabolic rate) and first-order kinetics at higher doses (rate proportional to levels). In general, this rate is in the range of 9 to 36 mg/dL/hr, with 20 mg/dL/hr being the accepted norm. At this point, there are no available agents to increase the metabolism of ethanol. "B" is incorrect because ethanol is too rapidly absorbed for charcoal to be of any benefit. "C," forced diuresis, will just result in an incontinent, sleeping patient and does not hasten metabolism.

 QUICK QUIZ: TOXICOLOGY 2

The best therapy for seizures secondary to an isoniazid overdose is:
A) Lorazepam
B) Phenytoin
C) Pyridoxine
D) Thiamine
E) Phenobarbital

The correct answer is "C." Isoniazid is a vitamin B6 antagonist. Thus, pyridoxine (in massive doses!) is the drug of choice in isoniazid-induced seizures. These seizures are often resistant to conventional therapy. Look for this type of overdose in patients who are being treated for active or latent tuberculosis; often these patients are immigrants and were exposed to TB in their country of origin.

▶ **CASE 1.5**

A family of four comes into your ED after being exposed to carbon monoxide (CO). They were in an idling car in the garage and were running the engine and heater to stay warm. You want to get a carboxyhemoglobin level on the whole family, but cannot get an arterial blood gas from the youngest child.

Question 1.5.1 What is your response?
A) Check pulse oximetry, and if the oxygen saturation is normal, be reassured
B) Check end-tidal carbon dioxide
C) Check a venous carboxyhemoglobin level
D) Check a venous carboxyhemoglobin and correct for the difference between venous and arterial samples

Answer 1.5.1 **The correct answer is "C."** A venous carboxyhemoglobin is just as accurate as an arterial carboxyhemoglobin—in fact, no correction is needed, which is why "D" is wrong—and, a venous gas much less painful to draw. "A" is incorrect because the pulse oximeter does not reflect hypoxia in carbon monoxide poisoning. Thus, standard pulse oximetry is useless in determining the carboxyhemoglobin level. "B" is incorrect because end-tidal carbon dioxide is measuring CO_2 and not CO.

Question 1.5.2 **When determining which patients need hyperbaric oxygen on the basis of a carboxyhemoglobin level, the level to rely upon is:**
A) The carboxyhemoglobin level on arrival to the ED
B) The carboxyhemoglobin level at 4 hours after exposure
C) The carboxyhemoglobin level projected to "time zero" (e.g., at the time of exposure)
D) None of the above

Answer 1.5.2 **The correct answer is "C."** A major consideration regarding the initiation of hyperbaric oxygen therapy is the patient's clinical situation. More severely ill patients with CO poisoning (e.g., severe acidosis, unconscious, unresponsive) should be considered candidates for hyperbaric oxygen, and some hyperbaric oxygen centers will treat regardless of measured carboxyhemoglobin level in these patients. If the treatment decision is made based on the carboxyhemoglobin level, the level projected to time zero gives the most accurate information about the degree of exposure. The rest of the answers are incorrect.

The father has a headache and a time zero carboxyhemoglobin level of 12%. The mother, who is pregnant, is asymptomatic and has a time zero carboxyhemoglobin level of 18%. Both of the children are asymptomatic. The 6-year-old has a time zero carboxyhemoglobin level of 18% while the 8-year-old has a level of 23%.

Question 1.5.3 The first step in the treatment of these patients is:
A) Start an IV and administer saline
B) Start *N*-acetylcysteine, which is a free radical scavenger
C) Start continuous positive airway pressure (CPAP) to maximize airflow by keeping the airways from collapsing
D) Administer 100% oxygen
E) Intubate the most severe patient, 100% oxygen for the others

Answer 1.5.3 **The correct answer is "D."** Because CO competitively binds to hemoglobin in place of oxygen and in fact has greater affinity for hemoglobin than oxygen, high-flow 100% oxygen is the cornerstone of treating CO poisoning. The half-life of CO in a patient breathing room air is approximately 300 minutes; this is reduced to 90 minutes when breathing high flow oxygen and reduced to 30 minutes when breathing 100% hyperbaric oxygen. Thus, *the first step in CO poisoning is to administer 100% oxygen*. The rest of the answers are incorrect. If the patient is not ventilating well and requires intubation, this would be appropriate, and the FiO_2 should be set to 100%, regardless of the patient's pulse oximetry or arterial oxygen readings. However, in our patients who are breathing without difficulty, there will be no advantage (and much higher risk) to intubation.

Question 1.5.4 Which of the following can be seen with carbon monoxide poisoning?
A) Rhabdomyolysis
B) Cardiac ischemia
C) Long-term neurologic sequelae, including dementia
D) Pulmonary edema
E) All of the above

Answer 1.5.4 **The correct answer is "E."** All of the above can be seen with carbon monoxide poisoning. Additional findings include lactic acidosis, seizures, syncope, and headache. "C" deserves a bit more discussion. Long-term neurologic sequelae can develop from days to months after the exposure and include cognitive deficits, focal neurologic deficits, movement disorders, and personality changes. It appears that using hyperbaric oxygen in the appropriate patient can reduce long-term neurologic sequelae.

Your closest diving chamber is about 90 minutes away and will hold only one patient at a time. You need to make a decision about who to send for hyperbaric oxygen.

Question 1.5.5 Which patient will benefit most from hyperbaric oxygen therapy?
A) Asymptomatic pregnant mother, time zero carboxyhemoglobin of 18%
B) Asymptomatic 6-year-old, time zero carboxyhemoglobin of 18%
C) Asymptomatic 8-year-old, time zero carboxyhemoglobin of 23%
D) Adult male with mild headache only, time zero carboxyhemoglobin level of 12%

Answer 1.5.5 **The correct answer is "A."** Generally accepted criteria for hyperbaric oxygen include: mental status changes, asymptomatic carboxyhemoglobin levels >25%, acidosis, cardiovascular disease, and age >60. Obviously, these are relative criteria. An otherwise normal 61-year-old with a mild exposure need not have hyperbaric oxygen. *Pregnancy is an indication for hyperbaric oxygen therapy* because fetal hemoglobin has a high affinity for carbon monoxide, with the fetus acting as a "sink" for CO. The high aerobic metabolic activity of fetal development is impacted greatly by exposure to the anaerobic environment created by carbon monoxide.

Question 1.5.6 All of the following are well-established consequences of hyperbaric oxygen EXCEPT:
A) Seizures
B) Psychosis
C) Myopia
D) Ear and pulmonary barotraumas
E) Direct pulmonary oxygen toxicity

Answer 1.5.6 **The correct answer is "B."** All of the rest are found as a result of hyperbaric oxygen. "C," myopia, is found in up to 20% of patients being treated with hyperbaric oxygen. It is due to direct toxicity of oxygen on the lens and usually recovers within weeks to months.

▶ **Objectives: Did you learn to …**
- Diagnose and manage patients with carbon monoxide poisoning?
- Describe complications of carbon monoxide poisoning?
- Identify patients who may benefit from hyperbaric oxygen therapy?
- Describe the complications of hyperbaric oxygen therapy?

▶ **CASE 1.6**

A 50-year-old man comes to your ED after being bitten by a stray dog outside your hospital. Apparently, there is a problem with roving packs of feral dogs in your part of town. The

bite was unprovoked and is on the abdomen. The patient has no other health history of note and has not taken antibiotics for over a year. There is a 3-cm laceration on the abdomen.

Question 1.6.1 All of the following are true about dog bites EXCEPT:

A) They tend to be primarily crush-type injuries
B) In general, the infection rate is similar to a laceration from any other mechanism (e.g., knife cut), except on the hands and feet
C) A common organism in infected dog bites is *Staphylococcus aureus*
D) Primary closure of dog bite wounds is an acceptable option (except perhaps on the hands and feet)
E) They always require antibiotics

Answer 1.6.1 The correct answer is "E." All of the rest are true statements. Dog bites (except, perhaps, for those from teacup poodles named Fifi) tend to be crush injuries (as contrasted with cat bites and Fifi, which are primarily puncture wounds). The infection rate is about the same as other lacerations. Bites on the hands and feet tend to have a higher rate of infection. Most dog bite infections are polymicrobial with mixed aerobic and anaerobic bacteria. *S. aureus* is often present, along with other organisms including *Pasteurella* and *Capnocytophaga* (say that one ten times fast). Other organisms include *Streptococcal* species and Gram-negative species. Dog bites do not generally require antibiotic prophylaxis, except under certain circumstances (e.g., presentation >9 hours after bite, immunocompromised, large, or complicated wound, perhaps hands and feet).

Question 1.6.2 You are concerned about rabies prophylaxis. Which of the following is the best next step?

A) Isolate the suspect animal for 3 days
B) Sacrifice the suspect animal and examine the liver
C) Administer rabies immune globulin IM
D) Administer rabies immune globulin IV followed by rabies vaccination series
E) Administer rabies immune globulin by infiltrating it around the wound followed by rabies vaccination series

Answer 1.6.2 The correct answer is "E." You should infiltrate rabies immune globulin around the wound and then begin the rabies vaccination series. Infiltrate as much of the immune globulin as possible around the wound and administer the remainder IM at a different site. **Do not give more than the recommended dose of immunoglobulin. This can reduce the immunogenicity of the vaccine.** "A" is incorrect because the animal needs to

be isolated for *10 days*, not 3. "B" is incorrect. If captured, the animal can be sacrificed, but the brain should be examined—not the liver. "C" and "D" are both incorrect methods of administering the vaccine and immune globulin. Note that the average incubation period of rabies is 85 days. So, immunizing up to 3 months (90 days) after the bite-event is indicated.

Question 1.6.3 Which of the following requires rabies prophylaxis in all cases?

A) Stray rabbit bites
B) Stray rat bites
C) Stray bat bites
D) Stray squirrel bites
E) Stray snake bites

Answer 1.6.3 The correct answer is "C." All bats should be considered rabid unless available for observation and testing. See Table 1-4 for detailed recommendations. Also, see the CDC or your state public health website for information about rates of infection in wild animals in your area. Of note, there have been rabid squirrels in Iowa City, our illustrious home: Google it.

HELPFUL TIP:
Patients should receive a tetanus booster every 10 years. For a contaminated wound, the tetanus booster should be within the last 5 years. Patients should receive at least one dose of Tdap (tetanus, diphtheria, and acellular pertussis) between ages 11 and 18 and a single dose between ages 18 and 64. In addition, healthcare workers and those > 65 years of age who will be around infants should receive a single dose of Tdap (for pertussis prophylaxis). Pregnant women should have a Tdap with every pregnancy to protect the infant (week 27–30 seems optimal; Healy CM et al. *JAMA* 2018 Oct 9).

HELPFUL TIP:
If a patient at risk for tetanus has not had a primary series of tetanus immunizations, administer tetanus immune globulin, *and* start the primary tetanus series. Children who have had at least 3 doses of their primary series (routinely given at age 2, 4, and 6 months) are considered "immune" and can be given a booster as needed as listed above. DTaP is appropriate for children aged 6 weeks to 7 years.

You decide to irrigate this patient's wound.

TABLE 1-4 GUIDELINES FOR RABIES PROPHYLAXIS	
General Rule	**Animals**
Always assume rabid unless available for testing	Foxes, bats, raccoons, skunks, dogs, cats, ferrets, other carnivores
Judge on an individual basis	Rodents (rats, mice, etc.), lagomorphs (rabbits, etc.), squirrels
Never require rabies prophylaxis	Non-mammals (snakes, lizards, etc.)

Question 1.6.4 Which of the following statements is true about irrigating a wound and subsequent risk of wound infections?

A) Povidone-iodine as a 50% irrigation solution (e.g., Betadine) in the wound will decrease the infection rate
B) Irrigation with normal saline is the only recommended method of cleaning a wound
C) Irrigation with normal saline and irrigation with tap water are equally effective in reducing wound infection rates
D) Use of lidocaine with epinephrine in a wound increases the rate of infection
E) Irrigation of a wound with either alcohol or hydrogen peroxide will reduce the rate of wound infection

Answer 1.6.4 The correct answer is "C." Infection rates (in the United States) are the same whether the wound is irrigated with normal saline or tap water. "A" is incorrect. Povidone-iodine is toxic to tissue and polymorphonuclear leukocytes and actually may **increase** infection rates unless a solution of 1% or less is used. Full strength povidone-iodine **can** be used on intact skin as a cleanser but should not be used in a wound. "B" is incorrect because other solutions (poloxamer 188, balanced salt solutions, etc.) can be used but are more expensive and do not offer any benefit in reduction in infection rates. "D" and "E" are both incorrect. Use of lidocaine with epinephrine ("D") may be warranted for local anesthesia for further wound exploration and/or closure. It has **not** shown to increase rates of infection. As with povidone-iodine, alcohol ("E") may be used for cleaning skin, but should be kept out of the wound. It is toxic to tissue and acts as a fixative. Hydrogen peroxide ("E") is also toxic to tissue and should not be used in open wounds—no matter what grandma says! Chlorhexidine can also be used on intact skin (not in the wound) and is more bactericidal than Povidone-Iodine.

Question 1.6.5 How long after a laceration occurs can the wound be closed primarily?

A) 6 hours
B) 12 hours
C) 18 hours
D) 24 hours
E) Any of the above can be correct depending on the wound

Answer 1.6.5 The correct answer is "E." There is no arbitrary time limit to when a wound can be closed. Facial wounds may be closed up to 24 hours after injury for cosmetic reasons, while you may not want to close other, contaminated wounds more than 12 hours after injury. Some wounds you may not want to close at all (e.g., bites to the hand, wounds contaminated with grease, wounds contaminated with manure, human bite wounds), rather allowing them to close by secondary intention.

▶ **Objectives: Did you learn to …**
 · Describe the indications for rabies prophylaxis?
 · Recognize the issues that arise with animal bites and indications for closure and/or prophylactic antibiotics?
 · List recommendations for tetanus prophylaxis and boostering?
 · Use various wound irrigation solutions for cleansing wounds?
 · Decide upon the time frame for wound closure?

▶ CASE 1.7

A 52-year-old male presents to your ED via ambulance complaining of a headache after a fall. He was working and fell approximately 10 ft. He notes no injury except for head and neck pain. A quick survey reveals that he has a BP of 128/86 mm Hg, pulse 100 bpm, and respirations of 12. There was no loss of consciousness at the scene. He "saw stars" and was clumsy, dazed, and cognitively slowed at the scene without any focal neurologic deficit. He is now back to his baseline.

Question 1.7.1 A concussion is defined as:

A) Any neurologic symptoms (e.g., clumsy, dazed, or slow, nausea, dizziness) after head injury
B) Loss of consciousness followed by return to baseline
C) Loss of consciousness with continued neurologic symptoms
D) Confusion after head trauma regardless of whether the patient lost consciousness or not
E) Any traumatic injury to the head

Answer 1.7.1 The correct answer is "A." A concussion is defined as *any* neurologic symptom after head trauma. **Note that a concussion does not require a loss of consciousness.** For this reason, "B" and "C" are incorrect. "D" is incorrect because manifestations of concussion are not limited to confusion, but also include protracted vomiting, transient amnesia, slowed mentation, "dizziness," and other neurologic symptoms. "E" is incorrect because by definition, a concussion requires neurologic symptoms.

Your patient opens his eyes spontaneously, follows commands, answers all orientation questions correctly, but appears unsteady when ambulating.

Question 1.7.2 His Glasgow Coma Scale (GCS) is:

A) 5
B) 10
C) 14
D) 15
E) 20

Answer 1.7.2 The correct answer is "D." The Glasgow Coma Scale (GCS) is a scale used to indicate the severity of neurologic dysfunction and is often applied to victims of head trauma. Remember, however, that it does not predict mortality or morbidity, but is only used as a descriptive scale of the patient's current state. Only the maximum score of 15 is considered a normal GCS. There are three components to the GCS, listed in Table 1-5.

TABLE 1-5   GLASGOW COMA SCALE

Eye opening Mnemonic: "4 eyes"	Spontaneous = 4 To speech = 3 To pain = 2 No response = 1
Verbal response Mnemonic: "Jackson 5"	Alert and oriented = 5 Disoriented conversation = 4 Nonsensical speech = 3 Moaning = 2 No response = 1
Motor response Mnemonic: "Six Cylinders"	Follows commands = 6 Localizes pain = 5 Withdraws from pain = 4 Decorticate flexion = 3 Decerebrate extension = 2 No response = 1

HELPFUL TIP:
Your chair and refrigerator each have a GCS of 3. Remember that *nothing* can have a GCS less than 3.

Question 1.7.3 **In patients with head injury, and independent of other factors, a GCS score of 15 indicates that:**
A) The patient does not require a head CT scan
B) There is essentially no possibility that this patient has an intracranial injury requiring surgical intervention
C) There is little or no possibility that this patient has any focal intracranial bleed
D) There is up to a 4% chance this patient will need neurosurgical intervention
E) None of the above

Answer 1.7.3 **The correct answer is "D."** In appropriately selected patients (e.g., those with a significant mechanism of injury), about 18% with a GCS of 15 will have some intracranial lesion, and up to 4% will eventually require neurosurgical intervention. These are generally patients who have a depressed skull fracture but a normal GCS. "A" is incorrect since a normal GCS in and of itself does not allow one to forgo head CT in patients with a significant mechanism of injury. "B" and "C" are also incorrect for the reasons noted earlier. Remember that the GCS is *not* linear; a GCS of 14 is bad. Patients with a GCS of 14 *must* have a CT scan—unless another factor in the clinical decision-making dictates otherwise (e.g., the finding is preexisting from dementia or otherwise).

Question 1.7.4 **In an adult patient with a significant head injury, which of the following is NOT an indication for a head CT scan?**
A) Intoxication with drugs or alcohol
B) Persistent vomiting
C) Amnesia or memory deficit
D) Age greater than 40
E) Seizure

Answer 1.7.4 **The correct answer is "D."** Older patients are at greater risk of developing serious intracranial injuries, and the age of 60 is usually considered an independent indication for a head CT *with significant injury*. While there is no "upper limit of normal" for vomiting after head trauma, the best data available suggest that any vomiting after head trauma in an *adult* indicates the need for a head CT. The currently recommended criteria for a CT of the head in various age groups are listed in Table 1-6.

You obtain the head CT and find a subdural hematoma. You arrange to transfer this patient for neurosurgical intervention in order to drain the subdural hematoma. It is about a 4-hour drive by ambulance to the nearest facility that has a neurosurgeon.

Question 1.7.5 **Which of the following is indicated as prophylaxis against increased intracranial pressure in this patient?**
A) Hyperventilation after intubation
B) IV mannitol
C) Trendelenburg position
D) IV dexamethasone
E) None of the above

Answer 1.7.5 **The correct answer is "E."** None of the above is indicated as prophylaxis for increased intracranial pressure. "A" is incorrect for two reasons. First, this patient does not need to be intubated. Second, routine hyperventilation as prophylaxis for increased intracranial pressure is of no benefit. This has been well studied. What happens is that hyperventilation *does* cause vasoconstriction reducing intracranial blood flow and therefore intracranial pressure. However, hyperventilation also causes ischemia around the area of the injury secondary to the vasoconstriction and may worsen outcomes. "B" is incorrect because prophylactic mannitol, like prophylactic hyperventilation, confers no benefit. "C" is incorrect. Trendelenburg positioning, or elevating the legs above the heart, would result in increased intracranial pressure. There is very limited data to support or

TABLE 1-6   INDICATIONS FOR HEAD CT BY AGE

Patient Age	Indications for Head CT after Trauma with a Significant Mechanism
Adult	Intoxication Age >60 Any memory deficit Vomiting (number of times undefined) Seizure Headache
PECARN Rules for Pediatric Head Trauma and Need for CT Scan (*The Lancet*. 2009;374(9696):1160–1170) **CT needed if:**	
Children >2 year	GCS <15 Signs of a basilar skull fracture Agitation, somnolence, slow responses, or perseveration Vomiting Loss of consciousness Severe headache Severe mechanism (Fall >5 ft, MVC with ejection, roll over, fatality) Bike/pedestrian vs. car without helmet High impact object If there are changes during observation (MS change, worsening headache, new or persistent vomiting), consider CT based on clinical judgment
Children <2 years	GCS <15 Palpable skull fracture Agitation, somnolence, slow responses, perseveration Scalp hematoma (except for frontal) LOC >5 seconds Severe mechanism (fall >3 ft, MVC with ejection, roll over, fatality) Bike/pedestrian vs. car without helmet High impact object If there are changes during observation (MS change, worsening headache, new or persistent vomiting), consider CT based on clinical judgment. If child <3 months of age, consider parenteral preference and consider scanning

refute prophylactic elevation of the head of the bed to *prevent* increased intracranial pressure; while this will reduce intracranial pressure, cerebral perfusion pressure will also be mildly reduced. For *treatment* of increased intracranial pressure, there is slightly more evidence for benefit of elevating the head of the bed (i.e., *reverse* Trendelenberg). "D" is incorrect since steroids are not useful acutely in head trauma. However, steroids are useful in cerebral edema secondary to tumor.

HELPFUL TIP:
About two-thirds of patients with a mild head injury (not deemed severe enough to obtain a CT scan) will have some measurable decrement in function at 1 month secondary to post-concussion syndrome. Symptoms include headache, dizziness, difficulty concentrating, personality changes, etc. (*J Emerg Med.* 2011;40:262).

▶ **Objectives: Did you learn to …**
- Use the GCS?
- Recognize which patients with head trauma are appropriate to obtain a head CT?

- Manage patients presenting with potential intracranial injuries?

▶ **CASE 1.8**

A 23-year-old male is in a bar fight. He only had "two beers" and was just standing there "minding my own business" when he was jumped by those infamous "two dudes" (how can those two dudes be in so many places at once?). He presents to you about 1 hour after the event with facial trauma. His vitals are normal and he is mentating well (with the exception of some impaired judgment secondary to the alcohol). His blood alcohol level is 150 mg/dL, showing that he is legally intoxicated. On examination, you notice that the patient has some epistaxis and a quite swollen nose. In addition, there is one avulsed tooth and one tooth that is displaced.

Question 1.8.1 The best way to transport an avulsed tooth is:
A) In sterile water
B) In the buccal mucosa after thorough washing with soap

C) In a glass of milk
D) Wrapped in saline-soaked gauze
E) Under a pillow

Answer 1.8.1 The correct answer is "C." The best way to transport an avulsed tooth is (1) in a glass of milk, (2) in Hanks' balanced salt solution (good luck finding this when you need it!), or (3) in the buccal mucosa or under the tongue in a patient in whom the risk of aspiration is not a concern. "A" is incorrect because sterile water is hypotonic and may damage the tooth root decreasing the success rate of reimplantation. "B" is incorrect because *washing the tooth with soap* is not appropriate. Again, you want to maintain the viability of the root if possible. "D" is incorrect as well. If this is the only option available to you, it is better than nothing, but a glass of milk or under the buccal mucosa is preferred. "E" is acceptable only if you are a tooth fairy.

You call the dentist who is (of course) out of town. A dentist will not be available for at least 12 hours.

Question 1.8.2 Your best course of action at this point is:
A) Continue to keep the tooth viable in a glass of milk
B) Continue to keep the tooth viable in the buccal mucosa
C) Clean the tooth and keep it sterile and dry for reimplantation in 12 hours realizing that a bridge will probably be needed to hold the tooth in position
D) Reinsert the tooth into the socket yourself

Answer 1.8.2 The correct answer is "D." If there is going to be any delay in reimplantation by a dentist, the best course of action is to reinsert the tooth into the socket yourself. "A," "B," and "C" are all incorrect because they will reduce the rate of successful reimplantation.

HELPFUL TIP:
Primary ("baby") teeth should NOT be re-inserted into the socket! They ankylose to the bone preventing the eruption of the permanent tooth and cause a cosmetic deformity.

HELPFUL TIP:
Any patient who is in the ED, says he only had three beers, and was "minding his own business" is probably not telling the truth on either account.

You now turn your attention to this patient's bloody nose and are trying to decide whether or not to get an x-ray.

Question 1.8.3 The BEST timing for a radiograph of the nose is:
A) As soon as possible after the trauma, once other injuries are stabilized and more important problems are addressed

B) As soon as possible to assure that there are no bone fragments threatening the brain
C) There is no need for a radiograph acutely. You can wait for 3 or 4 days
D) There is never any indication for nasal radiographs

Answer 1.8.3 The correct answer is "C." There is no need for radiographs acutely except in extraordinary circumstances. The reasons for a radiograph are to document a fracture *and* to assist in reduction. Because of swelling, it is difficult to get a good cosmetic result reducing a nasal fracture acutely. Thus, a radiograph is indicated in 3 to 4 days *only* if there is evidence of nasal deformity once swelling has resolved. If there is good cosmesis and the patient can breathe through his (they are almost always male) nose, a radiograph is unnecessary just to document a fracture. "A" and "B" are incorrect because, as noted earlier, there is no reason to do a radiograph at all unless there is evidence of deformity once the swelling is resolved. "D" is incorrect for the reasons noted earlier.

Question 1.8.4 You get the epistaxis stopped and examine the nasal mucosa. Which one of these is considered an emergency?
A) Closed nasal fracture
B) Septal hematoma
C) Trauma to Kiesselbach plexus
D) A deviated septum

Answer 1.8.4 The correct answer is "B." A septal hematoma is considered an emergency. The problem is that the perichondrium, which supplies nutrition to the septum, is no longer in contact with the septum because of the intervening hematoma. Thus, the septal cartilage can necrose leading to a perforated septum. Septal hematomas should be drained acutely and the nose packed to keep the perichondrium in contact with the septal cartilage. "A" is incorrect (see previous question). "C" is incorrect. Kiesselbach plexus is in the anterior nose and is a venous plexus. Bleeding is easily controlled and generally is self-limited. "D," a deviated septum, may indicate an underlying fracture but in and of itself is not an emergency.

You continue to evaluate this patient and note that he has the loss of upward gaze in the right eye, the side on which he was hit. All of the other extraocular motions are intact.

Question 1.8.5 The most likely diagnosis in this patient is:
A) Blowout fracture with entrapment of the inferior rectus
B) Blowout fracture with dysfunction of the superior rectus
C) Injury to cranial nerve III, which controls the superior AND inferior rectus muscles
D) Volitional refusal to perform upward gaze on the right side in this intoxicated patient

Answer 1.8.5 The correct answer is "A." The most likely diagnosis is blowout fracture with entrapment of the inferior rectus. The force of a blow to the globe is transmitted to the inferior orbital wall, which is the weakest point in the orbit. This can cause entrapment of the contents of the inferior orbit, including the inferior rectus, causing an inability to perform upward gaze. Due to disconjugate gaze, patients with entrapment of the inferior rectus muscle from a blowout fracture may complain of diplopia. "B" is incorrect because a blowout fracture generally refers to the inferior orbital wall, which would not entrap the superior rectus. In addition, patients with an entrapped superior rectus would have difficulty with downward gaze. "C" is incorrect because it is unlikely that being hit in the face would cause an injury to CN III. In addition, a CN III lesion would affect all extraocular muscles except for the lateral rectus (CN VI) and the superior oblique (CN IV). "D" is incorrect because it is impossible to move the eyes independently of one another unless you are a chameleon or particularly talented.

> **HELPFUL TIP:**
> Note that a blowout fracture may be a good thing. Having the fracture allows pressures to equilibrate and prevents orbital compartment syndrome (proptosis, visual loss, etc.). Proptosis with visual loss is a surgical emergency mandating an immediate lateral canthotomy (easy to do …. check YouTube).

The patient has had a long night of partying, and it is 3:00 AM Saturday morning when you call your consultant about the blowout fracture. The consultant is not happy and refuses to see the patient acutely. He wants you to send him to the office in 3 days (Tuesday morning).

Question 1.8.6 Your response is:
A) To call another consultant; a blowout fracture should be attended to immediately
B) Do nothing; evaluation in 2 to 3 days for a blowout fracture, even with inferior rectus entrapment, is appropriate
C) Start steroids to reduce muscle edema to facilitate the spontaneous release of the entrapped muscle
D) Start antibiotics and hospitalize the patient so that he can be seen in the morning when the consultant makes rounds
E) Stick pins in a voodoo doll of your consultant

Answer 1.8.6 The correct answer is "B." While blowout fractures with muscle entrapment require close follow-up, there is no need to intervene acutely. In fact, a decision to operate may be delayed for up to 14 days. If the entrapment spontaneously resolves when the swelling goes down (not uncommon) and there is no diplopia or other complicating symptoms, surgery is not needed. The other answers are all incorrect because acute intervention is not required in this patient. "E," however, may be of some benefit—depending on your voodoo skills.

> **HELPFUL TIP:**
> **Caveat to the above: In the pediatric population, immediate surgical repair should be undertaken in trapdoor fractures.** A trapdoor fracture is one in which

there is significant entrapment of the inferior rectus muscle. If the muscle is left entrapped in the pediatric population, restriction and fibrosis may occur, so immediate evaluation by a surgeon is warranted. **Oral steroids** at a dose of 1 mg/kg may decrease edema in the first 7 days limiting ultimate fibrosis. In patients with significant sinus disease, antibiotics may be considered, usually a penicillin or cephalosporin.

The patient mentioned above has a "friend" who was also in the altercation. He, too, was just "minding his business"—like everyone in the bar—until there was a gentleman's disagreement that could only be resolved with a broken beer bottle. He has a simple laceration of the chin, which you repair. This patient has a blood alcohol level of 150 mg/dL (the legal limit in most states is 80 mg/dL). Since he is intoxicated, the nurses are reluctant to allow the patient to leave because of liability issues. He seems initially very cooperative and competent. However, the nurse manager reminds you of the legal issues. The patient is getting more agitated; he wants to go home.

Question 1.8.7 Your response is:
A) Sedate the patient with haloperidol and observe him until sober
B) Sedate the patient with a benzodiazepine and observe him until sober
C) Call the police to remove this patient from your ED
D) Use restraints on the patient and observe him until sober, as sedative drugs may prolong time in the ED
E) Let the patient leave the ED with a competent adult

Answer 1.8.7 The correct answer is "E." The patient was initially cooperative and competent. Competence *is not* based on a blood alcohol level but rather on your judgment of the patient's ability to make rational decisions. We allow patients on narcotics to make decisions about their own care all of the time despite having narcotics on board. There are patients who will have capacity and are safe at a blood alcohol of 200 mg/dL and others who may be impaired at 80 mg/dL. So, judge capacity individually.

▶ **Objectives: Did you learn to …**
  · Treat acute dental trauma?
  · Diagnose and manage nasal and periorbital trauma?
  · Care for the intoxicated patient with minor trauma?

> ▶ **CASE 1.9**

A 17-year-old female fell asleep with her contact lenses in her eyes last evening. This morning she notes quite a bit of eye pain and photophobia. You evert the eyelids (something that should be done in all cases of possible foreign body) and find no evidence of a foreign body. When you stain her eye, you find a corneal ulcer.

Question 1.9.1 The treatment for this patient is:
A) Debridement with a burr and systemic antibiotics
B) Debridement with a cotton swab and systemic antibiotics
C) Topical antibiotics, topical cycloplegia, and ophthalmologic referral
D) Copious irrigation, systemic antibiotics, and cycloplegia

Answer 1.9.1 **The correct answer is "C."** This is an ophthalmologic emergency that requires topical antibiotics, cycloplegia (for pain control), and referral to an ophthalmologist. These ulcers can become quite deep and result in a ruptured globe.

You consult with your ophthalmologist who would like you start a cycloplegic agent in this patient prior to transfer.

Question 1.9.2 The drug you would choose for a cycloplegic agent is:
A) Pilocarpine eye drops
B) Timolol eye drops (e.g., Timoptic)
C) Tetracaine eye drops
D) Cyclopentolate eye drops

Answer 1.9.2 **The correct answer is "D."** Cyclopentolate is the only cycloplegic agent listed above. Cycloplegic agents paralyze the ciliary muscle dilating the pupil (midriasis) so that the eye cannot accommodate. Pilocarpine ("A") is a miotic agent. Timolol ("B") is a beta-blocker used in the treatment of glaucoma. Tetracaine ("C") eye drops are a topical anesthetic. Thus, "D" is the only correct answer. Other cycloplegic agents include homoatropine and atropine. However, these have a prolonged effect.

Question 1.9.3 If your patient just had a simple corneal abrasion, you would not have had to think so hard! Regarding corneal abrasions, you realize that:
A) Patching an eye after a corneal abrasion reduces pain and promotes healing
B) If a topical antibiotic is needed after a large corneal abrasion, gentamicin ophthalmic ointment is the drug of choice
C) Tetracaine is a good topical anesthetic and should be considered for home use in patients with a painful corneal abrasion
D) Patients should avoid wearing contact lenses until the eye has been healed for at least a week

Answer 1.9.3 **The correct answer is "D."** A is incorrect because patching an eye may actually increase pain and decrease healing. Whether or not to use a patch should be a matter of patient comfort only. "B" is incorrect because gentamicin ophthalmic ointment (as well as other topical aminoglycosides) actually reduces healing of the cornea, and antibiotics are not necessary unless there are signs of infection. "C" is incorrect because patients should never be sent home with a topical anesthetic. They reduce healing and can lead to further injury if the patient, whose eyes are now insensate, continues a harmful activity, rubs his/her eyes, etc. The thinking on this is changing a bit (*Ann Emerg Med.* 2018;71:767–778), but most still avoid sending a patient home with topical anesthetics.

HELPFUL TIP:
To differentiate a topical ophthalmologic problem from iritis, put in some tetracaine. If the pain resolves, it is likely, **but does not prove,** that the problem is superficial (e.g., corneal abrasion). Posttraumatic iritis is manifested by ciliary flare, anterior chamber cells, and marked photophobia. These patients really need a slit lamp examination.

▶ **Objectives: Did you learn to …**
· Recognize a corneal ulceration and treat it appropriately?
· Treat corneal abrasions?
· Understand the proper use of cycloplegic agents?

 QUICK QUIZ: EYE TRAUMA

You are on call for your group and a welder who was welding and grinding presents at 2:00 AM with severe bilateral eye pain. When he left work at 5:00 PM the day before, he did not notice any problem. He notes that he was wearing his dark goggles some of the time while he was welding but did quite a bit of work without goggles as well.

The most likely diagnosis in this patient is:
A) Foreign body
B) Ultraviolet (UV) keratitis
C) Globe penetration secondary to the welding and a foreign body
D) Iritis

The correct answer is "B." This patient likely has UV keratitis. The others are not likely because they generally present unilaterally. In addition, in the cases of "A" and "C," they should present directly after the event rather than 9 hours later, as in our patient. UV keratitis is found in patients who are welders or have been out in the sun for an extended period of time (at the beach, snow skiing ["snow blindness"], tanning bed, etc.). UV keratitis generally presents as severe, bilateral, eye pain about 6 to 10 hours following the activity. It is treated with cycloplegic agents and pain medication, often requiring narcotics.

HELPFUL TIP:
Patients who have a foreign body in the eye following a high-speed injury (e.g., grinding wheel) should be assumed to have a globe perforation until proven otherwise.

 QUICK QUIZ: ORTHOPEDIC EMERGENCIES

Which of the following is most commonly associated with significant vascular injury?
A) Pubic ramus fracture
B) Knee dislocation

C) Shoulder dislocation
D) Elbow dislocation
E) Ankle dislocation

The correct answer is "B." In up to 33% of knee dislocations (*not patellar dislocations*), a popliteal artery injury can be identified. It is debated as to whether all patients with knee dislocations require angiography or CT angiography or if physical examination and ankle-brachial indices are sufficient to rule out popliteal artery injury, but vascular injury is a major cause of limb loss and morbidity. "A" is incorrect because pubic ramus fractures are relatively minor injuries without vascular involvement, requiring only pain control. Shoulder dislocations ("C") are commonly associated with injury to the axillary nerve. Elbow dislocations ("D") can be associated with injury to the median nerve and brachial artery. However, arterial injuries are much less common than with knee dislocations. Ankle dislocations ("E") are rarely associated with vascular injury.

▶ CASE 1.10

A 55-year-old male farmer is injured by a grass-fed cow that pins him against a fence. His leg was trapped against the fence for several minutes. Being a typical Midwestern farmer, he ignores the injury until his wife convinces him later that afternoon to have it evaluated. He presents to your office complaining of severe pain in the calf area. A radiograph is normal, and the patient has normal distal pulses. The calf (his leg, not the cow) is tender with increased pain on passive stretch. His pain seems to be out of proportion to his injury. The calf (the cow) may also be tender and USDA grade prime.

Question 1.10.1 Which of the following is true?
A) Since the patient has excellent pulses, a compartment syndrome is not likely
B) Compartment syndrome is defined as compartment pressure >30 mm Hg
C) Compartment syndrome is only associated with significant crush injuries or fractures
D) Pain out of proportion to the injury is a red flag for compartment syndrome

Answer 1.10.1 **The correct answer is "D."** Pain out of proportion to the injury is a red flag for compartment syndrome. "A" is incorrect because pulses can be maintained until there is significant increase in compartment pressures and significant injury to muscle and nerves. "B" is incorrect because it is difficult to define a specific cutoff for compartment syndrome. Some patients tolerate higher pressures and others cannot tolerate 30 mm Hg (normal compartment pressure is zero). However, when the pressure gets above 20 to 30 mm Hg, strong consideration should be given to the presence of compartment syndrome. "C" is incorrect. Compartment syndrome can be due to a number of factors including electrical injury, excessive muscle use, tetany, reperfusion after ischemia, aggressive volume resuscitation, etc.

HELPFUL TIP:
The classic findings of arterial insufficiency (the "5 Ps" being pulselessness, paresthesia, pallor, pain, and paralysis) are often considered necessary for compartment syndrome to be diagnosed. This is incorrect. Of these, pain is often the only symptom; the second most frequent would be paresthesia. If your patient has compartment syndrome with the "5 Ps" present, there is likely extensive injury.

You decide that it is likely that this patient has a compartment syndrome.

Question 1.10.2 Which of the following labs will be the most helpful in guiding treatment for this patient?
A) CBC
B) Urinalysis
C) Glucose
D) Sodium
E) PT/PTT

Answer 1.10.2 **The correct answer is "B."** One of the major complications of compartment syndrome is rhabdomyolysis. This will manifest itself as a urine which is dipstick positive for blood, but with a negative microscopic examination for red blood cells. The positive dipstick is picking up myoglobin in the urine. Rhabdomyolysis can be confirmed by a serum level of creatine phosphokinase (CPK). CBC, glucose, sodium, and coagulation studies may be appropriate depending on the clinical situation, but are not useful in establishing the presence of myoglobinuria.

HELPFUL TIP:
Myoglobin can be measured in the urine. However, many laboratories have stopped doing this test favoring the positive dipstick/negative microscopic examination approach. **There can be other causes of a heme positive dipstick.** Thus, always check a CPK as well if rhabdomyolysis is a consideration.

The patient has a positive dipstick for blood with no red blood cells on microscopic examination (presumptive myoglobinuria). His serum CPK is 32,000 U/L, which is well above five times the upper limit of normal (the cutoff for consideration of rhabdomyolysis; although levels of >15,000 U/L are common when one has symptomatic rhabdomyolysis), so you make the diagnosis of rhabdomyolysis.

Question 1.10.3 The *most common* adverse consequence and greatest danger of rhabdomyolysis is:
A) Disseminated intravascular coagulation (DIC)
B) Acute kidney injury
C) Seizure from hypocalcemia

D) Acute gout from hyperuricemia

E) Cardiac arrhythmia from hyperkalemia

Answer 1.10.3 The correct answer is "B." Myoglobin precipitates in the renal tubules causing acute kidney injury. "A," DIC, can occur but is rare. "C," seizures from hypocalcemia, have not been reported in this condition, nor has "D," gout. The potassium elevation from rhabdomyolysis may reach a level sufficient to cause arrhythmias ("E"); however, this is not as common as "B"; this is exacerbated by possible coexistent hypocalcemia.

Question 1.10.4 The primary treatment for rhabdomyolysis is:

A) Mannitol infusion

B) Saline infusion

C) Furosemide

D) Dialysis

Answer 1.10.4 The correct answer is "B." The most important treatment for rhabdomyolysis is saline infusion. Lactated Ringers should be avoided as it contains potassium, which may further contribute to hyperkalemia as mentioned above. Previously, there has been debate over alkalinization of the urine (using IV sodium bicarbonate) and whether it has any additive benefit for preventing acute kidney injury over saline alone, but there is no evidence to support this practice. "A," mannitol, can be used to increase urine flow, but this is really a treatment that is secondary to good hydration and may cause hypovolemia compounding the problem. "C," furosemide, is controversial and has no outcome benefit but can be used for fluid overload. "D," dialysis, is what we are trying to avoid using saline.

 HELPFUL TIP:
In adult patients with rhabdomyolysis, the goal is to maintain urine output of 200 to 300 cc/hr.

The patient is able to maintain urine output after you institute saline.

Question 1.10.5 What treatment are you going to suggest for the underlying compartment syndrome?

A) Fasciotomy

B) Immobilization and traction

C) Hot packs and elevation of the affected limb

D) Ice and elevation of the affected limb

E) Below knee amputation

Answer 1.10.5 The correct answer is "A." The treatment of compartment syndrome is fasciotomy. A rapid surgical or orthopedic consultation is critical in the treatment of compartment syndrome. "E" is what we are attempting to avoid by urgent treatment with fasciotomy. The other options will not treat compartment syndrome and should not delay urgent treatment with fasciotomy.

The patient does well and everyone is happy ... except for the cow, who finds his way onto the table as the centerpiece of Christmas dinner.

▶ **Objectives: Did you learn to ...**
- Recognize manifestations of compartment syndrome and understand that compartment syndrome can be present with pain alone?
- Identify patients at risk for compartment syndrome and rhabdomyolysis?
- Manage compartment syndrome?
- Diagnose and treat rhabdomyolysis?

▶ **CASE 1.11**

A 24-year-old African-American male presents to the ED complaining of fever, chills, and dyspnea. He has chest pain that is respirophasic ("pleuritic") in nature. He is noted to be tachypneic with a respiratory rate of 36 and an oxygen saturation of 90% on room air. He has a history of sickle cell disease and has had a number of sickle cell crises in the past. He is up to date on immunizations, including *Streptococcus pneumoniae* and *Haemophilus influenzae* vaccines.

Question 1.11.1 The patient's current symptoms are MOST concerning for and suggestive of:

A) Pneumothorax

B) Pulmonary embolism

C) Acute chest syndrome

D) Sickle cell–related pericarditis

E) Thoracic aortic aneurysm dissection

Answer 1.11.1 The correct answer is "C." This patient likely has acute chest syndrome, which is associated with sickle cell anemia *and may be indistinguishable from pneumonia.* Acute chest syndrome is characterized by pleuritic chest pain, fever, cough, chills, dyspnea, rales, and rhonchi. The etiology is unknown, but it may be secondary to infarction of the lung and/or fat emboli. All of the other diagnoses should also be entertained at this point, but acute chest syndrome is most likely. Sickle cell–related pericarditis ("D") is a rare complication of the disease.

Question 1.11.2 All of the following are recommended in the initial treatment of acute chest syndrome EXCEPT:

A) Hydroxyurea

B) Oxygen

C) IV normal saline

D) Morphine

Answer 1.11.2 The correct answer is "A." Hydroxyurea, while useful for the chronic treatment of sickle cell anemia, is not indicated for the treatment of acute chest syndrome. However, it can reduce the incidence of acute chest syndrome by 50% when used chronically. Management of acute chest syndrome includes alleviating hypoxia ("B"), IV fluid resuscitation ("C"), and appropriate analgesia ("D"). Other treatments include IV antibiotics to cover for community-acquired pneumonia (although acute chest syndrome is *not bacterial*). It is prudent to cover these patients with antibiotics because adult patients with sickle cell are de facto splenectomized and the initial presentation of acute chest syndrome can be easily confused with pneumonia.

The patient continues to be hypoxic despite your therapy. His CBC shows a slight elevation in the WBC count and a hemoglobin of 9 g/dL. A chest radiograph indicates progression of infiltrates.

Question 1.11.3 **The next step in treating this patient is:**
A) Fresh frozen plasma
B) Pentoxifylline
C) Packed red blood cells
D) Exchange transfusion
E) Any of the above

Answer 1.11.3 **The correct answer is "D."** Patients with acute chest syndrome who remain hypoxic with progressing infiltrates are candidates for exchange transfusion to bring the level of HbS to <30% of the total. Simply administering blood ("C") will not resolve the problem because HbS will still be present in significant amounts. If this patient had a more significant anemia, packed red cell transfusion would be a more viable option. But transfusion at a level of 9 g/dL of hemoglobin is not indicated (generally the threshold is 7 g/dL in the hemodynamically stable patient). "A" and "B" are also incorrect. Fresh frozen plasma has no role in the treatment of acute chest syndrome, nor does pentoxifylline.

Your patient recovers from this episode. He has had numerous pain crises in the past, as well as hospitalizations for other reasons. You have an opportunity to provide some patient education. You answer a few of your patient's questions and then review potential manifestations of sickle cell disease.

Question 1.11.4 **Which of the following may be a manifestation of sickle cell disease?**
A) Joint and bone pain
B) Acute abdominal pain
C) Acute sequestration syndrome
D) Aplastic crisis
E) All of the above

Answer 1.11.4 **The correct answer is "E."** All of the above can be associated with sickle cell anemia (keep reading for additional information).

Question 1.11.5 **Which of the following infections is a common cause of aplastic crisis in sickle cell anemia?**
A) Parvovirus B-19
B) Influenza virus
C) CMV virus

D) Parainfluenza virus
E) None of the above

Answer 1.11.5 **The correct answer is "A."** Patients with sickle cell anemia can develop aplastic anemia in response to a parvovirus B-19 infection. Epstein–Barr virus and some bacteria have also been reported to cause aplastic crisis in patients with sickle cell anemia.

Question 1.11.6 **Acute sequestration syndrome is a manifestation of sickle cell anemia. In which group does acute sequestration syndrome occur?**
A) Younger than 5 years
B) 5 to 12 years old
C) 12 to 25 years old
D) Older than 25 years
E) Older than 65 years

Answer 1.11.6 **The correct answer is "A."** Acute sequestration syndrome occurs when the spleen sequesters red blood cells, leading to a drop in hemoglobin. The presentation can be quite dramatic with severe left upper quadrant pain, splenomegaly, and profound anemia, sometimes resulting in hypovolemic shock and death. Because it requires a functional spleen, it is most common in children younger than 5 years. Patient with sickle cell anemia who are older than 5 years generally do not have a functioning spleen; most often it is infarcted so that acute sequestration syndrome no longer occurs. The mortality of acute sequestration syndrome is 15% per episode and 50% recur.

HELPFUL TIP:
Exchange transfusions to reduce the percent of HbS to <30% is also indicated in stroke. Also, keep the hemoglobin >9 g/dL in those with a sickle cell–related stroke.

▶ **Objectives: Did you learn to …**
- Recognize acute chest syndrome?
- Manage a patient with acute chest syndrome?
- Use exchange transfusion in a patient with sickle cell anemia?
- Recognize various other manifestations of sickle cell anemia?

▶ **CASE 1.12**

A 52-year-old truck driver presents to your ED after being out in subzero temperatures for several hours trying to repair his truck. He is hypothermic when you use a low-reading rectal thermometer with appropriate calibration ("Thanks for getting the most accurate temperature, doc!"). His initial core temperature is noted to be 28°C. He has a pulse of 24 bpm, a BP of 70/30 mm Hg, and slowed mentation. However, he is awake, and thus able to joke about a thermometer in his rectum.

Question 1.12.1 The appropriate first-line treatment for this patient's profound bradycardia is:
A) Atropine
B) Epinephrine
C) Dopamine
D) Lidocaine
E) Re-warming

Answer 1.12.1 The correct answer is "E." The hypothermic heart is generally resistant to drugs. Thus, the best treatment for this patient is re-warming. Bradycardia from other causes can be treated with atropine 0.5 mg IV push or infusion of epinephrine or dopamine depending on the underlying rhythm.

Question 1.12.2 All of the following are acceptable methods of re-warming THIS patient EXCEPT:
A) Active external re-warming (e.g., hot packs)
B) Immersion in 40°C water
C) Passive external re-warming (e.g., blankets)
D) Heated, humidified oxygen
E) Thoracic lavage with warm fluids

Answer 1.12.2 The correct answer is "C." Patients with a temperature below 30°C generally do not have enough endogenous heat production to effectively re-warm themselves. Thus, external or internal *active* re-warming is indicated. All of the other options are acceptable methods of re-warming this patient. Extracorporeal blood warming via ECMO or dialysis along with thoracic cavity lavage via chest tubes and warm crystalloid are also effective. Gastric, rectal, and bladder lavage with warm fluids are generally not very effective because of the limited surface area involved. Plus, they can cause large electrolyte shifts.

Question 1.12.3 Rapid re-warming of the extremities is associated with:
A) Alkalosis, hypokalemia
B) Acidosis, hypokalemia
C) Acidosis, hyperkalemia
D) Alkalosis, hyperkalemia
E) Mixed acid–base disorder

Answer 1.12.3 The correct answer is "C." Re-warming of the extremities can lead to return of cold blood to the core leading to a paradoxical drop in body temperature. In addition, hypothermia causes lactic acidosis with hyperkalemia in the extremities. As the peripheral blood is re-warmed and peripheral vasodilation occurs, the hyperkalemic, acidotic blood is mobilized to the patient's central circulation, with resultant systemic metabolic acidosis and hyperkalemia.

Question 1.12.4 Which of the following is NOT associated with an increased risk of hypothermia?
A) Diabetes mellitus
B) Obesity
C) Alcohol use
D) Old age
E) Chronic illness

Answer 1.12.4 The correct answer is "B." In Iowa, we start to work on our winter fat layer in October for just this reason. Why do you think we eat all that candy corn? Obese patients have a smaller body surface area-to-mass ratio, which is somewhat protective for hypothermia. "C," alcohol use, causes patients to be relatively insensate to cold (thus the term "liquid jacket"), causes a peripheral vasodilatation, increasing heat loss, and causes poor choices (like not wearing a real jacket). Thermoregulation is impaired as we age. Thus, "D," old age, is associated with a greater propensity toward hypothermia. Diabetes ("A") and any chronic illness ("E") can also predispose to hypothermia.

....

The patient's mental status clears and he complains that his fingers and toes, which were numb and cold, are now quite painful. You note that there is probably freezing of tissue (frostbite).

Question 1.12.5 The best method of re-warming the frostbite is:
A) Slowly in tepid water
B) Rapidly in the hottest water he can stand (tested by you, of course, to ensure that there will be no burns)
C) Using a hot air source such as a hair dryer
D) Using moist heat via a heating pad
E) Wearing mittens

Answer 1.12.5 The correct answer is "B." Frostbitten parts should be re-warmed as quickly as possible in hot water between 37°C and 40°C. Water temperature cooler and hotter than this can lead to increased tissue loss. The other methods "A," "C," "D," and "E" are not recommended. *Do not re-warm parts that may become frozen again* (i.e., if you are in the field). Re-freezing will cause additional damage.

....

The patient has a lot of pain after thawing and reperfusion. You control the pain with morphine.

Question 1.12.6 Which of the following is the most appropriate dose of morphine in this hemodynamically stable 100-kg male?
A) 2 mg IV
B) 4 mg IV
C) 6 mg IV
D) 8 mg IV
E) 10 mg IV

Answer 1.12.6 The correct answer is "E." The appropriate dosing of morphine in acute pain is a never-ending source of amazement to our resident physicians who prefer to start with 1 to 2 mg IV. Nonetheless, the correct dose of IV morphine is 0.1 mg/kg or 10 mg in this 100-kg male. Similarly, the correct dose of fentanyl is 1 μg/kg (100 μg in a 100-kg adult) and the dose of hydromorphone is 0.015 mg/kg (1–2 mg in a 100-kg adult). However, there really is no "fixed" dose of narcotic pain medication in the ED. Titrate the dose until you obtain pain relief—with the patient still breathing.

It is 2 days later. The patient is noted to have black eschar on multiple fingers and toes. There is no obvious perfusion to these areas.

Question 1.12.7 **The best course at this point is:**
A) Debridement of the nonviable tissue
B) Skin grafting over open areas after debridement
C) Observation for a number of weeks despite the black eschar
D) Amputation of the nonviable distal digits

Answer 1.12.7 **The correct answer is "C."** It can take weeks for the proper demarcation line for debridement and grafting to become apparent. Thus, aggressive intervention at this point is counterproductive and may lead to additional tissue loss. For this reason, "A" and "D" are incorrect. Skin grafting is also not appropriate at this time because debridement of the eschar is not appropriate.

▶ **Objectives: Did you learn to …**
- Identify severe bradycardia in hypothermia and treat it appropriately?
- Manage a patient with hypothermia?
- Use methods of re-warming and identify complications of re-warming?
- Recognize risk factors for hypothermia?
- Diagnose and manage frostbite?

 QUICK QUIZ: DANGER IN THE LAUNDRY ROOM

Which of the following is true about the ingestion of household bleach?
A) Patients who drink household bleach are at a high risk of esophageal and gastric burns
B) Oral burns are a good predictor of esophageal burns
C) All patients who ingest household bleach should be referred for upper endoscopy to rule out burns
D) Household bleach ingestions are generally benign and require no treatment if the patient is not symptomatic

The correct answer is "D." Most **household** bleach ingestions are benign and need no therapy if the patient is asymptomatic. However, **this does not extend to industrial bleach or drain cleaner.** There is a high risk of esophageal and gastric burns with industrial bleach. "B" is incorrect. The oral mucosa may be normal in industrial bleach or drain cleaner ingestion and there may still be significant esophageal and gastric burns. For this reason, all patients with drain cleaner or industrial bleach ingestion should undergo upper endoscopy. "C" is incorrect; patients with household bleach ingestions do not require upper endoscopy unless symptomatic.

▶ **CASE 1.13**

An 18-year-old male was working outside in the heat and humidity. The outside temperature reached 105°F with 90%

humidity. He usually lives in northern Canada and works for the government tracking the migration of caribou—but he is here in Iowa on a job detasseling corn. (This is a real thing. Look at www.teamcorn.com—seasonal hard work that pays well.) His friends noticed that he became confused, complained of a headache and muscle cramps, and became light-headed. On arrival to your ED, he is not sweating and is lethargic. His rectal temperature is 41.5°C. He says with a smile, "Guess I just can't handle the heat, eh?"

Question 1.13.1 **All of the following are indicated in the treatment of this patient EXCEPT:**
A) Pack the patient in ice to reduce core temperature
B) IV fluids
C) Use a fan and spray water on the patient to promote evaporative cooling
D) Administer glucose if the patient is hypoglycemic

Answer 1.13.1 **The correct answer is "A."** Packing patients in ice is contraindicated. Total body immersion in **ice water** is useful but packing the person in ice actually reduces cooling for two reasons. First, it causes cutaneous vasoconstriction. Second, it does not allow conductive cooling such as would be seen in ice water submersion: solid ice does not have as much skin contact as water or the circulation to conduct away the heat. Remember that submersion in ice is also associated with causing **hypo**thermia. The appropriate treatment of heat exhaustion/heat stroke (heat stroke being defined as CNS dysfunction with a change in the level of consciousness) is cool water–soaked blankets and towels with fans aimed at the patient. This allows evaporative cooling and also conductive heat loss (to the water in the towels). Antipyretics are generally not effective because by this point, the patient's endogenous thermoregulation is kaput.

Question 1.13.2 **Which of the following IS NOT a contributing factor to heat exhaustion/heat stroke?**
A) Use of stimulants such as ephedra or amphetamines
B) Dehydration
C) Anticholinergic drugs
D) Thin body habitus
E) Extremes of age

Answer 1.13.2 **The correct answer is "D."** This is why Iowans start to work on their swimsuit figures in April—it's a matter of life-or-death, not narcissism. A thin body habitus is not a risk factor for heat stroke/exhaustion; the opposite is true. Obesity predisposes to heat stroke/exhaustion because there is less evaporative surface area per kilogram of weight. All of the others predispose to heat-related illness. "A" and "C" reduce sweating and, in the case of "A," increase metabolic rate. Both of these predispose to heat-related disease. Of particular note is "E." Small children sweat less readily than do adults. This predisposes them to heat-related disease but makes them less stinky than adults. The elderly do not have the same compensatory ability as younger adults.

HELPFUL TIP:
Up to 80% of patients with heat stroke will not have a prodrome of nausea, lightheadedness, confusion, headache, etc., which is seen in heat exhaustion. Make sure you check hepatic enzymes in patients in whom you suspect heat stroke. They are almost uniformly elevated (beware they may take several hours to rise) and normal liver enzymes should cause you to question your diagnosis.

▶ **Objectives: Did you learn to …**
· Recognize and manage heat exhaustion/heat stroke?
· Recognize risk factors for heat exhaustion/heat stroke?

▶ **CASE 1.14**

A 19-year-old female presents to the ED with complaints of wheezing. She has a history of asthma. You have been following her since her eighth birthday when her mother noticed that she couldn't blow out her candles. In general, she has mild asthma controlled with occasional albuterol and not requiring an inhaled steroid. However, over the past several months, things have accelerated, and she now uses her rescue inhaler daily. On examination, she is tachypneic, using accessory muscles of respiration with a respiratory rate of 30 and wheezing in all fields. Her oxygen saturation is 95% on room air. Pulse is 110 bpm with a normal BP. Her blood gas is as follows: pH 7.40, CO_2 40 mm Hg, O_2 80 mm Hg, and HCO_3 24 mEq/L.

Question 1.14.1 A normal blood gas in this patient suggests that:
A) This is a mild exacerbation that should respond well to therapy
B) She has a respiratory acidosis
C) She has a respiratory alkalosis
D) This is a severe exacerbation that will require aggressive therapy
E) She can safely be discharged

Answer 1.14.1 The correct answer is "D." A pH of 7.4 with a CO_2 of 40 mm Hg in a patient who is asthmatic and tachypneic is a bad sign. The CO_2 *should* be low in a tachypneic patient because they will be blowing off CO_2. Thus, a normal CO_2 and normal pH indicate that the patient is retaining CO_2. This is just another case where looking at the patient is more important than looking at the labs. Even though the blood gas itself is technically within normal limits, this patient clinically appears sick. "B" and "C" are both incorrect since the blood gas indicates neither an acidosis nor alkalosis.

Question 1.14.2 Which of the following tests are indicated in routine evaluation of a patient with an asthma exacerbation?
A) Chest x-ray
B) CBC
C) Arterial blood gas
D) All of the above
E) None of the above

Answer 1.14.2 The correct answer is "E." None of the above tests are indicated in the routine evaluation of an asthma exacerbation. A chest x-ray ("A") should be reserved for those patients in whom pneumonia or other pulmonary process is suspected. A CBC ("B") is not going to change your therapy in the routine asthma exacerbation and is not indicated. Likewise, an ABG ("C") is unnecessary in most asthma exacerbations. It can be used to assist in your clinical evaluation to determine whether or not the patient is retaining CO_2; however, even in the "crashing patient," an ABG is not necessary because **intubation is a clinical decision and should not be based on the blood gas**.

Question 1.14.3 You decide to initiate therapy for this patient. Of the following options, the *initial* treatment of this patient is:
A) Subcutaneous epinephrine
B) Albuterol MDI (metered-dose inhaler) with spacer
C) Nebulized ipratropium
D) Oral steroids
E) IV steroids

Answer 1.14.3 The correct answer is "B." The initial treatment for this patient—and any patient presenting with an asthma exacerbation—is a bronchodilator. A beta-agonist is preferred, in this case albuterol. It makes little difference whether this is via nebulizer or MDI, as long as one uses adequate doses. One albuterol nebulization is equal to about 8 to 10 puffs of an albuterol MDI with a spacer. "A" is incorrect because subcutaneous epinephrine is second or third line in the treatment of asthma. "C" is incorrect. While ipratropium *is* effective in asthma, it may be given with albuterol (Duoneb) and should not be given alone. "D" and "E" are incorrect. Steroids are indicated, but bronchodilator therapy is the primary treatment in acute asthma exacerbations.

There is no albuterol MDI available to you in your ED, so the patient receives nebulized albuterol. However, she continues to wheeze.

Question 1.14.4 How many albuterol treatments can this patient safely receive?
A) One every other hour
B) One per hour
C) Two per hour
D) Three per hour
E) Continuous nebulization of albuterol is safe

Answer 1.14.4 The correct answer is "E." Albuterol can be administered via nebulizer continuously if needed, even in the pediatric age group. Tachycardia, one of the main side effects of albuterol treatment, will often **improve** with continuous albuterol. This occurs because the patient's tachycardia is often driven by hypoxia. Once the asthma is adequately treated, oxygenation improves, and the pulse comes down.

The patient does not respond well to albuterol alone, so you add ipratropium. At this point, you also want to order steroids.

Question 1.14.5 Which of the following statements about steroid use in asthma exacerbation is true?
A) IV steroids are superior to PO steroids in the treatment of asthma
B) All patients who are steroid dependent should have additional systemic steroids even if they have already taken their dose for the day
C) The effective dose range for steroids in asthma is well established
D) Only patients requiring admission should have oral or parenteral steroids

Answer 1.14.5 The correct answer is "B." All patients who are steroid dependent should get steroids if they present to the ED with an acute exacerbation of asthma. "A" is incorrect. IV steroids and oral steroids have the same efficacy in acute asthma exacerbations. Thus, the choice of route depends mostly on convenience and cost. "C" is incorrect. Multiple steroid dosing regimens and ranges of doses have been used in asthma with success. "D" is incorrect. Discharged patients who have anything more than a minor asthma exacerbation should receive steroids.

HELPFUL TIP:
When compared with oral steroids, IV steroids *may increase* hospitalizations, cost, and treatment failure in those with chronic obstructive pulmonary disease. Use oral steroids whenever possible; the bioavailability is high (*JAMA.* 2010;303(23):2359–2367).

HELPFUL TIP:
Magnesium sulfate (2 g over 10 minutes in adults, 25 mg/kg in children) can be used in patients with status asthmaticus. Magnesium is a direct smooth muscle relaxant. Not all patients will respond, and in patients who do respond, you can expect a 60- to 90-minute effect. Avoid using magnesium in patients with renal failure since they may become toxic.

The patient responds to nebulizers and steroids. You decide to send her home.

Question 1.14.6 Which of the following is true?
A) You should discharge the patient on 2 puffs of an albuterol MDI via spacer to be used PRN
B) You should place the patient on a steroid, tapering the dose over 3 weeks
C) You should discharge the patient on 8 to 10 puffs of an albuterol MDI via spacer to be used every 6 hours around the clock

D) You should start the patient on a steroid inhaler
E) You should start the patient on a long-acting bronchodilator inhaler

Answer 1.14.6 The correct answer is "D." The patient should be started on a steroid inhaler to prevent recurrent exacerbations. She has been using her albuterol daily, indicating poor control. Overlapping this with oral steroids will give the inhaled steroid a chance to work while the patient is being covered with the oral steroids. "A" is incorrect. One nebulization is equal to 8 to 10 puffs of an MDI. If you simply go back to low-dose albuterol, the patient is more likely to do poorly. We tend to underdose albuterol inhalers; patients can safely take more than 2 puffs. "B" is incorrect because patients *do not need a steroid taper* if they are not on chronic steroids and will not be taking steroids for more than 10 days. You can simply treat the patient (e.g., with prednisone 40 mg PO QD for 5–10 days) and then stop. No taper is needed. *Note that this is not true for patients on chronic steroids who clearly do need a taper.* "C" is incorrect because scheduled albuterol is not as effective as PRN use. In addition, albuterol can certainly be used more than every 6 hours. "E" is incorrect because long-acting inhaled bronchodilator therapy should not be used alone in asthma due to the potential to increase mortality; it should only be used with an inhaled steroid.

▶ **Objectives: Did you learn to …**
- Recognize clinical and blood gas manifestations of a severe asthma exacerbation?
- Evaluate a patient presenting with an asthma exacerbation?
- Initiate treatment for asthma in the ED?
- Formulate a plan for discharging an asthma patient from the ED?

▶ **CASE 1.15**

A 7-year-old presents to the ED with wheezing and hives after being stung by a "bee." He was evidently throwing rocks at a yellow-jacket nest when he was stung, so hopefully, he at least learned something. On examination, the patient has hives and wheezing with a normal BP for his age. He is mildly tachycardic.

Question 1.15.1 Potentially useful treatments for this patient include all of the following EXCEPT:
A) IV diphenhydramine
B) Intramuscular (IM) epinephrine
C) Subcutaneous (SC) diphenhydramine
D) IV cimetidine

Answer 1.15.1 The correct answer is "C." Subcutaneous diphenhydramine can cause skin necrosis and is contraindicated. Either IV or IM diphenhydramine can be used. Of the others, *intramuscular* (not SC) epinephrine should be used in the patient with anaphylaxis; **epinephrine is the drug of choice for anaphylaxis.** Subcutaneous epinephrine is erratically absorbed. Remember that diphenhydramine will not reverse bronchospasm or hypotension. If hypotension persists despite IM epinephrine and IV fluids, IV epinephrine should be administered. Intravenous H2 blockers (e.g., cimetidine, ranitidine) *may be* effective in the treatment of anaphylaxis and should be used routinely in these patients.

> **HELPFUL TIP:**
> Only honeybees generally leave a stinger. Remove it by any means possible. The amount of envenomation is directly proportional to the amount of time the stinger is in the skin and *not* to how you remove it (credit card, forceps, etc.).

The patient responds well to the therapy. As you are going to discharge him and want to write his prescriptions.

Question 1.15.2 The patient should be discharged with which of the following?
A) Diphenhydramine every 6 hours for the next 48 hours
B) Cimetidine every 12 hours for the next 48 hours
C) An anaphylaxis ("bee sting") kit
D) All of the above medications

Answer 1.15.2 **The correct answer is "D."** Patients can have biphasic reaction mediated by "slow reacting substance of anaphylaxis," which is now believed to be a neutrophil chemotactic factor. This recurrence may occur up to 48 hours after the initial event. Thus, prescribing medications such as antihistamines (diphenhydramine) and H2 blockers (cimetidine) to prevent the recurrence is prudent ("A" and "B"). However, the rate of recurrence is <1% (*Ann Emerg Med.* 2014;63:736). Also, the patient should have a "bee sting" kit available ("C"), which should include a pre-filled syringe for epinephrine injection (e.g., Epi-Pen). It is recommended that patients have two syringes available at home as the failure rate with one injection is fairly high.

The parents are concerned about this child who likes to play outside. They worry that he will get stung again.

Question 1.15.3 You let them know that:
A) Any sting should be treated as an emergency
B) He will continue to be allergic to "bee stings" in the future
C) He should take prophylactic medication before going out to play in the woods or other areas where he might get stung
D) None of the above

Answer 1.15.3 **The correct answer is "D."** Here is why. Patients who are allergic to one species of hymenopteran are not necessarily allergic to others. In general, the allergy is species specific. Thus, most stings will be benign in an allergic patient **unless** it is a sting from the offending species. "B" is incorrect. Many children tend to "outgrow" "bee sting" allergies. This is in contrast to adults in whom reactions tend to get worse over time. "C" is incorrect. Obviously, the child should be careful not to irritate yellow jackets (did any of you hurl rocks at wasp nests as a kid?), but prophylactic treatment is not routinely indicated.

> **HELPFUL TIP:**
> Adults with a systemic allergic reaction to an insect sting have a 30% to 60% risk of experiencing another systemic reaction upon being stung again. Therefore, adults are more likely to benefit from venom testing and prophylaxis (which can reduce the risk to 5%). All patients with a history of anaphylaxis should be provided with an anaphylaxis kit.

▶ **Objectives: Did you learn to …**
- Describe the physiology and natural course of bee sting reactions?
- Treat a patient with an anaphylactic reaction to a bee sting?

▶ CASE 1.16

A 14-year-old otherwise healthy male presents to the ED with acute onset left testicular pain when running 1 hour prior to presentation. He denies any trauma to the region. He states that his pain is severe and only on the left. The pain is increased with ambulation and movement. He has had nausea and vomiting. He denies diarrhea, fever, chills, dysuria, hematuria, or penile discharge.

Vital signs: temperature 37°C, pulse 110 bpm, respirations 18, and BP 120/85 mm Hg. He is in distress secondary to pain. Abdomen: normal bowel sounds, nontender, soft, no masses. Genitourinary: circumcised male, no penile lesions, no discharge. The left testicle is tender to palpation and has a normal lay in the scrotum. The cremasteric reflex is normal bilaterally.

Question 1.16.1 What is the significance of the normal lay and cremasteric reflex?
A) The cremasteric reflex should be abnormal in epididymitis
B) The presence of a cremasteric reflex effectively rules out testicular torsion
C) The normal lay of the testicle in the scrotum effectively rules out testicular torsion
D) The presence or absence of a cremasteric reflex is not helpful in ruling out testicular torsion

Answer 1.16.1 **The correct answer is "D."** The presence or absence of a cremasteric reflex (cremasteric contraction with elevation of the testis in response to stroking of the same side upper thigh) is neither sensitive nor specific enough to confirm or rule out the presence of testicular torsion. Likewise, the lay of the testicle can be normal in patients with testicular torsion. An abnormal testicular lay and the absence of the cremasteric reflex may point toward testicular torsion. However, you cannot rely on these findings to rule out torsion.

Question 1.16.2 The LEAST likely diagnosis in this patient is:
A) Torsion of testis
B) Epididymitis
C) Torsion of appendix testis
D) Torsion of appendix epididymis
E) Testicular tumor

Answer 1.16.2 The correct answer is "E." Testicular torsion is characterized by acute onset of unilateral testicular pain, often during activity such as running. It has a bimodal age distribution, during the first year of life and again during puberty. The differential diagnosis is dependent on the patient's age. If the patient is younger than 15 years, the differential consists of testicular torsion, epididymitis, torsion of appendix testis or appendix epididymis, orchitis, hydrocele, and varicocele. In patients older than 15 years, the differential includes all of these diagnoses plus testicular tumor. However, testicular tumors are generally painless and should not present with acute symptoms.

Question 1.16.3 What is the most reliable method for diagnosing testicular torsion?
A) Doppler (Duplex color)
B) Radionuclide scan
C) Surgical exploration
D) X-ray
E) MRI

Answer 1.16.3 The correct answer is "C." *Every patient with suspected testicular torsion should have surgical exploration of the scrotum.* All of the other studies are adjunctive. For example, radionuclide scan ("B") may result in a false-negative and takes several hours to perform. Ultrasound ("A") is operator dependent and may miss cases of torsion. Surgical exploration is the only definitive diagnostic tool. The window of opportunity for surgery is about 6 hours, after which the testicle may not be salvaged. Orchiopexy should be performed on the involved and uninvolved sides to prevent torsion. Manual detorsion can be attempted and requires sedation and pain medications. Twist testis like you are opening a book (the right testis counterclockwise and the left clockwise). If pain resolves, you have detorsed the testis.

▶ **Objectives: Did you learn to …**
· Examine a patient presenting with acute scrotal pain?
· Generate a differential diagnosis for scrotal pain based on the patient's age?
· Evaluate a patient with suspected testicular torsion?

 QUICK QUIZ: UROLOGIC INFECTION 1

What is the most common agent causing epididymitis in a 21-year-old male?
A) *Escherichia coli*
B) *Neisseria gonorrhoeae*
C) *Chlamydia trachomatis*
D) *Pseudomonas* species
E) *Ureaplasma urealyticum*

The correct answer is "C." In young males, epididymitis is usually the result of sexually transmitted diseases. Of these, *C. trachomatis* is currently the most common etiologic agent. *N. gonorrhoeae* is second most common in this age group. It is therefore essential to treat for both agents when the diagnosis of epididymitis is suspected.

 QUICK QUIZ: UROLOGIC INFECTION 2

What is the most common agent causing epididymitis in a 55-year-old male?
A) *E. coli*
B) *N. gonorrhoeae*
C) *C. trachomatis*
D) *Pseudomonas* species
E) *U. urealyticum*

The correct answer is "A." Gram-negative rods are the most common cause of epididymitis in older men. Of these, *E. coli* is the most common etiologic agent, followed by *Klebsiella* and *Pseudomonas* species.

▶ **CASE 1.17**

A 22-year-old otherwise healthy female college student presents to the ED with dysuria and urinary frequency of 2 days duration. She denies any abdominal/pelvic pain, flank pain, hematuria, fever, chills, vaginal discharge, nausea, vomiting, or diarrhea. Her last menses was 2 weeks ago, and she states she is not sexually active. She is on oral contraceptives to treat menstrual cramps and denies any allergies.

Question 1.17.1 A urine beta-HCG is NOT indicated for which of the following patients who presents with abdominal pain?
A) A 32-year-old female who has had a tubal ligation
B) A 16-year-old female who by history has never been sexually active
C) A 25-year-old female who has had a normal period 1 week ago and swears on a stack of Bibles that she couldn't possibly be pregnant
D) A 24-year-old, married, professional female who is taking oral contraceptives and had a normal menses 1 month ago
E) A 25-year-old male

Answer 1.17.1 The correct answer is "E." Of course males do not need a pregnancy test (although the HCG may be elevated in testicular cancer). All female patients of reproductive age, except for those who have had a hysterectomy, must have a pregnancy test as part of the evaluation of abdominal pain. There are several reasons for this position. First, many patients may not be candid about their sexual activity. In fact, in one study, almost one-third of patients who said "they could not possibly be pregnant," including one who denied ever having intercourse, were pregnant. Second, the failure rate of tubal ligation is up to 5%

over 10 years depending on the technique used (laparoscopic tubal ligation is the least reliable). To raise your concern a little higher, almost all of the pregnancies in patients who have had a tubal ligation are ectopic.

HELPFUL TIP:
When examining a patient whose history is consistent with vulvovaginitis, remember that a KOH preparation is only 65% to 80% sensitive for *Candida* and treatment based on symptoms and physical findings is certainly reasonable. There are PCR and DNA probe tests available as well. The DNA probe has a rapid turnaround time and is less expensive than the PCR.

You get a urinalysis (UA) on this patient, mostly out of habit. The UA shows 5 to 10 WBCs/HPF, 2 + bacteria, 2 + leukocyte esterase, and 1 + nitrite.

Question 1.17.2 Which of the following antibiotic regimens IS NOT indicated for the treatment of simple cystitis?
A) 3-day course of trimethoprim–sulfamethoxazole (TMP–SMX)
B) 3-day course of a fluoroquinolone
C) 5-day course of nitrofurantoin
D) Single dose of fosfomycin

Answer 1.17.2 **The correct answer is "B."** The usual causative agents for uncomplicated cystitis are Gram-negative organisms such as *E. coli*. In areas that have high rates of resistance to TMP–SMX (>30% or more of isolated *E. coli* bacteria resistant), nitrofurantoin can be used. As to **"B," fluoroquinolones would be effective, but are not indicated for uncomplicated cystitis. There are several FDA warnings about systemic use of fluoroquinolones including concerns for tendinopathy, hypoglycemia, irreversible neurological symptoms, etc.** Cephalexin is effectively used in pregnant females, although a 7-day course is recommended. Fosfomycin has a lower cure rate than the other regimens and is more expensive.

HELPFUL TIP:
A false-negative urinalysis is common in women with uncomplicated cystitis. Empiric treatment of urinary tract infection (UTI) is reasonable in a female of childbearing years presenting with one or more typical symptoms (urgency, frequency, dysuria) and no vaginal symptoms. The sensitivity of symptoms is 90% while that of a dipstick is only 70%.

Question 1.17.3 All of the following patients with pyelonephritis should be admitted EXCEPT:
A) A 22-year-old G1 P0 female <24 weeks of gestation, hemodynamically stable
B) A 22-year-old female unable to tolerate PO fluids or medications

C) A 22-year-old female with unreliable social situation and/or compliance
D) A 22-year-old female with an unclear diagnosis or extreme pain

Answer 1.17.3 **The correct answer is "A."** The old adage that all pregnant patients with pyelonephritis must be admitted has gone out of favor. It is safe to send patients home who are <24 weeks of gestation, compliant, have stable vital signs, and are accessible by telephone. Patients should be given clear instructions to return for any complications. All of the other situations require in-hospital care.

▶ **Objectives: Did you learn to …**
- Decide which patients should have a urine beta-HCG in the ED?
- Provide appropriate antibiotic treatment to a patient with an uncomplicated UTI?
- Identify patients with pyelonephritis who require hospital admission?

▶ **CASE 1.18**

A 63-year-old male presents to the ED with a 2-day history of fever, urinary frequency, dysuria, and difficulty initiating the urinary stream. He also relates having some perineal pain. On examination, his vitals are stable except for a temperature of 38.5°C. His rectal examination is remarkable for a tender, warm, edematous prostate. There are no perirectal masses and the stool is heme negative. He has no penile lesions, discharge, scrotal masses, or tenderness. He does not exhibit any costovertebral angle tenderness. His UA is positive for 10 WBCs/HPF, 1+ nitrite, 1+ leukocyte esterase.

Question 1.18.1 What is the most likely diagnosis in this patient?
A) Pyelonephritis
B) Perirectal abscess
C) Epididymitis
D) Acute prostatitis
E) Cystitis

Answer 1.18.1 **The correct answer is "D."** This patient's symptoms most closely fit those of someone with acute prostatitis. Although his UA is also consistent with pyelonephritis or cystitis, his examination findings are more suggestive of acute prostatitis. He lacks costovertebral angle tenderness (pyelonephritis), and he has a significant temperature that argues against a simple cystitis. In the absence of scrotal tenderness, epididymitis is also quite unlikely.

Question 1.18.2 What should be included in the treatment regimen for this patient?
A) Oral fluoroquinolone or TMP–SMX for at least 3 weeks
B) Instructions for hydration, sitz baths, stool softeners, and nonsteroidal anti-inflammatory drugs (NSAIDs)
C) Admission for IV antibiotics if he appears toxic or hemodynamically unstable

D) Foley or suprapubic catheter if urinary retention is a problem
E) All of the above

Answer 1.18.2 The correct answer is "E." Patients with acute prostatitis should be treated for at least 3 weeks with oral antibiotics to prevent chronic prostatitis; some suggest up to 42 days. Treatment should be initiated with a fluoroquinolone while urine cultures are pending since sulfa resistance is high in some areas of the country.

While this patient is still in the ED, he develops acute urinary retention. A Foley catheter is placed without difficulty and 300 cc of slightly cloudy urine is obtained. Your patient feels much better and thanks you for alleviating his pain. You decide to discharge him home with the Foley catheter and a leg bag after discussion with a urologist and follow-up arrangement.

Question 1.18.3 Which of the following are causes of urinary retention in men?
A) Phimosis, urethral stricture, benign prostatic hyperplasia (BPH), calculi
B) Anticholinergics, sympathomimetics, narcotics, antipsychotics
C) Psychogenic
D) Cauda equina syndrome, diabetes, spinal cord injuries
E) All of the above

Answer 1.18.3 The correct answer is "E." All of the above can cause urinary retention in men. By far, the most common cause of acute urinary retention is BPH. The categories of acute urinary retention may be divided into neurogenic (spinal cord injuries, cauda equina syndrome, diabetes, syringomyelia, etc.), obstructive (BPH, phimosis, paraphimosis, calculi, urethral stricture, etc.), pharmacologic (anticholinergics, antihistamines, narcotics, antipsychotics, tricyclics, etc.), and psychogenic, which is a diagnosis of exclusion.

HELPFUL TIP:
Sending patients home on an alpha-blocker (e.g., doxazosin, tamsulosin) may reduce the need for re-catheterization after the catheter is removed.

▶ **Objectives: Did you learn to …**
- Recognize the clinical presentation of acute prostatitis?
- Treat a patient with acute prostatitis?
- Identify causes of urinary retention in a male?

 QUICK QUIZ: FORBIDDEN FORESKIN

Which of the following is characterized by a swollen, painful, retracted foreskin that cannot be reduced back to its normal position?
A) Phimosis
B) Paraphimosis

C) Balanoposthitis
D) Meatal stenosis

The correct answer is "B." Paraphimosis is a condition in which the foreskin is retracted, swollen, and unable to reduce into its normal position. Ice and steady manual compression often permit reduction. Surgery is indicated if manual reduction fails. "A," phimosis, is a condition in which the distal foreskin is too tight to be retracted to allow exposure of the glans. It is often confused with penile adhesions in those younger than 2 years. "C," balanoposthitis, is a form of cellulitis involving the foreskin and glans in the uncircumcised male associated with poor hygiene. Treatment is with warm soaks, antibiotics, and possible circumcision. The use of antibiotics is dictated by the nature of the disease. Bacterial balanoposthitis is usually related to streptococcal, staphylococcal, gonococcal, or chlamydial infection. Treat based on your clinical suspicion. Candida, etc., require only topical antifungals. Good hygiene is a must. "D," meatal stenosis, is common in *circumcised* males, associated with an inflammatory reaction involving the meatus. Symptoms that indicate the need for surgical treatment include spraying of the urine stream or dorsal deflection of the stream.

 QUICK QUIZ: FORESAKEN FORESKIN

Until what age is it normal to have adhesions between the glans and foreskin in uncircumcised males?
A) Adhesions are always abnormal
B) Age 6 months
C) Age 1 year
D) Age 2 years
E) Age 3 years

The correct answer is "E." Some adhesions are normal in young children. However, the foreskin should be fully retractable in uncircumcised males by the age of 3 to 5 years. Before this, no action need be taken.

▶ **CASE 1.19**

A 20-year-old female presents to your ED complaining of low abdominal pain. She is on "the ring" for contraception and has been faithfully using it. She has had regular menses and has not noticed any change in her pattern of menses. Her pain had a sudden onset but is not associated with any vaginal bleeding. On vaginal examination, you find marked cervical motion tenderness but no palpable adnexal mass.

Question 1.19.1 Based on this information you decide that:
A) The absence of an adnexal mass effectively rules out ectopic pregnancy
B) All forms of contraception reduce the risk of ectopic pregnancy (if the patient gets pregnant despite using contraception)

C) The fact the patient has had normal periods effectively rules out an ectopic pregnancy

D) Cervical motion tenderness effectively clinches the diagnosis of pelvic inflammatory disease

E) None of the above is true

Answer 1.19.1 The answer is "E," none of the above. "A" is incorrect because only 10% of patients with an ectopic pregnancy will have a palpable mass in the adnexa. "B" is incorrect because both intrauterine devices and tubal ligation *increase* the risk of ectopic pregnancy if the patient becomes pregnant. "C" is incorrect because 15% to 20% of patients with ectopic pregnancy have no history of missed menses. "D" is incorrect because cervical motion tenderness can be present not only in pelvic inflammatory disease but also in other illnesses such as ovarian torsion, ectopic pregnancy, etc.

Question 1.19.2 Risk factors for ectopic pregnancy include all of the following EXCEPT:

A) Prior ectopic pregnancy

B) Oral contraceptive use

C) History of pelvic inflammatory disease

D) Treatment for infertility

E) Current intrauterine device use

Answer 1.19.2 The correct answer is "B." All of the others increase the risk of an ectopic pregnancy. Other risk factors include cigarette smoking, recent elective abortion, previous tubal surgery, and tubal ligation.

You decide that this patient may have an ectopic pregnancy. A urine HCG test is positive for pregnancy.

Question 1.19.3 The significance of a positive pregnancy test is that:

A) An ultrasound will be able to detect an ectopic pregnancy if one is present

B) The serum level of HCG is *at least* 1,000 mIU/mL

C) Combined with the patient's abdominal pain and cervical motion tenderness, it effectively rules in an ectopic pregnancy

D) The urine HCG is 98% sensitive for pregnancy 7 days after implantation

Answer 1.19.3 The correct answer is "D." "A**"** is incorrect. The pregnancy test is positive very early and ultrasound may not be positive by an experienced operator until 6 weeks of pregnancy. "B" is incorrect. The urine may be positive at serum HCG levels of 25 to 50 IU/L. Patients may not have an HCG level of 1,000 IU/L until 6 weeks of pregnancy. "C" is incorrect because patients with a normal pregnancy may also have abdominal pain and cervical motion tenderness.

The patient's serum HCG is 440 IU/L. You order an ultrasound and find no evidence of an intrauterine or ectopic pregnancy.

Question 1.19.4 Your next step is to:

A) Reassure the patient that she does not have an ectopic pregnancy

B) Recheck the serum HCG in 48 hours

C) Refer for a laparoscopy to rule out ectopic pregnancy

D) Recheck an HCG in 1 to 2 weeks

E) Follow the patient clinically

Answer 1.19.4 The correct answer is "B." In a normal pregnancy, the HCG should double every 1.8 to 3 days. If the HCG *is not* doubling in this time frame, it is likely an ectopic pregnancy. Remember, the fact that you did not see an ectopic pregnancy on ultrasound is irrelevant. By an HCG of 6,500 IU/L, an experienced ultrasonographer should certainly be able to see an intrauterine pregnancy on ultrasound; if not seen, an ectopic should be reconsidered. "A" is incorrect because of the above. "C" is incorrect. This is invasive and not needed. "D" is incorrect because of the time frame; the HCG should be rechecked in 24 to 48 hours. An ectopic may well rupture within 1 to 2 weeks. "E" is incorrect. If you follow the patient clinically, you are basically saying that you will wait until the ectopic ruptures before addressing the problem.

Question 1.19.5 You recheck the HCG in 48 hours and it is now 1,000 IU/L (prior level 440 IU/L). Your interpretation is that:

A) This patient does not likely have an ectopic pregnancy

B) This patient has a molar pregnancy

C) This patient has a blighted ovum

D) The patient has fetal demise of an intrauterine pregnancy

E) All of the above are possible

Answer 1.19.5 The correct answer is "A." Since the HCG doubled as expected in a normal pregnancy, it is **not** likely that this is an ectopic pregnancy, a blighted ovum ("C") or intrauterine fetal demise ("D"). In all of these conditions, the HCG would not double. "B" is also not likely because in a molar pregnancy, the HCG would rise dramatically.

▶ **Objectives: Did you learn to …**
   · Evaluate a fertile female with pelvic pain?
   · Diagnose an ectopic pregnancy?

 QUICK QUIZ: TWISTED SISTER

Which of the following is typical of ovarian torsion?

A) Periumbilical pain gradually migrating to both the right and left quadrants

B) Sudden onset of colicky abdominal pain with vaginal bleeding

C) Sudden onset of colicky abdominal pain in one of the lower quadrants

D) Sudden low back pain with radiation to the perineum

The correct answer is "C." Patients with ovarian torsion present with sudden onset of severe lower abdominal pain. The pain is frequently colicky. Since only one ovary is involved, the pain is located in one side or the other. Spontaneous torsion/detorsion may also occur so that the pain may remit spontaneously. Ovarian torsion can be diagnosed by Doppler ultrasound that examines flow to the ovaries. However, many gynecologists consider this a clinical diagnosis, so obtain consultation early for suspected ovarian torsion cases. The treatment is surgical (think of it as equivalent to a torsed testis in a male).

▶ CASE 1.20

A middle-aged unresponsive, disheveled patient is brought by emergency medical services (EMS) to your ED. They had been called by his girlfriend who had seen him lying in the grass outside his home this morning. He has spontaneous respirations and shallow respirations of 20 per minute and a weak but palpable pulse at 110 beats per minute.

Question 1.20.1 What should be your first steps in assessment and treatment?
A) Oxygen by nonrebreather mask (NRB), stat serum glucose, naloxone, and thiamine
B) Oxygen by NRB, ECG, head CT
C) Oxygen by NRB, intubate, ECG, head CT
D) Intubate, ECG, head CT

Answer 1.20.1 The correct answer is "A." There are several causes of unresponsiveness that can be immediately corrected. A helpful algorithm to recall in the initial treatment for an unresponsive patient is "DON'T": **D**extrose, **O**xygen, **N**aloxone, **T**hiamine (the so-called "coma cocktail"). Answer "A" is correct because naloxone and oxygen are administered and glucose is checked. If a rapid blood sugar test is unavailable, empirical administration of dextrose would be appropriate. Rapid treatment of hypoxia, hypoglycemia, and narcotic overdose can improve mental status and thus avoid intubation. ECG and head CT ("B") may be indicated later in the evaluation. You could argue for intubation in this patient since he is unresponsive ("C" and "D"), but the next steps would not be ECG and head CT. So "A" is the most appropriate answer.

⋯⋯⋯⋯⋯⋯⋯⋯⋯⋯⋯⋯⋯⋯⋯⋯⋯⋯⋯⋯⋯

The patient is found to be hypothermic, hypoglycemic, and hypoxic. He is placed on oxygen and given warm normal saline, an amp of D50W, and naloxone. The patient now is saturating at 98% on NRB. He is responding to painful stimuli by moaning and withdrawing his extremities but is not opening his eyes. He has gurgling respirations and still has no gag reflex.

Question 1.20.2 What is your next step?
A) Intubate
B) Obtain head CT
C) Obtain ECG
D) Continue on an NRB
E) Obtain an ABG

Answer 1.20.2 The correct answer is "A." Although the patient has improved and has normal oxygen saturation, his level of consciousness is still too low to protect his airway. Thus, he should be intubated before further diagnostic studies are performed. A simple method to determine the need for intubation is the GCS (Table 1-5). Patients with a GCS of 8 or less should be intubated, as they cannot protect their airway from aspiration of oral secretions and/or emesis. The rhyme "GCS of 8, intubate" assists in recollection of this rule. Those with a GCS of > 8 may also require intubation. Remember, intubation is a clinical decision and not all patients will follow the "GCS of 8 intubate" rule (e.g., someone you expect to have a rapidly downhill course such as in a subarachnoid hemorrhage). This patient has a GCS of 7 (eyes 1, verbal 2, movement 4). He has gurgling respirations, and you cannot ensure he is able to protect his airway. Therefore, he should be intubated before other studies or interventions. "D" is incorrect because he cannot protect his airway. "E" is incorrect because the decision to intubate is a clinical one and not tied directly to the blood gas!

⋯⋯⋯⋯⋯⋯⋯⋯⋯⋯⋯⋯⋯⋯⋯⋯⋯⋯⋯⋯⋯

The girlfriend arrives and gives further history that the patient is an alcoholic and had told her he had quit drinking 2 days ago. She states he has had a seizure in the past when he stops drinking. As if she had uttered the magic words, he starts to seize before your eyes.

Question 1.20.3 What should you do now?
A) Give lorazepam and admit for probable delirium tremens (DTs)
B) Give lorazepam, obtain a head CT, blood cultures, and ECG
C) Give lorazepam, extubate, and admit for probable DTs
D) Give phenytoin and admit for probable DTs

Answer 1.20.3 The correct answer is "B," give lorazepam to abort the seizure. Even though it is easy to assume that the patient had a seizure from DTs, which may have resulted in hypoxia, hypothermia, and hypoglycemia, this kind of thinking can lead to errors. It is still possible that the patient has a spontaneous or traumatic brain hemorrhage, thus the need for a head CT. It is also possible that the patient is septic—remember that hypothermia can be seen with sepsis. Thus, blood cultures should be obtained and possibly an LP performed. Finally, an ECG can show a myocardial infarction or arrhythmia that may also result in seizure. "D" is incorrect because phenytoin is not the first drug of choice for an actively seizing patient, and phenytoin does not work in alcohol withdrawal seizures; a benzodiazepine such as lorazepam should be administered. New guidelines suggest up to 8 mg of lorazepam in a seizing patient (*Epilepsy Curr.* 2016;16(1):48–61). If you don't have an IV, give it IM. "C" is incorrect; the patient still has a GCS of less than 8 and is unable to protect his airway so he should not be extubated.

▶ **Objectives: Did you learn to …**
- Rapidly assess and treat an unresponsive patient?
- Use the GCS to determine need for intubation?

▶ CASE 1.21

You are working in a rural ED and get a call that the volunteer ambulance service is bringing an unresponsive, adult male patient status post motor vehicle collision. They bring the patient on a backboard with a c-collar.

Question 1.21.1 The primary survey of a trauma patient includes all of the following EXCEPT:
A) Check for pulses
B) Immobilize the c-spine, evaluate the airway, and listen for breath sounds
C) GCS
D) Abdominal examination
E) Unclothe the patient

Answer 1.21.1 The correct answer (and what you do NOT want to do in the primary survey) is "D." The primary survey is the initial evaluation performed on every trauma patient by the algorithm "ABCDE." **A:** Airway assessment includes c-spine immobilization; opening the airway by jaw thrust/chin lift; and, when indicated, bag-valve mask, intubation, or cricothyrotomy. **B:** Breathing includes listening for breath sounds, administering oxygen, and treating pneumothoraces. **C:** Circulation requires assessment of BP, checking pulses, and treatment of hypotension and tachycardia with crystalloids and blood. **D:** Disability is the rapid neurologic examination for potential cord injury and GCS. **E:** Exposure involves disrobing the patient and rolling them to assess any injury to the back.

On the primary survey, the patient was not protecting his airway and was intubated with an 8-mm endotracheal tube (ETT) with rapid sequence intubation (RSI). The patient is noted to have breath sounds on the right but no breath sounds on the left.

Question 1.21.2 What is the next best step in evaluation and treatment of this patient?
A) Remove the ETT; you must be in the esophagus
B) Get a chest x-ray to confirm tube placement
C) Do needle decompression of left chest
D) Insert a left chest tube
E) Check ETT for depth at the teeth and position

Answer 1.21.2 The correct answer is "E." This patient has breath sounds on the right; therefore, esophageal intubation is unlikely, making "A" incorrect. The most likely and easily recognizable source of absent breath sounds on the left is a right main stem bronchus intubation. Thus, looking at the depth of placement of the ETT at the teeth ("E") is the initial evaluation indicated. The ETT should be placed at about three times the size of the ETT (i.e., $3 \times 8 = 24$ cm) assuming that the size of ETT was correctly chosen. This is an important calculation to remember, as it also applies to pediatric patients. A chest x-ray can also evaluate for right main stem intubation but should not be the first step. A pneumothorax may be the cause of unilateral breath sounds, but right, or less commonly, left, main stem intubation should be considered first.

Question 1.21.3 You now note that there is an open chest wound to the left lateral rib cage. Funny … you didn't notice that before. What is the initial treatment of this new finding?
A) Needle thoracostomy
B) Chest tube placement
C) Occlusive dressing
D) Chest x-ray

Answer 1.21.3 The correct answer is "C." This patient has an open "sucking" chest wound. Each time the patient inspires, air can be sucked into the chest cavity acting as a one-way valve. This can result in a tension pneumothorax. Thus, the initial treatment is to apply an occlusive dressing to the wound (e.g., such as petrolatum gauze).

Following the placement of the occlusive dressing, the patient continues to have absent breath sounds on the left, is now hypotensive, and has distended neck veins. The presumed diagnosis is a tension pneumothorax.

Question 1.21.4 What should you do now?
A) Chest x-ray
B) Chest tube placement through wound
C) Chest tube placement through separate site
D) Remove occlusive dressing

Answer 1.21.4 The correct answer is "D." The occlusive dressing itself may cause a tension pneumothorax, so its placement should be immediately followed by chest tube placement. If a tension pneumothorax develops before the tube is placed, removing the dressing ("D") can usually alleviate the tension component. Emergency medical technicians will often place a dressing that is closed only on three sides to serve as a release valve and avoid this possibility. The diagnosis of tension pneumothorax is clinical. The time required to obtain a chest x-ray may result in the death of the patient. When placing a chest tube in a patient with an open wound, **never pass the tube through the wound**, as it is likely to follow the path of the initial penetration into lung parenchyma.

HELPFUL TIP:
Needle thoracostomy is useful in a tension pneumothorax and should be the initial step in most cases. You may need a long needle in an obese patients.

The patient now has a chest tube in place but remains hypotensive. Two large bore (18 gauge or larger) IVs were established. No external source of bleeding is identified.

Question 1.21.5 When should blood be administered?
A) Immediately
B) If patient is hypotensive
C) If persistent hypotension after 1 L of normal saline
D) If persistent hypotension after 4 L of normal saline
E) If FAST examination shows intra-abdominal free fluid

Answer 1.21.5 The correct answer is "C." If a patient arrives hypotensive with no signs of external bleeding, 1 L of crystalloid (normal saline) should be given immediately. The traditional teaching has been to start blood after hypotension unresponsive to 2 L of saline. This has changed in the most recent ATLS guidelines. If the patient continues to be hypotensive, packed red blood cells should be started along with additional normal saline. The FAST examination is a rapid bedside ultrasound to identify free fluid in the trauma patient's abdomen and pericardial sac. Persistent hypotension with positive FAST examination for intra-abdominal blood is an indication for emergent exploratory laparotomy.

▶ **Objectives: Did you learn to …**
- Employ the primary assessment of a trauma patient?
- Treat an open chest wound?
- Resuscitate an unstable trauma patient?

HELPFUL TIP:
Tranexamic acid 1 g can be used as a hemostatic agent in hypotensive trauma patients *who present within 3 hours of the initial injury*. It may worsen outcomes if given outside of the 3 hour window. If you are going to transfuse a large amount of blood, the best evidence suggests RBCs:FFP:platelets in a 1:1:1 ratio.

 QUICK QUIZ: CHEST PAIN

A 54-year-old female presents to your ED with a chief complaint of chest pain. She states it came on suddenly while she was trying to rid her garden of a plague of thistles (or garlic mustard—your choice). She describes it as "sharp" and it radiates through to her back. She reports difficulty breathing. Her past medical history is pertinent for hypertension, breast cancer, and obesity. She is a smoker.

Based on this history, what diagnosis can be excluded from your differential?
A) Acute myocardial infarction
B) Aortic dissection
C) Pulmonary embolism
D) Pneumothorax
E) None of the above

The correct answer is "E." The patient's history is most suggestive of pulmonary embolism with her complaint of sharp chest pain, trouble breathing, cancer history, and smoking. However, at this point in time, all of the etiologies listed—and more—must

be considered. Women often have atypical presentations of cardiac chest pain. In addition, patients often use the term "sharp" to describe "intense" or "strong" pain.

 QUICK QUIZ: AORTIC DISSECTION

In aortic dissection, the BP is different between the extremities in less than 30% of cases. If you diagnose thoracic aortic dissection, and the patient's BP is different in the upper extremities, what limb should you use to guide BP management?
A) Right arm
B) Left arm
C) Either lower extremity
D) The limb with the highest BP
E) The limb with the lowest BP

The correct answer is "D." An aortic dissection may impair the blood flow to certain extremities due to the false lumen. The BP should be maintained at a systolic BP of 100 to 120 mm Hg (or a bit lower) in the extremity with the highest BP. This will decrease the forces propagating the dissection.

HELPFUL TIP:
Patients with an aortic dissection should be started on an IV beta-blocker (e.g., esmolol) with a pulse goal of 60 BPM. Once this is achieved, add a vasodilator drip (e.g., nitroprusside, nitroglycerin) if the BP is still over 120 systolic. This minimizes stress to the aortic wall. The goal is a pulse of approximately 60 bpm and a systolic blood pressure of 100–120 mm Hg. Remember that lowering the pulse rate is just as important as reducing the blood pressure. The treatment of "Type A" dissection (dissection of the ascending aorta… the heart to left subclavian artery) is generally surgical. Descending aortic dissections ("Type B," distal to the left subclavian artery) can be managed medically. Either way, get your vascular or thoracic surgeon involved.

▶ **CASE 1.22**

A mother brings her 3-year-old child into the ED. She states that the child has been vomiting and complaining of abdominal pain all afternoon. He has had between 8 and 10 episodes of emesis; the last two have contained small amounts of bright red blood. He has had a little non-bloody diarrhea. He has not been tolerating fluids. On examination, you find the child to be moderately ill appearing with normal color, but he seems less interactive than you would expect. His vitals reveal a temperature of 36.5° C, a pulse of 170 bpm, a respiratory rate of 28, and a BP of 98/58 mm Hg. His abdomen is slightly and diffusely tender. He has dry mucous membranes.

Question 1.22.1 **In general (not specifically in this patient), what is the initial treatment of a moderately dehydrated child?**
A) 20 cc/kg bolus of D5 1/2 NS
B) 10 cc/kg bolus of isotonic crystalloid fluid
C) Oral challenge of a small amount of electrolyte solution
D) 12.5 mg promethazine suppository

Answer 1.22.1 **The correct answer is "C."** Many children who are vomiting and have diarrhea will be able to tolerate small (5 cc) sips of fluid administered every few minutes. Oral fluids should be attempted prior to IV therapy. One might also administer ondansetron to help reduce vomiting (2 mg in those <15 kg, 4 mg in those >15 kg). In children who are severely dehydrated, as evidenced by altered mental status or change in skin turgor, IV fluid resuscitation should begin immediately. If IV rehydration is considered appropriate, use normal saline in 20 cc/kg aliquots. Therefore, answers "A" and "B" are not correct. Promethazine ("D") is an antiemetic that has been used in children in the past. However, promethazine has received a "black box" warning from the FDA for children younger than 2 years, as there is a risk of respiratory depression. The black box warning goes on to say promethazine should be used with caution even in those children over 2 years of age.

You obtain some lab work and notice that the child has normal renal function but low serum bicarbonate, indicating a possible metabolic acidosis. In speaking with his mother, you discover that earlier in the day, he was playing unsupervised in the bathroom, where she keeps her prenatal vitamins. Upon questioning the child, he states that he ate a bunch of "candy" in the bathroom about 3 hours ago (all the more reason to keep things up high and away from children!).

Question 1.22.2 **What component of prenatal vitamins is most concerning for toxicity?**
A) Folic acid
B) Iron
C) Calcium
D) Vitamin D

Answer 1.22.2 **The correct answer is "B."** Folic acid, calcium, and vitamin D are all tolerated well in high doses, as their absorption from the GI tract is limited. Iron, however, can continue to be absorbed while the pills remain in the GI tract. Iron is a direct irritant to the GI mucosa (causing bloody emesis and diarrhea) and interferes with the electron transport chain and aerobic metabolism.

Question 1.22.3 **The nurse asks if you should add on an iron level to the blood that was drawn 3 hours after the ingestion. You respond:**
A) "No thanks. Iron levels are not helpful"
B) "No thanks. It's too early. We need to wait until at least 12 hours have elapsed"
C) "Yes, please. If it's normal, we don't need any further treatment"
D) "Yes, please. It may help us determine the severity of toxicity"

Answer 1.22.3 **The correct answer is "D."** The iron level between 2 and 4 hours after ingestion is the most accurate; beyond this period, the majority of the iron is moving intracellularly and cannot be measured. For slow-release iron, serum concentrations should be measured at 6 to 8 hours after ingestion. These measures will give you a peak serum iron concentration that correlates well with the severity of toxicity. *However, a low serum level of iron does not mean the symptomatic patient is OK. Treatment is based on clinical findings and NOT on serum iron levels.* Once the iron moves into the periphery, the serum levels can be low despite significant toxicity. You should also check LFTs and a glucose in addition to the BUN/Cr/electrolytes that you have already ordered.

Question 1.22.4 **How do patients with an iron overdose present?**
A) Abdominal pain, vomiting, and diarrhea
B) Hematemesis, shock, and coma
C) Relatively asymptomatic
D) All of the above

Answer 1.22.4 **The correct answer is "D."** Patients who have had an iron overdose classically pass through five different phases. The first phase is characterized by nausea, vomiting, diarrhea, and abdominal pain. There may be hematemesis and hematochezia as the GI mucosa becomes irritated. The second phase is a relatively asymptomatic period as the GI symptoms resolve. During this quiet phase, iron is absorbed and transported to the periphery where it causes the interruption of aerobic metabolism. In the next (third) phase, patients become hypotensive, acidotic, and can develop multisystem organ failure and coma. It is this shock that is the usual cause of death in iron toxicity. The fourth phase is heralded by hepatic necrosis. Liver failure, which does not occur in all patients, is the second most frequent cause of death in cases of iron toxicity. Finally, the patient may develop bowel obstructions 2 to 4 weeks or longer after the ingestion due to stricture formation at the site of mucosal irritation. See Table 1-7.

Question 1.22.5 **Abdominal films reveal radiopaque pills in the stomach. What is the best next step in treatment for this patient?**
A) Whole bowel irrigation with polyethylene glycol solution
B) Gastric lavage
C) Activated charcoal
D) Syrup of ipecac

Answer 1.22.5 **The correct answer is "A."** Gastric lavage and induced vomiting both entail a fair amount of risk (aspiration and pneumonitis) and neither has been shown to be beneficial. And, syrup of ipecac is no longer manufactured in the United States; therefore, "B" and "D" are not correct. Iron, lithium, and lead will not adsorb to activated charcoal; therefore, it is of no benefit in such cases, and "C" is incorrect. Treatment for iron

TABLE 1-7   MANIFESTATIONS OF IRON TOXICITY

First (or early) phase	Hours 0–6 (rarely > 6 hours)	Vomiting and diarrhea, often bloody Metabolic acidosis Shock
Second (or quiescent) phase	3–48 hours (time variable)	Resolving acidosis Resolving hypovolemia Frequently, asymptomatic
Third phase	12–48 hours (time variable)	GI hemorrhage Lethargy, coma, shock Cardiovascular collapse Metabolic acidosis Renal failure (variable)
Fourth phase	2 days or more	Hepatotoxicity Hepatic necrosis Coma
Fifth phase	2–4 weeks	GI obstruction due to strictures and scarring

toxicity involves whole bowel irrigation with polyethylene glycol solution to flush the iron out of the GI tract. There are various doses and rates of administration published, but 10 to 15 mL/kg/hr, up to 2,000 cc/hr, seems to be a reasonable place to start. This requires the placement of a nasogastric tube. If a patient does not tolerate the volume of the infusion, the rate should be decreased by 50%. The irrigation should continue until the rectal effluent is clear and there are no visible pill fragments. If follow-up radiographs demonstrate persistent iron tablets in the stomach, consider the possibility of a bezoar having formed, which may require endoscopic or surgical intervention for removal.

 HELPFUL TIP:
Patients who are *entirely* asymptomatic 6 hours after iron ingestion *and* do not have any radiographic evidence of iron in the GI tract are not at risk for toxicity. They can be safely discharged with close follow-up. The caveat is that chewable multivitamins are not radiopaque and will not show up on x-ray.

Question 1.22.6 The patient is symptomatic (vomiting and diarrhea), acidotic, and also has an iron level 650 μg/dL, which puts him at significant risk for toxicity. What is your next step?
A) Correction of acid–base disturbance and aggressive fluid resuscitation
B) EDTA
C) Deferoxamine
D) A and B
E) A and C

Answer 1.22.6 **The correct answer is "E."** In addition to symptoms and acidosis, an iron level >500 μg/dL and ingestion of more than 60 mg/kg of elemental iron are considered high-risk situations, and chelation with deferoxamine is warranted. Deferoxamine is used to chelate iron, while EDTA is a chelation

treatment for lead poisoning. Fastidious supportive care, with correction of the patient's volume and acid–base disturbances, is imperative. Ensuring that the patient is euvolemic is especially important when using chelation therapy, given that the major side effect of deferoxamine is hypotension. The dose of deferoxamine is 15 mg/kg/hr for 24 hours, but may be slowed down if the patient becomes hypotensive.

 HELPFUL TIP:
Dialysis does not remove iron from the blood stream nor the intracellular space, where the majority of it will be found. Dialysis may be indicated to treat renal failure or persistent profound acidosis.

 HELPFUL TIP:
The much touted "deferoxamine challenge" to see if there is free iron in the blood is not an accurate predictor of toxicity. The test is done by giving an individual a single challenge dose of deferoxamine and seeing if the urine changes to a "vin rose" color reflecting circulating free iron. However, this does not predict who needs therapy, since the iron may already be working its evil in the periphery.

▶ **Objectives: Did you learn to …**
• Rehydrate a child with GI symptoms?
• Recognize the manifestations of iron poisoning?
• Manage a child with an iron ingestion?

▶ **CASE 1.23**

A 25-day-old female newborn is brought to the ED by her parents. They state that she has not been breastfeeding well this morning and has felt warm. They measured her axillary temperature as 100.6°F with an axillary digital thermometer at home. They have not noticed any rhinorrhea, cough, or rashes. The baby is having five to six wet diapers per day and five to six yellow, seedy, stools per day. The child has not had any sick contacts. She slept normally last night but was a little hard to wake up from her morning nap today. The baby was the 7 lb 8 oz product of an uncomplicated term gestation, born via normal spontaneous vaginal delivery to a group B *streptococcus* (GBS)–negative mother. There were no complications in the early neonatal period, and the baby was discharged with the mother at 2 days of life after receiving routine neonatal care. At her 2-week weight check, she seemed to be gaining weight well and her doctor had no concerns.

Question 1.23.1 Which of these is NOT a common cause of serious infections in children younger than 1 month?
A) *Listeria monocytogenes*
B) *Neisseria meningitides*
C) Group B *Streptococcus* (GBS)
D) *Pseudomonas aeruginosa*

Answer 1.23.1 **The correct answer is "D." "A,"** *L. monocytogenes*, is an obligate intracellular anaerobe that is transmitted transplacentally from mother to child. "B," *N. meningitides*, is a Gram-negative diplococcus that colonizes the respiratory tract of up to 15% of healthy individuals. It is usually spread through close contact. "C," GBS, is a Gram-positive organism that colonizes the genital tract of normal healthy women. GBS may be the most common cause of bacterial infection in the newborn. The peak incidence of GBS disease is in the first 7 days of life, but there may be a delayed presentation out to 30 days. *Pseudomonas* ("D") infections are not commonly seen in the neonatal period.

HELPFUL TIP:
Look carefully for cold sores or other vesicular lesions on children with rashes. Also try to get a history of any close contacts between the patient and people with cold sores. Herpes virus infection can be devastating to the newborn, and they may require treatment with antiviral medication.

The child is seen in her father's arms. She appears to have normal color and tone. She is sleeping but arouses after some stimulation. She seems fussy but can be consoled by her parents. Vitals: temperature 38.7°C rectally, pulse 165 bpm, and respiratory rate 32. She appears to be well hydrated, and otherwise has a completely normal physical examination.

Question 1.23.2 What further evaluation is indicated now?
A) CBC, blood cultures, catheterized urine for analysis and culture
B) CBC, blood cultures, bag urine for analysis and culture
C) CBC, blood cultures, chest radiograph, catheterized urine for analysis and culture
D) CBC, blood cultures, catheterized urine for analysis and culture, lumbar puncture, and chest radiograph

Answer 1.23.2 **The correct answer is "D."** It is important that a complete evaluation and septic workup be performed on all febrile children younger than 28 days old without a definite source of infection. This includes CBC, blood cultures, catheterized urine specimens for analysis and culture, and a lumbar puncture. A chest x-ray need not be done in the patient without respiratory symptoms but is highly recommended. LP is mandatory. Even if you suspect a pneumonia or UTI, an LP should still be considered as it is impossible to tell if the bacteria have spread hematogenously to the meningeal space.

HELPFUL TIP:
Do not delay antibiotic therapy to obtain a lumbar puncture. Lumbar punctures performed within 2 to 4 hours of receiving antibiotics should still yield valid results.

HELPFUL (AND CONTROVERSIAL) TIP:
Some would argue that a bag urine should be done as the initial urine examination. While not as specific as a catheterized urine, it is more sensitive for UTI. If the bag UA comes back positive, a catheterized specimen should be sent for culture. About 13% of children with a UTI will not have pyuria; use clinical judgment (*Pediatrics*. 2016 July).

Question 1.23.3 You are awaiting lab results. Should you play World of Warcraft, Minecraft, or start antibiotics? You decide to start antibiotics. Which antibiotics are most appropriate for empiric therapy in this patient?
A) Ampicillin and gentamicin
B) Ceftriaxone
C) Valacyclovir
D) Amoxicillin with or without clavulanate
E) Any of the above are equally valid choices

Answer 1.23.3 **The correct answer is "A."** Ampicillin and gentamicin cover all of the common causes of serious bacterial infection in the newborn, and both antibiotics penetrate into the cerebrospinal fluid (CSF) well. Ceftriaxone also penetrates the CSF well, but is highly bound to albumin and may displace bilirubin. There have been case reports of kernicterus following the administration of ceftriaxone in newborns, so its use is not recommended in children younger than 1 month. If there is concern for a herpes virus infection, acyclovir IV would be preferred over valacyclovir, but neither of these is used on an empiric basis routinely. Amoxicillin, with or without clavulanate, does not penetrate the CSF as well as ampicillin and is thus not preferred when meningitis is a possibility.

Question 1.23.4 What is the appropriate disposition for this child?
A) Admission to the general pediatrics floor
B) Admission to the pediatric intensive care unit
C) Monitor for 3 hours in the ED, and decide based on laboratory results
D) Discharge with 24-hour follow-up

Answer 1.23.4 The correct answer is "A." This child does not look toxic and can probably be managed appropriately on a general pediatrics floor instead of an intensive care unit. This child should be admitted, regardless of what the laboratory results demonstrate. Some experienced practitioners will discharge a nontoxic febrile child from the ED if he or she is older than 2 months and has follow-up within 24 hours. However, there is some risk inherent in this practice—namely, that deterioration in the patient's condition may go unrecognized at home and that the family will fail to follow-up. The standard of care is to admit all children who have a fever when they are less than 30 days old.

HELPFUL TIP:
With the advent of the polyvalent pneumococcal vaccine and the implementation of universal screening for GBS, the incidence of occult serious bacterial infection is falling. It may be that in the near future, the way in which febrile infants younger than 3 months are evaluated and treated will change. However, the practice outlined in Table 1-8 represents the current standard of care.

HELPFUL TIP:
Even when present, otitis media **is not** considered a source of fever when evaluating the neonate. You should continue with your clinical and laboratory evaluation as if you did not even see the ears!

▶ **Objectives: Did you learn to …**
· Describe common bacterial agents causing infection in the early neonatal period?
· Evaluate the febrile newborn?
· Manage the febrile newborn?

▶ **CASE 1.24**

A 6-month-old male is brought to the ED by his father. He has had a little bit of rhinorrhea for the last 36 hours but no fevers. A few hours ago, he began coughing and seemed to be having some difficulty breathing. He has been taking his bottle and rice cereal well. His father states that there have been no changes in his stools. He is fully vaccinated, has no significant past medical history, and has had no known sick contacts.

Question 1.24.1 What is the most common cause of respiratory distress in a 6-month-old (and not necessarily the diagnosis in this child)?
A) Pneumonia
B) Foreign body aspiration
C) Bronchiolitis
D) Second-hand smoke exposure

TABLE 1-8   CURRENT RECOMMENDATIONS FOR EVALUATING THE FEBRILE CHILD

Age ≤28 days
• These neonates are assumed to have bacteremia and potential seeding of the CSF, even if a source is discovered.
• Workup should include cultures of blood, urine, CSF, and stool (if GI symptoms present) and CXR (if respiratory symptoms present).
• CBC and/or CRP can be obtained, but the decision about whether or not to proceed with evaluation should not be based on these results!
• The child should be admitted for IV antibiotics until cultures are negative.

Age 1–3 months
• It is safest to assume they are still unable to contain bacterial infections at this age.
• Patients at low risk of having a serious bacterial infection have the following labs:
  • WBC >5,000, <15,000/mm^3 with band count <1,500/mm^3
  • Normal urinalysis
  • Normal CSF
  • Stool microscopy <5 WBC/HPF if diarrhea present
• If no source is found on examination, it is reasonable for patients meeting these low-risk criteria to be managed with intramuscular ceftriaxone in the ED/clinic—if follow-up can be arranged to receive a second dose in 24 hours.
• It should be emphasized that these infants are still vulnerable to dissemination of bacterial infections. Therefore, those with an obvious source, those who appear clinically ill, or those who do not meet the low-risk criteria should be cultured and admitted for IV antibiotics until cultures are negative.

Age 3–36 months
• Management of fever in this group is somewhat controversial, as the advent of Prevnar (pneumococcal vaccine) and continued use of HIB vaccine will presumably reduce the risk of invasive bacterial disease.
• It is generally accepted that well-appearing children with fevers less than 39°C do not require further evaluation or antibiotics.
• Up to 5% of children with temperature >39°C who appear clinically well will have positive blood cultures (occult bacteremia), putting them at risk for serious infections. One approach is to obtain screening WBC on those with fevers >39°C. If WBC <5,000 or >15,000/mm^3 or bands >l,500/mm^3, then further evaluation of blood, urine, and CSF should be considered.

Answer 1.24.1 The correct answer is "C." Bronchiolitis is very common, especially in the winter months. It is usually caused by the respiratory syncytial virus, but can also be caused by parainfluenza, influenza, and human metapneumovirus. Bronchiolitis is usually associated with profuse rhinorrhea, bronchospasm, and mucus plugging of the bronchiole tree. Although, "A," pneumonia is a serious cause of respiratory problems, it is not terribly common in infants. "B," foreign body aspiration, is something that must be always considered in an infant, especially a 6-month-old who is becoming more mobile (and to whom everything looks like food). Second-hand smoke exposure can cause chronic irritation to the respiratory tract and can exacerbate bronchospasm, but it is infrequently the sole cause of respiratory distress.

As you examine the child, you note that he is mildly tachypneic with some suprasternal, subcostal, and intercostal retractions. He makes a whistling, wheezing sound on inspiration (stridor) that seems to get worse the harder he breathes. He also has a brassy-sounding cough that does not seem to be productive.

Question 1.24.2 What is the most likely diagnosis at this point?
A) Pneumonia
B) Croup
C) Laryngomalacia
D) Asthma

Answer 1.24.2 The correct answer is "B." Croup, or laryngotracheobronchitis, is a common infection of the upper and lower respiratory tract. It is most commonly caused by parainfluenza virus, but may also be caused by influenza and respiratory syncytial virus. Classically, croup affects children younger than 5 years, although it is occasionally seen in older children. As the glottis swells, children develop a wheeze/whistle on inspiration (inspiratory stridor) and a characteristic brassy "seal-like" barking cough. The vast majority of cases are mild. Occasionally, however, children may require control of the airway due to hypoxia. "A," pneumonia, is an infection of the lower airways that can be either bacterial or viral in nature. These children generally have a fever and productive cough. They may be tachypneic and have an increased work of breathing, but they usually do not have inspiratory stridor. "C," laryngomalacia, is a congenital disorder. These children usually develop symptoms at a few weeks of age and present with inspiratory stridor that gets worse with crying. It tends to be a little better when the child is calm and in the supine position. Laryngomalacia resolves spontaneously in the majority of children as the larynx becomes firmer and the airway diameter increases, but some children will require surgical intervention to facilitate feeding and growth. The child in this vignette is presenting with a new problem, as opposed to a chronic one, so this is not laryngomalacia. "D," asthma, is another disease of the lower airways, and wheezing is expiratory in nature.

You decide to do a radiograph of this child's neck to aid in the diagnosis (although this is certainly not necessary nor advocated in most cases—but this is a board review book, not real life).

Question 1.24.3 You are most likely to see which of the following on cervical radiograph?
A) Thumb sign
B) Quincke sign
C) Spine sign
D) Retropharyngeal space swelling
E) Steeple sign

Answer 1.24.3 The correct answer is "E." Radiographs in croup may show the "steeple sign," which is a subglottic narrowing of the trachea from edema, giving it a steeple-like appearance. "A," the thumb sign, is seen in epiglottitis. "B," Quincke sign, is incorrect, as it has nothing to do with radiology. Quincke sign is the ungual capillary pulsation associated with aortic insufficiency—it's rare, not seen in children, and nearly useless knowledge… but that is what you are paying us for! "C," the spine sign, is loss of progressive radiolucency of the spine on lateral chest radiograph. This is seen when something—classically an infiltrate indicative of pneumonia—is overlaying the lower thoracic spine, making the vertebral bodies appear more dense. Finally, "D," retropharyngeal space swelling, is seen in retropharyngeal abscess.

Question 1.24.4 What is the most appropriate definitive therapy for this patient at this time?
A) Epinephrine 0.01 mg SQ
B) Nebulized albuterol
C) Dexamethasone 0.6 mg/kg PO/IM/IV
D) High flow oxygen and prepare to intubate

Answer 1.24.4 The correct answer is "C." Corticosteroids help to decrease the glottic edema. One dose of dexamethasone 0.3 to 0.6 mg/kg (maximum of 10 mg) can be given via multiple routes (PO/IM/IV) and is usually sufficient to improve the airway swelling enough to allow the child to breathe comfortably. The advantage of dexamethasone over prednisone or another corticosteroid is that its long half-life obviates the need for further dosing at home. While waiting for the dexamethasone to work, epinephrine may be administered via nebulizer for severe cases. This usually leads to significant clinical improvement and gives time for the steroid to begin to take effect. Subcutaneous epinephrine is usually unnecessary. Albuterol, while helpful for bronchospasm, does not do anything to treat the glottic edema that is causing the majority of the respiratory distress. Intubation is not indicated at this point if the child is not in impending respiratory failure, hypoxic, or minimally responsive.

 HELPFUL TIP:
While classically we have used racemic epinephrine, the "d" isomer is inactive. In addition, racemic epinephrine is more expensive and must be kept refrigerated if a multidose vial is used. L-epinephrine, 5 cc of 1:1,000, delivered by nebulizer is as—if not more—effective,

than racemic epinephrine, is cheaper, and is the same dose for everyone (our favorite since we can't do simple math!).

You administer the appropriate dose of dexamethasone to the child along with a treatment of nebulized epinephrine. He improves markedly. You watch him for 2 hours. He is able to tolerate oral fluids well and is active and playful. He still has a brassy cough, but no inspiratory stridor.

Question 1.24.5 **What should his disposition be?**
A) Admit for 23 hours of observation
B) Administer second dose of racemic epinephrine and re-evaluate
C) Discharge to home with close outpatient follow-up
D) Administer albuterol and re-evaluate

Answer 1.24.5 **The correct answer is "C."** After administering dexamethasone and epinephrine, it is imperative to observe children for at least 2 hours. If the child redevelops stridor at rest, he should receive a second dose of epinephrine. Any child who needs a second treatment has more severe croup, is at higher risk of having complications, and should be considered for hospital admission. If the child is free of stridor 2 hours after nebulized epinephrine, he can be safely discharged with close outpatient follow-up (within 24 hours) as long as the parents are reliable, able to monitor the child, comfortable with the plan, and able to return if the child's condition should deteriorate.

> **HELPFUL TIP:**
> Remember that an oxygen saturation of less than 95% is singularly abnormal in a child.

▶ **Objectives: Did you learn to …**
  - Describe common causes of respiratory distress in children?
  - Manage pediatric airway problems?
  - Treat children with croup?

 QUICK QUIZ: FOREIGN BODY

A 3-year-old boy and his 5-year-old sister were being silly, avoiding bedtime, and jumping on their parent's bed. Naturally, the boy had a nickel in his mouth that he'd found on the floor. When their mother walked in to wrangle them into their pajamas, they predictably collided in mid-air and both fell off the bed and onto the floor. She was unable to find the nickel after the incident. Coincidentally, the 3-year-old feels like he has something stuck in his throat—something with Thomas Jefferson's head on it.

When the family arrives in your office, he takes liquids without much trouble but won't take anything solid. He says his "throat hurts." He's not drooling or having any trouble breathing.

How do you confirm that the coin is not in the airway?
A) CT of the larynx and chest without IV contrast
B) CT of the larynx and chest with IV contrast
C) AP and lateral plain films of the neck
D) Direct laryngoscopy
E) Call a pulmonologist for emergent fiberoptic bronchoscopy

The correct answer is "C." Fortunately coins are radiopaque—at least as of the printing of this book (maybe we'll have wooden coins again someday!). Some plastic toys legally contain barium and are radiopaque while others are inadvertently radiopaque (like those old toys contaminated with lead … a mixed blessing at best!). The esophagus tends to collapse from anterior to posterior when there is nothing in the lumen. Therefore, a coin in the esophagus should look round on an AP x-ray. By contrast, the trachea is supported by cartilaginous rings around most of its circumference. The posterior part of the trachea, however, abuts the esophagus and has no cartilage. Therefore, coins that fall into the trachea generally have an end-on appearance on AP radiographs and look like a disc on a lateral film.

The coin fell into the stomach on the way to x-ray and the little boy feels better.

What foreign bodies in the *stomach* need to be removed emergently?
A) A button battery
B) A paperclip that is folded in its original form
C) Two small magnets
D) A doll's shoe

The correct answer is "C." Two magnets can attract each other through opposing loops of bowel, causing bowel necrosis and perforation. One magnet should not cause any trouble, but two should be taken seriously. **Button batteries lodged in the esophagus need to be removed emergently. However, once a button battery transitions to the stomach, it will likely pass without causing any difficulty. However, it should be removed if it remains in the stomach for more than 48 hours or is ≥15 mm in size.** Other smooth or rounded objects are unlikely to cause any trouble. Even small sharp objects (e.g., pushpins) generally pass without causing perforation or other significant damage.

▶ **CASE 1.25**

A 67-year-old female with a history of end-stage renal disease on hemodialysis presents slumped over and complaining of generalized weakness. By the time she is in a room, her eyes are closed, she is nonverbal, withdraws from painful stimuli and does not follow commands but has a palpable pulse at 80 bpm. Her husband notes that she has been using "light salt," which contains potassium. You remember the "coma cocktail" from earlier in this chapter: glucose, naloxone, thiamine, and oxygen. You also remember that not all narcotic overdoses are associated with pinpoint pupils. You treat her appropriately. The patient's blood sugar is 211 mg/dL.

The patient's husband states that dialysis was not performed today. The patient also missed her last dialysis appointment 2 days ago because she felt ill at home. Her mental status is unchanged after the "coma cocktail"; she is unable to protect her airway. Husband confirms patient is full code. You decide to proceed with intubation.

Question 1.25.1 The best medications to use in this patient are (induction agent/paralytic agent):
A) Etomidate/succinylcholine
B) Etomidate/ketamine
C) Etomidate/rocuronium
D) An induction agent and a paralytic are unnecessary in this patient since she is only responsive to deep stimuli

Answer 1.25.1 The correct answer is "C." Rocuronium would be the paralytic of choice in this patient. In a patient with chronic kidney disease on hemodialysis, assume the presence of hyperkalemia until proven otherwise. Succinylcholine may cause hyperkalemia (and cardiac arrest) so it is contraindicated in patients with a high likelihood of hyperkalemia. Succinylcholine should also be avoided in crush injuries, neurologic injuries/myopathies, and burn patients where it may cause malignant hyperthermia. A sedative should be used for induction to prevent pain and either etomidate or ketamine may be used—not both.

You secure the airway. A STAT potassium returns at 7.9. Darn! You look at the monitor and notice the QRS is looking a little wide. Double darn!

Question 1.25.2 While you are waiting for an ECG to be obtained, you administer:
A) Kayexalate
B) Sodium bicarbonate
C) Calcium gluconate
D) Insulin/glucose
E) Albuterol nebulizer

Answer 1.25.2 The correct answer is "C." In hyperkalemia with evidence of ECG changes (peaked T waves, wide QRS, sine wave), calcium needs to be administered immediately. The calcium stabilizes cardiac cell membranes within 1 minute. Calcium gluconate 1 g or calcium chloride 1 g may be given. Calcium chloride is irritating to veins and may cause necrosis if it extravasates: central line administration is preferred. All of the other answers do lower potassium levels (including continuously nebulized albuterol), but when there is evidence of ECG changes, giving calcium is your top priority. The other agents may take as long as 30 to 60 minutes to act. As a note, bicarbonate may not be particularly effective in patients with chronic kidney disease, another reason to use calcium first in this patient.

After 2 doses of calcium gluconate, the QRS narrows and you want to get the excess potassium out of your patient's body.

Question 1.25.3 Which of the following removes potassium from the body?
A) Hemodialysis
B) Insulin/glucose
C) Kayexalate (sodium polystyrene)
D) Albuterol
E) A and C

Answer 1.25.3 The correct answer is "E." Both hemodialysis and sodium polystyrene will remove potassium from the body. Insulin/glucose will drive it intracellularly in 30 to 60 minutes, but does not rid the body of potassium. Be careful: sodium polystyrene exchanges sodium for potassium and thus may worsen congestive heart failure. **The use of sodium polystyrene with sorbitol is discouraged.** It is associated with bowel ischemia and necrosis. **In addition, be careful using sodium polystyrene in those with GI problems (ileus, stricture, etc.) for the same reason.** Note that patiromer (Veltassa), a second potassium binder is also available. However, it may not lower potassium for up to 7 hours after administration and is NOT approved for the acute lowering of potassium. Remember that *both* patiromer and sodium polystyrene (Kayexalate) bind many medications and reduce their bioavailability significantly. Finally, sodium zirconium cyclosilicate (Lokelma) has recently been released. It seems to work within 1 hour and will likely become the potassium binder of choice.

The patient does well and, in the future, knows to avoid "light" salt (KCl) (of course, "light" is now spelled "lite" for some unknown reason).

▶ **Objectives: Did you learn to …**
· Describe contraindications of succinylcholine in intubation?
· Treat hyperkalemia in the acute situation?

▶ CASE 1.26

A 24-year-old male presents to your ED complaining of "dental pain." He reports a long history of poor dental hygiene and has not seen a dentist in several years. He smokes two packs of cigarettes per day (and proudly wears a "Marlboro" hat) and admits drinking a 2-L bottle of "Hillbilly Holler (Sugared)" every day at work. (It includes a free coupon for dental service after 100 bottles, but he has never availed himself of this.) The pain is described as constant and throbbing in nature located in the right lower jaw area.

Question 1.26.1 What findings during your examination would raise your concern regarding the patient's clinical condition?
A) Large amounts of secretions
B) Decreased ability to open his mouth for the examination
C) Swollen and elevated tongue
D) Pain and decreased range of motion of the neck
E) All of the above

Answer 1.26.1 The correct answer is "E." If a patient is having trouble swallowing secretions ("A"), it should raise concern for swelling in the posterior pharynx which can compromise not only the ability to swallow one's saliva but can also signal a high risk for upper airway occlusion secondary to swelling. Trismus ("B") is also concerning because it may indicate deeper infection involving the muscles of mastication. "C," a swollen and elevated tongue, may indicate the development of Ludwig angina, a life-threatening infection of the floor of the mouth, which can spread to the deeper tissues of the submandibular and submaxillary spaces. "D," pain and decreased range of motion of the neck, could indicate the possibility of a retropharyngeal abscess.

HELPFUL TIP:
Adult epiglottitis often presents with sore throat and neck tenderness. So, if the patient has neck tenderness out of proportion to what you would expect, consider epiglottitis or a retropharyngeal abscess.

Luckily, the patient is otherwise clinically stable aside from the focal dental pain. Your examination shows the tissues around tooth number 29 (we can never remember that pesky numbering scheme either) to be swollen and inflamed with signs of fluctuance and severe tenderness on palpation. An orthopantogram shows a periodontal abscess.

Question 1.26.2 Which antibiotic is NOT an appropriate choice for this clinical condition?
A) Penicillin VK
B) Clindamycin
C) Amoxicillin/clavulanate
D) Trimethoprim–sulfamethoxazole

Answer 1.26.2 The correct answer is "D." Penicillin VK, clindamycin, and amoxicillin/clavulanate all provide good coverage for anaerobic bacteria including anaerobic Gram-negative cocci, which are the main culprits in dental infections. TMP–SMX has some Gram-negative coverage but lacks the anaerobic coverage needed to treat infections of the oral cavity.

The same gentleman returns to you 3 weeks later complaining of a sore throat. On examination, he looks toxic and has fever, chills, dyspnea/cough, and unilateral neck swelling. His throat looks similar to a streptococcal tonsillitis. However, the neck is tender, *and this guy really looks sick.* Pulse is 130 bpm and BP is 80/50 mm Hg. He was seen last week by someone else for a mild sore throat and given a "Z-Pak" (azithromycin—mostly on a whim). He has gotten progressively worse. Chest x-ray shows infiltrates and small abscesses.

Question 1.26.3 Your presumptive diagnosis is:
A) Mononucleosis
B) *Fusobacterium*
C) *Arcanobacterium hemolyticum*
D) Viral URI

Answer 1.26.3 The correct answer is "B." *Fusobacterium* is an anaerobic infection that has been found with increasing frequency in adolescent/college-age patients. It can initially present similarly to a strep throat but may go on to "Lemierre syndrome," which is a septic thrombophlebitis of the internal jugular vein. This can then lead to septic emboli to the lungs, sepsis, and multiorgan failure. The point here is that penicillin is still the drug of choice for strep throat, and it covers *Fusobacterium*, which the macrolides do not. As for the other answers, this is not likely mononucleosis ("A"), since the neck swelling is unilateral and patients with mono usually are not this toxic nor have infiltrate on chest x-ray. "C," *A. hemolyticum*, is also common in college-age students and is initially clinically indistinguishable from strep throat. However, 50% of patients will have a maculopapular or scarlatiniform rash starting on the extremities and involving the trunk and back but sparing the head; as opposed to the rash of scarlet fever, the rash does not peel. It rarely causes invasive disease such as pneumonia or meningitis. It will respond to erythromycin or clindamycin and less so to penicillin. "D" is obviously incorrect and if you chose this one, back to medical school for you!

The patient spends 3 weeks in the ICU and eventually succumbs to his disease. Not good (way for us to end on a "downer" you say, but at least you get the message that "Z-paks" aren't always the answer).

▶ **Objectives: Did you learn to …**
• Diagnose and treat a dental abscesses?
• Identify *Fusobacterium* and *Arcanobacterium* infections

▶ **CASE 1.27**

An 82-year-old female slumps over in church (it's always the bathroom or church—avoid these and you will live forever). Luckily, there is a nurse present who just happens to have a monitor/defibrillator. The nurse lets you know she can't feel a pulse. You quickly hook the patient up a cardiac monitor and see the rhythm in Figure 1-2.

Question 1.27.1 "Uh-oh," you think. You astutely identify the rhythm as:
A) Atrial fibrillation
B) Ventricular tachycardia
C) Ventricular fibrillation
D) PEA

Answer 1.27.1 The correct answer is "C." Note absence of p-waves, no complexes—just a sinusoidal pattern of rapid, irregular ventricular activity that results in no functional contractions (thus no cardiac output, and thus no pulse).

Question 1.27.2 Aside from starting CPR, the first-line treatment for this is:
A) Amiodarone
B) Epinephrine

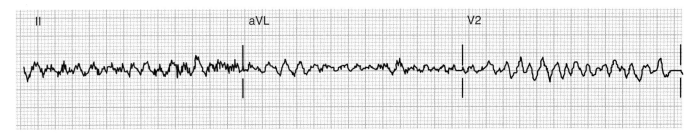

FIGURE 1-2. Rhythm strip for question 1.27.1.

C) Electrical defibrillation

D) Adenosine

Answer 1.27.2 **The correct answer is "C."** The initial treatment for ventricular fibrillation or pulseless ventricular tachycardia is electrical defibrillation. CPR should be in process as defibrillation is set up. Epinephrine ("B") and amiodarone ("A") are part of the algorithm but are not the first treatment. "D" is just wrong.

HELPFUL TIP: "SHOCKING!"

The "stacked defibrillations" (100J, 200J, 360J) are no more. Defibrillate at 360J once *or* 150 to 200J with a biphasic defibrillator.

Question 1.27.3 Shock delivered! Now what?

A) Check your rhythm

B) Check for a pulse

C) Perform CPR

D) Check rhythm and pulse at the same time

E) Intubate and check rhythm

Answer 1.27.3 **The correct answer is "C," perform CPR.** Current ACLS guidelines recommend 2 minutes of CPR following defibrillation (Not like the TV shows, where patients just jump up and walk out, right?). You can check for a pulse ("B") and check your rhythm ("A") after that 2 minutes of CPR is completed. Intubation ("E") may be considered during a code, *but if you are able to effectively bag a patient, it is more important to continue high-quality CPR.* Intubation is no longer considered mandatory—and, in fact, outcomes seem to be better *without* intubation.

As you are continuing CPR, you ask the nurse to give epinephrine 1 mg (vasopressin is out of the ACLS guidelines). The medication is administered. On next pulse check, you see sinus tachycardia on the monitor, but there is no pulse with palpation. You identify that the patient currently is in pulseless electrical activity (PEA).

Question 1.27.4 Now what?

A) Defibrillation

B) CPR and epinephrine

C) CPR and defibrillation

D) Call an end to the code

Answer 1.27.4 **The correct answer is "B," CPR and epinephrine.** Epinephrine should continue to be administered every 3 to 5 minutes. PEA Is NOT an indication for defibrillation ("A" and "C"). It seems a little premature to call the code ("D") at this time.

HELPFUL TIP:

When a patient is in PEA, always think through the potentials' causes. A mnemonic of "5Hs and 5Ts" will help you remember them all.

Hs: Hypovolemia, hypothermia, hypo/hyperkalemia, hypoxia, hydrogen ion (acidosis)

Ts: Tension pneumothorax, tamponade (cardiac), toxins, thrombosis (PE), thrombosis (coronary)

Success! On next rhythm check there is a pulse. Well done!

Clinical Pearls

○ Avoid CT scans in patients with known urolithiasis who have the same symptoms again unless you suspect a post-obstructive infection or have reason to believe it could be an aortic problem (e.g., at-risk patients over 50 years old).

○ Avoid the use of narcotics for migraine headaches if possible. Prochlorperazine or metoclopramide work well with prochlorperazine IV being the preferred agent.

○ Do not do a chest CT (or d-dimer) if a patient is PERC negative and is low risk for a PE. Besides the expense, the cancer risk for a 20-year-old female from a single 64-slice chest CT is approximately 1 in 250.

○ Do not do a head CT for patients with simple syncope: syncope is not a brain disease. It is generally a problem of CNS perfusion; you have to knock out both hemispheres simultaneously to lose consciousness.

○ Do not do a head CT in low-risk patients with head trauma. Use a prediction rule. However, it is reasonable to CT those on anticoagulants.

○ Do not do a head CT looking for the cause of vertigo; it is almost always useless. If you need imaging, do an MRI but recognize that an MRI will be negative for posterior circulation stroke in 30% of cases within the first 24 hours.

○ Do not do a head CT of children with a first uncomplicated seizure.

○ Do not get back imaging for acute low back pain unless there are red flags, such as fever, cancer history, significant trauma (not just twisting or picking something up), neurologic symptoms or signs.

○ Only give as much blood as is necessary. Giving one unit is fine. As a general rule, don't transfuse a stable patient with a hemoglobin of 7 g/dL or greater.

○ Phenytoin and fosphenytoin do not work for alcohol withdrawal seizures, seizures caused by drug overdose or withdrawal (in general). Use a benzodiazepine.

BIBLIOGRAPHY

American Academy of Pediatrics. Tetanus. In: Kimberlin DW, Brady MT, Jackson MA, Long SS, eds. *Red Book®: 2015 Report of the Committee on Infectious Diseases*. American Academy of Pediatrics; 2015; 773–778.

Benson BE, et al. American Academy of Clinical Toxicology; European Association of Poisons Centres and Clinical Toxicologists. Position paper update: gastric lavage for gastrointestinal decontamination. *Clin Toxicol (Phila)*. 2013;51(3):140–146.

Brown CV, et al. Preventing renal failure in patients with rhabdomyolysis: do bicarbonate and mannitol make a difference? *J Trauma*. 2004;56(6):1191–1196.

Carraro S, et al. Bronchiolitis: from empiricism to scientific evidence. *Minerva Pediatr*. 2009;61:217–225.

Diercks DB, et al. ACEP Clinical Policies Committee. Clinical policy: critical issues in the evaluation and management of adult patients with suspected acute nontraumatic thoracic aortic dissection. *Ann Emerg Med*. 2015;65:32–42.

Engebretsen KM, et al. High-dose insulin therapy in beta-blocker and calcium channel-blocker poisoning. *Clin Toxicol (Phila)*. 2011;49(4):277–283.

Frithsen IL, Simpson WM Jr. Recognition and management of acute medication poisoning. *Am Fam Physician*. 2010;81:316–323.

Green NE, Allen L. Vascular injuries associated with dislocation of the knee. *J Bone Joint Surg Am*. 1977;59:236–239.

Herz AM, et al. Changing epidemiology of outpatient bacteremia in 3- to 36-month-old children after the introduction of the heptavalent-conjugated pneumococcal vaccine. *Pediatr Infect Dis J*. 2006;25:293–300.

Huff JS, et al. ACEP Clinical Policies Committee. Clinical policy: critical issues in the evaluation and management of adult patients presenting to the emergency department with seizures. *Ann Emerg Med*. 2014;63:437–447.

Isbister GK, Kumar VV. Indications for single-dose activated charcoal administration in acute overdose. *Curr Opin Crit Care*. 2011;17:351–357.

Leung AK, Sigalet DL. Acute abdominal pain in children. *Am Fam Physician*. 2003;67:2321–2326.

Marx J, et al. *Rosen's Emergency Medicine Concepts and Clinical Practice*. 8th ed. St. Louis, MO: Mosby Elsevier Health Sciences; 2010.

Mokhlesi B, et al. Adult toxicology in critical care: Part II: Specific poisonings. *Chest*. 2003;123:897–922.

Moscati RM, et al. A multicenter comparison of tap water versus sterile saline for wound irrigation. *Acad Emerg Med*. 2007;14(5):404–409.

Nikkanen H, Skolnik A. Diagnosis and management of carbon monoxide poisoning in the emergency department. *Emerg Med Pract*. 2011;13:1–14.

Panju AA, et al. The rational clinical examination: is this patient having a myocardial infarction? *JAMA*. 1998;280:1256–1263.

Rogers RL, McCormack R. Aortic disasters. *Emerg Med Clin North Am*. 2004;22:887–908.

Steiner RW. Treating acute bronchiolitis associated with RSV. *Am Fam Physician*. 2004;69:325–330.

Toce MS, Burns MM. The poisoned pediatric patient. *Pediatr Rev*. 2017;38(5):207–220.

Touger M, et al. Relationship between venous and arterial carboxyhemoglobin levels in patients with suspected carbon monoxide poisoning. *Ann Emerg Med*. 1995;25(4):481–483.

Wolf SJ, et al. ACEP Clinical Policies Committee. Clinical policy: critical issues in the management of adult patients presenting to the emergency department with acute carbon monoxide poisoning. *Ann Emerg Med*. 2008;51:138–152.

Yucesoy K, Yuksel KZ. SCIWORA in MRI era. *Clin Neurol Neurosurg*. 2008;110:429–433.

Cardiology

2

Mark A. Graber and Jason K. Wilbur

We are going to start this chapter with a knock-down, drag-out, fight about blood pressure. What is this? Medicine or hockey? There is considerable controversy over what constitutes an appropriate blood pressure goal for a wide range of adult patients. In this chapter, we are following the recommendations of the Eighth Joint National Committee (JNC 8) which have been endorsed by the American College of Physicians and the American Academy of Family Physicians—and which we assume will be on the test (*Ann Intern Med.* 2017;166:430). The American College of Cardiology and the American Heart Association (ACC/AHA) disagree.

For the record, the ACC/AHA prefer the following:

Blood Pressure	Action	Further Action
<120/80 mm Hg	Reassess annually	
120/80–129/80 mm Hg	Life style modification	Reassess in 1 **month**
Hypertensive: 130–139/80–89 mm Hg	Calculate 10-year risk using the ACC/AHA ASCVD risk calculator (see: https://www.mdcalc.com/ascvd-atherosclerotic-cardiovascular-disease-2013-risk-calculator-aha-acc)	If >10% 10-year ASCVD risk, start antihypertensive; otherwise, life style changes
>140/90 mm Hg	Start antihypertensive pharmacotherapy	Reassess in 1 **month**
Goal blood pressure < 130/80 mm Hg for everyone		

Note that this table represents a simplification of the ACC/AHA guidelines. Much more detail is available in the full report (*J Am Coll Cardiol.* 2018;71:e127).

We are going to continue our fight with aspirin for **primary prevention**. Four words: **Don't do it routinely.** The consensus based on new data is that aspirin for primary prevention increases bleeding risk and does not reduce cardiovascular events, disability-free survival, or all-cause mortality (*N Engl J Med.* 2018;379:1519). **Continue to use it in patients *who have***

had **a cardiovascular event (angina, PVD, stroke, etc.)** where the benefit does outweigh the risk. To continue, omega-3s from fish oil still don't help prevent cardiac disease or cancer (*N Engl J Med.* 2019;380:23–32). Finally, there are competing 2013 and 2018 lipid guidelines. The ACP and AAFP have not endorsed the 2018 guidelines. However, we do discuss them toward the end of the chapter.

▶ CASE 2.1

A 35-year-old female presents with a 1-hour history of chest pain, which resolved spontaneously. The pain is described as a chest pressure radiating to both arms. The patient is a smoker but has no other risk factors (no family history of cardiac disease, hypertension, diabetes, hyperlipidemia, etc.). The patient is diaphoretic and has a normal blood pressure. Physical examination reveals that the patient has tenderness to palpation of the anterior chest wall that reproduces the chest pressure. She is now otherwise free of chest pain and all her lab assays, including cardiac enzymes, are normal.

Question 2.1.1 **Which of the following is true about this patient's physical findings and history?**
A) Pain radiating to both arms makes it unlikely that this patient's pain is cardiac
B) The physical findings that are most highly associated with an acute myocardial infarction (AMI) include hypotension, diaphoresis, and a new S3 gallop
C) The absence of risk factors makes it unlikely that this patient has cardiac disease
D) The fact that the pain is reproducible on palpation of the chest wall effectively rules out cardiac disease
E) Based on the information available, further cardiac evaluation is unnecessary

Answer 2.1.1 **The correct answer is "B."** The findings that are most likely to be associated with an AMI are hypotension, diaphoresis, and a new S3 gallop. "A" is not true because pain radiating to both arms can still be associated with cardiac disease. In fact, compared with left arm radiation, right arm radiation or bilateral arm radiation doubles the likelihood of the pain being cardiac (LR 2.3 for radiation to the left arm vs. LR 4.1–4.7 for radiation to the right or bilateral arms [*JAMA* 2005;294(20):2623–2629]). Women with AMI often present atypically and may experience more chest pain radiating to the right arm/shoulder and the anterior neck or with abdominal pain, as compared to men. "C" is incorrect. The absence of risk factors is only one consideration in the evaluation of this patient. Smoking, hypertension, family history, etc., **do not** change the prior probability of cardiac disease enough to allow them to be used to rule out or rule in cardiac disease. Of note, male gender and diabetes **do** increase the pretest probability of coronary artery disease (CAD). But luckily our patient is female! Evaluation of pretest probability is important in the diagnostic algorithm, but should be *used in addition to, not in exclusion of*, clinical judgment and findings. "D" is incorrect. It is true that chest pain reproduced by palpation of the chest wall makes cardiac disease less likely. However, 15% of patients with cardiac disease and 17% of patients with a pulmonary embolism (PE) will have their pain reproduced by chest wall pressure (*BMJ* 2005;330:452–453). This does not mean that you are making their cardiac pain worse. It is likely because of the patient's inability to discriminate between the types of pain (cardiac vs. chest wall).

....

You decide that further testing is warranted, including an ECG and cardiac enzymes.

Question 2.1.2 Which of the following statements is TRUE?
A) A normal initial ECG in the emergency department (ED) effectively rules out cardiac disease
B) Creatine phosphokinase MB fraction (CPK-MB) is more sensitive but less specific than troponin
C) Serum troponin is an unreliable marker of cardiac ischemia in patients with renal failure
D) The serum troponin is 100% specific for myocardial infarction
E) A normal high sensitivity troponin and ECG in the ED 3 hours after the pain began can be used to make decisions about who to admit

Answer 2.1.2 **The correct answer is "E."** Newer "rule out" protocols allow ED physicians to categorize chest pain patients into a low-risk pool within 3 hours after pain onset. If the patient is found to be at low risk using a validated risk assessment tool (see "HEART" calculator at: https://www.mdcalc.com/heart-score-major-cardiac-events) **and** has a normal ECG **and** has a negative *high-sensitivity* troponin at 3 hours after presentation, one can rule out myocardial infarction without an admission. Remember, these are low-risk patients to begin with, not the 70-year-old with a history of CAD who is puffing like chimney. Note that the HEART score incorporates the ECG and troponin. There is a 16% discordance in how physicians score the same low-risk patients vis-à-vis HEART (*Acad Emerg Med.* 2018 Nov 14). "A" is incorrect since 9% of patients with AMI will have a normal initial ECG in the ED. In fact, only about 50% of those with AMI have a diagnostic ECG in the ED. **Even a normal ECG**

obtained during chest pain does not reliably rule out AMI (*Acad Emerg Med.* 2009;16:495). "B" is incorrect since the CPK-MB is overall less sensitive and may have a later rise than a high-sensitivity troponin. CPK-MB and myoglobin add little, if anything, to the troponin. Eighty percent of AMIs will have one positive marker within the first 3 hours of ED arrival (but 20% will not). "C" is incorrect. Patients with renal disease may have a mildly elevated troponin at baseline due to poor clearance, but troponin can still be useful in these patients if it continues to rise. It helps to know the patient's baseline troponin in renal failure, but this is NOT an indication to start drawing a baseline troponin on all of your patients with renal failure. "D" is incorrect because we now know that other processes, such as PE, can elevate the serum troponin.

HELPFUL TIP:
Elevated troponin levels may be due to conditions other than AMI, including heart failure, PE, burns, sepsis or other critical illness, stroke, and more. In "atypical" patients (younger, female patients, like this one), also consider spontaneous coronary artery dissection (SCAD). Although uncommon, SCAD is more likely in women, especially those who have recently been pregnant or undergone highly aerobic activity, like running a marathon. SCAD should be considered in patients who present with symptoms of ischemia or infarct but who do not possess traditional cardiovascular risk factors.

HELPFUL TIP:
The new ultra-sensitive troponin may be positive within 3 hours. *You need to know what test your hospital is doing.* Troponin levels peak in about 36 hours after an infarct and may stay elevated for 7 to 10 days, so the infarct may have occurred anywhere within this time frame. Follow the trend of the troponin to help determine when the infarct occurred.

Question 2.1.3 All of the following statements are true EXCEPT:
A) All myocardial infarctions present with chest pain
B) Dyspnea may be the only presenting symptom of myocardial infarction
C) Patients with myocardial infarction can present with syncope
D) Females, the elderly, and diabetic patients are more likely to present with atypical symptoms of myocardial infarction

Answer 2.1.3 **The correct answer is "A."** As the saying goes, "Never say never, and never say always." Many elderly and diabetic patients ("D") will present with atypical symptoms or painless, "silent" myocardial infarctions. In fact, up to 30% of myocardial infarctions are pain free. "B" is a correct statement because, especially in the elderly, dyspnea may be the only presenting symptom due to left ventricular failure secondary to ischemia. "C" is a correct statement because syncope (as well as lightheadedness and fatigue) can be presenting symptoms of a myocardial infarction.

Her ECG shows nonspecific ST-T changes.

Question 2.1.4 Which of the following drug(s) is/are indicated in the initial management of this patient?
A) Aspirin
B) Thrombolytic such as tPA or streptokinase
C) Heparin
D) Glycoprotein IIb/IIIa inhibitor (e.g., abciximab [ReoPro])
E) All of the above

Answer 2.1.4 The correct answer is "A." Immediate therapy in the ED requires ASA 325 mg orally (chewed). Since we are not sure that this patient has AMI or unstable angina, there is no indication for thrombolytic therapy ("B"), heparin ("C"), or glycoprotein IIb/IIIa inhibitor ("D"). Since she is currently pain free, heparin carries more of a risk than a benefit at this juncture and is not recommended. However, all patients with possible angina or an AMI should have aspirin unless they are truly allergic (e.g., hives, anaphylaxis). "B" is incorrect because thrombolytics are indicated for acute ST elevation myocardial infarctions (STEMI), not for a simple chest pain evaluation.

HELPFUL TIP:
In med school, we learned "MONA (morphine, oxygen, nitroglycerin, aspirin) greets all patients." Snappy mnemonic, but is it right? Recent data suggests that there is no need for oxygen if the oxygen saturation is 94% or above. In fact, it might be harmful. Hyperoxia is clearly detrimental in the ICU setting. So, withhold oxygen unless the oxygen saturation is <94%. Morphine should be used only after a patient fails specific therapy, such as aspirin and nitroglycerin. And, nitroglycerin does not change infarct size, but it does improve chest pain.

HELPFUL TIP:
Current use of anticoagulants or aspirin should **not** preclude the administration of aspirin in the ED for a patient with chest pain that may be cardiac in origin. You never know whether the patient is actually taking it or not. So, unless there is a real allergy to aspirin, it must be given to chest pain patients with a possible cardiac etiology—even if they tell you that they took an aspirin that morning already.

HELPFUL TIP:
Why do we always say to chew the aspirin? Does it really make a difference? Yes. In a small study of healthy volunteers, chewed aspirin started to work in 5 minutes, as opposed to 12 minutes for regular swallowed aspirin. It also reached its peak effect quicker, too.

The patient tells you that she is allergic to aspirin, which causes hives and bronchospasm. She can, however, take other nonsteroidal anti-inflammatory drugs (NSAIDs) without difficulty. Oh, great. Now you need to go to plan B (no, not the "morning after pill").

Question 2.1.5 Which of the following is an acceptable substitute for aspirin in this situation?
A) Dipyridamole
B) Ticagrelor (Brillinta)
C) Ibuprofen or naproxen
D) Celecoxib (Celebrex)
E) Salsalate

Answer 2.1.5 The correct answer is "B." Ticagrelor (Brillinta) 180 mg as a loading dose is the correct choice. Alternatively, clopidogrel (Plavix) in a loading dose of 600 mg can be used as a substitute for aspirin in the setting of unstable angina or AMI. The other options are incorrect. "A" is incorrect because dipyridamole (in combination with aspirin) is indicated only for stroke prevention. Dipyridamole itself is a relatively weak platelet inhibitor. "C" is incorrect because ibuprofen and naproxen are reversible platelet inhibitors that do not give adequate platelet inhibition and have **NOT** been shown to be of benefit in angina/AMI. In addition, both ibuprofen and naproxen can block the effect of aspirin by making its binding sites on platelets unavailable. **In fact, stopping NSAIDs in any patient being admitted for possible CAD is considered good practice since they are known to increase the risk of a cardiac event.** "D" and "E" are both incorrect because celecoxib and salsalate have not been shown to inhibit platelets to a significant degree and thus would be of no use in this situation.

HELPFUL TIP:
Why not prasugrel (Effient) for AMI? While it is an option, it cannot be used in those over age 75 or in patients with a history of stroke or TIA. And the dose must be reduced in those weighing <60 kg. It also loses potency when stored. Don't even consider Zonivity (vorapaxar) … it has a 4-week washout period and no benefits over the other agents. Plus it must be used *with* aspirin.

HELPFUL TIP:
It is unclear which, if any, of the NSAIDS (except aspirin) is the safest in the setting of a history of CAD. Some data support the use of naproxen if an NSAID is required. Other data do not show any difference between the NSAIDS. Guidelines suggest stopping all NSAIDs (except aspirin) upon admitting a patient for an acute coronary syndrome (ACS) or a question of ACS. Do not use ketorolac to treat chest pain which is potentially ACS as this is also an NSAID (*BMJ* 2017;357:j190).

Well, not all chest pain is cardiac, and this patient may have another cause for hers.

Question 2.1.6 Which of the following is TRUE?
A) Giving a "GI cocktail" (e.g., combination of Maalox and viscous lidocaine) can reliably differentiate cardiac from esophageal/GI causes of chest pain
B) A normal chest radiograph and symmetrical pulses in the upper extremities reliably rules out a thoracic aortic dissection
C) Most patients with a spontaneous pneumothorax should be treated with a chest tube
D) If nitroglycerin relieves the chest pain, then the pain is certainly cardiac
E) Pain is a finding in only about 60% of patients with a PE

Answer 2.1.6 **The correct answer is "E."** Only a small majority (59%) of patients with pulmonary emboli have pain as a feature. "A" is incorrect because about 20% of patients with cardiac pain will have their pain relieved by a GI cocktail. Conversely, "D" is incorrect because nitroglycerin can relieve pain from esophageal spasm as it is a nonselective smooth muscle relaxer. "B" is incorrect because only 50% of patients with an aortic dissection will have unequal pulses and blood pressures, and only 75% will have an abnormal chest x-ray. The consideration of an aortic dissection mandates a chest CT scan with contrast, transesophageal echo, or angiogram. Remember that about 20% of the population will have unequal blood pressures in the upper extremities at baseline. "C" is incorrect because most patients with spontaneous pneumothorax can be treated with a "pigtail" catheter with a Heimlich valve. This type of treatment reduces the morbidity associated with a chest tube.

HELPFUL TIP:
Non-ionic CT contrast is safe even in those with an elevated creatinine (<4 mg/dL). Don't go hog wild (a real "thing" in Iowa). But if you really need that CT in a patient with a creatinine of 2 mg/dL (such as for dissection of PE) go for it (*Ann Emerg Med.* 2017;69:577 and others).

HELPFUL TIP:
Chest x-ray findings in patients with thoracic aortic dissection may include widened mediastinum, obliterated aortic knob, pleural "capping," tracheal deviation, depression of left main stem bronchus, esophageal deviation, and loss of the paratracheal stripe. But just do the contrast CT…you will sleep better.

The patient's pain recurs in the ED. You suspect that she is having a myocardial infarction, but do not yet have unequivocal proof, such as ECG changes or elevated cardiac enzymes. The patient becomes markedly hypotensive in response to another dose of sublingual nitroglycerin.

Question 2.1.7 Which of the following is TRUE?
A) Intravenous nitroglycerin is contraindicated in this patient
B) Hypotension caused by nitroglycerin is usually unresponsive to IV saline
C) Hypotension caused by nitroglycerin may be indicative of a right ventricular infarction, which is most commonly associated with an inferior wall myocardial infarction (IAMI)
D) Hypotension caused by nitroglycerin is diagnostic of cardiogenic shock, suggesting that this patient will have a poor outcome

Answer 2.1.7 **The correct answer is "C."** Hypotension in response to nitroglycerin may be indicative of a right ventricular infarct, which is most commonly associated with an inferior wall acute MI (IAMI). Since the right ventricle is dependent on filling pressure (preload), nitroglycerin, which drops the preload, will frequently result in hypotension in those with a right ventricular infarct. "A" is incorrect because hypotension from sublingual nitroglycerin is not a contraindication to additional nitrates *once the patient's blood pressure is stable.* A typical sublingual dose is 400 µg (0.4 mg). A typical IV dose starts at 20 µg/min. Thus, the sublingual dose is quite a bit larger than the IV dose. In such a situation, you could consider starting IV nitroglycerin at 10 to 20 µg/min and titrating up as the blood pressure allows. "B" is incorrect because hypotension from nitroglycerin will generally respond to a saline bolus. "D" is incorrect. Certainly, patients with cardiogenic shock will be hypotensive, but hypotension with nitroglycerin is a common result of the drug itself and does not define cardiogenic shock.

HELPFUL TIP:
Oral beta-blockers (metoprolol succinate, carvedilol (Coreg), bisoprolol) should be initiated in most patients with an AMI—generally within 24 hours of the infarct. Hold beta-blockers in those with hypotension, heart block, or heart failure (HF). Beta-blockers are still important in these patients but should not be started until the patient is hemodynamically stable and asymptomatic in terms of HF. Remember that beta-blockers will reduce cardiac output.
Consider holding beta-blockers in IAMI, as these patients often have bradycardia and heart block. Also, beware of atypical presentations of IAMI such as nausea, vomiting, and other GI symptoms.

Question 2.1.8 Which of the following is TRUE of patients with an IAMI?
A) They will likely continue to have problems with right ventricular functioning in the future
B) They will need to increase their salt intake in order to increase preload and right ventricular filling pressure
C) Their right ventricular function should return to normal or close to normal following their infarction
D) A and B

Answer 2.1.8 The correct answer is "C." Most patients will have return of right ventricular functioning following a myocardial infarction. "B" is incorrect because there will be no need to increase right ventricular filling pressure (which is what IV saline does acutely) once right ventricular function returns to normal.

....

The patient's pain continues despite treatment with nitroglycerin, and you obtain another ECG (Fig. 2-1).

Question 2.1.9 Which of the following is TRUE regarding this ECG?
A) This injury pattern on ECG is most consistent with an anterior wall MI
B) In this situation, percutaneous transluminal coronary angioplasty (PTCA) and stent placement is superior to tPA or other thrombolytic
C) This injury pattern on ECG is most consistent with pericarditis
D) This injury pattern on ECG proves that this patient does not have an aortic dissection
E) This pattern on ECG is totally fine. What, me worry?

Answer 2.1.9 The correct answer is "B." Intervention in the cath lab with PTCA and/or stent placement is superior to thrombolytic therapy in the treatment of AMI, provided that the "door to balloon" time is 90 minutes or less. In cases where the patient is located in a facility without a cardiac catheterization laboratory, the patient may receive thrombolytic therapy. "A" is incorrect because this pattern is indicative of an **inferior wall**, not an anterior wall, MI. You will note that this ECG shows ST elevations in leads II, III, and aVF (inferior leads) along with reciprocal ST-segment depression in leads V1 and V2. An anterior wall MI is defined by ST elevations in leads V3, V4, and V5, and an anteroseptal MI shows ST elevations in leads V1, V2, and V3. For IAMI concerning for RV infarction, consider "right-sided chest leads." "D" is incorrect because patients with pericarditis should have ST elevations in all leads (although an ECG is only 80% sensitive for pericarditis). "D" is incorrect because patients with an aortic dissection can present with an abnormal ECG that looks similar to an infarct pattern. So, ECG changes do not prove that the patient does not have an aortic dissection. "E" is just plain wrong and you **should be worried** if you see this pattern!

....

You now have all the evidence that you need to show that this patient is indeed having an ongoing myocardial infarction. Since your rural hospital is "just around the corner from nowhere," stenting is not going to happen within 90 minutes. You decide to initiate thrombolytic therapy.

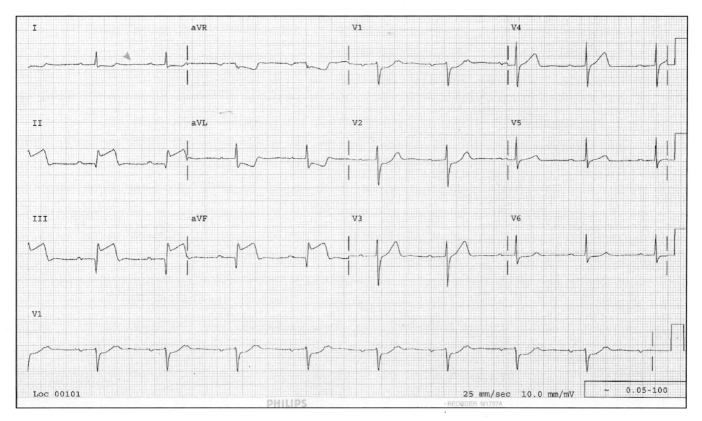

FIGURE 2-1. ECG for patient in question 2.1.9.

Question 2.1.10 **All of the following are true statements EXCEPT:**

A) Patients who are candidates for thrombolytics must have at least 1 mm of ST-segment elevation in at least 2 contiguous limb leads or at least 1 to 2 mm of ST-segment elevation in at least 2 contiguous precordial leads

B) Patients who are candidates for thrombolytics must have an absence of prior history of hemorrhagic stroke

C) Patients who are candidates for thrombolytics should have no active bleeding, including menstrual bleeding

D) Patients who are candidates for thrombolytics should have no history of recent head trauma

E) Patients who are candidates for thrombolytics should not be pregnant

Answer 2.1.10 **The correct answer is "C."** While active internal bleeding is a contraindication to the use of thrombolytics (or fibrinolytics, as these terms are used interchangeably), menstrual bleeding is not. While there are no controlled trials, anecdotal evidence suggests that thrombolytics are safe with menstrual bleeding. "A" is true. See Table 2-1A for more clarity on the definition of STEMI as the ST-segment definition depends on the sex of the patient, to some degree. For thrombolytics, patients with only ST-segment **depression** or a normal ECG, even with symptoms, do **not** benefit. "B," "D," and "E" are all true statements. Patients are not candidates for thrombolytics if they have recent head trauma, are pregnant, or have had a hemorrhagic stroke **ever**. See Table 2-1B for a more comprehensive list of contraindications.

HELPFUL TIP:
"Facilitated PCI," that is, administration of thrombolytics with the intent to perform PCI within 2 or more hours of giving thrombolytics has very mixed (and mostly negative) data. Outcomes are worse (and not just because PCI is a "rescue" technique at this point). It certainly is **NOT** the standard of care and, in fact, is no longer considered as part of the treatment algorithm. If thrombolytics versus primary PCI is being considered, it is valuable to contact the cardiologist at the cath center to determine whether he/she would like thrombolytics before transfer—timing (both from symptom onset and for transfer) is central to the decision-making process. "Rescue PCI" for failed reperfusion after thrombolytic therapy should be performed as soon as logistically possible, ideally within the first 24 hours, but NOT within the first 2 to 3 hours post thrombolytic therapy.

HELPFUL TIP:
Remember to repeat the ECG **after** thrombolytics to prove that ST elevations have resolved. Evidence of successful reperfusion after thrombolytics is suggested by: nearly sudden and complete relief of chest pain, >70% ST elevation resolution in the index lead showing the greatest degree of elevation, plus or minus the presence of reperfusion arrhythmia.

TABLE 2-1A ACC/AHA GUIDELINES FOR THE USE OF FIBRINOLYTIC THERAPY IN PATIENTS WITH ST-ELEVATION MYOCARDIAL INFARCTION: INDICATIONS

Definition of ST-segment elevation myocardial infarction is any ONE of the following ECG findings in a patient with a history suggestive of myocardial ischemia:
- ≥1 mm of ST-segment elevation in at least 2 contiguous limb leads
- In men, ≥2 mm of ST-segment elevation in at least 2 contiguous precordial leads
- In women, ≥1.5 mm of ST-segment depression in V2-3 or ≥1 mm of ST-segment depression in any other contiguous precordial leads
- **New** complete bundle branch block that obscures the ST-segment analysis

Class 1 recommendation for fibrinolytic therapy:
- In the absence of contraindications and when PCI cannot be performed within 120 minutes of first medical contact, fibrinolytic therapy should be given to patients presenting with STEMI and having onset of symptoms within prior 12 hours.

Class 2a recommendation for fibrinolytic therapy:
- In the absence of contraindications and when PCI is not available, it is reasonable to give fibrinolytic therapy in STEMI if there is clinical and/or ECG evidence of ongoing ischemia 12–24 hours after symptom onset, a large area of myocardium is at risk, or hemodynamic instability is found.

PCI, percutaneous coronary intervention.
Adapted from O'Gara PT, et al. 2013 ACC/AHA Guideline for the management of ST-segment elevation myocardial infarction. *J Am Coll Cardiol.* 2013;61(4):e78–140.

TABLE 2-1B ACC/AHA GUIDELINES FOR THE USE OF FIBRINOLYTIC THERAPY IN PATIENTS WITH ST-ELEVATION MYOCARDIAL INFARCTION: CONTRAINDICATIONS

Class 3 "Absolute" contraindications
Any prior intracranial hemorrhage
- Known structural cerebral vascular lesion
- Known intracranial neoplasm
- Ischemic stroke within 3 months (except acute stroke within 4.5 hours)
- Suspected aortic dissection
- Active internal bleeding (except menstrual bleeding)
- Significant closed-head or facial trauma within 3 months
- Intracranial or intraspinal surgery within 2 months
- Severe uncontrolled hypertension (unresponsive to emergency treatment)
- For streptokinase, prior treatment within the previous 6 months

Relative contraindications
- History of chronic, severe, poorly controlled hypertension
- Significant hypertension on presentation (>180/110 mm Hg)
- History of prior ischemic stroke > 3 months
- Dementia
- Known intracranial pathology not covered in absolute contraindications
- Traumatic or prolonged CPR (>10 min)
- Major surgery in prior 3 weeks
- Recent internal bleeding (prior 2–4 weeks)
- Noncompressible vascular punctures (e.g., subclavian line)
- Pregnancy
- Active peptic ulcer
- Oral anticoagulant therapy

Adapted from O'Gara PT, et al. 2013 ACC/AHA Guideline for the management of ST-segment elevation myocardial infarction. *J Am Coll Cardiol.* 2013;61(4):e78–140.

After conferring with your closest cath center, you give a thrombolytic—and cross your fingers. Unfortunately, the patient develops a new LBBB. In addition, the ECG shows evidence of a first-degree heart block (a prolonged PR interval), although the heart rate remains normal at 80 bpm.

Question 2.1.11 **The proper response to this is to:**
A) Insert a Swan–Ganz catheter to monitor central pressures
B) Insert a temporary pacemaker regardless of the heart rate
C) Administer atropine to this patient
D) Administer isoproterenol to this patient
E) Do nothing, other than observe this patient

Answer 2.1.11 **The correct answer is "B."** For patients with an AMI, a transvenous pacemaker should be inserted if the patient develops (1) complete heart block, (2) second-degree heart block type II (Mobitz II), or (3) new LBBB with first-degree AV block. See Tables 2-2 and 2-3 for more on arrhythmia and pacemakers in the setting of AMI. "A" is incorrect because a Swan–Ganz catheter will be of no help in arrhythmias. "C" is incorrect because atropine is indicated for symptomatic bradycardia and not for a bundle branch block. "D" is incorrect for the same reason as "C." In addition, isoproterenol is arrhythmogenic and is no longer recommended. "E" is incorrect because the patient may rapidly progress into a complete heart block. Of note and importantly, the placement of a transvenous pacemaker should not delay transfer for catheterization since a pacemaker may also be placed in the cath lab. However, apply an external pacemaker as required.

The patient requires heparin with the thrombolytic that you choose (and is indicated, by guidelines, for a minimum of 48 hours and preferably for the duration of the index hospitalization, up to 8 days or until revascularization is performed).

TABLE 2-2 TYPE OF HEART BLOCK ASSOCIATED WITH INFARCTION

Anterior myocardial infarction	Bundle branch blocks Mobitz type II second-degree heart block
Inferior myocardial infarction	Bradycardia from: • Mobitz type I second-degree heart block • Third-degree heart block

TABLE 2-3 CLASS I INDICATIONS FOR PACEMAKER IN PATIENTS WITH AN ACUTE MYOCARDIAL INFARCTION

New left bundle branch block + first-degree AV block
New right bundle branch block + left anterior or posterior fascicular block + first-degree AV block
Mobitz type II heart block
Third-degree heart block
Symptomatic bradycardia unresponsive to atropine.

Question 2.1.12 **Which of the following dosing regimens is the best accepted for use in AMIs?**
A) Enoxaparin 30 mg subcutaneously (SC) every 12 hours
B) Enoxaparin 1 mg/kg SC every 12 hours
C) Heparin 5,000 units bolus and a drip at 1,000 units per hour
D) Heparin 100 unit/kg bolus with a drip at 25 units/kg/hr
E) None of the above represents the best dosing option in this situation

Answer 2.1.12 **The correct answer is "B."** For anticoagulation in AMI, the dose of enoxaparin is 1 mg/kg SC every 12 hours. "A" is incorrect since 30 mg SC every 12 hours is the dose for DVT prophylaxis in post-op joint replacement patients, not for anticoagulation. "C" is incorrect. This is the classic way that heparin has been dosed but it **is not** the best option listed. "D" is incorrect as well. The **correct** dose for heparin **when given with a thrombolytic is** 60 units/kg bolus (maximum of 4,000 units) with a drip of 15 units/kg/hr (maximum dose of 1,000 units/hr), with rate adjusted to achieve an activated partial thromboplastin time (aPTT) of 1.5 to 2 times control (for 48 hours or until revascularization). The bottom line here is that either enoxaparin or heparin can be used in this setting, and they are more or less equivalent. If you choose to use heparin, *do not use fixed dose heparin but rather weight-based dosing*. **One advantage to unfractionated heparin** is that the half-life is 30 minutes, so it is rapidly cleared. Additionally, it can be reversed with protamine zinc. (Did you know that protamine was originally extracted from fish sperm? Who came up with that idea? It is now produced by recombinant technology.)

HELPFUL TIP:
Did you know that for ST-elevation MI, an initial dose of 30 mg of **IV enoxaparin** (that's right—intravenous) should be given with the **first (and only the first)** dose for those age <75 years. The IV dose should be given at the same time as the first 1 mg/kg subcutaneous dose. Do it!

The patient receives her thrombolytic, enoxaparin, and transvenous pacing, and she is admitted to the hospital to a monitored bed. You get a call from the nursing staff 5 hours later. The rhythm strip shows 3 PVCs per minute. Your patient remains pain free and is hemodynamically stable.

Question 2.1.13 **The nurse (who has more than a few gray hairs) would like an order for lidocaine. Your response is:**
A) "Do it. Give the lidocaine"
B) "Give amiodarone—it works better than lidocaine"
C) "Give no antiarrhythmic at this point in time"
D) "Check labs including potassium and magnesium"
E) C and D

Answer 2.1.13 **The correct answer is "E."** The use of lidocaine in this setting incurs no benefit and is proarrhythmic. The same is true for prophylactic amiodarone, which can cause torsades de pointes, albeit at a lower frequency than other antiarrhythmics (such as quinidine, procainamide, sotalol, and newer Class III antiarrhythmic agents). In the setting of AMI, antiarrhythmics may be indicated only for complex arrhythmias (PVC couplets, triplets, nonsustained ventricular tachycardia [<30 seconds], or >10 PVCs per minute). More than 90% of patients will have isolated PVCs in the peri-infarct period, and there is no association with increased mortality. Correcting hypokalemia and hypomagnesemia can help to reduce arrhythmias, and checking these labs is prudent.

....

The patient remains pain free while in the hospital. She is ready to be discharged 4 days later—but she's still getting enoxaparin for a total of 8 days, as recommended in the guidelines.

Question 2.1.14 Which of the following tests is the most appropriate for this patient prior to discharge?
A) Coronary angiography
B) Submaximal stress test plus echocardiography
C) Full Bruce protocol, symptom limited, stress test
D) Spiral CT to assess for coronary artery calcification
E) Ping test

Answer 2.1.14 **The correct answer is "B."** Submaximal stress testing is considered the standard of care; a noninvasive evaluation of left ventricular ejection fraction (e.g., echocardiogram or radionuclide study) is also indicated. Patients with a positive submaximal stress test should be referred for catheterization. Patients with a borderline stress test can be sent for a radionuclide study. Coronary angiography **is not** routinely recommended for all patients who have had a myocardial infarction unless they are considered to be at high risk (continued symptoms, positive screening test such as submaximal stress test, heart failure, cardiogenic shock, etc.). "C" is incorrect because a symptom-limited, full-protocol stress test should be done only 14 to 21 days after an infarction. Finally, spiral CT ("D") to assess for coronary artery calcification has no role in risk stratification after a myocardial infarction … their risk is 100%! Also, keep in mind that the weight of the clinical evidence **favors transfer for early catheterization**, especially for higher risk patients. "E," a ping test, is a test to see if your internet service is working.

Question 2.1.15 The patient passes her stress test with flying colors (and you pass your Board Examination). Patients after a myocardial infarction should be routinely discharged on all of the following medications EXCEPT:
A) Aspirin
B) Beta-blocker
C) Continuous nitroglycerin (e.g., patch or isosorbide)
D) HMG-CoA reductase inhibitor ("statin")
E) Sublingual nitroglycerin for PRN use

Answer 2.1.15 **The correct answer is "C."** There is no benefit to scheduled nitrates unless needed for a specific indication

(e.g., recurrent angina). All post-myocardial infarction patients should be discharged on aspirin, a beta-blocker, a statin, nitroglycerin PRN, and an angiotensin-converting enzyme (ACE) inhibitor—if they are tolerated, of course. A P2Y$_{12}$ inhibitor should be continued for up to 12 months in those with no stent (options include clopidogrel 75 mg daily, ticagrelor 90 mg BID). See "helpful tip" for treatment of those with a stent (after question **2.2.9**).

....

HELPFUL TIP:
All patients with an ST-elevation MI **or** non-STEMI/unstable angina should be discharged on an intensive lipid-lowering regimen with an HMG-CoA reductase inhibitor ("statin"), such as atorvastatin 40 to 80 mg per day, including those with a baseline LDL <70 mg/dL. Keep reading for more on statins below.

....

While this patient had a STEMI (or "Q-wave" MI), it is also important to recognize some of the differences between STEMI and non-STEMI.

Question 2.1.16 Regarding non-STEMI, which of the following statements is TRUE?
A) Patients with a non-STEMI have the same, or perhaps a bit worse, outcomes long term than do patients with a STEMI
B) Patients with a non-STEMI have worse in-hospital outcomes when compared with patients with a STEMI
C) Unstable angina and non-STEMI can be readily differentiated from one another on presentation
D) None of the above is true

Answer 2.1.16 **The correct answer is "A."** Patients with a non-STEMI actually have the same, or perhaps even slightly worse, outcomes long term when compared to patients with a STEMI. This makes sense; there is still myocardium left to infarct after a non-STEMI. As to the other answers, patients with a STEMI do have worse in-hospital outcomes, and unstable angina and non-STEMI look similar on ECG with T-wave inversion, etc., but without the ST elevations that are classically seen in a transmural infarction.

▶ **Objectives: Did you learn to …**
• Define the accuracy of the initial history, ECG, and labs in the diagnosis of cardiac disease in the ED or office?
• Recognize the role and significance (or lack thereof) of risk factors, such as diabetes, family history, smoking, and hypertension, in the decision of whether or not to admit a patient to the hospital for chest pain?
• Generate a differential diagnosis of chest pain?
• Identify the roles of various diagnostic tests in the evaluation of chest pain?
• Treat a patient with an AMI?

QUICK QUIZ: CORONARY CALCIUM

You are seeing a 42-year-old male patient. He is asymptomatic and presenting for a routine annual exam. The patient looks well-conditioned and admits (well, beams…the jerk) that he exercises daily without any chest pain. He smokes one pack of cigarettes per day and has a blood pressure of 135/87 mm Hg, total cholesterol of 179 mg/dL, and HDL of 30 mg/dL. He takes no medication. In order to better stratify his risk for atherosclerotic cardiovascular disease (ASCVD), he is wondering if he should get one of those fancy CT scans he's seen advertised on billboards in your town.

Which of the following is true regarding the role of a coronary calcium score in this patient?
A) A coronary calcium score may be a helpful tool in the evaluation of this patient if used in combination with an ASCVD risk score
B) A coronary calcium score is a helpful tool in the evaluation of this patient independent of his calculated ASCVD risk score and will help decide statin treatment for primary prevention
C) A coronary calcium score is only useful in evaluating this patient once he has had an echocardiogram
D) A coronary calcium score is only useful in the evaluation of ongoing anginal chest pain

The correct answer is "A." The patient presents with an ACC/AHA ASCVD risk score of 7.7% which places him in the 10-year intermediate-risk category (find calculator at https://www.mdcalc.com/ascvd-atherosclerotic-cardiovascular-disease-2013-risk-calculator-aha-acc). What to do in that category is in itself controversial, with ACC/AHA recommending statin therapy to all patients in that risk category and the USPSTF giving statins a "C" rating for individualizing the decision. In this circumstance, more information via a CT coronary calcium score **may** be useful. However, there is significant controversy over the utility of the calcium score with some evidence favoring its use, while the USPSTF states that the evidence is insufficient (*JAMA* 2018;320(3):271–280). Independently ("B"), a coronary calcium score is not helpful, as you would need to know other patient characteristics and risk factors in order to make a decision on primary prevention. "C" and "D" are incorrect because a coronary calcium score does not require an echocardiogram and it can be used to help stratify risk.

QUICK QUIZ: GLYCOPROTEIN IIB/IIIA INHIBITORS

You are seeing a patient in the ED with chest pain. The ECG shows elevated ST segments in leads V1, V2, and V3 with reciprocal changes inferiorly. You have run through the "standard" medications, but the patient continues to have pain. You consult a cardiologist who suggests the use of a glycoprotein IIb/IIIa inhibitor.

Which of the following is true about the glycoprotein IIb/IIIa inhibitors?
A) They are best used in patients who are not candidates for PTCA and stenting
B) They cause no increase in the rate of intracranial bleeding
C) They are useful in all groups of patients with ACS
D) They are most effective in patients going to PTCA and/or stenting

The correct answer is "D." The glycoprotein IIb/IIIa inhibitors are most effective in patients who are undergoing PTCA or stenting. The GUSTO V trial showed **NO** difference in 30-day mortality in patients **who were not** scheduled for catheterization. Thus, "A" is incorrect. "B" is incorrect because glycoprotein IIb/IIIa inhibitors do increase rates of intracranial and other bleeding. "C" is incorrect because patients who have an ACS that is well-controlled with other drugs (e.g., heparin, metoprolol, and ASA) are not likely to benefit from glycoprotein IIb/IIIa inhibitors.

HELPFUL TIP:
Since the arrival of potent P2Y$_{12}$ inhibitors (e.g., ticagrelor, prasugrel), which inhibit platelet degranulation upstream from the IIb/IIIA receptor, glycoprotein IIb/IIIa inhibitors are now only used in special circumstances for patients undergoing PTCA/stenting.

▶ CASE 2.2

A 53-year-old male with a history of hypertension and smoking, but no family history of cardiac disease, presents to your office complaining of a chest pain. The pain is substernal, radiates to his left arm, and is associated with exertion. The patient notes that this same pain has been going on for the last 6 months and has not changed at all in duration, intensity, or characteristic. It generally lasts 5 minutes or so and resolves with rest.

Question 2.2.1 You tell the patient that:
A) Without doing any test, you know that the probability that this pain is cardiac is greater than 85%
B) If his ECG in the office is normal, his pain is unlikely to represent cardiac disease
C) Even with risk factors, his probability of having CAD with "typical angina" is about 50%
D) The only interventions indicated at this point are lifestyle modifications (e.g., stop smoking) and addressing his cholesterol and hypertension
E) It is likely that he has unstable angina

Answer 2.2.1 The correct answer is "A." A 50-year-old male with "classic" angina symptoms has **greater than a 90%** probability of having CAD. "B" is incorrect because patients with angina who are pain free may have a normal electrocardiogram (as will many patients with active angina or even a myocardial infarction). Thus, his pain could still be cardiac in origin. "C" is incorrect because, based on demographic data, his risk of CAD is much higher than 50%. "D" is incorrect because he needs a further evaluation and treatment of his chest pain. "E" is incorrect since this pain represents "stable angina." There has been no change in quality, duration, amount of exertion required to bring on symptoms, etc., eliminating unstable angina as a diagnosis. Use of tools such as the TIMI Risk Score (https://www.mdcalc.com/timi-risk-score-stemi) and/or Grace Risk Model (https://www.mdcalc.com/grace-acs-risk-mortality-calculator) can assist in estimation of the level of risk and to help guide management decisions.

HELPFUL TIP:
Know your pretest probability of cardiac disease before embarking upon testing for chest pain. This varies by age and type of chest pain. An approximation of the probability of cardiac disease is as follows:
Male, *atypical angina*: age 30 to 39 = 34%, age 40 to 49 = 51%, age 50 to 59 = 65%, age 60 to 69 = 72%.
Male, *typical angina*: age 30 to 39 = 76%, age 40 to 49 = 87%, age 50 to 59 = 93%, age 60 to 69 = 94%.
Female, *atypical angina*: age 30 to 39 = 12%, age 40 to 49 = 22%, age 50 to 59 = 31%, age 60 to 69 = 52%.
Female, *typical angina*: age 30 to 39 = 26%, age 40 to 49 = 55%, age 50 to 59 = 73%, age 60 to 69 = 86%.

You send the patient home on aspirin with a prescription for sublingual nitroglycerin for PRN use and arrange for a stress test.

Question 2.2.2 All of the following are considered absolute contraindications to exercise stress testing EXCEPT:
A) Left bundle branch block (LBBB)
B) Presence of severe heart failure
C) Critical aortic stenosis
D) Myocarditis
E) Unstable angina

Answer 2.2.2 The correct answer is "A." An LBBB is a relative—not absolute—contraindication to stress testing. In the setting of LBBB, there are already repolarization abnormalities that limit the usefulness of the ECG component of a stress test. One should add an imaging modality, such as myocardial perfusion scanning or echocardiography, in cases of LBBB. The same holds for any baseline ECG pattern that would interfere with ST-segment interpretation (baseline ST changes, LVH with repolarization changes involving the ST-T wave, intraventricular conduction delay, paced rhythm, preexcitation, or ST-T changes due to digoxin therapy). The rest are all "absolute" contraindications to exercise stress testing. See Table 2-4 for a list of contraindications to stress testing.

Question 2.2.3 Exercise stress testing is best suited to which group of individuals?
A) Men with an intermediate probability of cardiac disease
B) Women with a high risk of cardiac disease
C) Men at a high risk of cardiac disease
D) Men at a low risk of cardiac disease
E) Women with a low risk of cardiac disease

TABLE 2-4 CONTRAINDICATIONS TO EXERCISE STRESS TESTING

Absolute contraindications	• Acute myocardial infarction within 2 days • Dissecting aneurysm • Recent pulmonary embolism • Active thrombophlebitis • BP > 200/120 mm Hg • Hemodynamically significant arrhythmias • Severe heart failure • Severe aortic stenosis • Active myocarditis, pericarditis, or endocarditis • Inability to complete test (e.g., severe knee arthritis) • Unstable angina
Relative contraindications	• Left bundle branch block • Moderate aortic stenosis • Hypertrophic cardiomyopathy • Electrolyte disturbance • High-grade AV block • Tachyarrhythmias or bradyarrhythmias including uncontrolled atrial fibrillation

Answer 2.2.3 The correct answer is "A." Stress testing is best suited to patients with an intermediate pretest probability of cardiac disease (between 25% and 75%). "B" and "C" are incorrect since patients with a high risk of cardiac disease should go directly to another study, such as nuclear myocardial perfusion imaging study (MPI, also sometimes termed "thallium stress testing") or stress echocardiography. "D" and "E" are incorrect since these are not the best groups in whom to use exercise stress testing; there will be a greater proportion of false-positive results in these low-risk patients. Exercise stress testing in these groups is best used to allay patient fears that they do not have cardiac disease, not to prove they do have cardiac disease. However, a false-positive stress test may lead to other unnecessary invasive testing!

You decide to do an exercise stress test on this patient. It turns out to be negative.

Question 2.2.4 Your next step is to:
A) Reassure the patient that he does not have cardiac disease
B) Suggest a chest CT scan to rule out possible aortic aneurysm
C) Schedule the patient for another cardiac test such as stress echocardiogram, exercise myocardial perfusion test, or angiography
D) Schedule the patient for endoscopy to rule out gastroesophageal disease as a cause of these symptoms
E) Start an anxiolytic to treat the panic disorder, which is the underlying cause of his chest pain

Answer 2.2.4 The correct answer is "C." This patient who is in his 50s and who has a "classic" history for angina has greater than a 90% pretest probability of cardiac disease. Thus, it is likely that the negative stress test is a **false** negative. What was the point of that stress test anyway? It probably should not have been done in this patient since a negative test just leads to further testing (as would have a positive test, probably resulting in angiography). For this reason, "A" is incorrect. "B," "D," and "E" are also incorrect because you have not yet eliminated a cardiac cause.

You are considering whether to order an MPI or a stress echocardiogram.

Question 2.2.5 Which of the following is true?
A) Stress echocardiography is more sensitive for cardiac disease than is an MPI
B) Stress echocardiography is more specific than is a stress MPI
C) MPI is more specific for cardiac disease than is stress echocardiography
D) None of the above is true

Answer 2.2.5 **The correct answer is "B."** Stress echocardiography is more specific for cardiac disease than is MPI. Alternatively, MPI is more sensitive. Table 2-5 summarizes this data. Remember that positive and negative predictive values of these tests will vary depending on the pretest probability of disease in the patient **and** severity of disease. Numbers given above are overall.

You decide to send the patient for an MPI. However, since you last saw him, he fell and sprained his ankle…just to help us write this case (taking one for the team). So, you decide to stress him chemically. The patient is taking theophylline (really—in the 21st century!) for chronic obstructive pulmonary disease (COPD).

Question 2.2.6 The LEAST desirable pharmacologic agent to administer for stressing this patient is:
A) Adenosine
B) Dobutamine
C) Dipyridamole
D) All of the above are equally acceptable methods of chemically stressing this patient
E) Neither A nor C is desirable

Answer 2.2.6 **The correct answer is "E."** Theophylline (and caffeine) interact with both adenosine and dipyridamole, attenuating their effect. Additionally, adenosine may precipitate

bronchospasm and should be avoided in patients with COPD or asthma. Thus, neither drug is a good choice for stressing this patient. Dobutamine is an acceptable method of chemically stressing those on theophylline or caffeine (like us), but it would only be used with an echocardiogram—not an MPI. On the other hand, COPD patients often have poor echocardiographic windows. Is this patient headed to a cath? We'll see…

You do your patient a big favor by tapering him off theophylline and getting him on a more modern inhaled COPD regimen. Good thing he came to see you. Indeed, his echocardiogram windows are suboptimal. Several studies have shown that regadenoson (Lexiscan®) appears safe in COPD (e.g., *J Nucl Cardiol.* 2008;15:319). So, finally, you order a regadenoson-based MPI (after completing a prior authorization, calling his insurance company, etc., etc.).

Question 2.2.7 The patient's MPI shows an antero-apical nonreversible ("fixed") defect. The best interpretation of this is that it indicates:
A) Attenuation artifact from breast tissue
B) Prior myocardial infarction
C) Angina
D) Anomalous cardiac circulation
E) It is not significant and therefore adds no value to this test

Answer 2.2.7 **The correct answer is "B."** A nonreversible ("fixed") defect suggests prior myocardial infarction. A reversible defect suggests inducible ischemia. "A" is incorrect since breast attenuation occurs mostly in women (but can also be seen in obese males, which is part of the rationale for performing PET imaging in patients with BMI > 35 kg/m^2 since PET uses a higher-energy isotope to mitigate soft tissue attenuation). Another advantage of a PET scan is that it can detect both cardiac perfusion *and* myocardium viability. "C" is incorrect since angina would likely be manifested by a reversible deficit.

Since a reversible defect was not found on the stress test, you conclude that there is no myocardium currently at risk. However, the patient continues to have chest pain and now at an increasing frequency with less exertion. He is asymptomatic when he presents to your office. He was noted at the last visit to have an elevated glucose at 350 mg/dL.

Question 2.2.8 What is the next step in the evaluation or treatment of this patient?
A) Stress echocardiogram to document what segments are involved
B) Start the patient on insulin to control his blood sugars
C) Proceed directly to cardiac catheterization
D) Since there were no reversible deficits on stress testing, schedule the patient to see a gastroenterologist
E) Give a trial of NSAIDs to help differentiate chest wall pain from other causes

TABLE 2-5 OVERALL SENSITIVITY AND SPECIFICITY OF NONINVASIVE CARDIAC TESTING

	Sensitivity (%)	Specificity (%)
Exercise stress testing	45–68	77
Myocardial perfusion imaging (thallium or SPECT)	88	77
Stress echocardiography	76	88
Cardiac CT	88–99%	64–83%

Answer 2.2.8 **The correct answer is "C."** Given that this high-risk patient has worsening angina and now is even at higher risk since he probably has diabetes, he should have the definitive test done. "A" is incorrect since we already have done a noninvasive test. We already know what segment was previously infarcted, as noted on the MPI. "B" is incorrect for two reasons. First, addressing his diabetes will not address the immediate problem of what you must presume is unstable angina. Second, insulin is not necessarily the first drug to use in this patient who presumably has type 2 diabetes. Certainly, the blood glucose needs to be addressed but so does the chest pain. Which is going to kill him first? "D" is incorrect. The sensitivity of MPI is in the 88% range (see Table 2-5), so it will miss 12% of disease. Thus, we still have not proven in this high-risk patient that he does not have treatable cardiac disease causing his chest pain. "E" is incorrect for the same reason.

....

The patient has a catheterization done that shows three-vessel disease including left main CAD. The cardiologist calls you with the report the next day and suggests PTCA with stenting, since, in his opinion, "This is the best modality for diabetics and diabetics are high-risk candidates when it comes to surgery."

Question 2.2.9 **Your opinion is that:**
A) Patients with stents generally have better outcomes in terms of control of angina with stenting when compared with coronary artery bypass grafting (CABG)
B) Diabetic patients do particularly well with stenting when compared with CABG
C) Medical control of symptoms is indicated as the best management in this diabetic patient with three-vessel disease
D) Diabetic patients do better with CABG when compared with stenting
E) You don't have an opinion. You just do what the nice cardiologist says

Answer 2.2.9 **The correct answer is "D."** This patient should probably have surgery for his three-vessel disease because diabetic patients generally have **worse** outcomes with stenting than do nondiabetic patients in terms of angina relief and need for repeat revascularization. "A" is incorrect because a proportion of patients with stents have to go on to have an open CABG due to in-stent restenosis or incomplete revascularization with percutaneous revascularization. "B" is incorrect. Diabetic patients have a much higher rate of in-stent restenosis or secondary occlusion (meaning a narrowing/stenosis somewhere else in the diseased vessel). "C" is incorrect. The indications for CABG are significant left main CAD (>50%), three-vessel disease with evidence of LV dysfunction (ejection fraction <50%), or origin/proximal LAD/LCX disease (left main equivalent). This patient has left main vessel disease and thus medical control is **NOT** the best option for this patient. He is also young and, from the available data, appears to be a good surgical candidate. Therefore, CABG is the guideline-recommended option for this patient. "E" is incorrect because you went to medical school and have a brain.

HELPFUL TIP:
Drug-eluting stents (DES) decrease overall re-occlusion rates in comparison to bare metal stents (BMS). Women who have multiple stents and multi-vessel disease are at a higher risk of restenosis, as are patients with a small post-stenting lumen size. Early re-occlusion secondary to thrombosis is higher with DES versus BMS, and the mortality risk due to stent thrombosis when it occurs is high (range 20–45%). This is because it takes the body longer to cover these stents with intima (i.e., re-endo-thelialization). Thus, clopidogrel, ticagrelor or prasugrel (not our favorite) for 1 year **PLUS** aspirin for life should be used in patients who have a DES inserted. For BMS, the recommendation is to use one of the antiplatelet agents for **3 to 6 months PLUS** aspirin for life. (Note: the risk of stent thrombosis with a bare metal stent is highest in the first 14–30 days.) Eighty-one milligrams of aspirin to Aspirin 81 mg seems to be the Goldilocks spot: not too much bleeding, adequate antiplatelet effect.

HELPFUL TIP:
A plea from your editors. Don't continue clopidogrel, etc., outside of the time frame in which they have been shown to be useful (3–6 months for a BMS, 1 year for a DES) unless there is ongoing ACS. The bleeding risk is increased for no or minimal benefit. Continue aspirin indefinitely, of course (*N Engl J Med.* 2014;371:2225–2226). For patients on warfarin or another oral anticoagulant, consideration should be given to reducing the duration of triple therapy (oral anticoagulant + ASA + clopidogrel, for example) due to bleeding risk without significant benefit. Drop one of the antiplatelet drugs. However, the optimum duration of therapy has not been established. It may be safe to stop triple therapy as early as 4 to 6 weeks after a DES (*J Am Coll Cardiol.* 2015;65:1619).

HELPFUL TIP:
The treatment of *stable* angina is somewhat controversial. Most data shows that conservative *optimized* medical treatment is just as good as stenting for both cardiovascular disease outcomes and symptom relief (*N Engl J Med.* 2015;373:1937; *Lancet* 2018;391(10115):31–40).

For those with unstable angina/MI/multivessel disease, CABG leads to overall better outcomes when compared to stenting. This is especially true in diabetics (*Lancet* 2018;391:939). However, with isolated *stable* left main CAD, stenting seems as good as CABG in **non**diabetics.

....

Your patient has a CABG and comes into your office complaining of chest pain and fever 3 weeks after the surgery. He has had the pain and fever for 4 days and does not seem to be getting any better. He has no cough, no sputum production,

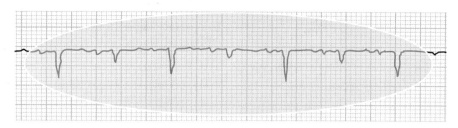

FIGURE 2-2. Electrical alternans. Note alternating voltages on ECG.

and the pain seems to be worse when he breathes or lies down. He reports no dyspnea and has 97% oxygen saturation on room air. The wound from the surgery is well healed, and a chest radiograph shows no evidence of abnormalities.

Question 2.2.10 Which of these studies is LEAST likely to be abnormal in this patient?
A) ECG
B) Ventilation/perfusion (V/Q) scan
C) Echocardiogram
D) Sedimentation rate (ESR)

Answer 2.2.10 **The correct answer is "B."** A V/Q scan is not likely to be positive in this patient. This patient is unlikely to have a pulmonary embolism (PE), given the duration of symptoms, the fact that the patient has chest pain that worsens with inspiration (found in only 59% of those with PE), fever, absence of dyspnea, and has normal oxygen saturation. Certainly, this **could** still be a PE, but it would be less likely than other, more plausible, explanations. The most likely diagnosis in this patient, given the lack of other symptoms, is post-pericardiotomy syndrome. This is similar to Dressler syndrome, which occurs after a myocardial infarction and presents with fever and chest pain several days to weeks after the inciting event. The white blood count is often elevated, as is the ESR. The ECG can be helpful as can an echocardiogram.

You obtain an ECG on this patient that shows a pattern consistent with pericarditis.

Question 2.2.11 Which of the following patterns can be seen in a patient with pericarditis?
A) Diffuse ST-segment elevation
B) Normal ECG
C) LBBB
D) A and B
E) All of the above

Answer 2.2.11 **The answer is "D."** Both diffuse ST-segment elevations and a normal ECG can be seen with pericarditis, as can electrical alternans (Fig. 2-2). A PR depression (Fig. 2-3) can also be seen in pericarditis and is almost pathognomonic. There is one caveat: If there are **only inferior wall ST elevations, isolated PR depression in aVL may be associated with an inferior wall MI.** The initial ECG is only 80% sensitive for pericarditis. Small (low voltage) QRS complexes or electrical

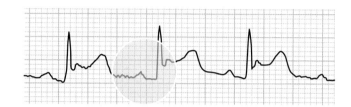

FIGURE 2-3. PR depression.

alternans can also be seen if there is a pericardial effusion. "C" is incorrect since bundle branch blocks have nothing to do with pericarditis.

After a complete history, physical examination, ECG, and echocardiogram, you determine that he has pericarditis.

Question 2.2.12 Which of the following drugs might be helpful in this patient?
A) Heparin
B) Warfarin
C) Furosemide
D) Colchicine

Answer 2.2.12 **The correct answer is "D."** Colchicine is the only drug in the list that is a treatment for pericarditis. It can be used first line with an NSAID such as aspirin, indomethacin, or naproxen (*Lancet* 2014;383(9936):2232–2237). Steroids are reserved for those who fail NSAIDs and colchicine. Do not use anticoagulation, either heparin or warfarin, in patients with pericarditis. This can cause bleeding into the pericardial space and tamponade. Thus, "A" and "B" are incorrect. "C" is incorrect because furosemide will likely make this patient worse. Patients with increased pericardial pressures are dependent on circulating preload volume in order to fill the right heart. Decreasing the preload may cause dyspnea in this patient.

The patient returns the next day and is now feeling short of breath. On examination, you notice JVD and peripheral edema. His blood pressure is 90/50 mm Hg with a pulse of 130 bpm. You rightly call an ambulance.

Question 2.2.13 The best initial treatment of this patient is:
A) Furosemide
B) Nitroglycerin
C) IV saline
D) Morphine

Answer 2.2.13 **The correct answer is "C."** This patient is in "pure" right heart failure secondary to possible cardiac tamponade. He is preload dependent. The treatment is to **increase** his preload by using IV saline. All the other options reduce the preload and will worsen this patient's symptoms.

He gets admitted to a cardiac inpatient bed and you give a bolus of 1 liter 0.9% saline IV on the way to the hospital. Despite this, he remains dyspneic with elevated neck veins and has a pulsus paradoxus of 14 mm Hg (normal <10 mm Hg).

Question 2.2.14 **The** *next step* **for this patient is:**
A) Change the patient to steroids from indomethacin
B) Perform a pericardiocentesis
C) Start a positive inotrope (e.g., dopamine) to improve right heart function
D) Start an afterload reducer to reduce cardiac demand

Answer 2.2.14 **The correct answer is "B."** The patient is clearly not doing well if he is getting more dyspneic and not responding to your treatment. The pulsus paradoxus is 14 mm Hg. This is indicative of possible cardiac tamponade, but it may be seen in constrictive pericarditis, severe asthma, or anything else that reduces right heart filling (e.g., tension pneumothorax). This patient's clinical picture is consistent with decompensated cardiac tamponade, and drastic action is indicated to relieve the symptoms of right heart failure. The definitive treatment is pericardiocentesis. "A" is incorrect because more drastic action is required. You would be correct to change the patient to prednisone or to add colchicine if not done already. "C" is incorrect since an inotrope will do little to help this problem. "D" is incorrect for two reasons: the first is that this is a right heart problem and reducing afterload (systemic vascular resistance) will not help the right heart, which pumps against pulmonary resistance; second, most drugs that reduce systemic vascular resistance will also decrease preload to some degree, worsening the symptoms of tamponade.

HELPFUL TIP:
Be aware that up to 25% of patients with cardiac tamponade will **NOT** demonstrate an elevated pulsus paradoxus. So, a normal pulsus paradoxus does not rule out cardiac tamponade.

HELPFUL TIP:
Measuring pulsus paradoxus: Pump up the BP cuff to greater than the systolic BP. Deflate the BP cuff slowly and listen for the first Korotkoff sound heard **only** during expiration; continue slowly deflating until you hear the Korotkoff sounds with inspiration as well. The difference is the pulsus paradoxus.

You perform a pericardiocentesis and the patient gets better. Of course, a good outcome never protected anyone from a lawsuit …

▶ **Objectives: Did you learn to …**
· Evaluate a patient with typical anginal chest pain?
· Describe the test characteristics of various types of noninvasive cardiac testing?
· Become familiar with the interpretation of noninvasive cardiac testing?
· Recognize various indications for PTCA with stent placement versus CABG?
· Understand the physiology, presentation, and treatment of post-pericardiotomy syndrome?
· Treat pericarditis and cardiac tamponade?

 QUICK QUIZ: CARDIAC CT SCAN

When planning treatment or diagnosing (i.e., "ruling out" ACS) based on a cardiac CT angiogram (CCTA), which of the following is TRUE?
A) In patients with stable CAD, CCTA is associated with reduced CAD mortality and overall mortality compared to other noninvasive tests (MPI, exercise testing, etc.)
B) The radiation exposure for CCTA is less than that of MPI
C) The downstream radiation exposure after MPI is less than that of CCTA
D) CCTA images are of best quality in patients with a pulse of 80 to 100 bpm
E) A creatinine of 1.6 mg/dL is a contraindication to the use of CCTA because of the contrast load

The correct answer is "B." The radiation exposure of CCTA is less than that of MPI, both initially and downstream (thus, "C" is wrong). More patients who have MPI go on to angiogram and additional radiation exposure. "D" is incorrect. The slower the heart rate, the better the images (within reasonable limits, of course, as pulse of 12 bpm isn't so good). So, patients are often pretreated with metoprolol to slow the heart rate before CCTA. "E" is also incorrect. It turns out that IV contrast is less of a factor in renal failure than we have thought (*Radiology* 2014;273(3):714; *Ann Emerg Med.* 2017 Aug 12). If you feel the patient really needs the CT and has a creatinine of 1.7 mg/dL or less, go ahead with the CT. What about option "A"? It turns out that even though CCTA is better at identifying cardiac disease (Table 2-5) and leads to more interventions than MPI and echo, its use is not associated with a reduction in cardiovascular or all-cause mortality. CCTA does reduce non-fatal MIs. Most of the benefit was from more aggressive medical management (e.g., statins, BP control) and not revascularization (*N Engl J Med.* 2018;379:924–933). So, treat your patients appropriately and you can bypass the CCTA in patients with stable CAD.

QUICK QUIZ: HYPERTENSION

According to the Eighth Joint National Committee (JNC 8), the blood pressure goal in a patient with diabetes is:
A) <100/50 mm Hg
B) <110/70 mm Hg
C) <130/80 mm Hg
D) <140/90 mm Hg
E) None of the above

The correct answer is "D." According to JNC 8, the goal for a diabetic patient (or any patient age 30–59 years, including those with chronic kidney disease) is <140/90 mm Hg. Tighter control does not seem to confer any benefit. The BP goal in those over age 60 is <150/90 mm Hg. These goals are consistent with the best current evidence at the time JNC 8 was published. In fact, tight blood pressure control in diabetics increases mortality (*JAMA* 2010;304(1):61–68). However, the American Diabetes Association continues to recommend more aggressive targets (e.g., <140/90 mm Hg in the 2018 *Standards* update, with the caveat that treatment should be individualized).

 HELPFUL TIP:
Recommendations for treating hypertension in the elderly vary a little based on the organization publishing the goals. For patients over age 80 years, there is universal agreement (ACC/AHA, JNC 8, ASH, ESH/ESC,

ACP, AAFP) that <150/90 mm Hg should be the goal. For patients age 60 to 79 years, JNC 8, ACP, and AAFP recommend a goal of <150/90 mm Hg while the other organizations recommend a goal of <140/90 mm Hg—but with a systolic pressure remaining greater than 115 mm Hg. Most of these guidelines also specifically state that standing blood pressure and/or 24-hour ambulatory blood pressures should be measured in older adults and considered in individualized blood pressure targets.

► **CASE 2.3**

A 24-year-old male presents to your clinic with a 50-hour history of an irregular heart rate. He is generally well but has a history of hypertension (too many super-jumbo burgers … with bacon … he's been "supersized"), which he has been trying to control with exercise and diet (he switched to tofu burgers yesterday). There is no prior history of cardiac disease or palpitations. He did "have a bit to drink" celebrating … well, whatever, just celebrating … who needs a reason! He was embarrassed about his drinking and thus waited 2 days to seek care. There is no family history of heart disease and the patient does not smoke. Vital signs reveal an irregular pulse of 130 bpm and a blood pressure of 160/100 mm Hg. The patient is afebrile and has normal respirations. He has no heart murmur. The ECG is shown below (Fig. 2-4).

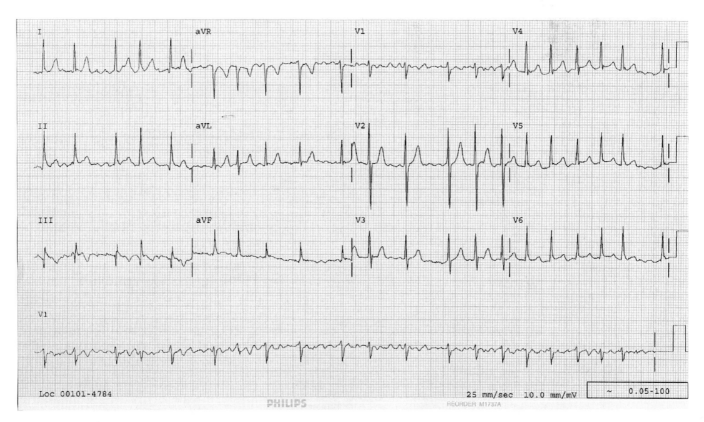

FIGURE 2-4. ECG for patient in question 2.3.1.

Question 2.3.1 The most appropriate diagnosis is:
A) Multifocal atrial tachycardia (MAT)
B) Wandering atrial pacemaker
C) Atrial fibrillation
D) Ventricular tachycardia
E) Accelerated junctional rhythm

Answer 2.3.1 The correct answer is "C," atrial fibrillation. This is characterized by the lack of P waves and an irregularly irregular rhythm. "A" and "B" are incorrect. While both MAT and a wandering atrial pacemaker are irregularly irregular, both have P waves. "D" is incorrect. Ventricular tachycardia is a wide complex tachycardia and is regular. "E" is incorrect. While there are no P waves, an accelerated junctional rhythm should be a regular, organized rhythm.

Question 2.3.2 What is the most likely cause of this patient's dysrhythmia?
A) Congenital prolonged QT syndrome
B) Hypertrophic cardiomyopathy
C) Alcohol use
D) Marijuana use
E) Ischemic cardiac disease

Answer 2.3.2 The correct answer is "C." The most likely cause of atrial fibrillation in this 24-year-old is alcohol. This is also known by the moniker "holiday heart." It occurs after episodes of significant alcohol intake. The underlying mechanism is not known, but alcohol is known to be cardiotoxic at higher doses which varies by individual. "A" is incorrect because prolonged QT typically causes polymorphic ventricular tachycardia (torsades de pointes). "B," hypertrophic cardiomyopathy, is unlikely since the patient has never had a murmur, and hypertrophic cardiomyopathy generally presents with signs of aortic outlet obstruction (syncope or angina with exercise) although a subset of patients do not have obstructive physiology. "D" is incorrect because marijuana is not implicated in causing atrial fibrillation, and "E" is incorrect because a patient who is 24 years old is unlikely to have ischemic cardiac disease.

Question 2.3.3 Other states that can cause atrial fibrillation include all of the following EXCEPT:
A) Valvular disease, especially mitral disease
B) Hyperthyroidism
C) Stroke
D) Heart failure
E) Pulmonary embolism (PE)

Answer 2.3.3 The correct answer is "C." Stroke does not generally cause atrial fibrillation but can be a result of atrial fibrillation. Certainly, stroke and other intracranial injuries can be associated with arrhythmias. However, these are generally isolated PVCs. Stroke may also be associated with heart failure and ischemic changes on the ECG (the etiology is unknown…call it "neurohumeral" and you will sound smart), but it is rarely an isolated cause of atrial fibrillation. Valvular heart disease, hyperthyroidism, heart failure, and PE have all been demonstrated to be causes of atrial fibrillation. Valvular heart disease, heart failure, and PE have a similar mechanism: stretching of the atrium leading to atrial irritability. Atrial fibrillation is found in 10% to 20% of those with hyperthyroidism, especially in the elderly.

The patient confides that he was indeed at a bachelor party several days ago (so that was what he was celebrating) and had a bit too much to drink. This is quite unusual for the patient. He generally drinks 2 to 3 beers per week, but on this particular night had 12 or more (hmm … now we're wondering). The patient's pulse increases to 160 bpm, but he remains asymptomatic.

Question 2.3.4 The INITIAL goal for this patient, suspected of having 50 hours of atrial fibrillation, is:
A) Anticoagulation
B) Immediate cardioversion (DCCV)
C) Rate control
D) Blood pressure lowering
E) Treatment of alcohol withdrawal

Answer 2.3.4 The correct answer is "C." Since this patient has had > 48 hours of atrial fibrillation, rate control is the goal. One should consider anticoagulation ("A"), but rate control is the most immediate concern. In real life, one would simultaneously address the patient's rate and anticoagulation needs, but—hey—a test isn't real life! If the onset of atrial fibrillation is indeterminate or >48 hours, one should withhold cardioversion due to the risk of thrombus formation in the atria and subsequent embolization; therefore, "B" is incorrect. "D" is incorrect because control of blood pressure is a secondary goal in this situation, and "E" is incorrect as this patient's tachycardia is not due to alcohol withdrawal.

The patient's heart rate remains elevated at 160 bpm with occasional forays into the 170 bpm range.

Question 2.3.5 Which of the following is the best drug to administer to this patient?
A) Digoxin
B) Lidocaine
C) Amiodarone
D) Adenosine
E) Diltiazem

Answer 2.3.5 The correct answer is "E." Of the options listed, diltiazem should be the first choice for rate control. "A" is incorrect. Digoxin will be of limited use since it takes at least 30 minutes to have an effect. As an aside, digoxin is associated with higher mortality rates in those with atrial fibrillation. Don't use it; we have better drugs. Digoxin can be used in those with atrial fibrillation secondary to heart failure but will still not significantly help with rate control—especially in younger patients with robust sympathetic tone. "B" is incorrect because lidocaine is indicated for a wide complex tachycardia. "C" is incorrect. Amiodarone will work as a treatment of atrial fibrillation but is a second-line drug because it can cause torsades de pointes. It can be used in patients with atrial fibrillation and congestive failure, where verapamil or diltiazem might be contraindicated. Amiodarone is considered to be advantageous in maintaining sinus rhythm, especially when given as pretreatment prior to cardioversion, but is not as efficacious in prompt heart rate control due to longer onset of action. Be aware that amiodarone can lead to "chemical cardioversion' with the attendant stroke risk. "D" is incorrect. Adenosine is ultra-short-acting, blocks the AV node, and can be used to convert a paroxysmal supraventricular tachycardia (PSVT) or slow down the rate of the arrhythmia temporarily if you are not sure what the diagnosis is (e.g., a rapid atrial flutter vs. PSVT). However, adenosine will not reduce the ventricular rate in atrial fibrillation since atrial fibrillation does not require the AV node to propagate. A beta-blocker could also be used in this situation.

Being the astute clinician that you are, you realize that 50% of atrial fibrillation will spontaneously convert to normal sinus rhythm, especially if present <72 hours. A transthoracic echocardiogram was performed and did not demonstrate any structural heart disease or vegetations. Thus, you choose to give verapamil and monitor the patient. At 24 hours, he still is in atrial fibrillation, although the rate is controlled well (90–110 bpm) with verapamil and he is normotensive. You discuss his case with your friendly neighborhood cardiologist who suggests that you plan cardioversion in 3 to 4 weeks.

Question 2.3.6 How would you anticoagulate this patient should you choose anticoagulation?
A) Start warfarin alone
B) Start heparin and rivaroxaban at the same time
C) Start heparin alone
D) Start aspirin alone

Answer 2.3.6 **The correct answer is "A."** If the onset of atrial fibrillation is indeterminate or >48 hours (as with this patient), one should withhold cardioversion and anticoagulate the patient for 3 weeks before cardioversion. A second strategy is to anticoagulate the patient and arrange for a trans-esophageal echocardiogram. If the trans-esophageal echocardiogram shows no vegetations, you can proceed with cardioversion. For those with <48 hours of atrial fibrillation, immediate cardioversion is a viable option. Since we now are planning to cardiovert this patient in the future, "A" is the most reasonable option provided. Some physicians will start heparin or low-molecular-weight heparin at the initiation of warfarin; however, the combination is not necessary in patients with nonvalvular atrial fibrillation. This scenario is much different than when patients have a PE/DVT. **For nonvalvular atrial fibrillation, starting warfarin (or a DOAC) alone is sufficient.** "B" is incorrect. There is no need to bridge patients starting rivaroxaban or apixaban with heparin; the anticoagulant effect is "immediate" and there is no transient hypercoagulable state. Dabigatran still requires 5 to 10 days of heparin, enoxaparin, etc. Heparin ("C") or aspirin ("D") alone would not be the best choices in this case.

HELPFUL TIP:
Note that the *Chest* guidelines, updated in 2018 (*Chest* 2018;154(5):1121), recommend a direct oral anticoagulant over warfarin for anticoagulation in atrial fibrillation. Rivaroxaban, apixaban (factor Xa inhibitors), and dabigatran (a direct fibrin inhibitor) are all approved for use in nonvalvular atrial fibrillation (although warfarin is less expensive, even when checking INRs). There may be some clinical advantages to apixaban, including fewer embolic phenomenon and less bleeding. But, there is no compelling evidence to favor one over the other. We now have reversal agents for dabigatran and the factor Xa inhibitors. In general, avoid edoxaban (Savaysa). The outcome data isn't as good as with other factor Xa inhibitors.

Question 2.3.7 All of the following can be used to cardiovert atrial fibrillation EXCEPT:
A) Ibutilide
B) Electrical cardioversion
C) Quinidine
D) Digoxin
E) Procainamide

Answer 2.3.7 **The correct answer is "D."** Digoxin does not work to cardiovert atrial fibrillation. Digoxin may facilitate cardioversion in patients with heart failure by reducing atrial stretching. However, it does not convert atrial fibrillation. All of the other answers are correct. Because of potential induction of arrhythmias with the other agents, electrical cardioversion is becoming the preferred method of restoring normal sinus rhythm.

▶ **Objectives: Did you learn to …**
- Recognize the clinical and ECG presentation of atrial fibrillation?
- Use rate-controlling drugs to treat a patient with atrial fibrillation?
- Appropriately employ anticoagulation in atrial fibrillation for a patient undergoing cardioversion?
- Identify appropriate situations for cardioversion of atrial fibrillation?

 QUIZ: ANTIHYPERTENSIVE AGENTS

A 70-year-old male complains of erectile dysfunction (ED) and requests medical treatment. You begin to discuss sildenafil (Viagra®—or whatever your phosphodiesterase-5 [PDE5] inhibitor of choice is). You believe his ED is secondary to vascular disease and that he is healthy enough to engage in sexual activity.

Which of the following antihypertensive drug classes can cause prolonged hypotension when used with PDE5 inhibitors?
A) Peripheral alpha-blockers
B) Calcium channel blockers (CCBs)

C) ACE inhibitors

D) Thiazide diuretics

E) Beta-blockers

The correct answer is "A." The peripheral alpha-blockers (doxazosin, prazosin, and tamsulosin) can cause symptomatic hypotension when combined with sildenafil or other drugs of this class (Cialis [tadalafil], Levitra [vardenafil]). This hypotensive effect is more severe when these drugs are combined with a nitrate. Nitrates should **not** be administered within 24 hours (or longer in patients with renal or hepatic dysfunction) of these drugs, as the combination has reportedly resulted in prolonged hypotension and strokes. None of the other drugs ("B"–"E") cause this hypotensive effect when combined with a PDE5 inhibitor.

▶ CASE 2.4

A 55-year-old male with a history of newly identified atrial fibrillation is referred to you for "medical clearance" for surgery. He has a history of hypertension and hypercholesterolemia (to calculate his CHA_2-DS_2-VASC score, see Table 2-6A). He has normal cardiac function otherwise with a normal ejection fraction and no valvular disease on echocardiogram. His atrial fibrillation has not been addressed since it was discovered by the surgeon at a pre-op visit. His heart rate is 80 bpm when you see him, his rhythm is irregularly irregular, and he has no signs of heart failure.

Question 2.4.1 Which of the following options would be appropriate for this patient?

A) Anticoagulate the patient with warfarin or a direct oral anticoagulant (DOAC) and allow him to stay in atrial fibrillation

B) Place the patient on aspirin and allow him to stay in atrial fibrillation

C) Give digoxin to cardiovert the patient

D) Recommend DC cardioversion immediately since sustained normal sinus rhythm yields the best long-term outcomes

E) A and B

Answer 2.4.1 The correct answer is "E." This patient's CHA_2-DS_2-VASC (see Table 2-6A) score is "1" allowing him to take aspirin *or* be anticoagulated with either a DOAC or warfarin. For a CHA_2-DS_2-VASC score of 1, it is still a matter of clinical judgment based on patient-specific risk factors (see Table 2-6B). Prior to deciding on an approach to anticoagulation in a particular patient, calculate a HAS-BLED score (https://www.mdcalc.com/has-bled-score-major-bleeding-risk) to determine risk of bleeding. Balance stroke and bleeding risk when making a decision. A CHA_2-DS_2-VASC score of "0" corresponds to what we used to call "lone atrial fibrillation" and does not necessitate anticoagulation. In a 2019 update to the ACC/AHA Guidelines for the Management of Patients with Atrial Fibrillation, it was recommended to initiate anticoagulation with a DOAC (preferred) over warfarin for nonvalvular atrial fibrillation in men with a CHA_2-DS_2-VASC score of ≥2 and for women with a score ≥3. Please see Tablet 2-6B for anticoagulation recommendations

based on CHA_2-DS_2-VASC score Renal and hepatic function should be evaluated at initiation of anticoagulation and at least annually. "C" is incorrect since this patient does not require rate control and digoxin is not effective for cardioversion. "D" is wrong. Long term, it is reasonable to allow most patients to remain in atrial fibrillation as long as they are properly anticoagulated based on the CHA_2-DS_2-VASC score. Outcomes of patients who stay in atrial fibrillation and are given appropriate therapy are the same (or a bit better) than in patients in whom one tries to maintain sinus rhythm with drugs such as amiodarone, etc.

HELPFUL TIP:

Other options for atrial fibrillation include ablation and closure of the left atrial appendage (LAA). Compared with anticoagulation, LAA closure reduces the stroke risk as much as anticoagulation but entails the risk of surgery (about 1:25 will have some significant complication).

The patient returns at age 75. He is 20 years older. You, however, have not aged a day because doctors are immortal, right? He is now hypertensive, and diabetic, and he requires a cholecystectomy. Apparently, he only sees you for pre-op exams. His CHA_2-DS_2-VASC score is now 4 and he has been on warfarin for the past 5 years.

TABLE 2-6A CALCULATING THE CHA_2DS_2-VASc SCORE

Criteria	Points	
Congestive heart failure	1	
Hypertension (treated or above 140/90 mm Hg)	1	
Age >75	2	
Diabetes	1	
Stroke, TIA or thromboembolic disease	2	**Score and Risk of CVA** (in %/yr) 0=0.2–0.6% 1= 0.6–1.3%/yr 2 = 2.2%/yr 3 = 3.2%/yr 4 = 4%/yr 5 = 7%/yr 6 = 10%/yr
Vascular disease (CAD, PAD, aortic plaque)	1	
Age 65–74	1	
Sex **C**ategory **F**emale[a]	1	

[a]New guidelines *do not* include female gender as a risk factor *unless* there is another risk factor present. So, women cannot have a score of "1." If they have *only* female gender, the score is zero. If they have another risk factor, they get +1 for gender + the points for the additional risk factor.

TABLE 2-6B TREATMENT OF NONVALVULAR ATRIAL FIBRILLATION BASED ON THE CHA_2DS_2-VASc SCORE

CHA_2DS_2-VASc Score	Recommended Treatment[a]
0	No anticoagulation indicated but use clinical judgment (0.5–0.7% stroke risk/yr)
1	Consider anticoagulation with a DOAC (preferred) or warfarin (0.6–1.3% stroke risk/yr). Use clinical judgment
2 or greater	Anticoagulation with a DOAC (preferred)[b] or warfarin (2.2% or > stroke risk/yr)

[a]Aspirin is no longer recommended for A-fib. The data does not support its use.

[b]DOAC, direct acting oral anticoagulant: Xarelto (rivaroxaban), Eliquis (apixaban) and Pradaxa (dabigatran), Savaysa (edoxaban). Apixaban has the best profile for bleeding versus prevention of stroke.

Question 2.4.2 Which of the following approaches is the best for controlling his anticoagulation, given that he needs surgery?

A) Stop the warfarin several days before surgery to allow his INR to normalize. Restart the warfarin after surgery

B) Hospitalize the patient a couple of days ahead of time and start heparin. Then stop his warfarin. Restart the warfarin after surgery

C) Use low-molecular-weight heparin at home and stop the warfarin once this is started. Restart the warfarin after surgery

D) Stop the warfarin several days before surgery to allow his INR to normalize. Start heparin after surgery and simultaneously restart warfarin

Answer 2.4.2 The correct answer is "A." For patients with nonvalvular atrial fibrillation who are undergoing surgery or invasive diagnostic procedures, it is reasonable to interrupt anticoagulation for up to 1 week without substituting heparin (assuming they haven't had a recent stroke or other thromboembolic event). "Bridge" therapy with IV heparin or low-molecular-weight heparin confers no benefit (*Circulation* 2015;131(5):488). The risk of perioperative bleeding with heparin is actually greater than the risk of thromboembolism from atrial fibrillation. "B," "C," and "D" are incorrect because the patient does not need heparin. Bridging therapy is typically indicated for patients at higher risk for thromboembolic events such as those with mechanical heart valves, prior stroke, or CHA_2DS_2-VASc score >5.

The 75-year-old patient has his surgery and returns to your clinic for a postoperative check-up 1 month after his surgery. You check his INR and it is noted to be 5.2. There is no active bleeding.

Question 2.4.3 The most appropriate action at this point is to:

A) Hospitalize the patient for observation since he is at a high risk of bleeding

B) Give the patient 5 mg of vitamin K orally

C) Give the patient 2 units of fresh frozen plasma to reverse his anticoagulation

D) Hold the next warfarin dose and reduce the maintenance dose

E) A, B, and C

Answer 2.4.3 The correct answer is "D." The risk of bleeding in a relatively healthy patient with an INR of 5.2 is very low. Thus, simply holding the next one to two doses of warfarin and reducing the maintenance dose of warfarin is appropriate. "A" is incorrect because the patient does not need hospitalization. "B" is incorrect because it will be difficult to anticoagulate the patient after vitamin K is administered. "C" is incorrect because there is no active bleeding.

The patient misunderstands your instructions and takes an extra dose of warfarin that evening and for the next 2 days. He returns to your clinic and his INR is now 13.

Question 2.4.4 What is the best option for therapy at this point?

A) Vitamin K 5 mg IV × 1

B) Fresh frozen plasma

C) Vitamin K 5 mg PO × 1

D) Vitamin K 10 mg IV × 1

Answer 2.4.4 The correct answer is "C." Giving this patient 5 mg of PO vitamin K is the best solution. This has been found to reduce the INR while still allowing the patient to be anticoagulated relatively easily after treatment. "B" is incorrect because there is no call for FFP in this asymptomatic patient. The other answers are incorrect because there is no advantage to higher doses or IV doses of vitamin K in this patient, and the higher doses will make continued anticoagulation more difficult.

HELPFUL TIP: REVERSING WARFARIN

In patients who are not bleeding:

- If the INR is <4.5 simply reduce the dose of warfarin or hold the next dose of warfarin.
- If the INR is 4.5 to 10 you have several options. If there is no bleeding: hold one or two doses of warfarin. **Routine vitamin K is not recommended.** If the patient will require surgery or is at high bleeding risk, administer vitamin K ≤ 5 mg with another 1 to 1.5 mg in 24 hours.
- If the INR is >10 administer 2.5 to 5 mg of vitamin K even if there is no bleeding.

In patients who are bleeding:

- Administer prothrombin complex concentrate (e.g., Kcentra® … should they buy a vowel? They can afford it!). This is preferred over fresh frozen plasma (FFP), which is second line. In addition, administer 5 to 10 mg of vitamin K. The INR of FFP is approximately 1.5. You won't get it lower no matter how much FFP you give. Tell your surgeon to chill.

▶ **Objectives: Did you learn to …**

- Weigh the advantages and disadvantages of rate control versus rhythm control strategies for atrial fibrillation?
- Manage anticoagulation and atrial fibrillation vis-à-vis surgery?
- Manage the over-anticoagulated patient?

▶ CASE 2.5

A 62-year-old female presents to your office with a history of occasional palpitations that are of great concern to her. She notes that she feels a racing heart that lasts for a matter of seconds and occurs every 7 days or so. However, when she has the symptoms, she will generally get four to five episodes during that day. She denies any chest pain, dyspnea, lightheadedness, or other associated symptoms. You order an event monitor and it shows that the patient is having nonsustained episodes of monomorphic ventricular tachycardia lasting 4 beats or less each. She is asymptomatic except for the palpitations.

Question 2.5.1 The best approach at this point is to:
A) Start an antiarrhythmic such as quinidine or mexiletine to control the heart rhythm
B) Refer the patient to a cardiologist for an electrophysiologic (EP) study to determine the best drug to control this rhythm
C) Implant an automatic defibrillator to prevent sudden death
D) Implant a pacemaker
E) Check serum potassium, magnesium, TSH, glucose, CBC

Answer 2.5.1 **The correct answer is "E."** The first step in determining the treatment of this patient is to make sure that there is not an underlying metabolic abnormality that could predispose to this rhythm abnormality.

You check a panel of laboratory studies including thyroid function tests, electrolytes, magnesium, glucose, and CBC. They are all within normal limits. You suggest that the patient avoid potential triggers such as caffeine and sympathomimetics. "Darn," she sighs. "I have to quit my crystal meth?"

Question 2.5.2 The next step for this patient is to:
A) Start an antiarrhythmic such as quinidine or mexiletine to control the heart rhythm
B) Refer the patient to a cardiologist for an EP study to determine the best drug to control this rhythm

C) Implant an automatic defibrillator to prevent sudden death
D) Start a beta-blocker
E) Order transthoracic echocardiogram to rule out structural heart disease

Answer 2.5.2 **The correct answer is "E."** Nonsustained ventricular tachycardia is associated with sudden cardiac death in the presence of structural heart disease such as hypertrophic cardiomyopathy or ischemic heart disease. An echocardiogram as well as stress test will be helpful in evaluating for these underlying conditions. There is no evidence that nonsustained, asymptomatic ventricular tachycardia worsens outcomes **as long as the patient has no underlying cardiac disease.** In an otherwise healthy, asymptomatic patient, the risk of using antiarrhythmic drugs to suppress ventricular ectopy leads to worse outcomes than doing nothing. Quinidine, mexiletine, amiodarone, and other antiarrhythmics all have proarrhythmic effects. In general, there is more sudden death in these patients if they are treated with antiarrhythmic drugs than if they are watched. Therefore, "A" is incorrect because these drugs will actually increase mortality. "B" is incorrect since the patient has asymptomatic, self-limited episodes. The reason to do an EP study is to determine if there is an inducible arrhythmia and to determine treatment. This patient does not (yet) need treatment. "C" is incorrect because this patient has asymptomatic nonsustained ventricular tachycardia. Thus, an implantable defibrillator is not indicated. *After your evaluation is complete,* you may prescribe a beta-blocker ("D") for relief from palpitations. A beta-blocker (metoprolol or carvedilol) is considered the first-line drug in this type of patient. You can add diltiazem or verapamil to this should she still feel palpitations. Amiodarone would be third line should she continue to be bothered by the palpitations after trying beta-blockers and calcium channel blockers.

The echocardiogram and stress test are normal, and the patient does well for the next 3 months but then becomes symptomatic with prolonged episodes of ventricular tachycardia. While all of the episodes are self-limited, the patient has had two episodes of syncope.

Question 2.5.3 Which of the following is the best next step in treating this patient?
A) Sotalol
B) Implantable defibrillator
C) Amiodarone
D) Electrophysiologic study
E) Tocainide (an oral lidocaine equivalent)

Answer 2.5.3 **The correct answer is "D."** An electrophysiologic study is indicated to induce and characterize the ventricular tachycardia. Certain types of ventricular tachycardia respond very well to radiofrequency ablation so this should be the next step. **Some of you may have answered "B." This is true in patients with ischemic heart disease, left ventricular dysfunction, and symptomatic ventricular tachycardia. These patients should get an implantable defibrillator as should** "all" heart failure patients with an ejection fraction of <30% to 35% (there are literally over 200 variations of this recommendation based on heart failure class, QRS duration, etc., but this is the basic idea). Our patient may yet get an implantable defibrillator since she is now symptomatic (syncope), but do the EP study first.

▶ **Objectives: Did you learn to …**
- Evaluate a patient with palpitations?
- Manage nonsustained, asymptomatic, ventricular tachycardia?

▶ CASE 2.6

A 22-year-old female presents to your office with a history of palpitations. You are able to capture the arrhythmia on the monitor in your office: the rhythm strip shows evidence of isolated premature atrial contractions (PACs). She is otherwise healthy and taking no medications, and there is no family history of heart disease.

Question 2.6.1 All of the following are salient points of the history with regard to PACs EXCEPT:
A) Aged cheese consumption
B) Caffeine use
C) Tobacco use
D) Alcohol use
E) COPD

Answer 2.6.1 The correct answer is "A." Aged cheese **can** cause problems in combination with monoamine oxidase inhibitors (MAOIs). In combination with an MAOI, aged cheese and other sources of tyramine can cause a hypertensive emergency. However, this patient is not taking any medications. All of the other conditions and drugs listed can cause PACs. While there are conflicting data about the strength of the association caffeine, it is clear that COPD, tobacco, and alcohol can all cause an increase in sympathetic tone, leading to PACs. Neurologic abnormalities (e.g., stroke) can also be associated with PACs, as can some drugs (e.g., theophylline).

HELPFUL TIP:
You have to eat 2 pounds of cheddar cheese in half an hour in order to develop a hypertensive crisis with an MAOI. In studies where there was free access to cheese, the maximum anyone was able to eat was 1.9 pounds in 2 hours. Believe it or not, someone studied this (probably somewhere in Wisconsin). And, banana peels (but not the fruit of the banana) are contraindicated with MAOIs…really (who eats the peel anyway?).

Question 2.6.2 Which of the following statements about PACs is true?
A) Mitral valve prolapse is associated with PACs
B) Mitral valve stenosis is associated with PACs
C) Bicuspid aortic valve is associated with PACs
D) None of the above is true

Answer 2.6.2 The correct answer is "B." Anything that can cause an increase in left atrial pressures (and therefore atrial wall stretching) is associated with an increase in the number of PACs. Mitral stenosis causes increased pressures in the left atrium, wall stretching, and enlargement and thus predisposes to PACs. "A" is incorrect. Even though multiple problems have been blamed on mitral valve prolapse, a study done as part of the Framingham study showed that the symptoms blamed on mitral valve prolapse (anxiety, PACs, tachycardia, etc.) are no more prevalent in those with mitral valve prolapse than in those without it. "C" is incorrect. A bicuspid aortic valve **may** cause PACs as a result of heart failure when the patient decompensates and has increased left-sided heart pressures. However, a bicuspid aortic valve itself is not a source of PACs. Similarly, hypertrophic cardiomyopathy, other causes of heart failure, drugs (e.g., theophylline and digoxin), and neurologic diseases can be associated with PACs.

This patient is bothered by her PACs. She is rather aware of them and finds them disconcerting.

Question 2.6.3 What is the best pharmacologic therapy to consider at this point?
A) Sotalol
B) Metoprolol
C) Trasylol
D) Amiodarone
E) Mountain Dew—lots of it

Answer 2.6.3 The correct answer is "B." A beta-blocker may help to reduce this patient's PACs. "A" is incorrect because, while sotalol can be used for both atrial and ventricular arrhythmias, it is proarrhythmic and can cause torsades de pointes. Thus, it should be initiated in the hospital with monitoring and reserved for those with severe arrhythmias. "C" is incorrect because Trasylol is the trade name for aprotinin, an enzyme that *was* used to reduce bleeding during surgical procedures. "D" is incorrect because, like sotalol, amiodarone is proarrhythmic, and its use should be limited to those with significant arrhythmias.

▶ **Objectives: Did you learn to …**
- Recognize causes of PACs?
- Treat a patient with bothersome PACs?

 QUICK QUIZ: VALVULAR DISEASE

Surgery is indicated in which of these patients with valvular disease?
A) An asymptomatic patient with severe mitral regurgitation and a left ventricular ejection fraction (LVEF) of less than 60%
B) An asymptomatic patient with a bicuspid aortic valve

C) Asymptomatic aortic regurgitation with an LVEF of less than 50% on echocardiogram

D) Only symptomatic valvular lesions should be approached surgically

E) A and C

The correct answer is "E." Once patients with mitral regurgitation and aortic regurgitation become symptomatic, the morbidity and mortality increases significantly. Thus, these patients should be operated on **before** they become symptomatic. Patients should have routine echocardiography yearly if they have severe valvular disease. In addition to evaluating the valve, echocardiography allows you to evaluate ventricular size and function. Importantly, proper management of patients with valvular heart disease depends on accurate diagnosis of the cause as well as proper staging of the disease process, which is based on valvular anatomy, valvular hemodynamics, severity of left ventricular dilation and systolic function, and patient symptoms. (NOTE: left ventricular systolic function and patient symptoms are only part of the decision-making process regarding management and timing of referral to surgery.)

 QUICK QUIZ: MINIMALLY INVASIVE VALVE REPLACEMENT

A 78-year-old female with syncope was found to have severe aortic stenosis on echocardiogram. She's worried about open-heart surgery and has heard about something called a "Transcatheter Aortic Valve Replacement" (TAVR). You counsel her on the risks, benefits, and alternatives. Which of the following is true?

A) TVAR is especially useful in those who are likely to be the most active after surgery since it is less invasive

B) A small leak at the side of TAVR is common and associated with a poor outcome

C) Stroke risk in 30 days is 8% to 10%

D) No anticoagulation is needed since it is a bioprosthetic valve

E) Mitral valve injury is a well-recognized complication of TAVR

The correct answer is "E". Mitral valve injury has been associated with TAVR procedures. "A" is wrong since TAVR is most useful in those who are not likely to be extremely active, such as elderly patients and/or those with multiple comorbidities. "B" is also incorrect. Small leaks are common *but are not associated with a worse outcome*. On the other hand, moderate or severe leaks do worsen outcome. Stroke risk is 2% to 5% and peri-procedure mortality is 1% to 4%. Bleeding is not uncommon at the site of vascular access. Finally, patients should be anticoagulated for at three (or more) months after TAVR and 6 months after an open bioprosthetic aortic valve replacement.

 HELPFUL TIP: TRANSCATHETER VALVE REPLACEMENT
Transcatheter mitral valve replacement for mitral regurgitation is not quite ready for prime time. Outcomes after the procedure are not different than the outcomes in those treated medically (*N Engl J Med.* 2018;379:2297–2306). For *mitral stenosis* transcatheter or open repair are both options depending on the valve anatomy. For aortic regurgitation (AR), TAVR has not been as successful or as widely used as it has been for aortic stenosis (AS); this may be due to the widely heterogeneous etiologies of AR as compared to AS, which occurs along a more predictable pathophysiologic pathway.

▶ **CASE 2.7**

A 74-year-old male presents to your office with a chief complaint of a "long cold" with an intermittent cough for 5 months. He has also noticed that he gets up to urinate twice a night although he has no trouble with his urine stream, starting urination, or dribbling afterward. He has been a bit more tired lately and notices that his exercise tolerance has decreased to several blocks, limited mainly by shortness of breath. He has not had any chest pain. He has no history of asthma or COPD and has not had any exposures to drugs or chemicals. He has a history of hypertension and noncompliance with medical recommendations. In fact, he is taking no medications except for an aspirin a day. His pulse is 100 bpm with a blood pressure of 160/95 mm Hg. He looks comfortable. On examination, you find only trace pitting edema of the lower extremities.

Question 2.7.1 Which of the following is NOT a possible cause of cough in this patient?
A) Heart failure
B) Asthma
C) Deconditioning
D) COPD
E) GERD

Answer 2.7.1 **The correct answer is "C."** Deconditioning may cause dyspnea on exertion but should not cause a cough. The purpose of this question is to point out the fact that a "chronic cold" or "chronic cough" in an elderly person can be due to a myriad of causes, including "occult" heart failure (systolic dysfunction (HFrEF) or diastolic dysfunction (HFpEF)). Do not make the assumption that the patient's diagnosis (e.g., a "chronic cold") is necessarily the correct diagnosis.

 HELPFUL TIP:
Systolic heart failure (secondary to infarction, etc.) is now termed "Heart Failure with a reduced Ejection Fraction" (HFrEF). Diastolic heart failure is now termed "Heart Failure with a preserved Ejection Fraction (HFpEF). In this book we use both the "old" and new notations.

You decide that this patient may have heart failure. An ECG shows no evidence of prior or ongoing ischemia. There are no signs of atrial enlargement or ventricular hypertrophy on the ECG.

Question 2.7.2 The proper conclusion from this is:

A) The patient does not have cardiac chamber enlargement or hypertrophy and therefore is unlikely to have heart failure
B) The absence of evidence for prior infarct makes heart failure unlikely
C) Regardless of the ECG results, clinical judgment alone is sufficient to make the diagnosis of heart failure, being correct 85% of the time
D) The patient's edema is likely from venous insufficiency
E) Despite a normal ECG, further testing is needed in this patient to evaluate for heart failure

Answer 2.7.2 The correct answer is "E." "A" is not correct because only 30% to 60% of moderate-to-severe left ventricular hypertrophy (LVH) is detectible on ECG. "B" is incorrect because patients with HFpEF (discussed later) may not have any evidence of prior ischemia or infarct. "C" is incorrect. The clinical diagnosis of heart failure is incorrect up to 50% of the time. For this reason, confirmation is required *before* embarking upon a therapeutic adventure for heart failure. "D" is unlikely, since the patient has other symptoms of heart failure (exertional dyspnea, cough, etc.) that make simple venous insufficiency unlikely. Plus, have you ever known "get further information" to be the wrong answer?

Question 2.7.3 You decide on further testing. Assuming every test is easily available to you (which might not be the case depending on the setting in which you work), what is the one best test that you would use to determine if this patient has heart failure?

A) Echocardiography
B) Brain natriuretic peptide (BNP) level
C) Chest radiograph looking for evidence of pulmonary edema (Kerley B lines, etc.)
D) SPECT myocardial perfusion imaging (MPI)
E) Positron emission tomography (PET) testing

Answer 2.7.3 The correct answer is "A." Echocardiography is the procedure of choice for the diagnosis of heart failure. This is for two reasons. First, you can assess left ventricular systolic function as well as look for diastolic dysfunction to determine if this is HFrEF or HFpEF. Second, you can evaluate the potential causes of heart failure including valvular heart disease, ischemic heart disease, pericardial disease, deposition disease (amyloidosis, hemochromatosis), etc. "B" is incorrect because the BNP will give you less concrete information about the patient compared to echocardiography. In this patient, with a high pretest probability of heart failure, BNP will most likely be elevated (though not always). "D" and "E" are incorrect because MPI and PET testing are best used to diagnose ischemia due to CAD.

HELPFUL TIP:
In a low-risk patient, a BNP of <100 pg/mL effectively rules out heart failure. A BNP of 100 to 500 pg/mL is indeterminate and may not be related to cardiac disease. A BNP of >500 pg/mL is relatively specific for heart failure (if other cardiac and noncardiac causes are excluded). Alternate cardiac causes of an elevated BNP include acute coronary syndromes, heart muscle disease, valvular heart disease, pericardial disease, atrial fibrillation, myocarditis, cardiac surgery, and status-post DC cardioversion.

(LESS) HELPFUL TIP:
Noncardiac causes of an elevated BNP include renal failure, anemia, advanced age, sepsis, pulmonary (obstructive sleep apnea, pulmonary hypertension, severe pneumonia), critical illness, severe burns, toxic/metabolic events (cancer, chemotherapy, envenomation). Obesity can cause a falsely low BNP.

BNP-directed therapy for heart failure does not seem to be any better than symptom directed therapy (*Eur Heart J.* 2014;35(1):16–24) (*JAMA* 2017;318:713). An elevated BNP *in the absence of heart failure* is still a marker for a worse outcome when compared to those with a normal BNP (*J Am Coll Cardiol.* 2018;71(19)).

The patient has an echocardiogram that shows a left ventricular ejection fracture (LVEF) of 35% and a regional wall motion abnormality (RWMA).

Question 2.7.4 This is the most consistent with a diagnosis of:

A) HFrEF secondary to myocarditis
B) HFrEF secondary to CAD
C) HFpEF secondary to hypertension
D) HFrEF secondary to constrictive pericarditis
E) Age-related changes; therefore, a normal variant

Answer 2.7.4 The correct answer is "B." A regional wall motion abnormality (RWMA) suggests that this patient has ischemic or infarcted myocardium. "A" is not the best choice since those with myocarditis (fulminant or acute) typically have global hypokinesis (although RWMA has been reported) and the patient would typically appear more clinically ill. "C" is incorrect by definition. HFpEF requires an LVEF of at least 50%, recognizing that this group may not have an entirely normal LVEF, but the major abnormality is not a reduction in LV systolic function. HFpEF is associated with a hypertrophied left ventricle and a **preserved** LVEF. HFrEF is defined by an LVEF of <40%. The echocardiogram in constrictive pericarditis ("D") generally shows normal left ventricular systolic function. It may reveal pericardial thickening, dilated inferior vena cava or hepatic veins, and abnormal mitral and tricuspid in-flow Doppler.

HELPFUL TIP:
Toxins such as methamphetamine, cocaine, alcohol, and antineoplastic chemotherapeutic drugs can cause a cardiomyopathy and should be considered as a possible etiology of heart failure in the appropriate patient.

Question 2.7.5 Which of the following is the most appropriate next strategy to work up this patient's HFrEF?
A) Cardiac MRI to assess myocardial viability
B) Coronary angiogram
C) Measure serial troponins to rule out acute coronary syndrome (ACS)
D) Electrophysiologic study to assess for inducible ventricular arrhythmia
E) CT to assess calcium scores

Answer 2.7.5 The correct answer is "B." Ischemic heart disease causes most HFrEF. If you can reverse the ischemia, mortality is decreased from 16% annually to 3.2% annually. Of all the options listed above, coronary angiography remains the gold standard to evaluate for CAD in this setting. Coronary angiograms provide information about anatomy and feasibility of revascularization but do not predict recovery of function after revascularization. This patient does not have chest pain or ECG changes to suggest ACS; therefore, "C" is incorrect. "D" is incorrect, as there is no indication for an electrophysiologic study in the absence of any arrhythmia. "E" is incorrect, because, as noted, the presence or absence of coronary calcification would not change the overall management plan for this patient. CT calcium scoring may be used as an additional risk stratification tool in intermediate-risk patients (similar to CRP, in addition to traditional risk factors such as hypertension, dyslipidemia, vascular or renal disease, etc.) but **not** in high-risk, symptomatic patients.

The coronary angiogram shows diffuse CAD; no coronary lesions are considered to be amenable to angioplasty and there are no vessels considered to be viable targets for bypass surgery. You decide to initiate medical therapy in this patient. In addition, you advise the patient regarding the nonpharmacologic therapies for heart failure treatment.

Question 2.7.6 Possible nonpharmacologic therapies for HFrEF include all of the following EXCEPT:
A) Fluid restriction of <2 L/day
B) Sodium restriction of <3 g/day
C) Dietary consultation
D) Cardiac risk factor modification
E) Monthly weight monitoring.

Answer 2.7.6 The correct answer is "E." The keystone of an effective heart failure treatment regimen is sodium and fluid balance as well as management of comorbidities ("A" and "B"). Cardiac risk factors, including hypertension, diabetes, hyperlipidemia, sleep apnea, obesity, sedentary lifestyle, smoking/

alcohol/drug use, etc. need to be treated with the same aggressiveness as in a patient with an ACS. Patients should be advised about **daily** weight monitoring rather than monthly monitoring ("E"). A weight gain of more than 3 to 5 lb may necessitate additional doses of a diuretic. **Note that significant fluid restriction to 1.5 to 2 L/day is typically, though not exclusively, reserved for Stage D advanced heart failure patients who are hyponatremic or diuretic resistant.** Conversion of patients in atrial fibrillation *via ablation (but not drugs)* to normal sinus rhythm is also of benefit and reduces mortality, hospitalizations, and improves left ventricular function (*N Engl J Med.* 2018;378(5):417–427).

HELPFUL TIP: PLEASE PASS THE SALT
Even though it is traditional, there is only weak evidence to suggest that salt restriction in CHF makes any real difference (*JAMA Intern Med.* 2018;178(12):1693–1700). European guidelines suggest limiting to no more than 6 grams of sodium per day (*Eur Heart J.* 2016;37(27):2129). We suspect the answer on the test will still be to restrict salt. But for your "real-life" patients, 1.5 to 2 gram sodium restriction per day may be excessive.

You wish to start an appropriate drug regimen for this patient's heart failure.

Question 2.7.7 All of the drugs below have been shown to reduce mortality in patients with HFrEF EXCEPT:
A) Digoxin
B) Metoprolol succinate
C) ACE inhibitors
D) Hydralazine and long-acting nitrates used in combination in patients intolerant of ACE inhibitors
E) Spironolactone

Answer 2.7.7 The correct answer is "A." Digoxin is an inotropic agent, and as such, would intuitively make sense as an effective drug for HFrEF. However, digoxin has **not** been shown to increase survival and in fact may worsen outcomes, especially in women and those with atrial fibrillation (*J Am Coll Cardiol.* 2018;71(10)). Its use is primarily for symptomatic relief. If using digoxin in HFrEF, the therapeutic target is a dose that achieves a plasma concentration of drug in the range of 0.5 to 0.9 ng/mL. The common daily dosage to achieve that target is typically 0.125 to 0.25 mg/day in patients <70 years of age with normal renal function and body mass. For patients with abnormal renal function, low body mass, or age >70, low doses (0.125 mg daily or every other day) are recommended initially with the dose titrated to the target therapeutic range. Digoxin **does** reduce hospitalizations and improve symptoms in those with HFrEF who are symptomatic despite use of maximal guideline-directed therapy. As noted above, digoxin *seems to worsen mortality* in those with atrial fibrillation, however. Avoid digoxin in patients with atrial fibrillation and significant sinus or AV nodal block unless they have a pacemaker. NOTE: Other cardiac medications such as amiodarone, dronedarone, verapamil, propafenone, and quinidine as well as noncardiac meds such as clarithromycin, erythromycin, itraconazole, and cyclosporine can increase the serum digoxin concentrations and may precipitate digoxin toxicity.

All of the other options, including the combination of isosorbide dinitrate and hydralazine, have been shown to reduce mortality. However, hydralazine and isosorbide dinitrate are generally reserved for those patients who are unable to tolerate ACE inhibitors or angiotensin receptor blockers (ARBs) or remain symptomatic despite maximal medical therapy with the other medications. This combination seems particularly effective in African Americans. However, enalapril reduces mortality by 28% when compared with hydralazine and nitrates. Thus, hydralazine and nitrates are second line. None of the "traditional" loop diuretics such as furosemide, bumetanide, etc., have been shown to positively affect mortality.

You start this patient on furosemide for diuresis and lisinopril for HFrEF. You also decide to initiate metoprolol succinate for its survival benefits. However, the patient's symptoms worsen.

Question 2.7.8 Which of these is true about the use of metoprolol succinate in HFrEF?

A) Metoprolol succinate is the only beta-blocker indicated for use in HFrEF

B) Metoprolol succinate is best used in those patients who are still symptomatic since it will help to control symptoms

C) Metoprolol succinate should only be initiated in patients with well-controlled HFrEF who are not currently having significant symptoms

D) Metoprolol succinate can lead to significant hypokalemia when combined with diuretics, so potassium levels should be monitored closely

E) Metoprolol succinate is contraindicated in patients who have both COPD and HFrEF

Answer 2.7.8 **The correct answer is "C."** Beta-blockers should **not** be initiated in patients who are significantly symptomatic or decompensated. While beta-blockers do reduce mortality, they can increase symptoms and further exacerbate heart failure. Therefore, they are best initiated in the stable patient (as an outpatient or 24 to 48 hours prior to hospital discharge and on a stable drug regimen). Even then some patients cannot tolerate the introduction of beta-blockers without worsening of symptoms, which may require additional diuresis, discontinuation of the beta-blocker, a reduction in dose, or other measures. "A" is incorrect. Long-acting metoprolol **succinate**, bisoprolol, and carvedilol all have a benefit in HFrEF. Specifically avoid atenolol which does not seem to improve outcomes. "B" is incorrect because beta-blockers may actually worsen heart failure symptoms. "D" is incorrect since beta-blockers do not cause hypokalemia. "E" is incorrect. Beta-blockers can be used in patients with COPD with the same caveats that apply to any other patient: if the patient is becoming more symptomatic on the beta-blocker, reduce the dose, or discontinue the drug. In fact, beta-blockers may improve survival in COPD.

HELPFUL TIP:
When starting a beta-blocker for HFrEF, start low and go slow! When starting digoxin for HFrEF, monitor for hypokalemia, hypomagnesemia, or hypothyroidism to avoid digoxin toxicity, even with low doses.

You reduce the dose of metoprolol succinate and consider starting this patient on another medication.

Question 2.7.9 Which of the following patients is/are good candidates for spironolactone?

A) A patient with NYHA Class I and Class II heart failure

B) A patient with NYHA Class III and Class IV heart failure

C) Both A and B

D) Neither A nor B

Answer 2.7.9 **The correct answer is "B."** Spironolactone has been shown to reduce mortality in patients with New York Heart Association (NYHA) Class III and Class IV heart failure. It has not been studied in Class I (thus "A" is wrong). However, it may be useful in symptomatic patients with Class II with an EF of <30%. Serum potassium needs to be monitored closely after initiation of spironolactone, especially since it will generally be used with an ACE inhibitor or ARB, both of which can increase the serum potassium. This drug should be avoided in patients with renal insufficiency or patients with serum potassium >5 mEq/L. Spironolactone is indicated for patients with NYHA Classes II–IV and who have LVEF ≤35% and a creatinine of <2.5 mg/dL in males or <2 mg/dL in females (or estimated GFR >30 mL/min/1.73 m^2). Eplerenone is another aldosterone inhibitor but is much more expensive with little, if any, advantage. *Remember that trimethoprim–sulfamethoxazole can lead to fatal hyperkalemia in those on an ACE/ARB/spironolactone and other potassium sparing drugs with even a couple of doses.*

HELPFUL TIP:
Aliskiren (Tekturna), a renin inhibitor, **is contraindicated** with an ARB or ACE inhibitor. It worsens outcomes and causes hyperkalemia. It also worsens outcomes in patients with diabetes. Another "don't use it" drug.

You treat this patient with metoprolol succinate, lisinopril, furosemide, atorvastatin, and aspirin. This regimen seems to help, and the patient's symptoms improve. However, a few weeks later, he presents to the ED with increased dyspnea. There have been no changes in his medications, and he assures you that he is taking his medications as directed. His examination reveals that he has elevated JVD, rales over the lower half of his lung fields bilaterally, and pedal edema.

Question 2.7.10 Common causes of decompensation in patients with otherwise stable heart failure include all of the following EXCEPT:
A) Inactivity
B) Fever
C) Arrhythmia
D) Dietary indiscretion
E) Ischemia

Answer 2.7.10 **The correct answer is "A."** Inactivity will not generally cause an exacerbation of heart failure (though may have been an underlying cause!). The major causes of acute exacerbations of chronic heart failure include dietary indiscretion (increased salt and fluid consumption), increased metabolic demand (e.g., from infection), anemia, medication noncompliance, arrhythmia, and ischemia. The inappropriate use of medications, such as some calcium channel blockers and the institution of beta-blockers when heart failure is decompensated, is also a common cause of exacerbations of HF.

The patient notes that he did have some chest pain earlier in the day. You want to initiate therapy. You take his vitals, and his pulse is 100 bpm, blood pressure 140/95 mm Hg, oxygen saturation 89% on room air, and respiratory rate 32.

Question 2.7.11 Besides oxygen, the one best drug to initiate first in the ED to treat this patient with an acute exacerbation of his chronic HFrEF is:
A) Furosemide
B) Digoxin
C) A positive inotrope, such as dobutamine
D) Nitroglycerin
E) An ACE inhibitor

Answer 2.7.11 **The correct answer is "D."** This patient will benefit from nitroglycerin for several reasons. First, the patient has told you that he had chest pain earlier today. Thus, it is possible that this patient's heart failure exacerbation is due to ischemic disease. Nitroglycerin will help this via vasodilation. The second reason is that the goal here is to restore normal cardiac function by causing vasodilation and decreasing preload and afterload. Nitroglycerin will do both of these. "A," furosemide, is also a good choice but not the one best choice. By inducing diuresis, furosemide will also significantly decrease preload and provide symptomatic relief. But remember not all heart failure patients are fluid-overloaded (such as with flash edema from ischemia). "B" is incorrect because it will take some time for digoxin to have a significant impact on this patient's symptoms. "C" is incorrect because dobutamine is a second-line drug reserved for those not responding to more conservative therapy for "cardiogenic shock," and it would not be indicated in active ischemia due to increasing myocardial oxygen demand. Norepinephrine would generally be the preferred alternative

if a positive inotrope is needed in cardiogenic shock. "E" is technically not incorrect, but it is not the best answer. There is ample evidence that ACE inhibitors, which work as afterload reducers, can be used in acute HF exacerbations either IV (e.g., enalapril) or sublingual (e.g., captopril). However, these drugs should be reserved as second-line therapy for patients who do not respond to more appropriate initial measures, and they would not be the first-line to address ischemia among choices listed.

You treat the patient with nitroglycerin, he improves, and you admit him to the floor. While in the hospital, the patient develops some additional chest pain that lasts for 10 minutes and responds to additional sublingual nitroglycerin. His BNP is noted to be elevated. His hemoglobin (Hb) is 7.2 g/dL and hematocrit (HCT) is 22%. He is still in congestive failure. The pathologist tells you that there is blood available in the blood bank to transfuse this gentleman if you so choose. There is a problem, of course: he is in heart failure, appearing fluid-overloaded, and now is somewhat tachycardic at 110 bpm.

Question 2.7.12 You tell the pathologist that:
A) Hb of 7.2 g/dL is not an indication for transfusion
B) Transfusing this gentleman is inappropriate since he is already in heart failure and may become more fluid-overloaded with a blood transfusion
C) You would like to go ahead with transfusing this patient
D) Making this patient's blood more viscous with a transfusion will increase the stress on his heart
E) Erythropoiesis-stimulating agents (ESAs), such as darbepoetin (Aranesp®) and erythropoietin, are safer and more effective than blood transfusions for patients with HF

Answer 2.7.12 **The correct answer is "C."** This patient should be transfused. Guidelines suggest triggering transfusion in heart disease when the Hb is <8 to 10g/dL and if the patient is symptomatic (i.e., tachycardic, chest pain). There is no benefit to transfusing patient with a higher Hb (*Ann Intern Med.* 2013;159:770). Use clinical judgment, of course, as there are no guidelines for transfusion in an individual with ACS. ESAs ("E") seems to increase thromboembolic events without providing any benefit in those with stable HF and mild-to-moderate anemia. They should generally be avoided in this population.

Regarding non-STEMI, there are no official ACC/AHA recommendations regarding transfusion. However, the mortality at 30 days is increased if the Hb is <11 mg/dL in a patient with a non-STEMI. Whether or not transfusion will help this is not known: it may just be that patients with anemia are sicker at baseline. Patients with an HCT of <20% to 24% likely benefit from a transfusion while those with an HCT >27% to 30% do not. For 25% to 26% use your judgment. HF is different. Blood transfusion should be reserved for patients with heart failure that are severely anemic and the transfusion be undertaken **slowly** and with the concurrent use of diuretics to avoid volume overload (*Am Heart J.* 2009;158:653–658). "A" and "B" are incorrect because this patient should be transfused carefully as noted above. "D" is incorrect since transfusing this patient to a normal Hb and HCT will not cause excess blood viscosity.

HELPFUL TIP:
Nesiritide (Natrecor), a BNP analog, can be used for HFrEF but is expensive, contributes to renal failure, and likely increases mortality. Nesiritide can produce prolonged hypotension, which limits the dose that can be used. This is a therapy of last resort … and that may be too charitable. Just don't use it.

▶ **Objectives: Did you learn to …**
- Recognize atypical presentations of heart failure with reduced ejection fraction in the elderly?
- Describe the sensitivity and specificity of an ECG for LVH?
- Evaluate a patient with heart failure with reduced ejection fraction?
- Manage a patient with heart failure with reduced ejection fraction and understand the role of beta-blockers, ACE inhibitors, ARBs, digoxin, and spironolactone in the treatment of HFrEF?
- Describe the role of BNP measurement in the evaluation of heart failure with reduced ejection fraction and of nesiritide in the treatment of heart failure?

 QUICK QUIZ: HEART FAILURE CLASSIFICATION

A 72-year-old male with a history of myocardial infarction, PTCA, and stenting is known to have heart failure with an EF of 35% per recent echocardiogram. He presents with shortness of breath with light activities for the last 2 weeks. The appropriate classification of his heart failure by ACC/AHA stage and NYHA class is, respectively:
A) A and II
B) B and II
C) C and II
D) C and IV
E) D and IV

The correct answer is "C." The NYHA classification system has been around for a long time and is based on heart failure symptoms and has some fluidity to it. Patients can move from one class to another and then back again. On the other hand, the ACC/AHA staging system is progressive. We might joke that "everyone has ACC/AHA stage A heart failure," since anyone at risk for heart failure is, by definition, stage A. Both the NHYA and ACC/AHA systems can and should be used together to categorize patients with heart failure. See the following table to review the classes/stages.

NHYA Heart Failure Classification System	ACC/AHA Heart Failure Staging System
I. Cardiac disease but no symptoms and no limitation with ordinary physical activity.	A. Patients at risk for heart failure who have not yet developed structural changes or symptoms (e.g., patients with diabetes, hypertension).
II. Mild symptoms and slight limitation with ordinary activity.	B. Patients with structural heart disease who have not yet developed symptoms.
III. Significant limitation in activity due to symptoms. Comfortable at rest.	C. Patients who have developed clinical heart failure.
IV. Severe limitations. Symptoms even while at rest.	D. Patients with refractory heart failure requiring advanced therapies.

▶ CASE 2.8

Your patient with heart failure does well and is discharged from the hospital after a couple of days. You are just beginning to think that the authors are tired of writing questions about heart failure … but you are wrong. The patient's 70-year-old wife shows up with shortness of breath. Her physical examination is consistent with heart failure. Since you have learned so much from the previous case already, you send her to get an echocardiogram. You also order the recommended tests: CBC, electrolytes, ECG, thyroid functions, etc.

Question 2.8.1 The results of the echocardiogram show a concentric thickening of the left ventricle with an ejection fraction of 75%. This is most consistent with:
A) Ischemic cardiomyopathy
B) HFpEF
C) Viral cardiomyopathy
D) Hypertrophic cardiomyopathy
E) None of the above

Answer 2.8.1 **The correct answer is "B."** "A" is incorrect since there would likely be evidence of RWMA if there had been an old myocardial infarction. Also, this patient has a preserved ejection fraction, which is consistent with HFpEF rather than the decreased ejection fraction associated with ischemic cardiomyopathy. "C" is incorrect. Viral cardiomyopathy is associated with a dilated ventricle rather than a hypertrophic one, and there would be global dyskinesia with decreased ejection fraction. "D" is incorrect; hypertrophic cardiomyopathy is usually associated with asymmetric hypertrophy, often septal, rather than concentric hypertrophy of the left ventricle. Hypertrophic cardiomyopathy *may* lead to HFpEF in addition to left ventricular outflow tract obstruction.

Question 2.8.2 HFpEF is associated with which of the following?
A) A prolonged history of untreated hypertension
B) Poor relaxation of the ventricular wall
C) Thyroid disease
D) A and B
E) B and C

Answer 2.8.2 The correct answer is "D." HFpEF is often associated with long-standing hypertension as well as a stiff ventricular wall that does not relax to allow good filling during diastole (therefore "diastolic dysfunction"). *For these reasons (and others), HFpEF is more common in the elderly.* "C" is not correct because hyper- and hypothyroidism are usually associated with a dilated cardiomyopathy.

Question 2.8.3 HFpEF represents approximately what percentage of HF?
A) <5%
B) Approximately 10%
C) Approximately 25%
D) Approximately 50%
E) >75%

Answer 2.8.3 The correct answer is "D." HFpEF represents between 40% and 60% of cases of HF when looking at the population as a whole. The other answers are incorrect. The point here is that, as discussed earlier, patients with HF need an echocardiogram to determine what type of heart failure they have.

Question 2.8.4 Which of the following drugs is the LEAST desirable in patients with HFpEF?
A) Diuretics
B) ACE inhibitors
C) Nitrates
D) Digoxin
E) Negative inotropes such as beta-blockers and CCBs

Answer 2.8.4 The correct answer is "D." Poor digoxin. It is not good for almost anything. Nesiritide, digoxin, and other positive inotropes (e.g., milrinone) are not very useful in HFpEF. This makes sense. The problem here is not a lack of contractility but alternatively a lack of muscle relaxation. While there has not been a superior therapeutic regimen identified by randomized control trials, the goals of therapy are blood pressure control, the use of diuretics to relieve congestion and edema, treatment of ischemia if present, and control of the heart rate to avoid tachycardia.

Question 2.8.5 Which of the following drugs or drug classes is theoretically the best choice for the treatment of HFpEF?
A) ACE inhibitors
B) Beta-blockers
C) Diuretics
D) Hydralazine
E) ARBs

Answer 2.8.5 The correct answer is "B." Beta-blockers, especially metoprolol succinate, are useful as initial therapy in HFpEF. Beta-blockers (1) slow down the heart to permit longer LV filling duration during diastole and (2) help to relax the myocardium to promote a less restrictive filling pattern. If a patient fails beta-blockers, try a CCB (e.g., verapamil, diltiazem). Unlike HFrEF, the treatments of HFpEF are not well established, and there is no convincing evidence that beta-blockers or ACE inhibitors reduce mortality.

HELPFUL TIP:
Heart failure is a terminal illness with a 5-year survival of only 50%. This is worse than many cancers.

▶ **Objectives: Did you learn to …**
· Understand the pathophysiology of HFpEF?
· Treat a patient with HFpEF?

▶ CASE 2.9

Your "congestive heart failure couple," as they now call themselves, are doing so well that the wife refers her cousin to you (… and we still aren't tired of writing heart failure questions). Her cousin, a 65-year-old male, arrives at your office and you immediately notice the smell of tobacco leaching from his clothing. The small burns in his sleeves confirm to you that he smokes, and he informs you that he has smoked three packs per day "since birth." He recently has noticed some swelling in his feet and increased shortness of breath. He denies a history of cardiac disease. An ECG performed in the office shows right-axis deviation and a right bundle branch block (RBBB). An echocardiogram shows that he has normal left ventricular function, but a hypertrophied right heart with paradoxical bulging of the ventricular septum into the left ventricle was noted.

Question 2.9.1 This clinical picture is most consistent with which of the following?
A) Constrictive pericarditis
B) Chronic mitral valve prolapse
C) Cor pulmonale
D) Old right ventricular infarction with subsequent dysfunction
E) Chiari network

Answer 2.9.1 The correct answer is "C." A typical picture of cor pulmonale is right ventricular hypertrophy (RVH) with paradoxical bulging of the septum into the left ventricle, right-axis deviation on ECG, and partial or complete RBBB. "A" is incorrect. Constrictive pericarditis is associated with pericardial thickening, dilated inferior vena cava or hepatic veins, and abnormal mitral and tricuspid flow. "B" is incorrect because mitral valve prolapse in the absence of severe mitral regurgitation is not likely to be hemodynamically significant. "D" is incorrect because with a right ventricular infarct, you would expect to see a poorly functioning right ventricle. "E" is incorrect because a Chiari network is normal vestigial variant in the right atrium and would not cause RVH.

Question 2.9.2 Cor pulmonale may result from all of these disease processes EXCEPT:
A) Sickle cell anemia
B) Left ventricular failure
C) Pulmonary embolus (PE)
D) Chronic obstructive lung disease
E) Interstitial lung disease

Answer 2.9.2 The correct answer is "B." Cor pulmonale is the term used for right heart failure caused by diseases primarily affecting the lungs and pulmonary vasculature. The chronic pressure overload of the right ventricle as it ejects in to the high resistance pulmonary vasculature results initially in RVH with normal RV systolic function but over time, the RV contractility declines leading to RV dilation and right-sided heart failure with associated significant tricuspid regurgitation and right atrial dilation.

Question 2.9.3 A possible finding on the ECG of this patient would include:
A) P-mitrale (an "m" shaped, notched P wave in lead II)
B) P-pulmonale (an enlarged, peaked, P wave in lead II)
C) Absent P waves
D) Inverted P waves

Answer 2.9.3 The correct answer is "B." Patients with cor pulmonale often have an enlarged and peaked P wave in lead II reflecting right atrial enlargement. "P-mitrale" is found in **left** atrial enlargement and is characterized by a prolonged and/or notched ("m-shaped") p-wave in lead II.

....

Pulmonary function testing and chest radiography support an underlying diagnosis of COPD. You counsel the patient to quit smoking, prescribe pulmonary rehabilitation, and treat him with bronchodilator therapy.

Question 2.9.4 Besides stopping smoking, the best treatment of this patient's cor pulmonale and pulmonary hypertension (PHTN) is:
A) Continuous prostacyclin infusion
B) Continuous, low-flow oxygen
C) Calcium channel blockers (CCBs)
D) Nitroglycerin
E) Antibiotics to reduce pulmonary inflammation secondary to infection

Answer 2.9.4 The correct answer is "B." In this patient who is a smoker *with cor pulmonale,* the best drug is continuous, low-flow oxygen. This will help to reverse the pulmonary vasoconstriction caused by chronic hypoxia. It should go without saying that you must do everything you can to get him to **stop smoking**. His disease process will progress much faster if he continues to smoke. "A" is incorrect because prostacyclin infusion is useful in primary pulmonary hypertension (PHTN), not this type of cor pulmonale. "C" is incorrect. In some cases of **primary** PHTN, CCBs, PDE5 inhibitors (e.g., sildenafil), and several other medications, which serve as direct vasodilators to dilate the pulmonary vascular bed, can be useful. However, this is not the best choice for this patient with COPD. "D" is incorrect because patients with cor pulmonale are dependent on high right heart–filling pressures to get blood through the pulmonary vasculature. Nitroglycerin will reduce preload, thereby lowering right ventricular pressure and resulting in worsening of his symptoms. "E" is also incorrect. Antibiotics might be needed in this patient for pneumonia, bronchiectasis, etc., but they are not going to help with the treatment of cor pulmonale.

HELPFUL TIP:
Remember sleep apnea as a cause of cor pulmonale. Nocturnal oxygen desaturation causes increased pulmonary vascular resistance causing elevated right ventricular pressure and possibly right-sided failure if severe and untreated.

HELPFUL TIP:
In a reversal of fortunes for home oxygen companies and fire fighters everywhere, oxygen for *COPD-related* mild hypoxia (baseline SpO_2 89–93%) or desaturation with walking to SpO_2 <90% for ≥10 seconds, but ≥80% for ≥5 minutes, has not been shown to improve survival or rate of hospitalization (*N Engl J Med.* 2016;375:1617). Note that this study did not include patients with resting saturations below 88%, which is when we usually employ home oxygen. Nor did these subjects have cor pulmonale (for which oxygen is indicated). We don't know what the right answer on the test will be, but keep this in mind.

▶ **Objectives: Did you learn to …**
· Diagnose cor pulmonale?
· Describe causes of cor pulmonale?
· Treat a patient with cor pulmonale?

▶ **CASE 2.10**

A 65-year-old male presents to your clinic for a complete history and physical examination. You notice that his abdominal examination reveals a pulsatile mass, which you suspect may represent an aortic aneurysm (*now we are tired of writing heart failure questions*). This finding is confirmed by ultrasound. The radiologist reports that the patient has a 3.5-cm abdominal aortic aneurysm without evidence of dissection or thrombus formation.

Question 2.10.1 The best advice to this patient is:
A) Have the aortic aneurysm fixed now while he is still healthy
B) Have a follow-up ultrasound every 3 months
C) Have a stent placed to prevent further aortic dilatation
D) Have an angiogram in the next several days to rule out vascular disease below the aorta (femoral arteries, iliac arteries, etc.)
E) Have a repeat ultrasound at 1 year

Answer 2.10.1 The correct answer is "E." Patients with an abdominal aortic aneurysm less than 4 cm in diameter should have an ultrasound yearly to check progression. Those with an aneurysm 4 to 5 cm in diameter should have an ultrasound every 6 months. An ultrasound on an every 3 to 6 months basis is also indicated for aneurysms that are growing >0.5 cm per year. Bottom line: the larger the aneurysm, the more frequently one should do an ultrasound. "A" is incorrect (see next question for an explanation). "C" is incorrect since a stent is not indicated at this point. "D" is incorrect. The only reason to do an angiogram at this point is if the patient is symptomatic or if you are planning surgical intervention.

Question 2.10.2 The patient is really worried that this aneurysm will rupture and kill him. You educate him that the benefit of having the aneurysm repaired is greater than the risk of the surgery when the aneurysm reaches:
A) ≥4.5 cm
B) 5 to 5.5 cm
C) 5.5 to 6 cm
D) >6 cm
E) No repair is indicated until the patient becomes symptomatic

Answer 2.10.2 The correct answer is "B." The risk of the surgery outweighs the benefits until the aneurysm reaches somewhere between 5 and 5.5 cm. The rest are incorrect. It would be an especially bad idea to wait until an aneurysm is symptomatic, as a ruptured aortic aneurysm can be lethal in a matter of minutes.

HELPFUL TIP:
Percutaneous endovascular stent graft repair is becoming the procedure of choice as compared to open repair. But there are tradeoffs: 30 day mortality from an endovascular graft is 1.6% versus 3.2% for open repair, but at 8 years rupture rate was 5.4% versus 1.4%. Overall 8-year mortality is the same (*N Engl J Med.* 2015;373:328).

HELPFUL (-ISH) TIP:
The rate of AAA rupture is higher in women, and there is some debate as to what the threshold should be for elective surgical repair for women. Should it occur when the AAA diameter is 5 cm or less? Maybe. But women also have higher rates of complications post-repair.

The patient goes to Texas (or Arizona or Florida—somewhere warmer than Iowa) for the winter as part of the re-establishment of human annual migration. When he returns, he calls you complaining of back pain that is somewhat sharp and radiating into his legs. You meet him in the ED and suspect that he is having a dissection of his aneurysm.

Question 2.10.3 All of the following are true regarding aortic dissection EXCEPT:
A) A substantial number of patients will have palpable pulses below the level of the dissection
B) Patients may have an elevated LDH and microangiopathic findings on RBC examination
C) Blood pressure should be kept on the high side to ensure perfusion below the area of the aneurysm
D) The pain may migrate down from the chest to the lower abdominal area over time
E) The pain may be episodic

Answer 2.10.3 The correct answer is "C." One does not want to keep the blood pressure on the high side. In fact, reducing the blood pressure is the initial treatment of choice for a dissecting aneurysm. "A," "B," "D," and "E" are all correct statements. Patients may have an elevated LDH and microangiopathic findings on RBC smear as a result of trauma and cell lysis. "D" is a correct statement, but patients often do not have this "classic" migrating pattern of pain. "E" is often true of pain in aortic dissection—it may be episodic.

The patient has a blood pressure of 160/105 mm Hg and a pulse of 115 bpm. Clearly, this is too high in a patient who has an ongoing dissection. You decide to treat this patient before transferring him to a tertiary care center where he can be surgically managed.

Question 2.10.4 The best medication(s) to use in this patient to control his blood pressure is/are:
A) Sublingual nifedipine plus metoprolol
B) Amlodipine
C) Intravenous hydralazine
D) Intravenous esmolol plus nitroprusside
E) Intravenous nitroglycerin

Answer 2.10.4 The correct answer is "D." The goal of therapy here is not only blood pressure reduction but also control of shear forces on the aorta, which requires the prevention of tachycardia. Intravenous beta-blockers such as labetalol, propranolol, metoprolol, or esmolol are the first-line agents. Esmolol is preferred because of the short half-life; you easily can turn it off if there is hypotension. Shoot for a pulse of 60 bpm. Nitroprusside (or our favorite, IV nitroglycerin) can be added if the blood pressure control remains suboptimal even after beta-blockade. In this scenario, nitroprusside should never be given without beta-blockade, as it may cause reflex tachycardia induced by vasodilation and thus further aortic shear stress. The same rationale is true for not using intravenous hydralazine without beta-blockers in this scenario. "A" is incorrect for two very good reasons. First, nifedipine should **never** be used sublingually. Syncope, heart block, MI, stroke, and other serious adverse consequences have been reported. Second, nifedipine increases heart rate causing an increase in shear forces on the aorta. "B" is incorrect since amlodipine does nothing to reduce heart rate, is not titratable to any useful degree, and the onset of action is too slow to be used when prompt blood pressure lowering is desired. "E" is incorrect because nitroglycerin alone causes reflex tachycardia.

HELPFUL TIP:
Screen for an aortic aneurysm **once** in men age 65 to 75 who have ever smoked 100 cigarettes or more (per USPSTF and ACC/AHA guidelines). Also, consider screening those *who have not smoked* age 65 to 75 based on comorbidities (e.g., DM, HTN, family history) and risk, realizing that guidelines in these groups vary considerably, and the best approach is an individualized one.

▶ **Objectives: Did you learn to …**
- Identify the treatment options and timing of treatment of an abdominal aortic aneurysm?
- Manage a patient with a dissecting aneurysm?

▶ CASE 2.11

A 60-year-old male presents with dizziness and palpitations. The patient has a blood pressure of 100/60 mm Hg and a pulse of 160 bpm. His ECG is shown in Figure 2-5.

Question 2.11.1 Which of the following interventions are appropriate options in the treatment of this patient?
A) Amiodarone, lidocaine, defibrillation, metoprolol
B) Amiodarone, lidocaine, defibrillation, diltiazem
C) Amiodarone, lidocaine, cardioversion, diltiazem
D) Procainamide, lidocaine, adenosine, defibrillation
E) Amiodarone, procainamide, lidocaine, cardioversion

Answer 2.11.1 The correct answer is "E." The rhythm is stable ventricular tachycardia. Procainamide, lidocaine, amiodarone, and *synchronized* cardioversion can all be used for ventricular tachycardia. "A" is incorrect for two reasons. The rhythm is ventricular tachycardia and is stable, and neither metoprolol nor defibrillation is appropriate. Defibrillation could be appropriate if the patient was unstable, pulseless (including pulseless ventricular tachycardia), or had ventricular fibrillation. "B" is incorrect because of the inclusion of diltiazem and defibrillation. "C" is incorrect because of the inclusion of diltiazem. "D" is incorrect because adenosine, which is used for atrial arrhythmias, is useless in ventricular arrhythmias and because, again, defibrillation is inappropriate.

HELPFUL TIP:
Procainamide is another option for ventricular tachycardia if you have time to load it.

The patient does not respond to IV amiodarone and you choose to cardiovert him.

Question 2.11.2 Which of the following is the recommended energy (in joules) for an initial attempt at synchronized cardioversion?
A) 200 joules, monophasic
B) 360 joules, monophasic
C) 300 joules, biphasic
D) 360 joules, biphasic
E) None of the above

Answer 2.11.2 The correct answer is "A." For cardioversion of stable ventricular tachycardia, start with 100 to 200 joules for monophasic waveforms and 100 to 200 joules for biphasic waveforms. The rest are incorrect.

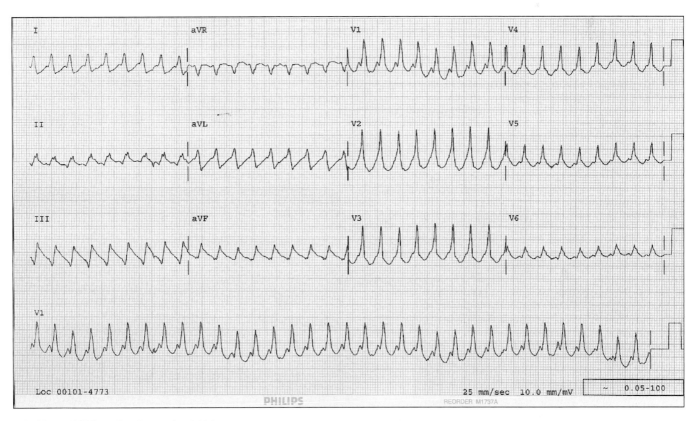

FIGURE 2-5. ECG for patient in question 2.11.1.

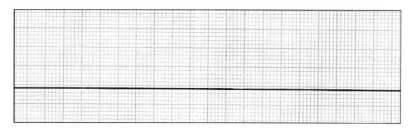

FIGURE 2-6. ECG for patient in question 2.11.3.

HELPFUL TIP:
For **defibrillation**, escalating doses of electricity are out of the new protocols. Start with a single shock at 360 joules with a monophasic defibrillator or 150 to 200 joules if using a biphasic defibrillator, depending on the manufacturer. See Chapter 1 for a "practice code."

HELPFUL (AND VERY IMPORTANT) TIP:
The 2010 and 2015 AHA guidelines for ACLS emphasize the importance of starting with chest compressions (Circulation–Airway–Breathing) and NEVER interrupting chest compressions during resuscitation (really that means minimizing interruptions—they feel that too often chest compressions are halted for less important interventions such as intubation, venous access, etc.).

You cardiovert the patient, and the rhythm in Figure 2-6 is on the monitor. Is it getting hot here, or is it just you?

Question 2.11.3 Of the following, what is the first step you will take (while maintaining good compressions and ventilations, of course)?
A) Re-shock the patient at the same energy level
B) Check another lead to assure the readout is accurate
C) Give epinephrine, 1 mg IV
D) Give atropine, 1 mg IV

Answer 2.11.3 **The correct answer is "B."** This rhythm is asystole. It is important to quickly check another lead and make sure that all of the leads are connected properly. "A" is incorrect because cardioversion/defibrillation is not routinely indicated in the treatment of asystole. "C" and "D" are incorrect because it is important to ensure that the patient actually is in asystole prior to treating with any medications.

HELPFUL TIP:
With regard to ACLS, doing compressions and ventilations are particularly important. There is no need to intubate the patient if he/she can be easily bagged. The correct number of ventilations (10–12/min) and compressions (100 bpm with 2 inches of depth) in a ratio of 15 compressions: 2 breaths for two provider CPR or 30:1 for single provider is important. The Bee-Gees "Staying Alive" has the correct rate for compressions. Queen's "Another One Bites the Dust" also has the correct rate but is considered less decorous in the code situation (of course, you don't have to sing it out loud!).

Question 2.11.4 The new lead placement continues to show asystole. Which of the following drugs and doses are considered appropriate in asystole?
A) Epinephrine 1 mg
B) Atropine 0.5 mg
C) Atropine 1 mg
D) Epinephrine 10 mg
E) A and C

Answer 2.11.4 **The correct answer is "A."** Atropine is no longer in the ACLS guidelines for asystole. Older ACLS recommendations for asystole included both epinephrine and atropine.

▶ **Objectives: Did you learn to …**
- Recognize and manage ventricular tachycardia and asystole?
- Apply the current American Heart Association's ACLS guidelines to a patient in asystole?

▶ **CASE 2.12**

A 75-year-old female presents to your office complaining of episodic palpitations with episodes of lightheadedness that are *not* concurrent with the palpitations. You perform an electrocardiogram in your office, and the rhythm is shown in Figure 2-7.

Question 2.12.1 What rhythm does this represent?
A) First-degree heart block
B) Second-degree heart block type I (Wenckebach)
C) Second-degree heart block type II
D) Third-degree heart block
E) Atrial flutter with variable block

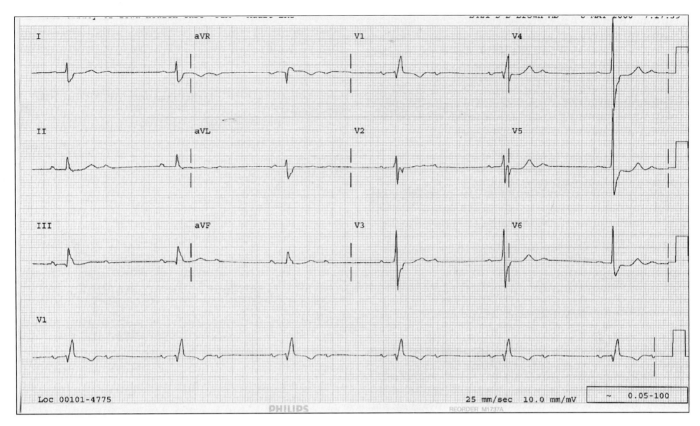

FIGURE 2-7. ECG for patient in question 2.12.1.

Answer 2.12.1 The correct answer is "C." Your patient's ECG shows a second-degree heart block, type II (Mobitz II). This is characterized by a **fixed PR interval** with an intermittently non-conducting *P* wave and resultant dropped beats. "A" is incorrect. First-degree heart block is characterized by a prolonged PR interval without any blocked beats (meaning every QRS is preceded by a *P* wave conducted with a long PR interval). The upper limit of normal of the PR interval is 0.2 seconds (and we admit that this one is darn close, but Mobitz II is the issue here). A second-degree heart block, Mobitz type I (Wenckebach), is defined by a progressively prolonged PR interval ending with a non-conducted *P* wave and a dropped beat. A third-degree heart block is characterized by no consistent pattern between the P waves and the QRS complex. "E" is incorrect because, by definition, atrial flutter is represented by a rapid atrial rate. In this patient, the rate is slow.

....

By the time the patient arrives at the hospital, she is having a rapid, chaotic rhythm, which appears to be atrial fibrillation on the monitor. It seems as though there are also episodes of atrial flutter with 2:1 block.

Question 2.12.2 The most likely diagnosis in this patient with varying rate is:
A) Sick sinus syndrome (bradycardia–tachycardia syndrome)
B) Hypothyroidism
C) Hyperthyroidism
D) Hyperkalemia

Answer 2.12.2 The correct answer is "A." The most likely diagnosis in this patient is "sick sinus syndrome," also known as "tachy–brady" syndrome and "bradycardia–tachycardia" syndrome. This syndrome is most common in elderly individuals and reflects the replacement of the SA node with fibrous tissue. "B" is incorrect because hypothyroidism should cause bradycardia without intermittent tachycardia. "C" is incorrect because hyperthyroidism should cause tachycardia without bradycardia. "D" is incorrect because hyperkalemia generally causes a widened QRS complex on ECG and eventually ventricular tachycardia. Note: With Mobitz type II second degree heart block, the problem is infra-nodal, below the AV node, and can result in complete heart block. Sick sinus syndrome is due to disease of the SA node.

Question 2.12.3 Which of the following is the definitive treatment of sick sinus syndrome?
A) Mexiletine
B) Hydralazine
C) Quinidine
D) Pacemaker
E) Implantable defibrillator

Answer 2.12.3 The correct answer is "D." In general, patients with sick sinus syndrome become symptomatic because of the bradycardia episodes. Thus, pacing is necessary. Note: A pacemaker would also be indicated in patients with Mobitz type II second-degree heart block without tachy–brady syndrome. "A" and "C" are incorrect because these two drugs are aimed primarily at ventricular arrhythmias; sick sinus syndrome is a problem with the SA node. "B" is incorrect because hydralazine is an afterload reducer with no direct effect on cardiac rhythm. "E" is incorrect because patients with sick sinus syndrome do not have ventricular fibrillation or ventricular tachycardia, and thus there is no need for a defibrillator.

 HELPFUL TIP:
In sick sinus syndrome, in addition to the pacemaker, it is often necessary to add a beta-blocker or a CCB (diltiazem or verapamil) to address the tachycardia (e.g., PSVT or atrial fibrillation).

▶ **Objectives: Did you learn to …**
  • Identify and differentiate second-degree heart blocks?
  • Diagnose and treat sick sinus syndrome?

▶ CASE 2.13

A 58-year-old male smoker with a history of type 2 diabetes mellitus presents with complaints of easy fatigability and pain in his thighs when exerting himself. The left leg is worse than the right. The pain resolves after resting and is no worse going downhill than uphill. He works as a carpenter, and the leg pain is now limiting his ability to work. He will not quit smoking ("It's the only thing I truly love, Doc"). The patient states that his symptoms are better when he hangs his leg over the side of the bed at night.

Question 2.13.1 The etiology of this patient's leg pain is most likely:
A) Peripheral venous disease (e.g., venous insufficiency, varicose veins)
B) Spinal stenosis
C) Diabetic neuropathy
D) Peripheral arterial disease (e.g., arterial stenosis)
E) None of the above

Answer 2.13.1 The correct answer is "D." Intermittent claudication is the classic presenting symptom of peripheral arterial disease. When rest pain is present, relief of symptoms occurs by making the affected area dependent (e.g., hanging the legs over the side of the bed), letting gravity help increase blood flow. The pain associated with diabetic neuropathy begins distally, has a burning quality, and is not typically relieved with rest. In fact, patients often notice it more at rest (e.g., during the night). Patients with peripheral venous disease will often have worsening of their symptoms when their legs are in a dependent position. Spinal stenosis is often made worse by walking downhill and better when walking uphill or leaning forward (a kyphotic/forward flexed position opens up the foramen, thereby decreasing nerve root compression).

His examination shows decreased pulses in the lower extremities bilaterally. You would like to confirm your suspicion that this patient has peripheral vascular disease.

Question 2.13.2 What is the first study you would order in this patient?
A) Spiral CT to confirm vascular calcification
B) Ankle-brachial index (ABI)
C) Color Doppler to assess flow
D) Catheterbased arteriography
E) None of the above.

Answer 2.13.2 The correct answer is "B." The ABI is sensitive and specific for peripheral arterial disease in the lower extremity. The pressure in the ankle should be higher than that in the brachial artery in a healthy person. The highest sensitivity is achieved by measuring pressures in both brachial arteries, both dorsalis pedis, and both posterior tibial arteries. Neither spiral CT or color Doppler are recommended as the initial screening test for the presence of peripheral vascular disease (although CT angiogram may be useful in the future to define the degree and location of narrowing in preparation for bypass or angioplasty). Catheter-based arteriography is an option but should be reserved for patients with known peripheral artery disease in whom intervention is being considered.

The ABI results are normal. However, you strongly suspect claudication.

Question 2.13.3 The next step should be:
A) Catheter-based arteriography
B) Repeat ABI after an exercise stress test
C) Magnetic resonance arteriography
D) CT arteriography
E) None of the above

Answer 2.13.3 The correct answer is "B." In patients in whom you strongly suspect peripheral vascular disease, ABIs after exercise can be positive when a resting test is negative. This would be the least invasive and most cost-effective test of the options given.

The post-exercise ankle-brachial indices are as follows: 0.9 in the right leg, 0.4 in the left leg.

Question 2.13.4 The proper interpretation of this information is:
A) 95% probability of some degree of occlusive disease in the right leg, severe occlusive disease in the left
B) No occlusive disease in the right leg, mild disease in the left
C) Moderate occlusive disease on both legs
D) No occlusive disease in either leg

Answer 2.13.4 The correct answer is "A." A normal ABI should be 0.95 to 1.29. An ABI of 0.9 is 95% sensitive for finding **some** degree of occlusive disease on arteriography (although it may not be hemodynamically significant). An ABI of 0.81 to 0.94 represents mild arterial disease that may or may not be associated with claudication. An ABI of 0.41 to 0.80 is classified as moderate arterial disease and is usually associated with some degree of claudication. An ABI of ≤0.4 represents severe disease and may be associated with rest pain. Paradoxically, an ABI > 1.30 represents noncompressible arteries and may be a marker for arterial calcification. In these cases, a toe-brachial index should be measured (really). (Don't ask us ... we don't know where to find a toe BP cuff either. Maybe you can use a full-sized gnome or pixie cuff. We'd love to sell you one.)

You decide to start the patient on a medication to help control his claudication.

Question 2.13.5 Which of the following statements is correct?
A) Pentoxifylline is relatively contraindicated in heart failure
B) Cilostazol is the best choice for claudication in patients with heart failure
C) Beta-blockers are good arterial dilators and are thus useful in claudication
D) The main mechanism of action of pentoxifylline and cilostazol is selective vasodilation
E) Tobacco smoking paradoxically alleviates claudication

Answer 2.13.5 The correct answer is "A." Cilostazol (Pletal®) and pentoxifylline (Trental®) are phosphodiesterase inhibitors. Their mechanism of action in improving walking distance is poorly understood. Other phosphodiesterase inhibitors (such as milrinone) increase mortality in patients with heart failure. Thus, pentoxifylline and cilostazol ("B") should be used with *extreme caution*, if at all, in patients with heart failure. Selective beta-blockers actually cause peripheral arterial constriction, not arterial dilation; therefore, "C" is also incorrect. The purported benefit of pentoxifylline is to increase RBC malleability and thus reduce the viscosity of blood in the microcirculation. It has no vasodilative effects. However, cilostazol does have some vasodilative effects. Therapeutic benefit with these drugs may take several weeks. A dedicated and supervised walking program is of paramount importance and underutilized. Given the strong association between smoking and peripheral artery disease, smokers should be encouraged to quit, so "E" is incorrect. Statins should also be initiated and have been shown to have benefit (*Cochrane Database Syst Rev.* 2007 Oct 17;(4):CD000123). Therapy of PAD should include antiplatelet therapy and cardiovascular risk factor modification.

HELPFUL TIP:
Remember that peripheral artery disease is considered a CAD equivalent with the same 10-year attendant cardiac risk even in the absence of CAD.

Question 2.13.6 In and of themselves, indications for further intervention for peripheral artery disease (e.g., bypass, stenting) include all of the following EXCEPT:
A) Rest pain
B) Persistent pain that interferes with day-to-day functioning
C) Tissue loss
D) 80% occlusion of the femoral artery

Answer 2.13.6 The correct answer is "D." Classic indications for invasive treatment of lower extremity PAD are (1) salvage of a threatened limb (rest pain, nonhealing ulceration, or gangrene) and (2) improvement in functional capacity. An 80% occlusion of the femoral artery, in and of itself, is not an indication for percutaneous or surgical revascularization in a patient who is asymptomatic. Endovascular therapy is generally preferred. Note that claudication is a marker for a high risk of mortality (up to 31% over 10 years). There is also an increased risk of limb loss.

The patient sees the light, but does not go into it, and quits smoking. The case ends happily ...

HELPFUL TIP:
No anticoagulation regimen seems to prevent re-occlusion of lower extremity arteries after stenting. Patients should, however, continue on their current antithrombotic regimen as indicated for cardiovascular disease (ASA, warfarin, DOACs, etc.).

▶ **Objectives: Did you learn to ...**
• Recognize symptoms and signs of peripheral vascular disease?
• Order appropriate diagnostic tests for a patient suspected of having peripheral vascular disease?
• Develop an understanding of the agents used to treat peripheral vascular disease?

▶ **CASE 2.14**

A 75-year-old male presents to your office for a complete physical examination before prostate surgery. On examination, you notice a 3/6 harsh, mid-systolic ejection murmur heard best at the upper right sternal border and radiating to the neck. S1 and S2 are normal. An echocardiogram demonstrates mild aortic stenosis. Currently he is asymptomatic.

Question 2.14.1 The indications for valve replacement surgery include:
A) Grade 4/6 murmur
B) Requirement for major, semi-elective surgery such as prostatectomy
C) Severe aortic stenosis without symptoms and normal LV function
D) Severe aortic stenosis in a patient undergoing coronary bypass grafting
E) All of the above

Answer 2.14.1 The correct answer is "D." As a general rule, aortic stenosis is repaired when it becomes symptomatic. Repair of *asymptomatic*, severe aortic stenosis is indicated in the following scenarios: undergoing CABG or other valve or aorta surgery, LVEF < 50%, hypotension in response to exercise, or high likelihood of rapid progression. "A" is incorrect because the loudness of the murmur does not always correlate with its functional significance. "B" is incorrect as well. As long as the lesion is not hemodynamically significant, the patient should tolerate prostate surgery. "C" is incorrect because surgery is not usually necessary even in severe valvular disease **without** symptoms as long as the left ventricular function is normal. Note that it is not uncommon that patients with severe aortic stenosis report that they are asymptomatic, but they have modified their activity to avoid symptoms which may have occurred gradually so that they don't recognize the decline.

> **HELPFUL TIP:**
> There is a move afoot to repair aortic stenosis before it becomes symptomatic. This is because the LV starts to fibrose prior to onset of symptoms, and the fibrosis is associated with worse long-term outcomes. This is not the standard yet, however (*Circulation* 2018;138:1935).

Question 2.14.2 The patient would like to know how often he should have a repeat echocardiogram given that he has mild disease. Your answer is:
A) Every 3 to 5 years
B) Every year
C) Every 6 months
D) When he develops symptoms
E) None of the above

Answer 2.14.2 The correct answer is "A." Patients with mild aortic stenosis who are asymptomatic can be followed by echocardiogram every 3 to 5 years. Patients with severe disease should have yearly echocardiography to evaluate for left ventricular dysfunction. See Table 2-7.

TABLE 2-7 RECOMMENDED INTERVALS FOR ECHOCARDIOGRAPHIC EVALUATION FOR VALVULAR DISEASE[a]

Lesion	Mild Disease	Moderate Disease	Severe Disease
Aortic stenosis	Every 3–5 years	Every 2 years	Every 6–12 months
Mitral stenosis	Every 3–5 years	Every 1–2 years	Every 1–2 years
Aortic regurgitation	Every 3–5 years	Every 1–2 years	Every 6–12 months
Mitral regurgitation	Every 3–5 years	Every 1–2 years	Every 6–12 months

[a]Recommendations vary.

Two years later, the patient returns for a checkup and states that he believes he has been having symptoms from his aortic stenosis.

Question 2.14.3 All of the following can occur with symptomatic aortic stenosis EXCEPT:
A) Left-to-right intracardiac shunt
B) Exertional dyspnea
C) Syncope
D) Angina
E) Lightheadedness

Answer 2.14.3 The correct answer is "A." Intracardiac shunts don't occur with aortic stenosis. If you got this one wrong, back to anatomy for you! An isolated, fixed valvular lesion as an adult cannot cause intracardiac shunting. Exertional dyspnea, lightheadedness (presyncope), syncope, and chest pain are common symptoms in severe aortic stenosis.

Question 2.14.4 Which of the following statements about aortic valve disease is INCORRECT?
A) Aortic stenosis can be treated quite effectively with balloon valvulotomy with good long-term outcomes
B) There are no known medical treatments that reduce the need for aortic valve replacement
C) Risk factors for the development of aortic stenosis are similar to CAD
D) Valve replacement surgery is the preferred treatment of symptomatic aortic stenosis

Answer 2.14.4 The correct answer is "A." Valvulotomy (balloon aortic valvuloplasty) is not a long-term solution for the management of severe symptomatic aortic stenosis. While it may be indicated as a "bridge" to definitive treatment (surgery or transcatheter aortic valve replacement [TAVR]), durability of the valvulotomy results are poor, only lasting 3 to 6 months. The procedure carries the attendant risk of cerebral embolism causing stroke, aortic rupture, or acute severe aortic insufficiency. The epidemiological risk factors for aortic stenosis and CAD are similar (as is the pathophysiology). Unfortunately, there are no drugs that are effective at reducing the need for valve replacement. You can provide symptomatic relief but that is all.

▶ **Objectives: Did you learn to …**
- Recognize symptoms of aortic stenosis?
- Manage a patient with aortic stenosis?
- Evaluate aortic valve disease and determine long-term follow-up vis-à-vis periodic echocardiograms?

▶ **CASE 2.15**

A 35-year-old male presents to the office with upper respiratory symptoms. He is taking no medications except for a bit of pseudoephedrine for his cold. You notice when looking at his vital signs that his blood pressure is 180/106 mm Hg. Repeat measurement confirms that the blood pressure is elevated at 175/105 mm Hg.

Question 2.15.1 What is your initial approach to this patient?

A) Start a chronic antihypertensive since he is at risk for a stroke within the next couple of days with a blood pressure at this level

B) Administer clonidine in the office to reduce the blood pressure to a safe level of about 150/100 mm Hg

C) Watch the patient over the next 2 weeks and get additional blood pressure readings before deciding what to do and instruct him to discontinue pseudoephedrine

D) Schedule the patient for outpatient labs and electro-cardiogram

E) Fire the patient from your practice. He's messing up your quality measures

Answer 2.15.1 The correct answer is "C." The diagnosis of hypertension requires two elevated blood pressures on two different occasions. This patient's elevated blood pressure could be situational, related to decongestants and current illness (though decongestants only increase systolic blood pressure by 2–3 mm Hg if at all). Neither "A" nor "B" is correct because a blood pressure of 175/105 mm Hg does not pose a risk of acute stroke, and the pressure need not be lowered acutely *unless there is evidence of end-organ injury* (e.g., angina, heart failure, hypertensive encephalopathy). "D" is incorrect because you cannot definitively establish that this patient has hypertension based on only one in office blood pressure measurement. As for "E"…really? Is this why we went into medicine?

....

The patient returns to your office with blood pressures measured six times over a period of 2 weeks at a local pharmacy. Only three of the six readings suggest that the patient is hypertensive. The patient states that the elevated blood pressures were while he was under stress at work.

Question 2.15.2 Your best response at this point is to:

A) Start an antihypertensive

B) Send the patient for a 24-hour ambulatory blood pressure measurement

C) Don't worry about the blood pressure since half of the readings were within a normal range

D) Get a nephrology consult to help in decision making

E) Make another office visit so you can buy that Porsche

Answer 2.15.2 The correct answer is "B." One way to determine if a patient with contradictory readings is hypertensive is to perform 24-hour ambulatory blood pressure monitoring. This can be useful in patients who have elevated blood pressures in the office but not at home or vice versa. It can also be used if you do not trust the blood pressure readings taken outside of your office. "A" is incorrect since we have not yet established that this patient is hypertensive. "C" is incorrect since we have not yet established that this patient is not hypertensive. "D" is incorrect because you are smarter than that and should be able to work through this kind of case yourself! As to "E," whoops, we forgot. We're family physicians, not radiologists. No Porsche for us!

Question 2.15.3 The following are all well-accepted indications for 24-hour ambulatory blood pressure monitoring EXCEPT:

A) Suspected white coat hypertension

B) Patients with difficult-to-control hypertension

C) Patients having hypotensive symptoms on their antihypertensive treatment

D) Follow-up after initiating antihypertensive treatment

E) Evaluation of patient for autonomic dysfunction

Answer 2.15.3 The correct answer is "D." One need not do 24-hour ambulatory blood pressure monitoring to document response to antihypertensive therapy in patients in whom most or all measurements post-treatment are normal. All of the other answer choices are considered reasonable indications for 24-hour ambulatory blood pressure monitoring.

....

Elevated blood pressure in response to stress (especially in the doctor's office) is called "white coat hypertension."

Question 2.15.4 Which of the following statements is true about white coat hypertension?

A) As long as the majority of blood pressure readings are normal, the patient does not require treatment because there is no increased risk of adverse cardiac outcomes

B) Patients with white coat hypertension have an intermediate risk for adverse outcomes when compared with patients with normal blood pressure and those with chronically elevated blood pressure

C) White coat hypertension is more common in young patients

D) Patients with white coat hypertension have an elevated left ventricular mass when compared to patients with normal blood pressures

E) B and D

Answer 2.15.4 The correct answer is "E." Patients with white coat hypertension have outcomes that are intermediate between normotensive and hypertensive patients. In addition, they have an elevated left ventricular mass. Surprisingly, white coat hypertension is more common in the elderly.

Question 2.15.5 Hypertension is defined as an ambulatory 24-hour monitor *average* blood pressure of:

A) 135/85 mm Hg during the day and 125/75 mm Hg at night

B) 140/90 mm Hg during the day and 130/85 mm Hg at night

C) 130/85 mm Hg over 24 hours

D) 140/90 mm Hg over 24 hours

Answer 2.15.5 The correct answer is "A." Hypertension is diagnosed via ambulatory monitoring when patients have an average blood pressure of >135/85 mm Hg during the day and >125/75 mm Hg at night, as defined by JNC 8. Another published criterion is a blood pressure of >140/90 mm Hg more than 40% of the time. The ACC/AHA would like to make things more difficult. Their criteria are 24-hour mean of 125/75 mm Hg, daytime average of >/=130/80 mm Hg or nighttime average of >/= 110/65 mm Hg.

The ambulatory blood pressure monitor reveals that the patient's blood pressure is >140/90 mm Hg more than 40% of the time, indicating that he is indeed hypertensive.

Question 2.15.6 The initial evaluation of the hypertension includes the following:
A) History, physical, CBC, urinalysis, glucose, BUN, creatinine, electrolytes, ECG, and lipids
B) History, physical, CBC, uric acid, glucose, BUN, creatinine, electrolytes, and lipids
C) History, physical, CBC, urinalysis, glucose, BUN, creatinine, electrolytes, ECG, lipids, and echocardiography
D) History, physical, and labs only as indicated by history and physical

Answer 2.15.6 **The correct answer is "A."** History, physical, CBC, urinalysis, glucose, BUN, creatinine, electrolytes, ECG, and lipids are the generally agreed-upon initial workup of the hypertensive patient. "C" includes echocardiography, which is not recommended as part of the routine evaluation but may be indicated if signs of cardiac disease are present.

The patient's ECG comes back showing evidence of LVH.

Question 2.15.7 This finding suggests that:
A) You should initiate this patient's therapy with an ACE inhibitor since ACE inhibitors prevent disadvantageous cardiac remodeling
B) The patient has heart failure
C) You should recommend an echocardiogram for this patient
D) You should order a BNP level to screen for LVH and early heart failure

Answer 2.15.7 **The correct answer is "C."** The sensitivity of ECG for LVH is only in the 30% to 60% range with a specificity of 80%. Thus, a "positive" ECG is not a strong enough indication to initiate therapy for LVH. For this reason, an echocardiogram should be done to confirm the diagnosis of LVH. "A" is incorrect since an ACE inhibitor is not necessarily the first drug one would start. In addition, we really don't know if this patient has LVH yet, though ACE inhibitors do prevent harmful cardiac remodeling. "B" is incorrect. Certainly, long-standing hypertension and significant LVH can cause heart failure. However, we cannot conclude that this patient has heart failure on the basis of an ECG, especially in the absence of symptoms. "D" is incorrect since the sensitivity of the BNP as a screening tool in an asymptomatic population is poor.

The echocardiogram is normal. You have decided to start this patient on treatment for his hypertension.

Question 2.15.8 Based on outcome data, which of the following is the LEAST effective drug to start on this patient?
A) An Angiotensin Converting Enzyme inhibitor (ACEI), such as lisinopril
B) An Angiotensin Receptor Blocker (ARB), such as losartan

C) An alpha-blocker, such as doxazosin
D) A thiazide diuretic, such as chlorthalidone
E) A Calcium Channel Blocker (CCB), such as amlodipine

Answer 2.15.8 **The correct answer is "C."** Alpha-blockers have worse outcomes in hypertension when compared to other antihypertensives. The JNC 8 recommendations suggest that the first-line agent, in the general non-Black population including those with diabetes, could appropriately be a thiazide-type diuretic, CCB, ACEI, or ARB. Notice that beta-blockers do not make the list of first-line antihypertensives. For the Black population (in general), including those with diabetes, the initial antihypertensive treatment should include a thiazide-type diuretic or a CCB.

Question 2.15.9 Time to digress a bit. Which of the following drugs is the _best_ choice as your initial agent for the treatment of hypertension in a patient with diabetes and known microalbuminuria?
A) Lisinopril
B) Metoprolol
C) Losartan
D) Verapamil
E) Amlodipine

Answer 2.15.9 **The correct answer is "A."** In a diabetic patient who has proteinuria, an ACE inhibitor is indicated to slow down the progression of renal disease. An ARB or non-dihydropyridine CCB (verapamil, diltiazem) is a viable alternative for those who cannot tolerate an ACE inhibitor. (Note: Some patients may not tolerate verapamil or diltiazem due to bradycardia or may not be candidates due to LV _systolic_ dysfunction). However, ACE inhibitors are still first-line. These recommendations stem from the renal and cardiac benefits of ACE inhibitors.

HELPFUL TIP:
Although thiazide diuretics decrease the left ventricular diameter (due to diuresis), beta-blockers, CCBs, and ACE inhibitors **all** reverse LVH.

HELPFUL TIP:
Experts (and the literature) go back and forth between choosing the old standby, hydrochlorothiazide (HCTZ), and the even older drug, chlorthalidone. Hypokalemia is more frequently seen with chlorthalidone than with HCTZ. Potassium should be monitored periodically with diuretics anyway, and hypokalemia often complicates hypertension.

Question 2.15.10 Digressing a bit further ... Which of the following drugs might you want to use as your initial agent for the treatment of hypertension in a 72-year-old male who you also diagnosed with symptomatic benign prostatic hypertrophy (BPH)?
A) Amlodipine

B) Doxazosin
C) Captopril
D) Losartan
E) Verapamil

Answer 2.15.10 The correct answer is "B." Doxazosin is an alpha-blocker that is useful in the treatment of symptomatic BPH. None of the other choices can be used for this indication. Of course, alpha-blockers are also antihypertensives, and thus serve a useful purpose by killing two birds with one stone (Why would you want to kill two birds? And why with stones? Isn't there a better way?). As noted above, alpha-blockers do not confer as much benefit for the hypertensive patient as other classes of drugs. Thus, alpha-blockers are not the best choice in general but could be used as the initial agent if you have a compelling reason.

The point of these digressions is that you should look at the patient's other underlying conditions when deciding what to recommend at initial therapy. Another example would be a patient with CAD and angina starting on a beta-blocker as initial treatment rather than a thiazide (since the beta-blocker may improve angina symptoms and is indicated for CAD). Recall that not all beta-blockers are created equal. Atenolol is least preferred and metoprolol succinate is among the best. If the patient has renal disease, consider an ACE inhibitor or ARB as first-line treatment for hypertension.

· ·

Remember the 35-year-old guy? You start him on chlorthalidone, but his blood pressure does not respond at a dose of 12.5 mg/day (have your patients cut the 25-mg tabs in half). His blood pressure on follow-up is 148/96 mm Hg.

Question 2.15.11 The best approach for such a patient is to:
A) Push his chlorthalidone to 25 mg daily before starting another medication
B) Stop the chlorthalidone and start another medication
C) Rely on exercise and diet to normalize the blood pressure
D) Start a second drug **before** you have maximized the dose of the first drug
E) Start a workup for secondary causes of hypertension
F) A or D

Answer 2.15.11 The correct answer is "F." Per the JNC 8 guidelines, both "A" and "D" are acceptable strategies; you could push up the dose of a first drug or add a second drug. There is a lack of randomized controlled trials to guide these recommendations. JNC 8 urges us to tailor therapy based on individual circumstances, clinician and patient preference, and drug tolerability. Low-dose chlorthalidone (12.5 mg) provides the greatest blood pressure reduction per mg of drug, and there is little clinical benefit of utilizing >25 mg daily of HCTZ or chlorthalidone. Higher doses are associated with increased adverse effects with minimal clinical gain in hypertension management. "B" is incorrect because a patient with this level of blood pressure elevation will generally require more than one drug to achieve a normalized blood pressure. "C" is

incorrect because the majority of patients are unable to maintain an adequate diet or exercise regimen to effectively treat blood pressure. Exercise and dietary change are certainly laudable goals and should be encouraged in all patients. However, they are not likely to normalize blood pressure in most hypertensive patients. "D" is also correct as it represents one of the acceptable JNC 8 guideline strategies to dose antihypertensive drugs. "E" is incorrect since this patient has not yet proven to be resistant to treatment.

> **HELPFUL TIP:**
> Another strategy for the *initial* treatment of hypertension, depending on the patient's blood pressure, is to start therapy with two drugs at submaximal doses (e.g., lisinopril 10 mg and HCTZ 12.5 mg), recognizing that most patients will eventually need two drugs.

· ·

You decide to start this patient on diltiazem as a second agent.

Question 2.15.12 Which of the following side effects is most characteristic of diltiazem and other CCBs?
A) Dehydration
B) Cough
C) Dependent edema
D) Hypokalemia
E) Elevated cholesterol

Answer 2.15.12 The correct answer is "C." As a class, CCBs tend to cause peripheral edema. Dehydration and hypokalemia can be caused by diuretics. Cough and hyperkalemia are characteristic of ACE inhibitors and ARBs (though cough is less common with ARBs). Diuretics can increase cholesterol, while beta-blockers can increase triglycerides.

· ·

Despite the fact that the patient is on two medications, he remains hypertensive. In fact, the blood pressure has barely moved. With your thorough history taking, you have ruled out excess alcohol intake (often an "occult" cause of hypertension). The patient is compliant with his medications.

Question 2.15.13 Further investigations that might be helpful in determining the cause of hypertension in this patient include all of the following EXCEPT:
A) Checking the potassium level *while the patient is taking his current medications* to rule out hyperaldosteronism
B) Assessing for renal artery stenosis (RAS)
C) Checking a 24-hour urine for glucocorticoids
D) Checking a 24-hour urine for catecholamines
E) Screening for obstructive sleep apnea

Answer 2.15.13 The correct answer is "A." Hypertension is secondary to another cause in about 1% of patients with mild hypertension but in 10% to 45% of those with severe, difficult to control hypertension. Secondary causes of hypertension include hyperaldosteronism, RAS, pheochromocytoma, Cushing disease, untreated obstructive sleep apnea, primary hyperparathyroidism, medications (e.g., oral contraceptives), and others. "A" is the thing to avoid because when checking the serum potassium level for hyperaldosteronism, the patient must be off all diuretic medications and have an unrestricted salt intake. All of the other choices *can* be a part of a workup for secondary hypertension caused by RAS ("B"), Cushing disease ("C"), and pheochromocytoma ("D"), respectively (see Table 2-8).

Question 2.15.14 **You decide to check this patient for RAS. The best choice for a screening test for RAS is:**
A) Doppler ultrasound
B) Captopril renal scan
C) Serum renin level
D) MR or CT angiography
E) Both A and D

Answer 2.15.14 **The correct answer is "E."** Per the ACC/AHA guideline for diagnosing RAS, duplex ultrasonography, CTA in patients with normal renal function, and MRA are the recommended screening tools for diagnosis of RAS (Class I Level of Evidence B). The captopril renal scintigraphy ("B"), selective renal vein renin measurements ("C"), plasma renin activity, and the captopril test (which includes measurement of plasma renin levels at baseline and after captopril administration) are considered Class III for screening tests for establishing the diagnosis of RAS.

HELPFUL TIP:
Consider an evaluation for RAS in a patient who has a "positive" clinical (inadvertent) "captopril challenge." If you start an ACE inhibitor and see a dramatic decline in renal function in a few days, RAS, especially bilateral RAS, may be the culprit.

Your patient does not have any identifiable cause for secondary hypertension. You add a third agent, and his blood pressure comes under control. Sometimes, you just have to be persistent!

TABLE 2-8 CAUSES OF SECONDARY HYPERTENSION

Drugs, including over-the-counter medications
Sleep apnea
Endocrine:
● Hyperaldosteronism
● Pheochromocytoma
● Thyroid disease
● Cushing syndrome (innate or iatrogenic)

Vascular:
● Renal artery stenosis
● Coarctation of the aorta
● Intrinsic renal disease

HELPFUL TIP:
Adding spironolactone to the regimen of a patient with difficult to control blood pressure can often be helpful even in the presence of another diuretic. It should be a part of any antihypertensive regimen which includes 4 drugs. The 4 drugs should include a diuretic, an ACE or an ARB, a CCB, and spironolactone. Watch for hyperkalemia when spironolactone is used with ACE inhibitors. Eplerenone is an acceptable alternative but is more expensive.

▶ **Objectives: Did you learn to …**
• Evaluate a patient with initial high blood pressure readings?
• Select initial antihypertensive therapy?
• Appropriately tailor the treatment of hypertension, based on patient-specific characteristics?
• Use and interpret 24-hour ambulatory blood pressure monitoring?
• Understand the concept of white coat hypertension?
• Generate a differential diagnosis and an appropriate evaluation of secondary hypertension?

▶ CASE 2.16

You have a patient who is mildly hypertensive and decide to check baseline labs. On no medications whatsoever, the patient's potassium is low at 3 mEq/L. You re-check the potassium before getting too excited. It is 2.9 mEq/L.

Question 2.16.1 **Of the following, the MOST LIKELY cause of low potassium in this hypertensive patient is:**
A) Hyperaldosteronism
B) Hypoaldosteronism
C) Spuriously low potassium because of an elevated glucose
D) Metabolic acidosis

Answer 2.16.1 **The correct answer is "A."** Hyperaldosteronism can cause **hypo**kalemia and hypertension. Aldosterone increases the secretion of potassium, which leads to hypokalemia. "B" is incorrect because **hypo**aldosteronism, such as that seen with adrenal failure secondary to adrenal destruction, causes **hyper**kalemia and **hypo**tension. "C" is incorrect because elevated glucose does not result in a spuriously low potassium; if you answered "C," maybe you were thinking of sodium (the sodium goes down by approximately 1.6 to 2 mEq/L for every 100 mg/dL increase in the glucose). Finally, "D" is incorrect because a metabolic acidosis should cause an elevated potassium rather than a low one.

HELPFUL TIP:
The serum potassium goes up by *approximately* 1 mEq/L for every 0.1 decrease in the pH from 7.4. Thus, the potassium would go from 4 to 6 mEq/L if the pH changes from 7.4 to 7.2.

You suspect that the patient has hyperaldosteronism.

Question 2.16.2 Which of the following is true?
A) Many patients with hyperaldosteronism have normal serum potassium
B) In hyperaldosteronism, the plasma aldosterone-to-renin ratio is usually high
C) All antihypertensives should be stopped before checking a plasma renin level
D) If a confirmatory 24-hour urine is done, the urine potassium should be low to confirm the diagnosis of hyperaldosteronism
E) A and B

Answer 2.16.2 The correct answer is "E." Many patients with hyperaldosteronism will have normal serum potassium levels. In addition, the plasma aldosterone-to-renin level is usually high. "C" is incorrect because, although ACE inhibitors and spironolactone (and perhaps all diuretics) should be stopped before renin and aldosterone levels are drawn, other antihypertensives (e.g., CCBs) will have little effect on plasma renin levels. "D" is incorrect because hyperaldosteronism causes potassium wasting, so the urine potassium should be elevated.

You diagnose this patient with hyperaldosteronism.

Question 2.16.3 The most common cause of hyperaldosteronism is:
A) Adrenal adenoma
B) Idiopathic
C) Pituitary adenoma
D) Aldosterone-secreting tumor such as small-cell carcinoma
E) Renal artery stenosis

Answer 2.16.3 The correct answer is "A." Adrenal adenomas are the most common cause of hyperaldosteronism. The second leading cause is idiopathic ("B").

Question 2.16.4 Accepted approaches to the treatment of hypertension caused by hyperaldosteronism include all of the following EXCEPT:
A) Unilateral adrenalectomy in the case of adrenal adenoma
B) Liberalized sodium intake
C) Use of a potassium-sparing diuretic
D) Use of a combination of amiloride and HCTZ

Answer 2.16.4 The correct answer is "B." Liberalizing sodium intake will actually cause volume expansion, which is counterproductive and can lead to further hypokalemia. Once the patient is hypervolemic, there will be a spontaneous diuresis (the so-called "aldosterone escape") leading to increased hypokalemia. The exact mechanism of aldosterone escape is not known, but it occurs after a weight gain of approximately 3 kg from fluid retention. If you want to seem smart, just say it is "neurohumeral." You will probably be right and it makes you sound cool.

▶ **Objectives: Did you learn to …**
· Identify laboratory abnormalities that occur in hyperaldosteronism?
· Evaluate a patient suspected of having hyperaldosteronism?
· Initiate treatment of hyperaldosteronism?

 QUICK QUIZ: ACE INHIBITORS

Which of the following side effects is/are associated with the use of ACE inhibitors?
A) Cough
B) Dependent edema
C) Hypokalemia
D) Angioedema
E) A and D

The correct answer is "E." Both chronic dry cough and angioedema (more common in African-American patients or those with hereditary angioedema) are side effects of ACE inhibitors. Hyperkalemia is another potential concern. These side effects may not occur immediately. Hence, you should be wary of these symptoms in *any* patient on an ACE inhibitor for *any* period of time.

▶ **CASE 2.17: RHYTHM STRIPS**

Question 2.17.1 What is the rhythm on the rhythm strip shown in Figure 2-8?
A) Second-degree heart block, type I
B) Second-degree heart block, type II
C) Third-degree heart block with junctional escape rhythm
D) Sinus rhythm with non-conducted PACs

Answer 2.17.1 The correct answer is "A." This is a Wenckebach block, also known as second-degree heart block type I or Mobitz type I AV block. Note the progressive prolongation of the PR interval before a non-conducted *P* wave on the rhythm strip in Figure 2-9 (*arrows* indicate P waves).

Question 2.17.2 The proper treatment of an asymptomatic patient with this rhythm is:
A) Treat any underlying causes identified and observe
B) Place temporary pacemaker followed by permanent pacemaker
C) Give atropine followed by permanent pacemaker
D) Refer for an electrophysiologic study

Answer 2.17.2 The correct answer is "A." Wenckebach/second-degree heart block type I can be treated with observation as long as any underlying cardiac disease is treated. You should also stop any medications that might be contributing to this rhythm disturbance, such as digoxin, beta-blockers and other AV node blocking agents. Pacemaker is appropriate for a few select patients, usually those with symptoms. Atropine is used in the emergent setting for treatment of bradycardia.

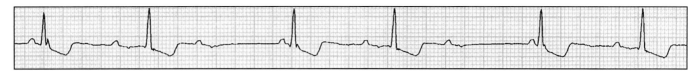

FIGURE 2-8. Rhythm strip for patient in question 2.17.1.

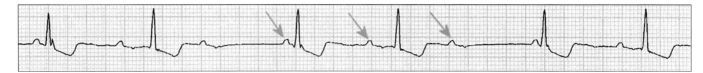

FIGURE 2-9. Arrows show P waves with progressively longer PR interval.

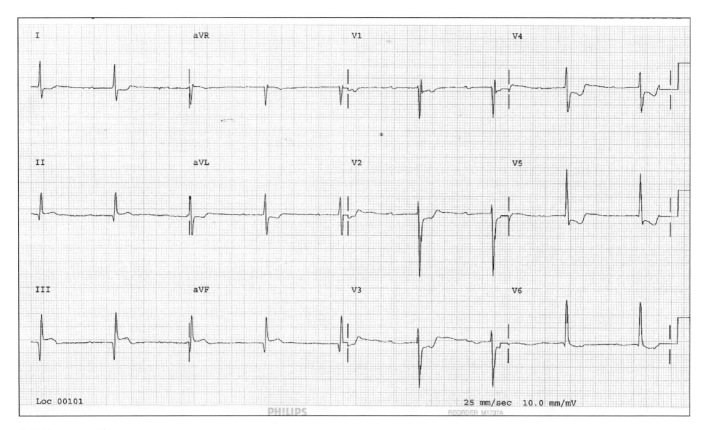

FIGURE 2-10. ECG for patient in question 2.17.3.

Question 2.17.3 What is the proper diagnosis of the ECG shown in Figure 2-10?
A) Anterior wall myocardial infarction
B) Posterior wall myocardial infarction
C) Pericarditis
D) Hyperkalemia
E) Inferior wall myocardial infarction (IMI)

Answer 2.17.3 **The correct answer is "E."** This is an IMI. Note the ST elevations in leads II and III, and aVF with reciprocal ST-segment depression in leads V2 to V5 (see indicator *arrows* in Fig. 2-11).

A patient presents with a history of lightheadedness when he stands and has the ECG shown in Figure 2-12.

Question 2.17.4 What is the rhythm?
A) Atrial flutter with 4:1 block
B) Atrial fibrillation with slow ventricular response
C) Atrial tachycardia with third-degree heart block
D) Mobitz type I (Wenckebach)

Answer 2.17.4 **The correct answer is "C."** This is an atrial tachycardia with a third-degree heart block. The P wave preceding

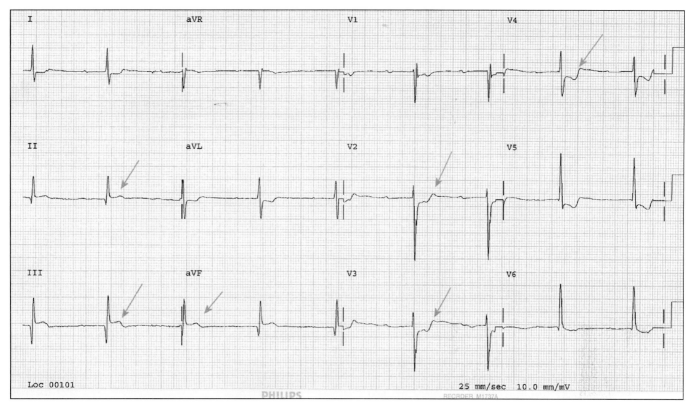

FIGURE 2-11. Arrows show ST-segment depressions in II, III, and aVF with reciprocal depressions in V2, V3, and V4.

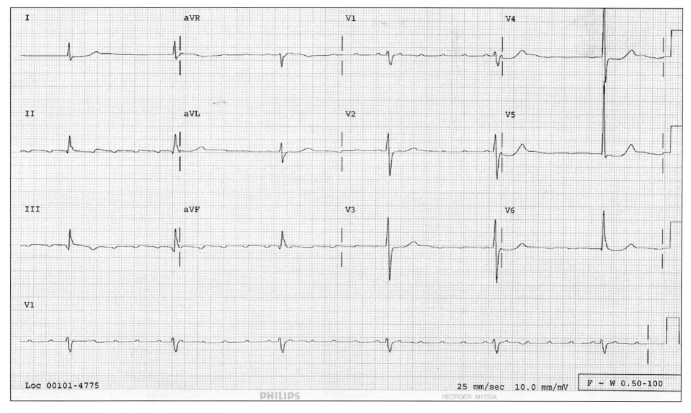

FIGURE 2-12. ECG for patient in question 2.17.4.

each QRS complex is indicated with an *arrow* on the ECG shown in Figure 2-13. Note that there is no consistent relationship between the P waves and the QRS complexes (i.e., the PR interval varies and there is no predictability), giving the diagnosis third-degree heart block.

Question 2.17.5 The appropriate treatment of this patient with atrial tachycardia and third-degree block is:
A) Pacemaker
B) Isoproterenol
C) Lidocaine
D) Atropine
E) No treatment needed

Answer 2.17.5 The correct answer is "A." The treatment of a third-degree heart block is a pacemaker. Atropine will increase the atrial rate, but that is not the problem here. The problem is AV conduction. Isoproterenol will increase the ventricular rate but is arrhythmogenic and may cause hypotension. Lidocaine is not indicated in this patient.

HELPFUL TIP FOR THE RHYTHM CONNOISSEUR:
Atrial tachycardia with block is "classic" for digitalis intoxication. If this patient were on digoxin, you would treat with Digibind.

Question 2.17.6 The drug of choice for the rhythm in Figure 2-14 is:
A) Atropine
B) Procainamide
C) Quinidine
D) Metoprolol
E) Lidocaine

Answer 2.17.6 The correct answer is "D." This is an **accelerated junctional rhythm** that generally occurs only in the setting of **cardiac ischemia**. Note the absence of P waves. Using a Class I antiarrhythmic can extinguish this rhythm, causing asystole (usually considered a bad outcome). The patient also has inferior wall ischemia (see Fig. 2-15, with indicator *arrows* showing depressed ST segments in the inferior leads). Slowing down this rhythm with metoprolol is acceptable, but you should treat the ischemia first. If the rhythm is not causing any problem, observation is good for now.

Question 2.17.7 The rhythm shown in Figure 2-16 is best described as:
A) Atrial flutter with 2:1 block
B) 2:1 second-degree heart block, Mobitz type II
C) Sinus bradycardia
D) Third-degree heart block

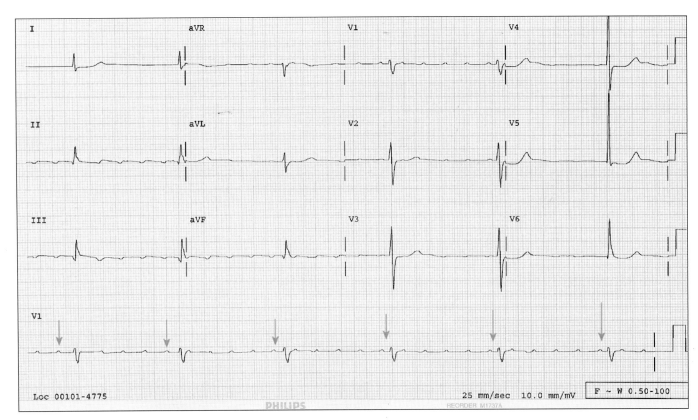

FIGURE 2-13. Arrows show P waves prior to each QRS. Note the unpredictable variation in PR intervals.

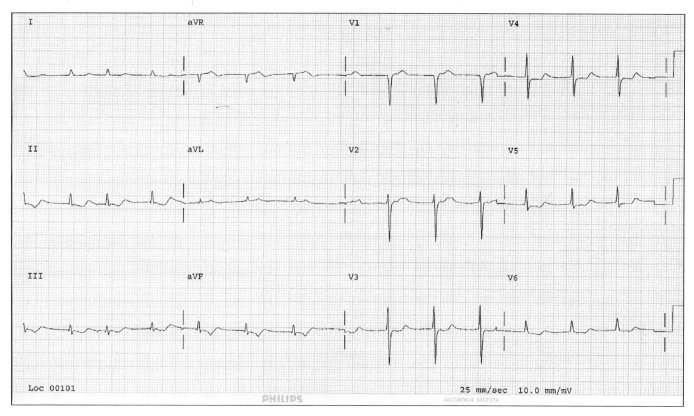

FIGURE 2-14. ECG for patient in question 2.17.6.

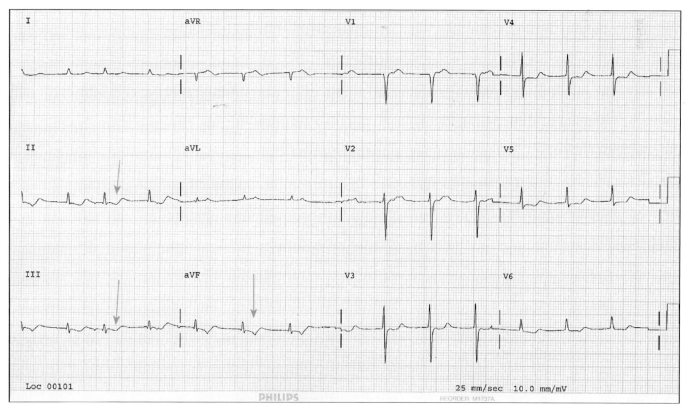

FIGURE 2-15. Accelerated junctional rhythm; arrows show inferior ST-segment depression.

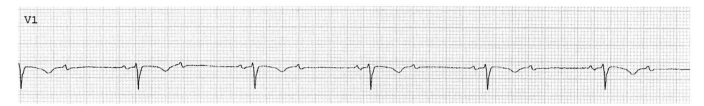

FIGURE 2-16. Rhythm strip for patient in question 2.17.7.

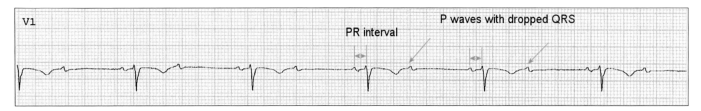

FIGURE 2-17. Second-degree heart block, Mobitz type II.

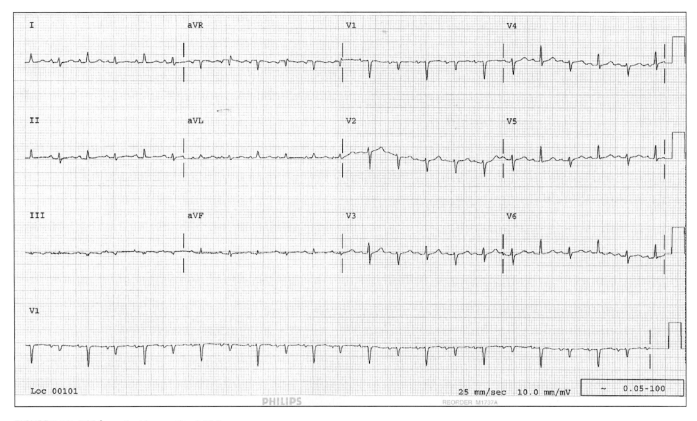

FIGURE 2-18. ECG for patient in question 2.17.8.

Answer 2.17.7 **The correct answer is "B."** This rhythm strip represents second-degree heart block, Mobitz type II. Notice that the PR interval is constant and there are dropped beats (see Fig. 2-17, with indicator *arrows* showing P waves with no associated QRS complexes). This patient needs a pacemaker.

Question 2.17.8 **The electrocardiogram shown in Figure 2-18 is consistent with which of the following?**
A) Pericardial effusion
B) Pneumothorax
C) Pulmonary embolus

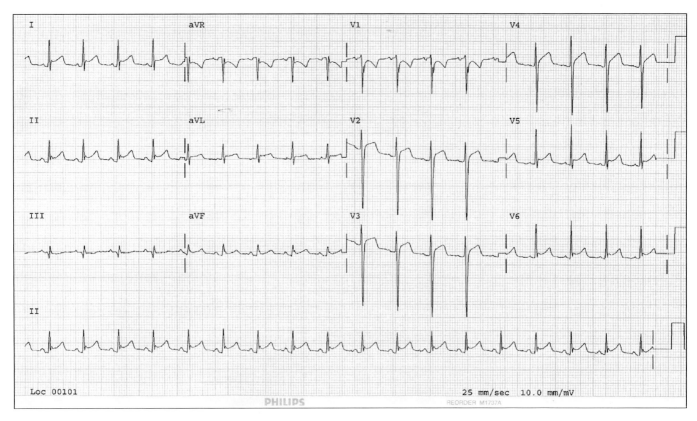

FIGURE 2-19. ECG for patient in question 2.17.9.

D) Cardiac contusion
E) None of the above

Answer 2.17.8 **The correct answer is "A."** This is an example of electrical alternans. Note the low QRS voltages that alternate in height from beat to beat. This type of pattern is seen with pericardial effusion. It is a late finding and one should be very concerned about tamponade.

Question 2.17.9 The ECG in Figure 2-19 is consistent with which of the following?
A) Anterior myocardial infarction
B) Anterolateral myocardial infarction
C) Pericarditis
D) Early repolarization
E) Total heart infarction

Answer 2.17.9 **The correct answer is "C."** This ECG is consistent with pericarditis. This ECG demonstrates several findings that indicate pericarditis, including sinus tachycardia, diffuse ST elevations, and PR depression, which are pathognomonic (see Fig. 2-20).

▶ **Objectives: Did you learn to …**
- Identify several types of cardiac arrhythmias, including heart block and junctional rhythm?
- Diagnose inferior MI by ECG?
- Describe ECG features of pericardial effusion and pericarditis?

▶ **CASE 2.18**

A 24-year-old female presents to the ED with a history of tachycardia and the rhythm strip shown in Figure 2-21. Her blood pressure is 115/70 mm Hg with an oxygen saturation of 98% on room air. There are no associated symptoms of chest pain, dyspnea, etc.

Question 2.18.1 The appropriate treatment of this patient is:
A) Adenosine 6 mg IV followed by 12 mg IV
B) Diltiazem 5 mg/kg IV
C) Verapamil 25 mg IV
D) Digoxin 0.5 mg IV
E) Defibrillation

Answer 2.18.1 **The correct answer is "A."** This rhythm is paroxysmal supraventricular tachycardia (PSVT). There are several treatment options for PSVT, which include adenosine, diltiazem, and verapamil. However, "B" and "D" are incorrect because the dose for diltiazem is 0.25 mg/kg IV, not 5 mg/kg, and the dose for verapamil is 2.5 to 5 mg IV, not 25 mg IV. While **cardioversion** is also an option in a hemodynamically stable patient, medication should be tried first. **Defibrillation** is never recommended for a perfusing rhythm.

You treat the patient with adenosine but there is no response. Thus, you choose to try a CCB. Unfortunately,

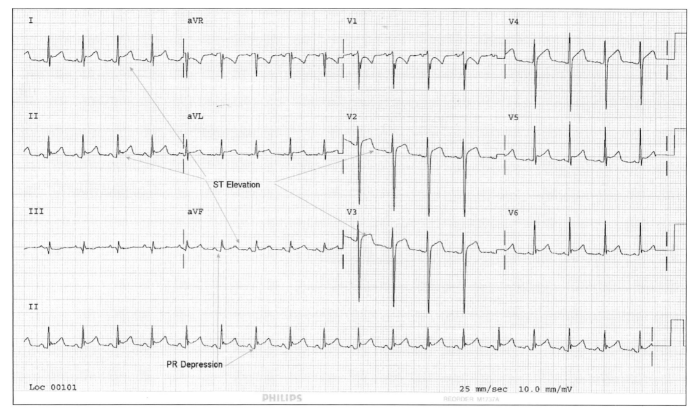

FIGURE 2-20. ECG consistent with pericarditis.

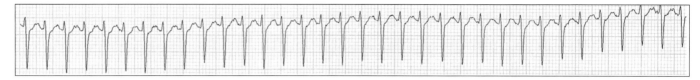

FIGURE 2-21. Rhythm strip for patient in question 2.18.1.

the patient rapidly deteriorates with the CCB, and her heart rate actually increases, so you successfully cardiovert the patient. The ECG done after cardioversion is shown in Figure 2-22.

Question 2.18.2 This ECG represents:
A) Normal ECG
B) Wolf–Parkinson–White (WPW) syndrome
C) Right bundle branch block
D) Right-axis deviation
E) Left ventricular hypertrophy

Answer 2.18.2 The correct answer is "B." This is an ECG demonstrating WPW pattern. When combined with documented tachyarrhythmia, it is referred to as WPW syndrome. Note the short PR interval as well as the delta wave (Fig. 2-23).

....

Let's say this patient comes back to the ED with atrial fibrillation in the upcoming week. This time you suspect WPW and want to choose a rate-controlling medication.

Question 2.18.3 Which is the BEST medication choice for this patient in light of her diagnosis of WPW?
A) Procainamide
B) Sotalol
C) Diltiazem
D) Verapamil
E) Metoprolol

Answer 2.18.3 The correct answer choice is "A." Patients with WPW deteriorate with beta-blockers and CCBs ("B"–"E"). The drug of choice is procainamide in patients with WPW who present with PSVT, including atrial fibrillation/flutter. The other alternative is ibutilide. Why are AV nodal blocking agents bad? The AV node is protective since it helps block most re-entrant conductions (for re-entrant arrhythmias that rely on the AV node). If you block the AV node with beta-blockers or CCBs, the re-entrant loop is allowed to go "wild" (just like you've probably seen that reality show, "Rhythms Gone Wild"). The clues to look for to help identify patients with WPW are a **young** patient with previous episodes of **palpitations**, rapid heart rate, or **syncope**.

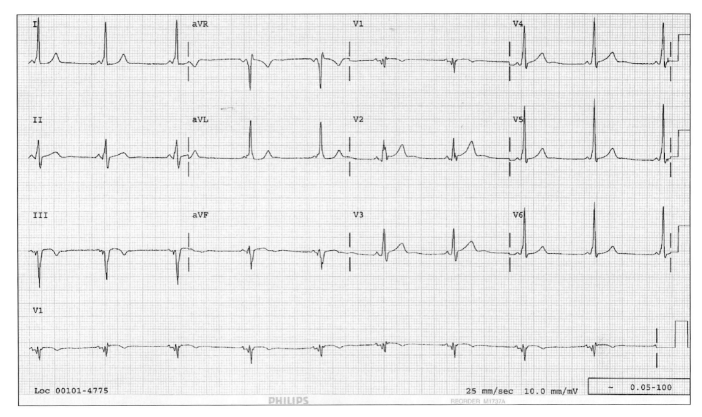

FIGURE 2-22. ECG for patient in question 2.18.2.

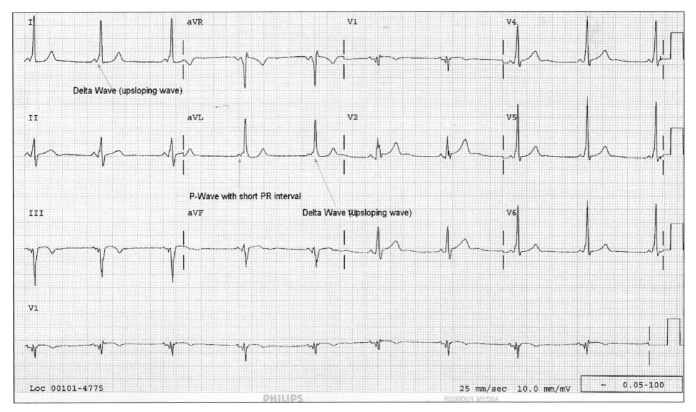

FIGURE 2-23. ECG consistent with Wolf–Parkinson–White syndrome.

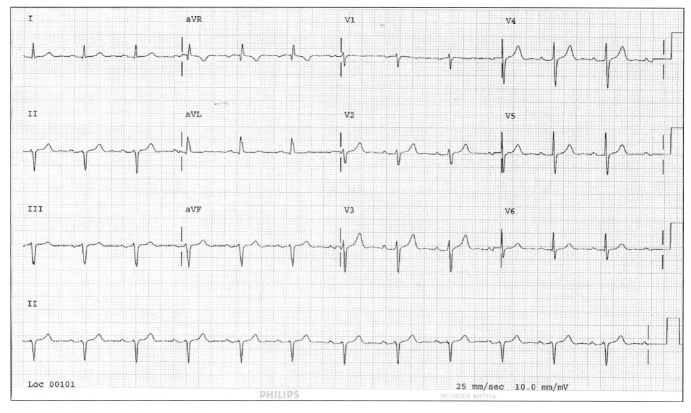

FIGURE 2-24. ECG for patient in question 2.18.4.

Question 2.18.4 The ECG shown in Figure 2-24 represents which of the following?
A) LBBB
B) RBBB
C) Left anterior fascicular block (LAFB)
D) Left posterior fascicular block
E) None of the above

Answer 2.18.4 The correct answer is "C." For those of us who are visually challenged, any patient with a net negative force in lead II will have left axis deviation and likely left anterior fascicular block (LAFB) (provided proper lead placement). Also, look for net negative deflection in leads III and aVF. For those who like the numbers, LAFB is present when the QRS axis is −45 to −90 degrees, there is an rS pattern (with small r waves) in leads II, III, and aVF and a qR pattern (with small q waves) in I and aVL. Because the QRS is narrow, neither LBBB ("A") nor RBBB ("B") can be correct. Left posterior block ("D") is quite uncommon due to the size of the posterior fascicle.

Question 2.18.5 The ECG shown in Figure 2-25 represents which of the following?
A) LBBB
B) RBBB
C) LAFB
D) Left posterior fascicular block
E) None of the above

Answer 2.18.5 The correct answer is "A." This ECG represents an LBBB. Criteria include QRS width ≥ 0.12 ms, upright (monophasic) QRS in leads I and V6, and a mostly negative QRS in V1.

HELPFUL TIP:
We don't suggest that you rely on this but … The R–R prime is on the **right** side of the ECG in an RBBB (V1, V2, V3). The R–R prime is on the **left** side of the ECG in an LBBB (lead I).

Question 2.18.6 The ECG shown in Figure 2-26 represents which of the following?
A) First-degree block
B) RBBB
C) LAFB
D) All of the above
E) None of the above

Answer 2.18.6 The correct answer is "D." This ECG represents a first-degree AV block, an RBBB, and an LAFB. The RBBB is defined by a QRS width of ≥0.12 ms (>3 small blocks) and an rsR ("rabbit ears") in chest leads V1–V3. This patient also has an LAFB (see question **2.18.4** for criteria).

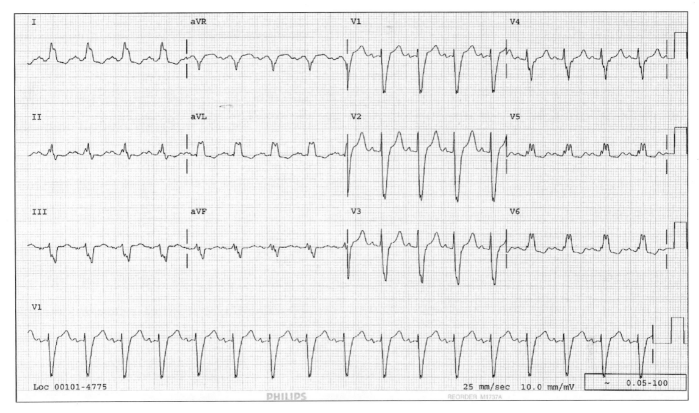

FIGURE 2-25. ECG for patient in question 2.18.5.

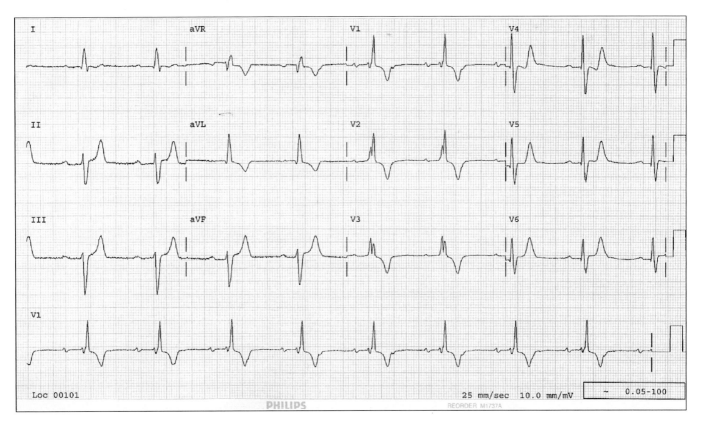

FIGURE 2-26. ECG for patient in question 2.18.6.

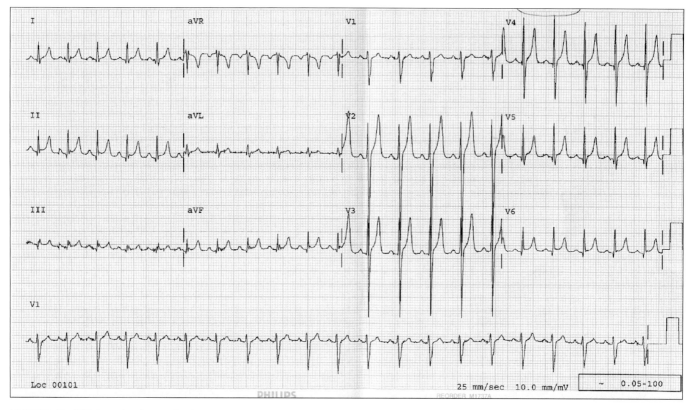

FIGURE 2-27. ECG for patient in question 2.19.1.

▶ **Objectives: Did you learn to …**

· Identify PSVT by ECG and prescribe initial treatment?

· Describe ECG findings of WPW?

· Differentiate between different types of heart block based on ECG findings?

▶ CASE 2.19

A 75-year-old patient with chronic kidney disease and diabetes presents to your ED for chest tightness, fatigue, and palpitations, and has the ECG shown in Figure 2-27.

Question 2.19.1 What is the most likely electrolyte abnormality in this patient?
A) Hypokalemia
B) Hyperkalemia
C) Hyponatremia
D) Hypermagnesemia
E) Hypercalcemia

Answer 2.19.1 The correct answer is "B," hyperkalemia. Note the peaked T-waves across the precordium. Note also that the patient has early repolarization. "A" is incorrect, and many of the opposite ECG findings occur with hypokalemia. ECG findings of **hypo**kalemia include decreased amplitude of T-waves, progressing to T-wave inversions associated with ST-segment depression, followed by increased PR interval and increased P-wave amplitude. The U-wave is a late and inconsistent finding of hypokalemia.

Question 2.19.2 All of the following are potential causes of this patient's hyperkalemia EXCEPT:
A) Metabolic acidosis
B) ACE inhibitors
C) ARBs
D) Renal failure
E) Furosemide

Answer 2.19.2 The correct answer is "E." Furosemide will cause **hypo**kalemia rather than hyperkalemia. All the other answer choices are potential causes of hyperkalemia. Other causes of hyperkalemia include a potassium load from muscle breakdown (e.g., rhabdomyolysis, burns, transfusion of old blood), tumor lysis syndrome, and other exogenous sources of potassium such as penicillin, potassium supplements, "lite" salt, and water softeners (those that use potassium). Consider also Addison disease and hypoaldosteronism. Digoxin toxicity is also a possibility.

Question 2.19.3 What is the rhythm shown in Figure 2-28?
A) Atrial fibrillation
B) Normal sinus rhythm with multiple PACs
C) Third-degree heart block with rapid rate
D) Multifocal atrial tachycardia (MAT)

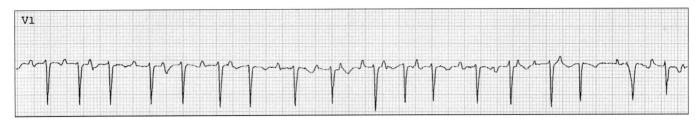

FIGURE 2-28. ECG for patient in question 2.19.3.

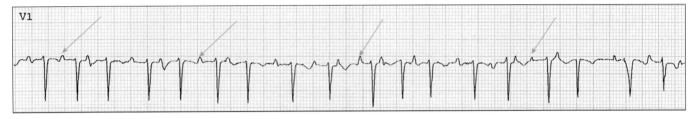

FIGURE 2-29. Arrows show P waves of varying morphology, consistent with MAT.

Answer 2.19.3 The correct answer is "D." This is a MAT. Note the multiple morphologies of the P waves indicated by *arrows* in Figure 2-29 as well as the irregularity of the rhythm. Here are helpful tips in diagnosing and treating MAT: three or more different P-wave morphologies with varying PR intervals. Causes include theophylline, pulmonary disease, and abnormal electrolytes (K^+ or Mg). Digoxin may worsen MAT! Rarely, AV nodal ablation with permanent pacing can be considered in refractory cases.

Question 2.19.4 All of the following are treatments of MAT EXCEPT:
A) Nondihydropyridine CCB (verapamil, diltiazem)
B) Beta-blocker
C) Magnesium
D) Improving pulmonary function and reducing hypoxia
E) Adenosine

Answer 2.19.4 The correct answer is "E." All of the others are indicated in the treatment of MAT. Adenosine may slow down the rhythm temporarily but is not considered a treatment of this rhythm.

▶ **Objectives: Did you learn to …**
 • Recognize ECG findings associated with hyperkalemia and hypokalemia?
 • Describe ECG findings and treatment options for MAT?

▶ **CASE 2.20**

A 28-year-old woman with no significant past medical history presents to clinic with complaints of progressive shortness of breath; she becomes dyspneic with less activity compared to 1 year ago. If she exerts herself beyond a brisk walk, she becomes lightheaded, pre-syncopal, and feels tightness in her chest. She also notes generalized fatigue. Your examination discloses a heart rate of 105 bpm and normal blood pressure.

Resting transcutaneous oximetry is 92% on room air. BMI is 24 kg/m². She has JVD but clear lungs. A grade 2/6 mid-systolic murmur is heard over the left upper sternal border. Electrocardiogram is shown (Fig. 2-30).

Question 2.20.1 What is the most likely diagnosis?
A) CAD
B) Pulmonary hypertension
C) Asthma
D) Congenital aortic stenosis
E) Mitral valve prolapse

Answer 2.20.1 The correct answer is "B." The physical examination is consistent with right ventricular pressure overload. This is supported by the electrocardiogram demonstrating right atrial enlargement, right-axis deviation, and RVH. CAD ("A") is almost unheard of in a woman younger than 30 years without any risk factors. Asthma ("C") may cause her symptom complex but is not supported by her examination. Aortic stenosis ("D") causes neither resting hypoxemia nor RVH. Because they have a fixed cardiac output (limited by lung vascular pressures), patients with pulmonary hypertension often get pre-syncopal with exertion.

Note: Findings that suggest RVH on the ECG: right-axis deviation, right atrial abnormality (*P*-wave >2.5 boxes tall in lead II), RVH (tall R in V1), and strain pattern in leads II and III *as indicated by arrows* in Figure 2-31. Often patients with pulmonary hypertension will have an intraventricular conduction delay with R–R′ in V1 (not shown on this electrocardiogram, Fig. 2-31).

Question 2.20.2 The following tests may be helpful in elucidating the cause of pulmonary hypertension EXCEPT:
A) Chest x-ray and pulmonary function studies
B) Chest CT scan
C) ANA, HIV antibody/antigen testing and liver function studies
D) Nasopharyngoscopy
E) Polysomnogram

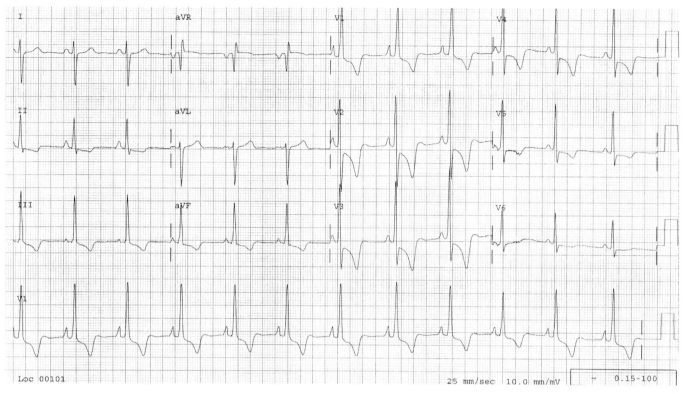

FIGURE 2-30. ECG for patient in question 2.20.1.

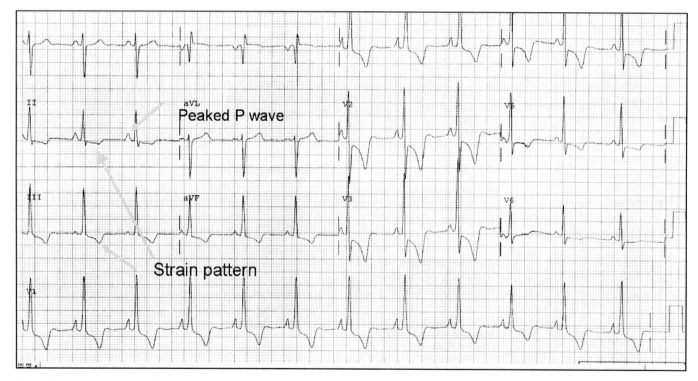

FIGURE 2-31. ECG consistent with RVH. Note large R wave in V1 and right-axis deviation.

Answer 2.20.2 The correct answer is "D." An important part of the workup for pulmonary hypertension is defining the etiology and potentially reversible causes. There is no cookbook approach, and diagnostic workup should be tailored by the history and physical examination. Chest radiography and PFTs ("A") can identify chronic lung disease causing (or contributing to) pulmonary hypertension. A CT scan ("B") is done to exclude chronic thromboembolic pulmonary disease and to evaluate for fibrosis, sarcoidosis, etc. Connective tissue disease, HIV, and cirrhosis ("C") are known to cause pulmonary hypertension. Sleep apnea ("E") is an important, treatable cause of PHTN. Nasopharyngoscopy has no role in this workup.

An echocardiogram confirms findings suggestive of severe pulmonary hypertension and changes consistent with right ventricular pressure overload (a right heart catheterization is required for diagnosis). No intracardiac shunt is identified by echocardiogram. The remainder of her diagnostic workup fails to identify a secondary cause of pulmonary hypertension. A right heart catheterization confirms severe pulmonary hypertension but fails to identify a shunt. A vasodilator challenge (with adenosine) is performed and no change in pulmonary pressure is elicited. She is given a diagnosis of idiopathic pulmonary arterial hypertension.

The treatment of pulmonary hypertension is, in general, very specialized and a cardiologist should be involved. Exceptions include pulmonary hypertension from chronic hypoxia (smoking, sleep apnea) that are amenable to primary care management. Chronic PE can also be managed by the primary care practitioner, although the patient should still follow with a cardiologist due to the potential for right heart failure.

HELPFUL TIP:
Additional therapy for pulmonary hypertension may include prostacyclin and phosphodiesterase inhibitors (e.g., sildenafil, tadalafil, vardenafil). Some patients require anticoagulation. Management should be directed by a pulmonary hypertension specialist.

▶ **Objectives: Did you learn to …**
- Diagnose and evaluate for pulmonary hypertension?
- Identify secondary causes of pulmonary hypertension?
- Explain the importance of co-management with a cardiology team for the treatment of pulmonary hypertension?

▶ **CASE 2.21**

A 54-year-old male presents to your clinic complaining of dyspnea and fevers. His temperature in the office is 38.5°C and heart rate is 113 bpm with pulse oximetry of 93%. On physical examination, you notice that he had nodules on his fingertips and notice a slight reddish discoloration under his fingernails.

On further questioning, he tells you that he recently moved here from a major city and had used IV drugs in the very distant past, by which he means as recently as last month.

Question 2.21.1 Your next step in management is:
A) Order a chest x-ray and start empiric levofloxacin
B) Order a chest x-ray and start empiric ceftriaxone and azithromycin
C) Order a chest x-ray, echocardiogram, draw blood cultures
D) Order a chest x-ray and start empiric piperacillin and vancomycin
E) Order a chest x-ray and do nothing, it is probably viral

Answer 2.21.1 The correct answer is "C." Although the chest x-ray is overkill for a case of endocarditis, it may identify other causes of fever and help evaluate for heart failure. The patient is presenting with IV drug use history, Osler nodes, and Janeway lesions (nail-bed hemorrhages), as well as fever. These easily meet three minor Duke criteria (see Table 2-9), qualifying for a "possible diagnosis of endocarditis." Now what you need is one major criterion to definitively diagnose endocarditis. A positive echocardiogram or blood culture would qualify. Once the blood cultures are drawn, if your suspicion is high, you may start empiric antibiotics for endocarditis.

Question 2.21.2 Which valve(s) are most commonly affected by endocarditis?
A) Aortic valve
B) Mitral valve
C) Pulmonic valve
D) Demonic valve
E) A and B

TABLE 2-9 REVISED DUKE CRITERIA FOR ENDOCARDITIS (DEFINITIVE DIAGNOSIS: TWO MAJOR CRITERIA OR ONE MAJOR + THREE MINOR CRITERIA. POSSIBLE DIAGNOSIS: ONE MAJOR + ONE MINOR CRITERION OR THREE MINOR CRITERIA)

Major Criteria	Minor Criteria
• Two positive blood cultures for organisms typical of endocarditis • Three positive blood cultures for organisms consistent with endocarditis • Serologic evidence of *Coxiella burnetii* • Echocardiographic evidence of endocardial involvement: Oscillating intracardiac mass on a heart valve, on supporting structures, in the path of regurgitant jets, or on implanted material without another anatomic explanation; cardiac abscess; new dehiscence of prosthetic valve; or new valvular regurgitation	• Predisposing heart disorder • IV drug abuse • Fever ≥ 38°C • Vascular phenomena: arterial embolism, septic pulmonary embolism, mycotic aneurysm, intracranial hemorrhage, conjunctival petechiae, or Janeway lesions • Immunologic phenomena: glomerulonephritis, Osler nodes, Roth spots, or rheumatoid factor • Microbiologic evidence of infection consistent with but not meeting major criteria • Serologic evidence of infection with organisms consistent with endocarditis

Answer 2.21.2 The correct answer is "E." The aortic and mitral valves are most commonly affected. There is no demonic valve, we hope, but there is the tricuspid, of course.

Question 2.21.3 Which of the following organisms is most common in acute endocarditis?
A) *Staphylococcus aureus* and group B streptococci
B) Alpha-hemolytic streptococci or enterococci
C) Enterovirus
D) Fungi
E) *Elmo muppetel (can you tell we are getting tired … the jokes are getting weaker)*

Answer 2.21.3 The correct answer is "A." Staph and group B strep are generally responsible for acute endocarditis while alpha-hemolytic streptococci and enterococci are more common with subacute endocarditis. Fungi may be present in IV drug abusers. As to *E. muppetel*, it is a new species recently described by us. We grovered it in Big Bird cultures.

▶ **Objectives: Did you learn to …**
  • Initiate evaluation and management of bacterial endocarditis?

 QUICK QUIZ: YET ANOTHER HEART FAILURE QUESTION (YOU THOUGHT WE WERE DONE…)

Cardiac resynchronization for heart failure is indicated in which of the following patients?
A) A patient who has an ejection fraction of 30% and is in atrial fibrillation that is rate-controlled
B) A patient who has an ejection fraction of 30% and is in atrial fibrillation that is *not* rate-controlled (say a rate of 110–115 bpm)
C) A patient who has an ejection fraction of 30% and in normal sinus rhythm who has an LBBB
D) A patient with an underlying arrhythmia such as PSVT who is symptomatic
E) A or B

The correct answer is "C." Bet we got you on this one, huh? The idea behind cardiac resynchronization is to put blood into the ventricle at the optimum time for function. This requires the atrium to be working properly. Thus, "A" and "B" are wrong. The concept is to pace the atrium and then also pace the ventricle so that the ventricle depolarizes at the optimum moment for blood ejection after the blood is sent to the LV by the atrium. This optimal blood ejection is disordered by an LBBB where depolarization of the ventricle is delayed causing a "dyssynchrony" (as it were) between the timing of atrial functioning and the timing of the ventricular depolarization. Cardiac resynchronization is "only" for patients with heart failure who are in normal sinus rhythm. So, the basic criteria for cardiac resynchronization include a QRS of >150 ms, with an LBBB, an LV ejection fraction of 30% or less, and sinus rhythm who have class III or

class IV heart failure (*J Am Coll Cardiol.* 2013;61(3):e6–75). It seems to improve the overall absolute survival by about 2%; it also reduces readmissions (*Ann Intern Med.* 2014;160:603).

 QUICK QUIZ: WHAT ARE YOU … A HEART FAILURE SPECIALIST?

Which of the following has been shown to improve mortality in patients with HFrEF?
A) Valsartan + Sacubitril (Entresto)
B) Ivabradine (Corlanor)
C) Azumumumab (Coregulator)
D) A and B
E) B and C

The correct answer is "A." First you need to know what these things are. Entresto combines an ARB plus a neprilysin inhibitor. Inhibiting neprilysin increases vasodilatation and sodium loss. It has been shown to be effective at reducing mortality from HFrEF. This can *replace* an ACE inhibitor or ARB. *Make sure the patient can tolerate an ARB or ACE* **before** starting Entresto. Use it in patients with NY class II–IV CHF, with an EF < 40%, no history of angioedema, and an adequate blood pressure. Also, it cannot be given with an ACE inhibitor because of the risk of angioedema. **Of course, you already know that an ACE inhibitor and an ARB should never be used together … right?**

Corlanor reduces heart rate without lowering BP and is *only* indicated in heart failure patients who do not reach their target heart rate with a beta-blocker. Corlanor would be added to an ACE inhibitor or ARB, a beta-blocker, and aldosterone antagonist. It *does not* replace the beta-blocker and *does not* improve mortality. It supplements the beta-blocker in patients with heart rate > 70 bpm after maximizing other medications (including a beta-blocker if tolerated). Corlanor can also be used in patients who do not tolerate a beta-blocker. We made up "C," although it wouldn't be a surprise to us if we see this drug name at some point in the future.

▶ **CASE 2.22**

A new patient presents for his annual examination and has some questions about cardiovascular disease risk. He also wants to chat about his favorite sports team (Iowa Hawkeyes, we hope), but you gently steer him back to the matter at hand.

Question 2.22.1 The following are all considered cardiac risk factors when calculating cardiac risk and need for statins per the ACC/AHA calculator (http://www.cvriskcalculator.com) EXCEPT:
A) Age
B) Relative with early heart disease
C) Smoking
D) Hypertension
E) Gender

TABLE 2-10 RISK FACTORS FOR CORONARY ARTERY DISEASE

- First-degree male relative with CAD or sudden death at age < 55 or first-degree female relative with CAD or sudden death at age < 65
- Smoking
- HDL < 40 mg/dL (HDL > 60 mg/dL is considered protective)
- Diabetes
- Hypertension (>140/90) or on antihypertensives
- Age: males >45, females >55
- Elevated LDL

Answer 2.22.1 The correct answer is "B." The ACC/AHA calculator includes the following risk factors for CAD: age, gender, "race," total cholesterol, HDL cholesterol, systolic and diastolic BP, diabetes, smoking and whether or not one is being treated for hypertension. Unlike many Caribbean resort destinations, the calculator is not all-inclusive. Many known risk factors for heart disease (e.g., family history, obesity) are not taken into account. The risk calculator is a tool; you must continue to apply clinical judgment. Also, the calculator, as well as the entire guideline, is not meant to be used to manage all forms of dyslipidemias. Remember from earlier in this chapter that peripheral vascular disease is considered a CAD equivalent.

See Table 2-10 for more details on risk factors.

· ·

This 55-year-old gentleman says, "All my friends take a medicine for cholesterol. Shouldn't I take one, too?" You are worried that he is susceptible to peer pressure, but you are also thinking about protecting him from atherosclerotic cardiovascular disease (ASCVD).

Question 2.22.2 According to the 2018 ACC/AHA Blood Cholesterol Guideline, all of the following *automatically* qualify as patients who would benefit from statin therapy EXCEPT:
A) A patient with known cardiovascular disease
B) A 40-year-old patient with an LDL of 200 mg/dL
C) A 55-year-old diabetic patient with an LDL of 130 mg/dL
D) A 55-year-old nondiabetic patient without known cardiovascular disease whose 10-year ASCVD risk is calculated as 10%
E) A 35-year-old smoker with hypertension

Answer 2.22.2 The correct answer is "E." The 35-year-old patient *might* be a candidate for a statin (HMG-CoA reductase inhibitor) but is not an *automatic* candidate based on the information given. All other options describe patients who would benefit from statin therapy according to the 2018 ACC/AHA guideline. The 2018 ACC/AHA guideline relies on a risk calculator for primary prevention. See Table 2-11 for a summary of the 2018 cholesterol guidelines. It is important to note that while the ACC/AHA guideline recommends moderate-to-high-intensity statin therapy starting at a 10-year ASCVD risk score of 7.5%, the USPSTF recommends **low-to-moderate** dose statin therapy at an **ASCVD risk score of 10%**. We cannot know for sure what answer the ABFM would use for the test, but they usually side with the USPSTF.

TABLE 2-11 2018 AMERICAN HEART ASSOCIATION (AHA)/AMERICAN COLLEGE OF CARDIOLOGY (ACC) LIPID GUIDELINES

Qualify for a high-dose statin	1. LDL >190 mg/dL *or* 2. History of CAD (or equivalent) *or* 3. DM and age 40–79
Qualify for a moderate-to-high dose statin (use risk calculator)*ᵃ*	Primary prevention if 10-year risk is >7.5% and the patient has an LDL of 70–189 mg/dL and age 40–75
Qualify for a low-dose statin	Those who qualify for a statin but don't tolerate high- or moderate-dose statin

Goals of Therapy
1. *The primary goal is to reach the appropriate dose of statin*
2. Reduction of LDL by 50% from baseline
3. There are no fixed LDL goals (such as past goals of LDL < 100 mg/dL)

Drug Doses
1. High-dose statin = atorvastatin 40–80 mg or rosuvastatin 20–40 mg
2. Low-to-moderate dose statin = atorvastatin 10–20 mg QD, pravastatin 40–80 mg BID, and rosuvastatin 5–10 mg QD, among others

*ᵃ*Find a cardiovascular risk calculator at http://tools.cardiosource.org/ASCVD-Risk-Estimator/.

· ·

The patient then asks you about something he read about "crap." A light bulb goes off and you realize he wants to know about C-reactive protein (CRP).

Question 2.22.3 Which of the following best represents the role of CRP in cardiac disease in 2015?
A) CRP should be measured in all patients in whom cardiac disease is suspected
B) CRP should be measured only in patients with intermediate cardiac risk factors (e.g., those with a 10-year risk of CAD of 10–20%)
C) CRP should be measured in patients with known heart disease in order to monitor inflammation and risk
D) CRP should be measured in low-risk (<10% risk of CAD in next 10 years) patients who have no known cardiac disease. An elevated CRP suggests that these patients should be treated with a lipid-lowering therapy
E) CRP has not been shown to be useful and does not contribute significantly to cardiac risk stratification

Answer 2.22.3 The correct answer is "E." Although, high-sensitivity CRP (hsCRP) was initially thought to be a possible biomarker for cardiac risk assessment, it has been shown to be of marginal benefit. The use of hsCRP led to minimal reclassification of patients (a maximum of 11% of intermediate patients were reclassified in one study). The Class IIa recommendation to use hsCRP was published by the AHA in 2003, prior to further studies that have questioned its usefulness.

 HELPFUL TIP:
We do not use hsCRP. However, if it were useful, it would be in the intermediate-risk patients.

Question 2.22.4 You may have noticed (we hope) that the risk calculator includes lipids as a risk factor. What does the USPSTF recommend in terms of screening for lipid disorders?

A) Screen all adults annually starting at age 25
B) Screen men age 35 years and older
C) Screen women age 45 years and older
D) Universal screening of all patients age 40 to 75

Answer 2.22.4 The correct answer is "D." USPSTF updated its lipid testing recommendations in 2016. Here is a summary:

Screen patients 40 to 75 years of age without CAD. Treatment is suggested for those 40 to 75 years of age with elevated lipids **and** one other risk factor for CAD (risk factors *for this purpose include* (LDL-C > 130 mg/dL or HDL-C < 40 mg/dL), diabetes, hypertension, and smoking) **and** >10% ten-year risk of having a cardiac event based on the ACA calculator.

Use low-to-moderate dose statins. For those with a risk of 7.5% to 10%, discuss pros and cons with the patient—which of course you do with all patients anyway (*JAMA.* 2016;316(19):1997–2007). **Note that the benefit of lipid treatment outweighs the risk of diabetes** (which can be seen with statins).

HELPFUL TIP:
Fasting lipids are out. Well, not entirely. But you don't have to have patients return for fasting lipids, that's for sure. Non-fasting is fine for making decisions about risk and starting therapy (*Eur Heart J.* 2016;37:1944–1953); fasting lipids serve as complementary data.

You obtain laboratory tests. The patient has normal electrolytes and the following cholesterol panel: total cholesterol 175 mg/dL, LDL 110 mg/dL, HDL 35 mg/dL, triglycerides 150 mg/dL. He is a 55-year-old African-American male, nonsmoker, and nondiabetic who takes no medications. His systolic blood pressure is 132/85 mm Hg. You plug all his data into the ASCVD risk calculator and generate a 10-year ASCVD risk of 7.5%.

Question 2.22.5 Given the ASCVD risk you calculated, and being consistent with the 2018 ACC/AHA guideline, you recommend:

A) No changes. Keep calm and carry on
B) A treadmill stress test
C) A high fiber diet
D) Low-intensity statin therapy (e.g., simvastatin 10 mg daily)
E) Moderate-intensity statin therapy (e.g., atorvastatin 10–20 mg daily)

Answer 2.22.5 The correct answer is "E." Did you think this patient was a candidate for moderate statin therapy prior to this guideline? If not, you are not alone. The 2018 ACC/AHA guideline has changed the way we determine risk, expanding the use of statins. Patients whose 10-year ASCVD risk is 7.5% or greater should be on moderate-to-high-intensity statin therapy. *As noted above, we have dueling guidelines.* Of course, you should discuss the pros and cons with every patient.

Question 2.22.6 Your astute patient appears to be goal-oriented and asks you what his target LDL should be. You reply:

A) "Targets are so 2012. The goal is to get you on a moderate-to-high-intensity statin. There is no specific LDL goal number"
B) "Your target LDL is <100 mg/dL"
C) "Your target LDL is about 70 mg/dL"
D) "Your target LDL is simply as low as we can get without causing rhabdomyolysis … . Well, maybe just a little rhabdo will be OK"

Answer 2.22.6 The correct answer is "A." The 2018 ACC/AHA guideline does not recommend treating to *specific* LDL targets. Instead, appropriate statin therapy should be selected based on risk category as previously indicated. Your goal is to get the patient to a maximal dose of statin and not a specific LDL. That said, the LDL should be reduced by 50% even if that is a starting point of 400 mg/dL and the patient ends up at 200 mg/dL.

HELPFUL TIP:
There is no evidence that "titrating up" the dose of a statin is necessary or helpful in preventing side effects. Just start the final appropriate dose of a statin on day 1 of treatment.

You advise your patient to start atorvastatin 20 mg daily. You check baseline transaminases, which are normal. When your patient returns 3 months later and sees your partner (because you took a "vacation" to study for the board examination), she checks his lipids and transaminases out of habit. If only you had been there! You know that the FDA no longer recommends periodic liver enzyme testing while on a statin. Statin-related hepatotoxicity is an idiosyncratic reaction that is extremely rare and completely unpredictable, so there is no point in routinely checking transaminases. Well, your partner didn't get the memo, and you return to find your patient's ALT and AST have both doubled while on atorvastatin and are now almost twice the upper limit of normal for your lab.

Question 2.22.7 When you find transaminases are twice the upper limit of normal while on a statin, the proper response is to:

A) Stop the statin because of the elevated liver enzymes
B) Start a different statin since this is not a "class effect"
C) Continue the statin and consider other causes for the elevated liver enzymes
D) Add cholestyramine to help ease the burden on the liver
E) Refer for liver biopsy to rule out other causes of elevated liver enzymes

Answer 2.22.7 The correct answer is "C." Statins can be continued as long as the elevation of liver enzymes is **less than three times the upper limit of normal**. Never assume that this is a drug effect if there is a reason to believe that the patient could have another disease, such as hepatitis C.

You are compelled to perform the requisite history and physical examination to assess for other causes of liver disease. In the course of your investigations, other labs and imaging may be in order. However, liver biopsy ("E") would be taking your fiduciary duty to the extreme. "A" is incorrect since the levels are only two times the upper limit of normal. "B" is incorrect for two reasons. First, there is no need to act to change the drug at this point. Second, *elevated liver enzymes are a class effect.* "D" is incorrect because you do not need to add another drug at this time, and cholestyramine will do nothing to "ease the burden on the liver," whatever that means.

....

After a thorough history, examination, appropriate lab and imaging tests, you determine that the liver enzyme elevation was due to fatty infiltration. A month later the enzymes have come down to the upper limits of normal. When you see your patient back, he complains of pain and tenderness in his legs, shoulders and back. He also reports generalized fatigue and weakness.

Question 2.22.8 What is the most appropriate next step in the evaluation and management of this complaint?
A) Stop his atorvastatin and replace it with rosuvastatin
B) Double the dose of atorvastatin
C) Check liver enzymes
D) Check creatine phosphokinase (CPK) level
E) Start coenzyme-Q10 (ubiquinone)

Answer 2.22.8 The correct answer is "D." This patient is presenting with symptoms that may be attributable to statin-induced myopathy. Statins have been associated with myalgia and rhabdomyolysis. Prior to making any decisions about therapy, the next step would be to confirm your suspicions by checking the CPK level. If this patient has statin-induced muscle symptoms, he is unlikely to improve by switching to rosuvastatin ("A"); hence, increasing the statin dose ("B") is the wrong thing to do. While it may be reasonable to check liver enzymes ("C") due to his complaint of fatigue, myopathy is more likely, given his constellation of symptoms. Of course, in your real medical practice, you could order liver enzymes and CPK, but an examination is not real life! Finally, "E" is incorrect. Coenzyme Q10 has not been shown to prevent or treat statin-related myopathy (*Mayo Clin Proc.* 2015;90:24). But vitamin D may be useful in patients who are deficient.

....

You check a CPK level, and it is ... normal. Darn. You thought you had this mystery wrapped up.

Question 2.22.9 From this normal CPK, you can conclude that:
A) He does not have statin-induced myopathy since the CPK is within normal limits
B) His fatigue and aches are a manifestation of depression and sleep disturbance
C) You can safely increase the dose of his statin

D) He still may have statin-induced myopathy despite a normal CPK
E) Your lab has a serious quality control issue

Answer 2.22.9 The correct answer is "D." He still may have statin-induced myopathy despite a normal CPK, so "A" is incorrect. There are several crossover trials that demonstrate myopathy in patients with normal muscle enzymes. The mechanism is thought to be a mitochondrial dysfunction. "B" is incorrect, and the reverse may actually be true (myopathy causing poor sleep and anhedonia). "C" is incorrect because he may indeed have a myopathy, and a trial off one or both drugs is warranted. Remember that gemfibrozil (and less so fenofibrate), which you might prescribe for hypertriglyceridemia, interact with statins to increase the risk of statin-induced myopathy/rhabdomyolysis. Remember also that there is no evidence that treating with gemfibrozil or fenofibrate improves cardiovascular outcomes.

....

You stop his atorvastatin. A few weeks later, he returns and feels great! You consider starting a different agent to treat his lipids.

Question 2.22.10 Which of the following is classified as a bile acid sequestrant?
A) Ezetimibe
B) Colestipol
C) Colesevelam
D) B and C
E) All of the above

Answer 2.22.10 The correct answer is "D." Ezetimibe (Zetia) is not a bile acid sequestrant but rather reduces cholesterol absorption by blocking at the brush border of the small intestine. This is a mechanism that is different from any of the other lipid-lowering agents. It is relatively safe but expensive and less potent than the statins. You could also try pravastatin and fluvastatin, which are less likely to cause myopathy.

HELPFUL RANT: "DO NOTHING THAT IS OF NO USE" (MIYAMOTO MUSASHI)
Don't feel obligated to "just do something." There is no data suggesting that any anti-lipid drugs other than the statins, ezetimibe, and PCSK9 inhibitors (see below) reduce cardiovascular outcomes. Some, such as niacin, may actually worsen outcomes.

HELPFUL TIP:
Evidence for ezetimibe is weak, including a much-touted 2015 study (*N Engl J Med.* 2015;372:2387). First, the study is flawed and looks at a very narrow group of patients (those hospitalized with known CAD, therefore secondary prevention). It says nothing about primary prevention. Second, many of the patients were not even on a statin, the standard of care. *Finally, you have to treat 50 patients for 7 years to prevent one cardiovascular event*—not a glowing endorsement, especially since they weren't on a statin.

You find yourself staring out the examination room window, ruminating on cholesterol medications.

Question 2.22.11 Side effects of ezetimibe include which of the following?
A) Diarrhea
B) Arthralgia
C) Angioedema
D) Liver enzyme elevation
E) All of the above

Answer 2.22.11 **The correct answer is "E."** "C" deserves special mention. As with ACE inhibitors, angioedema has been reported with the use of ezetimibe during post-marketing research. The rate of occurrence is not known. However, it can be life-threatening although no deaths have been reported to date. All of the other side effects are known to occur at a rate greater than with placebo.

Your patient is now OK taking maximal dose of a statin, but he has questions about a "cholesterol shot" his friend is taking. Apparently, his friend's LDL is 300—kind of high. You assume that he is talking about a PCSK9 (proprotein convertase subtilisin kexin type 9) inhibitor, which prevents the binding and the degrading of LDL receptors (thus, there are more LDL receptors to uptake LDL from the blood).

Question 2.22.12 The indications for the use of a PCSK9 inhibitor (Praluent® [alirocumab] and Repatha® [evolocumab]) in a patient on statins includes which of the following?
A) Ongoing angina regardless of the percent decrease of LDL on a maximal dose of a statin
B) Less than a 50% reduction from baseline of LDL after maximal dose statin + ezetimibe
C) An absolute LDL of >190 mg/dL after maximal dose statin regardless of the starting LDL
D) A cardiovascular event while on a maximal dose statin plus a bile acid sequestrant

Answer: 2.22.12 **The correct answer is "B."** Indications for the use of a PCSK9 inhibitor include the following: (1) Failure to reduce the baseline LDL by 50% on a maximal dose of a statin *and* ezetimibe, **or** (2) a patient who has a cardiovascular event while on a statin *plus* ezetimibe **and** an LDL of ≥50 mg/dL (not a bile acid sequestrant as in "D"), **or** a very high LDL secondary to familial hypercholesterolemia. These drugs are expensive (>$10,000/year), and prevent one cardiovascular even for every 74 patients treated for 2 years.

HELPFUL (BUT ABSURD) TIP:
Did you notice the 50 mg/dL LDL goal in the question answer above? That is not a typo. There are yet more 2018 guidelines from the AHA/ACC and these have

brought LDL targets back into favor. **For patients with ASCVD,** they recommend:
1) Aim for a 50% lowering of baseline cholesterol using a statin (as in the old guidelines) in patients with ASCVD
2) For "very high risk" ASCVD patients on maximal statins add ezetimibe if the LDL is >70 mg/dL. If the LDL remains >70 mg/dL, add a PSCK9 inhibitor
3) In those with an LDL > 190 mg/dL at baseline, don't use the calculator. Just start them on a high-intensity statin with a goal of <100 mg/dL. If you don't meet this goal and the patient has multiple risk factors, proceed as in #2 above to add ezetimibe and a PSCK9 inhibitor with a goal of <100 mg/dL

There are 7 more recommendations. They can be found at: https://www.ahajournals.org/doi/10.1161/CIR.0000000000000625. *Note that these have not been endorsed by the AAFP nor the ACP (American College of Physicians). They are based on "expert opinion" and not clear science. We don't know which recommendations will be on the test.*

HELPFUL TIP:
Metamucil or other psyllium products are useful in reducing serum cholesterol and provide a "nondrug" alternative. However, at least 7 g of soluble fiber daily is required.

▶ **Objectives: Did you learn to …**
· Determine risk factors for ASCVD?
· List the screening recommendations for lipid disorders?
· Describe the role of lipid-lowering therapy in the prevention of cardiac disease?
· Identify some of the potential side effects of lipid-lowering medications?

Clinical Pearls

○ A false-positive troponin can be caused by a PE, heart failure, burns, sepsis, stroke, and more.

○ A normal ECG during chest pain does not rule out ACS. In fact, 10% of patients with an MI will have an initially normal ECG with pain.

○ Aggressive blood pressure lowering in patients with diabetes may be harmful. Use the same goal as for almost everyone else, <140/90. The JNC 8 report suggests a goal of <150/90 in those 60 years of age and older.

○ Avoid the combination of a statin and gemfibrozil or fenofibrate; it can cause rhabdomyolysis. The risk is lower with fenofibrate, however.

○ Do not continue nonaspirin antiplatelet agents (e.g., clopidogrel) indefinitely after stent placement. Determine a target end date (e.g., 1 year of dual aspirin–clopidogrel after placement of a DES).

○ Do not do routine stress testing for asymptomatic patients preoperatively. In fact, don't perform stress testing in any asymptomatic patients.

○ Do not use beta-blockers alone as antihypertensive therapy unless there is another indication (e.g., post-MI, heart failure).

○ Do not use hsCRP to assess cardiac risk.

○ Do not use nonstatin drugs to lower cardiac risk in patients until statins have been maximized or are not tolerated (and then only as *secondary prevention*).

○ If using a beta-blocker preoperatively to reduce cardiac risk, start it well in advance of the surgery and get the patient on a stable dose before surgery.

○ Perform an echocardiogram when considering the diagnosis of heart failure. It will differentiate HFrEF from HFpEF.

○ Perform ECG and administer aspirin 325 mg immediately to all patients presenting with symptoms of acute coronary syndrome.

○ Prescribe ACE inhibitors over ARBs in patients with hypertension, cardiovascular disease, and/or chronic kidney disease.

○ Prescribe statins for all patients with a history of CAD. The 2018 ACC/AHA guideline eliminated an LDL goal, although the 2018 guidelines reinstated them (but these have not been endorsed by AAFP or ACP at the time of publication). The goal is to use high-dose statins in those who are high risk (e.g., history of myocardial infarction).

○ Stop all NSAIDs (except for aspirin) when admitting a patient for possible ACS. NSAIDs increase cardiac risk.

○ Use the CHA_2-DS_2-VASC score when determining the need for anticoagulation in atrial fibrillation. Women with a score of 2 and men with a score of 1 are candidates for anticoagulation.

BIBLIOGRAPHY

Adan V, Crown LA. Diagnosis and treatment of sick sinus syndrome. *Am Fam Physician*. 2003;67(8):1725–1732.

Amsterdam EA, et al. 2014 AHA/ACC Guideline for the management of patients with non–ST-elevation acute coronary syndromes: a report of the American College of Cardiology/American Heart Association Task Force on Practice Guidelines. *J Am Coll Cardiol*. 2014;64(24):e139–e228.

Body R, et al. Do risk factors for chronic coronary heart disease help diagnose acute myocardial infarction in the emergency department. *Ann Emerg Med*. 2007;49:145.

Eagle KA, et al. Perioperative cardiac evaluation for noncardiac surgery update. 2002. Available at: www.acc.org/clinical/guidelines/perio/update/periupdateindex.htm.

Fihn SD, et al. 2012 ACCF/AHA/ACP/AATS/PCNA/SCAI/STS guideline for the diagnosis and management of patients with stable ischemic heart disease: a report of the American College of Cardiology Foundation/American Heart Association Task Force on Practice Guidelines, and the American College of Physicians, American Association for Thoracic Surgery, Preventive Cardiovascular Nurses Association, Society. *J Am Coll Cardiol*. 2012;60(24):e44–e164.

Garty M, et al. Blood transfusion for acute decompensated heart failure—friend or foe? *Am Heart J*. 2009;158:653–658.

Gershon CA, et al. Inter-rater reliability of the HEART score. Acad Emerg Med. 2019 May;26(5):552–555.

Gibbons RJ, et al. Management of patients with chronic stable angina update. Available at: http://www.acc.org/clinical/guidelines/stable/update_index.htm.

Goyle KK, Walling AD. Diagnosing pericarditis. *Am Fam Physician*. 2002;66(9):1695–1702.

Gregoratos G, et al. ACC/AHA/NASPE 2002 Guideline update for implantation of cardiac pacemakers and antiarrhythmia devices. Available at: www.acc.org/clinical/guidelines/pacemaker/incorporated/index.htm.

Harris GD. Heart disease in children. *Prim Care*. 2000;27(3):767–784.

Hebbar AK, Hueston WJ. Management of common arrhythmias: Part I. Supraventricular arrhythmias. *Am Fam Physician*. 2002;65(12):2479–2486.

Hebbar AK, Hueston WJ. Management of common arrhythmias: Part II. Ventricular arrhythmias in special populations. *Am Fam Physician*. 2002;65(12):2491–2496.

James PA, et al. 2014 Evidence-based guideline for the management of high blood pressure in adults. Report from the Panel Members Appointed to the Eighth Joint National Committee (JNC 8). *JAMA*. 2014;311(5):507–520.

January CT, et al. 2014 AHA/ACC/HRS Guideline for the management of patients with atrial fibrillation: executive summary: a report of the American College of Cardiology/American Heart Association Task Force on practice guidelines and the Heart Rhythm Society. *J Am Coll Cardiol*. 2014;64(21):2246–2280.

January CT, et al. 2019 AHA/ACC/HRS Focused update of the 2014 AHA/ACC/HRS guideline for the management of patients with atrial fibrillation: a report of the American College of Cardiology/American Heart Association Task Force on the practice guidelines and the Heart Rhythm Society. *Circulation*. 2019;140:e125–e151.

Laussen PC. Neonates with congenital heart disease. *Curr Opin Pediatr*. 2001;13(3):220–226.

Moodie DS. Diagnosis and management of congenital heart disease in the adult. *Cardiol Rev*. 2001;9(5):276–281.

Nishimura RA, et al. 2014 AHA/ACC Guideline for the management of patients with valvular heart disease: a report of the American College of Cardiology/American Heart Association Task Force on Practice Guidelines. *J Am Coll Cardiol*. 2014;63(22):e57–e185.

O'Gara PT et al. 2013 ACCF/AHA Guideline for the management of ST-elevation myocardial infarction: a report of the American College of Cardiology Foundation/

American Heart Association Task Force on Practice Guidelines. *J Am Coll Cardiol.* 2013;61(4):e78–e140.

Stone NJ, et al. 2013 ACC/AHA guideline on the treatment of blood cholesterol to reduce atherosclerotic cardiovascular risk in adults. *J Am Coll Cardiol.* 2014;63(25 Pt B):2889–2934.

Taylor AL, et al. Combination of isosorbide dinitrate and hydralazine in blacks with heart failure. *N Engl J Med.* 2004;351(20):2049–2057.

Wilson PW, et al. C-reactive protein and risk of cardiovascular disease in men and women from the Framingham Heart Study. *Arch Intern Med.* 2005;165(21):2473–2478.

Yancy CW, et al. 2013 ACCF/AHA guideline for the management of heart failure: a report of the American College of Cardiology Foundation/American Heart Association Task Force on Practice Guidelines. *J Am Coll Cardiol.* 2013;62(16):e147–e239.

Pulmonology

Rachel R. Butler

3

► **CASE 3.1**

A 42-year-old male who works in a hog confinement area presents to your office complaining of cough, fever, wheeze, and dyspnea. He and some other workers were cleaning the confinement area with high-pressure hoses (which aerosolized hog waste, yum), and they *all* developed the same symptoms, which started between 4 and 8 hours after work. On examination, he is febrile with a respiratory rate of 28. He is able to talk in complete sentences. There are slight crackles when you auscultate the lungs. His chest x-ray is normal.

Question 3.1.1 **The most likely diagnosis is:**
A) Farmer's lung (hypersensitivity pneumonitis)
B) Organic dust toxicity syndrome
C) Reactive airway disease
D) Hydrogen sulfide poisoning
E) Bronchiolitis obliterans

Answer 3.1.1 **The correct answer is "B."** Organic dust toxicity syndrome (ODTS) occurs when moldy or decomposed hay and other organic material (such as hog manure) is moved. Endotoxins are aerosolized and inhaled, leading to the symptoms. The tip off here is that everyone on the job site was affected. Since hypersensitivity pneumonitis ("A") is specific to the individual, generally only one worker at the site will have symptoms. Compared with ODTS, hypersensitivity pneumonitis may present with an abnormal chest x-ray with micronodular or reticular opacities. "C" is incorrect because everyone is involved, which would be highly unusual with reactive airway disease. "D" is not correct. Hydrogen sulfide poisoning presents as a toxic pneumonitis with pulmonary edema, dyspnea, hypoxia, and loss of consciousness. Hydrogen sulfide also acts as a direct cellular toxin that binds to cytochrome oxidase system, similar to cyanide. In addition, hydrogen sulfide exposure comes from cleaning manure pits (as anyone in Iowa would know). Finally, "E," bronchiolitis obliterans, is a chronic illness rather than an acute

one. Of note, there is a strong association between ODTS and subsequent development of chronic bronchitis.

Question 3.1.2 **Appropriate treatment for this patient includes:**
A) Antibiotics
B) Intubation and mechanical ventilation
C) Supportive care
D) A and B
E) A and C

Answer 3.1.2 **The correct answer is "C."** Supportive care is the usual treatment of ODTS. Antibiotics are not needed because the syndrome is mediated by endotoxins rather than direct infection. "B" is incorrect because this patient is not in significant respiratory distress.

HELPFUL TIP:
Remember that other work exposures can cause fever, including "metal fume fever" which is caused by zinc. Patients are febrile by the end of the work week, improved over the weekend, only to reoccur in the middle of the next work week.

Keep reading to get to the objectives for this case.

► **CASE 3.2**

This patient's brother, who also works on a farm, notes that every time he unloads hay he has fever, cough, dyspnea, and sputum production. It tends to resolve in 2 to 5 days but reoccurs when he is re-exposed to hay. Does he wear a mask? Well, no. He would look silly and the guys would poke fun at him. Besides, none of the other workers on the farm are affected, and they are beginning to wonder if he is malingering. His examination reveals tachypnea and fine rales. There is no

wheezing present. A chest radiograph shows bilateral interstitial opacities.

Question 3.2.1 The most likely cause of this patient's
symptoms is:
A) *Thermoactinomyces candidus* (an actinomyces species)
B) *T. sacchari*
C) *Botrytis cinerea*
D) *Cryptostroma corticale*
E) None of the above

Answer 3.2.1 The correct answer is "A." This patient presents with classic symptoms of hypersensitivity pneumonitis or,
in this case, "Farmer's lung." This is caused by exposure to the
Actinomyces species. Acute findings include fever, chills, cough,
dyspnea, and chest tightness. X-ray findings are variable and
tend to be transient early on in the disease. High-resolution
chest computed tomography (CT) should be obtained, which
commonly shows centrilobular micronodules and ground-glass
opacification in a mid-to-upper zone predominance. "B," *T. sacchari*, is involved in hypersensitivity pneumonitis from sugarcane
(so-called Bagassosis). "C," *Botrytis cinerea*, is involved in hypersensitivity pneumonitis from grapes (so-called Spatlese lung).
Finally, "D," *Cryptostroma corticale*, is involved in "Maple bark
stripper's lung," another type of hypersensitivity pneumonitis—
though why anyone would want to strip maple bark is beyond us.

Question 3.2.2 The correct treatment for this patient with
Farmer's lung includes:
A) Antibiotics
B) Inhaled steroids
C) Oral steroids
D) Leukotriene inhibitors
E) Bronchoalveolar lavage (BAL)

Answer 3.2.2 The correct answer is "C." Oral steroids are effective in the treatment of hypersensitivity pneumonitis. Neither
antibiotics ("A") nor inhaled steroids ("B") are of any benefit.
"E," bronchoalveolar lavage, is not a treatment. However, it can
be used as a diagnostic tool. One would expect to see lymphocytes on BAL.

Question 3.2.3 You would advise this patient to:
A) Get a new job
B) Apply for disability
C) Use a respirator at work and avoid exposure to this toxin if
possible
D) Sue the employer
E) Take up worm farming or monoculture in rhubarb

Answer 3.2.3 The correct answer is "C." Wearing an appropriate respirator at work can be beneficial. Avoiding exposure is
even better. As for the other answers, you are a doctor not a
lawyer or career counselor. Stick with what you know!

The patient is unable to change jobs or wear a respirator because it itches and he "keeps forgetting it." But he's

persistent (or brave or thickheaded or unable to learn a new
skill), and keeps farming. Three years later, he returns with a
chronic cough, weight loss, dyspnea, fatigue, and clubbing of
the fingers.

Question 3.2.4 Further evaluation will most likely reveal:
A) Bronchogenic carcinoma
B) Air space disease (e.g., a pneumonia-like picture)
C) Decreased DLCO (**D**iffusing capacity of the **L**ungs for **CO**
[Carbon Monoxide])
D) Markedly abnormal bronchoalveolar lavage (BAL) with
lymphocytosis
E) Obstructive changes on pulmonary function testing

Answer 3.2.4 The correct answer is "C." Hypersensitivity pneumonitis can become chronic if exposure is not limited. In these
cases, patients will generally have systemic complaints such as
fatigue and possibly weight loss. Fever will be absent *as may a
history of prior episodes of acute hypersensitivity* pneumonitis.
Dyspnea and clubbing of the fingers are also generally noted,
reflecting chronic pulmonary disease. Along with this finding,
pulmonary fibrosis can occur and the DLCO may be decreased.
"A" is incorrect. Hypersensitivity pneumonitis does not lead to
lung cancer. "B" is incorrect. While acute hypersensitivity pneumonitis causes an alveolitis, chronic hypersensitivity pneumonitis
causes pulmonary fibrosis with an occasional micronodular pattern. "D" is incorrect. BAL in chronic hypersensitivity pneumonitis does not contain the markedly elevated lymphocyte count
that is seen with *acute* hypersensitivity pneumonitis. Finally, "E" is
incorrect. One would see a restrictive pattern on pulmonary function testing reflecting the fibrosis and not an obstructive pattern.

HELPFUL TIP:
If you have a patient with recurrent "pneumonia," consider hypersensitivity pneumonitis. It has many causes
in addition to farming, and it is idiopathic up to 25%
of cases.

▶ **Objectives: Did you learn to …**
  • Recognize the clinical presentations of ODTS and
    hypersensitivity pneumonitis?
  • Manage patients with lung disease related to agricultural
    exposures?

 QUICK QUIZ: ASTHMA

**All of the following populations are at increased risk for
developing asthma EXCEPT:**
A) Obese children
B) Female children
C) Children exposed to tobacco
D) Children with atopy
E) City children

The correct answer is "B." Male children have a greater prevalence of asthma. Interestingly, adult women "catch up" so

that there is gender equity in young adulthood. After age 40, the prevalence is higher in females. Of note, frequent respiratory infections seem to be *protective*. There is an inverse association between children living on farms and asthma incidence (another feather in the cap of Iowa). Presumably, this is related to the greater variety of antigen exposure.

▶ CASE 3.3

A 20-year-old woman with no significant past medical history presents with a 2-month history of episodic shortness of breath. These symptoms began with an upper respiratory tract infection. She has fits of coughing and trouble catching her breath with exertion. She states that her breath "sounds like whistles" at times. She tried a friend's albuterol inhaler and an over-the-counter epinephrine inhaler (Primatine... yes, it is back on the market) with some improvement and wonders if she has asthma. On examination, she is breathing comfortably at 16 times per minute and her oxygen saturation is 96% on room air. Her lungs are clear to auscultation, and the remainder of her examination is unremarkable. You want to better categorize this patient's disease.

Question 3.3.1 **Which of the following tests is most appropriate to order now?**
A) Spirometry
B) Chest x-ray
C) Arterial blood gas (ABG)
D) Methacholine challenge
E) Chest CT

Answer 3.3.1 **The correct answer is "A."** Since this patient has symptoms of bronchospasm, spirometry will be essential in determining if there is objective evidence of obstructive lung disease. However, spirometry results are often normal in mild cases of asthma, especially when the patient is asymptomatic. Bronchoprovocation testing, with methacholine or histamine, may be useful in such cases, but should follow basic spirometry. Although chest radiography (x-ray or CT) may reveal an occult process, it is not indicated in otherwise healthy patients with symptoms of bronchospasm. Bacterial pneumonia is a potential precipitant of bronchospasm that may be diagnosed on chest x-ray, but this patient has no constitutional symptoms (like fever) associated with serious bacterial infection. Obtaining an ABG (or better yet a venous blood gas) may be helpful when a patient presents with respiratory distress but certainly not in the office setting.

HELPFUL TIP:
A normal blood gas in a patient with an asthma exacerbation and tachypnea is an ominous sign that signals impending respiratory failure. The carbon dioxide ($PaCO_2$) should be low in a patient with tachypnea. Thus, a normal appearing ABG with a normal carbon dioxide level is an indication of respiratory muscle fatigue and early respiratory failure.

Question 3.3.2 **If this patient has mild asthma, which of the following pulmonary function test results would you expect to find?**
A) Forced vital capacity (FVC) 50% of predicted
B) Forced expiratory volume in 1 second (FEV_1) 100% of predicted
C) FEV_1/FVC ratio <0.7
D) Total lung capacity (TLC) 50% of predicted
E) FEV_1/TLC <0.7

Answer 3.3.2 **The correct answer is "C."** Patients with asthma will have a decreased FEV_1. The FVC may fall as well, but FEV_1 falls first and to a greater degree as the lung becomes obstructed. The ratio of FEV_1/FVC is very sensitive to airflow limitations, and FEV_1/FVC <0.7 (just the raw ratio of the two numbers) is generally considered diagnostic of obstructive airway disease. The rest are incorrect. TLC is not measured by spirometry (which is why "D" and "E" are incorrect); but if it were, TLC may be increased in patients with obstructive airway disease due to air trapping.

Your patient's office spirometry shows the following:
Normal FVC
FEV_1 82% predicted
FEV_1/FVC 0.68

Question 3.3.3 **These findings are most consistent with which of the following?**
A) Normal spirometry
B) Obstructive lung disease
C) End-stage emphysema
D) Interstitial fibrosis
E) Obesity-hypoventilation syndrome

Answer 3.3.3 **The correct answer is "B."** Always go first to the FEV_1/FVC ratio. In this case, it is <0.70, which is suggestive of airway obstruction. The information provided here lacks data regarding DLCO which should be decreased in emphysema, so you could not really differentiate between chronic obstructive pulmonary disease (COPD) and asthma. But this is clearly not end-stage emphysema, so "C" is incorrect. "D" is incorrect. Interstitial fibrosis is generally marked by a restrictive pattern on spirometry and decreased TLC. Both flow rate (e.g., FEV_1) and FVC are decreased in interstitial lung diseases but in proportion to each other. Thus, the FEV_1/FVC is often normal or elevated. See Table 3-1 for more on interpreting spirometry results.

Six months after you discuss her findings and prescribe inhaled beta-agonist therapy, she returns with complaints of continued wheezing and difficulty breathing. Her symptoms are brought on by cold weather and exercise and she uses her inhaler two times per week or less. She woke up two nights over the last 6 months with shortness of breath and coughing. Her albuterol still works for these symptoms, but she finds them bothersome and asks, "Why haven't I gotten over this?"

TABLE 3-1   GENERAL INTERPRETATION OF PULMONARY FUNCTION TEST RESULTS COMPARING OBSTRUCTIVE AND RESTRICTIVE DISEASE (MAY NOT BE APPLICABLE FOR ALL FORMS OF LUNG DISEASE)

PFT Result	Obstructive Pattern	Restrictive Pattern
FEV_1	<80% predicted	Decreased in proportion to loss of lung volume
FVC	Decreased	<80% predicted
FEV_1/FVC	<0.7	>0.7
FEF25–75%	<60% predicted	Decreased in proportion to loss of lung volume
TLC	Normal or elevated	Decreased
DLCO	Normal or elevated in asthma; normal or decreased in COPD	Decreased in intrinsic restrictive lung disease; normal in neuromuscular or musculoskeletal restrictive disease

COPD, chronic obstructive pulmonary disease; DLCO, diffusing capacity of the lung for carbon monoxide; FEF_{25-75}, forced expiratory flow at 25–75% vital capacity; FEV_1, forced expiratory volume in 1 second; FVC, forced vital capacity; TLC, total lung capacity.

Question 3.3.4 How would you categorize this patient's respiratory state?

A) Intermittent asthma
B) Mild persistent asthma
C) Moderate persistent asthma
D) Severe persistent asthma
E) Recurrent lower respiratory tract infections

Answer 3.3.4 **The correct answer is "A."** As of 2019—and incredibly—there have been no updates to the NHLBI National Asthma Education and Prevention Program (NAEPP) 2007 guidelines. According to those guidelines (Table 3-2), your patient meets the criteria for intermittent asthma. In such patients, mild symptoms correspond to an FEV_1 that is greater than 80% predicted—not to be confused with the FEV_1/FVC

TABLE 3-2   CATEGORIZATION OF SEVERITY OF ASTHMA AND STEPWISE APPROACH TO THERAPY

Determine Severity When Initiating Therapy

Components of Severity		Classification of Asthma Severity (≥12 years of age)			
		Intermittent	Persistent		
			Mild	Moderate	Severe
Impairment (Normal FEV_1/FVC)	Symptoms	≤2 days/week	>2 days/week but not daily	Daily	Throughout the day
	Nighttime awakenings	≤2×/month	3–4×/month	>1×/week but not nightly	Often 7×/week
	SABA[a] use for symptom control (not prevention of EIB[b])	≤2 days/week	>2 days/week but not daily and more than 1× on any day	Daily	Several times per day
	Interference with normal activity	None	Minor limitation	Some limitation	Extremely limited
	Lung function	• Normal EFV_1 between exacerbations • EFV_1 > 80% predicted • EFV_1/FVC normal	• EFV_1 > 80% predicted • EFV_1/FVC normal	• EFV_1 > 60% but <80% predicted • EFV_1/FVC reduced 5%	• EFV_1 < 60% predicted • EFV_1/FVC reduced > 5%
Risk	Exacerbations requiring oral systemic corticosteroids	0–1/year	≥2/year		
		Consider severity and interval since last exacerbation Frequency and severity may fluctuate over time for patients in any severity category			
		Relative annual risk of exacerbations may be related to FEV_1			
Recommended step for initiating therapy See bar chart in Figure 3–1 for treatment steps		Step 1	Step 2	Step 3 and consider short course of oral systemic corticosteroids	Step 4 or 5
		In 2–6 weeks, evaluate level of asthma control that is achieved and adjust therapy accordingly.			

[a]SABA, short-acting inhaled beta-2 agonist.
[b]EIB, exercise-induced bronchospasm.
Reproduced from Guidelines for the Diagnosis and Management of Asthma. National Asthma Education and Prevention Program, National Institutes of Health. Expert Panel Report 3, pages 305–310, 343–345. http://www.nhlbi.nih.gov/guidelines/asthma.

ratio which diagnoses obstructive lung disease but is not used to categorize severity.

Question 3.3.5 Which of the following is most appropriate for this patient given that she has intermittent asthma?
A) Add theophylline
B) Add montelukast
C) Continue albuterol as needed
D) Schedule albuterol every 4 hours
E) Prednisone 5 mg daily

Answer 3.3.5 **The correct answer is "C."** As already discussed, this patient appears to have intermittent asthma. She is in no respiratory distress, is oxygenating normally, and is still responding well to albuterol by her report. Although there is some debate about the role of inhaled steroids in intermittent asthma, the NAEPP and most experts do not recommend their use. Oral prednisone is certainly not indicated in this case. She should be continued on a short-acting inhaled beta-2 agonist, such as albuterol, without the addition of another medication. "D" is incorrect. Scheduled albuterol actually yields *less effective* symptom control than does PRN use. As to "A," a pox on those still prescribing theophylline.

Your patient goes on to develop more frequent recurrent symptoms, such that she is using her albuterol inhaler more than three times per week, although her nighttime symptoms are rare.

Question 3.3.6 Which medication is the most appropriate next step in treating this patient's asthma?
A) Inhaled triamcinolone
B) Inhaled salmeterol
C) Inhaled cromolyn sodium
D) Inhaled ipratropium
E) Oral montelukast

Answer 3.3.6 **The correct answer is "A."** Your patient now has mild persistent asthma and should be started on an inhaled steroid. When asthma symptoms become more persistent (i.e., when they occur >2 days per week or the patient awakens from sleep >2 times per month), the inflammatory component of the disease should be addressed while simultaneously treating the bronchospastic component with short-acting beta-2 agonists. Anti-inflammatory drugs are the mainstay of chronic asthma therapy, and inhaled corticosteroids are the most efficacious with the fewest side effects. Although ipratropium, cromolyn sodium, and montelukast have a place in asthma treatment, none of these medications is a first-line agent. Ipratropium is an anti-cholinergic that works through its bronchodilatory effects, while cromolyn sodium is a mast cell stabilizer. Montelukast is a leukotriene inhibitor. The long-acting inhaled beta-2 agonists, such as salmeterol, are only recommended at Steps 3 and higher of persistent asthma control (Table 3-2, Fig. 3-1; NHLBI recommendations, 2007).

 HELPFUL TIP:
Remember the "rule of twos": any patient who has >2 asthma exacerbations per week requiring rescue medication or who wakes with nocturnal symptoms >2 times per month should be on an anti-inflammatory drug, preferably an inhaled corticosteroid. Asthma classification and treatment has gotten ridiculously complex. You

Intermittent Asthma	Persistent Asthma: Daily Medication
	Consult with asthma specialist if Step 4 care or higher is required. Consider consultation at Step 3.

Step 1
Preferred
SABA* PRN

Step 2
Preferred
Low-dose ICS†
Alternative
Cromolyn, LTRA,‡ nedocromil, or theophylline

Step 3
Preferred
Low-dose ICS + LABA§
OR
Medium-dose ICS
Alternative
Low-dose ICS + either LTRA, theophylline, or zileuton

Step 4
Preferred
Medium-dose ICS + LABA
Alternative
Medium-dose ICS + either LTRA, theophylline, or zileuton

Step 5
Preferred
High-dose ICS + LABA
AND
Consider omalizumab for patients who have allergies

Step 6
Preferred
High-dose ICS + LABA + oral corticosteroid
AND
Consider omalizumab for patients who have allergies

Step up if needed (first, check adherence, environmental control, and comorbid conditions)
Assess control
Step down if possible (and asthma is well controlled at least 3 months)

Patient Education, Environmental Control, and Management of Comorbidities at Each Step
Consider subcutaneous allergen immunotherapy for patients who have allergic asthma at Steps 2 through 4

Quick-Relief Medication for All Patients
• SABA as needed for symptoms. Intensity of treatment depends on severity of symptoms: up to 3 treatments at 20-minute intervals as needed. Short course of oral systemic corticosteroids may be needed
• Use of SABA >2 days a week for symptom relief (not prevention of EIBⱽ) generally Indicates inadequate control and the need to step up treatment

* Short-acting inhaled beta₂-agonist.   † Inhaled corticosteroid.   ‡ Leukotriene receptor antagonist.   ‡ Long-acting inhaled beta₂-agonist.   ⱽ Exercise-incluced bronchospasm.

FIGURE 3-1. NHLBI recommended stepwise approach to asthma therapy.

may want to review this Asthma Care Quick Reference revised in September 2012 located at https://www.nhlbi.nih.gov/files/docs/guidelines/asthma_qrg.pdf.

HELPFUL TIP:
The leukotriene inhibitors (e.g., montelukast, zafirlukast) add little or nothing to maximized inhaled steroid therapy. In fact, they are clearly not as effective as inhaled steroids. They should be used only once a patient has failed inhaled steroids and should be added to the regimen; they are not a substitute for inhaled steroids.

Your patient does quite well over the next year, having very few exacerbations. During one of her visits, you note slightly edematous nasal mucosa and nasal polyps. You prescribe intranasal steroids. Then, one night when you are on call, she comes in severely dyspneic with audible wheezing. She talks in two- or three-word phrases. She reports a headache today, which she treated with aspirin (something she never takes, but a friend gave it to her thinking it was acetaminophen). Her asthma attack started about an hour after the aspirin dose. She has been otherwise well. She denies fever, rhinorrhea, nasal congestion, and sore throat. Her respiratory rate is 40, heart rate 120 bpm, and oxygen saturation 88% on room air. She has poor air movement on auscultation of her lung fields.

Question 3.3.7 Which of the following is the most likely reason for this patient's acute exacerbation of asthma?
A) Viral upper respiratory infection (URI)
B) Sinusitis
C) Noncompliance with inhaled albuterol
D) Sensitivity to aspirin
E) Noncompliance with nasal steroids

Answer 3.3.7 The correct answer is "D." It is likely that this patient has aspirin sensitivity. Up to 10% of adults with asthma have the clinical triad of asthma, aspirin sensitivity, and nasal polyposis. Patients with asthma should be warned about the potential for exacerbations resulting from consumption of aspirin and nonsteroidal anti-inflammatory drugs (NSAIDs). The drug-induced bronchial constriction caused by these medications can have an abrupt onset with severe symptoms. Patients with aspirin sensitivity can be desensitized with daily administration of small amounts of aspirin, but this should be done carefully with close supervision. Although viral URIs frequently cause exacerbations of asthma, your patient did not report antecedent symptoms of such an infection. Further discussion of the treatment of an acute asthma exacerbation can be found in Chapter 1, "Emergency Medicine."

After a brief hospitalization, your patient recovers nicely. Prior to this incident involving aspirin, she had been free of exacerbations for about a month.

Question 3.3.8 In addition to a short course of oral steroids, which of the following medication regimens do you prescribe for this patient with *aspirin sensitive* asthma at discharge?
A) Inhaled triamcinolone and inhaled albuterol as a "rescue"
B) Inhaled triamcinolone, oral montelukast, and inhaled albuterol as a "rescue"
C) Oral montelukast and inhaled albuterol as a "rescue"
D) Inhaled albuterol as a "rescue"
E) Inhaled salmeterol and inhaled triamcinolone

Answer 3.3.8 The correct answer is "B." Leukotriene inhibitors (e.g., montelukast, zafirlukast) have demonstrated effectiveness in reducing symptoms and improving peak flow in patients with **aspirin sensitive asthma**. Leukotriene inhibitors should be used only in asthma patients who are already using a corticosteroid inhaler—or those who cannot tolerate inhaled corticosteroid therapy. Therefore, "C" is not an appropriate choice. "D" is incorrect because there is no anti-inflammatory drug. Although "E" offers an anti-inflammatory agent, there is no rescue inhaler, and patients with asthma must always have access to a short-acting inhaled bronchodilator.

HELPFUL TIP:
Other NSAIDs have been implicated in "aspirin-exacerbated" asthma. The theory is that there is an imbalance between pro- and anti-inflammatory mediators that is exacerbated acutely by COX-1 inhibition.

Question 3.3.9 Which of the following medications, when used alone as maintenance therapy in persistent asthma, is associated with an increased risk of asthma-related mortality?
A) Inhaled fluticasone
B) Inhaled salmeterol
C) Oral zafirlukast
D) Oral prednisone

Answer 3.3.9 The correct answer is "B." Inhaled salmeterol, when used alone as a controller agent for asthma, has been associated with a two- to fourfold increase in the risk of death related to asthma or other respiratory conditions. Thus, the Food and Drug Administration (FDA) has mandated a "black box" warning be applied to salmeterol-containing products. It is not known whether inhaled steroid therapy is protective, but NHLBI/NAEPP guidelines recommend adding long-acting inhaled beta-agonists only after inhaled steroids are already in use.

HELPFUL TIP:
The importance of patient education in asthma cannot be overstated. Patients diagnosed with asthma should receive a written plan of action, detailing when to increase beta-2 agonist use and when to start an oral steroid. While there is no proven benefit to home peak

flow monitoring, this may serve to get patients more involved in management of their illness. A home peak flow meter can be used as a part of the educational process and to enhance communication between the healthcare practitioner and the patient.

HELPFUL TIP:
Asthma research is expanding the therapies available for severe asthmatics. For patients with severe asthma, frequent exacerbations despite guideline-based therapy, and an eosinophilic phenotype, new add-on therapies include anti-interleukin (IL)-5 antibodies (e.g., mepolizumab [Nucala] or reslizumab [Cinqair]), the anti-IL-5 receptor antibody benralizumab (Fasenra), or the anti-IL4 subunit alpha antibody dupilumab (Dupixent). Of note, these therapies are administered subcutaneously or intravenously and should be done in conjunction with an asthma expert.

▶ **Objectives: Did you learn to …**
- Identify triggers of bronchospasm?
- Evaluate symptoms of wheezing and dyspnea?
- Classify asthma?
- Prescribe appropriate medications for intermittent and mild persistent asthma?
- Describe the triad of asthma, aspirin sensitivity, and nasal polyposis?

 QUICK QUIZ: SPIROMETRY

A 60-year-old female who smokes two packs of cigarettes per day complains of shortness of breath and fullness in her throat. You obtain spirometry in the office and the results are given along with the flow/volume loop (Fig. 3-2).

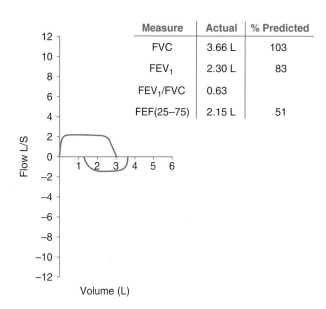

Measure	Actual	% Predicted
FVC	3.66 L	103
FEV$_1$	2.30 L	83
FEV$_1$/FVC	0.63	
FEF(25–75)	2.15 L	51

FIGURE 3-2. Spirometry results for patient in "Quick Quiz: Spirometry".

How do you interpret these findings?
A) Chronic obstructive lung disease
B) Restrictive lung disease
C) Fixed upper airway obstruction
D) Poor patient effort
E) Within normal range

The correct answer is "C." The flattened flow/volume loop is consistent with a fixed upper airway obstruction (e.g., laryngeal mass lesion). In this case, FEV$_1$ and the FEV$_1$/FVC ratio may look like other obstructive diseases (i.e., asthma, COPD), so you have to look at the flow/volume loop (always a good idea). Some examples of flow/volume loops are given below (Fig. 3-3).

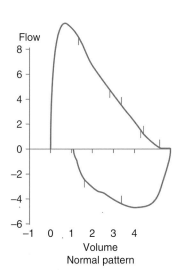

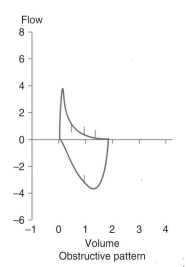

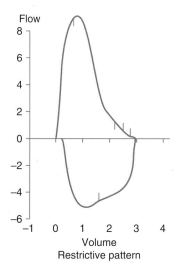

FIGURE 3-3. Typical spirometry results in normal lungs compared to lungs with obstructive or restrictive disease.

▶ CASE 3.4

You are seeing a 65-year-old male in the emergency department (ED) where he presented with complaint of increasing shortness of breath. He has obvious difficulty breathing and cannot speak in full sentences. However, you are able to elicit that he has been having increasing respiratory problems over the last 3 to 4 days. He has known COPD with FEV$_1$ of "less than one" (normal FEV$_1$ is about 4 L for a 50-year-old male and 3 L for a 50-year-old female; for calculations based on age, etc., see www.hankconsulting.com/RefCal.html *or* http://www.webcitation.org/75KGIXvSb). He has been using his inhalers much more than usual but with minimal improvement. He has smoked one pack per day since age 18 (but proudly points out he quit 2 days ago) and has a past medical history of high cholesterol, obesity, and hypertension.

On examination, he has a respiratory rate of 26 to 28, heart rate of 100 bpm, blood pressure of 130/90 mm Hg, and temperature of 37.7°C. His O$_2$ saturation is 84% on room air. On auscultation, you do not appreciate much due to his body habitus, but you still manage to hear some wheezing. He has a normal cardiac examination and no lower extremity edema.

Question 3.4.1 What is the next best step to help this patient?
A) Perform emergent endotracheal intubation
B) Administer supplemental O$_2$ via nasal cannula
C) Administer methyloprednisolone (Solu-Medrol), 1 g IV
D) Start antibiotics IV
E) Obtain a chest x-ray

Answer 3.4.1 **The correct answer is "B."** This patient is hypoxic, and your first priority should be to improve his oxygenation. There exists a theory that oxygenating patients with COPD will suppress their respiratory drive. The classical teaching (mostly incorrect) is that COPD causes a switch from carbon dioxide levels driving respiration to oxygen levels driving respiration. While this may be partly true, further study has suggested that the main reason COPD patients are at risk of worsening hypercapnia is due to loss of hypoxic pulmonary vasoconstriction and worsening ventilation–perfusion mismatch that occurs with excess oxygen delivery. Regardless of that, you need to first worry about this patient's oxygenation. He is not going to thrive with an 85% O$_2$ saturation.

"A" is incorrect. The patient is protecting his airway and you have not attempted improving his oxygenation with less invasive methods yet. Administering steroids, IV or PO, will have no immediate effect on his respiratory status. In fact, IV steroids *might* be worse than PO steroids (there is question of whether higher IV doses cause immunosuppression and subclinical myopathy; see *Am J Respir Crit Care Med.* 2014;189:1052). Antibiotics and a chest x-ray may be reasonable, but with low O$_2$ saturations, your priority is to quickly improve your patient's oxygen status.

HELPFUL TIP:
Patients admitted to a hospital for a COPD exacerbation (characterized by increased dyspnea, sputum production, and sputum purulence) should be treated with corticosteroids (oral prednisone is equivalent to IV steroids), an antibiotic that covers respiratory tract pathogens (numerous antibiotics are acceptable, including azithromycin, moxifloxacin, doxycycline, among others) and inhaled bronchodilators. Supportive therapy with supplemental oxygen and ventilation is often required as well.

Question 3.4.2 When initiating supplemental oxygen by nasal cannula, you instruct the nurse to keep the patient's oxygen saturation:
A) Between 96% and 100%
B) Between 90% and 95%
C) Between 85% and 89%
D) At whatever saturation he looks most comfortable

Answer 3.4.2 **The correct answer is "B."** The primary goal of supplemental oxygen is to reduce the risk of tissue hypoxia. Maintaining oxygen saturations above 90% (or PaO$_2$ 60–65 mm) will ensure tissue oxygenation. Higher oxygen saturations may result in CO$_2$ retention and hypercapnia, as noted earlier. Also, aiming at 100% with excessive levels of O$_2$ supplementation takes away an important patient assessment parameter because now you cannot tell easily whether his O$_2$ needs are going up or down. "D" is of special note. Patients with COPD who look comfortable may be developing hypercapnia and CO$_2$ narcosis. Thus, while comfort is a goal, it may not be the best judge of clinical status in patients with COPD exacerbations. To assess CO$_2$ levels, you will need an ABG or VBG.

Your patient is now on 5 liters per minute (LPM) of oxygen via nasal cannula. You obtain an ABG: pH 7.29, PCO$_2$ 74 mm Hg, PO$_2$ 58 mm Hg. The patient is awake and alert but says that he still feels "like dirt." He remains tachypneic, in obvious respiratory distress, with a respiratory rate of 28. Albuterol and ipratropium are given via nebulizer.

Question 3.4.3 What is the best next step?
A) Clearly, he is failing therapy—emergently intubate
B) Increase his O$_2$ to 100% via face mask
C) Initiate noninvasive positive pressure ventilation (e.g., BiPAP)
D) Start IV antibiotics
E) Obtain a chest CT with PE protocol

Answer 3.4.3 **The correct answer is "C."** This patient is retaining CO$_2$ despite tachypnea and is in impending respiratory failure. He is also not oxygenating well despite low-flow oxygen. Noninvasive positive pressure support (BIPAP) can relieve hypercapnia and improve oxygenation by decreasing work of breathing without requiring intubation and its associated morbidity. Often IV antibiotics ("D") are used for empiric therapy in severe exacerbations of COPD, but again, improving the respiratory status comes first. He is hypoxic, but his main problem is CO_2 retention—increasing his O_2 delivery will not alleviate that (thus, "B" is incorrect). Although his respiratory status is tenuous, he is not in imminent respiratory failure, and intubation ("A") is not warranted at this time. Chest CT ("E") can rule out a PE in this hypoxic patient and may confirm COPD changes including emphysema, but will greatly delay treatment and would not change your immediate course of action—in other words, you would be barking up the wrong bronchial tree.

After several hours of noninvasive positive pressure ventilation, your patient is doing well, and he is transferred out of the intensive care unit (ICU). When you see him the next day his medications include inhaled bronchodilators, ceftriaxone, azithromycin, and prednisone. A chest x-ray shows no evidence of infiltrate. He is weaned from the positive pressure support to oxygen by nasal cannula and then, 2 days later, to room air. At discharge, he appears comfortable, with a respiratory rate of 14 and an oxygen saturation of 92% on room air.

Question 3.4.4 **As you write his home-going prescriptions, what would be the best ongoing treatment for him?**
A) Inhaled long-acting beta-agonist (LABA) + albuterol
B) Inhaled steroid + albuterol
C) Inhaled steroid + LABA + albuterol as needed
D) Albuterol
E) Albuterol and theophylline

Answer 3.4.4 **The correct answer is "C."** This is a bit tricky, but due to the severity of his exacerbation, "C" is the best choice. Compared to patients with asthma, where long-acting bronchodilators are not indicated as first-line therapy, COPD patients have a clear symptomatic benefit from long-acting bronchodilators. The two available choices are anticholinergics (LAMAs, or long-acting muscarinic agents [e.g., tiotropium, umeclidinium]

or LABAs [e.g., salmeterol or formoterol]). Either choice is fine, and some prefer a LAMA as first line. An inhaled steroid does not modify the long-term decline in FEV_1 in patients with COPD. However, it will reduce the frequency of exacerbations and thus improve health status. Current guidelines recommend addition of inhaled steroids with $FEV_1 < 50\%$ predicted and frequent exacerbations (e.g., 3 exacerbations in the last 3 years). See Table 3-3 for more on guideline-directed treatment. It is important to recognize there are adverse effects of inhaled corticosteroids (ICS) therapy including dysphonia, skin bruising, and oral candidiasis. In addition, ICS therapy may increase the incidence of pneumonia and cataracts, as well as diminish bone density. Therefore, for patients with COPD, other therapies are recommended (bronchodilators, smoking cessation, pulmonary rehabilitation), if possible, prior to ICS therapy. For patients who have persistent symptoms, repeated exacerbations, or severe exacerbations despite optimal long-acting bronchodilator regiment, ICS therapy is recommended.

HELPFUL TIP:
We hate cats. So, what is this CAT and MMRC deal with the GOLD criteria? These are two ways of gauging the severity of COPD. A handy pocket card for the MMRC Dyspnea Scale and CAT scale (COPD Assessment Test) can be found at https://mdspiro.com/image/data/articles/COPD%20Pocket%20Consultant.pdf. These should be used periodically to assess how your patient is doing.

HELPFUL TIP:
American Thoracic Society (ATS) guidelines categorize obstructive airway disease based on the percent predicted FEV_1 of the patient. The response to bronchodilator is also categorized by ATS. To state that there was significant response to bronchodilator, there has to be an increase of *both* 200 cc and an increase of at least 12% in the FEV_1.

TABLE 3-3 GLOBAL INITIATIVE FOR OBSTRUCTIVE LUNG DISEASE (GOLD) COPD TREATMENT GUIDE

	GOLD COPD Treatment Guidelines			
Type of COPD	Exac/yr	FEV1	MMRC Score or CAT Score	Treatment
A	≤1	FEV1 ≥80%	0–1 and CAT <10	SABA PRN
B	≤1	FEV1 50%–80%	≥2 and CAT <10	LABA or LAMA→ combine if still symptomatic or add SABA
C	≥2	FEV1 30%–50%	0–1 and CAT <10	ICS + LABA +/or LAMA
D	≥2	FEV1 <30%	≥2 and CAT >10	ICS + LABA or LAMA or if FEV1 <50% + chronic bronchitis roflumilast **or** if former smoker azithromycin 250 mg/day

CAT, COPD Assessment Test; Exac/yr, exacerbations per year; ICS, inhaled corticosteroid; LABA, long-acting beta agonist; LAMA, long-acting muscarinic agent; MMRC, dyspnea scale; SABA, short-acting beta agonist. See https://goldcopd.org/gold-reports/ for more details.

Holding his inhalers and smiling toothlessly, your patient asks, "Which of these is going to keep me alive—just in case I can't afford them all?"

Question 3.4.5 Which of the following medication regimens has demonstrated decreased mortality in the treatment of stable COPD?
A) Inhaled tiotropium (LAMA)
B) Inhaled salmeterol (LABA)
C) Inhaled ipratropium
D) Inhaled corticosteroid
E) None of the above

Answer 3.4.5 The correct answer is "E." Aside from oxygen, no medical therapy has clearly demonstrated a mortality benefit for stable COPD. Again refer to Table 3-3 for stage of COPD and appropriate treatment. Another therapy to consider in advanced COPD is pulmonary rehabilitation (PR). While having no definite effect on survival, PR improves dyspnea and quality-of-life scores while reducing the number of hospitalizations and days in hospital. Also, there are oral phosphodiesterase inhibitors (e.g., roflumilast [Daliresp]) for *severe* COPD. As you probably already know, your authors are curmudgeons who don't like anything new. *But roflumilast is particularly on our bad list*. It increases FEV_1 by 45 mL over placebo. It has no effect on quality of life and exacerbations are 1.3/year with placebo and 1.2/year with roflumilast. It also causes diarrhea and depression/suicidality. Nonetheless, you should know about it. Another therapy for COPD patients with recurrent exacerbations despite optimal therapy is chronic azithromycin, which may reduce the frequency of exacerbations (*Int J Chron Obstruct Pulmon Dis.* 2018;13:3813–3829). However, this should be avoided in patients with a long QT interval or if there are major concerns about hearing loss. This therapy needs to be carefully considered as studies have revealed that during 5 days of azithromycin therapy, there was a small absolute increase in cardiovascular deaths among patients with high baseline risk of cardiovascular disease (*N Engl J Med.* 2012;366:1881–1890).

> **HELPFUL TIP:**
> Note that inhaled steroids should be used in those patients in group C or D (previously severe to very severe) COPD based on the Global Initiative for Obstructive Lung Disease (GOLD) guidelines. There is no benefit in patient group A or B (previously mild–moderate COPD) and there is a downside (an increase in pneumonia).

Later that year, the same patient gets admitted to the hospital for community-acquired pneumonia. During his stay in the hospital, the hospitalist orders a CT chest "to rule out other things." The patient recovers from his infection and returns to you with the CD of his CT chest images. The reading of the CT chest describes a 2-cm pulmonary nodule in the right upper lobe along with extensive subcarinal lymphadenopathy.

Question 3.4.6 What is the next best step in management of this patient?
A) Repeat CT chest in 3 months
B) Repeat CT chest in 6 months
C) Refer for bronchoscopy with endobronchial ultrasound-guided biopsy
D) Refer to an oncologist
E) Refer for a mediastinoscopy

Answer 3.4.6 The correct answer is "C." This patient probably has a malignant disease and tissue is needed to either diagnose it or rule it out (see more later in this chapter). Bronchoscopy with endobronchial ultrasound (EBUS) guided fine-needle biopsies is a minimally invasive procedure that can relatively safely obtain a tissue sample for the pathologist. There is good evidence that EBUS has high sensitivity and specificity compared with PET scanning. "A" and "B" are incorrect as this patient has a nodule that is larger than 1 cm along with mediastinal lymphadenopathy. This needs to be worked up and cannot wait 3 to 6 months. "D" is incorrect. Your patient will likely need to see an oncologist, but you need to first provide a tissue diagnosis. "E," mediastinoscopy, would likely provide you with the diagnosis, but it is a far more invasive procedure than bronchoscopy and carries higher mortality and morbidity.

> **HELPFUL TIP:**
> It turns out that up to **half** of patients **treated** for COPD don't actually have it. Sad but true. Check PFTs to confirm the diagnosis (*Chest.* 2015;147(2):369–376).

Your patient returns with increasing dyspnea now at rest. His biopsy was negative. Despite both of you being blue in the face, he has not quit smoking.

Question 3.4.7 Criteria for the use of continuous low-flow oxygen in those with COPD include all of the following EXCEPT:
A) PO_2 <55 mm Hg
B) Oxygen saturation <88%
C) PO_2 of <59 mm Hg with evidence of cor pulmonale
D) Episodic sleep apnea-related desaturations at night

Answer 3.4.7 The correct answer is "D." Episodic sleep apnea–related oxygen desaturations, while a cause for concern and amenable to treatment (e.g., CPAP), are not one of the criteria for the use of continuous low-flow oxygen. The other choices are correct. "C" deserves some special attention. Evidence of cor pulmonale can include "p-pulmonale" on ECG, peripheral edema, or a hematocrit >55%.

Question 3.4.8 Concerning hypoxemic patients with COPD (resting oxygen saturation of <88%), which of the following is true?
A) Patients on continuous, low-flow O_2 become oxygen dependent and cannot function without it

B) Continuous low-flow O_2 used for at least 8 hours a day helps to reverse pulmonary hypertension

C) Concurrent smoking is a contraindication to the prescribing continuous low-flow home O_2 because patients are spontaneously combusting right and left (like Spinal Tap drummers)

D) Low-flow O_2 used at least 15 hours a day significantly enhances survival

E) Low-flow O_2 is a well-tolerated and effective treatment for obstructive sleep apnea

Answer 3.4.8 The correct answer is "D." Patients who use continuous low-flow O_2 at home have an improved rate of survival. Patients should be encouraged to use O_2 at least 15 hours a day, if possible, to obtain this benefit. "B" is incorrect because patients need at least 15 hours of O_2 per day to have any significant benefit with regard to pulmonary hypertension. "C" is incorrect. Clearly, smoking while on O_2 is not a good idea, but patients can turn off their O_2 supply while smoking.

HELPFUL TIP:
Data suggests that up to 20% of patients hospitalized with a COPD exacerbation of unknown origin may actually have a PE. Don't narrow your differential too soon!

▶ **Objectives: Did you learn to ...**
- Recognize a patient presenting with signs and symptoms of COPD?
- Describe diagnostic and staging criteria for COPD?
- Develop a plan to manage hypoxemia and hypercapnia?
- Manage medications for acute exacerbations of COPD?
- Direct therapy for chronic COPD?
- Identify causes of dyspnea other than COPD presenting in a patient with known COPD?

 QUICK QUIZ: COPD

In a patient with COPD, a lung transplantation referral can be considered:
A) Once the patient requires oxygen
B) When you feel you have run out of interventions
C) Once insurance accepts your referral
D) After the patient meets strict criteria for the referral
E) If the patient's family keeps asking for the referral

The correct answer is "D." The International Society for Heart and Lung Transplantation created a set of criteria for when to consider transplantation and, more importantly, when should you consider *referral* for a lung transplant consultation. In COPD patients, the indication for *referral* is easy to remember and consists of BODE index >5 (BODE stands for **B**ody-mass-index, airflow **O**bstruction, **D**yspnea, and **E**xercise, which are the characteristics used in the index). The BODE index is an alternative to the GOLD criteria. The BODE index incorporates functional criteria such as breathlessness and 6-minute walking distance. Find a BODE calculator here: http://www.qxmd.com/calculate-online/respirology/bode-index. Criteria for *transplantation* in COPD are more complex and are beyond the scope of this book.

▶ **CASE 3.5**

Ms. Sarah Bellum (if you're not smiling, try saying the name out loud or the joke is just lame . . .) is a 32-year-old female who presents to your ED with shortness of breath. She just flew home from the International Conference on Balance and Coordination in London. Immediately after walking through her front door, she became acutely short of breath. This is associated with some moderately sharp chest pain located along the left side of her chest. The pain seems worse when she attempts to breathe deeply.

Question 3.5.1 Which important question(s) do you next ask Ms. Bellum?
A) Do you smoke cigarettes?
B) When was your last menstrual period?
C) Have you had surgery recently?
D) Do you have a history of kidney disease?
E) All of the above.

Answer 3.5.1 The correct answer is "E." Each of these questions addresses risk factors associated with pulmonary embolism (PE) and/or deep vein thrombosis (DVT). Smoking cigarettes and recent surgery are strong risk factors, as is an active pregnancy. Addressing a patient's menstrual cycle serves as a natural segue to a discussion about the use of oral contraceptives, which, too, is a prominent risk factor. As for renal disease, nephrotic syndrome has been associated with an increased risk of PE.

....

After further verbal probing, you discover that Ms. Bellum recently completed her menstrual cycle. The other presented questions turned up no risk factors. However, your smooth segue did reveal that she takes low-dose estrogen for birth control. You also learn that her aunt had a blood clot in her leg once. She has no further details but does not think that her aunt had any further complications from this condition. Regardless, PE just took a violent leap to the top of your differential. You glance at her vitals (temperature 37.1°C, heart rate 92 bpm, blood pressure 129/68 mm Hg, respiratory rate 21, SpO$_2$ 95% on room air) and notice that she appears mildly uncomfortable but not in any acute distress. Her physical examination is entirely unremarkable. You order an ECG to evaluate for potential cardiac etiologies for her symptoms.

Question 3.5.2 Assuming Ms. Bellum does have a PE, what is *her* ECG most likely to show?
A) $S_1Q_3T_3$
B) Nonspecific ST-T wave changes
C) Sinus tachycardia

D) Normal sinus rhythm
E) Multifocal atrial tachycardia

Answer 3.5.2 The correct answer is "D." The most common ECG finding associated with the diagnosis of PE remains normal sinus rhythm. With that said, the most common *arrhythmia* found in patients with a PE is sinus tachycardia. But alas, Sarah had a normal heart rate. The other choices can certainly be found with this condition but are far less frequent. Of note, the "textbook" $S_1Q_3T_3$ ECG rarely occurs and historically traces back to a handful of patients in the 1930s that had massive pulmonary emboli. Even if you do spot this pattern on an ECG, it is not specific enough to confirm the diagnosis. In the end, the clinical signs attributed to pulmonary emboli (such as the shortness of breath and chest pain) are more valuable than any abnormal ECG finding.

As you attempt to rule out other potential etiologies for the patient's symptoms (e.g., pneumonia, atelectasis, and pneumothorax), you order a trusty old chest radiograph.

Question 3.5.3 What is the *most common* radiographic finding in a patient with a PE?
A) Pleural effusion
B) No acute cardiopulmonary processes
C) Westermark sign
D) Hilar/mediastinal enlargement
E) Hampton hump

Answer 3.5.3 The correct answer is "B." Admittedly, this one is a bit tricky. Approximately 75% of the chest radiographs in the setting of PE are abnormal. However, there are numerous causes for these abnormalities and none of them individually surpass the frequency of the normal chest radiographs. Specifically, the "textbook" findings of Westermark sign (loss of peripheral vascular markings) and Hampton hump (a wedge-shaped opacity due to pulmonary infarction) are infrequent, and both have a low sensitivity and low specificity. In short, all the other options can be seen as the result of a PE, but none is more frequent than a normal chest radiograph.

ECG and chest radiograph in hand, you turn your attention toward ordering the appropriate laboratory tests to solidify your presumptive diagnosis. You are working with a medical student who suggests a number of lab tests. You agree with most of them but shoot him down on one.

Question 3.5.4 Which test should you AVOID ordering?
A) CBC
B) D-dimer
C) PT/PTT
D) Basic metabolic panel (Na^+, K^+, Cl^-, CO_2^-, BUN, Cr^-, and glucose)
E) Urine pregnancy test

Answer 3.5.4 The correct answer is "B." The D-dimer can be a blessing for some but is the bane of existence for others. In this

patient, a D-dimer is not useful. This test has great sensitivity but poor specificity. It is positive in far more conditions than PE. Used as a "rule-out" test for PE, it only applies in low-risk patients. Ms. Bellum is not a low-risk patient as suggested by the **P**ulmonary **E**mbolism **R**ule-out **C**riteria (aka, "PERC"; see Helpful Tip) due to her use of exogenous estrogen. The Wells criteria for PE place her in the moderate-risk group (16.2% risk of PE). As such, even a negative D-dimer is insufficient for ruling out the diagnosis. As for the other tests, they all serve a valuable role in her evaluation. For instance, the CBC ("A") could provide evidence of anemia, while the PT/PTT ("C") may reveal a coagulopathy. Assessing her renal function ("D") may be needed for her evaluation and treatment planning, and the same can be said for verifying her gestational status ("E"). Plus, a urine pregnancy test is performed on almost every woman in an ED. It might as well be part of the triage process.

That pesky med student seemed to know a lot about the PERC rules and Wells criteria. But when he listed the Wells criteria, he got one wrong.

Question 3.5.5 The Wells criteria for PE include all of the following EXCEPT:
A) Estrogen use
B) Pulse >100 bpm
C) Previous history of venous thromboembolism
D) Clinical symptoms and signs consistent with PE
E) Hemoptysis

Answer 3.5.5 The correct answer is "A." While an important risk factor for PE, estrogen use is not included in the Wells criteria. All the others count in the Wells criteria (Table 3-4). Using a medical calculator website, such as www.mdcalc.com, is most helpful.

TABLE 3-4 WELL'S SCORE FOR PEA	
Clinically suspected DVT	3 points
No alternative diagnosis more likely than PE	3 points
Tachycardia >100	1.5 points
Immobilization for ≥3 days or surgery in the previous 4 weeks	1.5 points
History of DVT or PE	1.5 points
Malignancy within 6 months	1 point
Presence of hemoptysis	1 point

Score >6: high probability of PE (78%)
Score 2–6: moderate probability of PE (27.8%)
Score <2: low probability of PE (<3.4%).
[a]D-dimer is *only* useful to rule out the low-probability patient. Otherwise, the post-test probability with a normal D-dimer does not change enough to get you to a low-enough risk to rule out a PE.

HELPFUL TIP:
The PERC rules are a validated set of rules that allow categorization of a patient into a low-risk group to rule out
PE clinically. If the patient meets **all** of the following, PE
is ruled out (*assuming you believe the patient is low risk to
begin with*). Find a calculator here: https://www.mdcalc.
com/perc-rule-pulmonary-embolism.

1) Age <50 years
2) Heart rate <100 bpm
3) SaO_2 >94% on room air
4) No unilateral leg swelling
5) No hemoptysis
6) No recent history of trauma or surgery
7) No prior DVT or PE
8) No hormone use

HELPFUL TIP:
Remember not to get a D-dimer on *no-risk* patients. This
simply increases the CT rate and exposure to unnecessary radiation. The *fatal* cancer rate in a 20-year-old
female undergoing a *single* 64-slice chest CT is 1:142
(*JAMA.* 2007;298(3):317–323)! Plus, 25% of "positive"
CTs are false positive, damning them to the hell of anticoagulation (*Am J Roentgenol.* 2015;205:271). This is
especially common in low-risk patients and single sub-
segmental PEs.

The CBC, coagulation studies, and basic metabolic panel all
return within normal limits. In addition, Ms. Bellum is not
pregnant. Thus, you wish to (finally) solidify that diagnosis
you have suspected for quite some time.

Question 3.5.6 Since you do not put her in the low-risk
category by your clinical judgment, what diagnostic study
should you order?
A) VQ (ventilation–perfusion) scan
B) CT scan of the chest without contrast
C) CT scan of the chest with contrast
D) Pulmonary angiogram
E) Compressive Dopplers of the lower extremities

Answer 3.5.6 **The correct answer is "C."** The American College
of Radiology (ACR) lists the CT scan of the chest with contrast
(i.e., CT angiography or CTA) as the modality of choice in stable patients with a suspected PE. Its benefits: it is noninvasive,
cheaper than pulmonary angiography, and far more available
than VQ scans. It should be noted that pulmonary angiography still remains the "gold standard" for diagnosing pulmonary
emboli, but that is more of an academic point. As for VQ scans,
they are not available in many locales and often return nondiagnostic. However, they can be used in a patient *with a normal
chest x-ray.* A V/Q scan is likely to be non-diagnostic in those
with an abnormal chest x-ray (e.g., COPD patients). A chest CT
without contrast ("B") will not enhance the pulmonary arteries,

making the diagnosis of a PE far more difficult, if not impossible. Since most pulmonary emboli are believed to arise from the
lower extremity venous system, "E," Dopplers of the legs, could
be considered if the patient was a poor candidate for both CTA
and VQ scan (e.g., COPD and Stage 4 chronic kidney disease).
But this approach is obviously not diagnostic of PE; it would
just help you determine if the patient has an active thrombosis,
and you would manage the same whether she has a PE or DVT
or both.

HELPFUL TIP:
In pregnancy, both chest CT and V/Q scanning are
acceptable imaging options and involve acceptable
radiation levels (*Obstet Gynecol.* 2011;118(3):718–729).

**As keenly suspected, Ms. Bellum's CTA of the chest reveals
a moderate-sized pulmonary embolus in the left pulmonary
artery. Her vital signs are still stable and her pain is well-controlled with oral hydrocodone. She is surprised by the diagnosis you give her but appears to be taking it in stride.**

Question 3.5.7 What is the optimal management plan for
the patient moving forward?
A) Bolus her with unfractionated heparin (UFH), start her on
oral warfarin, and discharge her to home
B) Start the patient on low-molecular-weight heparin (LMWH),
initiate oral warfarin therapy, and admit the patient to the
family medicine service
C) Start apixaban (Eliquis) or rivaroxaban (Xaralto) and discharge to home
D) Start her on oral warfarin and discharge her to home with
primary care follow-up in the next 2 to 3 days
E) B or C

Answer 3.5.7 **The correct answer is "E."** Let's dissect why. "A"
and "D" are both incorrect because they do not include adequate anticoagulation. Certainly "B" is the classic approach.
However, this patient meets the "HESTIA" criteria for early
discharge from the ED (see Table 3-5), and need not be admitted, so many physicians now would choose discharge on a
direct anticoagulant. Early discharge has been found to be safe
in low-risk patients [those with all HESTIA criteria negative
and a low Pulmonary Embolism Severity Index (*Ann Intern
Med.* 2018;169(12):855–865 and *Acad Emerg Med.* 2018 Sep;
25(9):997–1003]. To calculate the PESI, use an online calculator, such as https://www.mdcalc.com/pulmonary-embolism-
severity-index-pesi. With regard to selecting an anticoagulant,
current evidence does not support the use of one agent over
another; UFH, LMWH, and fondaparinux followed by warfarin
are all appropriate as are the newer agents (e.g., apixaban, dabigatran, and rivaroxaban). Both warfarin and dabigatran require
an overlap with heparin. With UFH, LMWH, or fondaparinux
transitioning to warfarin, continue these drugs until the patient's
INR has been therapeutic (INR of 2–3) for at least 24 hours and
the overlap is for **at least 5 days**. Dabigatran requires 5 days of

TABLE 3-5 MODIFIED HESTIA CRITERIA FOR DISPOSITION OF PATIENT WITH A PULMONARY EMBOLISM

Modified HESTIA criteria: Any POSITIVE response mandates admission for PE treatment. If all are negative, check the Pulmonary Embolism Severity Index (PESI).

- Hemodynamically unstable by clinician judgment
- Thrombolysis or embolectomy needed
- Active bleeding or high risk for bleeding: GI bleeding or surgery ≤2 weeks ago, stroke ≤1 month ago, bleeding disorder or platelet count <75/L, uncontrolled HTN (sBP >180 or dBP >110)
- Oxygen needed to maintain $SaO_2 > 90\%$
- PE diagnosed while on anticoagulation
- Requiring IV pain medication
- Medical or social reason for admission (e.g., concurrent infection, poor/no support system)
- Creatinine clearance <30 mL/min by Cockcroft–gault formula
- Severe liver impairment
- Pregnant
- Known history of heparin-induced thrombocytopenia

heparin overlap (and of course we don't check the INR). Avoid edoxaban (Savaysa) if possible. It can only be used in those with a CrCl of **less than** 95 mL/min. Also, it requires dose adjustment for those with a CrCl of between 50 and 15 mL/min (do not use under CrCl 15 mL/min).

Question 3.5.8 How long are you going to maintain this patient on anticoagulation?
A) 3 months
B) 6 months
C) 9 months
D) Lifetime

Answer 3.5.8 **The correct answer is "A."** For a PE that has a reversible cause (oral contraceptive pills in this patient with a long airplane trip), 3 months of anticoagulation is adequate. For those with a second PE, lifetime anticoagulation is warranted. For those with a cryptogenic PE or PE from an acquired or inherited thrombophilia (e.g., Factor V Leiden), recommendations are all over the place from 3 months to life. Nine months is likely adequate for a patient with a PE from an irreversible cause, *although patients go back to their pre-treatment risk as soon as you stop anticoagulation.* And, a first PE trumps everything else in terms of risk factors for a second PE—including all those fancy thrombophilia tests! So, finding a thrombophilia does not necessarily help your decision-making process. Note that some guidelines suggest anticoagulation for life after a first cryptogenic/unprovoked PE if benefit seems to outweigh risks. This should be decided after 3 months of anticoagulation (*Chest.* 2016;149(2):315–352).

HELPFUL TIP:
An elevated A–a gradient suggests a ventilation/perfusion mismatch and occurs in a number of conditions, including atelectasis, right-to-left shunt, acute respiratory distress syndrome (ARDS), air embolism, resolving severe asthma, COPD with oxygen treatment, and

bronchiectasis with impaired gas exchange. Thus, an elevated A–a gradient is not specific for PE. Likewise, a normal A–a gradient and normal oxygen saturation do not rule out PE! In fact, in patients without underlying lung disease, the PIOPED study found no difference in the oxygen saturation and A–a gradient among patients with and without PE.

HELPFUL TIP:
Only 88% of patients with a PE are hypoxic, 70% have dyspnea or tachypnea, 65% have pleuritic pain, and as few as 30% are tachycardic. The point here is to have a high clinical suspicion in the right situation despite the lack of the classic triad. To make things worse, the troponin and BNP can be elevated in patients with a PE.

HELPFUL TIP:
Compression stockings may prevent post-thrombotic syndrome, the recurrent swelling and edema often found after a DVT—or may not! Evidence is conflicting. Consider prescribing compression stockings routinely in these patients.

Thrombolysis is generally not indicated for a DVT unless there is impending gangrene (phlegmasia). It will prevent post-thrombotic syndrome with a number needed to treat (NNT) of 7 for proximal DVTs but doesn't change quality of life. This comes at the number needed to harm (NNH) of 1 in 22 patients requiring a blood transfusion, NNH of 1 in 11 developing a PE, and **NNH of 1 in 5 requiring a vena cava filter** (*JAMA Intern Med.* 2014;174(9):1494–1501).

Your patient does well, completes her course of apixaban, and has no further episodes over the next 2 years. She develops gallstones and plans to have an elective laparoscopic cholecystectomy. A surgeon colleague sends her back to see you for a preoperative evaluation. You find no evidence of cardiac, pulmonary, or hematologic disease. She is no longer on warfarin and is doing well.

Question 3.5.9 Which of the following postoperative management strategies do you recommend?
A) Aspirin 81 mg PO daily
B) Warfarin 5 mg PO daily
C) UFH 5,000 units subcutaneously daily
D) Enoxaparin 40 mg subcutaneously daily
E) No antiplatelet or anticoagulant drugs

Answer 3.5.9 **The correct answer is "D."** Even for a relatively minor surgical procedure where anesthesia is used for 30 minutes or less and the postoperative recovery is usually quick, your patient is at moderate risk for venous thromboembolism. Her history of PE puts her in a higher risk category, and she requires prophylaxis. Of the choices available, enoxaparin would be the most appropriate. LMWH and UFH are both acceptable for prevention of DVT/PE in the postoperative period, but "C" is wrong because UFH must be dosed every 8 to 12 hours rather than daily. "A" is incorrect. Aspirin is sometimes used postoperatively, but the dose should be 160 mg/day or greater. Also, compared with heparin and its derivatives, aspirin is less efficacious in the prevention of thrombus. "B" is incorrect. Warfarin alone is not appropriate in this setting due to its slow onset of action. Of course, early ambulation is also indicated.

HELPFUL TIP:
The optimal length of time that patients require prophylaxis for venous thromboembolism after surgery is unknown. Arguments can be made for prophylaxis until the patient is ambulating several hundred feet per day.

▶ **Objectives: Did you learn to …**
- Recognize risk factors for a PE?
- Understand the variability of symptoms and signs in PE?
- Appreciate the PERC rules and Wells criteria and how they can be used to rule out a PE?
- Implement treatment and prevention for PE?
- Understand the A–a gradient?

 QUICK QUIZ: VENA CAVAL FILTERS

Which statement best describes the use of vena caval filters in preventing PE?
A) Vena cava filters reduce the risk of PE but only in patients who are maintained on anticoagulation
B) Retrievable vena caval filters have been shown to have a *short-term* advantage while the patient is in the hospital; they should be removed as soon as possible
C) Vena cava filters unequivocally reduce PE risk in both anticoagulated and non-anticoagulated patients
D) One need not workup a patient for a PE in the presence of a vena cava filter, which is almost 100% effective.

The correct answer is "B." All of the rest are wrong. All evidence suggests that vena caval filters are essentially useless in preventing PE (*JAMA.* 2015;313(16):1627). In addition, they can break with strut migration to the heart or through the vena cava. The 2016 ACCP guidelines recommend against vena caval filters in patients who can be anticoagulated even after a recurrent PE. And, they may increase mortality in those who have contraindications to anticoagulation (*JAMA Netw Open.* 2018;1(3):e180452). They may have some short-term benefit for inpatients such as with trauma. For patients with a recurrent DVT/PE while on anticoagulation, the proper approach is to accelerate the anticoagulation: if they are on warfarin, apixaban, dabigatran, or rivaroxaban, switch (at least temporarily) to enoxaparin; if they are on enoxaparin, increase the dose by 1/4–1/3.

▶ **CASE 3.6**

A 50-year-old male who is a heavy drinker with a history of squamous cell carcinoma of the neck presents to your office complaining of abdominal pain. He has been coughing and expectorating bloody sputum and notes a low-grade fever, chills, and mild dyspnea starting about 1 week ago. He denies nausea, emesis, and chest pain. His squamous cell carcinoma was treated with external beam radiation several years ago. Examination reveals an afebrile male in mild distress. His vital signs are normal, and his lungs sound clear. The abdominal examination reveals only mild epigastric tenderness.

The chest x-ray is available for your review (see Fig. 3-4). Your colleague, who is on call today, walks by and asks if you have any admissions for her.

Question 3.6.1 You consider this 50-year-old with a cough and reply:
A) "Yes. This gentleman will need the ICU"
B) "Yes. This gentleman will need a respiratory isolation room"
C) "No. I'm sending this gentleman home with metronidazole"
D) "No. I'll workup this gentleman as an outpatient"

Answer 3.6.1 The correct answer is "B." Because he is expectorating bloody sputum and has a cavitary lesion on chest x-ray (right upper lobe), this patient should be admitted to a respiratory isolation room until tuberculosis is ruled out. He will need further evaluation and possibly intravenous antibiotic therapy, both of which may be accomplished during his hospitalization. "A" is incorrect. There is no need to send this patient to the ICU based on his current picture. "C" is also incorrect. Metronidazole alone is not an appropriate therapy for this patient even if this is bacterial.

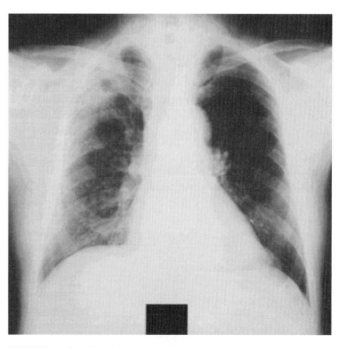

FIGURE 3-4. Question 3.6.1 patient's chest x-ray.

Question 3.6.2 What is the best next step in the diagnosis of this process?
A) Bronchoscopy
B) Sputum cultures
C) Blood cultures
D) Chest CT
E) Open-lung biopsy

Answer 3.6.2 The correct answer is "D." The chest x-ray demonstrates a cavitary lesion in the right upper lobe. Chest CT is warranted for further characterization of the lesion. From history, examination, and chest x-ray, it is not possible to determine whether the lesion is an abscess or a malignant process. An indolent course with low-grade fever is characteristic of lung abscess. However, the pre-existing squamous cell carcinoma has potential to have spread to the lungs, and squamous cell carcinoma is known to cause cavitations. Culture of sputum and blood, including evaluation of first morning sputum for acid-fast bacilli (AFB), will be an essential part of the assessment but may not yield as much information as chest CT, and sputum culture should be done in conjunction with cytology and Gram stain. Bronchoscopy should be postponed until CT results are available. Bronchoscopic biopsy is potentially detrimental if the lesion is an abscess since the airway could flood with pus if the entire cavity wall is penetrated.

Chest CT further confirms a parenchymal abscess in the right upper lobe with cavitation and air within the cavity. Bronchoscopy reveals pus in the airway and extrinsic compression of the bronchi. A lavage sample is obtained, but biopsies are not taken due to the clinical impression that this is a lung abscess.

Question 3.6.3 What organisms are most commonly isolated in lung abscesses?
A) Anaerobic bacteria
B) Aerobic bacteria
C) Tuberculosis
D) Mixed aerobic/anaerobic bacteria

Answer 3.6.3 The correct answer is "A." Anaerobes are isolated most often, followed by mixed anaerobic/aerobic bacteria, followed by aerobic bacteria alone (especially staphylococci).

Gram stain of sputum demonstrates Gram-positive cocci and Gram-negative rods. Cultures are pending. Tuberculin skin test is negative.

Question 3.6.4 What is the most appropriate therapy for this patient?
A) Refer for surgical drainage
B) Oral levofloxacin
C) Intravenous clindamycin
D) Intravenous metronidazole
E) Intravenous ceftriaxone

Answer 3.6.4 The correct answer is "C." Most lung abscesses are polymicrobial, but the most important aspect in treatment appears to be the use of an antibiotic active against anaerobes. Intravenous clindamycin is the usual choice for lung abscess due to its coverage of anaerobes and *Streptococcus pneumoniae*. Metronidazole is less effective, failing in up to 50% of cases of putrid lung abscess. A beta-lactam with beta-lactamase inhibitor (e.g., piperacillin/tazobactam) is another good choice. Ceftriaxone and levofloxacin offer poor coverage of anaerobes. Surgical drainage of lung abscesses is needed in only 5% to 10% of cases. Most resolve with just antibiotics.

▶ **Objectives: Did you learn to …**
· Recognize the presence of a cavitary lesion on chest x-ray?
· Identify the common causes of cavitary lesions?
· Manage a patient with a lung abscess?

▶ CASE 3.7

A 53-year-old male is accompanied by his wife to your office and complains of a cough for 6 weeks. It is worse at night and any time he lies down. He denies sputum production, shortness of breath, chest pain, and wheezing. He takes an antacid once or twice per day to settle his stomach and notes very bad heartburn. He smoked three packs of cigarettes per day until 1 year ago, when he quit "cold turkey." He takes only hydrochlorothiazide for hypertension. He has no cardiac disorders. His wife reports that he snores at night, and she adds, "He's always hacking and clearing his throat—all night." The review of systems is negative. In order to sleep better, he has recently started having a shot (or 2 . . . or 3 . . .) of whiskey before going to bed.

Question 3.7.1 What is the most likely cause for the cough?
A) Gastroesophageal reflux
B) Lung cancer
C) Antihypertensive medication
D) Alcohol abuse
E) Congestive heart failure (CHF)

Answer 3.7.1 The correct answer is "A." This patient appears to have a chronic cough that is most likely due to gastroesophageal reflux disease (GERD). He takes antacids and exhibits throat clearing, which can be a subtle sign and is not typically identified by patients as reflux. In addition, he drinks alcohol at bedtime, further predisposing to reflux. He has a history of smoking, which does place him at increased risk for developing a bronchogenic carcinoma, but a lung mass would not be a common cause for cough. Hydrochlorothiazide is not known to cause cough (although angiotensin-converting enzyme [ACE] inhibitors are). Also, it is unlikely that symptoms would be isolated to nighttime if his cough were medication-related.

HELPFUL TIP:
Remember that ACE inhibitors may cause cough in 5% to 20% of patients taking them. For patients who develop a cough and are on an ACE inhibitor, a brief trial off the medication may save a costly workup for chronic cough. Usually, symptoms resolve within 1 week but may persist for 1 month. Cough due to an ACE inhibitor may first occur up to 6 months after starting the ACE inhibitor.

HELPFUL TIP:
Asymptomatic reflux disease does not exacerbate asthma. So, don't blame asthma on *asymptomatic* nocturnal reflux (*Am J Respir Crit Care Med*. 2009;180(9):809–816 and *N Engl J Med*. 2009;360(15):1487–1499).

On physical examination, you note a mildly overweight male in no distress. His vital signs are normal. His lungs are clear to auscultation. The nasal and oropharyngeal mucosae are intact, moist, and not inflamed. The remainder of the examination is unremarkable. Chest x-ray shows flattened diaphragms but is otherwise negative. You suspect GERD, but also entertain other diagnoses.

Question 3.7.2 Which of the following is your next step in managing this patient's cough?
A) Start a proton pump inhibitor
B) Start an inhaled steroid
C) Order 24-hour esophageal pH monitoring
D) Obtain spirometry
E) Obtain a chest CT

Answer 3.7.2 The correct answer is "A." An empiric trial of an effective gastric acid-suppressing medication in this *symptomatic patient* is likely to relieve the cough if the diagnosis is accurate. The ACCP recommends starting therapy with a proton pump inhibitor rather than an H_2-blocker. The usual antireflux measures, such as avoiding fatty foods, alcohol, and food before bedtime, should be instituted as well. Prescribers must be aware that sometimes a complete resolution of cough takes months. A 24-hour pH monitor ("C") is invasive and often not necessary if an empiric trial of gastric acid suppression resolves the problem. Starting the evaluation of chronic cough with a chest x-ray is part of the ACCP recommendations, but CT scan ("E") is not indicated with a negative chest x-ray. If the cough does not resolve with empiric therapy, spirometry should be considered.

He does not respond after 2 months of empiric treatment, and he is becoming more concerned. The examination is unchanged. Spirometry is normal with a normal flow volume loop.

Question 3.7.3 Which of the following management options is LEAST likely to benefit this patient?
A) Combination antihistamine and decongestant
B) Inhaled corticosteroid
C) Inhaled beta-2 agonist
D) Antibiotics

Answer 3.7.3 The correct answer is "D." This patient has no signs or symptoms of sinusitis or bacterial pulmonary infection, so treating with an antibiotic is inappropriate and unlikely to help. However, some form of empiric therapy might be tried. He could have postnasal drainage without signs on physical examination, and empiric therapy with combination antihistamine and decongestant may improve the cough. Inhaled corticosteroids and beta-2 agonists are the mainstay of chronic asthma therapy and may help relieve this patient's chronic cough. This patient could yet have "cough-variant asthma" despite normal spirometry results.

Question 3.7.4 The three most common causes of chronic cough (cough lasting longer than 8 weeks) are:
A) Postnasal drip, asthma, GERD
B) GERD, COPD, congenital lung disease
C) Lung cancer, postnasal drip, COPD
D) Obstructive sleep apnea, respiratory infections, asthma

Answer 3.7.4 The correct answer is "A." Epidemiologic studies have demonstrated that most cases of chronic cough are due to postnasal drainage (often termed "upper airway cough syndrome"), asthma, or symptomatic GERD. Most cases of chronic cough seem to have only a single cause, although some will have more than one cause. Empiric therapy should be aimed at these top three causes. Of course, infection (pertussis in particular), malignancy, and other causes of cough are important to consider—and potentially rule out—as well.

The evaluation of chronic cough should proceed in a logical manner. Usually, history and physical examination will find the cause. If this is unrevealing, consider a stepwise evaluation addressing each of the chronic etiologies in Table 3-6 in order. If this still does not give you an answer, consider a methacholine challenge test to see if you can reproduce the symptoms that would lead you to a presumptive diagnosis of asthma with normal spirometry.

TABLE 3-6 SELECTED COMMON CAUSES OF ACUTE AND CHRONIC COUGH	
Acute	URI, pertussis, allergic rhinitis, COPD exacerbation, asthma, acute sinusitis
Chronic	GERD, postnasal drip, asthma, chronic sinusitis, allergic/vasomotor rhinitis, ACE inhibitors, eosinophilic bronchitis, chronic bronchitis, postinfectious asthma

ACE, angiotensin-converting enzyme; COPD, chronic obstructive pulmonary disease; GERD, gastroesophageal reflux disease; URI, upper respiratory infection.

HELPFUL TIP:
Look in the ears—cerumen impaction can cause a chronic cough and is often overlooked. Remember medications, especially ACE inhibitors (as above); other drugs that can cause cough include amiodarone, ARBs (lower risk than ACEIs), olanzapine, and some asthma medications (e.g., albuterol, montelukast).

▶ **Objectives: Did you learn to ...**
- Recognize the most common causes of chronic cough?
- Evaluate a patient with chronic cough?
- Develop a management plan for chronic cough?

▶ CASE 3.8

You see a 38-year-old female in follow-up for a recent episode of sinusitis. The illness has been present for about 6 weeks and has not responded to 2 weeks of appropriate antibiotics. She continues to have intermittent nosebleeds, fatigue, arthralgias, low-grade fevers, and night sweats. Two new complaints have surfaced: she has a cough productive of white sputum and she occasionally expectorates quarter-sized clots of blood. She has pleuritic chest pain, but denies dyspnea, tobacco use, and cardiac or pulmonary disease.

She is afebrile with a respiratory rate of 16, blood pressure 120/74 mm Hg, and pulse rate 92 bpm. Her oxygen saturation is 98% on room air. There is dried blood in the nares, but the oropharynx is clear. Cardiac and pulmonary examinations are unremarkable.

Question 3.8.1 Which initial test is most appropriate?
A) Chest x-ray
B) Sputum cytologic analysis
C) Bronchoscopy
D) Chest CT
E) CBC

Answer 3.8.1 The correct answer is "A." Hemoptysis is alarming to the patient and the physician—we hope. A stepwise approach is warranted with chest x-ray as the first step. Sputum for cytology might help if the suspicion for lung cancer was substantial, but the yield is likely to be low here. She may eventually require bronchoscopy if suggested by initial studies. Chest CT is likely to be part of the evaluation, but a chest x-ray should be performed first. Obtaining blood for a CBC is also important, although likely to be normal in the setting of minor hemoptysis.

You obtain the chest x-ray pictured in Fig. 3-5.
    You obtain the following laboratory results:
    CBC: Leukocytosis, thrombocytosis, and normochromic, normocytic anemia
    ESR: 70 mm/hr
    Urine dipstick: Positive for protein, heme, and red cells

Question 3.8.2 Which of the following tests will best assist you in the diagnosis of this patient?
A) Antineutrophil cytoplasmic antibody (ANCA)
B) Antiglomerular basement membrane antibody
C) Antinuclear antibody (ANA)
D) A and B
E) A and C

Answer 3.8.2 The correct answer is "D." This patient is presenting with the classic triad of granulomatosis with polyangiitis (GPA), a disease of the upper respiratory tract, lower respiratory tract, and kidneys, formerly known as Wegener's granulomatosis (as a response to Wegener's association with the Nazi Party, professional bodies and journals have replaced his name

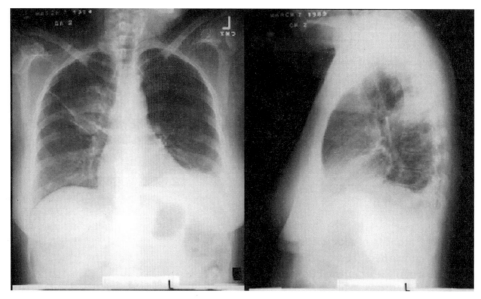

FIGURE 3-5. Patient's chest x-ray.

with a descriptive name). She has some of the additional signs and symptoms associated with GPA, as well. Common findings include pleuritic chest pain, myalgias, arthralgias, ptosis, fever, weight loss, and purpuric skin lesions, among others.

ANCA, and especially c-ANCA that is more specific for GPA, is present in up to 90% of patients with GPA. An ANA is not helpful in diagnosing GPA. An antiglomerular basement membrane antibody (anti-GBM) may be helpful in diagnosing Goodpasture syndrome (named for an American pathologist—not a Nazi—so he gets to keep the eponym). Goodpasture syndrome can be clinically easily confused with GPA; they both present with respiratory and renal involvement. Thus, anti-GBM antibody will be helpful in differentiating these two. However, about 10% of patients with Goodpasture syndrome will also have GPA—just to add to the confusion. For a partial list of causes of hemoptysis, see Table 3-7.

Question 3.8.3 Which of the following is NOT a radiographic finding of granulomatosis with polyangiitis?
A) Nodules that may be cavitary
B) Alveolar opacification
C) Pleural opacities
D) Widened mediastinum

Answer 3.8.3 **The correct answer is "D."** A widened mediastinum is not one of the classic findings in GPA. However, one may, on occasion, see hilar adenopathy. All of the other choices can be found in GPA. In the patient's x-ray (Fig. 3-5), a right upper lobe mass is easily distinguished. In a young, non-smoking female presenting with these symptoms, such a lung mass should lead to the consideration of GPA or possibly an infectious process. She is less likely to have a malignant process.

HELPFUL TIP:
A major, and probably the most common cause, of hemoptysis is bronchitis. This is especially true in smokers and the elderly.

The diagnostic evaluation is in progress. Laboratory tests are pending, and a chest CT is scheduled. You have arranged for a pulmonologist to see her. When you are on call, the physician covering the ED calls you to admit her for "massive hemoptysis." When you arrive, the patient looks comfortable and has normal vital signs. She begins a fit of coughing, expectorating several ounces of bright red blood. Her systolic blood pressure falls to 80 mm Hg. Her respiratory rate is 40. Her work of breathing has increased considerably. The situation does not improve after 5 minutes of observation, and her O_2 saturation is now 83% on room air.

Question 3.8.4 Remembering the movie *Moulin Rouge* (which has nothing to do with this case except for hemoptysis), what is your first action in this situation?
A) Arrange emergent bronchoscopy
B) Transfuse 2 units of blood
C) Perform endotracheal intubation
D) Provide bolus IV normal saline

Answer 3.8.4 **The correct answer is "C."** Massive hemoptysis is variably defined as 100 to 600 mL of blood expectorated per day, and it can result in hemodynamic compromise and asphyxiation. Quantification of the blood loss by the patient is usually unreliable. The main cause of mortality with hemoptysis is not hypovolemia but rather asphyxiation from blood in the lungs. As with any patient in acute respiratory distress, the airway must be controlled first. The best choice here is to perform intubation. Since this patient is known to have a potential source for bleeding in the right lung, intubation of the left mainstem bronchus may protect the left lung from the blood. Also, placing this patient on her right side (so that the bleeding source is dependent) may protect the left lung. If available, emergent bronchoscopy may allow identification of the bleeding site and selective lung intubation. However, bronchoscopy is not well suited for stopping the hemorrhage. The most that a bronchoscopist can do is place an endobronchial blocker and seal off the bleeding lobe. Interventional radiology should usually be the first treatment once the bleeding site has been localized. Emergent surgery is indicated if the bleeding remains brisk and not responsive to other interventions. Fluid resuscitation is important. However, before any of these other measures is undertaken, the airway must be protected.

HELPFUL TIP:
It is important to understand that patients with hemoptysis do not die of exsanguination but rather drown in their own blood—which is such a more pleasant image. The volume of blood needed to cause asphyxiation is surprisingly low and nowhere near the volumes that GI bleeders lose. Of note, small volume hemoptysis may be clinically significant in patients with underlying lung disease such as COPD due to less reserve and increased dead space. Also, a low oxygen saturation will occur long before you notice any change in the hemoglobin. Therefore, serial hemoglobins make little sense in hemoptysis patients.

TABLE 3-7 CAUSES OF HEMOPTYSIS

Vascular	PE, vasculitides (Goodpasture syndrome, granulomatosis with polyangiitis), arteriovenous malformation
Neoplastic	Bronchogenic carcinoma, metastatic disease
Connective tissue	Lupus, rheumatoid arthritis
Cardiac	CHF, mitral stenosis
Infectious	TB, bronchitis, pneumonia, abscess
Drugs	Anticoagulants, cocaine, solvents
Miscellaneous	Trauma, foreign body, epistaxis, hematemesis

CHF, congestive heart failure; PE, pulmonary embolism.

The patient stabilizes in the ICU. You plan to start treatment for her granulomatosis with polyangiitis. She does better and is discharged in 2 days.

 HELPFUL TIP:
The 5-year mortality of untreated granulomatosis with polyangiitis is 90%. These patients need aggressive treatment. Cyclophosphamide + steroids or rituximab + steroids seem to be the best combinations.

▶ **Objectives: Did you learn to …**
  · Perform an appropriate evaluation on a patient with hemoptysis?
  · Recognize the major causes of hemoptysis?
  · Diagnose granulomatosis with polyangiitis?
  · Identify and treat massive hemoptysis?

▶ CASE 3.9

A 35-year-old African-American female presents with dyspnea worsening over the last 2 months. She also complains of cough, generalized fatigue, and intermittent low-grade fevers. She does not smoke. Chest x-ray shows hilar adenopathy and small bilateral pleural effusions. Spirometry is consistent with a restrictive pattern.

Question 3.9.1 Of the following, which is the most likely diagnosis?
A) Granulomatosis with polyangiitis
B) Sarcoidosis
C) Bronchogenic carcinoma
D) Pneumonia
E) Microscopic polyangiitis

Answer 3.9.1 The correct answer is "B." The findings of hilar lymphadenopathy and a restrictive pattern on spirometry are most consistent with sarcoidosis. The chest x-ray findings do not support the diagnosis of granulomatosis with polyangiitis. Besides, it can't be "A"—we just did that case (and when would you see two GPA cases in a row on a test—let alone in your career?). "E" is incorrect. Microscopic polyangiitis is a systemic vasculitis related to GPA, presenting with similar features as GPA but without granulomatous disease. Bronchogenic carcinoma ("C") is unlikely in this relatively young non-smoker who does not demonstrate findings of carcinoma on x-ray. The clinical history is not typical of pneumonia ("D"), and chest x-ray shows no infiltrate. Tuberculosis (TB), although not an answer option, should also be considered, and the appropriate history and testing should be completed. In fact, TB and sarcoidosis often present in a similar fashion as may some fungal diseases and others.

Question 3.9.2 Which of the following is NOT commonly associated with sarcoidosis?
A) Hypercalcemia
B) Elevated ACE levels
C) Reduced diffusion capacity
D) Hypothyroidism
E) Facial or peripheral nerve palsy

Answer 3.9.2 The correct answer is "D." Sarcoidosis is marked by the presence of non-caseating granulomas. While sarcoid can infiltrate the thyroid, it rarely, if ever, causes hypothyroidism. Pulmonary sarcoidosis includes a decreased diffusion capacity and decreased vital capacity. Other laboratory findings include hypercalcemia, hypercalciuria, elevated liver and pancreatic enzymes, and elevated ACE levels. Neurologic involvement occurs in up to 5% of patients and frequently presents as facial paralysis but may present as any central nervous system lesion. Peripheral nerves may also be involved.

Question 3.9.3 Which of the following is NOT found as a part of sarcoidosis?
A) Erythema nodosum
B) Myocardial infarction
C) Cardiac arrhythmias
D) Elevated liver enzymes
E) Vision loss

Answer 3.9.3 The correct answer is "B." Sarcoidosis does not cause myocardial infarctions. While there is cardiac involvement with sarcoidosis, the manifestations are bundle branch block, cardiac arrhythmias, and sudden death. Many organs can be affected by sarcoidosis, including the skin, eye (iritis), heart, lung, liver, nervous system—essentially anywhere granulomas form.

Question 3.9.4 Which of the following is true about ACE levels in sarcoidosis?
A) An elevated ACE level is specific for sarcoidosis
B) ACE levels often correlate with disease severity in sarcoidosis
C) ACE inhibitors are effective in the treatment of sarcoidosis
D) All of the above

Answer 3.9.4 The correct answer is "B." One can follow ACE levels to track the progress of the disease. However, since treatment is based on symptoms, following ACE levels is not recommended. "A" is incorrect. ACE levels may be elevated in silicosis, miliary TB, and asbestosis, among others. "C" is incorrect. ACE inhibitors are not used to treat sarcoidosis.

This patient is found to have only pulmonary sarcoidosis with some mild systemic symptoms.

Question 3.9.5 Which of the following is the best initial choice for management?
A) Observation
B) Oral corticosteroids
C) Oral antibiotics
D) Inhaled corticosteroids
E) Methotrexate

Answer 3.9.5 The correct answer is "A." This patient has apparent pulmonary-limited disease and has minimal systemic symptoms. Nearly 50% of patients with sarcoidosis may have spontaneous resolution of their symptoms without treatment. In fact, treatment may actually prolong the disease process. If her pulmonary or systemic symptoms worsen or are causing major life problems, she should be started on oral steroids. Systemic corticosteroid therapy is the mainstay of treatment for sarcoidosis. Methotrexate and other immune-modulating drugs may be employed as well and offer a steroid-sparing effect, but these are not first-line agents. Evidence for the use of inhaled corticosteroids is lacking. Antibiotics are not effective.

▶ **Objectives: Did you learn to …**
- Recognize the clinical manifestations of sarcoidosis?
- Manage a patient with mild sarcoidosis?

▶ CASE 3.10

A 57-year-old male with no prior medical history comes in to clinic with a 1-week history of right rib pain and low-back pain. The rib pain is worse with deep breaths and especially bothers him at night. There has been no trauma. He has lost 20 lb in the last 3 months. He has a cough productive of white sputum. He denies any other symptoms. He smokes one to two packs of cigarettes per day but does not drink alcohol.

Vital signs: temperature 36.5°C, pulse rate 95 bpm, blood pressure 110/70 mm Hg, respiratory rate 16. On room air, his oxygen saturation is 96%. There is no adenopathy. His lung sounds are clear on the left and decreased on the right. There is dullness to percussion and decreased tactile fremitus over the right lower lung field.

Question 3.10.1 Based on this patient's history and physical examination, what do you expect to find on chest x-ray?
A) Normal chest x-ray
B) Cavitary lung lesion
C) Pleural effusion
D) Expanded lung fields
E) Pneumothorax

Answer 3.10.1 **The correct answer is "C."** This patient's findings suggest pleural effusion. Everything is diminished in pleural effusion: there is dullness to percussion, decreased breath sounds, decreased tactile fremitus, and decreased voice transmission. A cavitary lung lesion presents with either a normal examination or findings similar to an infiltrate (e.g., crackles, increased fremitus, and dullness to percussion). Expanded lung fields on chest x-ray are often seen in patients with COPD or asthma, and examination findings include prolonged expiratory phase, wheezing, and resonance to percussion. Pneumothorax presents with hyperresonance to percussion, decreased breath sounds, and decreased fremitus.

HELPFUL TIP:
Chest radiographs have a low sensitivity for rib fractures. However, this is really not a problem. The presence or absence of a rib fracture is generally immaterial. What we are interested in is whether or not there is anything underlying the rib fracture, such as a pulmonary contusion or hemothorax.

Your suspicions are confirmed. The chest x-ray shows obliteration of the right hemidiaphragm, and the posterior costophrenic angle is obscured on the lateral view, consistent with pleural effusion. There is also a right upper lobe lung mass.

Question 3.10.2 Which of the following will provide the most information and guidance for your thoracentesis?
A) Supine chest x-ray
B) Chest CT
C) Lateral decubitus chest x-ray
D) Chest ultrasound
E) Apical view chest radiograph

Answer 3.10.2 **The correct answer is "D."** Prior to performing a thoracentesis, you must know whether the effusion is loculated or freely flowing. Portable ultrasound has become a validated and widely accepted modality to diagnose and assess pleural effusion. Also, ultrasonography has been found to be more sensitive for detection of pleural fluid than a chest radiograph. Chest CT is somewhat more sensitive but more cumbersome, exposing the patient to additional radiation, and does not allow a bedside diagnosis and treatment. A decubitus film, with the affected side down, would allow you to see the effusion "layer out" unless it is loculated but again is less sensitive. A supine chest x-ray may cause the effusion to "layer out" too, but you will not be able to see it as well, which is why effusions may be missed when a patient is unable to stand or sit upright for his x-ray.

Question 3.10.3 Relative and absolute contraindications to thoracentesis include all of the following EXCEPT:
A) Herpes zoster in the area of needle placement
B) Coagulopathy
C) Diaphragmatic rupture
D) Positive pressure ventilation
E) History of recurrent laryngeal nerve injury or compromise

Answer 3.10.3 **The correct answer is "E."** Absolute contraindications include chest wall compromise (e.g., burn, cellulitis, herpes zoster, ruptured diaphragm) and cases where chest tube thoracostomy would be more appropriate. Relative contraindications are poor patient cooperation, coagulopathy, anticoagulation therapy, very small effusions (<10 mm on decubitus film view), positive pressure ventilation, and pleural adhesions.

Question 3.10.4 On ultrasound, the effusion appears free flowing and not loculated. What is the most appropriate next step?
A) Referral for surgical drainage
B) Place a chest tube to drain the effusion

C) Perform an ultrasound-guided diagnostic thoracentesis at the bedside

D) Order two pizzas, one for you and one for the patient (you have both had a long day and are hungry)

Answer 3.10.4 **The correct answer is "C."** The patient has a relatively large pleural effusion. Ultrasound-guided thoracentesis is a good first step in evaluating this effusion. Ultrasound guidance is quickly becoming the standard of care as it has been shown to decrease complications of pneumothorax as well as the number of unsuccessful clinical attempts or "dry taps." Referral to a thoracic surgeon ("A") may eventually be necessary, but this would not be the first step. Placing a chest tube ("B") into an effusion is not recommended at this point, and the diagnostic study should be obtained first.

. . . .

Ultrasound-guided thoracentesis is successful in obtaining fluid. The fluid is amber and cloudy, with a pH 7.3, lactate dehydrogenase (LDH) 800 IU/L, glucose 65 mg/dL, total protein 5.5 g/dL, WBC 1,300/mm³, RBC 50,000/mm³. _Serum studies done the same day include LDH 155 IU/L, glucose 99 mg/dL, and total protein 7 g/dL. Cytology, Gram stain, and culture of the pleural fluid are pending._

Question 3.10.5 **Which of the following is the most accurate statement regarding the pleural fluid analysis?**
A) The fluid is due to infection
B) The fluid is due to cancer
C) The fluid is a transudate
D) The fluid is an exudate

Answer 3.10.5 **The correct answer is "D."** Pleural effusions are broadly categorized as exudates and transudates (see Tables 3-8 and 3-9). Such a categorization helps to narrow the differential diagnosis. In this case, several elements of the pleural fluid are consistent with an exudate. LDH and protein can be used to determine whether the pleural fluid is transudative or exudative. Per Light's criteria, a pleural effusion is _suggestive_ of an exudative process if two of any of the following criteria are met: pleural fluid LDH >2/3 the upper limit of normal serum LDH, a pleural LDH:serum LDH ratio of >0.6, and a pleural protein:serum protein ratio of >0.5. All three of these indicators point to an exudate in this case. Also, exudative effusions tend to have a higher degree of cellularity than transudative effusions. With the information given, it is difficult to determine if the effusion is related to infection, cancer, or some other process.

. . . .

TABLE 3-8 CATEGORIZATION OF PLEURAL FLUID AS AN EXUDATE OR TRANSUDATE

Exudate characterized by
- Pleural fluid to serum protein ratio >0.5
- Pleural fluid to serum LDH ratio >0.6
- Pleural fluid LDH greater than 150 mg/dL (two-thirds the upper limit of normal serum LDH)

TABLE 3-9 CATEGORIZATION OF PLEURAL EFFUSIONS BY CLASS (TRANSUDATE VERSUS EXUDATE)A

Type of Effusion	Potential Causes
Transudative effusions	Heart failure, cirrhosis, nephritic syndrome, atelectasis, myxedema, pulmonary embolism, urinothorax
Exudative effusions	Bronchogenic carcinoma, metastatic neoplasm, mesothelioma, pneumonia, TB, chylothorax, pancreatitis, esophageal rupture, collagen vascular diseases (rheumatoid arthritis, Sjögren syndrome), trauma, drugs (nitrofurantoin, amiodarone, methotrexate), heart failure with diuretic therapy, pulmonary embolism

Note: Heart failure and pulmonary embolism can cause exudative and transudative effusions.
ᵃSee _exudate_ criteria (Table 3-8). Everything else is a transudate.

. . . .

The pleural fluid cytology comes back negative. The patient's symptoms and examination have not changed. Repeat radiograph still shows an upper lobe mass.

Question 3.10.6 **What is the most appropriate next step in approaching this pleural effusion?**
A) Await pleural fluid culture results
B) Perform bedside chest tube drainage of the effusion
C) Refer for surgical evacuation of the effusion
D) Refer for bronchoscopy
E) Place a chest tube for chemical pleurodesis

Answer 3.10.6 **The correct answer is "D."** The effusion is clearly exudative, and the patient appears to have a lung mass. Biopsy of the lung mass via bronchoscopy is indicated. A negative pleural fluid cytology does not rule out lung cancer. Positive cytology indicates advanced stage lung cancer. Chest tube drainage of a pleural effusion is not recommended except under extraordinary circumstances. Intermittent thoracentesis is preferred and has lower morbidity. Surgical evacuation of the fluid would be indicated if the patient were symptomatic, and the effusion was loculated and/or related to infection. If the effusion grows, or is drained and recurs, it may respond to pleurodesis. Otherwise, pleurodesis is not indicated at this time.

HELPFUL TIP:
Patients with malignant pleural effusions are not likely to benefit from surgery since the tumor is not localized and is not resectable by this point. Long-term outcomes with a malignant pleural effusion are bleak.

. . . .

Now that you have gained expertise with ultrasound of a pleural effusion, your colleague sends you a patient that has a pleural effusion on chest x-ray. Your colleague asks you

whether you could "tap" the fluid for him as he does not feel comfortable with the portable ultrasound. Also, he has a tee time in 30 minutes.

Question 3.10.7 **On ultrasound, you quickly visualize the chest and see a septated and loculated pleural effusion. What is the best next step?**
A) Return the patient back to his doctor—the effusion is too small to access
B) Perform ultrasound-guided needle thoracentesis
C) Refer to a thoracic surgeon
D) Place a small-bore chest tube
E) Head to the golf course with your colleague. Nothing you can do here

Answer 3.10.7 **The correct answer is "C."** A loculated and septated pleural effusion can very often be seen in empyema and evacuation usually requires surgical intervention. Thoracentesis would unlikely be successful and would expose the patient to an unnecessary procedure after which he would still need to see a surgeon. Placing a chest tube blindly into a loculated pleural effusion is unsafe. That procedure should be done under visualization; most commonly, video-assisted thoracic surgery would be utilized. Intrapleural fibrinolytics may improve outcomes but should be done in consultation with a thoracic surgeon or pulmonologist.

▶ **Objectives: Did you learn to …**
- Recognize the historical and physical examination findings of pleural effusion?
- List potential etiologies of pleural effusion?
- Narrow the differential diagnosis based on pleural fluid findings?
- Decide when to perform diagnostic and therapeutic thoracentesis?
- Decide when to perform chest tube drainage?

▶ CASE 3.11

A 60-year-old male presents to the ED for a cough. His symptoms began with a cold 2 weeks ago, and the other symptoms have improved, but the cough has persisted. He has mild production of white sputum with no hemoptysis. The patient denies fevers, night sweats, chills, and weight loss. He's had no chest pain or dyspnea. He smokes one pack of cigarettes per day, works in construction, and does not have a regular doctor. In fact, with some pride, he says, "I haven't seen a doctor in over 30 years." On physical examination, you find a fit-appearing male in no acute distress. His vital signs are normal. His lung sounds are diminished bilaterally, but the remainder of the examination is unremarkable. While breathing ambient air, the patient's oxygen saturation is 94%. You obtain a chest x-ray, which is shown in Fig. 3-6.

Question 3.11.1 **Your next step is to:**
A) Prescribe a 5-day course of azithromycin
B) Refer the patient to a pulmonologist

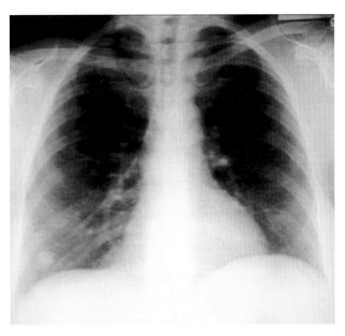

FIGURE 3-6. Question 3.11.1 patient's chest x-ray.

C) Order a high-resolution CT scan of the chest
D) Have the patient return to you in 3 months to repeat a chest x-ray
E) Reassure the patient and have him return as needed

Answer 3.11.1 **The correct answer is "C."** The chest x-ray in Fig. 3-6 shows a single nodule in the right lower lobe. The nodule is round, less dense than bone, and appears to be >1 cm in diameter. These are sometimes called "coin lesions." There are no other abnormalities. The most appropriate next step in the evaluation is to order a high-resolution CT scan of the chest. Treatment with azithromycin is inappropriate in this setting, as this patient has no signs of pulmonary infection on examination or chest x-ray. Referral to a pulmonologist is premature without first investigating the nodule by CT scan. Delaying further imaging and evaluation is also inappropriate since 15% to 75% of solitary pulmonary nodules (SPNs) ≥8 mm are ultimately diagnosed as cancer.

Question 3.11.2 **Which of the following is NOT considered a benign pattern of calcification on CT scan?**
A) Diffuse, homogeneous calcification
B) Central calcification
C) Laminar calcification
D) Spiculated, irregular calcification
E) "Popcorn" calcification

Answer 3.11.2 **The correct answer is "D."** We are accustomed to thinking of calcified nodules as being benign, but that is not always the case. Irregular, spiculated calcification is not reassuring. The other options are considered indicative of a benign lesion. Two patterns on CT are relatively specific for cancer: a scalloped border and the corona radiata sign, which is composed of fine linear strands extending out from the nodule.

Question 3.11.3 All of the following are useful to help assess the risk of cancer in a patient with a solitary pulmonary nodule (SPN) EXCEPT:
A) Smoking status
B) Age
C) Diameter of the nodule
D) Gender

Answer 3.11.3 The correct answer is "D." Determining the probability of cancer in patients with an SPN is an inexact science. The risk of cancer is generally assessed as low, intermediate, or high based on patient and radiograph characteristics. Although men are slightly overrepresented in lung cancer diagnoses, this is generally thought to be due to greater smoking rates in men and to occupational hazards. Gender itself does not help to risk-stratify patients with an SPN. Smoking increases the risk of an SPN being cancer, with greater use increasing the risk of cancer. As with most cancers, increasing age is associated with a higher risk. The diameter of the nodule is also important. If the diameter is <8 mm, the risk of cancer is low. When the diameter is ≥3 cm, the SPN is now referred to as a "pulmonary mass" and is highly likely to be cancerous. An SPN >3 cm in diameter should be considered cancer until proven otherwise.

The Fleischner Society has published an updated set of widely accepted recommendations regarding follow-up of incidentally found pulmonary nodules in 2017. The guideline does not apply to patients <35 years or with a history of cancer or immunosuppression (see Table 3-10).

HELPFUL TIP:
There is a calculator to help you determine the risk of malignancy for SPNs: http://reference.medscape.com/calculator/solitary-pulmonary-nodule-risk (this is the Mayo Clinic model). Another calculator based on the Fleischner criteria is at MD-Calc.

Later that week, your patient returns with his CT scan in hand. His cough is somewhat better (therapeutic CT scan radiation therapy … you know, like those CT scans in California that were mis-programmed and cooking people's brains accidentally? Really …). You review the CT scan with him. It shows a round, smooth nodule measuring 2 cm in diameter and located in the periphery of the right lower lobe. There are no calcifications in the nodule and no other abnormalities.

Question 3.11.4 Which of the following is the most appropriate next step?
A) Referral for bronchoscopy
B) High-resolution CT scan every 3 months
C) Chest x-ray every 3 months
D) Bone scan
E) Referral to a thoracic surgeon

Answer 3.11.4 The correct answer is "E." This patient needs a biopsy. There are several factors that put your patient at higher

TABLE 3-10 FLEISCHNER SOCIETY 2017 GUIDELINES FOR MANAGEMENT OF INCIDENTALLY DETECTED PULMONARY SOLID NODULES IN ADULTS

Nodule Type	Size			Comments
	<6 mm (<100 mm³)	6–8 mm (100–250 mm³)	>8 mm (>250 mm³)	
Single				
Low risk	No routine follow-up	CT at 6–12 months, then consider CT at 18–24 months	Consider CT at 3 months, PET/CT, or tissue sampling	Nodules <6 mm do not require routine follow-up, but certain patients at high risk with suspicious nodule morphology, upper lobe location, or both may warrant 12-month follow-up (recommendation 1A).
High risk	Optional CT at 12 months	CT at 6–10 months, then CT at 18–24 months	Consider CT at 3 months, PET/CT, or tissue sampling	Nodules <6 mm do not require routine follow-up, but certain patients at high risk with suspicious nodule morphology, upper lobe location, or both may warrant 12-month follow-up (recommendation 1A).
Multiple				
Low risk	No routine follow-up	CT at 3–6 months, then consider CT at 18–24 months	CT at 3–6 months, then consider CT at 18–24 months	Use most suspicious nodule as guide to management. Follow-up intervals may vary according to size and risk (recommendation 2A).
High risk	Optional CT at 12 months	CT at 3–6 months, then at 18–24 months	CT at 3–6 months, then at 18–24 months	Use most suspicious nodule as guide to management. Follow-up intervals may vary according to size and risk (recommendation 2A).

Notes: These guidelines apply to newly detected indeterminate nodules in persons 35 years of age or older. Low-risk patients have minimal or absent history of smoking and no other known risk factors. High-risk patients have a history of smoking or of other known risk factors.

risk of having a malignant cause for the SPN, including his age and tobacco use. These put him into an intermediate- to high-risk category for cancer. Although the nodule is smooth on CT, its size is >8 mm and there are no calcifications. This patient should be referred for transthoracic fine-needle biopsy or open biopsy. "A" is tempting but incorrect. Bronchoscopy is insensitive in the peripheral lung, especially when the lesion is relatively small. "B" and "C" are also wrong here but are appropriate in other settings. In this case, repeat imaging over time may delay a diagnosis of malignancy. Without symptoms of bone pain or confirmation that the SPN is a cancer that might metastasize to bone, a bone scan will have a very low yield.

Your patient returns from the surgeon much relieved. Fine-needle biopsy proved the SPN to be a hamartoma. Now your patient wants to quit smoking for good, and he thinks that he will need some assistance. You recommend nicotine replacement products and bupropion, but your patient claims to have had an allergic reaction to bupropion. Fortunately, you know of an effective alternative.

Question 3.11.5 To assist with tobacco cessation, you prescribe which of the following?
A) Varenicline
B) Fluoxetine
C) Olanzapine
D) Metoprolol
E) Clonidine

Answer 3.11.5 The correct answer is "A." Randomized trials have demonstrated the effectiveness of the nicotine partial agonist, varenicline (Chantix). This FDA-approved medication appears to be at least as effective as bupropion as an aid to smoking cessation. It had been thought that varenicline caused psychiatric side effects. This has been disproven in randomized, post-marketing, trials. Varenicline seems safe even for those with psychiatric disorders. However, the FDA still suggests that patients who develop depression, aggressive behavior, etc., stop varenicline and contact their provider. Fluoxetine and other selective serotonin reuptake inhibitors have not demonstrated a benefit. In schizophrenic patients, the use of atypical antipsychotic medications may aid in smoking cessation when compared with typical antipsychotics. Clonidine is sometimes used to help patients who are withdrawing from narcotics, and it may have some limited role in smoking cessation but is not very effective. You can also combine therapies: varenicline + nicotine replacement therapy (NRT) or use two types of NRT, such as gum + patch (*BMC Public Health*. 2015 Jul 22;15:689).

As you are walking out of your patient's room, your patient says, "Hey Doc, my brother smokes too, is there a test you can do to make sure he doesn't have lung cancer?"

Question 3.11.6 You respond:
A) "Sure, I'll put in an order for him to get an outpatient chest x-ray"
B) "Tell him to make an appointment and we will discuss the risks/benefits of low-dose CT scan"
C) "Here have him expectorate in this cup, and I'll send his sputum for cytology"
D) "Nah, we don't recommend lung cancer screening at this time"
E) "Yes. We just need a Ouija board and a magic 8-ball"

Answer 3.11.6 The correct answer is "B." In 2013, the USPTF issued a grade B recommendation for annual lung cancer screening with low-dose CT scan in adults aged 55 to 80 years who have a 30 pack-year smoking history and currently smoke or have quit within the past 15 years. Screening should be discontinued once a person has not smoked for 15 years or develops a health problem that substantially limits life expectancy or the ability or willingness to have curative lung surgery. These recommendations are based on the National Lung Screening Trial that showed that for every 1,000 people who got screening for lung cancer, 3 fewer died of lung cancer because of screening. About 300 people need to be screened to save one life from lung cancer. Patients should be given the risks/benefits of lung cancer screening since approximately 365/1,000 patients will have a false-positive result (usually because of a benign pulmonary nodule) that leads to more CT scans (extra radiation), more invasive procedures (biopsies and surgeries), and patient stress and anxiety. Confused yet? Don't worry, the American Thoracic Society has developed a patient decision guide found at https://www.thoracic.org/patients/patient-resources/decision-aid-for-lung-cancer-screening-with-ct.php. It is important to stress that this lung cancer screening should not take the place of efforts to stop smoking! Of note, "A" and "C" are incorrect because neither plain chest radiographs nor sputum cytology have been shown to improve lung cancer mortality.

▶ **Objectives: Did you learn to …**
- Weigh risk factors when evaluating an SPN?
- Develop a plan for evaluating an SPN?
- Assist a patient with smoking cessation?
- Learn the risks/benefits of lung cancer screening in the appropriate patient population?

▶ CASE 3.12

A 74-year-old male presents to your ED for weakness, cough, and fatigue. His wife relates an incomplete recovery since his myocardial infarction last year. He continues to have poor appetite and listlessness, and she thinks that he may be depressed. He is short of breath and confused. His wife says that yesterday he developed a fever, chills, and a new cough productive of white sputum. His past medical history is otherwise remarkable for a cholecystectomy. He is taking aspirin (secondary prevention, not primary!), metoprolol, and atorvastatin.

Vitals: temperature 39°C, respiratory rate 30, pulse 90 bpm, blood pressure 140/80 mm Hg. Oxygen saturation on room air is 90%. He is thin, pale, and oriented to person only. The lung examination is remarkable for rales in the left lower field, with dullness to percussion and increased tactile fremitus. The remainder of the examination is normal.

The chest x-ray shows a left lower lobe infiltrate. Other laboratory data currently available: hemoglobin 12.4 g/dL, WBC 14,100/mm³, platelets 340,000/mm³, creatinine 1.9 mg/dL, BUN 50 mg/dL, and normal electrolytes, troponin, and CK. An ECG shows normal sinus rhythm.

Question 3.12.1 What is your next step in managing this patient's medical condition?

A) Place a chest tube on the left
B) Perform chest CT
C) Administer inhaled bronchodilators
D) Administer parenteral antibiotics
E) Perform intubation and mechanical ventilation

Answer 3.12.1 **The correct answer is "D."** Given the clinical picture and chest x-ray findings, the patient most likely has community-acquired pneumonia. Therefore, the administration of parenteral antibiotics is the best choice. "A" is incorrect. Since there is no effusion, a chest tube would be useless. "B" is incorrect. CT is not required in this straightforward case of pneumonia. "C" is incorrect. The patient is not wheezing and there is no indication for bronchodilators at this time. As for "E," since your patient's respiratory status is stable, he does not require intubation.

HELPFUL TIP:
Remember that it is impossible to tell a "typical" versus an "atypical" pneumonia by radiograph. Do not base your therapy for community-acquired pneumonia on the radiographic appearance. Atypical organisms can cause lobar consolidation and typical pneumonias can appear diffuse. Note that treatment guidelines make no mention of radiographic appearance.

HELPFUL TIP:
There are several scoring systems to help decide on whether a patient with pneumonia needs to be admitted, their likely mortality rate, etc. Some of the popular ones include the Pneumonia Severity Index and the CURB-65. Both are available at MD-Calc.

HELPFUL TIP:
The variables for CURB-65 include:
Confusion (based on a specific mental test or disorientation to person, place, or time)
Urea (BUN) >20 mg/dL
Respiratory rate >30 breaths/min

Blood pressure <90/60 mm Hg
Age >**65** years
Patients with a score of 0 or 1 have a low risk of death and are generally safe for outpatient management.

Question 3.12.2 Based on patient-specific characteristics and your knowledge of causative factors involved in pneumonia, which of the following is LEAST likely to be the agent causing this patient's infection?

A) *Mycoplasma pneumoniae*
B) *S. pneumoniae*
C) *Haemophilus influenzae*
D) *Pseudomonas aeruginosa*

Answer 3.12.2 **The correct answer is "D."** When a pathogen is identified in adult community-acquired pneumonia, it is usually *S. pneumonia* ("B"). In fact, *S. pneumoniae* makes up 40% to 60% of all cases of community-acquired pneumonia in the elderly. Non-typeable *H. influenzae* ("C") composes about 5% to 10% of cases. *Mycoplasma* pneumoniae ("A") is implicated in 5%, and it is more common in young adults. *P. aeruginosa* pneumonia is uncommon in healthy elders and more likely to occur in patients with serious underlying lung disease or immunodeficiency (think cystic fibrosis). Approximately 5% of patients or more are infected with multiple agents.

Question 3.12.3 On the basis of your assessment of his risk, you decide to admit this patient to the hospital. An IV is in place. Which of the following IV antibiotic regimens do you choose?

A) Penicillin
B) Azithromycin
C) Penicillin and gentamicin
D) Azithromycin and ceftriaxone
E) Piperacillin/tazobactam and ciprofloxacin

Answer 3.12.3 **The correct answer is "D."** The 2007 Infectious Disease Society of America/American Thoracic Society (IDSA/ATS) guideline for community-acquired pneumonia (*still* not updated as of the writing of this book) recommends that for community-acquired pneumonia treated in the hospital setting, the optimal antibiotic regimen must offer good coverage of *S. pneumoniae, H. influenzae,* and atypical organisms such as *Mycoplasma* and *Chlamydia* species. Most *S. pneumoniae* bacteria are resistant to penicillin ("A") and about 20% to 30% are resistant to macrolides such as azithromycin ("B"). Therefore, these agents should not be used alone in the treatment of pneumonia in hospitalized patients. Gentamicin ("C") has no activity against *S. pneumoniae* but has a role in *P. aeruginosa* infections. Ceftriaxone offers good Gram-negative coverage and activity against *S. pneumoniae.* Azithromycin covers atypical organisms. For these reasons, "D" is the best choice. An alternative regimen would be monotherapy with a respiratory fluoroquinolone, such as moxifloxacin or levofloxacin (remembering the cautions associated with fluoroquinolones). The combination of piperacillin/tazobactam with ciprofloxacin ("E") is reserved for patients with more severe pneumonia, requiring ventilation and ICU care.

....

Initial blood cultures grow *S. pneumoniae.* Sputum Gram stain and culture are negative. The patient initially does well and defervesces after 2 days of IV antibiotics. However, on day 3, he again spikes a fever. He looks moderately ill. Your examination reveals increased dullness to percussion on the left. There is no jugular venous distention (JVD) or peripheral edema. The radiograph is shown in Fig. 3-7.

Question 3.12.4 The most likely diagnosis at this point is:
A) Anaerobic abscess
B) Development of resistant *S. pneumoniae*
C) Parapneumonic effusion
D) Transudate secondary to heart failure
E) Drug-induced transudate

Answer 3.12.4 **The correct answer is "C."** The most likely problem in this patient is a parapneumonic effusion. "A," an anaerobic abscess, is unlikely given that there are no air/fluid levels and the fact that the fluid appears to be in the pleural space. "B" is unlikely. Development of resistance should take more than 3 days, especially since this patient is on two drugs. "D" is unlikely given that this patient does not have a history of heart failure, is febrile, and has no JVD, etc. "E" is unlikely. None of the drugs that he is on is known to cause pleural effusions.

....

You place a chest tube to drain the pleural effusion (free flowing on ultrasound) and continue the current antibiotic regimen. The patient does well and is discharged 1 week later on clarithromycin after sensitivities conclude that his organism is susceptible to it.

Six weeks after the onset of illness, he returns for follow-up to ensure clearing of the chest x-ray. He is feeling well. He is alert and oriented, and his lung examination is now normal. There is no lymphadenopathy in the neck or supraclavicular areas. The x-ray still shows left lower lobe infiltrate, unchanged in size from the initial x-ray. The pleural effusion has resolved.

Question 3.12.5 Which of the following is the most appropriate next step in the evaluation and management of this patient?
A) Chest CT
B) Chest x-ray in 2 weeks
C) Chest x-ray in 6 weeks
D) Prescribe amoxicillin/clavulanate
E) Refer for bronchoscopy

Answer 3.12.5 **The correct answer is "C."** There are no clear guidelines regarding follow-up chest x-ray in patients who had pneumonia. The British Thoracic Society published recommendations in 2007 where it advised repeating chest x-ray in 6 weeks in patients with a smoking history. The reason for that recommendation is a chance that the infiltrate would obscure an underlying malignancy. Those over age 50 should also have follow-up x-ray. Bacteremic pneumococcal pneumonia has been associated with very slowly clearing x-rays, up to 3 to 5 months in some cases. Thus, repeating the chest x-ray in 2 weeks is unlikely to show resolution, so "B" is incorrect. In elderly patients, the chest x-ray takes longer to normalize than in younger patients.

The patient is clinically doing well and does not require treatment for a persistent pulmonary infection, so "D" is incorrect. Chest CT ("A") and bronchoscopy ("E") would give more information, but in the absence of systemic symptoms, such as weight loss, persistent cough, hemoptysis, or fever, they are not

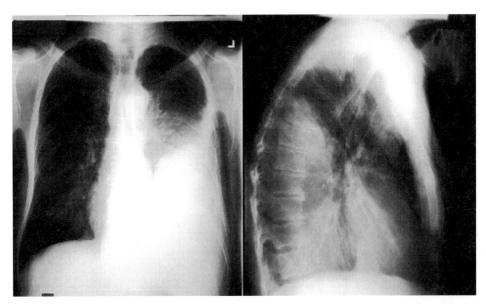

FIGURE 3-7. Question 3.12.4 patient's chest x-ray.

indicated. It is important to consider the fact that this "infiltrate" may represent a neoplastic process if it does not resolve within several months.

HELPFUL TIP:
Even with extensive evaluation (blood culture, sputum culture, etc.), an infectious agent is only identified in 50% of cases of pneumonia. Thus, treatment is usually empiric. Sputum cultures do not alter antibiotic therapy or disease outcome in most patients with pneumonia, and 30% of patients with pneumonia are not able to produce sputum. Blood cultures are of little or no value in pneumonia, but are still recommended in most guidelines for hospitalized patients. If possible, do blood cultures before initiating therapy.

HELPFUL TIP:
"Health care associated pneumonia" (HCAP) is no more (e.g., pneumonia acquired in a nursing home, in patients on hemodialysis, with recent IV therapy, within 90 days of a prior admission, etc.). The application of HCAP guidelines has not resulted in better outcomes and in most settings has led to harm through significant overuse of anti-MRSA and antipseudomonal antibiotics (*Clin Chest Med*. 2018;39(4):765–773). **Hospital Acquired Pneumonia (HAP) is still a thing and comprises a pneumonia that occurs >48 hours after admission.**

So what's to do? Despite the limitations of HCAP criteria, two findings are consistent. The first is that prior detection of MRSA or *Pseudomonas* predicts a much higher risk of these pathogens causing pneumonia. Physicians should cover empirically for these pathogens if they are known to have been identified in the past (vancomycin + piperacillin/tazobactam). The second is that the implications for missing these pathogens is of most concern in patients with significant sepsis and/or requiring intensive care. These patients should still have MRSA and *Pseudomonas* coverage (as above). Finally, *hospital acquired pneumonia (HAP) and ventilator-associated pneumonia* should both be treated empirically with a regimen that covers *MRSA, Pseudomonas*, and other Gram negatives. Non-invasive cultures should be collected and the antibiotic regimen adjusted according to the results (*Clin Infect Dis*. 2016;63(5):e61–e111).

HELPFUL TIP:
Proton pump inhibitors and H$_2$-blockers are associated with an increased risk of pneumonia. Stop them when you can.

HELPFUL TIP:
Steroids *may* be helpful in hospitalized patient with community-acquired pneumonia who are not severely immunosuppressed, are not on chronic steroids, and don't have uncontrolled diabetes (a relative contraindication to steroids). The dose is prednisone 40 mg daily for 3 to 7 days. See *Lancet*. 2015;385(9977):1511–1518 and *Clin Infect Dis*. 2018;66:346 if you want to try this at home (well, in the hospital).

In one of life's funny little coincidences, the next day you diagnose this patient's 36-year-old healthy son with a community-acquired pneumonia. He has a fever, cough, and left lower lobe infiltrate on chest x-ray, but he is hemodynamically stable. You determine that he's fit for outpatient management.

Question 3.12.8 Which of the following drug regimens is appropriate for the treatment of this patient in the outpatient setting?
A) Cephalexin 250 to 500 mg PO QID for 10 days
B) Penicillin V 250 mg TID for 10 days
C) Clarithromycin 500 mg BID for 10 days
D) Doxycycline 100 mg BID for 10 days
E) C or D

Answer 3.12.8 The correct answer is "E." The treatment of community-acquired pneumonia requires coverage of "typical" and "atypical" organisms. Neither "A" nor "B" covers atypical organisms. Guideline-recommended choices for the outpatient treatment of community-acquired pneumonia include doxycycline and macrolides such as clarithromycin (doxycycline has the least resistance). Additional options include the respiratory fluoroquinolones such as moxifloxacin, gemifloxacin, or levofloxacin. However, respiratory fluoroquinolones should not be used in all cases. The IDSA/ATS consensus guidelines recommend that respiratory fluoroquinolones be reserved for patients with serious underlying disease (e.g., COPD, diabetes, immunocompromised states). Of the appropriate regimens, doxycycline and erythromycin are the least expensive, but erythromycin is associated with a high rate of gastrointestinal intolerance.

HELPFUL TIP:
2007 IDSA/ATS guidelines for Community-Acquired Pneumonia recommend treating patients with community-acquired pneumonia for the minimum duration of 5 days. However, prior to discontinuation of treatment, they should also be afebrile for 48 to 72 hours and should have no more than one of the following criteria of instability: heart rate >100 bpm, respiratory rate >24, systolic blood pressure <90 mm Hg, O$_2$ saturation <90% on room air, PaO$_2$ <60 mm Hg on room air, inability to maintain oral intake, confusion. Should

the patient have more than one of these criteria, longer antimicrobial therapy is indicated (and hopefully you do not still have them in the community!).

▶ **Objectives: Did you learn to …**
- Recognize the clinical presentation of community-acquired pneumonia in different patient populations?
- Determine the appropriate disposition for a patient with community-acquired pneumonia?
- Initiate outpatient and inpatient treatment for community-acquired pneumonia?

▶ CASE 3.13

While you are covering the ED, a 60-year-old female comes in by ambulance. She is unresponsive, and her husband states that he found her 30 minutes ago surrounded by bottles of pills and an empty bottle of vodka. She has a history of COPD, hypertension, osteoarthritis, and depression. The EMTs brought in her pill bottles, which include lorazepam, acetaminophen/hydrocodone, hydrochlorothiazide, aspirin, and sertraline. Only a few tablets are left in the bottle of hydrochlorothiazide. She is wearing a nonrebreather facemask with 50% oxygen. Her respirations are shallow with a rate of 8. The remainder of her vitals: temperature 36°C, blood pressure 90/50 mm Hg, and pulse rate 90 bpm. Oxygen saturation is 88% and increases to 94% with some assisted breaths. One nurse is obtaining a blood gas while another gives naloxone. You decide that this patient cannot protect her airway and choose to intubate her. The blood gas drawn just before intubation shows pH 7.16, $PaCO_2$ 60 mm Hg, and PaO_2 40 mm Hg.

Question 3.13.1 These findings imply which of the following processes?
A) Metabolic acidosis
B) Metabolic alkalosis
C) Respiratory alkalosis
D) Mixed metabolic/respiratory acidosis
E) Mixed metabolic/respiratory alkalosis

Answer 3.13.1 **The correct answer is "D."** The pH is acidotic (<7.4). In a patient whose baseline $PaCO_2$ is not known to you, you might assume her $PaCO_2$ is usually 40 mm Hg, which is the accepted normal for most patients.

If the acidosis is purely due to acute respiratory changes and CO_2 retention, a rise in $PaCO_2$ of 10 should be accompanied by a fall in pH equal to 0.08. In this case, the change in $PaCO_2$ is 20. So, $20/10 \times 0.08 = 2 \times 0.08 = 0.16$ resulting in a pH of $7.4 - 0.16 = 7.24$.

However, this patient's pH is measured at 7.16, lower than expected for a pure respiratory acidosis presenting acutely. Thus, you can determine that the acidosis is both metabolic (perhaps from lactic acidosis from hypoperfusion) and respiratory.

HELPFUL TIP:
It is clear that low tidal volumes are protective in patients with acute respiratory distress syndrome/acute lung injury (ARDS/ALI) and prevent VILI (ventilator-induced lung injury). It is unclear whether the same strategy should be employed for all the patients. There is data that shows that even slightly injured lung is more prone to VILI, so it is reasonable to aim for a tidal volume of 6 to 8 mL/kg of predicted body weight in all patients. In addition, patients with asthma or COPD can quickly develop dynamic hyperinflation with higher tidal volumes. Ventilated patients with obstructive disease generally need more time for exhalation.

Your patient is on assist-control mode of ventilation. A nasogastric tube, 2 IVs, and a bladder catheter are in place. She is given IV *N*-acetylcysteine. Her blood pressure improves to 112/67 mm Hg, and her oxygen saturation is 99%. Her chest x-ray shows an endotracheal tube terminating 3 cm above the carina and no infiltrates. Thirty minutes after you intubated her, with the ventilator rate at 14 breaths/min, FiO_2 100%, and tidal volume at 400 mL, you obtain another ABG: pH 7.35, $PaCO_2$ 45 mm Hg, PaO_2 130 mm Hg. She takes 6 to 8 spontaneous, assisted breaths, while the ventilator provides the remaining breaths. She appears to be perfusing her periphery well.

Question 3.13.2 Your next action is to:
A) Decrease the tidal volume to allow for permissive hypercapnia
B) Increase the tidal volume to achieve a pH of 7.45 to 7.50
C) Reduce FiO_2 while maintaining oxygen saturations at or above 90%
D) Change to pressure support ventilation

Answer 3.13.2 **The correct answer is "C."** Your patient is perfusing well, and her PaO_2 and measured oxygen saturation are much improved. You should now decrease the FiO_2, with the goal being to achieve an FiO_2 of less than 60% while maintaining adequate perfusion and oxygen saturation. An FiO_2 of 100% is somewhat toxic and can lead to airway injury. "A" is incorrect. However, permissive hypercapnia (allowing CO_2 to rise to >80 mm Hg as long as the patient tolerates it) may be useful in ventilated patients with COPD, ARDS, or asthma; it allows you to reduce tidal volumes and pressures without doing harm. But remember that you still need to maintain oxygenation. "B" is incorrect. Your patient is doing reasonably well with her slightly acidotic pH, which has corrected very quickly. It may be inadvisable to attempt to increase her pH beyond 7.40, as she may develop respiratory alkalosis that can then lead to cardiac arrhythmias. Because of her low respiratory rate, she should remain on some type of assisted volume-cycled ventilation. "Pressure support ventilation," as its name implies, only augments patient-triggered breaths with increased airway pressure.

This pressure is in addition to the background positive end-expiratory pressure (PEEP); PEEP is used to prevent alveolar collapse and subsequent lung injury.

HELPFUL TIP:
Permissive hypercapnia is an approach to the ventilated patient where the provider allows CO_2 build up and decrease in pH (even down to levels of 7.1) in order to provide long expiratory times and low minute ventilation to prevent hyperinflation and barotrauma.

Question 3.13.3 In this patient, which of the following ventilator management techniques will unequivocally decrease her FiO₂ requirement?
A) Increase the respiratory rate
B) Increase the positive end-expiratory pressure (PEEP)
C) Decrease the tidal volume
D) Addition of inhaled nitric oxide (NO)

Answer 3.13.3 The correct answer is "B." Two standard techniques are usually employed to improve a patient's oxygenation: increasing FiO_2 and PEEP. PEEP maintains positive pressure in the airways at the end of expiration. Its use increases lung compliance and decreases ventilation/perfusion mismatching, resulting in better oxygenation. Since FiO_2 >60% over periods longer than 48 hours may result in oxygen toxicity, PEEP may be employed to reduce the need for high levels of FiO_2. "A" and "C" are incorrect. Increasing respiratory rate or tidal volume will cause increases in minute ventilation, which reduces $PaCO_2$, but has little effect on PaO_2. Decreasing minute ventilation, through decreased respiratory rate or tidal volume, causes CO_2 retention and increased $PaCO_2$. "D" is incorrect. Nitric oxide has been shown to improve oxygenation in select patients with severe pulmonary hypertension and ARDS, but *does not improve overall outcomes and is potentially nephrotoxic.*

You follow the patient during her hospitalization. The next day she is more alert and is able to follow commands. Her ventilator requirements have decreased. You consider extubation.

Question 3.13.4 All of the following parameters predict a poor outcome for attempted weaning from ventilation EXCEPT:
A) Minute ventilation supplied by ventilator is <10 L/min
B) PaO_2 <55 mm Hg while on FiO_2 >35%
C) Rapid shallow breathing index (RSBI) of 140
D) Physical examination findings of increased respiratory effort

Answer 3.13.4 The correct answer is "A." Preparing to withdraw a patient from mechanical ventilation—typically called weaning or liberation—relies considerably on judgment, but a few objective parameters can be helpful. In general, the patient to be liberated must be awake, alert, and cooperative. She should have reasonably good oxygenation on a lower FiO_2, have

PEEP <8 cm H_2O, and be able to generate adequate inspiratory pressures. Minute ventilation from the ventilator of less than 10 L/min is associated with greater success with weaning.

Poor prognostic indicators include a minute ventilation from the ventilator >10 L/min, PaO_2 <55 with FiO_2 >35%, and RSBI >105 (see Helpful Tip). Patients with poor cardiopulmonary reserve or who have significant underlying disease may also have difficulty weaning. Allow patients a period of breathing on their own (e.g., a T-piece) before extubating. This way, if the patient fails, you can simply hook her back up to the ventilator.

HELPFUL TIP:
Rapid Shallow Breathing Index (RSBI) is one of the predictors of successful extubation. It is calculated by dividing respiratory rate by tidal volume in liters while patient is maintained on pressure support ventilation with minimal settings (pressure of 5–10, PEEP 5–8). For example, patient breathing 20 times per minute with 500 mL of tidal volume has RSBI of 20/0.5 = 40. Patient breathing 34 times per minute with tidal volume of 210 mL has RSBI of 34/0.21 = 161 and is obviously not ready to be extubated.

HELPFUL TIP:
ICU setting is much different than OR; extubations in the ICU carry higher risk of failure. Do not feel bad if your patient needs to be re-intubated. There is no perfect predictor of successful ICU extubation and data show that up to 15% of ICU patients will require re-intubation despite good predictors of successful extubation.

HELPFUL TIP:
Minute ventilation (for the patient) is calculated by multiplying respiratory rate by tidal volume. Thus, a person getting 20 breaths/min from the ventilator at 400 mL/breath generates a minute ventilation = (20 breaths/min × 400 mL/min)/1000 = 8 L/min.

▶ **Objectives: Did you learn to …**
- Recognize a mixed respiratory/metabolic acidosis?
- Calculate expected pH changes in acute respiratory acidosis?
- Institute ventilation with appropriate initial ventilator settings?
- Identify potential complications of ventilation?
- Wean a patient from the ventilator?

▶ **CASE 3.14**

A 52-year-old male smoker presents for a 3-month history of productive cough. He reports multiple episodes of pneumonia, but continues to produce copious sputum between episodes of pneumonia. Chest x-ray is unremarkable. Chest

CT shows enlarged peripheral airways with thickened airway walls in the lower lobes bilaterally. Sputum culture grows several types of bacteria, including *P. aeruginosa.*

Question 3.14.1 Which of the following do you recommend as initial therapy?
A) Corticosteroids
B) Antibiotics
C) Chemotherapy
D) Supplemental oxygen
E) Wedge resection of the affected lung tissue

Answer 3.14.1 **The correct answer is "B."** This patient's findings are consistent with the diagnosis of bronchiectasis, a chronic inflammatory disease of the medium-sized bronchi. Appropriate initial therapy consists of prolonged courses of antibiotics, usually 2 weeks of a narrow-spectrum antibiotic followed by reassessment. Doxycycline, amoxicillin, clarithromycin, amoxicillin/clavulanate, and trimethoprim/sulfamethoxazole are often used. Respiratory quinolones demonstrate some limited use in patients with *Pseudomonas.* Patients should be directed to discontinue tobacco use and take inhaled bronchodilators. Resection of the affected lung tissue may be necessary but should not be the initial therapy. Supplemental oxygen therapy is used if oxygenation is poor. Chemotherapy and prolonged oral corticosteroids are not used to treat bronchiectasis.

HELPFUL TIP:
Patients with acute exacerbations of bronchiectasis are often treated with prolonged courses of antibiotics tailored to previous sputum cultures. For those with recurrent exacerbations (2–3 per year), preventative therapy with a macrolide antibiotic is recommended, after cultures exclude nontuberculous mycobacterial (NTM infection) due to the concern for development of resistance. For those with recurrent exacerbations and *Pseudomonas aeruginosa* in their sputum, a trial of inhaled antibiotics (such as tobramycin) may be used. It is also recommended patients regularly use airway clearance techniques to help remove airway secretions. Pulmonary rehabilitation may also offer a benefit to patients with moderate-to-severe airflow limitation on pulmonary function testing.

Question 3.14.2 In most adults with bronchiectasis, its cause is:
A) Genetic
B) *Pseudomonas* infection
C) Tobacco smoking
D) Allergic bronchopulmonary aspergillosis (ABPA)
E) Unknown

Answer 3.14.2 **The correct answer is "E."** There are limited data regarding the etiology of bronchiectasis, but many conditions and environmental exposures seem to have an association.

In most patients, no cause is identified. Children are more likely than adults to have an identified etiology of their bronchiectasis, and the most common causes in kids are foreign body aspiration, cystic fibrosis, and gastroesophageal reflux. Identified etiologies in adults include those mentioned for children and pulmonary infections, ABPA, COPD, rheumatic or other inflammatory diseases, immunodeficiencies, and cigarette smoking.

▶ **Objectives: Did you learn to …**
• Identify findings consistent with bronchiectasis?
• Treat a patient with bronchiectasis?

 QUICK QUIZ: DYSPNEA

A 75-year-old gentleman presents to your office with emphysema diagnosed elsewhere. He reports dyspnea on exertion after 1 to 2 blocks. He smokes 10 cigarettes per day and does not have underlying cardiac disease. Physical examination is remarkable for fine crackles in both lung bases. Chest x-ray shows increased interstitial markings in the lower lobes. He has no pulmonary function testing on record.

Of the following tests, which is the most likely to confirm or alter the diagnosis?
A) Spirometry, diffusing capacity, lung volumes
B) Spirometry, ABG, diffusing capacity
C) ABG, diffusing capacity, lung volumes
D) ABG, lung volumes, chest CT

The correct answer is "A." This case demonstrates a commonly seen phenomenon: patients who smoke and have dyspnea are assumed to have obstructive lung disease, particularly emphysema. However, pulmonary function tests are required to make the diagnosis of obstructive disease. Furthermore, this patient's chest x-ray shows increased interstitial markings in the lower lung fields suggesting interstitial lung disease. This disease process is associated with a restrictive pattern on pulmonary spirometry. Lung volumes and diffusing capacity will provide a more complete picture. Thus, spirometry, diffusing capacity, and lung volumes would allow you to make the diagnosis. In interstitial lung disease, spirometry shows a FEV_1/FVC ratio >0.7, a decreased diffusing capacity, and decreased total lung capacity (the hallmark of restrictive lung disease). ABG is unlikely to help differentiate restrictive from obstructive lung disease, so options "B" through "D" are not correct.

HELPFUL TIP:
The diffusing capacity, as measured by DLCO, is low in the following disease states: emphysema, interstitial lung disease (e.g., sarcoid, alveolitis, pulmonary radiation, pulmonary toxicity from drugs such as amiodarone, pulmonary fibrosis), *Pneumocystis* pneumonia, and pulmonary vascular disease. Anemia will also cause a low DLCO—so a hemoglobin or hematocrit should always be ordered with DLCO.

HELPFUL TIP:
DLCO can be *increased* by pulmonary hemorrhage, polycythemia, massive obesity, left-to-right intracardiac shunting, asthma, and left heart failure (increase capillary volume in the lungs).

QUICK QUIZ: PULMONARY INFECTIONS

A 72-year-old woman you admitted to the hospital for pneumonia is having worsening dyspnea and hypoxemia. She is decompensating despite 3 days of antibiotic therapy with intravenous levofloxacin. According to her husband, the couple had been working on their Iowa farm, and made a trip to an old barn to collect manure *a week before the patient developed a cough and fever* (so this is not hypersensitivity pneumonitis, nor organic dust toxicity syndrome). The barn was noted to be the home of numerous birds. Her respiratory rate is 32, and her oxygen saturation is 89% on 5 L/min of oxygen by nasal cannula. Chest x-ray reveals a diffuse interstitial infiltrate, enlarged mediastinal nodes, and normal heart size.

Which of the following is the most likely culprit for the cause of her current illness?
A) *S. pneumoniae*
B) *H. influenzae*
C) *Coxiella burnetii*
D) *Histoplasma capsulatum*
E) *Blastomyces dermatitidis*

The correct answer is "D." The case described here is classic for an environmental exposure to a large dose of *Histoplasma* organisms. Histoplasmosis is often transmitted by bird or bat droppings. *Histoplasma* occurs most commonly in the Mississippi and Ohio River valleys, causing a self-limited disease in most persons. Patients who have *Histoplasma* infection frequently develop calcified mediastinal lymph nodes after resolution of the infection. Diagnosis can be made by urinary antigen or bronchoscopic biopsy. The bacterial causes are unlikely to be important factors here, as she was on a broad-spectrum antibiotic for 3 days with no improvement. *C. burnetii*, the agent causing Q fever, is rare and tends to affect workers exposed to fresh animal material, such as placentas. *Blastomyces* is found in the same regions as *Histoplasma*, but the site of exposure tends to be more moist, unlike the dry environment inside a barn. We all have granulomas from histoplasmosis on CXR in Iowa.

► CASE 3.15

A 42-year-old female comes to your office with a history of asthma that has been difficult to control. She relates symptoms that have been worsening over the last 4 to 6 weeks. She received two courses of oral corticosteroids during that time. Her symptoms improved with this therapy but quickly returned after completing the steroids. She denies fever, chills, and night sweats, but complains of a chronic cough productive of brownish-colored sputum. She is a homemaker in a suburban area and has no pets. Physical examination reveals wheezing throughout all lung fields but is otherwise normal. Laboratory evaluation includes CBC with increased eosinophils, normal C-reactive protein, and an elevated IgE level of 1250 ng/mL. A high-resolution CT scan of the chest reveals central bronchiectasis.

Question 3.15.1 What is the most likely diagnosis?
A) Hypersensitivity pneumonitis
B) Acute eosinophilic pneumonia
C) Allergic bronchopulmonary aspergillosis (ABPA)
D) Bacterial pneumonia
E) Churg–Strauss vasculitis

Answer 3.15.1 The correct answer is "C." This patient's history points to the diagnosis of ABPA, which is characterized by the presence of severe asthma, brownish mucus plugs, peripheral eosinophilia above 10%, elevated serum IgE, and central bronchiectasis. IgE elevation is required to be greater than 1,000 ng/mL. "A" is unlikely but a bit tricky. First, there is no history of exposure to a causative agent. Second, let's focus on symptoms. Constitutional symptoms—often fever—are present in the acute form of hypersensitivity pneumonitis. However, they need not be present in the subacute and chronic forms of the disease. So, based on symptoms, this could be hypersensitivity pneumonitis. However, the radiologic findings of hypersensitivity pneumonitis would include interstitial lung disease, rather than central bronchiectasis. Thus, this is not likely hypersensitivity pneumonitis.

"B" and "D" are incorrect. Note that she has no significant constitutional symptoms that might be more typical of acute eosinophilic pneumonia or bacterial infection. You would also expect an infiltrate on the chest CT. "E" is incorrect. Churg–Strauss vasculitis is characterized by transient patchy interstitial infiltrates, fever, weight loss, elevated sedimentation rate, abnormal liver enzymes, and a peripheral blood eosinophilia >1,000 cells/μL. This is often related to using an oral steroid and a leukotriene inhibitor simultaneously. It is not related to inhaled steroid use. Extrapulmonary manifestations (CHF, pericarditis, tender subcutaneous nodules, peripheral neuropathy—most commonly mononeuritis multiplex) distinguish Churg–Strauss from other eosinophilic pulmonary conditions.

Question 3.15.2 Which of the following would be the next best step in confirming the diagnosis?
A) Sputum cultures
B) Transbronchial biopsy
C) Methacholine challenge
D) Allergy skin testing for *Aspergillus* species
E) p-ANCA

Answer 3.15.2 The correct answer is "D." Most but not all of the following criteria (Table 3-11) need to be present in order to make the diagnosis of ABPA. Transbronchial biopsy is unnecessarily invasive, and the other tests will not help to confirm the diagnosis.

TABLE 3-11 CRITERIA FOR THE DIAGNOSIS OF ALLERGIC BRONCHOPULMONARY ASPERGILLOSIS (ABPA)

- Asthma
- Central bronchiectasis
- Elevated total serum IgE >1,000 ng/mL
- Immediate skin test reactivity to *Aspergillus*
- Elevated serum-specific IgE and/or IgG to *Aspergillus fumigatus*
- Peripheral blood eosinophilia >10%
- Pulmonary infiltrates

Question 3.15.3 The most appropriate treatment for this patient with ABPA would include which of the following?
A) Antibiotics
B) Oral corticosteroids
C) Leukotriene receptor antagonist
D) Itraconazole
E) Inhaled ipratropium bromide

Answer 3.15.3 The correct answer is "B." Oral corticosteroids are the treatment of choice for ABPA. Patients are typically treated for several months with tapering doses rather than short courses of steroids. Serum IgE levels and chest x-rays are used to monitor response to treatment. Please note that "D" is incorrect, and azoles are *not* the mainstay therapy in ABPA. The goal of treatment is suppression of the immune system responding to the fungal antigen. There are studies that show benefit of adding an antifungal agent as a steroid-sparing agent. However, there are risks associated with concomitant use of steroids and azoles, namely, marked adrenal suppression. Hence, oral corticosteroids should be your first choice.

▶ Objectives: Did you learn to …
  • Identify the clinical presentation of ABPA?
  • Diagnose and treat a patient with ABPA?

▶ CASE 3.16

A 16-year-old female comes to your office with complaints of sneezing spells, itchy watery eyes, and nasal congestion for the past 2 years. These symptoms are worse during the spring and fall and when she plays with her cat. She denies any other constitutional symptoms and has no other past medical history. She has tried over-the-counter loratadine without relief. She has lived in the same residence for the past 6 years and denies any other environmental exposures. Her examination reveals pale nasal mucosa and swollen nasal turbinates bilaterally. Her lungs and skin are clear.

Question 3.16.1 You are not clear if this is allergic rhinitis or nonallergic rhinopathy (previously known as vasomotor rhinitis). The most effective way to determine if this is allergic is to:
A) Do a methacholine challenge test
B) Do a Hansel stain of nasal mucus

C) Check overall IgE levels
D) Perform a nasal mucus electrophoresis to visualize allergic bands
E) Waft hot peppers under her nose…see what happens

Answer 3.16.1 The correct answer is "B." The best way to tell if this is allergic is to do a Hansel stain of the nasal mucus. This will show eosinophils if it is allergic. If this is nonallergic rhinopathy, eosinophils will be absent. If it is infectious, there will likely be a predominance of neutrophils. "A" is incorrect. A methacholine challenge test is helpful in diagnosing asthma, not allergic rhinitis. Neither "C," IgE levels, nor nasal mucus electrophoresis have any use here (and nasal mucus electrophoresis has no use anywhere that we know of… and it is disgusting). IgE is only elevated in 40% of patients with allergic rhinitis. Does anyone ever actually do a Hansel stain? Probably not, but once again, this is for the Board Examination, not real life.

Question 3.16.2 The Hansel stain shows eosinophils. "Eureka!" you shout. Which of the following would be the most appropriate next step in managing her symptoms?
A) Recommend allergen-impermeable encasements for mattress and pillow
B) Use topical decongestant sprays
C) Change classes of antihistamines
D) Refer for allergy evaluation, including percutaneous aeroallergen skin testing
E) Recommend a high-efficiency particulate air filter for the home

Answer 3.16.2 The correct answer is "C." Although all of the above choices may provide relief for allergic symptoms, the best first step would be to try changing the class of antihistamines. Antihistamines (and NSAIDs for that matter) are grouped into classes based on chemical structure. One class may be helpful for a patient when another class does not work.

The other choices are suboptimal. Without skin testing, avoidance measures may be needless, costly, and ineffective. Skin testing alone ("D") would not immediately improve her symptoms, and you would still need to do something with therapy (we hope) while waiting 3 months to see an allergist. Allergen-impermeable encasements ("A") are currently recommended for patients with dust mite allergy. Although filters ("E") are often recommended for pet allergies, the data regarding their effectiveness in reducing allergic symptoms is contradictory. Topical decongestant sprays ("B") are an inappropriate choice secondary to the addictive nature of these medications and the risk of causing rebound symptoms. Removing a pet from the bedroom may reduce—but not eliminate—allergen exposure. Further evaluation should be performed prior to recommending any such lifestyle modifications. Another reasonable option would be a trial of intranasal corticosteroid. Finally, you could also put an allergen impermeable encasement around the cat …

Your patient's 17-year-old brother is in the next examination room. He is a Boy Scout who just returned from a backpacking trip in the four corners area of New Mexico, Arizona,

Colorado, and Utah. He has noted myalgias, fever, and chills. He knows that you are reviewing pulmonary medicine for your upcoming Board Examination, so he presents to your office complaining of dyspnea that has been getting markedly worse over the past several days. He has no URI symptoms such as coryza, rhinorrhea, ear pain, etc. Additionally, he has nausea, vomiting, and diarrhea with severe abdominal pain. His respiratory rate is 40 with an oxygen saturation of 88% on room air. ("See," he says, "I told you I'm sick.") You place him on nasal oxygen and order a chest x-ray, which shows bilateral pulmonary edema.

Question 3.16.3 Based on the epidemiology and chest x-ray appearance, your best guess at this point in the disease is:
A) Plague
B) Coccidiodomycosis
C) Hantavirus from Sin Nombre (No Name) strain
D) Noncardiogenic pulmonary edema from smoking paraquat (you never know what is going on at those Boy Scout camps)
E) Ischemic cardiomyopathy from cocaine use (you never know what is going on at those Boy Scout camps)

Answer 3.16.3 The correct answer is "C." This is a typical history and physical examination for hantavirus. The absence of URI symptoms, the presence of GI symptoms, and the noncardiogenic pulmonary edema are all symptoms/signs of hantavirus. In fact, it may present as an acute abdomen. It is spread by aerosolization of mouse excrement or urine. "B" is incorrect. Although coccidiodomycosis, "Valley Fever," is found in the same geographical region, it presents with lower respiratory symptoms, a thin walled cavitary lesion, erythema nodosum (10%), and eosinophilia. Coccidiomycosis is generally a low-grade, subacute process that lasts weeks to months. It does not cause non-cardiogenic pulmonary edema. "A," pneumonic plague, while also found in the same area, causes high fever, bloody sputum, pleuritic chest pain, and develops over hours to days. It can be rapidly fatal if not recognized and treated within the first day. "D" and "E" are wrong for so many reasons that we won't bother to enumerate them here, but you never *do* know what goes on at camp.

Question 3.16.4 Laboratory findings suggestive of hantavirus include all of the following EXCEPT:
A) Thrombocytopenia
B) Leukocytosis with a left shift
C) A lymphocytic predominance
D) An immunoblast count <10%

Answer 3.16.4 The correct answer is "D." In fact, thrombocytopenia, a 10% or **greater** immunoblast count, and a left shift constitute the so-called diagnostic triad in a patient with appropriate clinical findings. Immunoblasts are the most immature cell in the lymphocyte line (they still enjoy scribbling on walls and drinking irresponsibly). Overall, case fatality rate of hantavirus is up to 50%. Care is supportive. Extra-corporeal membrane oxygenation may be used in seriously ill patients. There is often

an oliguric phase that needs careful management to prevent fluid overload. This can be problematic because patients are often hypotensive and there is a proclivity toward giving them fluids.

▶ **Objectives: Did you learn to …**
- Assess and treat allergic rhinitis?
- Diagnose and manage a hantavirus infection?

Clinical Pearls

○ A normal CO_2 on a blood gas in a dyspneic patient suggests CO_2 retention and portends a declining respiratory status.

○ A venous blood gas has essentially the same values as an arterial blood gas except for the O_2 which you can get from a transcutaneous monitor. Venous gases hurt less.

○ Always use spirometry to diagnose COPD. Only 55% of those diagnosed using clinical signs and symptoms have COPD; the rest have a different underlying cause for their dyspnea.

○ Asymptomatic GERD does not cause asthma exacerbations.

○ Be judicious when treating sarcoid with steroids; use them only when symptoms are severe or intolerable by the patient. They can prolong the course of the disease.

○ Blood cultures are not generally helpful in pneumonia (but someone will want them).

○ Do not use a long-acting beta-agonist in asthma without an inhaled steroid. It worsens outcomes.

○ Do not use inhaled steroids in mild-to-moderate COPD. They increase pneumonia and confer no benefit.

○ For COPD patients, initiate treatment in symptomatic patients with a short-acting inhaled bronchodilator (e.g., albuterol), then add a long-acting inhaled bronchodilator (e.g., tiotropium) if symptoms are not controlled.

○ It is impossible to reliably differentiate a "typical" from an "atypical" pneumonia by x-ray.

○ When discharging a patient on oxygen, make sure there is still an oxygen requirement and it was not a function of the acute illness that brought the patient to the hospital.

BIBLIOGRAPHY

American College of Chest Physicians. *Pulmonary Medicine Board Review*. Northbrook, IL: ACCP; 2009;167–173.

American Lung Association Asthma Clinical Research Centers, et al. Efficacy of esomeprazole for treatment of poorly controlled asthma. *N Engl J Med.* 2009;360(15): 1487–1499.

Bashir R, et al. Comparative outcomes of catheter-directed thrombolysis plus anticoagulation vs. anticoagulation alone to treat lower extremity proximal deep vein thrombosis. *JAMA Intern Med.* 2014;174(9): 1494–1501.

Blum CA, et al. Adjunct prednisone therapy for patients with community-acquired pneumonia: a multicentre, double-blind, randomised, placebo-controlled trial. *Lancet.* 2015;385(9977):1511–1518.

Briel M, et al. Corticosteroids in patients hospitalized with community-acquired pneumonia: systematic review and individual patient data metaanalysis. *Clin Infect Dis.* 2018;66:346.

Cahill K, et al. Nicotine receptor partial agonists for smoking cessation. *Cochrane Database Syst Rev.* 2007;24(1):CD006103.

Celli BR, et al. The body-mass index, airflow obstruction, dyspnea, and exercise capacity index in chronic obstructive pulmonary disease. *N Engl J Med.* 2004;350:1005–1012.

Chang PH, et al. Combination therapy of varenicline with nicotine replacement therapy is better than varenicline alone: a systematic review and meta-analysis of randomized controlled trials. *BMC Public Health.* 2015;15:689.

Collins BF, et al. Factors predictive of airflow obstruction among veterans with presumed empirical diagnosis and treatment of COPD. *Chest.* 2015; 147(2):369–376.

Cui Y, et al. Long-term macrolide therapy for the prevention of acute exacerbations in COPD: a systematic review and meta-analysis. *Int J Chron Obstruct Pulmon Dis.* 2018;13:3813–3829.

Daniels JM, et al. Antibiotics in addition to corticosteroids for acute exacerbations of chronic obstructive pulmonary disease. *Am J Respir Crit Care Med.* 2010;181:150–157.

Decramer M, et al. for Global Initiative for Chronic Obstructive Lung Diseases. Global strategies for the diagnosis, management, and prevention of chronic obstructive pulmonary disease: GOLD executive summary. 2018.

DiMango E, et al. Effects on asymptomatic proximal and distal gastroesophageal reflux on asthma severity. *Am J Respir Crit Care Med.* 2009;180(9):809–816.

Ege MJ, et al. Exposure to environmental microorganisms and childhood asthma. *N Engl J Med.* 2011;364:701–709.

Einstein AJ, et al. Estimating risk of cancer associated with radiation exposure from a 64 slice computed tomography coronary angiography. *JAMA.* 2007;298(3):317–323.

Frank Peacock W, et al. Emergency department discharge of pulmonary embolus patients. *Acad Emerg Med.* 2018 Sep; 25(9):995–1003.

Gibson PG, et al. Allergic bronchopulmonary aspergillosis. *Semin Respir Crit Care Med.* 2006;27(2):185–191.

Hutchinson BD, et al. Overdiagnosis of pulmonary embolism by pulmonary CT angiography. *Am J Roentgenol.* 2015;205(2):271.

Irwin RS, Madison MJ. The diagnosis and treatment of cough. *N Engl J Med.* 2000;343(23):1715–1721.

James A; Committee on Practice Bulletins—Obstetrics. Practice bulletin number 123: thromboembolism in pregnancy. *Obstet Gynecol.* 2011;118(3):718–729.

Kalil AC, et al. Management of adults with hospital-acquired and ventilator-associated pneumonia: 2016 clinical practice guideline by the Infectious Diseases Society of America and the American Thoracic Society. *Clinical Infectious Diseases.* 2016;63(5):e61–e111.

Kearon C, et al. Antithrombotic therapy for VTE disease. *Chest.* 2016;149(2):315–352.

Kiser TH, et al. Outcomes associated with corticosteroid dosage in critically ill patients with acute exacerbations of chronic obstructive pulmonary disease. *Am J Respir Crit Care Med.* 2014;189:1052–1064.

Lacasse Y, et al. Clinical diagnosis of hypersensitivity pneumonitis. *Am J Respir Crit Care Med.* 2003;168: 952–958.

Laszlo G. Standardisation of lung function testing: helpful guidance from the ATS/ERS Task Force. *Thorax.* 2006;61:744–746.

Mandell LA, et al. Infectious Diseases Society of America/ American Thoracic Society consensus guidelines on the management of community-acquired pneumonia in adults. *Clin Infect Dis.* 2007;1(44 Suppl 2):S27–S72.

Maurelus K, et al. Focus on Ultrasound for Thoracentesis. 2013. Available at https://www.acepnow.com/article/ultrasound-thoracentesis/. Accessed June 21, 2015.

Mismetti P, et al. Effect of a retrievable inferior vena cava filter plus anticoagulation vs. anticoagulation alone on risk of recurrent pulmonary embolism: a randomized clinical trial. *JAMA.* 2015;28;313(16):1627–1635.

National Asthma Education and Prevention Program. Expert Panel Report 3 (EPR-3): Guidelines for the diagnosis and management of asthma—Summary Report 2007. *J Allergy Clin Immunol.* 120;2007:S94–S138. Available at http://www.nhlbi.nih.gov/files/docs/guidelines/asthsumm.pdf. Accessed January 28, 2019.

Palareti G, et al. D-Dimer testing to determine the duration of anticoagulation therapy. *N Engl J Med.* 2006;355:1780–1789.

Paramothayan S, Jones PW. Corticosteroid therapy in pulmonary sarcoidosis: a systematic review. *JAMA.* 2002; 287(10):1301–1307.

Pasteur MC, et al. British Thoracic Society guideline for non-CF bronchiectasis. *Thorax.* 2010;65:i1–i58.

Ray WA, et al. Azithromycin and the risk of cardiovascular death. *N Engl J Med.* 2012;366:1881–1890.

Steinberg KP, Kacmarek RM. Respiratory controversies in the critical care setting. Should tidal volume be 6 mL/kg predicted body weight in virtually all patients with acute respiratory failure? *Respir Care.* 2007;52: 556–564.

Tillie-Leblond I, et al. Pulmonary embolism in patients with unexplained exacerbation of chronic obstructive pulmonary disease: prevalence and risk factors. *Ann Int Med.* 2006;144:390–396.

Turner TE, et al. Association of inferior vena cava filter placement for venous thromboembolic disease and contraindication to anticoagulation with 30-day mortality. *JAMA Netw Open.* 2018;1(3):e180452.

U.S. Preventive Services Task Force. Lung Cancer Screening Guidelines. 2013. Available at http://www.uspreventiveservicestaskforce.org/Page/Topic/recommendation-summary/lung-cancer-screening. Accessed June 23, 2015.

Vinson DR, et al. Increasing safe outpatient management of emergency department patients with pulmonary embolism: a controlled pragmatic trial. *Ann Intern Med.* 2018;169(12):855–865.

Von Essen SG, et al. After exposure to the hog barn environment. *J Swine Health Prod.* 2005;13:273–276.

Von Essen SG, et al. Organic dust toxic syndrome: a noninfectious febrile illness. *J Toxicol Clin Toxicol.* 1990;28(4):398–420.

Waterer GW. Health-care associated pneumonia: is it still a useful concept? *Clin Chest Med.* 2018;39(4):765–773.

Wilbur J, Shian B. Diagnosis of deep venous thrombosis and pulmonary embolism. *Am Fam Physician.* 2012;86(1):913–919.

Yasufuku K, et al. Comparison of endobronchial ultrasound, positron emission tomography, and CT for lymph node staging of lung cancer. *Chest.* 2006;130:710–718.

Zodang W, et al. Outpatient patient treatment in patients with acute pulmonary embolism. *J Thromb Haemost.* 2011;9:1500–1507.

Allergy and Immunology

4

Wendy W. Shen

▶ CASE 4.1

A 15-year-old girl has a history of acute difficulty breathing when playing basketball. Her symptoms include *inspiratory* wheezing/stridor, increased respiratory rate, throat tightness, and chest discomfort. Premedication with adequate doses of albuterol has no effect.

Question 4.1.1 What is the most likely diagnosis?
A) Exercise-induced asthma inadequately treated
B) Gastroesophageal reflux disease
C) Musculoskeletal chest pain
D) Hyperventilation
E) Vocal cord dysfunction

Answer 4.1.1 **The correct answer is "E."** Vocal cord dysfunction (VCD) is one of the most common asthma mimics. Patients with VCD present with hoarseness, coughing, dyspnea, and loud *inspiratory* **(and/or expiratory) wheezing/stridor**, along with other symptoms as mentioned above. Although laryngoscopy is the gold standard for the diagnosis of paradoxical vocal cord motion, pulmonary function testing (PFT) often is performed first due to asthma being in the differential diagnosis, and spirometry may indicate airway obstruction due to an extrathoracic component. The PFTs should show evidence of paradoxical inspiratory vocal cord adduction during symptoms which causes airflow restriction at the level of the larynx, and results in a flattened inspiratory loop on flow–volume diagram (see Chapter 3). VCD presents a diagnostic challenge, and often leads to unnecessary treatment for the misdiagnosis of asthma. In this patient, a β_2-agonist was ineffective, even though she displays symptoms with exertion. This argues against answer "A." The distinction between VCD and asthma may be less clear in other patients, since the two disorders sometimes coexist. The clinical history does not support the diagnoses of gastroesophageal reflux disease ("B"), musculoskeletal chest pain ("C"), or hyperventilation ("D").

You make the diagnosis of VCD. However, the patient also complains of rhinorrhea, itchy eyes, sneezing, and itchy nose that worsen in the spring and fall. Because you realize that we need to discuss it in this book, you kindly refer her for allergy testing (thank you!).

Question 4.1.2 With regard to radioallergosorbent testing (RAST) for allergic rhinitis, which of the following is true?
A) RAST is less expensive than traditional skin testing
B) RAST is more sensitive than traditional skin testing
C) RAST has a limited role in testing those with allergic rhinitis
D) Antihistamine use is a contraindication to the use of RAST

Answer 4.1.2 **The correct answer is "C."** RAST will be negative in up to 25% of those with a positive skin test, has poorly reproducible results, and is more expensive. Thus, skin testing remains the procedure of choice for identifying allergens. RAST can be used if skin testing is unavailable.

Question 4.1.3 Which of the following medications does NOT need to be discontinued prior to aeroallergen skin testing?
A) Intranasal steroid spray
B) Atenolol
C) Amitriptyline
D) Cyproheptadine
E) Azelastine nasal spray

Answer 4.1.3 **The correct answer is "A."** Intranasal steroid sprays do not need to be discontinued prior to skin testing as they do not interfere with immediate-type hypersensitivity reactions. Antihistamines, on the other hand (amitriptyline ["C"], cyproheptadine ["D"], or azelastine ["E"] and others), may blunt dermal reactivity. Although azelastine is administered as a nasal spray, its administration may interfere with skin test reactivity within 2 days of usage. Beta-blockers, such as atenolol ("B"), have been shown to affect skin test reactivity and should be avoided in patients undergoing skin testing.

Aeroallergen skin prick and intradermal testing reveals positive reactions to dust mites, cat, ragweed, and tree pollens.

The patient relates that she gets considerable nasal congestion and has tried over-the-counter decongestants with no relief.

Question 4.1.4 Which of the following interventions would provide the most relief for her nasal symptoms?
A) Diphenhydramine 25 mg PO BID
B) Montelukast 10 mg PO QHS
C) Intranasal steroid spray daily
D) Ipratropium bromide nasal spray BID
E) Getting rid of the cat. No one should have a cat. They are evil.

Answer 4.1.4 The correct answer is "C." Intranasal corticosteroids would provide the most relief in this patient by addressing nasal congestion in addition to the other nasal symptoms mentioned. Although antihistamines are very helpful in relieving nasal symptoms such as rhinorrhea, nasal itching, and sneezing, they are generally not as effective for nasal congestion. Likewise, montelukast is a leukotriene modifier, which is approved for the treatment of allergic rhinitis, but studies suggest that intranasal steroids are superior. In addition, nasal steroids are not systemic (although a bit may be absorbed). Ipratropium ("D") is mainly effective for rhinorrhea only, not nasal congestion. Nasal saline irrigations may be beneficial as they promote thinning of nasal secretions and drainage. However, it may not predictably improve nasal congestion. As to "E," yes, cats are evil and shed. But as family doctors we are supposed to be accepting of our patient's quirks.

HELPFUL (AND REALLY COOL) TIP:
Intranasal steroids also improve ocular symptoms. Whether some of the drug gets up the nasolacrimal ducts or is otherwise aerosolized into the eye is unclear. Obviously, do not put intranasal steroids directly in the eye. For moderate-to-severe allergic rhinitis, a combination of intranasal steroid and intranasal antihistamine is more effective than either alone.

She returns to you a year later, having tried intranasal steroid sprays and high-dose antihistamines, without gaining significant relief. She has instituted appropriate avoidance measures during the interim (there goes the cat…thankfully), also without improvement in symptoms. Because you know we need to address it in this book, you recommend allergen immunotherapy.

Question 4.1.5 All of the following statements are true regarding allergen immunotherapy EXCEPT:
A) Patients should carry emergency epinephrine to all immunotherapy shot appointments
B) It is unnecessary to stop beta-blocker therapy prior to starting immunotherapy
C) Patients should be observed in the office for at least 30 minutes after immunotherapy injections
D) At least 3 years of immunotherapy should be given to avoid recurrence of symptoms

Answer 4.1.5 The correct answer is "B." It has been shown that patients taking beta-blockers may be at increased risk of having more severe systemic reactions to immunotherapy. Patients should be treated with an alternative antihypertensive during immunotherapy. The current practice parameters for allergen immunotherapy recommend that emergency epinephrine should be readily available for the treatment of systemic allergic reactions associated with immunotherapy ("A"). To monitor for these immediate reactions, patients should be observed in the office setting for at least 30 minutes after immunotherapy shots are administered ("C"). Based on studies of seasonal symptom scores, the beneficial effects of allergen immunotherapy begin during the first year of therapy and continue throughout the treatment period. It is generally recommended that the initial course of allergen immunotherapy should last for 3 to 5 years in order to ensure maintenance of therapeutic effects (and a reliable revenue stream for allergists).

You are also seeing your patient's brother, who has a history of ragweed and grass allergy. He states that he is "allergic" to needles, too (funny guy). Accordingly, you decide to use sublingual (SL) desensitization instead of subcutaneous (SQ) routes. Luckily, there are FDA-approved sublingual preparations for desensitization to ragweed, Timothy grass and a 5-grass combination as well as for dust mites.

Question 4.1.6 Which of the following is true regarding SL desensitization?
A) It is more effective than SQ desensitization
B) It is overall safer than SQ desensitization; there are fewer adverse systemic reactions than with SQ desensitization
C) It can cause airway obstruction by causing tongue and pharynx edema
D) It is well studied as a combination therapy with SQ desensitization
E) B and C

Answer 4.1.6 The correct answer is "E." SL desensitization causes fewer anaphylactic reactions but can cause airway obstruction from local edema. "A" is incorrect. The majority of studies show that SQ desensitization is more effective than SL desensitization. "D" is also incorrect. The use of SL therapy in combination with SQ desensitization is contraindicated and may increase the rate of anaphylactic reactions. As a final note, most patients who require desensitization need treatment for more allergens than just Timothy grass *or* ragweed *or* the 5-grass combination limiting the usefulness of SL therapy. Patients are often also allergic to tree pollen, animal dander, and other allergens that cannot be treated with SL therapy.

HELPFUL TIP:
Beta-blockers should be stopped in patients with a history of anaphylaxis if possible. Beta-blockers amplify anaphylaxis and make it more difficult to treat.

▶ **Objectives: Did you learn to ...**
- Recognize symptoms of vocal cord dysfunction?
- Recognize symptoms of allergic rhinitis?
- Provide appropriate management for allergic rhinitis?
- Describe the role of immunotherapy in treating allergic rhinitis?

 QUICK QUIZ: ALLERGIC REACTIONS

A 52-year-old man with common variable immunodeficiency (CVID) receives his first infusion of intravenous immunoglobulin (IVIG) therapy. Ten minutes into the infusion, he complains of difficulty breathing and generalized pruritus.

Based on the traditional classification of hypersensitivity reactions, which of the following best categorizes this patient's reaction?
A) Type I—Immediate hypersensitivity reaction
B) Type II—Cytotoxic reaction
C) Type III—Immune complex reaction
D) Type IV—Delayed-type reaction

The correct answer is "A." Based on the clinical history and timing of the above event, you should suspect an immediate hypersensitivity reaction (Type I). Type I reactions typically occur within seconds to minutes after exposure to the offending agent and are due to cross-linkage of IgE antibodies that are bound to surfaces of mast cells or basophils, with subsequent release of mediators such as histamine. Pruritus, urticaria, angioedema, laryngeal edema, and possible generalized anaphylaxis can occur. To see why Types II to IV are incorrect, refer to Table 4-1 for definitions of the immunologic reaction types.

 QUICK QUIZ: CAN I HAVE THAT BANANA OR NOT?

A slightly deranged patient of yours has a serious latex allergy and wants to play "fruit roulette."

You tell her that all of the following may be associated with cross-reactivity in latex allergic patients EXCEPT:
A) Celery
B) Banana
C) Avocado
D) Kiwi

The correct answer is "A." Celery is so boring; it can't even cause an allergic reaction in those with latex allergy. Symptoms of oral allergy syndrome can include oral pruritus with or without angioedema of the lips, tongue, palate, and posterior oropharynx. Cross-reactivity has been reported between:
- Ragweed antigens: May result in sensitization to the gourd family and banana.
- Birch pollen allergy: May result in sensitivity to apple, carrots, parsnips, celery, hazelnuts, and potatoes.
- Latex-fruit cross-reactivity: May occur with banana, avocado, passion fruit, kiwi, and chestnut, but not celery. Your patient should be warned about these potential reactions.

 HELPFUL TIP:
The vast majority of patients who report penicillin (and other) allergies are not truly allergic. In the case of penicillin, 0.5% of those with reported penicillin allergy had skin reactions during testing and less than 10% had **any** reaction to a full dose of penicillin. Many patients misinterpret an adverse reaction (such as nausea) as an allergy.

TABLE 4-1 CLASSIFICATION OF IMMUNOLOGIC REACTIONS

Reaction Type	Mechanism	Clinical Features	Timing
Type I—Immediate	Antigen exposure causes cross-linkage of IgE antibodies that are bound to surfaces of mast cells and basophils, with subsequent release of mediators such as histamine.	Anaphylaxis Angioedema Bronchospasm Urticaria	Less than an hour after exposure
Type II—Cytotoxic	IgG or IgM antibodies are directed against antigens on the individual's own tissues, and subsequent complement activation leads to cell destruction.	Graft rejection Hemolytic anemia Neutropenia Thrombocytopenia	At least 5 days but sometimes many weeks after exposure
Type III—Immune complex	IgG or IgM antigen–antibody complexes form and deposit within blood vessels and tissues, causing complement activation and neutrophil recruitment, ultimately resulting in tissue damage.	Localized arthus reaction Serum sickness	1 week or more after exposure
Type IV—Delayed	Antigen exposure to sensitized T cells causes a reaction.	Contact dermatitis Stevens–Johnson syndrome	24–72 hours after exposure

HELPFUL TIP:
There is essentially no cross-reactivity between penicillin and third-generation cephalosporins (but there is with first- and second-generation cephalosporins, up to 5%). As long as the patient did not have true anaphylaxis, feel comfortable using third-generation cephalosporins in penicillin-allergic patients.

QUICK QUIZ: CONTRAST ALLERGY

A 57-year-old man with chest pain is scheduled for an elective cardiac catheterization. You remember that the patient has a history of generalized urticaria with lip and tongue angioedema shortly after receiving contrast dye for a CT scan several years back.

Which of the following interventions should be recommended for this patient prior to undergoing the planned procedure?
A) Use of higher-osmolality radiocontrast media if possible
B) Give a test dose of radiocontrast media and proceed as usual if testing is negative
C) Administration of prednisone and diphenhydramine as premedications
D) Percutaneous and intradermal skin testing with radiocontrast media
E) Desensitization procedure for radiocontrast media

The correct answer is "C." Anaphylactoid reactions to radiocontrast material are typically non–IgE-mediated; however, they look very similar to a Type I immunologic reaction and can be severe and life threatening. This patient will require premedication for this elective procedure. The appropriate premedication regimen for contrast dye allergy includes (1) diphenhydramine 50 mg IM/PO 1 hour before the procedure and (2) prednisone 50 mg PO 13 hours, 7 hours, and 1 hour before the procedure. "A" is incorrect. The use of **lower-osmolality** radiocontrast media is associated with fewer adverse reactions and is appropriate for contrast-allergic patients. "B" is incorrect. Test dosing for radiocontrast media should **NOT** be done; patients with no reaction to test doses have had severe reactions to full doses. In addition, test doses themselves have been reported to result in fatalities. Skin testing ("D") **can** be done, especially within a window of a few months after the reaction for retrospective evaluation, but the current consensus is that it has no clinical utility in predicting hypersensitivity reactions. There is no desensitization procedure available.

HELPFUL TIP:
There is no cross-reaction between shellfish and iodine-based contrast material. The allergy to seafood is an allergy to the protein (tropomyosins) in the seafood, not the iodine. Think about it for a second. How many people have you seen dropping dead from an anaphylactic reaction to iodized salt?

▶ CASE 4.2

An 18-month-old boy comes to clinic with a history of eczematous rash covering his extremities and face. His parents state that it worsens after the ingestion of certain foods. He has had increased fussiness over the last several months, as well as some difficulty gaining weight. Food allergy is suspected.

Question 4.2.1 Which of the following foods is NOT commonly implicated in food allergy?
A) Milk
B) Corn
C) Wheat
D) Soy
E) Egg

Answer 4.2.1 The correct answer is "B." Corn is not often implicated in food allergies (a good thing too, since we are writing this in Iowa, surrounded by corn). Although many foods are potentially antigenic, the great majority of food allergies involve only a few foods. Studies have shown that eight foods account for 93% of reactions, and these foods are, in order of frequency: egg, peanuts, milk, soy, tree nuts, fish, crustacean, and wheat. Although these food allergies may be outgrown, sensitivity to peanuts, tree nuts, fish, and crustaceans tend to be life-long.

HELPFUL TIP:
The peak incidence of food allergies occurs around age 1 year, with most allergies identified by the age of 2 years. Cow's milk and egg allergies tend to resolve by adulthood. The 2017 addenda to the Guideline for the Prevention of Peanut Allergy in the United States from the American Academy of Allergy, Asthma and Immunology recommended introduction of highly allergenic foods such as peanut products as early as 4 months of age. This recommendation was based on the data from landmark Learning Early About Peanut (LEAP) trial, which showed a statistical decrease in the prevalence in peanut allergies in those infants with severe eczema and/or egg allergy with early introduction of peanut products at age 4–11 months (*N Engl J Med*. 2015;372:803–813).

Two months later, this patient required an emergency room visit after developing increased work of breathing, wheezing, and an urticarial rash after eating. You refer him for testing. He is tested by both percutaneous skin testing and RAST and is found to have egg allergy.

Question 4.2.2 Which of the following vaccinations should NOT be given to this patient in light of his egg allergy?
A) MMR vaccine
B) Inactivated polio vaccine
C) Influenza vaccine
D) Conjugated pneumococcal vaccine (Prevnar)
E) All of the above should be provided without concern

Answer 4.2.2 The correct answer is "E." This patient should receive all of the above vaccinations without concern. "A" is incorrect. It had been common practice to withhold measles vaccination from children with a history of anaphylactic reaction to egg; the measles vaccine is prepared in chick-embryo fibroblast cultures. However, the MMR is safe to use in children with an egg allergy. Options "B" and "D" do not contain egg-related products and can therefore be given safely to this patient. Option "C" needs particular mention. It was previously common practice to provide an "egg free" influenza vaccination such as Flucelvax or Flublok to egg-allergic patients. As of 2016, the CDC recommends that individuals with a history of an egg allergy *of any severity receive any recommended age-appropriate influenza vaccination* as there is little cross-reactivity with egg allergies. If the patient has a history of a severe reaction to egg (anaphylactic reaction of symptoms other than hives), it is recommended for the individual to receive their influenza vaccination in a monitored healthcare setting under the guidance of a provider trained to recognize and treat severe allergic reactions (this can be a pharmacist). If a patient has a reaction to the influenza vaccine, it is contraindicated for the patient to receive the influenza vaccine in the future.

▶ **Objectives: Did you learn to …**
- Identify common food allergens?
- Recognize important associations between food allergy and selected vaccines?

▶ **CASE 4.3**

A 34-year-old female establishes care in your clinic. Her medical history consists of intermittent colicky, abdominal pain, and episodes of angioedema in the past with an unclear etiology. She has not noticed urticaria with those episodes. She has received multiple laparoscopic procedures that were unrevealing. During the initial interview, she relates several past episodes of lip and tongue swelling, for which she has not sought medical assistance. She has tried diphenhydramine without significant improvement. The swelling episodes resolve without intervention after 3 to 4 days.

Question 4.3.1 Which of the following laboratory tests would be most helpful in establishing the diagnosis in this patient?
A) ANA
B) C3 complement level
C) C4 complement level
D) Complete blood count (CBC)
E) SS-A and SS-B

Answer 4.3.1 The correct answer is "C." This patient's presentation should raise concern for hereditary angioedema (HAE). This entity is clinically characterized by recurrent episodes of angioedema involving any part of the body. Thus, it can present with laryngeal angioedema (the major cause of death) or recurrent abdominal pain (generally with a normal white count and

"always" without peritoneal signs). Urticaria is **NOT** a feature of this disorder. HAE is caused by a C1-esterase inhibitor deficiency; C1-esterase is a protease that normally acts to degrade C4. If there is an absence of C1-esterase *inhibitor*, C4 levels will be low as C1-esterase will continue to degrade C4. It is possible that a patient with HAE will have a normal level of C1-esterase inhibitor but will have a nonfunctional allele. So always check a C-1 esterase inhibitor level and C-1 esterase activity as well as a C4 level. If there is a nonfunctional allele, the C-1 esterase inhibitor level will be normal but C-1 esterase inhibitor function will be decreased.

While awaiting the test results, you discuss HAE with your patient.

Question 4.3.2 In order to minimize future attacks of angioedema, you recommend which of the following?
A) Avoidance of estrogen containing medications
B) Avoidance of ACE inhibitors
C) Testing and treatment of *Helicobacter pylori*
D) All of the above

Answer 4.3.2 The correct answer is "D." Education is the cornerstone of treatment of HAE. Patients need to know what triggers to avoid and how to identify symptoms early. Most attacks are precipitated by trauma (often head and upper airway trauma), medical procedures (dental and oral surgery in particular), emotional stress, infections, menstruation, or the use of medications, especially oral contraceptives and ACE inhibitors. Interestingly, *H. pylori* infection has been associated with HAE, and *H. pylori* eradication reduces the frequency of angioedema attacks.

Your patient is ultimately diagnosed with HAE.

Question 4.3.3 In this particular patient, which medication would be most helpful in preventing future episodes?
A) Emergency epinephrine
B) Oral diphenhydramine
C) Fresh frozen plasma (FFP)
D) Androgens (e.g., danazol)
E) No prophylactic treatment is available

Answer 4.3.3 The correct answer is "D." Emergency epinephrine and antihistamines are not generally effective, as HAE is not allergic in nature. Prophylactic treatment in the form of attenuated androgens (danazol) is available. Attenuated androgens appear to work by up-regulating the synthetic capability of hepatic cells that make C1-esterase inhibitor, thus decreasing the effect of C1 esterase and raising the C4 level. This, in turn, reduces the number and severity of acute exacerbations.

A subcutaneous C1 inhibitor (Takhzyro') was approved by the FDA in 2017 for prophylaxis in patients 12 years and older. *Treatment* of acute episodes of HAE includes FFP that contains C1-esterase inhibitor, the C1-esterase inhibitor replacement protein products (e.g., Ruconest, Berinert; Cinryze; Haegarda), and bradykinin/kallikrein inhibitors (ecallantide and icatibant). FFP would not be a long-term preventive measure, so "C" is incorrect.

HELPFUL TIP:
Make sure patients with HAE receive the hepatitis B vaccination series as they may require blood products for acute treatment of angioedema.

▸ **Objectives: Did you learn to ...**
· Identify a patient presenting with hereditary angioedema?
· Manage a patient with hereditary angioedema?

▸ CASE 4.4

Your patient's sister presents to clinic the next day with a similar history of angioedema symptoms, only less frequent and less severe.

Question 4.4.1 What is the likelihood that she has HAE as well?
A) Infinitesimally small because HAE is a rare disorder
B) About 25% because HAE is autosomal recessive
C) About 50% because HAE is autosomal dominant
D) Almost 100% because you can tell that she's got bad luck
E) Unknown because multiple gene involvement renders a simple calculation impossible

Answer 4.4.1 **The correct answer is "C."** HAE is transmitted in an autosomal dominant fashion with incomplete penetrance, which may be why the patient's sister is less symptomatic. New mutations do arise and cause a minority of cases.

Later that same night, you are called to the ED to see a patient with facial swelling. "Really?" you ask. "Yeah, really. Get in here." This patient is a 35-year-old female friend of your patient with HAE (so, her BFF not her biologic sister). She is worried that she too has HAE. This is the first ever episode of lip and face swelling, associated with itching in her mouth and a few hives on her arm and torso. She had shrimp gumbo for dinner, but has never had a reaction to shrimp before. She denies any recent trauma, surgery, or medication use. She is in no respiratory distress. Her O_2 saturation is 99% on room air and BP is 118/76 mm Hg. On lung examination, there is no stridor or wheezing.

Question 4.4.2 The most appropriate next step in the treatment of this patient is:
A) Supportive care and monitoring overnight in the intensive care unit (ICU)
B) Administration of FFP
C) Administration of epinephrine IM × 1
D) Administration of diphenhydramine, cimetidine, and prednisone PO
E) Prophylactic intubation

Answer 4.4.2 **The correct answer is "D."** This patient is different from your HAE patient. It is unlikely that she has HAE for several reasons: she's never had this reaction before, she has urticaria associated with the angioedema, and she did not experience an inciting event. This episode of angioedema and urticaria is more likely to have been caused by a typical allergic reaction and mast-cell release. For these types of reactions, antihistamines and steroids are the mainstay of therapy. However, the efficacy of steroids, antihistamines, and epinephrine is limited in angioedema (but it is worth a try). "A" is incorrect because it is overkill to admit her to the ICU, and you should be treating her rather than just monitoring her. "B" is incorrect because FFP treats HAE not allergic angioedema. "C" is incorrect because this patient is not having a full anaphylactic reaction. Epinephrine would be appropriate if she had wheezing, airway compromise, or hypotension. If you chose "E" for a walking, talking patient with no airway compromise, well . . . that just makes us sad. Note that steroids do not seem to add anything to the treatment of **urticaria** (vs. levocetirizine alone) (*Ann Emerg Med*. 2018;71(1):125–131), but should be reserved for patients with angioedema.

▸ **Objectives: Did you learn to ...**
· Differentiate HAE from allergic angioedema?
· Manage an anaphylactoid reaction?

Warning: The next section is about immunodeficiency syndromes. As Dante would say: "Abandon hope all ye who enter here." (One of the editors has a dog named Dante and she [the dog] says this all the time . . . to squirrels). See Table 4-2 for a quick review.

The main points and **the most important cases** are mentioned below. For those of you who are gluttons for punishment (gluttony is only Dante's third circle), look at the table.

The main points:
· Rule out the obvious: Does the patient have HIV, cancer, diabetes, lupus, or other chronic disease or is he/she on immunosuppressing drugs that predispose to recurrent infections?
· 1% to 3% of patients are heterozygous for an IgG subtype deficiency, the most common type of immunoglobulin deficiency. These patients may be asymptomatic or may present with recurrent sinusitis, otitis, skin infections, etc. IgG deficiency can be diagnosed by immunoglobulin electrophoresis. These patients often do not have an appropriate response to vaccinations.
· 1 in 700 patients are IgA deficient. Most are hereditary, but it can also be caused by several drugs (including captopril and thyroxine). Usually this resolves upon stopping the drug. Most patients with IgA deficiency are asymptomatic, although some have recurrent sinus and GI infections. Also, these patients frequently develop autoimmune disease and may have anaphylaxis to blood products.

TABLE 4-2 IMMUNODEFICIENCY SYNDROMES

Syndrome	Age of Onset	Defect/Laboratory Findings	Manifestations	Organisms Likely to Cause Infection
Humoral				
X-linked agammaglobulinemia	Late first year of life but up to age 50 (in very mild disease)	Low IgG, almost undetectable IgM, IgD, IgE, and IgA. No B cells	Multiple, recurrent infections (generally start at 6–18 months) especially lung, sinuses, ears, CSF. Eventually bronchiectasis and pulmonary insufficiency	Streptococcus, Haemophilus, Giardia
Common variable immunodeficiency	Variable but >2 years of age and mostly by age 30. May be older	Low levels of serum immunoglobulins	Sinus and respiratory infections. GI infections especially Giardia. Enhanced chance of lymphoma as adult. Autoimmune disorders	Pneumococcus, Haemophilus, Mycoplasma, Giardia
Hyper IgM syndrome	First 2 years of life	Elevated IgM, no IgG, IgA, IgE (although few may have very low level IgA, IgE)	Recurrent severe sinopulmonary infections. Autoimmune disorders	Encapsulated bacteria, Giardia, Pneumocystis, Cryptosporidium, Histoplasmosis
IgA deficiency	Not before age of 6 months; more severe disease presents by age 5	Low IgA levels, normal immunoglobulins otherwise	Most asymptomatic. May have respiratory tract infections. Watch for anaphylaxis with blood products	Haemophilus, Pneumococcus
Cellular				
Myeloperoxidase deficiency	Variable	Poor phagocytic killing	None except in the presence of other defects (e.g., diabetes), systemic candidiasis	Candida
Chronic granulomatous disease	Infant, toddler but occasionally in late life	Neutrophil dysfunction measured by nitroblue tetrazolium testing (and other tests)	Recurrent life-threatening illnesses especially pulmonary, hepatic, skin, and lymphatic abscesses	Staphylococcus, Aspergillus
Leukocyte adhesion deficiency	Early (poor separation of umbilical stump) or later if mild disease. Those with mild disease rarely have life-threatening illnesses	Poor adhesion of leukocytes to endothelium, etc.	Periodontal and dental infections, recurrent infections of skin, upper and lower airways, bowel, perirectal area	Pseudomonas and other gram-negative rods, Staphylococcus
Hyper IgE (Job syndrome)	First weeks to month of life	Elevated IgE levels, poor leukocyte chemotaxis	Facial abnormalities (hypertelorism; prominent, protruding triangular mandible; broad, somewhat bulbous nose). Eczema, mucocutaneous candidiasis, sinus, pulmonary, and skin infections. Recurrent "cold abscesses" in skin secondary to lack of inflammation	Multiple organisms, but especially Staphylococcus, Haemophilus, Candida
Wiskott–Aldrich	Early. Fatal by age 10 without bone marrow transplant	Low IgM, diminution of cellular immunity ability to respond to polysaccharide capsules	Eczema, thrombocytopenia with purpura, recurrent infections	Encapsulated organisms
Severe combined immunodeficiency syndrome	Early, by 6 months. Death by 2 years	Leukopenia, no mature T cells, low serum immunoglobulin levels	Colon and lung infections including diarrhea and abscesses	Multiple organisms, including viruses
DiGeorge syndrome	Early—in infancy	Absent thymus, reduced T3 + cells	Recurrent infections but variable in penetrance. Some have normal or near-normal immune function. Craniofacial abnormalities, congenital heart disease, chromosomal abnormalities, and hypocalcemia	Pneumococcus, Haemophilus

• Symptomatic immunoglobulin deficiencies can be treated with IVIG. The most common side effects of IVIG administration include renal failure, anaphylaxis, and thromboembolic disease.

▶ CASE 4.5

A 35-year-old male is seen by you in the hospital setting, after being admitted for pneumonia. Blood cultures reveal *Streptococcus pneumoniae.* The patient was well until age 25 when he began having recurrent infections and developed an autoimmune hemolytic anemia. He also relates frequent sinus infections (real ones … not the kind we so often see) requiring antibiotics 8 to 10 times a year. His last bout of pneumonia required a stay in the ICU.

Question 4.5.1 You suspect an immunodeficiency in this individual. What is the most useful test in making the diagnosis in this patient?
A) Complement levels
B) Immunoglobulin levels
C) CBC and differential
D) Bone marrow biopsy
E) Nitroblue tetrazolium test

Answer 4.5.1 **The correct answer is "B."** The clinical picture for this patient is most consistent with common variable immune deficiency (CVID). CVID, or acquired agammaglobulinemia, is similar to X-linked agammaglobulinemia, but generally has a later age of onset. In addition, it is associated with various gastrointestinal disorders, autoimmune disorders, and malignancy. Immunoglobulin levels are decreased secondary to inadequate B-cell differentiation. Therefore, the most useful laboratory test for the diagnosis of CVID would be serum immunoglobulin levels. With regard to the other options and other tests you might do to evaluate otherwise unexplained immunodeficiency:

• Immunodeficiency can be secondary to complement disorders and complement levels will be low in these patients.
• Nitroblue tetrazolium test will be abnormal in patients with phagocytic disorders.
• Response to vaccines will be muted or absent in humoral immunodeficiency (e.g., immunoglobulin deficiency).
• Delayed hypersensitivity skin testing (e.g., candida and mumps) may indicate a T-cell defect.

Question 4.5.2 Which of the following is the most appropriate treatment plan for this patient?
A) Prophylactic antibiotics
B) Bone marrow transplantation
C) Gene therapy
D) IVIG replacement
E) No treatment needed

Answer 4.5.2 **The correct answer is "D."** The treatment of choice for CVID includes replacement IVIG, especially in this patient who has a history of life-threatening infections. Prophylactic antibiotics may be required in addition to IVIG in some patients. Gene therapy is not currently possible because the genetic defect has not been identified. Although bone marrow transplantation is useful in other immunodeficiency states, it is not indicated in CVID.

HELPFUL TIP:
Patients with CVID may develop lymphoproliferative disorders (e.g., non-Hodgkin lymphoma). New adenopathy should be taken seriously.

▶ **Objectives: Did you learn to …**
· Describe presenting symptoms of common variable immunodeficiency?
· Recognize treatment options for CVID?

 QUICK QUIZ: IGA DEFICIENCY

A 37-year-old female is incidentally found to have an IgA level of 3 mg/dL (below the normal range).

What is the most likely clinical picture in this patient?
A) Pyogenic infections
B) Thrush
C) Cold abscesses
D) Aphthous ulcers
E) No clinical abnormalities

The correct answer is "E." IgA deficiency is present in approximately 1 in 700 Caucasians in the United States and is the second most common immunodeficiency described. Most of these patients are asymptomatic, but some IgA-deficient patients may present with an increased rate of respiratory tract infections.

HELPFUL TIP:
The evaluation of immunodeficiency should NOT stop when IgA deficiency is discovered since IgA deficiency is often asymptomatic and may be accompanied by a more serious form of immunodeficiency.

 QUICK QUIZ: IVIG

Which of the following patients is most likely to develop an anaphylactic reaction in response to the administration of IVIG?
A) A patient with IgA deficiency
B) A patient with IgG deficiency
C) A patient with sickle cell anemia
D) A patient with graft-versus-host disease
E) A pregnant patient

The correct answer is "A." Patients with IgA deficiency have pre-formed IgG or IgE antibodies against IgA, and thus may develop an anaphylactic reaction in response to IVIG (as well as blood and FFP, for that matter). Patients with IgG deficiency may have a similar problem, but it is much less common. Not all patients with IgA deficiency will develop anaphylaxis, but the risk is high enough to be prepared and to reduce the risk by using IgA-depleted IVIG and giving the IVIG slowly.

Clinical Pearls

○ An extensive evaluation for an underlying cause of chronic urticaria is very low yield and should not be done. Target the evaluation to the patient.

○ Beta-blockers should be used with caution in patients with a history of a severe anaphylactic reaction (e.g., requiring epinephrine). Beta-blockers increase the incidence and severity of anaphylaxis and blunt the response to therapeutic doses of epinephrine.

○ Do not use non-targeted IgE testing in the evaluation of asthma. Do testing for specific antigens as indicated based on the patient's history.

○ IgA immunodeficiency is often asymptomatic and should not be considered the cause of immunodeficiency unless no other cause is found.

○ Intranasal steroids are first line for allergic rhinitis and will also improve allergic eye symptoms (when given intranasally).

○ It is generally safe to use third-generation cephalosporins in a patient with penicillin allergy—as long as the reaction was not anaphylaxis.

○ RAST testing for allergy has a 25% false-negative rate. Skin testing remains the gold standard.

○ The great majority of patients who are reportedly "allergic" to penicillin do not have a true penicillin allergy.

○ There is no cross-reactivity between shellfish and iodinated radiocontrast.

○ Vocal cord dysfunction is an asthma mimic. Patients usually have inspiratory stridor.

BIBLIOGRAPHY

Azar AE. Evaluation of the adult with suspected immunodeficiency. *Am J Med*. 2007;120(9):764.

Bowen T, et al. 2010 International consensus algorithm for the diagnosis, therapy and management of hereditary angioedema. *Allergy Asthma Clin Immunol*. 2010;6(1):24.

Calderon MA, et al. Allergen injection immunotherapy for seasonal allergic rhinitis. *Cochrane Database Syst Rev*. 2007, Issue 1. Art. No.: CD001936.

Cooper MA. Primary immunodeficiencies. *Am Fam Physician*. 2003;68(10):2001–2008.

Du Toit G, et al. Randomized trial of peanut consumption in infants at risk for peanut allergy. *N Engl J Med*. 2015;372:803–813.

Quillen DM. Diagnosing rhinitis: Allergic versus non-allergic. *Am Fam Physician*. 2006;73(9):1583–1590.

Raje N, et al. Overview of immunodeficiency disorders. *Immunol Allergy Clin North Am*. 2015;35(4):599–623.

Scurlock AM. Food allergy in children. *Immunol Allergy Clin North Am*. 2005;25(2):369–388, vii–viii.

Nephrology

5

Melissa L. Swee

▶ CASE 5.1

A 49-year-old female with a 5-year history of type 2 diabetes mellitus presents for an initial visit. She has no known complications of diabetes. She takes metformin, glyburide, and aspirin. On examination, you find a pleasant, obese female in no distress. Her blood pressure is 136/86 mm Hg. As you discuss monitoring her diabetes, you recommend screening for early kidney disease.

Question 5.1.1 Which of the following approaches is the recommended way to screen for diabetic kidney disease?
A) Obtain a 24-hour urine collection for albumin now and again in 3 years
B) Obtain a spot urine albumin every year
C) Obtain a spot urine albumin/creatinine ratio every year
D) Obtain a urinalysis every year
E) Obtain a serum creatinine every year

Answer 5.1.1 The correct answer is "C." Moderately increased albuminuria (previously known by the misnomer "microalbuminuria") is a marker for increased risk of future kidney disease in diabetic patients. The best test to evaluate for moderately increased albuminuria is the urine albumin/creatinine ratio. Its advantages include ease of use, relatively low cost, and good correlation with 24-hour urine collections. Some of you may have chosen "B." A "spot microalbumin" (now a spot albumin) is a common but less accurate way to provide screening and may still be in use in some areas. As a practical matter, many physicians use urine albumin alone as a method of screening, but this method does not allow for corrections for variations in urine volume and dilution. A random spot urine albumin/creatinine ratio is normally less than 30 mg/g. Values above 30 mg/g are consistent with 24-hour measures showing abnormal amounts of albumin in the urine. Answers "D" and "E" offer measures of kidney function that simply are not sensitive enough to use for screening purposes.

HELPFUL TIP:
Note on terminology. The term "microalbuminuria" has been replaced with "moderately increased albuminuria," but the definition remains the same (30–300 mg protein in the urine per 24 hours). Compare this to "severely increased albuminuria," defined as greater than 300 mg of protein in the urine per 24 hours.

Question 5.1.2 Her albumin/creatinine ratio is 42 mg/g. The next step to confirm moderately increased albuminuria is:
A) Repeat urine albumin/creatinine ratio
B) Urine dipstick for protein
C) 24-hour urine collection for total protein excretion
D) Serum creatinine
E) Referral to a nephrologist

Answer 5.1.2 The correct answer is "A." Verification by repeat urine albumin/creatinine ratio is sufficient for a diagnosis of moderately increased albuminuria, so 24-hour urine collection ("C") need not be performed for confirmation. Of note, the diagnosis of moderately increased albuminuria requires 2 of 3 urine specimens showing >30 mg/g albumin/creatinine over a 6-month period. Since protein excretion must exceed 300 to 500 mg/day for a urine dipstick to detect proteinuria, urinalysis ("B") is not sensitive enough to be diagnostic. Serum creatinine ("D") elevation may be a marker for diabetic kidney disease, but it would develop late in the process. Nephrology referral ("E") is premature—you went to medical school; you can do this!

Question 5.1.3 Which of the following can cause a false-negative albumin/creatinine ratio?
A) Vigorous exercise
B) Fever
C) Cachexia
D) Poor glycemic control
E) Large muscle mass

Answer 5.1.3 The correct answer is "E." Patients with a large muscle mass have a high rate of creatinine excretion, which may decrease the albumin/creatinine ratio. Cachectic patients have the opposite problem, with low amounts of creatinine excretion, resulting in false-positive albumin/creatinine ratio. Fever, vigorous exercise, heart failure, and poor glycemic control can also cause transient increases in albuminuria, potentially resulting in false-positive albumin/creatinine ratios.

. . . .

Your patient's other laboratory studies reveal the following: hemoglobin A_{1c} 6.4%, serum creatinine 1.4 mg/dL, and normal electrolytes. A month later, your patient returns. Her blood pressure is 138/84 mm Hg. Her urine albumin/creatinine remains elevated on a second measurement. According to an eye examination yesterday, she has nonproliferative diabetic retinopathy.

Question 5.1.4 Because your patient has type 2 diabetes mellitus and moderately increased albuminuria, you realize that her likelihood of progressing to overt nephropathy is:
A) Almost zero
B) About half that of a similar patient with type 1 diabetes
C) Nearly equal to that of a similar patient with type 1 diabetes
D) More than twice that of a similar patient with type 1 diabetes
E) Absolutely certain (100% chance)

Answer 5.1.4 The correct answer is "C." Although earlier studies showed a greater progression to overt nephropathy in type 1 diabetics, more recent studies demonstrate a nearly equal rate of progression in types 1 and 2. About 20% to 40% of Caucasian patients with diabetes type 2 and moderately increased albuminuria will progress to diabetic nephropathy. The rate of progression to nephropathy in non-Caucasian populations is even higher.

Question 5.1.5 What is the most appropriate next step in the evaluation and management of this patient's moderately increased albuminuria?
A) Start an angiotensin-converting enzyme (ACE) inhibitor
B) Start an angiotensin receptor blocker (ARB)
C) Order renal ultrasound with Doppler of the renal arteries
D) Start insulin
E) Order a 24-hour urine collection for total protein

Answer 5.1.5 The correct answer is "A." ACE inhibitors should be the first-choice drugs unless there is a contraindication to their use. "B," ARBs, are considered second-line choice if the patient cannot tolerate an ACE inhibitor. "C," a renal ultrasound, is not indicated at this point in time since it is unlikely to change therapy. The choice to start insulin, "D," is also not necessarily dependent on albuminuria. Your patient already has good glucose control (HbA_{1c} of 6.4%). As previously stated, a 24-hour urine collection is not necessary for diagnosis.

HELPFUL (AND VERY IMPORTANT) TIP:
An ARB is *not* just an ACE inhibitor without the cough. A large meta-analysis showed that ARBs, while lowering blood pressure, *have no appreciable effect on MI or cardiovascular mortality* **versus placebo** (*BMJ.* 2011;342:d2234; *JAMA Intern Med.* 2014;174:773). But that's heart disease in diabetics (which is kind of important). Back to renal disease . . . The only study (to date) to directly compare an ACE inhibitor (enalapril) to an ARB (telmisartan) for renal protection in diabetes did not demonstrate a statistically significant difference between the two, although there was a trend in favor of the ACE inhibitor (*N Engl J Med.* 2004;351(19):1952). However, this was a small study (250 individuals) with a high dropout rate. Another study of 4,000 subjects showed that while *ARBs do reduce proteinuria, they have no benefit on mortality* (*N Engl J Med.* 2011;364:907-917), which is what we really care about.

. . . .

The patient has a full urinalysis to rule out renal inflammation (e.g., nephritis) and overt proteinuria (nephrotic syndrome). The urinalysis is entirely negative.

Question 5.1.6 What further investigations must your patient undergo to eliminate other potential causes of proteinuria?
A) Renal biopsy
B) Renal ultrasound with Doppler of the renal arteries
C) ANA, ESR, CRP
D) All of the above
E) None of the above

Answer 5.1.6 The correct answer is "E." No further evaluation is necessary in this patient with moderately increased albuminuria. The combination of diabetic retinopathy (a marker for diabetic renal disease), hypertension (BP >140/90 mm Hg in a diabetic patient), and abnormal protein in the urine as measured by the urine albumin/creatinine ratio is sufficient to make the diagnosis of early diabetic nephropathy. Renal biopsy ("A") is quite invasive and unlikely to change management. ANA, ESR, CRP ("C"), and ultrasound ("B") are unlikely to offer new information. If things do change (e.g., nephritic urine and gross proteinuria), then further evaluation may be indicated.

. . . .

You continue to follow this patient for several years. She ultimately is admitted for chest pain, rules out for myocardial infarction, but has a positive stress test. She will need to have a cardiac catheterization. Her creatinine is now 1.5 mg/dL, and her glomerular filtration rate is in the range of stage 3 chronic kidney disease.

Question 5.1.7 In addition to holding her metformin, which of the following interventions would be most

likely to reduce her risk of developing contrast-induced nephropathy?

A) *N*-acetylcysteine and IV saline
B) *N*-acetylcysteine and mannitol
C) IV saline
D) Sodium bicarbonate and mannitol
E) Mannitol and IV saline

Answer 5.1.7 **The correct answer is "C."** For patients at risk of contrast-induced nephropathy, contrast studies should be avoided *if possible* (see helpful tip below). If a contrast study must be done, stop aggravating medications like nonsteroidal anti-inflammatory drugs (NSAIDs—this patient shouldn't be on these anyway since she has CKD!). Hydration, usually with IV saline, should be given if there are no contraindications (e.g., heart failure). Nonionic lower osmolality (or even iso-osmolar) contrast agents should be used. Additionally, we recommend discussing these cases individually with your radiologist, cardiologist, or whomever is performing the procedure. Sodium bicarbonate and *N*-acetylcysteine do not have good evidence for effectiveness, but they also do not appear to do harm. The diuretics (mannitol, furosemide, etc.) may be associated with an *increased* risk of nephropathy, and mannitol in particular has an undesirable side effect profile.

HELPFUL TIP:
The old teaching about renal toxicity and iodinated contrast has recently been called into question (*Radiology*. 2014;273(3):714–725; *Radiology*. 2014;271(1):65–73). These studies have suggested that the risk of renal injury is low. However, few patients in these studies had a creatinine of >3 mg/dL. In short, don't go hog wild; try to avoid using contrast in renal disease, but it may not be as doom-and-gloom as once thought. If you really need to rule out that PE or aortic dissection, go for it. See also N Engl J Med 2019; 380: 2146-2155 DOI: 10.1056/NEJMra1805256

HELPFUL TIP:
Hemofiltration and hemodialysis have been studied in the prevention of contrast-induced nephropathy for patients at risk. There does not appear to be a benefit over more conservative approaches. Also, there is a move to dialyze patients who are already on dialysis within 24 hours of a contrast study. There is no good data, however, and studies show potential harm.

HELPFUL (AND VERY IMPORTANT) TIP:
The use of MRI contrast (gadolinium) in patients with renal disease has been associated with a scleroderma-like syndrome (nephrogenic systemic fibrosis). Gadolinium should be avoided in those with a CrCl of <30 mL/min. The data are less compelling in those with a CrCl of 30 to 60 mL/min. Since nephrogenic systemic fibrosis can affect more than just the kidneys, early dialysis may help prevent this disease by reducing the half-life of the gadolinium. Further, gadolinium may remain in the CNS and form deposits. What affect this has on cognition is unknown but is being investigated. For these reasons, the FDA suggests minimizing repeated gadolinium-enhanced MRIs, especially closely spaced MRIs. Patient-specific characteristics, such as pregnancy and anticipated lifetime exposure to gadolinium, should be weighed when deciding on imaging.

....

Upon cardiac catheterization, she is found to have several lesions. She undergoes coronary artery bypass grafting and is discharged. Her creatinine remains stable at 1.5 mg/dL.

A few months later, she presents with gradually increasing dyspnea and cough. Her urine output is reported to be normal. Her vitals show temperature 37°C, pulse 76 bpm, respiratory rate 24, and blood pressure 92/46 mm Hg. You note crackles at both lung bases. Her heart rhythm is regular and an S4 is audible. She has JVD of 9 cm and 2+ pitting pretibial edema.

The ECG shows sinus tachycardia but no evidence of potassium toxicity (peaked T-waves, prolonged QT). Laboratory results: troponin-T and CK normal, BUN 70 mg/dL, Cr 2.0 mg/dL (her baseline was 1.5 mg/dL), Na 128 mEq/L (reference range 135–145), K 5.5 mEq/L (reference range 3.5–5.0), HCO$_3$ 19 mEq/L, WBC 14,500 per mm^3, remainder of the CBC is normal. Urinalysis shows protein and glucose with a specific gravity >1.030, but there are few cells and no casts. Cultures and a chest x-ray are pending.

Question 5.1.8 **You suspect that her elevated creatinine is primarily due to which of the following processes?**

A) Adverse toxic effects of drugs on the kidney
B) Heart failure or other prerenal cause of renal failure such as dehydration
C) Sudden progression of diabetic nephropathy
D) Urinary obstruction
E) Urinary tract infection

Answer 5.1.8 **The correct answer is "B."** Your patient has clinical evidence of heart failure (HF), including edema and rales. With a BUN/Cr ratio greater than 20 and an elevated urine-specific gravity, she appears to have a prerenal azotemia, likely secondary to insufficient cardiac output. Drugs ("A") may play a role in her volume depletion, but the BUN/Cr ratio of >20 argues against a renal cause of her elevated creatinine. Therefore, the most likely culprit is HF. Diabetes should not cause a sudden worsening of renal disease. Although it has not been eliminated as a cause, urinary obstruction ("D") is less likely since she has good urine output. Answer "E" is incorrect since the urinalysis does not support diagnosis of infection, and heart failure explains the overall clinical picture much better.

Question 5.1.9 Given her diabetes and renal disease, which of the following is the most likely cause of her hyperkalemia?
A) Renal tubular acidosis (RTA) type 1
B) RTA type 2
C) RTA type 3
D) RTA type 4
E) RTA type 5

Answer 5.1.9 **The correct answer is "D."** RTA type 4 is due to aldosterone deficiency or the kidney's resistance to the activity of aldosterone. (Does the kidney truly possess free will and choose to exercise it to resist aldosterone? Sure… if it helps to think of it that way.) The most common cause of RTA type 4 is hyporeninemic hypoaldosteronism, which is often seen in diabetic nephropathy. The disorder is recognized by hyperkalemia and mild acidosis. RTA types 1 and 2 usually are *hypokalemic* and these forms of RTA are not associated with diabetes. RTA type 3 is very rare and is a combination of types 1 and 2. RTA type 5 does not exist.

Question 5.1.10 In an effort to *reduce* her serum potassium level (not temporize), you should do which of the following?
A) Temporarily hold her furosemide and ACE inhibitor
B) Increase her furosemide and temporarily hold her ACE inhibitor
C) Administer IV calcium gluconate
D) Bolus IV normal saline 1 to 2 L
E) Give albuterol by nebulizer

Answer 5.1.10 **The correct answer is "B."** Ah, test-taking—clearly not real life! The best answer here is to increase renal clearance of potassium with furosemide while holding the ACEI. Because ACE inhibitors can increase serum potassium, you should stop hers. "But what about her heart failure?" you ask. Well, good question. Given that her potassium is only slightly elevated, the ACEI could be continued while monitoring her serum potassium. "A" is incorrect; stopping the furosemide may lead to worsening HF symptoms and worsening hyperkalemia. In hyperkalemia, calcium gluconate ("C") is used to protect cardiac conduction, but it is not effective for reducing potassium concentrations. A bolus of normal saline ("D") is contraindicated in a patient with an acute HF exacerbation. Albuterol ("E") is a temporizing measure, reducing serum potassium by forcing potassium into the intracellular space.

You administer intravenous furosemide. The night after admission she starts vomiting, and your partner inserts a nasogastric tube, which is inadvertently left to continuous suction overnight (don't do this . . . there is almost no indication for an NG tube—especially on continuous suction). The next morning, your patient's laboratory results are as follows: BUN 49 mg/dL, Cr 2.0 mg/dL, Na 132 mEq/L, K 3.5 mEq/L, and HCO_3 38 mEq/L (reference 23–29 mEq/L).

Question 5.1.11 On the basis of history and laboratory data provided, you strongly suspect:
A) Metabolic acidosis
B) Respiratory acidosis
C) Metabolic alkalosis
D) Respiratory alkalosis

Answer 5.1.11 **The correct answer is "C."** Loss of gastric acid, through emesis or gastric suction, can result in a metabolic alkalosis. Although no pH is available to confirm alkalosis, you are able to infer the diagnosis based on the elevation in serum HCO_3. This is one of the many reasons that you should avoid nasogastric tubes unless there is a compelling reason, such as bowel obstruction. Even there, the usefulness is limited unless they are vomiting.

Your patient recovers surprisingly well from her heart failure. Her creatinine returns to baseline (1.5 mg/dL). You try to re-challenge the patient with an ACE inhibitor. However, her hyperkalemia recurs and she is unable to tolerate either ACEI or ARB. With beta-blocker and loop diuretic therapy, her average blood pressure is 130/80 mm Hg. At a follow-up visit, you find no signs or symptoms of HF.

Question 5.1.12 You want to lower your patient's risk of progressing to end-stage renal disease. To reduce proteinuria, which of the following strategies is best?

A) Add isosorbide dinitrate
B) Add a nondihydropyridine calcium channel blocker (e.g., diltiazem, verapamil)
C) Add a dihydropyridine calcium channel blocker (e.g., amlodipine, nifedipine)
D) Restrict protein in the diet
E) Aim for a higher A1C target, around 8%

Answer 5.1.12 The correct answer is "B." Nondihydropyridine calcium channel blockers reduce protein excretion in diabetic patients with nephropathy and slow down the progression of renal disease—but not to the degree of ACE inhibitors. "A," a long-acting nitrate, would be effective for angina and will lower blood pressure but does not demonstrate an effect on diabetic nephropathy. The dihydropyridine calcium channel blockers ("C") do **not** slow down progression to nephropathy to the same degree as some other antihypertensive drugs. The effect of protein restriction ("D") on nephropathy is controversial and not clearly beneficial; therefore, more effective therapies should be initiated first. Finally, "E" is incorrect since better glycemic control is associated with renal protection.

HELPFUL TIP:
For diabetic nephropathy, always start with an ACE inhibitor and try to maximize the dose. Full-dose ACE inhibitor treatment is associated with improved survival in diabetic nephropathy compared with low-dose therapy. The dose of ACE inhibitor may be limited by serum potassium level or the patient's blood pressure. Sodium restriction added to an ACE inhibitor is actually more effective than adding an ARB for proteinuria and blood pressure control (*BMJ*. 2011;343:d4366). In this study, the actual sodium in the diet was 2,500 mg (although the goal was 1,200 mg). Despite initial enthusiasm (or drug company marketing), an ARB plus an ACE is **not** useful in essentially any patient and results in increased side effects; this combination should be avoided.

Question 5.1.13 At a follow-up visit, you find that her estimated glomerular filtration rate (GFR) has declined to 40 mL/min/1.73 m² (from a previous baseline of 50 mL/min/1.73 m²). With this new information, you should discontinue which of the following medications?

A) Insulin
B) Metoprolol
C) Metformin
D) Aspirin
E) None of the above

Answer 5.1.13 The correct answer is "E." Per the FDA, as long as the GFR is greater than or equal to 30 mL/min/1.73 m², metformin is safe—with the following caveat. If a patient's GFR declines below 45 during treatment with metformin, the dose should be reduced by 50%. Additionally, do **not** start metformin unless the GFR is greater than 45 mL/min/1.73 m². Metformin actually seems to improve outcomes in those with renal disease and compensated heart failure even when the GFR (or creatinine clearance) is low.

HELPFUL TIP:
A rough estimate of the creatinine clearance can be calculated using the Cockcroft–Gault formula:

Estimated creatinine clearance = (140 − age[year])(body weight[kg])/(72 (serum creatinine [mg/dL]))

For women, multiply this figure by 0.85. One caveat is that this formula may not reflect early renal injury because of compensatory hypertrophy of the remaining glomeruli. **Normal** for healthy adult is 94 to 140 mL/min for men and 72 to 110 mL/min for women.

HELPFUL TIP:
There is no perfect equation for calculating the GFR. The abbreviated modified diet in renal disease (MDRD) calculation is increasingly used because it seems to be an accurate representation of kidney function in adults with renal disease. Unlike the Cockcroft–Gault equation, the MDRD makes an adjustment for African-American race but does not take weight into account. Both equations adjust for gender. Although the equation is a little complicated, many labs now calculate the MDRD GFR. If you want to calculate it yourself, there are multiple free sites and apps that you can access (e.g., www.mdcalc.com, www.niddk.nih.gov, etc.). From the authors' perspective, any of these are OK. We just want you to think about GFR!

Over the next year, your patient experiences increasing difficulties with glycemic control. Despite your efforts, her proteinuria and serum creatinine increase. As you discuss referral to a nephrologist, she asks about dialysis.

Question 5.1.14 Which of the following is NOT an indication for dialysis?

A) Severe hyperkalemia due to renal failure
B) Accelerated hypertension
C) Weight loss
D) Persistent nausea and vomiting despite treatment
E) Bleeding secondary to uremia

Answer 5.1.14 The correct answer is "C." In chronic renal failure due to any cause, *absolute* **clinical indications for initiating dialysis include** pericarditis, pleuritis, uremic encephalopathy, or other life-threatening situations such as severe volume overload, drug toxicities (e.g., lithium), severe electrolyte disturbances (such as hyperkalemia), and refractory metabolic acidosis. "C," weight loss, is not an indication in and of itself. However, declining nutritional status may improve with dialysis. Persistent nausea and vomiting may be due to uremia.

HELPFUL (AND VERY IMPORTANT) TIP:
Counter to what you might expect, early dialysis increases mortality (or at least is of no benefit). Do not initiate dialysis until the GFR is 5 to 7 mL/min/1.73 m² **or** the patient is having clinical problems that cannot be otherwise managed (*N Engl J Med.* 2010;363(7):609–619). Patients on early dialysis die from infection, complications from dialysis (hypotension), problems with their grafts (again leading to infection), etc. This does not mean avoid nephrologists. Dialysis planning should start when dialysis is anticipated to be needed in the future.

▶ Objectives: Did you learn to ...
- Screen for moderately increased albuminuria in diabetic patients?
- Evaluate and treat moderately increased albuminuria and overt proteinuria in diabetic patients?
- Identify prerenal acute kidney injury?
- Describe the features of RTA type 4?
- Identify gastric suctioning as a cause of metabolic alkalosis in the hospital?
- Discuss when to initiate dialysis in a patient with chronic renal failure?

▶ CASE 5.2

A 49-year-old African-American female with type 2 diabetes mellitus, hypertension, and hyperlipidemia returns for a follow-up visit. She's had diabetes for 15 years, and her control has been variable over that time. Now, her glycosylated hemoglobin is 8%. She has developed moderately increased albuminuria and diabetic retinopathy. You tell her that her renal function has progressively declined, which alarms her since her mother is on hemodialysis. Her creatinine was 1.2 mg/dL 3 years ago, and now it is 1.9 mg/dL. Her GFR is 36 mL/min/1.73 m². She weighs 100 kg, and her blood pressure is 120/76 mm Hg.

Question 5.2.1 Which of the following is the most appropriate description of her renal function?
A) Stage 1 chronic kidney disease (CKD)
B) Stage 2 CKD
C) Stage 3 CKD
D) Stage 4 CKD
E) Stage 5 CKD

Answer 5.2.1 **The correct answer is "C."** She has stage 3 CKD. Table 5-1 defines the various stages of CKD. Not all patients will

progress through all of the stages of CKD. On the basis of age alone, many elderly patients may be classified as having stage 1 or 2 CKD, and they may never progress. Knowledge of a patient's CKD stage is useful in determining how to treat, what drugs to avoid, etc.

HELPFUL TIP:
Patients with CKD, with or without diabetes, are at increased risk of coronary artery disease, so other risk factors for heart disease should be treated aggressively. In fact, many experts believe that CKD should be treated as a "coronary artery disease equivalent." At the least, CKD is an independent risk factor for CAD.

You increase the patient's insulin and lisinopril doses, confirm that she is taking aspirin, and convince her to quit smoking (you are very persuasive—not to mention good looking and strong . . . and humble). One month later, your patient returns with typical symptoms of a urinary tract infection (UTI) without systemic symptoms (e.g., fever, nausea). Her urine culture grows *Escherichia coli* resistant to trimethoprim/sulfamethoxazole but susceptible to all other antibiotics tested.

Question 5.2.2 Out of the following, the most appropriate antibiotic regimen for this patient's UTI is:
A) Ciprofloxacin 250 mg PO every other day for two doses
B) Ciprofloxacin 250 mg PO once
C) Ciprofloxacin 250 mg PO BID for 3 days
D) Levofloxacin 750 mg PO daily for 7 days

Answer 5.2.2 **The correct answer is "C."** This patient's GFR is 36 mL/min/1.73 m² and her creatinine clearance is 56 mL/min (using the Cockcroft–Gault equation). Therefore, the usual

Stage	GFR (mL/min/1.73 m2)	Comments
1	≥90	Stage 1 defined by evidence of kidney damage (e.g., structural damage, albuminuria) with normal GFR
2	60–89	Mild decline in renal function; about 5.4% of US population
3	30–59	Moderate decline in renal function; about 5.4% of US population (yes, same percentage as stage 2)
4	15–29	Severe decline in renal function; approaching need for dialysis
5	<15	End-stage disease

TABLE 5-1 STAGES OF CHRONIC KIDNEY DISEASE

GFR, glomerular filtration rate.

ciprofloxacin dose of 250 mg PO BID for UTI is safe and appropriate. Less frequent dosing may be required for a lesser GFR. The important thing here is to recall that CKD may require dosage adjustments for many medications. Numerous drugs are renally cleared, so it's always prudent to know the GFR or creatinine clearance and check for dosage adjustments before prescribing. Remember, however, that fluoroquinolones are not indicated for cystitis so other choices would be better if they were an option.

....

You assume the UTI cleared because you do not hear from her for a few months. Then her sister brings her in for an acute illness including nausea, emesis, confusion, and generalized weakness. These symptoms began yesterday. The only other thing new with her health is heartburn which she has been self-treating with increasingly larger amounts of Tums® (calcium carbonate), taking "handfuls" over the past few days. Her laboratory results now include creatinine 2.5 mg/dL, calcium 14 mg/dL (reference 8.9–10.5 mg/dL), and HCO₃ 37 mEq/L (reference 22–28 mEq/L).

Question 5.2.3 **The most appropriate treatment for her now includes:**
A) Hydrochlorothiazide (HCTZ)
B) Furosemide
C) Normal saline IV
D) A and C
E) B and C

Answer 5.2.3 **The correct answer is "C."** Your patient is now presenting with milk-alkali syndrome. The diagnosis should be recognized by the triad of hypercalcemia, metabolic alkalosis, and renal insufficiency in combination with the history of typical symptoms (described in the case) and excessive calcium carbonate ingestion. Treatment includes removal of the offending agent and treatment of the hypercalcemia with IV saline (to improve renal perfusion and metabolic alkalosis). "A," thiazide diuretics, results in reabsorption of calcium—the opposite of what you want to achieve in a patient with hypercalcemia. "B," furosemide, has fallen out of favor and may worsen hypovolemia further.

HELPFUL TIP:
Compared with loop diuretics, thiazide diuretics are generally better at lowering blood pressure. However, at a GFR < 30 mL/min/1.73 m², thiazides are less effective as antihypertensive agents. For patients with CKD stage 4 or stage 5, especially those with hypervolemia, consider using a loop diuretic or metolazone (which acts at multiple renal sites) instead of a thiazide.

....

You get the patient through her episode of hypercalcemia and advise her to lay off the calcium-based antacids, favoring an H₂-antagonist instead. As your patient's renal disease progresses over the years, you find that she has become anemic with a hemoglobin of 9.9 g/dL. She takes a multivitamin. Her iron studies are consistent with anemia of chronic disease and her screening colonoscopy last year was normal. The anemia is normocytic and normochromic.

Question 5.2.4 **If you were to treat her with an erythropoietic agent (e.g., erythropoietin or darbepoetin), her target hemoglobin would be:**
A) 8 to 9 g/dL
B) 10 to 11 g/dL
C) 13 to 14 g/dL
D) >15 g/dL

Answer 5.2.4 **The correct answer is "B."** For patients with CKD and anemia of chronic disease (when other causes of anemia have been ruled out and/or treated), erythropoietic agents should **not** be used to achieve "near normal" hemoglobin levels. Target levels are determined on an individual basis but in general will be between 9 and 11 g/dL. Higher hemoglobin levels—in particular, attempts to "normalize" the hemoglobin concentration—are associated with a greater risk of adverse events, including increased risk of mortality, need for dialysis, heart failure, graft thrombosis, uncontrolled hypertension, etc. These findings are consistent with a similar finding in cancer patients. If the patient is an appropriate candidate, the initial erythropoietin dose is approximately 50 to 100 U/kg per week. Because of the need to preserve veins for future hemodialysis access, experts recommend that erythropoietin be administered subcutaneously (and avoid PICC lines for the same reason). The FDA suggests withholding erythropoietin for hemoglobin >12 g/dL or if the hemoglobin increases by >1 g/dL in any 2-week period.

▶ **Objectives: Did you learn to ...**
· Stage CKD?
· Adjust medication doses based on renal function?
· Recognize and treat milk-alkali syndrome?
· Recognize appropriate targets for the treatment with erythropoietic agents?

▶ **CASE 5.3**

A 55-year-old male presents to your office for evaluation of blood in his urine discovered incidentally during a life insurance physical. The urinalysis showed 2+ blood on urine dipstick and 2 RBC/hpf. The remainder of the urinalysis and microscopic examination was normal.

Question 5.3.1 **After an appropriate history and physical examination, your first step in the evaluation of this urine abnormality is to:**
A) Repeat the urinalysis and microscopic examination
B) Obtain urine for culture
C) Order a renal ultrasound
D) Order a CT scan of the abdomen
E) Order an intravenous pyelogram (IVP)

Answer 5.3.1 **The correct answer is "A."** According to the urinalysis, there is a small amount of blood in your patient's urine, but the number of RBCs is actually normal (<3 RBC/hpf). Your first step should be to repeat the urinalysis and urine microscopic examination to determine if this patient actually meets the criteria for microscopic hematuria (≥3 RBC/hpf on 2 of 3 properly collected urine specimens, according to the American Urological Association [AUA]). A urine culture may prove useful later in the evaluation process but is not necessary now. Likewise, ordering imaging studies is premature because the diagnosis of microscopic hematuria has not been made.

HELPFUL TIP:
Kidney stones are a very common cause of gross and microscopic hematuria. However, recall that 20% of patients with kidney stones will have no blood in their urine and have a normal urinalysis. IgA nephropathy is one of the most common intrinsic renal diseases to cause microscopic hematuria; kidney cysts, including polycystic kidney disease, are common causes as well. Neoplastic diseases, in particular, bladder cancer and renal cell carcinoma, may also be discovered during the investigation of microscopic hematuria.

HELPFUL TIP:
Compared with microscopic hematuria, **gross hematuria** is more commonly associated with malignancy and, once confirmed, should prompt a thorough evaluation. Benign causes of **microscopic hematuria** in adults include: vigorous exercise, menstruation, sexual activity, viral illness, and trauma.

Further history reveals that he smokes one to two packs of cigarettes per day. He has a normal blood pressure and the remainder of the physical examination is unrevealing. Two urine samples reveal microscopic hematuria, with 5 RBC/hpf on each sample. The rest of the urinalysis is normal, and there are no red cell casts.

Question 5.3.2 **In your evaluation of this patient, you include all of the following tests EXCEPT:**
A) Urine cytology
B) CBC
C) Serum creatinine
D) CT scan of the abdomen and pelvis with particular note of the kidneys
E) Renal biopsy

Answer 5.3.2 **The correct answer is "E."** In most cases of microscopic hematuria, renal biopsy is not indicated. However, if an intrinsic renal cause of hematuria is suspected, renal biopsy may prove necessary. Intrinsic renal disease is more likely if there is proteinuria, hypertension, elevated serum creatinine, or an active urinary sediment (e.g., nephritic, dysmorphic red cells, red cell casts).

There is no evidence-based approach to evaluate microscopic hematuria in a standardized manner, and recommendations vary depending on the organization. Most experts, including the AUA guidelines, recommend a serum creatinine and usually include CBC, coagulation studies, and serum chemistries. Depending on the patient's age and risk factors, further studies may be indicated. For patients older than 35 years, you should consider studies to evaluate for urinary tract cancers. Urine cytology has low sensitivity but high specificity for bladder cancer and may be quite useful in conjunction with cystoscopy. Imaging of the urinary system is an absolute requirement in the workup of microscopic hematuria in older patients (generally, those over age 35 years). CT scan appears to have the greatest sensitivity for detecting masses, but ultrasound, IVP, or the combination of the two may also be employed. Cystoscopy should be considered in addition to CT, since CT is poor at visualizing bladder abnormalities. See Table 5-2 for a suggested workup for microscopic hematuria.

Question 5.3.3 **The US Preventive Services Task Force recommends which of the following screening strategies for detecting microscopic hematuria?**
A) Annual urinalysis after age 50
B) Urinalysis every 2 years after age 50
C) Annual urinalysis after age 65
D) Annual urinalysis in all high-risk patients older than 65 years
E) No screening at any age

Answer 5.3.3 **The correct answer is "E."** The USPSTF recommends *against* routine screening for microscopic hematuria to detect urinary tract cancers. In one-time urine specimens in healthy adults, the presence of abnormal numbers of RBCs (≥3 RBCs/hpf) can be as high as 39%. In up to 70% of patients, even after imaging of the upper and lower urinary tract, the source of microscopic hematuria cannot be found. In a low-risk population, the false-positive rate of microscopic hematuria found on urinalysis would be unacceptably high. Also, there is no evidence that early detection of urinary tract cancers through screening urinalysis improves prognosis.

TABLE 5-2 EVALUATION OF MICROSCOPIC HEMATURIA

After microscopic hematuria has been identified (2 of 3 urine samples with 3 or more RBC/hpf), the American Urological Association (AUA) recommends the following evaluation:
- Infection identified → treat with antibiotics and repeat urinalysis
- RBC casts, proteinuria, or elevated creatinine → begin evaluation for glomerulonephritis and consider referral to a nephrologist
- No infection or primary renal disease identified in first 2 steps → urine cytology, bladder cystoscopy (if at risk for bladder cancer based on environmental exposures and/or age >40), and CT scan (helical CT if stones suspected, contrast-enhanced CT if stones not suspected)
- If entire thorough diagnostic evaluation negative → follow-up urinalysis, urine cytology, blood pressure, and serum creatinine every 6–12 months

Your patient returns to discuss his laboratory and radiology results. His serum creatinine is 1.1 mg/dL, and his CBC, chemistries, and coagulation studies are normal. His urine cytology was negative, as was cystoscopy performed by your friendly neighborhood urologist. CT scan of the abdomen and pelvis reveals normal size kidneys and no masses, but three stones, measuring 2 to 3 mm in diameter, are noted in the left renal pelvis. There does not appear to be any obstruction. Your patient denies any history of renal colic.

Question 5.3.4 Regarding the finding of stones in the left renal pelvis, which of the following interventions is warranted at this time?
A) Observation
B) Lithotripsy
C) Ureteral stent placement
D) Ketorolac and fluids by IV
E) Prophylactic nephrectomy

Answer 5.3.4 The correct answer is "A." The incidental finding of stones during the evaluation of microscopic hematuria is common. The stones may be the reason for your patient's hematuria. Since the stones are small, they may pass without intervention. Stones less than 5 mm in diameter are likely to pass spontaneously. No further intervention is warranted in asymptomatic patients. "D" is of particular note. Ketorolac and other NSAIDs are effective in treating the pain of urolithiasis. However, fluid is not helpful in treating acute ureteral colic (unless the patient is dehydrated). Fluid does nothing to "push" the stone out: fluid increases pain by further dilating the renal pelvis and the body simply shifts the excess fluid to the non-obstructed kidney.

HELPFUL TIP:
Desmopressin (DDAVP), which decreases urine production and thus stretch on the renal pelvis, can be used to control pain in those with urolithiasis although we don't recommend it for routine use—there are plenty of good analgesics out there.

Your patient does well for a year. When you see him next, he presents to your office as a late afternoon add-on and complains of severe abdominal pain that woke him from sleep at 3 AM. He describes the pain as "sharp" or "crampy," occurring in his left lower quadrant and radiating to the left testicle. Although the pain has waxed and waned, it has never resolved completely. He is also nauseated and has been vomiting. On examination, he is afebrile and tachycardic and has a blood pressure of 110/56 mm Hg. He appears uncomfortable and is writhing in pain. There is left lower quadrant, flank, and costovertebral angle tenderness.

Question 5.3.5 Your next action is to:
A) Prescribe oral ibuprofen and morphine and arrange follow-up tomorrow
B) Give IM ketorolac and arrange follow-up tomorrow

C) Bolus 1 L IV saline, administer IV ceftriaxone, and arrange follow-up tomorrow
D) Send him to the emergency department (ED) for pain management, fluids, and possible admission

Answer 5.3.5 The correct answer is "D." In a patient with known kidney stones presenting with classic findings of urolithiasis, the most likely diagnosis is renal colic due to stones. This patient is nauseated and vomiting frequently and may not do well at home overnight. He is unlikely to tolerate oral medications and could become dehydrated. In addition, we don't have a urinalysis, and a postobstructive UTI is an indication for admission and possibly stenting. For these reasons, the most appropriate action is aggressive pain management and further workup, which can be accomplished in the ED. If the patient is unable to tolerate oral pain medications after treatment in the ED, admission to the hospital is warranted. Narcotic analgesics, IV NSAIDs (e.g., ketorolac), and IV fluids to maintain euvolemia are all appropriate. The role of antibiotics will depend on urinalysis findings, but most cases of acute renal colic do not require antibiotics.

HELPFUL (AND VERY IMPORTANT) TIP:
Urolithiasis and abdominal aortic aneurysm can have the same presenting symptoms and signs (including hematuria). For that reason, imaging is mandatory in the older individual in whom an abdominal aortic aneurysm is a consideration. Also, keep testicular torsion on the differential for younger male patients presenting with renal colic symptoms—these patients need a genital examination (but you knew that, right?).

You admit the patient to the ED and start IV saline to maintain hydration; and administer narcotics, NSAIDs (ketorolac), and antiemetics. CT scan shows a 5-mm stone in the proximal ureter. There is no hydronephrosis. Serum electrolytes, BUN, creatinine, and CBC are all normal. Urinalysis reveals 2+ blood, 1+ leukocyte esterase, trace protein, pH 6, specific gravity 1.025, 20 RBC/hpf, few calcium oxalate crystals, and otherwise normal.

Question 5.3.6 Which of the following is the most appropriate management at this point in time?
A) Add antibiotics to the current therapy
B) Continue the current therapy and observe
C) Refer for extracorporeal shock wave lithotripsy
D) Refer for endoscopic lithotripsy

Answer 5.3.6 The correct answer is "B." There is no reason to change management at this point in time. Many 5 mm stones will pass spontaneously. Although leukocyte esterase is detected on the urine dipstick, there is no compelling evidence of infection (e.g., fever, elevated WBC count, and WBCs on microscopic examination), so antibiotics are not necessary. But culturing the urine would be prudent.

HELPFUL TIP:
Stones of 6 mm or greater will pass spontaneously only 10% of the time and those 4 to 6 mm 50% of the time. Those less than 4 mm pass the great majority of the time. If pain persists or the stone does not pass within 72 hours, consider urologic intervention such as nephrostomy, stent placement, and/or lithotripsy. Renal injury from obstruction generally does not occur for at least 72 hours (and, amazingly enough, there is only a 20% chance of complications if a non-obstructing stone remains for 4 weeks).

HELPFUL TIP:
Patients discharged from the ED with urolithiasis should be placed on an NSAID in addition to a narcotic. This reduces pain and "bounce back" visits.

Question 5.3.7 Your patient—a man possessing incredible foresight—asks how he can avoid kidney stones in the future. Which of the following tests will be most useful in determining the treatments that may prevent future stone formation?
A) Urine culture
B) Stone recovery and analysis
C) Urinary calcium excretion
D) Urinary oxalate excretion
E) Serum uric acid

Answer 5.3.7 **The correct answer is "B."** The prevention of further stone formation is aided by knowledge of the stone type. Always attempt to recover the stone and send it for analysis—unless the patient is a well-known stone former and the composition of the stones is already known. The other studies listed may have value. Struvite stones form during bacterial infections of the urinary tract and a urine culture ("A") will help direct therapy when these stones are identified. Calcium oxalate stones are the most common and 24-hour urine collection to determine calcium and oxalate excretion ("C") can lead to diagnoses of metabolic disturbances (hyperoxaluria and hypercalciuria). Patients with uric acid stones ("D") should be evaluated for symptoms of gout and undergo serum uric acid measurements ("E").

Your patient passes the stone, his pain completely resolves, and he is discharged from the hospital within 24 hours of his admission. The stone is pure calcium oxalate. Studies of his 24-hour urine collection are pending.

Question 5.3.8 In order to reduce his risk of forming more stones, you tell him to incorporate all of the following lifestyle changes EXCEPT:
A) Restrict calcium intake
B) Restrict oxalate intake (e.g., leafy green vegetables, chocolate)
C) Increase daily water intake
D) Add a glass of orange juice daily
E) Decrease sodium intake

Answer 5.3.8 **The correct answer is "A."** To prevent recurrent urolithiasis, restricted calcium intake was encouraged in the past. Moderate calcium intake (1 g/day) is recognized as beneficial and should be encouraged. Patients should take calcium with meals, which will bind oxalate and prevent its absorption. A low-calcium diet actually leads to an *increased* risk of urolithiasis. Increase in urine oxalate greatly increases the risk of stone formation. Restriction of oxalate ("B") in the diet may help to reduce the risk of recurrent urolithiasis. Foods high in oxalate include spinach, rhubarb, nuts, chocolate and legumes. Unfortunately, oxalate is also the end product of numerous metabolic pathways, and significant reduction in urinary oxalate levels often proves difficult (good news for you rhubarb fans! We like rhubarb pie *and* chocolate . . . say, I feel a stone coming on).

Increased fluid intake ("C") to achieve a urine volume >2 L/day reduces stone formation. Water and citrus juices ("D") are traditionally recommended (hypocitraturia is associated with stone formation), but most fluids consumed are associated with a positive effect, including drinks with caffeine.

Decreasing sodium intake ("E") is always a good piece of advice to patients with kidney disease. With stones in particular, increased sodium intake increases calcium excretion and decreases citrate excretion. Both of these increase the risk of recurrent stones.

Question 5.3.9 Your patient is wondering if he should have his urolithiasis worked up to determine an etiology. All of the following are reasons to pursue a further evaluation in this patient EXCEPT:
A) A strong family history of stones
B) African ancestry
C) Chronic diarrhea
D) Hypertension
E) Bariatric surgery

Answer 5.3.9 **The correct answer is "D."** Simply having hypertension is not a reason to work up a patient for renal stones. All of the other choices are correct. Of note is "B." Patients of African ancestry are *less likely* to have stones. Therefore, the workup is more likely to reveal a pathologic process in these patients. "C" and "E" are also of note. Anything that can cause malabsorption including bowel surgery, history of inflammatory bowel disease, etc., can increase the risk of stones. Thus, evaluation is indicated in these patients.

Because of his strong family history, you decide to proceed with evaluation. Results of your patient's 24-hour urine have returned and are as follows (reference ranges):
Volume 1.6 L.
pH 6.5.
Creatinine clearance normal.
Calcium 410 mg (100–300 mg).

Uric acid 410 mEq (250–750 mEq).
Oxalate 42 mg (7–44 mg).
Citrate 560 mg (100–800 mg).
Magnesium 3.1 mEq (3–5 mEq).

Question 5.3.10 Which of the following medications is most likely to reduce his risk of developing kidney stones in the future?
A) Allopurinol
B) Potassium citrate
C) Hydrochlorothiazide
D) Sodium bicarbonate
E) Furosemide

Answer 5.3.10 **The correct answer is "C."** According to the 24-hour urine studies, your patient has hypercalciuria, suboptimal urine volumes (the goal for urine output in urolithiasis should be 2 L/day or more), and no other abnormalities. Patients with urolithiasis and hypercalciuria may benefit from the long-term treatment with thiazide diuretics, such as hydrochlorothiazide, which decrease calcium excretion and therefore stone formation. Furosemide increases calcium excretion and has the potential to increase stone formation.

Even though it seems counterintuitive, patients with **calcium** stones and **hyperuricosuria** (not this patient) may benefit from allopurinol. It is thought that hyperuricosuria predisposes to calcium stones. Also, allopurinol is useful in the treatment of patients with uric acid stones. Patients with uric acid stones and hyperuricosuria may benefit from alkalinization of the urine with sodium bicarbonate or potassium citrate. In general, dietary citrate should be maximized. Oral potassium citrate is indicated for patients with hypocitraturia.

The patient is wondering whether he can expect to get another stone.

Question 5.3.11 All of the following are true EXCEPT:
A) The peak incidence of kidney stones occurs at age 30
B) Kidney stones are more common in men than in women
C) The probability of a second kidney stone is 60% to 80%
D) Only people who become dehydrated can expect to have a second stone
E) Living in a hot climate can predispose to a second stone

Answer 5.3.11 **The correct answer is "D."** While dehydration predisposes patients to a second stone (and thus "E"), maintaining optimal hydration lowers the risk but is not a foolproof remedy. Kidney stones are more common in men and have a peak incidence at age 30. About 60% to 80% of patients with a kidney stone will suffer a recurrence.

Question 5.3.12 Which of these patients with urolithiasis requires hospitalization?
A) A patient with a high-grade obstruction
B) A patient with intractable pain or vomiting
C) A patient with an associated urinary tract infection
D) A patient with a solitary kidney or transplanted kidney
E) All of the above

Answer 5.3.12 **The correct answer is "E."** All of the patients listed above should be admitted. Obviously, patients having uncontrollable pain or vomiting will do poorly as outpatients. Urolithiasis with a coexistent UTI is a significant problem due to the risk of abscess formation, bacteremia, and renal parenchymal destruction. These patients require IV antibiotics and immediate urologic consultation, particularly in the presence of comorbidity. Patients with solitary or transplanted kidneys or in whom the diagnosis of renal colic is unclear should be admitted for monitoring of renal function and further evaluation.

HELPFUL TIP:
Recent high-quality data suggest that alpha-blockers (e.g., tamsulosin, doxazosin) are not helpful if the stone is <5 mm (most pass anyway). In stones 5 to 10 mm, there seems to be a benefit (*Cochrane Database Syst Rev.* 2018;4: CD008509; *JAMA Intern Med.* 2018;178(8):1051–1057). This recommendation seems to change yearly…

HELPFUL TIP:
Remember that multiple drugs can form radiolucent stones that will not show up on a CT scan. Among these are indinavir, acyclovir, and triamterene. Ultrasound should be the first modality, anyway. It detects hydronephrosis which is what we care about acutely and avoids radiation.

▶ Objectives: Did you learn to …
- Define microscopic hematuria?
- Evaluate a patient with microscopic hematuria based on risk and differential diagnosis?
- Describe the difficulties inherent in employing urine studies to screen for urinary tract cancers?
- Evaluate a patient with urolithiasis?
- Identify causes of urolithiasis based on the characteristics of the stone?
- Manage a patient with symptomatic urolithiasis?
- Use strategies to prevent stone formation based on the characteristics of the stone?

▶ CASE 5.4

A 19-year-old female presents to your office concerned about protein in her urine. As a college student, she has a part-time job in a medical laboratory. She "repurposed" a few urine dipsticks from the laboratory—you know, "just checking her urine"—and found that she had 2+ protein on urine dipstick. She has no urinary symptoms and denies fever, weight changes, and edema. She is afebrile with a blood pressure of 118/68 mm Hg. Examination is otherwise unremarkable. Repeat urinalysis in the office confirms 2+ protein, specific gravity 1.020, pH 6.5, and no blood. The urine microscopic examination is normal.

Question 5.4.1 Which of the following is the most appropriate next action in evaluating this patient?
A) Repeat urinalysis and urine culture
B) Ultrasound of the kidneys
C) 24-hour urine collection for protein and creatinine
D) Random urine protein/creatinine ratio

Answer 5.4.1 **The correct answer is "D."** Did you go for "C"? A random urine is much easier than collecting a 24-hour urine and correlates well with 24-hour collections. You *could* ask the patient to collect urine for 24 hours for protein and creatinine measurements, but why? Who wants to lug around a jug of their own urine all day? What will she tell her friends and coworkers?

Your patient already has protein on urinalysis twice. Another urinalysis ("A") will not help to determine if this is truly a worrisome finding or not. There is no evidence of a UTI (no leukocyte esterase, nitrites, etc., and no symptoms); thus, culture would be very low yield. There is no indication for renal ultrasound ("B") at this point.

HELPFUL TIP:
Concentrated or alkaline urine can result in overestimation of urine protein on dipstick. Note that this patient's urine specific gravity was normal.

Question 5.4.2 Which type(s) of protein are detected on a urine dipstick?
A) Albumin
B) Amino acids
C) Immunoglobulin light chains
D) A and B
E) A and C

Answer 5.4.2 **The correct answer is "A."** The urine dipstick only detects large–molecular-weight proteins—generally this means albumin. Amino acids are not detected. Immunoglobulin light chains, such as Bence Jones proteins, are also not detected on urine dipstick.

Her urine protein/creatinine ratio is equivalent to 1 g of urine protein per day. Creatinine clearance is normal. Serum creatinine, BUN, albumin, glucose, and electrolytes are normal.

Question 5.4.3 Which of the following is the best next step in your evaluation and management?
A) Start her on a low-protein diet
B) Order CT scan of abdomen and pelvis
C) Measure recumbent urine protein level
D) Refer for renal biopsy

Answer 5.4.3 **The correct answer is "C."** Proteinuria may be either transient or persistent. Transient proteinuria is often due to fever, exercise, or other causes and is not associated with significant kidney disease. Transient proteinuria is found in 7% of women and 4% of men. It often resolves spontaneously, and subsequent urine tests will probably be negative. However, at this point you don't know if this case will be transient or persistent proteinuria.

Orthostatic proteinuria is a common type of transient proteinuria seen in young, healthy persons. Up to 5% of adolescents have orthostatic proteinuria, and young adults may present with it as well. Protein is spilled in the urine when the patient is upright, but not when recumbent. There are two ways to determine recumbent urine protein: an easy way and a hard way. The easy way is to have the patient void before going to bed, stay supine all night (8 hours), and collect urine immediately upon waking. This urine is checked for protein/creatinine ratio. Another urine sample must be checked for protein/creatinine ratio after the patient has been upright. If the upright is abnormal and the recumbent is normal, you have diagnosed orthostatic proteinuria (and impressed your colleagues). The "hard way" involves splitting a 24-hour urine collection—two jugs of urine and the required arithmetic. Orthostatic proteinuria is a benign condition that usually resolves as the patient ages, requiring no additional evaluation.

A finding of 1 g of protein in a 24-hour urine collection is abnormal (normal <0.15 g/day), but it does not yet reach the nephrotic range (>3 g/day). Regardless, a low-protein diet ("A") is not helpful. CT scan of the abdomen and pelvis ("B") is unlikely to add any new information. Referring for renal biopsy ("D") is premature.

The patient collects urine in upright and recumbent positions, and both have abnormal amounts of protein. You refer the patient to a nephrologist who recommends follow-up rather than biopsy. Annual follow-up will include blood pressure, serum creatinine, and spot urine protein/creatinine ratio.

Question 5.4.4 In order to prevent worsening proteinuria, the nephrologist also recommends which of the following medications?
A) Amlodipine
B) Diltiazem
C) Furosemide
D) Benazepril
E) Aspirin

Answer 5.4.4 **The correct answer is "D."** Patients with proteinuria tend to respond well to ACE inhibitors. ACE inhibitors have been shown to reduce proteinuria by 35% to 40%. This effect is true in nondiabetic patients with proteinuria as well as in diabetic patients. ACE inhibitors appear to be superior to other antihypertensives, including calcium channel blockers ("A" and "B"). Furosemide ("C") would be indicated if your patient develops edema, but loop diuretics should not be used primarily for the treatment of hypertension or proteinuria. Aspirin ("E") may be indicated for protection against coronary artery disease in patients with risk factors, including CKD, but it is not a primary treatment of proteinuria or hypertension. Remember that NSAIDs can adversely affect renal function.

 HELPFUL (AND IMPORTANT) TIP:
While ACE inhibitors are first-line treatments for proteinuria, they also can cause effects on the fetus during pregnancy. Use is not contraindicated within women of child-bearing age, but should be undertaken with caution. Ensure she is on a reliable source of contraception (perhaps long-acting reversible contraception such as IUD or Nexplanon) and that she is counseled on the risks to the fetus if she were to get pregnant. If she does become pregnant, she must discontinue the ACE inhibitor right away.

Unfortunately, over the next few years, your patient develops hypertension. You maximize the dose of benazepril and need to add another drug to control her pressure. Her proteinuria increases to 3.5 g/day, and her plasma creatinine increases to 2 mg/dL. She develops edema, and her serum albumin is 2.8 g/dL. The urine shows only protein and no inflammatory components.

Question 5.4.5 This patient's current clinical condition is most appropriately described as:
A) Hypertensive nephropathy
B) Acute renal failure
C) Focal nephritic glomerulonephritis
D) Nephrotic syndrome
E) Floating kidney

Answer 5.4.5 **The correct answer is "D."** While identifying no specific disease state, the term "nephrotic syndrome" refers to a constellation of signs and laboratory abnormalities. A number of diseases may lead to nephrotic syndrome (keep reading for more on this). When urine protein exceeds 3 to 3.5 g/day, it is often referred to as "nephrotic range" proteinuria. "Complete" nephrotic syndrome consists of edema, heavy proteinuria (>3 g/day or 3.5 g/day) and hypoalbuminemia (<3 g/dL). Please note that we are not writing "3 or 3.5 g/day" to confuse you. That's just what the experts say. Basically, there's way more albumin in the urine than there should be. Additional associated abnormalities include hyperlipidemia and thrombosis (Table 5-3).

TABLE 5-3 CRITERIA FOR NEPHROTIC SYNDROME

Required for the diagnosis of nephrotic syndrome
- Albuminuria >3 g/day
- Hypoalbuminemia (serum albumin of <3 g/dL)
- Peripheral edema

Other (nondiagnostic but supportive) findings
- Hyperlipidemia
- Thrombotic events

Question 5.4.6 Which of the following findings in urine sediment is associated with nephrotic syndrome?
A) Red cell casts
B) White cell casts
C) Oval fat bodies
D) Uric acid crystals
E) Granular casts

Answer 5.4.6 **The correct answer is "C."** Urine sediment in nephrotic syndrome is typically bland. There is little cellular matter. Oval fat bodies and fatty casts occur in the urine of patients with heavy proteinuria and hyperlipidemia. Fat bodies reflect the increased permeability of the glomeruli and suggest some type of glomerular disease (including nephrotic syndrome) albeit not necessarily active disease. However, fat can also be seen in patients with polycystic kidney disease and fat embolism syndrome.

Red cell casts ("A"), the hallmark of nephritic syndrome, are absent in nephrotic urine. White cell casts ("B") are associated with interstitial nephritis and pyelonephritis. Uric acid crystals ("D") are sometimes seen in gout, hyperuricemia, and urate stone disease. Granular casts ("E") are not specific to any particular pathologic process and may be found in acute tubular necrosis, glomerulonephritis, and other renal diseases. See Table 5-4 for more details on urine sediment.

Question 5.4.7 Nephrotic syndrome is not a specific disease entity, but can be the end result of a number of processes. Which of the following cause(s) nephrotic syndrome?
A) Diabetes
B) Minimal change disease
C) Amyloidosis
D) Systemic lupus erythematosus
E) All of the above

TABLE 5-4 URINE SEDIMENT FINDINGS AND ASSOCIATED CONDITIONS

Sediment Finding	Associated Condition
Epithelial cell casts	ATN, acute glomerulonephritis
Fat bodies, fatty casts	Massive proteinuria (nephrotic syndrome), fat emboli, polycystic kidney disease, glomerular disease (may not be active as in nephrotic syndrome)
Granular casts	Nonspecific—many renal disorders
Hyaline casts	Concentrated urine, diuretic use, normal finding
Red cell casts	Glomerulonephritis, vasculitis (very specific to these)
Waxy casts	Advanced renal failure
White cell casts	Pyelonephritis, acute interstitial nephritis, various glomerular diseases

ATN, acute tubular necrosis.

Answer 5.4.7 The correct answer is "E." All of the above can be a cause of **nephrotic** syndrome. Remember that many causes of nephrotic syndrome can present initially with **nephritic** urine. Causes of nephrotic syndrome are summarized in Table 5-5.

Question 5.4.8 Which of the following tests is NOT indicated in most patients with nephrotic syndrome?
A) Hepatitis B and C serology
B) ANA
C) Serum and urine protein electrophoresis
D) HbA1c
E) CA-125 antigen

Answer 5.4.8 The correct answer is "E." Evaluation for cancer should be done if there is a specific reason to believe the patient has a malignancy (weight loss, mass on examination, etc.). CA-125 is a marker for ovarian cancer (among others . . . colon, pancreatic, etc.) and need not be done routinely. Plus, it's not a useful screening test for ovarian cancer. In addition to a thorough history and physical examination, consider obtaining the following in patients with nephrotic syndrome (as well as those with nephritic urine):

• Hepatitis B and C serology
• ANA
• Serum and urine protein electrophoresis
• ASO titer
• Cryoglobulins
• Serum complement levels
• ANCA
• Serum calcium (to rule out sarcoid)
• Antiglomerular basement membrane antibodies

Use clinical judgment to guide your workup. However, this evaluation will find the cause in many cases of nephritis and/or nephrotic syndrome.

The diagnosis in your patient is unclear despite the workup noted above. It is time to consider a renal biopsy.

TABLE 5-5 CAUSES OF NEPHROTIC SYNDROME

• Diabetes
• Amyloidosis
• Systemic lupus erythematosus
• Minimal change disease ("Nil" disease)
• Diffuse glomerulonephritis
• Membranous nephropathy
• IgA nephropathy
• Postinfectious glomerulonephritis (e.g., post-streptococcal GN)
• Membranoproliferative glomerulonephritis
• Various neoplastic diseases (lymphoma, multiple myeloma, lung cancer, etc.)
• Preeclampsia
• Familial kidney disease (Alport disease, Fabry disease)
• Focal and segmental glomerulosclerosis
• Medications (NSAIDs)
• Miscellaneous

Question 5.4.9 Absolute contraindications to renal biopsy include which of the following?
A) Hypertension
B) Use of an anticoagulant for atrial fibrillation
C) Perinephric abscess
D) Solitary renal cyst
E) All of the above

Answer 5.4.9 The correct answer is "C." The presence of renal or perirenal infection is a contraindication to renal biopsy. None of the others are absolute contraindications. However, **uncontrollable** hypertension, **irreversible coagulopathy, multiple bilateral cysts**, hydronephrosis, small kidneys (indicative of chronic, irreversible disease), known renal tumor, and lack of consent **are** additional contraindications to renal biopsy. Simply being on warfarin or another anticoagulant, which can be stopped or reversed, is not a contraindication to biopsy.

Question 5.4.10 Which of the following is an indication for renal biopsy?
A) Persistent hematuria in a patient with normal renal function and an otherwise negative workup
B) Persistent low-grade proteinuria (1–2 g/day range) with normal blood pressure and creatinine
C) Suspected case of IgA nephropathy
D) Nephrotic syndrome likely from diabetes mellitus
E) Persistent low-grade proteinuria with elevated blood pressure and/or elevated creatinine

Answer 5.4.10 The correct answer is "E." Patients with low-grade proteinuria and elevated serum creatinine and/or hypertension should have a renal biopsy in order to determine the etiology of their disease. Indications for biopsy are listed in Table 5-6.

▶ **Objectives: Did you learn to ...**
• Evaluate and follow a healthy-appearing patient with proteinuria?
• Define and diagnose orthostatic proteinuria and understand its significance?
• Manage a patient with progressive proteinuria?
• Define and evaluate nephrotic syndrome?
• Identify causes of nephrotic syndrome?

TABLE 5-6 INDICATIONS FOR RENAL BIOPSY

• Nephrotic syndrome **without** a systemic etiology found on other testing
• Hematuria from a glomerular source **with** hypertension or increasing creatinine
• Persistent low grade proteinuria **with** hypertension or increasing creatinine
• Nephritis **without** a systemic explanation (e.g., no lupus, drug exposure)
• Suspicion of granulomatosis with polyangiitis (formerly Wegener disease) or polyarteritis nodosum where other tissue is not available
• Acute or subacute renal failure without another explanation (although history will usually result in a presumptive diagnosis)

▶ CASE 5.5

While covering the ED, a 62-year-old female you have known for several years presents with her husband. She appears lethargic and is unable to give a coherent history. Her husband tells you that she began having stomach pain, nausea, and diarrhea 2 days ago. Although she has not been vomiting, she has been unable to drink or eat much due to nausea. She takes furosemide for edema and albuterol/ipratropium (Combivent) for chronic obstructive pulmonary disease (COPD). She smokes a pack of cigarettes per day.

On physical examination, her respiratory rate is 30, pulse 104 bpm, blood pressure 112/64 mm Hg, and temperature 37.9°C. She is somnolent and disoriented. Oral mucosa is dry. Lung examination demonstrates diminished air movement bilaterally. Her abdomen is diffusely tender, but there is no rebound. Rectal examination is negative for occult blood.

The first laboratory test you have available is a room air arterial blood gas (although venous would have been fine, right?): pH 7.12, $PaCO_2$ 33 mm Hg, PaO_2 80 mm Hg, HCO_3 10 mEq/L, and oxygen saturation 92%.

Question 5.5.1 This blood gas is most consistent with which of the following processes?
A) Compensated metabolic acidosis
B) Compensated respiratory acidosis
C) Poorly compensated metabolic acidosis
D) Poorly compensated respiratory acidosis
E) Pure respiratory alkalosis

Answer 5.5.1 **The correct answer is "C."** This patient is clearly acidotic, as her pH is well below the normal range of 7.35 to 7.45. So, whatever she has, it will be poorly compensated, ruling out "A" and "B." Based on the bicarbonate (HCO_3) level and the history of gastrointestinal losses due to diarrhea, you would suspect a metabolic acidosis. In order to have appropriate respiratory compensation, the $PaCO_2$ should fall 12 points for every 10-point drop in the HCO_3 below the normal level (normal HCO_3 is around 24 mEq/L).

In this case, the HCO_3 is 10 mEq/L (14 points below normal); therefore, the $PaCO_2$ is expected to drop by about ($1.2 \times 14 = 16.8$) or approximately 17. However, the $PaCO_2$ is not 23 mm Hg; it is 33 mm Hg (close to the normal range of 35–45). The patient's $PaCO_2$ is too high to appropriately compensate for her metabolic acidosis, and she thus has a poorly compensated metabolic acidosis.

There is another way to do this:

The pH should change by 0.08 for every 10 change in CO_2. So, if a patient's CO_2 is 50, the pH should be 7.32 if it is an uncompensated respiratory acidosis. If they are more acidotic (e.g., 7.24), they have a mixed respiratory and metabolic acidosis. If they are less acidotic (e.g., 7.39), they have a compensated respiratory acidosis.

While you are providing supportive care, the patient's laboratory results are completed: Na 134 mEq/L (reference range 135–145 mEq/L), K 2.1 mEq/L (3.5–5.0 mEq/L), Cl 112 mEq/L (98–107 mEq/L), HCO_3 10 mEq/L (23–29 mEq/L), BUN 29 mg/dL (5–20 mg/dL), Cr 1.1 mg/dL (0.6–1.2 mg/dL), Ca 9.1 mg/dL (8.5–10.2 mg/dL); CBC: WBC 16,100 cells/mm³, Hgb 13.9 g/dL, platelets 167,000 cells/mm³; urinalysis: specific gravity 1.030, remainder normal. Troponin-T, CK, and liver enzymes are normal.

Question 5.5.2 All of the following may be contributing to hypokalemia in this patient EXCEPT:
A) Hypomagnesemia
B) Furosemide
C) Acidosis
D) Beta-agonists such as albuterol
E) Diarrhea

Answer 5.5.2 **The correct answer is "C."** Acidosis should cause a spurious elevation in potassium—not hypokalemia. Magnesium ("A") depletion promotes potassium loss. Thus, hypomagnesemia can contribute to hypokalemia. "B," furosemide and other loop diuretics, causes renal potassium wasting. "D," beta-agonists transiently shift potassium into cells, thereby lowering the serum potassium. Diarrhea ("E") causes direct gastrointestinal losses of potassium.

Other causes of hypokalemia include thiazide diuretics, metabolic alkalosis (often from protracted emesis—although this represents a shift of potassium intracellularly and not a true hypokalemia), hyperaldosteronism, and RTA types 1 and 2.

Question 5.5.3 Since your administration likes to keep the hospital at 99% capacity, there are currently no cardiac-monitored beds available for this patient. The most appropriate initial therapy to correct her hypokalemia (2.1 mEq/L) is to give your patient:

A) KCl 40 mEq orally
B) KCl 80 mEq orally
C) KCL 20 mEq per hour IV
D) KCl 20 mEq *push* IV
E) KCl 60 mEq per hour IV

Answer 5.5.3 **The correct answer is "C."** Remember that this patient is nauseated and lethargic and has been unable to eat. Thus, oral potassium replacement is unlikely to work. Couple this with the fact that she is profoundly hypokalemic, and IV replacement becomes the treatment of choice. One should not give more than 20 mEq KCl IV per hour without a cardiac monitor. It should be given through a large bore peripheral IV or a central line due to venous irritation. If you chose "D," you just failed your test. IV push KCl is fatal.

Most commonly, the chloride salt of potassium (KCl) is administered to replete potassium stores. In the conscious patient with a functional gastrointestinal tract, oral KCl should be administered. Oral and intravenous bioavailability is very similar, but oral doses greater than 40 to 60 mEq may not be well tolerated.

HELPFUL TIP:
There are no reliably reproducible ways to gauge potassium depletion and amount needed to make a patient eukalemic. The best thing to do is start replacing with KCl and monitor serum potassium levels, adjusting the KCl dose as you go. Be careful when ordering potassium replacement: *hyper*kalemia is most commonly iatrogenic.

Question 5.5.4 In addition to KCl repletion, which of the following interventions do you initiate now in an attempt to correct the acidosis?

A) Bolus normal saline
B) Sodium bicarbonate
C) Bolus 5% dextrose
D) Intubation and mechanical ventilation

Answer 5.5.4 **The correct answer is "A."** On the basis of history, physical examination, and BUN/creatinine ratio, your patient is dehydrated. The first step is to correct the dehydration with intravenous fluids. Normal saline is preferred over dextrose ("C"), which might lead to further hyponatremia and hypokalemia. In addition, dextrose will not stay intravascular and will actually precipitate a diuresis by making the serum hypotonic. "B" is incorrect. There is no evidence that bicarbonate improves outcomes in metabolic acidosis (though some will try it if the patient's pH is 6.9–7.0). The best initial approach is to correct the underlying problem. In most cases, volume replacement

will lead to improvement in acidosis without needing to resort to bicarbonate. Although she is oxygenating well now, if your patient's respiratory condition deteriorates, she may require intubation ("D") and ventilator settings could be adjusted to aid in correcting the acid/base disorder.

▶ **Objectives: Did you learn to ...**
- Define acidosis and distinguish compensated from poorly compensated acidosis?
- Discuss causes of hypokalemia?
- Manage a patient with metabolic acidosis and hypokalemia?

 QUICK QUIZ: RHABDOMYOLYSIS

The primary mechanism by which renal failure occurs in rhabdomyolysis is:

A) Glomerular destruction
B) Acute tubular necrosis (ATN)
C) Interstitial nephritis
D) None of the above

The correct answer is "B." Myoglobin deposits in the renal tubules, causing local damage and ischemia, which results in acute tubular necrosis. Findings in the urinary sediment that support acute tubular necrosis include renal tubular epithelial cells and dark brown casts of granular material ("muddy" brown casts).

HELPFUL TIP:
Patients with rhabdomyolysis with creatine kinase (CK) <5,000 U/L and clear urine are unlikely to develop acute tubular necrosis, but should be monitored to assure dropping CK and adequate renal function.

 QUICK QUIZ: LUMPY KIDNEYS

Which of the following is/are associated with autosomal-dominant polycystic kidney disease (ADPKD)?

A) Liver cysts
B) Cerebral aneurysms
C) Colonic diverticula
D) Cardiac valvular disease
E) All of the above

The correct answer is "E." All of the above are associated with polycystic kidney disease. Of particular importance is the possibility of cerebral aneurysms (5–20%) leading to subarachnoid hemorrhage. However, aneurysm rupture remains fairly rare, but it does seem to run in families—and seems to result in a really bad day for your patient. Currently, screening for subarachnoid aneurysms in asymptomatic, low-risk patients with ADPKD is not recommended. ADPKD occurs in 1 in every 400 to 2,000 live births and is, as the name implies, autosomal dominant. Common extrarenal manifestations of ADPKD include cerebral aneurysms, hepatic cysts, cardiac valve disease, colonic diverticula, and abdominal and inguinal hernias.

 QUICK QUIZ: TOO SALTY

A 79-year-old female nursing home resident with moderate dementia presents for worsening confusion over the last 2 days. She just finished antibiotics for a urinary tract infection. Her temperature is 37.1°C, pulse 110 bpm, respiratory rate 18 breaths/minute, and blood pressure 108/56 mm Hg. She is disoriented and lethargic. Examination of the heart, lungs, and abdomen is unremarkable.

Laboratory studies are as follows: Na 165 mEq/L, K 4.6 mEq/L, Cl 118 mEq/L, HCO_3 28 mEq/L, BUN 31 mg/dL, Cr 1.1 mg/dL. Urine specific gravity is >1.030 and urine osmolality is 700 mmol/kg (elevated, reflecting reabsorption of free water). Her CBC is normal.

Initial treatment for this patient should be:
A) Normal saline IV bolus
B) Dextrose 5% IV bolus
C) Sterile water IV bolus
D) Furosemide 40 mg IV.
E) DDAVP

The correct answer is "A." Demented or delirious patients with an acute febrile illness may not be able to consume enough free water to avoid hypernatremia. Several mechanisms may be at work: free water loss due to illness, impaired thirst, and inability to respond to thirst due to cognitive or physical impairments.

Just as with hyponatremia, the hypernatremic patient should not be corrected too quickly. Sudden changes in plasma sodium may result in cerebral edema. Although there are no standardized guidelines to direct the correction of hypernatremia, most authorities recommend a maximal correction of 0.5 to 1 mEq/L/hr. In this patient who appears hypovolemic, the primary concern is to give volume. The administration of normal saline will allow you to administer volume while lowering her plasma sodium. Dextrose 5% solution will likely lower the sodium too quickly. Sterile water should never be administered IV because it will cause massive local hemolysis.

"D" is incorrect since she is dehydrated, based on history and lab findings. "E" is incorrect. This patient's kidney function is appropriate for her hypernatremia. She is concentrating her urine, as evidenced by her high urine specific gravity and urine osmolality. Therefore, she does not have diabetes insipidus, which is characterized by large volumes of dilute urine. DDAVP is an appropriate treatment for central diabetes insipidus. See Table 5-7 for more on causes of hypernatremia.

 HELPFUL TIP:
Generally, regulatory mechanisms will maintain a normal serum sodium. However, this requires access to free water. Immobile patients (especially the elderly) are particularly prone to problems because of their limited mobility and inability to independently access water.

TABLE 5-7 CAUSES OF HYPERNATREMIA
- GI loss of water
- Osmotic diuresis
- Excess exercise and sweating
- Diabetes insipidus
- Decreased access to free water

 HELPFUL TIP:
Calculators are available to estimate free water deficit in hypovolemic hypernatremic patients. There are several equations and it's not clear which one is superior to another. However, these must be viewed as rough guides. As fluids are replaced, reassess the patient frequently using clinical and laboratory measures.

▶ CASE 5.6

A surgical colleague asks you to consult on a patient because of increasing creatinine (yes, we know this will never happen with a surgeon—just consider this a thought experiment). A 63-year-old woman was admitted for an elective cholecystectomy. She is on postoperative day 3 and has fever with delirium. Her current medications are morphine, cefotetan, and acetaminophen as needed. She takes nothing by mouth, but has intravenous fluids (5% dextrose/0.45% saline) running at 100 cc/hr . . . continuously . . . since surgery. Plasma studies from the day of surgery and this morning are available:

Laboratory Test	Day Before Surgery	Day of Consultation
Sodium (mEq/L)	138	130
Potassium (mEq/L)	4.5	5.8
Chloride (mEq/L)	103	105
HCO_3 (mEq/L)	24	18
BUN (mg/dL)	15	30
Creatinine (mg/dL)	1.1	2.0

Question 5.6.1 **The BUN/Cr ratio on the day of consultation suggests that:**
A) She is hypovolemic
B) She has a prerenal cause of her increased creatinine, such as heart failure
C) Intrinsic kidney disease is more likely than a prerenal cause of her increased creatinine
D) Pyelonephritis is the most likely cause of her increased creatinine

Answer 5.6.1 **The correct answer is "C."** A BUN/Cr ratio <20 generally indicates an intrinsic renal cause of renal failure (increasing Cr) while a BUN/Cr ratio >20 indicates a prerenal cause such as hypoperfusion (e.g., heart failure, volume depletion, liver failure). In this patient, the BUN/Cr ratio is 15, suggesting—but not confirming—intrinsic renal disease.

Question 5.6.2 Which of the following is the most appropriate first step in determining the nature of this patient's elevated creatinine?
A) Give a trial bolus of normal saline
B) CT scan of the abdomen
C) Determine volume of urine output
D) Obtain urine for culture
E) Give a trial dose of furosemide

Answer 5.6.2 **The correct answer is "C."** Currently, all you know about this patient's kidney function is that it has declined since her admission and that it is not likely from a prerenal cause. It is important to know if this patient is oliguric/anuric or has adequate urine output. This is important because it can affect the treatment. For example, oliguric or anuric patients may become volume overloaded easily in response to IV fluids. Although hospital measurements of intake and output are often plagued by errors, you should start this evaluation by analyzing the patient's urine output, as well as fluid intake. Urine culture and CT scan may eventually play a role in your evaluation. The decision to give fluids or diuretics cannot be made until more information is gathered.

HELPFUL TIP:
Relatively small changes in serum creatinine may reflect acute kidney injury (previously termed "acute renal failure"). A patient with a baseline creatinine of 0.7 mg/dL has lost **half** her renal function when her creatinine increases to 1.4 mg/dL, even though this number may still be in the normal range for a particular lab—thus, the need to calculate a creatinine clearance and/or MDRD GFR. There are a number of definitions of acute kidney injury (e.g., RIFLE, AKIN, and KDIGO criteria), but the basic premise is that by some objective measure (e.g., creatinine, urine output), kidney function has rapidly declined.

HELPFUL TIP:
Like acute kidney injury, there is no single number that defines oliguria. However, one commonly used definition of oliguria is: less than 1 mL/kg/hr in infants, less than 0.5 mL/kg/hr in children, and less than 500 mL/day for adults. Of course, anuria is defined as no urine output (or less than 50 mL/day for adults).

Vital signs, intake, and output have been recorded by the nurses for each shift since admission and are provided in Table 5-8.

Question 5.6.3 You have now determined that your patient has become oliguric. Which of the following is most likely

to help you narrow the differential diagnosis of renal failure?
A) Calculation of creatinine clearance
B) Arterial blood gases
C) CT scan of the abdomen
D) Fractional excretion of sodium (FENa)
E) Furosemide challenge

Answer 5.6.3 **The correct answer is "D."** In this patient, you know that her BUN/Cr ratio is <20, pointing you toward intrinsic renal disease. But this ratio is not specific enough to rely upon. In oliguric renal failure, the FENa is a useful tool to help differentiate prerenal causes of renal failure from intrinsic renal causes. If the FENa is less than 1%, the kidney is functioning appropriately to conserve sodium and water to better perfuse the kidney, and a prerenal cause of failure is more likely such as hypoperfusion from shock, dehydration, heart failure, etc.

If the FENa is greater than 1%, salt and water losses are excessive, suggesting intrinsic kidney dysfunction. This calculation is **most meaningful** in oliguric renal failure (urine output <500 cc/day), but can also be used with any acute kidney injury in order to help determine the possible underlying cause. Also, FENa may be inaccurate in the elderly, patients receiving diuretics, and in chronic renal failure. The equation used to calculate FENa is:

$$FENa(\%) = [(urine\ Na/plasma\ Na)/(urine\ Cl/plasma\ Cr)] \times 100$$

HELPFUL TIP:
What if the patient is on a diuretic and you cannot make use of the FENa? Use the FEUrea, as urea excretion is not affected by diuretics. Here's the equation:

$$FEUrea(\%) = [(urine\ urea/plasma\ urea)/(urine\ Cr/plasma\ Cr)] \times 100$$

If the FEUrea is <35%, a prerenal cause is more likely. If FEUrea is >50%, acute tubular necrosis is more likely. Caveat: hyperglycemic diuresis increases excretion of urea even in hypovolemic states (e.g., 3 + glucose in the urine can give you a falsely high FEUrea).

On examination, you find a mildly disoriented female in no acute distress. She has lower extremity and sacral edema. You obtain urine studies, showing a specific gravity of 1.020, pH 6, 3 RBCs/hpf, 2 WBCs/hpf, and muddy brown granular casts. The urine creatinine is 6.5 mg/dL and the urine sodium is 45 mEq/L. You calculate the FENa at 10.65%.

Question 5.6.4 Given the clinical course and urine findings, which of the following is the best diagnosis?
A) Acute tubular necrosis (ATN)
B) Acute interstitial nephritis (AIN)
C) Vasculitis
D) Heart failure (HF)
E) Lactic acidosis

Answer 5.6.4 **The correct answer is "A."** ATN is a major cause of acute kidney injury in hospitalized patients. ATN is the result

TABLE 5-8 VITAL SIGNS, INTAKE, AND OUTPUT

	Day 1	Day 1	Day 1	Day 2	Day 2	Day 2	Day 3	Day 3	Day 3
	Shift 1	Shift 2	Shift 3	Shift 1	Shift 2	Shift 3	Shift 1	Shift 2	Shift 3
BP (mmHg)	118/60	117/63	102/57	80/42	92/48	102/67	105/60	102/61	102/79
Pulse (bpm)	84	82	92	124	117	106	100	102	93
Temp (°C)	37.3	37.0	37.7	40.0	39.1	37.1	38.0	36.9	36.8
RR	12	14	13	15	20	18	20	12	12
IV in (cc)	1,800	800	800	800	800	800	800	800	800
Urine out (cc)	1,650	1,000	750	850	600	400	180	100	80

of toxic and/or ischemic effects on the kidney tubules. Metabolic derangements in ATN include progressive hyponatremia, hyperkalemia, and metabolic acidosis with a high anion gap, all of which are present in this case. Typically patients with ATN have a FENa >1% (or FEUrea >50%) and a urine sodium >40 mEq/L. Remember, the functioning kidney should be retaining sodium to increase its perfusion if the source of the problem is extrinsic to the kidney or "prerenal." This is not happening here, so it is an intrinsic renal problem. In this case, FENa is 10.65%. In addition, "muddy" brown casts (renal tubular cell casts) are often found in the urinary sediment of patients with ATN. All of these findings point to ATN as the cause of renal failure in this patient.

Question 5.6.5 Based on the available data (including the vital signs in Table 5-8 and urine values), you suspect that ATN in this patient is the result of:
A) Acetaminophen
B) Hypotension
C) Intrinsic renal infection
D) Cefotetan
E) Any of the above is equally likely

Answer 5.6.5 **The correct answer is "B."** As you review the vital signs, intake, and output, you will notice that the patient had a hypotensive period associated with tachycardia and fever (day 2, shifts 1 and 2). She then developed progressively lower urine output despite stable IV intake. It is likely that she has had an ischemic insult to her kidneys as a result of hypotension and decreased perfusion. While many medications can cause ATN, cefotetan and acetaminophen are relatively safe. However, cephalosporins may cause acute interstitial nephritis (fever, rash, white cell casts, and perhaps eosinophils in the urine and peripheral blood).

 HELPFUL TIP:
In addition to hypoxic insult (shock, hypoperfusion, HF, etc.), common causes of ATN include medications such as tacrolimus, NSAIDs, ACE inhibitors, gentamicin, tobramycin, cyclosporine, and more.

When you go to check on the patient later in the afternoon, she has become more tachypneic and has rales on examination.

Question 5.6.6 Which of the following recommendations do you make for this patient's continuing care?
A) Administer "renal dose" dopamine
B) Increase IV fluids to 200 cc/hr, using 5% dextrose/0.45% saline
C) Consult nephrology for hemodialysis
D) Administer hydrochlorothiazide
E) Administer furosemide

Answer 5.6.6 **The correct answer is "E."** The treatment of acute kidney injury due to ATN is largely supportive. In this oliguric patient with signs of volume overload, a trial of a loop diuretic is appropriate. Intravenous furosemide dosed at 40 to 100 mg every 6 to 12 hours is a reasonable way to start. Of note, furosemide will often improve the symptoms of volume overload even if there is no diuresis; it has some direct vasodilating effect which decreases pulmonary artery pressure. "A," dopamine, is not effective in the treatment of ATN (it is not "renal sparing" and does not increase GFR). "B," more fluid, is clearly not indicated in this patient who is already fluid overloaded. Why not dialysis you ask ("C")? Early dialysis in ATN has been associated with greater mortality and increased kidney damage from hypotension, infection, and complement activation in the kidney. "D," hydrochlorothiazide, is also a diuretic but less effective than furosemide in the setting of a low GFR.

 HELPFUL TIP:
While traditionally taught, trying to "convert" oliguric to nonoliguric renal failure (by flogging the kidneys with diuretics) is not helpful and is possibly harmful. There is a trend toward greater mortality in patients who are treated this way. There's more: loop diuretics can cause deafness (eh?), vertigo, and tinnitus. Remember, it doesn't help to flog a dead horse or ailing kidneys. Why did we think it worked in the past? Probably the people who were able to produce urine in response to diuretics were less sick to begin with.

Your patient has very little response to furosemide, but you match her input and output and she has enough insensible loss to resolve her rales. She begins to eat, and you monitor her fluid intake carefully. You match her fluid intake with output, giving normal saline to match her urine output and suspected insensible losses. You treat her hyperkalemia with sodium polystyrene sulfonate *without sorbitol* (Kayexalate), which is effective. Her BUN and creatinine continue to rise over the next 2 days and reach 60 and 4 mg/dL, respectively. The plasma HCO_3 is 18 mEq/L.

Question 5.6.7 You now recommend:
A) Hemodialysis
B) Sodium bicarbonate
C) Strict protein restriction
D) Continuing to match intake and output
E) All of the above

Answer 5.6.7 **The correct answer is "D."** At this point, there is no reason to change your therapeutic approach. In particular, hemodialysis is not necessary. Indications for hemodialysis in this patient might include symptomatic uremia (e.g., coma, pericarditis), severe hyperkalemia or acidosis unresponsive to other therapies, and complications of volume overload (e.g., pulmonary edema). **Dialysis ("A") is actually associated with worse outcomes and prolonged renal disease (complement fixation in the kidney produces additional injury, episodic hypotension from dialysis increases kidney injury).** Sodium bicarbonate ("B") is used orally in patients with significant chronic acidosis in end-stage renal disease, but many patients can tolerate the temporary mild acidosis associated with acute kidney injury. Dramatic protein restriction ("C") will probably lower BUN but this should not be your primary goal. Your patient is recovering from surgery and was probably septic. She requires good nutrition to continue to heal.

> **HELPFUL TIP:**
> Acute kidney injury due to ATN typically lasts 7 to 21 days, with renal function returning as the tubular cells regenerate. However, the course is highly variable and depends on the patient's general health and the length and degree of the initial injury.

Question 5.6.8 In patients with acute tubular necrosis, the most common cause of death is:
A) Hemorrhage
B) Adverse event of hemodialysis
C) Infection
D) Transfusion reaction
E) Heart failure secondary to fluid overload

Answer 5.6.8 **The correct answer is "C."** In patients with ATN who die, infection is the usual culprit. Unfortunately, serious infection resulting in sepsis is one of the most common causes of ATN. It's the circle of life . . . or death, in this instance.

Ten days after her surgery, your patient's urine output increases markedly. Her BUN and creatinine return to their premorbid levels. The National Kidney Foundation makes you an honorary nephrologist and awards you the Bronze Nephron.

▶ **Objectives: Did you learn to …**
· Evaluate a hospitalized patient for acute kidney injury?
· Use urine studies, including urine sodium and FENa, to assist in the diagnosis of acute kidney injury?
· Identify acute tubular necrosis?
· Describe common causes of acute tubular necrosis, its treatment, and its prognosis?

▶ CASE 5.7

While on call, you admit a 75-year-old female for confusion. One month ago, she started hydrochlorothiazide (HCTZ) for hypertension. Her medications include HCTZ 25 mg daily, levothyroxine 125 mcg daily, aspirin 81 mg daily, sertraline (Zoloft) 50 mg daily, and atorvastatin (Lipitor) 40 mg daily. She has a 50-pack-year history of tobacco use and continues to smoke.

On examination, you find an irritable and confused female in no acute distress. Her admission vitals are BP 100/60 mmHg, P 120 bpm, RR 12 breaths/minute, T 36.1°C, weight 50 kg. Her oral mucosa is dry and she has poor skin turgor. She has clear lungs, an S4 on heart examination, and no edema. Her neurological examination is nonfocal.

Laboratory results: Na 110 mEq/L (135–145 mEq/L), K 3.0 mEq/L (3.5–5.0 mEq/L), Cl 70 mEq/L (98–107 mEq/L), HCO_3 33 mEq/L (23–29 mEq/L), BUN 30 mg/dL (5–20 mg/dL), Cr 1.0 mg/dL (0.6–1.2 mg/dL), glucose 110 mg/dL. Plasma osmolality 220 mOsm/L (270–299 mOsm/L).

Question 5.7.1 Which of the following statements is true regarding the etiology of her hyponatremia?
A) She has pseudohyponatremia
B) She has isovolemic hyponatremia
C) She has hypovolemic hyponatremia
D) She has hypervolemic hyponatremia

Answer 5.7.1 **The correct answer is "C."** The definition of hyponatremia is a plasma sodium concentration below 135 mEq/L. The evaluation of hyponatremia begins with the determination of the validity of the plasma sodium measurement. First question: is this pseudohyponatremia ("A")? Look at the measured serum osmolality. If it is low (as it is here), the patient does not have pseudohyponatremia. Pseudohyponatremia is caused by either hyperlipidemia or hyperproteinemia decreasing the water content of plasma. This distinction was more important in the past; newer laboratory techniques compensate for pseudohyponatremia.

Hyperglycemia and severe uremia can cause hyponatremia. In an instance where a patient's measured sodium concentration is hyponatremic and his glucose is 800 mg/dL, the measured serum osmolality may be **normal or elevated** (due to the elevated glucose, which "counts" as osmoles) and should be compared to the calculated osmolality using the equation:

$$\text{Osmolality} = 2(\text{sodium}) + \text{glucose}/18 + (\text{BUN}/2.8)$$

If the calculated osmolality approximates the measured osmolality, then much of the "hyponatremia" will autocorrect when the hyperglycemia is corrected. Therefore, you would not want to aggressively correct the serum sodium concentration without consideration of the patient's hyperglycemia. When in doubt, frequent sodium monitoring is advisable.

The next step in the evaluation of hyponatremia is to determine the patient's volume status. This patient has no signs of volume overload, such as edema or crackles, making hypervolemia ("D") less likely. She is tachycardic with a low blood pressure, dry mucous membranes, and a BUN/Cr ratio greater than 20, suggesting she is hypovolemic. Most likely, she has a hypovolemic hyponatremia.

HELPFUL TIP:
Always consider "beer potomania" (one of our favorite disease names . . . not to mention one of our favorite food groups). Here is what happens: too much beer (or any alcohol) plus too little solute equal poor free water excretion and hyponatremia.

Question 5.7.2 **What further information will help you narrow the differential diagnosis of hyponatremia in this patient?**
A) FENa
B) Urine osmolality and urine sodium concentration
C) Urine creatinine concentration
D) Urine potassium and calcium concentration

Answer 5.7.2 **The correct answer is "B."** Urine osmolality can be used to distinguish between impaired water excretion caused by SIADH (syndrome of inappropriate secretion of antidiuretic hormone), and pathologic water intake (polydipsia). In SIADH, the urine will be inappropriately concentrated with urine osmoles of >100 mosmol/kg (the patient is unable to retain sodium). FENa ("A") is discussed earlier; although the word "sodium" is in it, FENa is not helpful for discovering the etiology of hyponatremia. Concentration of potassium and calcium ("D") is not likely to add any useful information.

You order urine studies. Urinalysis: specific gravity 1.025, pH 5.0, trace protein, 0 to 1 RBC/hpf, 0 to 1 WBC/hpf, otherwise negative. Spot urine Na 70 mEq/L (elevated) and urine osmolality = 700 mmol/kg (elevated).

Question 5.7.3 **Given the patient's history, urine studies, and hypovolemic status, what is the most likely diagnosis?**
A) Syndrome of inappropriate secretion of antidiuretic hormone (SIADH)
B) Heart failure (HF)
C) Diuretic-induced hyponatremia
D) Hyponatremia due to reset osmostat
E) Potato chip deficiency (hypopringlism)

Answer 5.7.3 **The correct answer is "C."** In order to be useful in the diagnosis of hyponatremia, urine studies must be viewed in the context of volume status, plasma osmolality, and electrolyte levels. This patient's laboratory results are consistent with SIADH. However, patients with SIADH should be euvolemic or slightly hypervolemic. In fact, if a patient is hypovolemic, ADH levels should be appropriately elevated. Thus, her laboratory results and clinical picture are most consistent with diuretic-induced hyponatremia. Note that she also has a chloride-depletion alkalosis (formerly called contraction alkalosis).

The appropriate response of the kidney to hypoosmolality is to make maximally dilute urine (retain sodium to correct the hypoosmolality). Thus, the urine should have a specific gravity less than 1.005 and osmolality less than 100 mmol/kg.

Inappropriately concentrated urine (osmolality >100 mmol/kg) occurs when there is limited excretion of fluid and may be observed in SIADH, HF, cirrhosis, and renal failure. This is also reflected in the urine sodium. If the kidneys respond to hyponatremia as expected, urine sodium concentration should be low, typically less than 20 mmol/L and often less than 10 mmol/L. In the setting of hypovolemia, if the urine sodium concentration is inappropriately high, something is inappropriately spurring the kidney to excrete sodium (e.g., diuretic use, hypoaldosteronism). In this patient, the elevated urine sodium is likely due to the diuretic. Diuretic use is the most common cause of hypovolemic hypoosmolality, and thiazides are more commonly associated with hyponatremia than are loop diuretics (furosemide, etc.). Your patient is hypovolemic and hyponatremic, with a high urine sodium concentration and the history of diuretic use: most likely, her hyponatremia is diuretic induced.

"D," a reset osmostat, requires special mention. A reset osmostat, which is responsible for 20% to 30% of hyponatremia, occurs when the patient's body "adapts" to hyponatremia and "gives up" trying to correct the problem: the kidneys just throw in the towel. Patients with a reset osmostat will present like SIADH (hyponatremia, euvolemia or slight hypervolemia, and inappropriately concentrated urine) but will be resistant to treatment. If a patient with apparent SIADH does not respond to the usual treatment, consider a reset osmostat. Patients with a reset osmostat generally have mild hyponatremia (125–130 mg/dL). Newer research suggests that these patients have higher rates of morbidity and mortality, and correction of their sodium levels is often very difficult.

HELPFUL TIP:
When you encounter a patient with hyponatremic hypoosmolality, also look at the plasma potassium concentration. Diuretic use is a common cause of hyponatremia, hypokalemia, hypochloremia, and hypoosmolality occurring simultaneously.

Question 5.7.4 **In addition to discontinuing her diuretic, which of the following approaches is the best initial therapy for her hyponatremia?**
A) Saline 0.9% 1 L bolus followed by 150 cc/hr
B) Fluid restriction to 1,500 cc/day
C) Saline 3% 100 cc/hr for 24 hours

D) Furosemide 20 mg IV

E) A large bag of potato chips with a tomato juice chaser

Answer 5.7.4 The correct answer is "A." This patient is hypotensive and tachycardic and thus needs volume somewhat quickly to address her abnormal vital signs. If this patient was not hemodynamically compromised, you could forgo the fluid bolus. Excessively rapid correction of hyponatremia may lead to osmotic demyelination syndrome (formerly called central pontine myelinolysis).

Sodium concentrations less than 120 mEq/L are considered severe hyponatremia. Patients with acute, severe hyponatremia are almost always symptomatic as a result of the low sodium. By definition, acute hyponatremia has been present for 48 hours or less and chronic hyponatremia for more than 48 hours. As previously discussed, your patient's hyponatremia is due to a diuretic, which she started 1 month ago. Therefore, her hyponatremia is more likely to be chronic.

As a general rule, hypovolemic hyponatremia should be corrected by volume infusion, usually with 0.9% (normal) saline. Fluid restriction ("B"), while good treatment for SIADH, is not appropriate in this patient who is already volume depleted. Likewise, a loop diuretic is not appropriate ("D"). Both "C" and "E" will provide more sodium but will not provide the necessary volume.

Your patient has chronic hyponatremia, which needs to be corrected more slowly than acute hyponatremia. Chronic hyponatremia should be corrected no faster than 0.5 mEq/hr or 10 to 12 mEq/day. For significantly symptomatic patients with acute hyponatremia, sodium can be corrected more quickly.

In order to determine how quickly sodium concentrations will rise, you must know the concentrations of the solution being infused and the patient's plasma sodium. A liter of saline will affect the serum sodium by the following calculation:

$$Na \text{ increase} = (solution\ Na - plasma\ Na) / (total\ body\ water + 1)$$

$$Patient's\ Na = 110\ mEq/L$$

$$Na\ in\ 3\%\ saline = 513\ mEq/L$$

$$Na\ in\ 0.9\%\ saline = 154\ mEq/L$$

$$Total\ body\ water = weight\ (kg) \times 0.5\ (females)\ or\ 0.6\ (males)$$

When using 3% saline solution, 1 L will increase the plasma sodium as follows:

$$Na \text{ increase} = (513 - 110) / [(50 \times 0.5) + 1]$$

$$= 15.5\ mEq/l$$

At 100 cc/hr, the plasma sodium will increase at a rate of 1.55 mEq/hr.

This correction is too rapid for chronic hyponatremia.

When using normal saline (0.9%), 1 L will increase the plasma sodium as follows:

$$Na \text{ increase} = (154 - 110) / [(50 \times 0.5) + 1]$$

$$= 1.7\ mEq/L$$

Therefore, it is expected that 1 L of normal saline will increase the plasma sodium by 1.7 mEq initially, and 150 cc/hr will increase the plasma sodium by 0.25 mEq/hr, well within the safe range.

HELPFUL TIP:
Whenever correcting sodium, whether with moderate-to-severe hyponatremia or hypernatremia, check serum sodium concentrations frequently—every 2 to 4 hours is reasonable in the initial treatment period.

Question 5.7.5 In addition to HCTZ, which medication should you discontinue because of its potential role in hyponatremia in this patient?

A) Aspirin

B) Atorvastatin

C) Levothyroxine

D) Sertraline

Answer 5.7.5 The correct answer is "D." Serotonin reuptake inhibitors (SSRIs) and tricyclic antidepressants, among other medications, can stimulate the release of ADH from the pituitary gland, ultimately causing hyponatremia with an SIADH-type presentation. The association between SSRIs and hyponatremia is strong enough to consider measuring plasma sodium levels in elderly patients before and after starting an SSRI. The other medications are not associated with hyponatremia to any significant degree.

Your patient does well, recovers from her hyponatremia, and is discharged. In place of HCTZ, you start an ACE inhibitor for hypertension. You next see her a few months later when she starts to have problems with mild confusion. Her family reports that she is definitely not taking any diuretics. Her vitals are normal. Clinically, she appears euvolemic, and her examination is nonfocal. Her plasma sodium is 120 mEq/L, creatinine 1.1 mg/dL, plasma osmolality 240 mmol/kg, and urine osmolality 320 mmol/kg. Urinalysis shows specific gravity of 1.030 but is normal otherwise.

Question 5.7.6 In addition to the laboratory tests already available to you, which of the following laboratory tests should be done in patients with hyponatremia?

A) CBC

B) ESR

C) TSH

D) Liver enzymes

E) ADH

Answer 5.7.6 The correct answer is "C." Hyponatremia with hypoosmolality and a normal volume status is often the result of SIADH. However, SIADH is a diagnosis of exclusion. Both hypothyroidism and glucocorticoid deficiency present with similar features and should be ruled out. Hypothyroidism is more common, and at a minimum you must check TSH. Of special note is option "E." Most of the time, ADH levels are not helpful in the diagnosis of SIADH because up to 20% of patients with diagnosable SIADH do not have elevated plasma ADH levels. In fact you may see the designation change from SIADH to SIAD (syndrome of inappropriate diuresis) depending on what you are reading. SIADH is diagnosed on clinical grounds, with characteristic laboratory data, and lack of a better explanation.

HELPFUL TIP:
In any given patient with hyponatremia, what makes SIADH likely? All of the following data are used to support the diagnosis of SIADH: decreased plasma osmolality; inappropriately concentrated urine (e.g., a urine osmolality of >100 mosmol/kg); clinical euvolemia or mild hypervolemia; elevated urine sodium excretion (urine sodium >20 mEq/L); and the absence of diuretic use, hypothyroidism, and adrenal dysfunction.

You order a number of laboratory tests, including TSH, CBC, and electrolytes. In addition to the laboratory tests mentioned above, abnormal tests include plasma Cl 90 mEq/L (low), urine Na 50 mEq/L (high) (and urine osmoles, as noted above, are 320 mmol/kg). Thyroid function tests are normal. You diagnose SIADH.

Question 5.7.7 As initial treatment, you prescribe:
A) Demeclocycline
B) Lithium
C) Saline 0.9% bolus
D) Furosemide
E) Water restriction

Answer 5.7.7 **The correct answer is "E."** The laboratory results and clinical picture are consistent with SIADH (euvolemia, elevated urine sodium excretion, elevated urine osmolarity). Water restriction is the mainstay of therapy in SIADH. Free water should be restricted to 1 to 2 L/day. Demeclocycline ("A") and lithium ("B") interfere with the activity of ADH at the collecting tubules, but these drugs are reserved for SIADH patients with severe hyponatremia unresponsive to first- and second-line treatments. Saline infusion ("C") corrects hypovolemic hyponatremia. Furosemide ("D") is used in hypervolemic hyponatremia (e.g., CHF, renal insufficiency) and sometimes in more severe cases of SIADH in order to promote more dilute urine.

Question 5.7.8 The patient fails water restriction. The *next* step in the treatment of this patient is:
A) Demeclocycline
B) Lithium
C) Sodium chloride tablets
D) IV urea
E) None of the above

Answer 5.7.8 **The correct answer is "C."** Increasing salt intake and adding a loop diuretic are other ways to treat SIADH in patients who cannot or will not maintain fluid restriction. The aggressiveness of the intervention will depend on patient-specific factors, including symptoms and comorbidities. In an outpatient who is minimally symptomatic or asymptomatic, oral salt supplementation is most reasonable. IV urea ("D"), which

causes an osmotic diuresis, could be considered as the next step after sodium chloride tablets. Demeclocycline and lithium should be reserved for patients who fail the other treatments. In more severe hyponatremia and those with significant symptoms, admission for more aggressive therapy may be warranted.

HELPFUL TIP:
Conivaptan (Vaprisol®) and tolvaptan (Samsca®) both are ADH antagonists that can be used for SIADH. They are third-line agents. Potential problems include exacerbations of heart failure, orthostatic hypotension, and hypokalemia. *They must be started in the hospital because of the potential side effects and rapid serum sodium changes.*

▶ **Objectives: Did you learn to ...**
· Generate a differential diagnosis for hyponatremia?
· Identify medications that are commonly associated with hyponatremia?
· Use urine osmolality to identify impaired renal water handling?
· Calculate sodium correction using different concentrations of saline?
· Diagnose, evaluate, and treat a patient with SIADH?

▶ **CASE 5.8**

A 65-year-old male with a new diagnosis of heart failure returns to your office after starting several new medications within the last month. A cardiologist at Ivory Tower Academic Medical Center 100 miles away started these medications but never sent a note, and neither you nor your patient knows what drugs he's taking ("Well, there's a little white one and a pink one and . . ."). Over that same time period, he states that he has felt "worse than I did after my heart attack." At first he was just fatigued, but in the last few days, he has developed nausea, vomiting, and body aches.

On examination, his vitals are T 37.1°C, P 70 bpm, RR 8 breaths/minute, BP 100/58 mm Hg. He has trace pedal edema. His lungs are clear, and his abdomen is diffusely tender. When you stand him up to check his blood pressure, he loses consciousness but quickly recovers when placed supine (fortunately, you are strong and possess quick reflexes and caught him on the way down).

Your nurse draws blood, starts an IV, and obtains a venous blood gas on room air. VBG: pH 7.52, $PaCO_2$ 49 mm Hg, PaO_2 40 mm Hg, and HCO_3 39 mEq/L. His oxygen saturation on monitor is 95%.

Question 5.8.1 The blood gas is consistent with the diagnosis of:
A) Metabolic alkalosis with respiratory compensation
B) Respiratory alkalosis with metabolic compensation
C) Mixed metabolic/respiratory alkalosis
D) Mixed metabolic alkalosis and respiratory acidosis

Answer 5.8.1 The correct answer is "A." Your patient appears to have a pure metabolic alkalosis with respiratory compensation. His pH is above the upper limit of normal (range 7.35–7.45), and his plasma bicarbonate is elevated as well. In metabolic alkalosis, you can expect the $PaCO_2$ to rise in proportion to the rise in HCO_3. $PaCO_2$ should increase by 0.5 to 0.75 times the increase in HCO_3 from baseline (about 24 mEq/L). In this case, the HCO_3 has increased by 15 (39 – 24 = 15), and the $PaCO_2$ has appropriately increased by 9 (9/15 = 0.6). And remember, you cannot overcorrect your pH (although it is quite possible simultaneously to have two processes—an acidosis and an alkalosis resulting in a normal pH). Thus, the primary process has to be an alkalosis.

Question 5.8.2 Which of the following urine tests will aid in determining the cause of this patient's metabolic alkalosis?
A) Urine sodium
B) Urine potassium
C) Urine chloride
D) Urine bicarbonate
E) Urine creatinine

Answer 5.8.2 The correct answer is "C." You can approach the differential diagnosis of metabolic alkalosis by measuring the urine chloride (see next question). The other urine studies are less useful in metabolic alkalosis. Of course, an appropriate history and physical as well as plasma tests are required to determine the correct diagnosis and treatment.

You have admitted the patient and are on your way to the hospital to see him when the laboratory tests return (you aren't driving and talking on the phone at the same time, are you?). Plasma studies: Na 140 mEq/L (135–145 mEq/L), K 2.5 mEq/L (3.5–5.0 mEq/L), Cl 102 mEq/L (98–107 mEq/L), BUN 18 mg/dL (5–20 mg/dL), creatinine 0.9 mg/dL (0.6–1.2 mg/dL), Ca 9.5 mg/dL (8.5–10.5 mg/dL), Mg 1.4 mg/dL (1.7–2.2 mg/dL).

Urine studies: specific gravity 1.025, chloride 45 mEq/L (elevated).

Question 5.8.3 Of the following choices, which is NOT likely to contribute to metabolic alkalosis in this patient?
A) Corticosteroids
B) Diuretics
C) Hypokalemia
D) Vomiting

Answer 5.8.3 The correct answer is "D." This makes intuitive sense. If there is vomiting (or NG suctioning), the patient will have low plasma chloride and thus will have little in the urine, where it is being reabsorbed. All of the rest of the answers will cause an **elevated** urine chloride and thus are consistent with this patient's picture. With mineralocorticoid excess (aldosterone or extrinsic corticosteroids), "A," one excretes potassium, causing hypokalemia. Hypokalemia prevents the kidneys from optimally reabsorbing chloride ("C"). See Table 5-9 for more on causes of metabolic alkalosis.

TABLE 5-9 CAUSES OF METABOLIC ALKALOSIS DIVIDED BY URINE CHLORIDE LEVELS

Low Urine Chloride (<25 mEq/L)	High Urine Chloride (>40 mEq/L)
Vomiting	Hypokalemia (severe)
Nasogastric suctioning	Diuretics (loop or thiazide; early effect)
Factitious diarrhea (laxative abuse)	Alkali load
Cystic fibrosis	Bartter/Gitelman syndromes
Low chloride intake	Primary mineralocorticoid excess (hyperaldosteronism, corticosteroids)
Posthypercapnia	
Diuretics (loop or thiazide; late effect)	

It only took your nurse 40 minutes, but now you have the cardiologist's notes and the medication list. Your patient started taking atorvastatin, captopril, furosemide, isosorbide dinitrate, aspirin, and metoprolol in the last month—and you are not surprised he has orthostatic hypotension.

Question 5.8.4 All of the following are appropriate interventions in this patient EXCEPT:
A) Discontinue furosemide
B) Administer potassium chloride
C) Administer hydrochloric acid through an NG tube
D) Infuse normal (0.9%) saline
E) Administer ranitidine

Answer 5.8.4 The correct answer is "C." Chloride-responsive metabolic alkalosis is usually secondary to volume contraction. Your patient has renal salt and water losses due to a diuretic and has gastrointestinal volume losses due to emesis. Physical examination (except trace edema—but remember that he has heart failure) and laboratory findings support hypovolemia. The diuretic should be discontinued and volume should be replaced. An isotonic solution, such as normal saline, is an appropriate choice. However, you must monitor your patient's volume status closely due to his heart failure. Because his potassium is low, he requires KCl. An H_2-blocker, like ranitidine, is a good choice for a patient with alkalosis and gastrointestinal illness: it will reduce acid secretion in the stomach (and thus further acid loss) and may offer some symptomatic relief as well.

Hydrochloric acid is an option in severe metabolic alkalosis unresponsive to other therapies. However, it is not given by NG tube. HCl is very corrosive and should only be infused centrally.

Question 5.8.5 Your patient is not responding to the KCl you are administering. You give which of the following electrolytes to aid in repleting his potassium stores?
A) Sodium
B) Bicarbonate

C) Calcium
D) Phosphate
E) Magnesium

Answer 5.8.5 The correct answer is "E." Give magnesium before giving more potassium. Recall that his plasma magnesium level was slightly low at 1.7 mg/dL. Even if a patient's magnesium is only slightly low or even low-normal, continued hypokalemia in the face of KCl repletion may indicate whole-body magnesium depletion. Serum magnesium levels may not accurately reflect whole-body magnesium stores, especially in patients with heart failure. Furosemide causes further magnesium wasting. None of the other electrolytes listed earlier is as important to potassium repletion.

With correction of fluid and electrolyte status, your patient recovers quickly. You try to convey to the cardiologist the importance of good communication. However, as noted by George Bernard Shaw, "The single biggest problem in communication is the illusion that it has taken place."

▶ **Objectives: Did you learn to …**
- Identify metabolic alkalosis?
- Utilize urine chloride in the evaluation of metabolic alkalosis?
- Recognize various causes of metabolic alkalosis?
- Recognize the role of hypomagnesemia in treating hypokalemia?

 QUICK QUIZ: HEMATURIA

A 25-year-old male medical student presents with blood in his urine. When asked further about this finding, he admits that he was using urine dipsticks at home to check his urine. (Did you know that 20% of medical students meet the criteria for somatization disorder—now known as "somatic symptom disorder" in DSM V—at some time during medical school? It's true.) He has no gross hematuria, just 1+ blood on his urine self-test. He has no symptoms otherwise. His major concern is that his father had a renal transplant at age 30 for Alport syndrome.

Given that his father had Alport syndrome, what is the probability that this student has it?
A) Certain (100% chance)
B) One in two
C) One in four
D) Less than 1 in 20

The correct answer is "D." Alport syndrome, also known as hereditary nephritis, typically presents with microscopic hematuria and progresses to complete renal failure. Alport syndrome has a heterogeneous inheritance pattern: 80% of cases are due to X-linked disease, about 15% are autosomal recessive, and about 5% are autosomal dominant. Since most cases are X-linked, males are affected more severely and earlier than females. If

your medical student's father had Alport syndrome, it was most likely X-linked, and the patient could not possibly have inherited it. However, there is a 5% chance that the father had autosomal-dominant disease and then a 50% chance that the trait was passed on to the patient; therefore, "D" is correct.

▶ **CASE 5.9**

A 33-year-old male presents to the ED complaining of shortness of breath and cough of 10 days duration. He now sleeps in a chair due to orthopnea. He has severe fatigue and a mild, diffuse headache. Four days ago, he was seen in an urgent care clinic and diagnosed with bronchitis. He reports no medical problems or surgeries. He quit smoking 1 year ago and denies alcohol and drug use. He has a strong family history of hypertension. The review of systems is otherwise negative.

On physical examination, his vitals are T 36.8°C, P 104 bpm, RR 16 breaths/minute, and BP 200/118 mm Hg. There are bibasilar crackles with dullness to percussion at the lung bases. The heart, abdomen, and extremities are otherwise unremarkable.

His chest x-ray shows cardiomegaly, cephalization of lung markings, and bilateral small pleural effusions. An ECG shows sinus tachycardia with left atrial enlargement and left ventricular hypertrophy. Laboratory results: troponin-T negative, hemoglobin 9.1 g/dL (low), WBC count and platelets normal, Na 136 mEq/L, K 4.4 mEq/L, Cl 96 mEq/L, HCO_3 19 mEq/L (low), BUN 108 mg/dL (high), Cr 11.9 mg/dL (high), glucose 104 mg/dL, calcium 7.8 mg/dL (low), albumin 4 g/dL (normal).

Question 5.9.1 Which of the following is the most appropriate next step?
A) Prescribe levofloxacin and discharge patient with follow-up the next day
B) Prescribe furosemide and discharge patient with follow-up the next day
C) Administer a bolus of normal saline intravenously and admit the patient
D) Administer furosemide intravenously and admit the patient
E) Perform thoracentesis for diagnostic purposes

Answer 5.9.1 The correct answer is "D." The proper disposition of this patient is the hospital. His uremia is quite severe, and he is symptomatic from his renal failure. He needs further diagnostic tests and requires further monitoring. He has signs and symptoms of volume overload, and he may yet respond to loop diuretics. A trial of IV furosemide is reasonable. Even if it doesn't cause a diuresis, furosemide can decrease pulmonary capillary wedge pressure. The initial diagnosis of bronchitis was most likely erroneous and switching to another antibiotic ("A") will only perpetuate that error. As he is volume overloaded, you certainly do not want to administer more volume ("C"). If you are willing to attribute his pleural effusions to volume overload due to kidney failure, a thoracentesis ("E") is not necessary.

Question 5.9.2 The patient's ECG is normal. How should the low calcium be approached in the ED?
A) Administer calcium gluconate intravenously
B) Obtain a serum parathyroid hormone level
C) Monitor for signs and symptoms of hypocalcemia
D) Obtain an ionized calcium level

Answer 5.9.2 The correct answer is "C." Currently, your patient does not have signs and symptoms of hypocalcemia; therefore, he does not need IV calcium replacement in the ED ("A"). He should be observed for the development of signs and symptoms. Symptoms are mostly neurological—generalized seizures, perioral paresthesias, and carpopedal spasms. The two best-known signs of hypocalcemia are Chvostek and Trousseau signs. Chvostek sign is present if a grimace occurs in response to tapping the facial nerve. Trousseau sign is evoked by inflating a blood pressure cuff above the systolic pressure for 3 minutes and observing for hand spasms.

Since you expect that the patient's hypocalcemia is secondary to renal disease and hyperphosphatemia and you will treat him symptomatically, serum PTH level ("B") is not required. It is not necessary to measure ionized calcium ("D"). Since you have access to both the total serum calcium level and the serum albumin, you can calculate the corrected calcium. In addition, no correction is required since the albumin level is normal.

> **HELPFUL TIP:**
> If the patient does not respond to furosemide, IV nitroglycerin will likely be successful at reducing this patient's pulmonary edema by decreasing preload and afterload.

Your patient is admitted. Initially, his urine output increases slightly with loop diuretics, but then he becomes oliguric. You ask for a nephrology consult to assist in management of this case. The nephrologist plans to place an IV catheter for dialysis and is considering a renal biopsy. If the patient develops bleeding with these procedures, hemostasis may be impaired because of his uremia.

Question 5.9.3 Which of the following treatments is LEAST likely to reduce the risk of bleeding in this patient?
A) Hemodialysis
B) DDAVP
C) Cryoprecipitate
D) Platelet transfusion
E) Conjugated estrogens

Answer 5.9.3 The correct answer is "D." The cause of bleeding dysfunction in uremia appears to be the effect of uremic toxins on platelet function. Giving a uremic patient more platelets—especially when there is no thrombocytopenia—will not improve the situation, as the platelet dysfunction due to uremia will occur with the new platelets as well. "A," hemodialysis, will remove toxins related to uremia, improving platelet function. "B," DDAVP, is often the first-line treatment in a bleeding patient with uremia. DDAVP is not generally toxic and quickly reduces bleeding time. It acts by causing the release of factor VIII:vWF multimers from endothelial storage sites. Unfortunately, patients rapidly develop tachyphylaxis to DDAVP; once the multimers are depleted from the endothelial cells, DDAVP will not work until these multimers are replaced (usually a process of several days). "C," cryoprecipitate, enhances platelet aggregation and will reduce bleeding time for about 24 hours after administration. Estrogen is another option for renal failure–related bleeding and has been used for short durations and seems to be effective and well tolerated.

Question 5.9.4 In order to reduce the risk of renal osteodystrophy (elevated serum parathyroid hormone with mobilization of calcium from bone), which of the following medications will you prescribe initially?
A) Calcium carbonate
B) Aluminum hydroxide
C) Magnesium hydroxide
D) Sevelamer (Renagel®)
E) Vitamin D

Answer 5.9.4 The correct answer is "A." Renal osteodystrophy occurs when parathyroid hormone levels are elevated and bone is mobilized. This occurs because patients with renal failure cannot clear phosphate. The body tries to compensate by increasing parathyroid hormone secretion, which reduces phosphate and increases serum calcium. However, it also is detrimental to bone and leads to demineralization.

Gastrointestinal binding of phosphate requires large doses of a cation such as calcium (2 g/day). Calcium carbonate is associated with the least potential toxicity; therefore, it is the initial choice for treating hyperphosphatemia to reduce the risk of renal osteodystrophy. Also, you may consider calcium acetate, which is as safe as calcium carbonate and is a more potent phosphate binder but more expensive. Avoid aluminum and magnesium products ("B" and "C") in renal failure as these ions accumulate and can cause toxicity.

Sevelamer ("D") is a cationic polymer that binds phosphate in the gastrointestinal tract and avoids the problems that can occur with the calcium, magnesium, and aluminum compounds. It is expensive so calcium products should be tried first in the setting of hypocalcemia. Newer studies suggest that Sevelamer may have better cardiovascular outcomes, so practices may change in the near future.

Patients with chronic renal failure or end-stage renal disease on dialysis should also receive vitamin D ("E"). However, vitamin D causes **increased** gastrointestinal absorption of phosphate, so it should be given only after hyperphosphatemia has been controlled.

> **HELPFUL TIP:**
> Whenever prescribing calcium for renal osteodystrophy, have patients take it with meals—otherwise it will not bind phosphate. Also, calcium is absorbed better when taken with food.

HELPFUL TIP:
Cinacalcet (Sensipar®) is another option for treating renal osteodystrophy. By mimicking calcium in the parathyroid, it "fools" the parathyroid into thinking that the serum calcium is normal and thus reduces the output of parathyroid hormone. It sounds cool, but there's a price for being cool—in this case several thousand dollars per month (in 2018). There are several other new phosphate binders including ferric citrate (Auryxia®), which also increases serum iron levels, and lanthanum carbonate (Fosrenol®), which requires fewer pills than other options, but must be chewed completely (making it a less attractive option for your patients without teeth). Both of these are relatively expensive (approximately $800/month).

▶ **Objective: Did you learn to ...**
- Anticipate complications of renal failure, including hypervolemia, hypocalcemia, platelet dysfunction, and renal osteodystrophy?

▶ CASE 5.10

A 10-year-old male presents with his mother, who appears very anxious. She reports several episodes of red-brown urine this morning. The patient reports feeling a bit tired, but otherwise has no complaints. His past medical history is unremarkable and he takes no medications. On review of systems, he reports about 10 days of a sore throat that completely resolved a few days ago.

On examination, you find a pleasant young male in no acute distress. He is afebrile. His blood pressure is 140/94 mm Hg, and he has trace pretibial edema. The remainder of the examination is unrevealing.

Question 5.10.1 All of the following tests are likely to be helpful in the workup of this patient EXCEPT:
A) Urinalysis
B) Abdominal X-ray
C) CBC
D) Plasma electrolytes
E) BUN and creatinine

Answer 5.10.1 The correct answer is "B." Abdominal plain films are not useful in almost any situation unless looking for bowel obstruction. X-ray is not indicated and can be misleading in constipation. (What did you say? Free air? An upright chest is the most sensitive film for free air—save for CT.) If this patient had a presentation consistent with urolithiasis, an abdominal CT scan may be indicated, although an ultrasound would be the preferred first study for urolithiasis in most patients. All of the other laboratory tests should be ordered.

Urinalysis shows 2+ blood, 2+ protein, specific gravity 1.015, and numerous red blood cells with red cell casts. BUN is 35 mg/dL and creatinine is 1.8 mg/dL. CBC, coagulation studies, and electrolytes are pending.

Question 5.10.2 At this point, all of the following should be considered in the differential diagnosis EXCEPT:
A) Minimal change disease
B) Henoch–Schönlein purpura
C) Post-streptococcal glomerulonephritis
D) IgA nephropathy
E) Membranoproliferative glomerulonephritis

Answer 5.10.2 The correct answer is "A." Minimal change disease usually presents with clinical signs and symptoms of nephrotic syndrome and not gross hematuria. All of the other diseases are associated with hematuria, either microscopic or gross. Henoch–Schönlein purpura, post-streptococcal glomerulonephritis, IgA nephropathy, and membranoproliferative glomerulonephritis all have more "nephritic" features with "active" urinary sediments (dysmorphic red cells, red cell casts, white cells, and protein in the urine). These diseases also have a similar pathologic process in which immune complexes deposit in the glomeruli, resulting in glomerulonephritis.

CBC, coagulation studies, and electrolytes are all normal. You are suspicious that he may have had streptococcal pharyngitis that was unrecognized.

Question 5.10.3 Which of the following statements best describes the usual course of post-streptococcal glomerulonephritis?
A) Most patients progress to renal failure
B) After resolution of the initial episode, recurrent episodes of gross hematuria are common
C) In most cases, hypertension and uremia subside within 1 to 2 weeks after onset.
D) In most cases, hypertension is persistent and requires treatment
E) Adults tend to recover more quickly than children

Answer 5.10.3 The correct answer is "C." Post-streptococcal glomerulonephritis, characterized by immune complex deposition in the glomeruli, is a self-limited disease in most patients. There is a latent period, averaging 10 days, between pharyngitis and the development of hematuria. Recovery is expected to start within in 1 to 2 weeks. Recurrent episodes of gross hematuria are rare in post-streptococcal glomerulonephritis. Post-streptococcal glomerulonephritis is more common in children and tends to be more severe when it affects adults. Hypertension and uremia resolve relatively quickly, but microscopic hematuria may persist for 6 months.

HELPFUL TIP:
Renal biopsy is rarely indicated in children with nephritic urine and mild renal failure because the differential diagnosis can be narrowed by the clinical presentation and because many of the diseases are self-limited. In more severe cases, renal biopsy may be necessary to diagnose and treat appropriately. See Table 5-10 for a partial list of causes of hematuria in children.

TABLE 5-10 CAUSES OF GROSS HEMATURIA IN CHILDREN

Idiopathic (usually benign with resolution over time)
Urinary tract infection
Trauma
Congenital anomaly
Urethral irritation or trauma
Nephrolithiasis
Sickle cell disease/trait
Coagulopathy
Glomerular disease (e.g., post-streptococcal glomerulonephritis)
Malignancy (e.g., Wilm tumor)
Medications (e.g., hemorrhagic cystitis from cyclophosphamide)

▶ **Objectives: Did you learn to …**
- Evaluate a child with gross hematuria?
- Generate a differential diagnosis for hematuria and proteinuria in a child?
- Describe the usual course of post-streptococcal glomerulonephritis?

▶ CASE 5.11

The parents of a 2-year-old female bring her in to your office for a week-long history of diarrhea. Initially, her stools were loose and watery, but over the last 2 days, they have become bloody. The patient has appeared to have abdominal pain on occasions, and her appetite is depressed. Despite bloody diarrhea, her parents attempted to care for her at home until she became more lethargic (well, that didn't work . . . probably the same parents who refused vaccines). They are also worried about some bruising on her extremities.

Vital signs: T 37.2°C, P 145 bpm, BP 88/47 mm Hg, RR 40 breaths/minute. The patient appears pale, with slight scleral icterus. You note petechiae and purpura on the extremities. Her abdomen is diffusely tender. She responds to commands but appears very lethargic.

While you are arranging her admission to the hospital, some laboratory tests return: Hgb 8 g/dL, Hct 24%, WBC 14,000/mm³, platelets 50,000/mm³, Na 128 mEq/L, K 3.9 mEq/L, HCO₃ 14 mEq/L, BUN 38 mg/dL, creatinine 2.1 mg/dL. The peripheral blood smear shows schistocytes, "Burr" cells, and grossly reduced number of platelets.

Question 5.11.1 Which of the following is the most appropriate initial management of this patient?
A) Intravenous fluids
B) Dialysis
C) Platelet transfusion
D) Corticosteroids
E) Antibiotics

Answer 5.11.1 The correct answer is "A." The proper initial management consists of supportive therapy. This patient has signs of dehydration, which would be expected from the history of prolonged diarrhea. She is hyponatremic, and isotonic (0.9%) saline is the IV fluid of choice. Use 20 cc/kg boluses until her blood pressure stabilizes. This patient may also require an RBC transfusion given her anemia. Although she has had diarrhea, her potassium is currently in the normal range, probably due to decreased glomerular filtration. Given her renal failure, potassium should not be in her IV fluids.

Consideration of dialysis ("B") is premature. A platelet count of 50,000 is adequate for hemostasis, so answer "C" is incorrect. The schistocytes suggest a microangiopathic hemolytic anemia. Steroids are not generally helpful for this, so "D" is incorrect. Finally, antibiotics ("E") may (or may not) be beneficial if the patient has bacterial enteritis, but IV fluids should be administered first.

Question 5.11.2 Based on the available information, which of the following is the most likely diagnosis?
A) Thrombotic thrombocytopenic purpura
B) Hemolytic uremic syndrome
C) Postinfectious glomerulonephritis
D) Henoch–Schönlein purpura
E) Autosomal-recessive polycystic kidney disease

Answer 5.11.2 The correct answer is "B." Hemolytic uremic syndrome (HUS) is the most likely diagnosis. This patient presents with a classic history of uremia, hemolysis, and thrombocytopenia preceded by 5 to 7 days of diarrhea. Patients tend to become oliguric and sometimes anuric.

"A," thrombotic thrombocytopenic purpura (TTP), is related to HUS but is rare in children. The average age of a patient with TTP is 41 years with women making up about 70% of all cases. African-American ancestry is also a risk factor for TTP. In contrast to HUS, patients with TTP may present with the classic pentad: thrombocytopenia, fever, mental status changes, renal insufficiency, and hemolytic anemia. Usually, there is a prodrome viral illness with TTP but diarrhea occurs only rarely. See Chapter 6 for more details.

"C," postinfectious glomerulonephritis, usually occurs after pharyngitis or skin infection with group A beta-hemolytic streptococci. Common symptoms include edema and hematuria but not thrombocytopenia or diarrhea. "D," Henoch–Schönlein purpura (HSP), is a (usually) transient IgA vasculitis following upper respiratory infections in children and adolescents. HSP is not associated with a microangiopathic hemolytic anemia, thrombocytopenia or coagulopathy. Autosomal-recessive polycystic kidney disease ("E") is a rare disorder that presents early in childhood with abdominal masses, hypertension, urinary tract infections, and renal failure but not hemolytic anemia.

HELPFUL TIP:
HUS may occur without diarrhea. This atypical subtype of HUS occurs less frequently, is associated with *Streptococcus* infections or complement deficiencies, and carries a worse prognosis.

Question 5.11.3 **From the blood culture, you expect to find:**
A) *Shigella species*
B) *E. coli*
C) *Streptococcus pneumoniae*
D) *Haemophilus influenzae*
E) None of the above

Answer 5.11.3 **The correct answer is "E."** Although HUS is the result of bacterial enteritis, patients are not bacteremic. Instead, the endothelial damage and hemolysis are caused by Shiga toxin, released from *E. coli* or *Shigella dysenteriae*.

Question 5.11.4 **All of the following are true regarding Shiga toxin HUS in children EXCEPT:**
A) If dialysis is needed, renal function rarely returns
B) Half or more of the cases occur in the summer months
C) Ingestion of contaminated meat is a common source of *E. coli* O157:H7 infection
D) Cattle are the main vectors of *E. coli* O157:H7
E) Antibiotics do not reduce the risk of HUS in patients with confirmed *E. coli* O157:H7 infections

Answer 5.11.4 **The correct answer is "A."** All the other statements are true. The prognosis of Shiga toxin HUS in children is generally quite favorable, even if renal failure requires dialysis. While 50% will have some residual renal damage, only 4% go on to require long-term dialysis. HUS is more common in rural areas and in the summer. Cows are the culprits—they get the blame for everything. "E" is of special note. There is controversy over whether or not antibiotics may **increase** the risk of HUS developing in patients with *E. coli* O157:H7 infections; however, it is fairly clear that antibiotics do not reduce the risk. The idea is that bacterial death from antibiotics releases more Shiga toxin leading to HUS. Remember that most cases of bacterial gastroenteritis—*E. coli* O157:H7 included—will clear without antibiotic therapy.

> **HELPFUL TIP:**
> Other subtypes of *E. coli* as well as *Shigella* can be responsible for HUS. The absence of the O157:H7 subtype of *E. coli* does not rule out HUS.

▶ **Objectives: Did you learn to …**
• Evaluate and manage a child with hypovolemia and renal failure?
• Recognize a clinical history and laboratory findings suggestive of hemolytic uremic syndrome?
• Identify causes of hemolytic uremic syndrome?

▶ **CASE 5.12**

A 45-year-old female presents to your clinic complaining of urinary frequency, "bladder" pain, and urinary urgency. There is no dysuria, however. She has had hematuria on dipstick several times with urinalysis showing microscopic hematuria on more than three occasions. This has been going on for several months and other practitioners (less skilled than yourself) have treated with a number of antibiotics without any relief. On questioning, she also notes bladder pain during intercourse and some chronic, vague, lower pelvic pain distinct from the bladder pain. At this visit, urinalysis and pelvic examination are unremarkable except for tenderness over the bladder area.

Question 5.12.1 **The MOST IMPORTANT next step is:**
A) Urine culture
B) Trial of 4 weeks of antichlamydial therapy
C) Pelvic ultrasound
D) Psychiatry consult and/or SSRI therapy for somatization disorder (now called somatic symptom disorder)

Answer 5.12.1 **The correct answer is "C."** This patient is describing typical symptoms of "painful bladder syndrome," the disease formerly known as "interstitial cystitis." Painful bladder syndrome does not involve inflammation. Therefore, "interstitial cystitis" is, and always has been, a misnomer. Painful bladder syndrome consists, appropriately enough, of pain referable to the bladder that cannot be attributed to another cause. Patients generally note pain with filling of the bladder and relief of symptoms after urination. The pain may be described as urethral, as a suprapubic pressure, as a pressure or a burning pain. Painful bladder syndrome is a diagnosis of exclusion and now treated as a chronic pain syndrome. It is critical to rule out other pelvic pathology that might cause the same symptoms such as an enlarged uterus sitting on the bladder, fibroids, or ovarian cancer. Other causes of similar symptoms could be bladder irritants (caffeine, alcohol), a urethral diverticulum, a sexually transmitted infection, etc. While less common, painful bladder syndrome can be seen in men. In such cases, prostate pathology must be ruled out.

Question 5.12.2 **All of the following are mandatory at this point EXCEPT:**
A) Urine cytology in a high-risk patient (smoker, etc.)
B) Postvoid residual
C) Cystoscopy and hyperdistention of the bladder
D) Ruling out a bladder stone

Answer 5.12.2 **The correct answer is "C."** Cystoscopy and hyperdistention are NOT required in order to make the diagnosis of painful bladder syndrome. As noted above, painful bladder syndrome is a clinical diagnosis of exclusion: Is there anything else causing the symptoms? If not, as Sherlock Holmes said, "Once you eliminate the impossible, whatever remains, no matter how improbable, must be the truth." It is important to rule out tumor (if indicated), stones, and neurogenic bladder (thus the postvoid residual).

> **HELPFUL TIP:**
> Treatment of painful bladder syndrome may include referral to a pain clinic, support groups, treatment of any other underlying problems (inflammatory bowel

disease, etc.), tricyclics, gabapentin, intravesicular DMSO, recurrent hydrodistention of the bladder, etc. What about pentosan polysulfate sodium (Elmiron®)? It is very expensive, may take up to 6 months to work, and the benefit is modest at best.

HELPFUL TIP:
Why not chronic phenazopyridine (e.g., Pyridium) for painful bladder syndrome? Well, you can consider it. But there is a danger of methemoglobinemia.

▶ **Objectives: Did you learn to ...**
- Evaluate and manage a patient with painful bladder syndrome?

 QUICK QUIZ: ACID–BASE DISORDER

While covering your local ED, a 15-year-old female presents with her father. He reports that he came home from work, found her asleep on the couch, and had difficulty in waking her up. She is lethargic and complains of nausea, dizziness, and abdominal pain. Apparently, she had muscle aches after gymnastics practice and then took "handfuls" of aspirin to relieve her pain. She was taking three to four tablets every hour today but is not sure about her total ingestion. She denies other ingestions.

On physical examination, her vitals are: T 39°C, P 110 bpm, RR 18 breaths/minute, BP 104/68 mm Hg. She is diaphoretic. The neurological examination is nonfocal, but she becomes progressively more lethargic during the examination. A venous blood gas on room air shows pH 7.38 (normal), $PaCO_2$ 23 mm Hg (low), PaO_2 40 mm Hg (low, but her oxygen saturation is 98% on transcutaneous monitoring), and HCO_3 15 mEq/L (low). Other laboratory data: Na 140 mEq/L, K 3.1 mEq/L, Cl 101 mEq/L, HCO_3 15 mEq/L (low), BUN 19 mg/dL, creatinine 1.1 mg/dL.

The venous blood gas results are best described as:
A) Metabolic acidosis
B) Metabolic acidosis and metabolic alkalosis
C) Metabolic acidosis and respiratory alkalosis
D) Metabolic alkalosis and respiratory acidosis
E) Just dandy! Look at the pH, professor

The correct answer is "C." Although the pH is in the normal range, there is an acid–base disorder present. First, there appears to be a metabolic acidosis with an elevated anion gap. The measured HCO_3 is 15 mEq/L, consistent with an acidosis, and the anion gap is 24 (based on the calculation of $Na - (Cl + HCO_3)$, in this case: $140 - (101 + 15) = 24$). This patient has taken an inadvertent overdose of aspirin. In salicylate overdoses, a high anion gap metabolic acidosis is often observed. Since salicylates directly stimulate the CNS respiratory center, there is usually a concurrent respiratory alkalosis.

In a compensated metabolic acidosis, the $PaCO_2$ should drop by 1.25 mm Hg for every 1 mEq/L drop in HCO_3. In this case,

the serum HCO_3 is 9 mEq/L below normal (if the normal is counted as 24), so $PaCO_2$ should be about 29 mm Hg ($40 - (9 \times 1.25)$). However, the measured $PaCO_2$ is 23 mm Hg, indicating the presence of a respiratory alkalosis. Also, the pH is nearly normal despite the presence of a disturbance in measured HCO_3, **which only occurs when a mixed disorder is present.**

HELPFUL TIP:
It is impossible to overcorrect a metabolic abnormality. Thus, a patient with a metabolic acidosis will not become alkalotic or normal unless there is another primary process present (e.g., respiratory alkalosis). Likewise, a patient with a respiratory acidosis from the retention of CO_2 will not become alkalotic or normal unless there is a secondary primary process going on (e.g., metabolic alkalosis).

Proper treatment of salicylate overdoses includes supportive therapy, urine alkalinization with sodium bicarbonate, and possibly hemodialysis.

 QUICK QUIZ: DYSURIA

Your nurse comes to you with a patient request. A 25-year-old female called in complaining of 2 days of burning with urination, urgency to urinate, and increased frequency. She has no fever, nausea, abdominal pain, flank pain, or vaginal discharge. The patient wants to know, "Can't I just get some antibiotics?" She's sure this is a bladder infection, just like the one she had last year. Oh, by the way, she's leaving for Europe tomorrow for her honeymoon.

Your response is to:
A) Prescribe ciprofloxacin 500 mg BID for 3 days
B) Prescribe trimethoprim/sulfamethoxazole BID for 14 days
C) Ask her to come in for a urinalysis
D) Ask her to come in for a urine culture
E) Prescribe nitrofurantoin 100 mg BID x 5 days

The correct answer is "E." Although you could argue that the diagnosis of UTI should be confirmed by urinalysis, there is plenty of evidence that history alone is sufficiently accurate in the right population (in this case, women of child-bearing years—but **not** children, pregnant women, men, or the elderly). If a woman complains of dysuria and increased frequency without vaginal discharge, the likelihood ratio of UTI is about 25 and "pretest" probability is greater than 90% that she has a urinary tract infection (*JAMA*. 2002;287(20):2701–2710). If her urinalysis were completely normal, she may still have an infection and likely has a false-negative dipstick urine (only 70% sensitive). Thus, symptoms and historical elements are more useful than urinalysis ("C"). For this patient, empiric antibiotic therapy with an appropriate antibiotic (nitrofurantoin for 5 days or trimethoprim/sulfamethoxazole for 3 days are reasonable options). Fourteen days of trimethoprim/sulfa-methoxazole ("B") is overkill. Why not "A"? The FDA has issued several warnings about fluoroquinolones including hypoglycemia, *permanent* neurologic/CNS problems, psychiatric disturbances, etc. So, fluoroquinolones should not be used for cystitis unless there is an overwhelming reason to do so. Plus, the dose is wrong. For simple cystitis, the dose of ciprofloxacin is 250 mg BID for 3 days. Of course, urine culture is the gold standard for diagnosing UTI, but she will be in Europe by the time you get the results—and we're pretty sure your medical license does not extend to Paris (though maybe she needs someone to carry her bags). Additionally, increasing fluid intake may be helpful. Adding 1.5 L/day reduces the risk of UTI recurrence (*JAMA Intern Med.* 2018;178(11):1509–1515). The benefit of cranberry juice beyond just adding fluid is questionable. Finally, other options for cystitis include amoxicillin/clavulanate, cephalexin (for pregnancy), fosfomycin, cefixime, and cefpodoxime. Amoxicillin alone is not recommended because of resistance.

HELPFUL TIP:
With typical UTI symptoms (e.g., dysuria, frequency) and a negative urine culture or no response to antibiotics, consider other causes: painful bladder syndrome, chlamydia urethritis, prostatitis (in men), pelvic inflammatory disease (in women), pelvic mass, herpes genitalis, and drugs (e.g., diuretics, caffeine, and theophylline).

▶ CASE 5.13

You are asked to consult on a patient who is hospitalized by an orthopedic surgeon (consulted by a surgeon twice in a chapter—congratulations!). The patient is a 25-year-old female who has a history of osteomyelitis from an open fracture sustained in a skiing accident. She has recently begun to spike a fever to 38.5°C and have a rapid increase in her creatinine.

Medications: nafcillin, ibuprofen, morphine, lactated Ringer solution IV 100 cc/hr.

Labs: Cr 3.5 mg/dL, BUN 25 mg/dL.

CBC shows mild WBC count of 12,500/mm³ and differential shows eosinophilia.

Question 5.13.1 **Considering prerenal versus renal causes, you calculate the FENa, and what would you expect to find?**
A) FENa >2%, urine sodium <20 mg/dL
B) FENa <1%, urine sodium <20 mg/dL
C) FENa >2%, urine sodium >40 mg/dL
D) FENa <1%, urine sodium >40 mg/dL

Answer 5.13.1 **The correct answer is "C."** Remember . . . her BUN/Cr <20; therefore, it is likely **not** prerenal disease (and she's receiving volume and has no history of heart failure). Thus, the patient likely has intrinsic kidney disease. This means that the FENa should be >2% and the urine sodium >40 mg/dL. In this scenario, the kidney is not trying to hold on to sodium in an attempt to correct a prerenal cause of increasing creatinine.

TABLE 5-11 COMMON DRUGS ASSOCIATED WITH ACUTE INTERSTITIAL NEPHRITIS

- Penicillins
- Aspirin
- Ciprofloxacin (and likely other fluoroquinolones)
- Allopurinol
- NSAIDs
- Some ACE inhibitors
- Proton Pump Inhibitors
- Erythromycin

ACE, angiotensin-converting enzyme; NSAIDs, nonsteroidal anti-inflammatory drugs.

TABLE 5-12 SYMPTOMS/SIGNS/LABORATORY FINDINGS IN ACUTE INTERSTITIAL NEPHRITIS

- Fever
- Rash (variable, may not be seen in all)
- Acute rise in plasma creatinine
- Active urine sediment that includes white cell casts
- Peripheral eosinophilia and urine eosinophils (in most cases)
- Renal tubular acidosis

Note: Interstitial nephritis secondary to NSAIDs may occur without fever, rash, or eosinophilia.

The patient's examination shows a diffuse rash and the urine contains white cell casts. There are no red cells in the urine.

Question 5.13.2 **The most likely diagnosis is:**
A) Acute tubular necrosis (ATN)
B) Acute interstitial nephritis
C) Renal infarction
D) Glomerulonephritis
E) Nephrotic syndrome

Answer 5.13.2 **The correct answer is "B."** The combination of fever, rash, mild eosinophilia, exposure to a new drug (nafcillin), and white cell casts in the urine essentially makes the diagnosis of acute interstitial nephritis. "A" is incorrect. The patient with ATN may have the same FENa and urine sodium as this patient, but should have renal tubular cells and/or granular casts in the urine. Also, **ATN does not cause fever, eosinophilia, or rash.** "C," renal infarction, is unlikely in a young patient and the rest of the clinical picture is more consistent with acute interstitial nephritis. "D," glomerulonephritis, is a possibility (e.g., lupus could cause a rash and fever). However, glomerulonephritis is associated with **red cell casts** and not white cell casts. Finally, as you already learned above, nephrotic syndrome presents with a bland urinary sediment. See Tables 5-11 and 5-12 for more details.

Question 5.13.3 **How long after drug exposure does acute interstitial nephritis generally begin?**
A) 2 to 3 days
B) 10 to 14 days
C) Several months
D) A and B
E) Any of the above

Answer 5.13.3 The correct answer is "E." Patients can develop acute interstitial nephritis anywhere from 1 day to several months after beginning a drug. Rifampin can cause acute interstitial nephritis on day 1. Interstitial nephritis can begin within 2 to 5 days if there has been a prior exposure to the drug, will typically begin within 10 to 14 days on **first** exposure to a drug, and may be delayed for months in the case of NSAID exposure.

HELPFUL TIP:
Patients with acute interstitial nephritis will often have eosinophils in the urine and peripheral smear, but eosinophils may be absent especially in those with NSAID-induced acute interstitial nephritis. Treatment is to stop the offending drug. If this doesn't work, steroids or cytotoxic drugs may be needed.

▶ **Objectives: Did you learn to ...**
- Recognize the presenting symptoms of acute interstitial nephritis?
- Describe causes and prognosis of acute interstitial nephritis?

HELPFUL TIP:
ACE inhibitors have been shown to be useful in reducing progression of renal disease even when the patient's creatinine is 5.0 mg/dL. But be very careful in this group. Start low, go slow, and check potassium and creatinine. In patients with CKD stage 3 or 4 started on an ACE inhibitor, a mild increase in creatinine is typical and expected and should not result in discontinuation of the ACE inhibitor.

Clinical Pearls

- ACE inhibitors are the drugs of choice for renal protection. ARBs and nondihydropyridine CCBs such as verapamil or diltiazem are other options.
- Avoid NSAIDs in patients with chronic renal disease from any cause, as well as in patients with heart failure or hypertension.
- BUN/Cr ratio >20 generally indicates that an acute kidney injury is secondary to extrarenal causes (poor perfusion from dehydration or CHF, etc.). This rule does not apply to children, those with GI bleeds, patients on high-dose steroids, and other exceptions.
- Calcium (dietary or supplemental) taken with meals reduces the risk of calcium oxalate stones by binding oxalate in the GI track.
- Gadolinium can cause a scleroderma-like disease in those with a creatinine clearance <30 mg/mL/min.
- In an otherwise healthy female without a vaginal discharge, the symptoms of dysuria, frequency, and urgency have a 90% positive predictive value for UTI, better than that of a UA.
- Patients with urolithiasis should have an NSAID as part of their pain control regimen unless it is contraindicated.

- Replace magnesium in the hypokalemic patient who is not responding as expected to treatment. The same is true in the patient with hypocalcemia.
- Sodium bicarbonate and *N*-acetylcysteine do not protect the kidneys from iodinated contrast. However, the risk of renal injury with contrast is small; hydrate the patient with normal saline.
- The early initiation of dialysis in patients with chronic kidney disease leads to worse outcomes. Start dialysis only when indicated.

BIBLIOGRAPHY

Azadi R, et al. Hemolytic uremic syndrome caused by Shiga toxin-producing *Escherichia coli* 0111. *J Am Osteopath Assoc.* 2010;110(9):538–544.

Bangalore S, et al. Angiotensin receptor blockers and risk of myocardial infarction: meta-analyses and trial sequential analyses of 147020 patients from randomised trials. *BMJ.* 2011;342:d2234.

Barnett AH, et al. Angiotensin-receptor blockade versus converting-enzyme inhibition in type 2 diabetes and nephropathy. *N Engl J Med.* 2004;351(19):1952–1961.

Bent S, et al. Does this woman have an acute uncomplicated urinary tract infection? *JAMA.* 2002;287(20):2701–2710.

Blair HA. Patiromer: a review in hyperkalaemia. *Clin Drug Investig.* 2018;38(8):785–794

Brookhart MA, et al. Comparative mortality risk of anemia management practices in incident hemodialysis patients. *JAMA.* 2010;303(9):857–886.

Campschroer T, et al. Alpha-blockers as medical expulsive therapy for ureteral stones. *Cochrane Database Syst Rev.* 2018;4:CD008509.

Cheng J, et al. Effect of angiotensin-converting enzyme inhibitors and angiotensin II receptor blockers on all-cause mortality, cardiovascular deaths, and cardiovascular events in patients with diabetes mellitus: a meta-analysis. *JAMA Intern Med.* 2014;174(5): 773–785.

Cooper BA, et al. A randomized, controlled trial of early versus late initiation of dialysis. *N Engl J Med.* 2010;363(7):609–619.

Gill N, et al. Renal failure secondary to acute tubular necrosis: epidemiology, diagnosis, and management. *Chest.* 2005;128(4):2847–2863.

Haller H, et al. Olmesartan for the delay or prevention of microalbuminuria in type 2 diabetes. *N Engl J Med.* 2011;364:907–917.

Hoorn EJ, et al. Diagnosis and treatment of hyponatremia: compilation of the guidelines. *J Am Soc Nephrol.* 2017;28(5):1340–1349.

Hooton TM, et al. Effect of increased daily water intake in premenopausal women with recurrent urinary tract infections: a randomized clinical trial. *JAMA Intern Med.* 2018;178(11):1509–1515.

Hou FF, et al. Efficacy and safety of benazepril for advanced chronic renal insufficiency. *N Engl J Med.* 2006;354:131–140.

Kellum J, et al. Acute renal failure. *Am Fam Physician.* 2007;76(3):418–422.

Kohlstadt I, at al. Treatment and prevention of kidney stones: an update. *Am Fam Physician.* 2011;84(11):1234–1242.

Komaba H, et al. Initiation of sevelamer and mortality among hemodialysis patients treated with calcium-based phosphate binders. *Clin J Am Soc Nephrol.* 2017;12(9):1489–1497.

Lalau JD, et al. Metformin treatment in patients with type 2 diabetes and chronic kidney disease stages 3A, 3B, or 4. *Diabetes Care.* 2018;41(3):547–553.

Levey AS, et al. K/DOQI clinical practice guidelines for chronic kidney disease: evaluation, classification, and stratification. *Am J Kidney Dis.* 2002;39(suppl 1):S1–S266. Available at https://www.kidney.org/sites/default/files/docs/ckd_evaluation_classification_stratification.pdf. Accessed March 9, 2019.

Martinez-Bianchi V, Halstater BH. Urologic chronic pelvic pain syndrome. *Prim Care.* 2010;37:527–546.

McDonald JS, et al. Risk of intravenous contrast material-mediated acute kidney injury: a propensity score-matched study stratified by baseline-estimated glomerular filtration rate. *Radiology.* 2014;271(1):65–73.

McDonald RJ, et al. Intravenous contrast material exposure is not an independent risk factor for dialysis or mortality. *Radiology.* 2014;273(3):714–725.

Meltzer AC, et al. Effect of tamsulosin on passage of symptomatic ureteral stones: a randomized clinical trial. *JAMA Intern Med.* 2018 Aug 1;178(8):1051–1057.

Miller NL, Lingeman JE. Management of kidney stones. *BMJ.* 2007;334(7591):468–472.

Pfeffer MA, et al. A trial of darbepoietin alfa in type 2 diabetes and chronic kidney disease. *N Engl J Med.* 2009;361:2019–2032.

Phrommintikul A, et al. Mortality and target haemoglobin concentrations in anaemic patients with chronic kidney disease treated with erythropoietin: a meta-analysis. *Lancet.* 2007;369:381–388.

Pickar R, et al. Medical expulsive therapy in adults with ureteric colic: a multicentre, randomised, placebo-controlled trial. *Lancet.* 2015;386(9991):341–349.

Schena FP. Management of patients with chronic kidney disease. *Intern Emerg Med.* 2011;6(suppl 1):77–83.

Simerville JA, et al. Urinalysis: a comprehensive review. *Am Fam Physician.* 2005;71(6):1153–1162.

Slagman MC, et al. Moderate dietary sodium restriction added to angiotensin converting enzyme inhibition compared with dual blockade in lowering proteinuria and blood pressure: randomised controlled trial. *BMJ.* 2011;343:d4366.

Sterns RH, et al. Ion-exchange resins for the treatment of hyperkalemia: are they safe and effective? *J Am Soc Nephrol.* 2010; 21(5):733–735.

Strippoli GF, et al. Angiotensin converting enzyme inhibitors and angiotensin II receptor antagonists for preventing the progression of diabetic kidney disease. *Cochrane Database Syst Rev.* 2006;(4):CD006257.

Tarr PI, et al. Shiga-toxin-producing *Escherichia coli* and haemolytic uraemic syndrome. *Lancet.* 2005;365:1073–1086.

Vincendeau S, et al. Tamsulosin hydrochloride vs placebo for management of distal ureteral stones: a multicentric, randomized, double-blind trial. *Arch Intern Med.* 2010;170(22):2021–2027.

Whitmore KE, Theoharides TC. When to suspect interstitial cystitis. *J Fam Pract.* 2011;60(6):340–348.

Hematology and Oncology

6

Maresi Berry-Stoelzle and Jason K. Wilbur

▶ CASE 6.1

A 6-month-old boy presents to your office after his mother notices swelling and ecchymosis over his anterior right thigh. She does not recall any trauma to the area. The mother denies any history of bleeding problems, including during his circumcision. On physical examination the child has a large hematoma over his thigh. There are no obvious bony deformities and the child otherwise looks well. You suspect the child may have an inherited coagulation disorder.

Question 6.1.1 Which of the following statements is NOT correct?
A) Child abuse should be included in the differential diagnosis
B) The child did not bleed during circumcision, so the possibility of hemophilia need not be considered
C) A careful family history is important in the workup
D) Coagulation studies (PT, PTT) and CBC should be obtained

Answer 6.1.1 The correct answer (and untrue statement) is "B." The absence of bleeding during circumcision in no way rules out hemophilia. Up to half of patients with hemophilia do not bleed with circumcision. Depending on the severity of factor deficiency, the diagnosis may not be made until the child is very active or even in adulthood, after surgery, etc. Whenever you encounter unexplained bruising in a child or dependent adult—especially in locations that would be unusual for accidental trauma, such as the posterior thighs or back—child abuse ("A") should be included on your differential diagnosis. Since bleeding disorders in children are often inherited rather than acquired, a thorough family history ("C") is important. The initial workup for this patient would include blood counts and coagulation studies ("D").

Question 6.1.2 Which of the following is NOT TRUE about hemophilia A?
A) It is an X-linked disorder
B) It is the result of factor VIII deficiency

C) It generally leads to mucosal bleeding
D) It occurs most often in males
E) It can be treated with factor VIIa

Answer 6.1.2 The correct answer (and untrue statement) is "C." Hemophilia A is an X-linked deficiency of factor VIII, which presents with hematomas, bleeding, and hemarthrosis (and not generally mucosal bleeding or petechiae). Deficiency of factor IX, or hemophilia B, also known as "Christmas Disease," is also X-linked but is much less common. "D" deserves special mention. Hemophilia rarely occurs in females but can occur in three situations: (1) the female patient is a heterozygote who has early inactivation of the second X chromosome during embryogenesis; (2) both parents are carriers, in which case the father would have the disease overtly; (3) acquired factor VIII deficiency. This is generally found in individuals over 50 or those who are pregnant or postpartum. The most common underlying conditions include pregnancy, postpartum, malignancy, rheumatoid arthritis, medications, and connective tissue disorders. Some have no identifiable trigger. It is caused by factor VIII antibodies. "E" is true—and not a typo. Factor VIIa can be used in most cases of hemophilia A *and* B to stop bleeding. It is mostly used in patients who have factor inhibitors in the blood (developed as a response to repeated exposure to factor VIII or factor IX).

HELPFUL TIP:
Generally speaking, petechiae and mucosal bleeding result from platelet problems (e.g., mild von Willebrand disease [VWD] and thrombocytopenia), while hemarthrosis and hematomas result from factor deficiency. Severe VWD may present with hemarthrosis and hematomas.

HELPFUL TIP:
Von Willebrand disease (VWD) may be autosomal dominant (Type I), variable (Type II), or autosomal recessive (Type III). There is often a family history of Von

Willebrand factor (vWF) deficiency or bleeding, but a percentage of cases occur spontaneously.

Question 6.1.3 Which of the following is indicated when evaluating for a suspected inherited coagulopathy?
A) Prothrombin time (PT)
B) Partial thromboplastin time (PTT)
C) Platelet count
D) PFA-100
E) All of the above

Answer 6.1.3 The correct answer is "E." The PTT is actually the most sensitive test for hemophilia. "D" deserves special mention. The PFA-100 (**P**latelet **F**unction **A**nalyzer) tests for (appropriately enough) platelet functioning and will be abnormal in diseases of platelet dysfunction, such as VWD. While the PFA-100 can help make a diagnosis of VWD, it does not correlate directly with the risk of clinically meaningful bleeding.

....

You diagnose this patient with hemophilia A, and he grows up under your excellent tutelage (along with some guidance from your friendly neighborhood hemophilia treatment center, since overall outcomes are better with multidisciplinary care through a hemophilia center). As a junior high school student, he attends summer camp for hemophiliacs in Transylvania. For some bizarre reason, the counselors decide to have the kids play tackle football (crazy, but a true story that happened to one of your authors). The patient presents to the ED with bleeding into his right knee and left elbow.

Question 6.1.4 What is the initial step in the management of this patient's hemarthroses?
A) Joint aspiration
B) Desmopressin
C) Factor VIII infusion
D) Heparin infusion
E) Leeches

Answer 6.1.4 The correct answer is "C." While joint aspiration and desmopressin may be helpful, this patient needs to be treated with factor VIII in order to stop the bleeding. Joint aspiration ("A") may play a role in preventing blood-induced arthritis, a risk with recurrent joint bleeds. Desmopressin ("B") is useful in some cases of VWD and in some mild cases of hemophilia. Desmopressin releases vWF from platelets transiently increasing circulating vWF, which may be helpful in VWD but will not accomplish anything in this case. Antifibrinolytic therapy may also be of use: tranexamic acid or aminocaproic acid is commonly used to prevent clot breakdown. Heparin infusions ("D") would lead to prolonged bleeding and would be counterintuitive. Leeches ("E") are not indicated to treat hemarthroses.

Question 6.1.5 What factor level target is appropriate when treating this patient?
A) 5% to 10%
B) 40% to 50%

C) 75% to 80%
D) 100%

Answer 6.1.5 The correct answer is "B." For a hemarthrosis (except for the hip joint, which is a special case) or other "minor" bleeding, maintain a factor level of 40% to 50% for 72 hours. For more serious bleeding (e.g., intracranial), maintain a level of 80% to 100% for 10 days. If planning a procedure, such as joint aspiration, raise the factor level to 80% to 100%.

HELPFUL TIP:
Von Willebrand disease Type I will respond to desmopressin (as noted above). Type II has variable response to desmopressin. A trial at the time of diagnosis is recommended. Type III VWD requires infusion of factor VIII and vWF (e.g., Humate-P, Alphanate). Remember that factor VIII is not enough, you need a preparation that also includes vWF. If you do not have a VIII + vWF factor available, or if the bleeding continues after replacement therapy, you can always transfuse normal platelets as a last option. These will have adequate vWF.

Question 6.1.6 As your patient grows and enters adulthood, he is likely to encounter which of the following?
A) Hemarthrosis with significant arthritis and joint dysfunction
B) A historically low risk of HIV/AIDS from multiple transfusions, as compared to the 1990s
C) Maturational delay if antifactor antibodies are present
D) Reduced risk of coronary artery disease (CAD)
E) All of the above are found with hemophilia

Answer 6.1.6 The correct answer is "E." "A" is true. Patients still get recurrent hemarthroses leading to arthritis and joint dysfunction. "B" is true. Screening and the use of recombinant factor VIII has led to a marked reduction in HIV in hemophiliacs from a high of 50% in the 1990s. Patients with hemophilia do have delayed maturation ("C"), especially if antifactor antibodies are present. And finally, they do have a **reduced risk** of CAD ("D"). This is also seen in carriers of hemophilia genes.

▶ **Objectives: Did you learn to …**
• Suspect and test for a bleeding disorder in the appropriate setting?
• Use laboratory testing to assist in the diagnosis of a bleeding disorder?
• Identify and treat hemophilia A?

▶ **CASE 6.2**

A 4-year-old girl is brought to you after she is noted to have small pink spots on her lower extremities and bleeding from her gums. She had a URI a couple of weeks ago. She also recently received her second dose of her MMR vaccine (mom particularly wants to make sure she is protected from the recent resurgence in measles and mumps—thank you, anti-vaxers).

You note petechiae on her lower extremities and purpura in her oropharynx. The mother and patient deny any other bleeding. You obtain a CBC, which is normal except for a platelet count of 15,000/mm³. You suspect immune thrombocytopenic purpura (ITP, also known as idiopathic thrombocytopenic purpura).

Question 6.2.1 Which of the following may have led to this patient's ITP?

A) MMR vaccine
B) Infection
C) Food allergy
D) A and B
E) All of the above

Answer 6.2.1 The correct answer is "D." Both infections ("B") and the MMR ("A") vaccine have been linked to ITP (not autism . . . got that? . . . **NOT autism**). Food allergy ("C") does not cause ITP.

Question 6.2.2 Which of the following is NOT likely to lead to a sustained (let's say at least 2 days) increase in the patient's platelet count?

A) IVIG
B) Steroids (e.g., prednisone)
C) Platelet transfusion
D) Splenectomy

Answer 6.2.2 The correct answer (and what will not yield a sustained increase in platelet count) is "C." Transfused platelets will just be "chomped up" by "Mr. Spleen." However, platelets can be used to temporize if a patient must go to the OR, etc. **Most children can simply be observed. The only indication for treatment is bleeding.**

All of the treatments have a downside. Splenectomy ("D") is associated with a risk of sepsis. If possible, delay splenectomy until after the child is over 5 years old. Of note, failure of ITP to respond to splenectomy may be due to the presence of an accessory spleen, which can often be identified by a liver–spleen radionuclide study. Steroids ("B") may cause behavioral problems and long-term problems such as avascular necrosis. IVIG ("A") leads to a temporary increase in platelets that may last several weeks, but can be associated with renal injury and anaphylaxis among other possible adverse effects.

> **HELPFUL TIP:**
> If a child suspected of having ITP looks sick, you need to expand your differential diagnosis. Sepsis with disseminated intravascular coagulopathy (DIC) and thrombotic thrombocytopenic purpura—hemolytic uremic syndrome (TTP–HUS) is also in the differential. ITP is most common in children between the ages of 2 and 4 years, with a small peak incidence in adolescence. ITP often resolves without specific therapy; 80% to 90% of pediatric patients are back to normal within a few months, and fewer than 20% of children will remain thrombocytopenic for greater than 12 months. Only 0.1% to 0.5% develop intracranial bleeding.

> **HELPFUL TIP:**
> Do not bother checking for antiplatelet antibodies in those with ITP. Patients **without** ITP may have antiplatelet antibodies and the presence of these antibodies is not predictive of outcome.

> **HELPFUL TIP:**
> For **adults** with ITP, treatment is generally indicated. Treatment includes (in order) steroids, Rho(D) immunoglobulin **for Rh-positive patients**, IVIG (which causes a transient rise in platelet numbers), and splenectomy. Other treatment options for refractory cases include rituximab or various immunosuppressive agents. The thrombopoietin-receptor agonists, romiplostim (Nplate) and eltrombopag (Promacta) (real names and not Icelandic vocabulary words), stimulate platelet production and can also be used in ITP.

▶ **Objectives: Did you learn to …**
· Describe the natural history of ITP?
· Describe the treatments available to treat ITP?
· Understand the benefits and risks of the treatments for ITP?

▶ **CASE 6.3**

A 24-year-old female G1 P0 at 39 weeks of gestation presents to your office with a bruise on her anterior tibia, which she noticed after bumping into a coffee table. She has been healthy before and during her pregnancy and takes only prenatal vitamins. Her physical examination is unremarkable with the exception of an 8-cm bruise over her right anterior tibia. Her vital signs are normal. Her physical examination is remarkable for a gravid abdomen consistent with 39 weeks of gestation, fetal heart tones auscultated at 140 bpm, absence of right upper quadrant pain, and absence of peripheral edema. You obtain the following laboratory tests: CBC, which demonstrates white blood cell (WBC) 9,000/mm³, hemoglobin (Hgb) 11.8 g/dL, and platelet count 95,000/mm³; normal PTT and PT/INR; negative urinalysis; and normal liver enzymes.

Question 6.3.1 What is your next step?

A) Recommend immediate delivery by cesarean section as the infant likely has thrombocytopenia as well and is at high risk for intracranial hemorrhage
B) Recommend immediate delivery by cesarean section as this disorder will likely progress to eclampsia
C) Recommend close observation and reassure the patient that this is typically a self-limited condition
D) Start prednisone, 1 mg/kg daily, and taper slowly over the next 6 weeks
E) Recommend splenectomy as soon as possible after delivery

Answer 6.3.1 The correct answer is "C." This patient likely has gestational thrombocytopenia, a condition that occurs in up to 5% of pregnant women. It is characterized by mild thrombocytopenia occurring in late gestation, without other CBC abnormalities or physical findings; the platelet count is usually >70,000/mm³ (two-thirds are between 130,000/mm³ and 150,000/mm³). The condition resolves after delivery and is not associated with severe neonatal thrombocytopenia. No specific change in routine obstetrical care is warranted, although the anesthesiologist placing an epidural may want a follow-up platelet count closer to the time of delivery.

Question 6.3.2 You can reassure this patient that an adequate platelet count for clotting is typically as low as:
A) Minimum of 150,000/mm³
B) Minimum of 100,000–110,000/mm³
C) Minimum of 20,000–50,000/mm³
D) Minimum of 5,000/mm³
E) Minimum of 1. One platelet—that's it. It's just gotta be a big one.

Answer 6.3.2 The correct answer is "C." A platelet count of >20,000 to 50,000/mm³ is generally considered adequate for achieving clotting.

▶ **Objectives: Did you learn to …**
- Recognize gestational thrombocytopenia?
- Define the lower limit of platelet count appropriate for clotting?

 QUICK QUIZ: COAGULATION STUDIES

Which of the following conditions should be considered if both the PT and PTT are prolonged in a patient noted to be oozing from a surgical incision?
A) Severe liver disease, DIC, factor X deficiency
B) Heparin effect, VWD, factor XII deficiency
C) Warfarin effect, factor VII deficiency, vitamin K deficiency
D) All of the above

The correct answer is "A." The three factor deficiencies that may prolong both PT and PTT are II, V, and X. Both PTT and PT may be prolonged due to both **severe liver disease** and DIC. Mild vitamin K deficiency or **mild liver disease** generally affects the PT only. Generally, heparin affects PTT, and warfarin affects PT. Remember that the direct oral anticoagulants (rivaroxaban, dabigatran, etc.) cause bleeding without prolonging the PT or PTT.

 HELPFUL TIP:
Why does vitamin K work to improve the PT in liver disease? Because most alcoholics and others with liver failure are vitamin K deficient (poor absorption, poor nutritional intake, antibiotic use—recall that vitamin K is made in the gut by bacteria). Paradoxically, those with *liver failure* are often hypercoagulable even in the face of an elevated PT leading to thrombotic complications such as hepatic vein thrombosis. See the GI chapter for more details.

▶ **CASE 6.4**

A 42-year-old male presents to the ED with a gastrointestinal (GI) bleeding due to ibuprofen use. His Hgb is 6.8 g/dL and he is hemodynamically unstable at this point. You are confident that this patient should receive a transfusion, but you remember that blood transfusions actually increase mortality if used incorrectly.

Question 6.4.1 Which of the following is an indication for transfusion?
A) Hemodynamic instability in a trauma patient due to bleeding unresponsive to no less than 3 L of saline
B) Preoperative Hgb of 7 to 8 g/dL with expected intraoperative blood loss
C) Hemoglobin of 9.5 g/dL in a patient with angina
D) A stable ICU patient with an Hgb of 8.7g/dL
E) All of the above

Answer 6.4.1 The correct answer is "B." In general, a restrictive policy for blood transfusion has been shown to improve outcomes. "A" is incorrect because blood should be given to the hemodynamically unstable trauma patient after at most 2 L of saline (and per the ATLS recommendations after 1 L of saline). "B" is correct. A restrictive preoperative transfusion policy which limited transfusions to those with an Hb of <8 g/dL has shown survival benefit. "C" is incorrect. Transfusion should be considered in the patient with CAD only when the hemoglobin reaches 7 to 8 g/dL. Finally, "D" is incorrect. Transfusions should be withheld from a nonbleeding, hemodynamically stable ICU patient until the hemoglobin reaches 7 g/dL. A more liberal transfusion policy is associated with higher mortality. As an aside, some would transfuse postoperative patients with a hemoglobin of less than 10 g/dL if they are at high risk for ischemic disease (ischemic bowel, CAD, etc.). **Transfusion for indications other than these is not beneficial and has been proven harmful.** See Table 6-1 for a list of transfusion indications.

You decide to transfuse one unit of packed red blood cells (PRBCs). After 30 minutes, the patient complains of dyspnea and back pain. Repeat examination of this patient reveals a diaphoretic man with a pulse of 130 bpm and BP of 88/50 mm Hg. His lung fields are clear. Initial vitals before the transfusion were a pulse of 110 bpm and BP of 94/52 mm Hg.

Question 6.4.2 What is your next step?
A) Stop the blood transfusion and begin normal saline through the IV
B) Increase the rate of transfusion
C) Administer acetaminophen 650 mg PO
D) Administer furosemide 40 mg IV
E) Place a nasogastric tube for lavage

Answer 6.4.2 The correct answer is "A." *The transfusion must be stopped.* The patient is exhibiting signs and symptoms of a hemolytic transfusion reaction, which is generally the result of

TABLE 6-1 BLOOD TRANSFUSION INDICATIONS

Indication	Transfusion Threshold
Otherwise stable adult and pediatric intensive care patients	Hgb ≤7 g/dL
Hemodynamically stable postoperative patients	Hgb ≤8 g/dL **OR** for symptoms of chest pain, orthostatic hypotension, tachycardia unresponsive to IVF boluses, or CHF
Hemodynamically stable patients with preexisting cardiovascular disease	Hgb ≤8 g/dL **OR** for symptoms of chest pain, orthostatic hypotension, tachycardia unresponsive to IVF boluses, or CHF
Hemodynamically stable patients with acute coronary syndrome (ACS)	Unable to make a recommendation against liberal or restrictive transfusion.

Adapted from Carson JL, Grossman BJ, Kleinman S, et al. Red blood cell transfusion: a clinical practice guideline from the AABB. *Ann Intern Med.* 2012;157(1):49–58.

an ABO incompatibility. Patients may exhibit nausea, flushing, dyspnea, oliguria, back pain, and hypotension. Other findings include markers of hemolysis: hemoglobinuria, elevated serum-free hemoglobin, reduced haptoglobin, and elevated bilirubin. Patients are positive for direct antiglobulin test (i.e., Coombs). Therapy includes IV saline at a high enough rate to initiate a brisk diuresis to prevent hemoglobin from precipitating in the kidneys causing acute tubular necrosis. In evaluating the dyspnea, it is important to distinguish between transfusion-associated circulatory overload (TACO) and transfusion-related acute lung injury (TRALI). This may require a chest x-ray and assessment of oxygenation status (pulse oximetry or arterial blood gas measurement). TACO is more likely in patients who have received high volumes of fluids or are more sensitive to high fluid volume, such as those with underlying cardiac disease. Hypertension, hypoxemia, and pulmonary edema support the diagnosis of TACO. These patients should be treated with diuresis. TRALI may have a more sudden onset and will present with symptoms out of proportion to the volume of fluid or volume of transfusion. They will also require supportive care and consult to the transfusion service for further workup.

HELPFUL TIP:
Additional transfusion reactions include:
- Anaphylaxis (especially in those with IgA deficiency)
- Febrile, nonhemolytic reactions (which respond to meperidine and acetaminophen—"Finally, a use for meperidine!" you exclaim)
- Don't forget that fluid overload from transfusions may cause dyspnea

HELPFUL TIP:
Why did we always order "2 units of packed red cells?" In a non-bleeding patient, the transfusion of one unit of

PRBCs can be expected to raise the hematocrit by 3% to 4% (1 g/dL for Hb). Current guidelines recommend giving one unit and reassessing the patient. Every unit of blood has its own risk of mismatch, contagion, adverse reaction, etc.

▶ **Objectives: Did you learn to …**
- Decide when blood transfusion is appropriate?
- Recognize hemolytic transfusion reactions?

▶ CASE 6.5

A 56-year-old male presents to the ED with an acute abdomen, likely from a perforated diverticulum. He is taking warfarin for a DVT that occurred after a total knee arthroplasty. He weighs 65 kg. You are evaluating him for surgery and find the following laboratory results: Hgb 14.3 g/dL, platelet count 478,000/mm³, INR 3.5, and PTT 28 seconds.

Question 6.5.1 Which of the following statements about his preoperative management is correct?
A) Platelet transfusion perioperatively will produce the most immediate reduction in risk of bleeding from warfarin
B) Fresh frozen plasma (FFP) transfusion will produce the most immediate reduction in risk of bleeding from warfarin
C) Vitamin K administration orally (PO) will produce the most immediate reduction in risk of bleeding from warfarin
D) Vitamin K administration subcutaneously (SC) will produce the most immediate reduction in risk of bleeding from warfarin
E) Cryoprecipitate transfusion will produce the most immediate reduction in risk of bleeding from warfarin

Answer 6.5.1 **The correct answer is "B."** The patient above would benefit most immediately from the administration of FFP. FFP contains all the soluble plasma proteins found in whole blood, including the vitamin K-dependent factors that are depleted by warfarin. If a more sustained reversal is desired, the simultaneous administration of vitamin K is effective. **The preferred route of administration of vitamin K is oral.** Giving vitamin K IV is second best—this lowers the INR the same degree as oral vitamin K at 24 hours; the IV route may be preferred in instances where GI absorption is questionable. Avoid vitamin K SC or IM, which are less effective than PO and IV routes. The effects of FFP rarely last 24 hours; the effects of vitamin K are usually not apparent for 12 to 24 hours. The use of cryoprecipitate will not provide the appropriate factors depleted by warfarin. Cryoprecipitate contains vWF, factor VIII, factor XIII, and fibrinogen. Platelet transfusion would not benefit this patient since warfarin does not affect platelet function.

HELPFUL TIP: REVERSING WARFARIN
The most recent recommendations suggest using a 4-factor prothrombin complex concentrate (e.g., Kcentra) for reversing life-threatening bleeding

secondary to warfarin. A 3-factor prothrombin complex concentrate **plus** FFP is an alternative; 3-factor prothrombin complex concentrates lack factor VII. If these are not available, FFP is still an option.

HELPFUL TIP:
The INR of FFP is 1.5. No matter how hard you try, you cannot reduce the INR to less than 1.5 with FFP. Tell your surgeon to chill. Giving more FFP won't help.

▶ Objectives: Did you learn to …
 · Treat warfarin-induced hypocoagulability?

▶ CASE 6.6

A 20-year-old female with acute myeloid leukemia completed her second cycle of consolidation chemotherapy 5 days ago. She presents to the ED complaining of fatigue and fever. She denies cough, dysuria, abdominal pain, sinus drainage, or redness around her Hickman catheter. Her physical examination reveals a temperature of 38.4°C, pulse 100 bpm, BP 120/58 mm Hg, and respirations 14 breaths per minute. Her examination is otherwise unremarkable, including no redness or tenderness at the Hickman site. Your magic crystal ball tells you she does not have a line infection. Her laboratory results reveal the following: WBC 1300/mm³ (absolute neutrophil count 500 cells/mm³), Hgb 9 g/dL, hematocrit 27%, and platelet count 47,000/mm³. Blood cultures have been drawn.

Question 6.6.1 **What is your next step, and what is your rationale?**
A) Administer IV amphotericin B; a Candida urinary tract infection is most likely
B) Administer IV cefepime; she requires empiric coverage for both Gram-negative and Gram-positive organisms
C) Administer IV nafcillin; a Gram-positive bacterial infection is most likely and broader antibiotic coverage will encourage growth of resistant bacteria
D) Administer IV vancomycin; she most likely has an MRSA sinus infection
E) Close observation; there is no focus of infection and she looks well

Answer 6.6.1 **The correct answer is "B."** This patient has a neutropenic fever, which is a medical emergency. Prompt treatment with broad-spectrum antibiotics has drastically improved the survival of patients with neutropenic fever. Antimicrobial treatment should be started within 60 minutes of triage. Neutropenia is usually defined as neutrophils plus bands (absolute neutrophil count, ANC) <500/mm³ or <1,000/mm³ when the nadir has not been reached. Most myelosuppressive chemotherapeutic agents produce a reduction in WBCs 4 to 10 days after completion and nadir at 10 to 14 days. Fever is defined as

a **single** oral temperature >101°F (38.3°C) or a temperature >100.4°F (38°C) persisting for 1 hour or more. This patient does not need vancomycin since the absence of a line infection was stipulated in the history (via crystal ball that always works in our experience). Broad-spectrum coverage of Gram-positive and Gram-negative organisms, including *Pseudomonas*, is the cornerstone of therapy with specific therapy for any localizing symptoms or risk signs. See Table 6-2 for common antibiotic regimens.

TABLE 6-2 SUGGESTED ANTIBIOTIC REGIMENS FOR NEUTROPENIC FEVER

High-Risk Patients (ANC ≤ 100/mm³ or expected duration of neutropenia >7 days or significant comorbidity)

Comorbidities = hypotension, pneumonia, new onset abdominal pain or neurologic changes

Single Agents

Antipseudomonal β-lactam
 · Cefepime
 · Ceftazidime
 · Piperacillin-tazobactam
 · Carbapenem
 · Imipenem-cilastatin
 · Meropenem

Combination Agents

Add one of the following to the above regimen for management of complications or suspected/proven resistance:
 · Aminoglycoside
 · Fluoroquinolone (ciprofloxacin or levofloxacin)
 · Vancomycin

Additional considerations:
 · Add vancomycin if a line infection is suspected, MRSA is likely, skin or soft tissue infection, patient is clinically more ill (hypotension, hemodynamically unstable, etc.), or if no improvement after 3–5 days of empiric therapy.
 · Add linezolid or daptomycin for VRE, or patient intolerance to vancomycin.
 · Add metronidazole for abdominal symptoms or suspected *Clostridium difficile* infection.
 · Add antifungal (fluconazole, voriconazole, amphotericin B) if still febrile 4–7 days after a broad-spectrum antibacterial regimen and no identified source of fever. The risk of fungal infection is increased by this point.
 · Add acyclovir and/or fluconazole if there is oral ulceration.

Low-Risk Patients (anticipated neutropenia <7 days, able to take PO, hemodynamically stable, no comorbid conditions, able to comply with daily follow-up):
 · PO ciprofloxacin and amoxicillin-clavulanate
OR
 · Hospital admission and any of the above regimens for persistent fever or worsening symptoms.

Data from Infectious Diseases Society of America. Freifeld AG, et al. Clinical practice guideline for the use of antimicrobial agents in neutropenic patients with cancer: 2010 update by the Infectious Diseases Society of America. *Clin Infect Dis*. 2011;52(4):e56–e93.

HELPFUL TIP:
Patients with a neutropenic fever can have any infection seen in normal hosts, but you should also consider IV catheter infections, perirectal infections and abscesses, and necrotizing enteritis (aka "typhlitis"). Remember that they may not have an inflammatory reaction around a catheter site, abscess formation, infiltrate on chest x-ray, or WBCs in the urine because of the neutropenia. The absence of signs or symptoms should not dissuade you from starting empiric antibiotic therapy. Similarly, **the absence of fever in a neutropenic patient with focal infection should be approached as a high-risk situation**.

▸ **Objectives: Did you learn to …**
· Identify and treat a neutropenic fever?

▸ **CASE 6.7**

A 63-year-old male with a diagnosis of non–small cell lung cancer, undergoing weekly chemotherapy and radiation to a left upper lobe mass, presents to your office. He complains of dull, non-radiating back pain in the lower thoracic/upper lumbar area. He denies trauma or any new activities. He has no associated weakness or paresthesias. He denies difficulties with bowel or bladder function but does notice he is tripping more.

Question 6.7.1 What is your initial diagnostic and/or therapeutic approach to this patient?
A) MRI of thoracic and lumbar spine
B) Plain films of the thoracic and lumbar spine and a COX-2 inhibitor with a 2-week follow-up
C) Plain films of the thoracic spine and NSAIDs
D) Prescription for physical therapy and NSAIDs
E) Urinalysis with culture and antibiotics

Answer 6.7.1 The correct answer is "A." This is not your average back pain. Any patient with active malignancy complaining of back pain should be investigated for metastasis. While a plain film of the spine may be useful, the gold standard is MRI. This patient gives a history of "tripping" which, beyond the reference to the 1960s, may indicate lower extremity weakness, foot drop, etc. The real emergency is spinal cord impingement. Spinal cord compression may occur from direct extension of metastatic disease from the vertebrae or extension from retroperitoneal or paravertebral disease. Frequently, the pain predates neurological symptoms, and because of the potential for severe, adverse outcomes, you want to catch the disease early to prevent chronic impairment.

The patient undergoes MRI of the spine, which demonstrates a lesion compressing the cord at L1.

Question 6.7.2 Which of the following is NOT an appropriate therapeutic modality?
A) Decompression surgery
B) Dexamethasone 10 mg bolus IV, followed by 6 mg every 6 hours
C) Observation with pain control (e.g., with morphine PCA)
D) Radiation therapy to the affected area

Answer 6.7.2 The correct answer is "C." Patients with spinal cord compression who have aggressive interventions are more likely to retain function, including ambulation and bowel and bladder control. Steroids ("B") will help reduce edema surrounding the tumor and hopefully will relieve pressure on the cord. Radiation ("D") can often provide symptomatic relief and reduce the likelihood that the tumor will spread locally to impinge on the cord. Surgical decompression ("A") is another option. Of course, if this patient opted for a palliative care approach and had decided upon hospice, "C" might be appropriate, but he is still getting active therapy, and his remaining time could be spent with less pain and better function if one of the other options were chosen. Additionally, radiation can be seen as symptom-directed palliative care.

▸ **Objectives: Did you learn to …**
· Recognize and treat neoplastic spinal cord injury?

▸ **CASE 6.8**

A 32-year-old woman presents to your office with complaints of dyspnea, constipation, menorrhagia, and fatigue that are new over the past few weeks. She has a distant history of Hodgkin lymphoma treated with chemotherapy and radiation to the chest. Her physical examination reveals a well-developed woman, who appears comfortable at rest with normal vital signs. She has no adenopathy and the remainder of her examination is unremarkable. Her CBC with WBC differential is normal.

Question 6.8.1 Which of these diagnoses can be absolutely ruled out based on this patient's history?
A) Coronary ischemia
B) Hypothyroidism
C) Lung cancer
D) Relapse of the Hodgkin lymphoma
E) None of the above

Answer 6.8.1 The correct answer is "E." The point here is that patients with a history of Hodgkin lymphoma and chest radiation are at risk for a wide range of complications—even years after the disease has been successfully treated. Even though 80% of Hodgkin lymphoma patients have long-term disease-free survival, one in six patients can be expected to die from late effects of therapy. The key late effects of radiation therapy for Hodgkin lymphoma include secondary malignancy ("C"), including breast cancer, lung cancer, leukemia, sarcoma, and non-Hodgkin lymphoma, and accelerated cardiac disease ("A") at a younger age (5 to 10 times that of age-matched controls).

Other delayed complications that have been associated with radiation therapy include thyroid dysfunction, predominantly hypothyroidism ("B"), pulmonary fibrosis, non-coronary atherosclerotic disease, and muscle atrophy.

....

The patient has a normal chest radiograph and ECG. However, her TSH is markedly elevated, and you start her on levothyroxine. You plan to see her back in 8 weeks for re-evaluation and will provide additional counseling at that time.

Question 6.8.2 Which of the following preventative health issues is/are necessary to address at follow-up?
A) Early intervention by a fertility specialist if the patient desires pregnancy
B) Smoking cessation
C) Yearly mammograms
D) Yearly skin exams
E) All of the above

Answer 6.8.2 The correct answer is "E." Female patients who were treated for Hodgkin lymphoma with chemotherapy and radiation prior to age 20 have up to a 35% incidence of breast cancer by the age of 40. The typical latency period is 15 years. National guidelines recommend that annual breast cancer screening of Hodgkin lymphoma survivors treated with chest irradiation should begin 5 years post-treatment (no earlier than age 25), or age 40, whichever comes first. Breast cancer screening for these high-risk patients includes breast MRI in addition to mammography, although the evidence for this approach is scant. Smokers with a history of Hodgkin lymphoma have a 20-fold increased chance of developing lung cancer when compared to nonsmokers with a history of Hodgkin lymphoma. At least yearly skin exams are recommended along with the routine physical examination. Also, female patients with Hodgkin lymphoma have a 69% incidence of premature ovarian failure if treated for their cancer before the age of 29 and up to 96% if treated after the age of 30. While these statistics are improving with newer chemotherapy regimens, a patient should seek early referral to a fertility specialist if she desires pregnancy but is unable to conceive.

▶ **Objectives: Did you learn to …**
- List late complications of young adult lymphoma survivors?

▶ **CASE 6.9**

A 40-year-old male who has just received his first course of chemotherapy for non-Hodgkin lymphoma (NHL) presents to your ED complaining of weakness, cramps, and decreased urine output. He has no other medical problems and takes no medications except for prochlorperazine as needed for nausea. He has been eating and drinking well. His physical examination reveals a tired-appearing male, with normal vital signs. His head-and-neck examination reveals bilateral palpable cervical lymph nodes (2 cm). His lungs are clear in the upper lung fields with crackles bilaterally at the bases.

Muscle strength is normal, and reflexes are 3+ and symmetric. He exhibits 6 beats of clonus at the ankles. Chest radiograph shows evidence of early pulmonary edema.

Question 6.9.1 What is the most likely set of laboratory values you will find for this patient (reference ranges: potassium 3.5–5 mg/dL, phosphate 2.4–4.1 mg/dL, uric acid 3.5–7.2 mg/dL, calcium 8.5–10.2 mg/dL).
A) Potassium 2.3 mEq/L, phosphorus 3.1 mg/dL, uric acid 4 mg/dL, calcium 9 mg/dL
B) Potassium 2.6 mEq/L, phosphorus 6 mg/dL, uric acid 5 mg/dL, calcium 12 mg/dL
C) Potassium 6.5 mEq/L, phosphorus 7 mg/dL, uric acid 18 mg/dL, calcium 6 mg/dL
D) Potassium 6 mEq/L, phosphorus 6.8 mg/dL, uric acid 5 mg/dL, calcium 6.7 mg/dL
E) Potassium 4.5 mEq/L, phosphorus 3.2 mg/dL, uric acid 9 mg/dL, calcium 8 mg/dL

Answer 6.9.1 The correct answer is "C." This patient most likely has tumor lysis syndrome, which can occur in a patient with a highly responsive leukemia or a bulky lymphoma being treated with chemotherapy (it rarely occurs without treatment). Tumor lysis syndrome occurs when there is rapid release of intracellular contents into the bloodstream. It is characterized by high potassium, high phosphorus, high uric acid, and low calcium. Patients may experience renal failure, arrhythmias, fatigue, muscle cramps, and tetany.

....

The patient is found to have a creatinine of 8 mg/dL.

Question 6.9.2 What is the most likely cause of this patient's renal failure?
A) Dehydration
B) Heart failure
C) Hemoglobinuria
D) Rhabdomyolysis related to chemotherapy
E) Uric acid nephropathy

Answer 6.9.2 The correct answer is "E." Patients with tumor lysis syndrome may have renal failure secondary to uric acid nephropathy. This is caused by the precipitation of uric acid in the kidney. It can be prevented by starting allopurinol prior to the administration of chemotherapy. Although dehydration ("A") is not the cause of renal failure, it certainly will exacerbate the situation.

Question 6.9.3 Which of the following is MOST LIKELY to help this patient's current condition?
A) Allopurinol 300 mg orally
B) Calcium carbonate 500 mg orally
C) Emergent hemodialysis
D) IV D5W with 2 amps bicarbonate
E) IV normal saline 200 mL/hr

Answer 6.9.3 The correct answer is "C." The horses are already out of the barn, and in fact they're probably over the hills and through the woods. Allopurinol and oral calcium will not help this situation. The patient already has renal failure from his tumor lysis syndrome. While he may benefit from preventive measures, including aggressive hydration and allopurinol **prior to undergoing chemotherapy**, none of these measures are going to help his current renal failure. In addition, the patient may develop worsening pulmonary edema if given too much volume with IV fluids.

While awaiting hemodialysis, you should treat the patient's hyperkalemia. Treatment may include IV calcium gluconate, insulin and dextrose, and oral sodium polystyrene sulfonate (Kayexalate). Note that sodium bicarbonate for hyperkalemia has fallen out of favor.

HELPFUL TIP:
Rasburicase has also been approved for the prevention of tumor lysis syndrome. It converts uric acid into a nontoxic, excretable metabolite allantoin. It can also be used after tumor lysis syndrome has started. It has several black box warnings including: anaphylaxis, hemolysis, and methemoglobinemia. Its use is considered high risk in pregnancy. Except for the side effects noted above, it is well-tolerated, acts rapidly, and is effective. The need of dialysis secondary to tumor lysis syndrome has substantially declined since the introduction of rasburicase.

▶ **Objectives: Did you learn to …**
  · Diagnose and initiate treatment of tumor lysis syndrome?

 QUICK QUIZ: TOO MUCH OF A GOOD THING

A 60-year-old gentleman presents to your office with complaints of fatigue. He has a history of alcoholic cirrhosis, diet-controlled diabetes, and hypertension. He currently takes hydrochlorothiazide, enalapril, and monthly testosterone injections. He smokes two packs of cigarettes daily and consumes 6 to 8 beers nightly. His physical examination reveals an obese, ruddy-faced man with a temperature of 37°C, pulse 90 bpm, BP 164/80 mm Hg, and respirations 14 bpm. He is found to have a hematocrit of 54%.

Which of the following items in his history is LEAST likely to explain the elevated hematocrit?
A) Alcoholic cirrhosis
B) Diabetes
C) Antihypertensive medications
D) Testosterone injections
E) Smoking

The correct answer is "B." Diabetes should not cause an elevated hematocrit and often causes anemia secondary to renal disease and reduced responsiveness to erythropoietin. Approach an elevated hematocrit with two questions: (1) Is it due to increased RBC mass or decreased plasma volume? (2) Is it primary erythrocytosis or secondary?

This patient has many potential secondary causes of an elevated hematocrit. "A," alcoholic cirrhosis can lead to hepatocellular carcinoma which, along with other malignancies (e.g., renal cell carcinoma), can result in overproduction of erythropoietin, causing an elevated hematocrit. Diuretics ("C") decrease plasma volume, causing an elevation of hematocrit which is **not** a true polycythemia. Testosterone injections ("D") may cause polycythemia. Finally, he has a significant smoking history ("E") that may produce a secondary polycythemia due to hypoxia and cor pulmonale.

▶ **CASE 6.10**

A 30-year-old female presents to your office for a routine visit. She was hospitalized for an appendectomy and at the time of surgery, her platelet count was found to be 1,400,000/mm³, which her surgeon felt was most likely reactive. She has no other past medical history, is asymptomatic, and exercises three times per week. You repeat the CBC, showing WBC 5,000/mm³, Hgb 13 g/dL, and platelet count 800,000/mm³.

Question 6.10.1 What is your next step in managing this patient?
A) Anticoagulation with warfarin to a goal INR of 2 to 3
B) Counseling against becoming pregnant
C) Initiation of hydroxyurea 500 mg BID
D) No further evaluation or follow-up necessary
E) Observation and periodic evaluation of her CBC

Answer 6.10.1 The correct answer is "E." This patient likely has essential thrombocythemia (ET), which is the most common myeloproliferative disorder in the United States. ET is more common in females. Patients are typically older when diagnosed with median age of 60. It is rare in children younger than 14 years of age. Patients with ET have a higher rate of mortality than matched controls due to risk of thrombosis (arterial > venous) and bleeding events. In order to diagnose ET, other causes of thrombocytosis (e.g., inflammation, iron deficiency, recent surgery, infection, bleeding, and malignancy) must be excluded. A bone marrow biopsy may be helpful in establishing the diagnosis by demonstrating adequate iron stores and ruling out chronic myelogenous leukemia (CML) or myelodysplasia.

"A" is incorrect. Warfarin would not be appropriate prophylactic therapy and would not be used unless the patient had a thromboembolic event. Aspirin *can* be used especially for the vasomotor symptoms associated with essential thrombocythemia (erythromelalgia [a burning pain in the hands and feet], acral paresthesias, headache, lightheadedness, etc.). Aspirin should also be considered if the platelet count is greater than 1,500,000/mm³. "B" is incorrect. Although patients with ET have a high rate of spontaneous abortion, many can have normal, healthy pregnancies. The patient should be counseled regarding pregnancy risks. "C" is also incorrect. The patient is at low risk for thromboembolic events (platelet count <1,500,000/mm³, young age, no comorbid illness, or prior events). Hydroxyurea could be considered if the patient was at high risk for thrombo-embolic events or symptomatic.

HELPFUL TIP:
The most common cause of an abnormally high platelet count is reactive thrombocytosis, which can result from iron deficiency, infection, inflammation, or malignancy. There is no increase in bleeding or clotting risk in patients with reactive thrombocytosis. The diagnosis of ET can only be made once reactive thrombocytosis and the presence of other chronic myeloproliferative disorders are ruled out.

▶ **Objectives: Did you learn to …**
· Recognize the presentation and implication of essential thrombocytosis?

▶ CASE 6.11

A 15-year-old female presents to your office complaining of fatigue. She reports menarche at age 13 and complains of heavy menses. Her physical examination reveals a well-developed, well-nourished, pale female. You find no hepatosplenomegaly. Her laboratory results reveal a WBC 6,000/mm³, Hgb 8.9 g/dL, hematocrit 27%, platelet count 400,000/mm³, MCV 72 fL (low), red blood cell distribution width (RDW) 16 (high). You order more laboratory tests.

Question 6.11.1 What are the expected findings in this patient?
A) Increased iron, decreased ferritin, increased total iron binding capacity
B) Decreased iron, decreased ferritin, decreased total iron binding capacity
C) Increased iron, increased ferritin, increased total iron binding capacity
D) Decreased iron, increased ferritin, decreased total iron binding capacity
E) Decreased iron, decreased ferritin, increased total iron binding capacity

Answer 6.11.1 The correct answer is "E." This patient likely has iron deficiency anemia related to her heavy menses. Iron deficiency anemia is characterized by anemia along with a decreased serum iron, decreased ferritin, increased total iron binding capacity (TIBC), and decreased transferrin saturation. The decrease in serum ferritin is proportional to the decrease in total body iron stores. Hypochromic microcytic RBCs are found on peripheral smear. See Table 6-3 for a general guide to the causes of anemia based on red cell indices.

HELPFUL TIP:
The prevalence of VWD in women with menorrhagia ranges from 5% to 20%. Always make sure to take a good personal and family bleeding history.

TABLE 6-3 CAUSES OF ANEMIA BY RED CELL VOLUME

Low MCV (usually <80 fL)	Normal MCV (usually 80–100 fL)	High MCV (usually >100 fL)
Anemia of chronic disease Copper deficiency Iron deficiency anemia Lead poisoning Sideroblastic anemias Thalassemias	Acute blood loss Anemia of chronic disease Chronic renal insufficiency Early iron deficiency Endocrine (e.g., hypothyroidism) Primary bone marrow disorders	Alcohol effects B12 deficiency Drug effect (e.g., Hydroxyurea, AZT) Folate deficiency Hemolytic anemia Hypothyroidism (less commonly macrocytic, usually normocytic) Liver disease Primary bone marrow disease Reticulocytosis (hemolytic anemia, response to blood loss)

HELPFUL TIP:
Even if it looks like iron deficiency anemia, always consider other causes of anemia such as B12 deficiency, folate deficiency, and thalassemia. Often patients will have more than one cause for their anemia. Mixed vitamin B12 and iron deficiencies may present with normocytic anemia with an elevated RDW.

You start iron supplementation therapy in this patient.

Question 6.11.2 Which of the following tests will be the first to indicate that you have instituted appropriate therapy and that the patient is responding?
A) Increase in hematocrit
B) Increase in reticulocyte count
C) Increase in serum-free hemoglobin
D) Decrease in ferritin
E) Decrease in transferrin saturation

Answer 6.11.2 The correct answer is "B." The patient's reticulocyte count will increase first—before the hematocrit ("A"). This should start soon after treatment and maximize at 7 to 10 days. Pica (if present) should also resolve fairly early. "C" is incorrect. Only in exceptional circumstances (intravascular hemolysis) will there be free hemoglobin in the blood. "D" is incorrect because the ferritin is low in iron deficiency anemia and should increase with therapy. Finally, transferrin saturation ("E") should increase in patients once you start to treat their anemia, but the reticulocyte count increases first.

HELPFUL TIP:
Ferritin is not a useful test for iron deficiency in hospitalized patients or in those who are chronically ill. Ferritin is

an acute-phase reactant and thus may be elevated in these patients even when the patient has iron deficiency anemia (where the ferritin should be low). However, you can check a soluble transferrin receptor. See below for more.

HELPFUL TIP:
There may be no reticulocytosis with treatment of iron deficiency if the patient is simply iron deficient without anemia.

Question 6.11.3 How long should you continue iron supplementation once the patient's labs have normalized?
A) Stop immediately once anemia has resolved
B) Continue 3 to 6 months after the anemia has resolved
C) Continue for 1 year after the anemia has resolved
D) Indefinite iron supplementation is indicated

Answer 6.11.3 The correct answer is "B." Continue iron for 3 to 6 months once the anemia has resolved. Also address the underlying problem. In this patient, treat her heavy menstrual periods, which may respond to hormonal contraception, tranexamic acid, etc.

The patient returns in 2 months but her labs, if anything, are worse than at first presentation. The patient swears that she has been taking the iron faithfully.

Question 6.11.4 Which of the following can lead to a failure of iron therapy for iron deficiency anemia?
A) Proton pump inhibitors (PPIs)
B) Incorrect diagnosis
C) Oral antacids (e.g., calcium carbonate)
D) Atrophic gastritis, celiac disease, or *Helicobacter pylori* infection
E) All of the above

Answer 6.11.4 The correct answer is "E." Anything that neutralizes the stomach pH will interfere with iron absorption, including PPIs, antacids, and loss of acid-producing cells (e.g., pernicious anemia). Other GI diseases (e.g., celiac disease, *H. pylori*) can also interfere with iron absorption. Tea and some green leafy vegetables can also reduce iron absorption.

HELPFUL TIP:
Vitamin C (supplements or orange juice) enhances iron absorption and should be considered if a patient is not responding to iron therapy. Meat can also increase iron absorption (which we hate to say because one of us is a vegetarian … however, the truth hurts).

HELPFUL TIP:
A widened RDW and an elevated platelet count are typical of iron deficiency anemia. Conversely, the RDW will be normal in thalassemias.

The patient returns to your office and finally admits she has not been able to take the iron because of side effects. She has started a prenatal vitamin for the folate. Her hemoglobin is now down to 7.2 g/dL. She still feels fatigued. The patient will not agree to take any further iron orally. However, she is willing to consider other suggestions.

Question 6.11.5 What is your next step?
A) Encourage the patient to take the iron preparation along with calcium carbonate (Tums) to reduce the GI side effects
B) Continue her prenatal vitamin only and encourage her to eat more red meat
C) Give iron sucrose 200 mg IV weekly for 4 weeks
D) Transfuse 2 units of PRBCs immediately

Answer 6.11.5 The correct answer is "C." If oral iron preparations are not tolerated, IV iron preparations are available. Intramuscular preparations are best avoided due to pain at the injection site, skin discoloration, and risk for infection. The most commonly used options for IV replacement include iron dextran and iron sucrose. Iron dextran carries a risk of anaphylaxis in 0.6% to 2.3% of patients and other side effects in up to 25% of patients, including: bronchospasm, flushing, headache, fever, urticaria, nausea, vomiting, hypotension, seizures, myalgias, arthralgias, and increased thromboembolic events. Iron sucrose has a lower incidence of side effects—typically nausea, constipation, diarrhea, or a transient minty taste—and may be given to patients who have had a previous reaction to iron dextran.

There have been more recent developments of dextran-free infusions that can be provided more quickly and over a two-dose administration. Ferric carboxymaltose (Injectafer) and ferumoxytol (Feraheme) IV are other options to use for iron deficiency anemia in patients intolerant to iron or in those with CKD. Ferric carboxymaltose (Injectafer) is provided as 750 mg infusion over 15 minutes with repeat dose in 7 days. Ferumoxytol (FeraHeme) is provided as 510 mg infusion over 15 minutes with repeat dose in 3 to 8 days. Most common adverse reactions are: hypersensitivity, diarrhea, headache, nausea, dizziness, and hypotension.

"A" is incorrect because calcium will interfere with iron absorption. Additionally, she has dug in on her position of not taking oral iron, so it's time to try a different approach. "B" is incorrect because she needs more iron than can be provided through prenatal vitamins and her diet. Finally, "D" is incorrect as transfusion carries potential risks that could be avoided if she responds to IV iron replacement.

HELPFUL TIP:
Every other day iron seems to be just as effective as daily iron and may help to minimize side effects. In fact, iron absorption is higher with every other day iron (*Lancet Haematol.* 2017;4(11):e524).

▶ **Objectives: Did you learn to …**
· Obtain a thorough history in an anemic patient?
· Use laboratory parameters to identify the etiology of anemia?
· Initiate treatment for iron deficiency anemia?

▶ CASE 6.12

A 52-year-old woman with a history of rheumatoid arthritis is in your clinic for a 1-month follow-up after having a knee prosthesis removed secondary to a joint infection and osteomyelitis (*Staphylococcal aureus*). You obtain a CBC, revealing a WBC 8,000/mm³, Hgb 9.5 g/dL, hematocrit 28%, platelet count 450,000/mm³, and MCV 83 fL (normal). Serum iron levels are low with a normal serum transferrin receptor and increased ferritin.

Question 6.12.1 What is the most likely diagnosis?
A) Iron deficiency anemia due to rheumatoid arthritis
B) Anemia of chronic disease due to rheumatoid arthritis and osteomyelitis
C) Hemolytic anemia induced by antibiotics
D) Acute blood loss during surgery
E) Myelodysplastic syndrome (MDS) associated with rheumatoid arthritis

Answer 6.12.1 The correct answer is "B." Anemia of chronic disease is a hypoproliferative anemia that occurs in the setting of chronic infection, inflammation, malignancy, heart failure, diabetes, and other serious health conditions. The anemia is usually mild and characterized by low serum iron, increased ferritin (remember that ferritin is an acute-phase reactant and these patients often have inflammation), decreased serum transferrin, normal (or low) serum soluble transferrin receptor level, and decreased transferrin saturation (see below for more on the soluble transferrin receptor). In addition, reticulocyte count is typically low, erythropoietin may be mildly elevated, and peripheral smear may show hypochromic, microcytic RBCs, or normochromic, normocytic RBCs. If differentiation between iron deficiency anemia and anemia of chronic disease is not apparent, a bone marrow biopsy can be obtained to assess iron stores.

▶ **Objectives: Did you learn to …**
· Recognize a typical presentation of anemia of chronic disease/inflammation and the expected laboratory findings?

▶ CASE 6.13

A previously healthy 3-year-old female with a history of anorexia and irritability for 3 days is brought to your ED by her mother. On the day of admission, the child is difficult to arouse. You learn that her 6-year-old brother has had some difficulty reaching appropriate developmental milestones and is a "fussy eater."

Physical examination reveals a slightly pale-appearing child, who responds to tactile stimuli but not to voice. Vitals are normal and her examination is unremarkable except for her decreased level of consciousness. Laboratory studies include a WBC 8,000/mm³, Hgb 10 g/dL, platelet count 300,000/mm³, and MCV 75 fL (microcytic). Her urine dipstick is normal, except for 1 + glucose; there are no ketones in the urine. Her blood chemistries are within normal limits, with the exception of a phosphorous of 2 mg/dL (low). Her peripheral blood smear shows red cells with coarse basophilic stippling.

Question 6.13.1 What is the best working diagnosis at this time?
A) Acute lead poisoning
B) Anemia of chronic disease
C) Early diabetic ketoacidosis (DKA)
D) Severe iron deficiency anemia
E) Unrecognized bacteremia secondary to pyelonephritis

Answer 6.13.1 The correct answer is "A." Lead poisoning should be considered in a child presenting with symptoms of encephalopathy and anemia with basophilic stippling on RBCs. Basophilic stippling occurs when ribosome precipitates litter the RBCs. Basophilic stippling can be seen in alcohol abuse, thalassemias, and heavy metal poisoning. This child's brother also shows some symptoms consistent with lead poisoning with delayed developmental milestones and "picky eating" (anorexia). A child presenting in this manner should have a blood lead level checked to rule out elevated lead levels as an underlying cause. "B," anemia of chronic disease, is unlikely because this illness is acute. "C," DKA, is unlikely because urine ketones are 99% sensitive for DKA and her urine ketones are normal. "D" is unlikely because there should be no neurologic symptoms associated with iron deficiency anemia. "E," pyelonephritis, is unlikely because the patient is afebrile and has a normal white count and negative urine. We could have tipped you off to the answer with a "Flint, Michigan" reference but that would have been no fun.

HELPFUL TIP:
Lead levels >10 mcg/dL may cause developmental delay, loss of milestones (especially language), encephalopathy, seizures, cerebral edema, and cognitive impairment. CNS effects are especially problematic in children < 6 years old who have an incomplete blood–brain barrier. Lead paint in houses built before the 1970s and use of imported products such as pottery, solder, cosmetics, and crayons (and some toys made in China) still provide sources of lead ingestion. Children born in a foreign country and/or with recent foreign residence may also be at risk.

HELPFUL TIP:
Other symptoms of lead intoxication include: anorexia, decreased activity, irritability, insomnia, hearing loss, peripheral neuropathy, SIADH, decreased renal function, and anemia. Laboratory findings may include: anemia, signs of hemolysis, coarse basophilic stippling on RBCs, glycosuria, hypophosphatemia, positive qualitative urine coproporphyrin, and moderate increases in free erythrocyte protoporphyrin.

The patient's lead level is 70 mcg/dL. Because of your concern about acute lead intoxication and resulting encephalopathy, you decide to admit the child and treat her with dimercaprol and calcium disodium edetate (CaNa2EDTA).

Question 6.13.2 **All of the following are true EXCEPT:**
A) Dimercaprol should not be given if the child has a peanut allergy
B) The child's diet should be monitored for adequate intake of calories, iron, and calcium
C) The child's sibling should be tested, and arrangements should be made for close follow-up for both children
D) The dose of dimercaprol should be tripled for patients with glucose-6-phosphate dehydrogenase (G6PD) deficiency

Answer 6.13.2 **The correct answer is "D."** Dimercaprol is a lead chelator used to treat elevated lead levels. It is administered

intramuscularly, is water insoluble, and must be given in a peanut oil vehicle; hence, it should be avoided in individuals with a peanut allergy ("A"). **It may cause hemolysis in individuals with G6PD deficiency**, so these patients should be monitored closely and not receive larger doses of dimercaprol. It is important to test siblings of an affected child ("C"), because the source of lead is often in the house. Close follow-up of affected children is essential to monitor for increasing blood lead levels after treatment, which may indicate the source of lead has not been removed. The absorption of lead can be made worse by malnutrition, iron deficiency, and poor intake of calcium ("B"). Iron deficiency frequently occurs in affected patients and may worsen anemia. Other chelating agents include calcium disodium EDTA and d-penicillamine and succimer. It is recommended to use a combination of dimercaprol and EDTA for children with severe lead intoxication.

HELPFUL TIP:
A large percentage of lead is absorbed into bone with a half-life of greater than 25 years. In periods of physiologic stress, the inert pool of lead can be mobilized and released into the bloodstream, producing signs and symptoms of lead intoxication years after the initial exposure.

▶ **Objectives: Did you learn to …**
· Recognize the presentation of lead poisoning and the attendant changes in blood counts and cell indices?
· Initiate treatment for lead poisoning?

▶ **CASE 6.14**

A 6-month-old male infant is brought to you for a well-baby check-up. His mother reports that the child has had difficulty with feeding, has frequent colds, and is often irritable. She has noted recurrent episodes of jaundice, especially when he is sick. His physical examination reveals a small child, faintly jaundiced. His temperature is 37.5°C, pulse 160 bpm, BP 85/50 mm Hg, and respirations 30 bpm. His abdomen is soft with palpable splenomegaly. The remainder of the examination is unremarkable. Laboratories reveal a WBC 13,000/mm³, Hgb 9 g/dL, platelet count 260,000/mm³, and MCV 60 fL (low). He is noted to have target cells on peripheral blood smear.

Question 6.14.1 **Which one of the following is the most appropriate next step?**
A) Order PT/PTT
B) Order hemoglobin electrophoresis
C) Transfuse with 1 unit of PRBCs
D) Test for G6PD deficiency
E) Test for sickle cell anemia

Answer 6.14.1 **The correct answer is "B."** The clinical and laboratory presentation is consistent with a hereditary hemoglobinopathy, most likely a thalassemia. The splenomegaly, significant anemia, target cells, and the profoundly low MCV are all suggestive of thalassemia; patients with thalassemia often have recurrent episodes of jaundice reflecting hemolysis. He has no history of abnormal bleeding, so "A" would not be indicated. Also, as the child does not appear to be in distress, "C" would be an incorrect answer. G6PD-deficient patients experience episodes of hemolytic anemia. Peripheral smear review at that time may reveal bite or blister cells, rather than target cells, so "D" is not the right answer. "E" is incorrect since the peripheral smear would reveal sickle cells if the patient had sickle disease.

Beta thalassemia major is confirmed by hemoglobin electrophoresis.

Question 6.14.2 Which of the following regarding his management is NOT true?
A) Untreated, mortality may approach 80% by 5 years of age
B) Frequent blood transfusions may be required
C) The condition will improve with age
D) The child is likely to have growth retardation and delayed sexual maturation
E) Without iron chelation therapy, there is a high incidence of mortality with this disease

Answer 6.14.2 **The correct (and not true) answer is "C."** Beta thalassemia refers to the disease state in which there are mutations in both genes that code for beta globin. Without treatment, mortality from thalassemia major approaches 80% by 5 years of age. Patients with beta thalassemia will eventually develop iron overload, even without blood transfusions. The use of transfusions and concurrent chelation therapy with deferoxamine has reduced long-term complications related to the disease. Deferasirox (Exjade, Jadenu), an oral chelating agent, is available as an alternative to deferoxamine. Bone marrow transplant can be curative. Therapies to improve erythropoiesis and gene therapy are also being studied. Beta thalassemia minor (or beta trait) is much less severe and occurs when only one of the genes is defective.

HELPFUL TIP:
The FDA has approved deferiprone (Ferriprox) as an alternative chelating agent in transfusion-acquired iron overload. It is second line but can be administered orally. It can be considered when deferasirox is not effective and the patient is unable to use deferoxamine, the parenteral option.

HELPFUL TIP:
Alpha thalassemia has a more variable course. There are four alpha globin genes. If all four genes are defective, intrauterine fetal demise is the rule. When one gene is defective, there is a silent carrier state. When two genes are defective, there is a mild microcytic anemia. Here is

a memory aid: there are four alpha globin genes and "4" looks kind of like the Greek letter alpha; beta is the second letter in the Greek alphabet and beta globin has two genes.

HELPFUL TIP:
Because of the persistence of fetal hemoglobin (HbF) in the circulation up to 6 months of age, hemoglobinopathies might not be apparent until that time.

HELPFUL TIP:
Thalassemias may be erroneously diagnosed as iron deficiency anemia due to a low MCV. Consider testing for thalassemia in a patient with microcytic anemia, normal or increased iron levels, a normal RDW (less reliable), and appropriate ethnic background (e.g., Mediterranean or African descent).

HELPFUL TIP:
In other Hgb synthesis related news ... when you see that middle-aged patient with abdominal pain and psychiatric symptoms for the tenth (or twentieth or thirtieth) time, think of acute intermittent porphyria before you make the diagnosis of somatization disorder.

▶ **Objectives: Did you learn to ...**
• Recognize symptoms and RBC indices associated with thalassemia?

▶ **CASE 6.15**

A woman brings her 10-week-old female infant for evaluation. The child is colicky and irritable after feeding. She was born full term but has not been gaining weight appropriately. The patient's sister has sickle cell trait, so you obtain an Hgb electrophoresis, which ultimately demonstrates SS genotype.

Question 6.15.1 Which of the following is INCORRECT regarding the child's care?
A) The patient should remain on prophylactic antibiotics until the age of 5 years due to a high risk of pneumococcal sepsis
B) The child may develop splenomegaly and lymphadenopathy related to her disease
C) The disease provides protection against infection with parvovirus
D) The child may not develop pain crisis until she is older due to protection from HbF
E) The child is likely to have a delay in puberty

Answer 6.15.1 **The correct (actually "incorrect") answer is "C."** The patient has homozygous SS sickle cell disease. This child's mother should be counseled regarding the importance of continuing antibiotic prophylaxis until the age of 5 years ("A"), because her child is at high risk for pneumococcal sepsis. Sickle cell disease is protective against malaria, not parvovirus ("C"). In fact, parvovirus infection can be life-threatening in these patients due to the development of aplastic anemia.

During infancy, children may be noted to have reticulocytosis, hemolytic anemia, and sickling by 10 to 12 weeks. At 5 to 6 months, splenomegaly may be noted, and lymphadenopathy ("B") may be prominent between 6 months and 5 years. The earliest pain crisis often involves hands and feet (dactylitis) and occurs after the HbF decreases to adult values ("D"); this usually does not occur until after the age of 4 years. The spleen involutes by 5 to 8 years. Puberty is delayed by an average of 2.5 years ("E").

HELPFUL TIP:
Sickle trait, the condition in which a patient is heterozygous for Hb S, is associated with a normal life expectancy and no symptoms other than occasional hematuria and inability to concentrate urine. Pain crises are extremely rare and occur only in the settings of a low oxygen atmosphere (e.g., very high altitude) or extreme physical activity (e.g., running a marathon).

The child follows regularly with you for years, and she begins to develop more frequent pain crises in college. She is found to have an elevated C-reactive protein, increased LDH, and decreasing Hgb. You explain to her that some measures can be taken to reduce the frequency of pain crises.

Question 6.15.2 These measures include all of the following EXCEPT:
A) Initiation of hydroxyurea therapy
B) Avoidance of hot showers
C) Prompt treatment of infections
D) Adequate hydration and nutrition
E) Avoidance of emotional stress

Answer 6.15.2 **The correct (rather "incorrect") answer is "B."** Two main features of sickle cell disease are shortened RBC survival and vasoocclusion due to poorly deformable RBC membranes. Pain episodes occur due to acute episodes of tissue hypoxemia and microinfarction. Crises can be precipitated by stress, fatigue, cold weather (not hot showers, which cause problems in multiple sclerosis patients), infection, dehydration, acidosis, and poor nutrition (options "C–E"). The use of hydroxyurea ("A") promotes increased levels of HbF, and HbF is associated with decreased frequency and severity of pain crises.

HELPFUL TIP:
Acute chest syndrome (ACS) should be suspected when a sickle cell patient presents with fever, cough, chest pain, and pulmonary infiltrates on chest x-ray. ACS may be due to infection or pulmonary infarction. Treatment involves

aggressive pain management, antibiotics for respiratory pathogens, supplemental oxygen, cautious hydration, venous thromboembolism prophylaxis, and blood transfusion if the patient is significantly anemic. Exchange transfusion may also be required in more severe cases.

HELPFUL TIP:
For patients with sickle cell disease, simply replacing volume is usually appropriate. However for primary and secondary stroke prevention, transfuse/exchange transfuse so that the HbS is <30%. For presurgical patients, simply getting the Hbg to 10 g/dL seems adequate.

Since you first met that little baby girl, 22 years have elapsed, and she is getting married—and you are getting old (the alternative is worse, of course). She is concerned about significant illness related to her disease. You counsel her regarding the most common causes of morbidity and mortality.

Question 6.15.3 All of the following statements are true EXCEPT:
A) ACS and pain crises are the most common causes for hospital admission for patients with sickle cell disease
B) Eighty percent of patients develop cholelithiasis by the age of 35 years
C) Strokes may occur in 8% of patients by the age of 14 years, may be either symptomatic or clinically silent, and tend to be recurrent
D) Heart failure, pulmonary fibrosis, pulmonary hypertension, and renal failure complicate fluid management, transfusions, and maintenance of adequate oxygenation
E) Pregnancy should be avoided under any circumstance

Answer 6.15.3 **The correct answer (and exception) is "E."** The average life expectancy in patients with Hb SS is 42 years for men and 48 years for women. Maternal mortality occurs in about 1% of pregnancies. All of the rest are true including cerebrovascular events causing seizures and possible cognitive difficulty early in life. Of particular note, renal failure may be the cause of death in up to 10% of cases. Avascular necrosis and osteomyelitis (classically as a result of *Salmonella* infection), chronic skin ulcers, and priapism are also common.

▸ **Objectives: Did you learn to …**
• Recognize the presentation and implication of sickle cell disease?
• Initiate management of sickle cell disease?

QUICK QUIZ: THE CURIOUS CASE OF THE MISSING VITAMIN

A 72-year-old gentleman is brought to your office because a home health nurse noted he was becoming progressively weaker and more fatigued. He has a history of celiac disease for which he follows a strict gluten-free diet, but he has not been eating well. He also has a history of a seizure disorder and takes phenytoin. His review of systems is positive for dyspnea on exertion and mild anorexia. He has no other symptoms.

Physical examination reveals a thin, pale-appearing man with normal vital signs. His conjunctivae are pale and his tongue is smooth, with moist mucosa and no oropharyngeal lesions. The remainder of the examination is unremarkable. A CBC reveals a WBC 4,500/mm^3, Hgb 9 g/dL, hematocrit 28%, platelet count 140,000/mm^3, MCV 102 fL, RDW 14, and B12 level 900 ng/L (normal).

Which of the following statements is most likely FALSE?
A) The patient may have a high homocysteine level
B) The patient's condition could be made better with a trial of folate replacement
C) The patient may have a low RBC folate level
D) The patient's condition will likely require chronic blood transfusions
E) The patient may have a normal serum folate level

The correct (and False) answer is "D." This patient likely has folate deficiency, given a normal B12, macrocytic anemia, and risk factors for folate deficiency—old age, poor diet, avoidance of gluten (flour is normally fortified with folate), use of phenytoin, and possible malabsorption due to GI disease (celiac disease in this case, but also any other infiltrating or inflammatory process of the bowel). Dietary deficiency is uncommon in the United States due to supplementation of grain products with folate. Foods naturally high in folate include melons, bananas, leaf vegetables, asparagus, and broccoli. The recommended intake is 400 μg/day, and the body stores approximately a 4-month supply. If he has had recent adequate folate intake, the serum folate level may be normal, but the RBC folate will still be low, reflecting the deficiency (think of it as the HbA1C of folate).

To differentiate folate from B12 deficiency, check serum homocysteine and methylmalonate levels. Both will be elevated with B12 deficiency, while only homocysteine will be elevated in folate deficiency. Remember, you must exclude B12 deficiency before replacing folate because folate replacement can reverse the anemia, but will permit progression of neurologic effects of B12 deficiency, so "B" is true.

HELPFUL TIP:
Folate replacement is dosed as 1 to 5 mg daily for 1 to 4 months or until complete hematologic recovery occurs. If macrocytic anemia persists, other causes must be considered.

 QUICK QUIZ: REMEMBER THAT TAPEWORM FROM MEDICAL SCHOOL? HERE IT IS AGAIN!

A 47-year-old woman presents to your office complaining of tongue soreness, fatigue, and dyspnea with exertion. She denies unusual bleeding, weight loss, fevers, and night sweats. Her past medical history includes hypothyroidism, for which she takes levothyroxine. She does not drink alcohol or smoke. Physical examination reveals a tired-appearing woman with lemon-yellow colored skin, temperature 37°C, pulse 110 bpm, BP 120/74 mm Hg, and respirations 12 bpm. The examination is otherwise unremarkable. A CBC demonstrates a WBC count 4,000/mm^3, Hgb 9 g/dL, platelet count 140,000/mm^3, and an MCV of 105 fL. Her B12 level is 100 pg/mL (normal >300 pg/mL) and folate 40 ng/mL.

Which of the following historical elements is LEAST likely to contribute to her condition?
A) History of working as a park ranger in Canada
B) History of Zollinger–Ellison syndrome
C) History of hypothyroidism
D) History of new vegetarian diet started last month
E) History of GI surgery

The correct answer is "D." Most likely, this woman has pernicious anemia caused by B12 deficiency. Pernicious anemia is caused by immune destruction of parietal cells in the stomach, resulting in decreased absorption of B12. It typically develops in people over the age of 40 and is more common in people of northern European descent or in African Americans, as well as people with type A blood. Laboratory findings include anti-parietal cell antibodies in 90% of affected patients (5% of normal individuals also have the antibody) and antibodies to intrinsic factor in 70% of patients. Individuals commonly have other autoimmune diseases such as thyroid disease, diabetes, and vitiligo. Individuals may complain of paresthesias, GI symptoms, sore tongue, or weight loss. The lemon-yellow appearance of the skin is due to anemia and mild jaundice.

Other causes of cobalamin (B12) deficiency include gastrectomy, Zollinger–Ellison syndrome (inability to alkalinize the small intestine), blind loop syndrome, bacterial overgrowth from previous surgery, and ingestion of undercooked fish infested with the tapeworm *Diphyllobothrium latum* (found in Canada, Alaska, and the Baltics—hence, the history of working as a park ranger). Although a strict vegetarian diet can cause B12 deficiency, there are sufficient stores to last 3 to 5 years (in other words, more than 1 month).

 QUICK QUIZ: SAY, DID HE SWALLOW A PENNY?

A 21-year-old college student is brought to the ED by his friends because of bizarre behavior. His friends state that he has been acting "a little odd" lately, but they are unaware of any drug abuse. He does drink alcohol but is not known as a binge drinker—at least not by modern NCAA Division I drinking standards. His friends do not know his medical history but state he was taking a prescription drug for a "metabolic disorder," which he stopped several months ago. He is uncooperative, paranoid, and disoriented. You note brownish pigmentation of his corneas on physical examination. This may be the first—and last—case of Wilson disease you have ever seen.

Regarding this patient, which of the following is INCORRECT?

A) The patient has likely had episodes of hemolytic anemia in the past
B) The patient has likely discontinued penicillamine
C) The patient likely has an elevated ceruloplasmin level on blood test
D) The patient likely has hepatolenticular degeneration
E) The patient is at risk for hepatic failure

The correct answer is "C." This patient likely has Wilson disease (an autosomal-recessive defect in cellular copper export), which presents with **decreased** levels of ceruloplasmin, increased liver enzymes, and signs of hemolysis (from the direct toxic effect of copper on the cell). Symptoms typically present in the teens and early 20s. Presenting symptoms may include Kayser–Fleischer rings (golden-brown pigmentation of the cornea), hemolytic anemia, or neurologic symptoms, often mimicking psychiatric illness. Treatment of the disease includes lifelong therapy with penicillamine or trientine (chelating agents) and should be considered even for asymptomatic individuals known to have the disease. By the way, pennies are primarily zinc and contain little copper.

 QUICK QUIZ: "HOLE-Y BONES"

A 50-year-old man presents to your office with low-back pain of 8 weeks duration. He denies any history of trauma or overexertion. He notes the pain is constant and does not improve with positioning. Also, he has noticed some fatigue. He has no other complaints.

Physical examination reveals a well-nourished male with normal vital signs. His neurologic examination is normal. On musculoskeletal examination, he has midline point tenderness over T12. Plain films reveal a compression fracture at T12. A serum total protein level is 9 mg/dL (elevated), but the remainder of an evaluation for endocrine causes of osteoporosis is normal.

All of the following are necessary for the diagnosis of this patient EXCEPT:

A) Bone scan
B) Serum and urine protein electrophoresis with immunofixation
C) Bone marrow aspirate and biopsy
D) Quantitative immunoglobulins
E) Skeletal survey

The correct answer is "A." A spontaneous vertebral fracture in a 50-year-old male is definitely not normal. Multiple myeloma should be considered in patients with this presentation. Multiple myeloma is a clonal disorder of plasma cells. Risk factors include African-American race, male sex, and advancing age (median age of 60–65 at presentation). Workup for the diagnosis of multiple myeloma requires a serum and urine protein electrophoresis with immunofixation ("B"). This will help to identify a monoclonal protein. Quantitative immunoglobulins ("D") will help to assess whether this patient has an elevation of immunoglobulins in the range required for the diagnosis of multiple myeloma. A skeletal survey ("E") and bone marrow biopsy ("C") complete the diagnostic workup. A bone scan is not useful because the lytic lesions characteristic of multiple myeloma take up radioisotope only 20% of the time.

▶ CASE 6.16

On a routine insurance physical examination, a 55-year-old man was found to have a total protein of 9 g/dL (elevated). The remainder of his serum chemistries and his CBC were normal. He is active, feels well, and is not taking any medications. His physical examination is unremarkable. You order a serum and urine electrophoresis with immunofixation and quantitative immunoglobulins. He has a monoclonal spike with 1,400 g/dL of IgG kappa (elevated). His other immunoglobulins are within normal limits. A skeletal survey demonstrates no lytic lesions, and his bone marrow aspirate and biopsy demonstrate 6% plasma cells (normal is 1–4%). After the bone marrow biopsy, the hematologist sends him back to you for follow-up.

Question 6.16.1 **What is your next step in the management of this patient?**

A) Monitor blood, including serum immunoglobulins, every 3 to 6 months and, if stable after 1 year, annually thereafter
B) Monitor blood, including serum immunoglobulins, every 4 weeks indefinitely
C) Start on chemotherapy for multiple myeloma
D) Obtain yearly bone marrow biopsy and skeletal survey
E) No follow-up is necessary

Answer 6.16.1 **The correct answer is "A."** This patient has monoclonal gammopathy of undetermined significance, or MGUS, which is found in up to 3% of asymptomatic older (over 50 years old) individuals, mostly in Caucasians. A bone marrow biopsy indicating 10% plasma cells is required to make the diagnosis of multiple myeloma; this patient only has 6%. In addition, this patient has a normal CBC and is asymptomatic (no fatigue, bone pain suggestive of lesions, etc.). Thus, this patient has MGUS. Patients with MGUS typically do well, with only 1% per year progressing to multiple myeloma.

While patients should be reassured of the typically benign nature of this condition, up to 30% will have complications (multiple myeloma, amyloidosis, and other myeloproliferative disorders). After several unchanged immunoglobulin levels and normal CBCs within the 6 months of the initial diagnosis, annual or biannual evaluation should be adequate. Any changes in the patient's condition, such as unexplained anemia, increased immunoglobulin levels, renal insufficiency, or bony pain, should prompt further evaluation. An increase in immunoglobulin does not necessarily mean the monoclonal protein is increasing, and a serum protein electrophoresis and immunofixation should be obtained. Repeat bone marrow biopsy is indicated only if the clinical picture is confusing.

▶ **Objectives: Did you learn to ...**
  · Diagnose monoclonal gammopathy of undetermined significance?

▶ **CASE 6.17**

A 63-year-old woman presents to your office with complaint of fatigue. She states she felt like she spent the winter taking antibiotics because she developed "one infection after the other." Prior to this past winter, she had been well and did not take any prescription drugs regularly. Physical examination demonstrates a slightly pale, thin woman. Her temperature is 37.5°C, pulse 90 bpm, BP 120/58 mm Hg, and respirations 12 bpm. Her oropharynx demonstrates purpuric lesions. Her abdominal examination shows no organomegaly, and the remainder of the physical examination is unremarkable.

You obtain blood tests: WBC 2,100/mm³, Hgb 8.4 g/dL, and platelet count 20,000/mm³. A bone marrow aspirate and biopsy are obtained, which demonstrate a hypercellular marrow with 4% blasts, 4% ringed sideroblasts, and megakaryocytes. You talk to the hematologist, who suspects that your patient has a myelodysplastic syndrome (MDS).

Question 6.17.1 Which of the following statements is INCORRECT?
A) The small number of blasts in the bone marrow indicates a good prognosis
B) The patient cannot have MDS because she has pancytopenia
C) The patient may benefit from administration of erythropoietin
D) The patient may develop acute myeloid leukemia
E) The patient's gender may result in a better prognosis

Answer 6.17.1 The correct (rather "incorrect") answer is "B." Patients with MDS can be pancytopenic. MDS includes a number of clonal stem cell disorders characterized by dysplasia and ineffective hematopoiesis of one or more cell lines. The disease is typically one of older adults, with a median age of 65 to 70 years at onset; however, a better prognosis is associated with age <60 years and female gender. There is an increased risk of MDS in smokers, those exposed to benzene or alkylating agents, and with some hereditary disorders. Prognosis depends on the number of blasts, the number of lineages affected, and cytogenetic abnormalities. Median survival ranges from 10 to 66 months, and progression to acute leukemia ranges from 6% to 33% of patients, depending on the subtype of MDS.

Depending on the age and overall performance status of the individual MDS patient, treatment can range from supportive care with blood or platelet transfusions, to treatment with granulocyte colony stimulating factor (GCSF), to chemotherapeutics such as azacytidine, or even to bone marrow transplantation.

▶ **Objectives: Did you learn to ...**
  · Identify pancytopenia as a presentation of MDS?

 QUICK QUIZ: IT'S JUST KIDS' STUFF

All of the following are accurate statements about neutrophil counts in children EXCEPT:
A) African-American children may have a normal ANC of 1,000/mm³
B) Children over the age of 6 should be expected to have a normal ANC of 1,500 to 8,000/mm³
C) Neonates typically have a normal ANC of <500/mm³ at birth
D) Infants typically have 20% to 30% neutrophils on WBC differential
E) Five-year-old children have 50% neutrophils on WBC differential

The correct answer is "C." In the pediatric population, neutropenia is typically described as an ANC of <1,500/mm³. Up to 30% of African-American children have an *asymptomatic* ANC of <1,000/mm³ (e.g., no increased risk of infection). At birth, neutrophils make up the majority of the WBC differential (thus, more than 500, which is why "C" is an incorrect statement), decreasing to 20% to 30% after the first few days of life. At 5 years of age, neutrophils comprise approximately 50% of the differential, and this reaches 70% by puberty.

▶ **CASE 6.18**

A 49-year-old male presents to your office complaining of joint pain, fatigue, and increased urination. There is a family history of cirrhosis of the liver, apparently not related to alcohol. He does not take any medications and does not smoke but drinks two glasses of wine each night. Physical examination reveals a thin male with tanned skin (in the dead of winter in Iowa, so he is either rich or sick, take your choice) and normal vital signs. His heart and lung examinations are unremarkable. The abdomen is soft, nontender, and nondistended, and his liver edge is palpable 2 cm below the costal margin. He has pain with range of motion in his hips, knees, and MTP joints. The remainder of the examination is unrevealing. Serum electrolytes are normal, but his glucose is 282 g/dL. His transaminases are elevated.

Question 6.18.1 Of the following, what is the most likely diagnosis?
A) Alcoholic hepatitis
B) Colon cancer
C) Hemochromatosis
D) Vitamin B12 deficiency

Answer 6.18.1 The correct answer is "C." This patient presents with a "classic" history of hemochromatosis. Symptoms start during or after the fifth decade of life, are initially mild, and progress slowly. "Bronze diabetes" (bronze or tan skin color due to iron deposition accompanied by hyperglycemia) is sometimes noted. Most organs can eventually be involved, but most commonly symptoms are due to liver, cardiac, joint, and testicular involvement. "A," alcoholic hepatitis, is a consideration, but his reported use is unlikely to result in disease. You also would not expect to see some of the other symptoms (e.g., diabetes and arthritis) in relation to alcoholic hepatitis. "B," colon cancer, is unlikely to present in this way. "D," vitamin B12 deficiency, typically presents with anemia and neurologic symptoms.

Question 6.18.2 Which of the following laboratory values are most consistent with this patient's presentation?
A) Decreased iron, decreased ferritin, decreased transferrin saturation
B) Decreased iron, decreased ferritin, increased transferrin saturation
C) Increased iron, decreased ferritin, increased transferrin saturation
D) Increased iron, increased ferritin, decreased transferrin saturation
E) Increased iron, increased ferritin, increased transferrin saturation

Answer 6.18.2 **The correct answer is "E."** All of these iron studies (serum iron level, ferritin and transferrin saturation) are elevated in patients with hereditary hemochromatosis. A normal person maintains approximately 3 to 4 g of iron in the body. Normal individuals absorb about 1 mg/day of iron (10% of what is ingested), which is precisely balanced with loss through sweat, sloughing of cells, and GI losses. In hereditary hemochromatosis, 2 to 4 mg of iron is absorbed daily, resulting in the accumulation of iron.

The patient's diagnosis is confirmed, and you counsel him regarding his disease.

Question 6.18.3 All of the following statements are true EXCEPT:
A) This is an autosomal-dominant disease
B) Affected females typically present later in life due to increased iron losses
C) Patients may benefit from phlebotomy even after development of symptomatic disease
D) Patients are susceptible to unusual infections
E) Patients are at high risk for hepatocellular carcinoma

Answer 6.18.3 **The correct answer (or exception) is "A."** Hereditary hemochromatosis is an autosomal-**recessive** disorder. Approximately 10% of Caucasians are heterozygous, and 5/1,000 are homozygous for the gene mutation. Patients are at increased risk for infections ("D") due to *Listeria*, *Vibrio vulnificus* (sorry, no sushi!), and *Yersinia enterocolitica*. Affected females may present later in life due to increased iron losses from menstruation, pregnancy, and lactation ("B").

Treatment includes phlebotomy ("C") or chelation therapy if phlebotomy is contraindicated. Patients should be monitored closely for development of hepatoma, since therapy does not reduce the risk of hepatocellular carcinoma once cirrhosis is present ("E"). Family members should be screened for the disease so they can be started on therapy early, in order to prevent the development of cirrhosis.

HELPFUL TIP:
Hemochromatosis is a genetic disease; therefore, identifying a defect in the HFE gene makes the definitive diagnosis. Patients may have high ferritin levels for many reasons, including many causes of inflammation and liver disease. To confirm the diagnosis, test for the two genetic defects known to cause the disease: C282Y and H63D. In persons of northern European descent, heterozygosity is remarkably prevalent with about 10% of these patients carrying C282Y and 15% to 20% carrying H63D. However, the disease is autosomal recessive and will only manifest with two copies of C282Y or one copy of each (C282Y/H63D). H63D alone (and other mutations) appear less deleterious compared to C282Y.

HELPFUL TIP:
Other causes of iron overload include thalassemia, sideroblastic anemia, and frequent blood transfusions (such as with sickle cell anemia).

▸ **Objectives: Did you learn to …**
· Describe symptoms and signs of hemochromatosis?
· Recognize complications related to iron overload?

▶ CASE 6.19

A 56-year-old man undergoes a laryngoscopy. In an outdated move that is generally not recommended now, his doctor used extra doses of benzocaine spray (like gallons of the stuff) to overcome a strong gag reflex. The patient tolerated the procedure well, but afterward he started to have cyanosis around the lips. You are now seeing him in the ED, and he has a bluish discoloration of his lips and fingertips and is complaining of a headache. You administer oxygen by nasal cannula with no improvement in his cyanosis. You draw venous blood for labs and find that it has an unusual chocolate color.

Question 6.19.1 All of the following statements are likely to be true about this patient EXCEPT:
A) A measured arterial blood gas will demonstrate a normal PaO₂
B) The pulse oximeter will show high-normal oxygen saturation
C) The patient may require therapy with methylene blue
D) The patient should not be treated with methylene blue if he has a history of G6PD deficiency
E) Additional doses of benzocaine can be lethal

Answer 6.19.1 **The correct answer (and exception) is "B."** This patient has methemoglobinemia, which in his case was likely a result of the benzocaine spray. Methemoglobinemia results when iron in hemoglobin is oxidized from the ferrous to the ferric state and the hemoglobin becomes incapable of binding and transporting oxygen. The blood gas oxygen may look normal ("A") because the RBCs cannot release oxygen (and thus remain oxygenated). However, the pulse oximeter will show a low O_2 saturation. **So, there is often a gap between what you see on the blood gas and what the pulse oximeter suggests.**

In a normal patient, less than 1% of hemoglobin is found in the methemoglobin form. Depending on the percentage of methemoglobin, presentations will vary. At methemoglobin levels of 10% to 20%, patients present with cyanosis refractory to oxygen. The arterial blood gas may show a normal PaO_2 with low oxygen saturations. When methemoglobin levels are >30%, patients present with headache, dizziness, dyspnea, and tachypnea (signs of moderate hypoxemia). At >50%, patients develop stupor and obtundation (signs of severe hypoxemia), and levels >70% may be lethal.

Certain drugs such as nitroprusside, sulfonamides, some local anesthetics (in this case benzocaine "E"), and acetaminophen have been found to cause methemoglobinemia.

Treatment of methemoglobinemia is methylene blue ("C"). However, patients with G6PD deficiency should not be given methylene blue, and hyperbaric oxygen therapy should be considered instead ("D"). Remember, when patients have been exposed to cyanide, you want to **cause** methemoglobinemia. The exact mechanism by which this protects against cyanide is unknown, since patients begin to improve prior to the presence of methemoglobinemia.

HELPFUL TIP:
Children with diarrhea may develop methemoglobinemia, although it is rarely clinically significant.

HELPFUL (AND SOMEWHAT USEFUL) TIP:
Methylene blue is, a potent inhibitor of monoamine oxidase, and can cause a serotonin syndrome if used in those on SSRIs or other serotoninergic drugs.

▶ **Objectives: Did you learn to …**
- Describe findings and treatment of methemoglobinemia?

▶ **CASE 6.20**

A 16-year-old sub-Saharan African male presents to your office for progressive fatigue and dyspnea over the past few days. He also has some mild upper respiratory symptoms that are being "treated" with sulfamethoxazole—trimethoprim. (The doctor down the street is known to treat all respiratory infections with antibiotics.) On examination, you find a well-nourished male in no distress. He is afebrile but slightly tachycardic. You note mild scleral icterus and pallor of the palmar creases, but the remainder of the examination is unremarkable. A CBC shows normal WBC count and platelets, with Hgb 10.2 g/dL. On peripheral smear, "bite cells" and rare Heinz bodies are reported. The LDH and bilirubin are elevated and the serum haptoglobin is low, but the other serum chemistries are normal.

Question 6.20.1 Which of the following is the most likely diagnosis?
A) Hereditary spherocytosis
B) G6PD deficiency
C) Sickle cell disease (homozygous)
D) Sickle cell trait (heterozygous)
E) Iron deficiency anemia

Answer 6.20.1 **The correct answer is "B."** The most likely cause of this patient's anemia is G6PD deficiency. He appears to have a hemolytic anemia, as evidenced by the elevated LDH, bite cells, elevated bilirubin, low haptoglobin, and the acute onset of symptoms. Heinz bodies are inclusions in red cells seen on peripheral smear within the first few days of an oxidative stress in patients with G6PD deficiency. Bite cells are formed as the red cells pass through the spleen and the Heinz bodies are removed. The other diagnoses are less likely. Hereditary spherocytosis ("A") is caused by an inherited defect in the red cell membrane, and episodes of hemolytic anemia may be brought on by environmental stress. However, patients generally have a baseline anemia, and spherocytes should be seen on peripheral smear. Sickle cell disease and trait are discussed in more detail elsewhere. "E," iron deficiency anemia, does not generally present acutely and is not associated with findings of hemolysis.

HELPFUL TIP:
G6PD deficiency is the most common inherited RBC enzyme defect, affecting 10% of males of sub-Saharan African descent. It occurs more commonly in African and Mediterranean populations.

Hemolytic anemia in G6PD deficiency is caused by oxidative stress on red cells, most commonly as the result of infection or administration of certain drugs.

Question 6.20.2 Which of the following can precipitate a hemolytic crisis in G6PD deficiency?
A) Sulfa antibiotics
B) Fresh fava beans
C) Nitrofurantoin
D) Some antimalarial drugs
E) All of the above

Answer 6.20.2 **The correct answer is "E."** All of the above can cause a hemolytic crisis in G6PD deficiency. Multiple other drugs can be involved as well, including vitamin C, salicylates, isoniazid, and phenytoin.

HELPFUL TIP:
Fresh fava beans aren't worth the bother. First you have to shell them and then *peel each and every bean*. After all that work, you just end up with a hemolytic crisis if you have G6PD deficiency. Get the canned ones.

Question 6.20.3 Which of the following is the most appropriate intervention for this patient with G6PD deficiency at this point?
A) Admit to the hospital and observe
B) Admit to the hospital and transfuse 2 units of packed red cells
C) Recommend supportive care and follow-up in a few days
D) Recommend splenectomy and refer to a general surgeon

Answer 6.20.3 The correct answer is "C." The hemolytic anemia of G6PD deficiency is self-limited and will resolve. This is because in most cases of G6PD deficiency, only about 25% of the RBCs (the older cells) are susceptible to oxidative stress. Severe episodes should be treated in the hospital setting, but most episodes can be managed as an outpatient. Patients should be educated on the drugs and stressors that may precipitate an episode of hemolytic anemia. Splenectomy may limit hemolysis in patients with more severe disease.

HELPFUL TIP:
If you check a G6PD level during or just after a hemolytic crisis, it will likely be normal even in those with G6PD deficiency. The cells that have low levels of G6PD have hemolyzed. The younger cells that are left (those that are tested) have normal levels of G6PD.

▶ **Objectives: Did you learn to …**
• Identify clinical and laboratory manifestations of G6PD deficiency and describe its management?

 QUICK QUIZ: TOO MANY LYMPHOCYTES

A 72-year-old man presents to your office for follow-up after a recent hospitalization for pneumonia. While he was in the hospital, he had an increased WBC with lymphocytosis. You repeat his CBC and find a WBC of 22,000/mm³, with 80% lymphocytes, Hgb of 14 g/dL, and a platelet count of 200,000/mm³. You review office records from a visit 1 year ago and find a WBC of 14,000/mm³ with 76% lymphocytes. You send his peripheral blood for flow cytometry, which is consistent with a diagnosis of chronic lymphocytic leukemia (CLL).

Which of the following statements about this patient is INCORRECT?
A) This patient is at risk for the development of hemolytic anemia
B) This patient is at risk for serious infection

C) This patient is likely to experience a relatively benign disease course
D) This patient should be started on chemotherapy
E) This patient may develop "B symptoms" (fever, night sweats, weight loss)

The correct (or rather "incorrect") answer is "D." CLL is characterized by progressive accumulation of long-lived lymphocytes. It is more common in men and tends to be a disease of older adults (median age at diagnosis is 65 years); however, up to 20% of cases occur in patients <60 years of age. Diagnosis is made if a patient has >5,000/mm³ mature-appearing lymphocytes in the blood representing a clonal line. With the use of immunophenotyping, bone marrow biopsy is not necessary for diagnosis, but may be useful for prognosis.

This patient has a low-stage CLL (the only finding is lymphocytosis) and does not require immediate treatment with chemotherapy. He should be monitored every 6 to 12 months or sooner if he develops symptoms, such as infections, fatigue, bulky lymphadenopathy, or bleeding. Patients with CLL are at risk for developing autoimmune diseases, including hemolytic anemia, autoimmune thrombocytopenia, pure red cell aplasia, and autoimmune neutropenia.

 QUICK QUIZ: TOO MANY NEUTROPHILS

A 46-year-old woman presents to your office for a preoperative evaluation. She is planning an elective hysterectomy for uterine fibroids. She has no significant past medical history. Her review of systems is positive only for night sweats. Her physical examination is unremarkable except for a palpable spleen tip. You obtain a CBC, showing a WBC 50,000/mm³, Hgb 11 g/dL, and a platelet count 350,000/mm³. On her peripheral blood smear, she has mostly neutrophils and bands, with some metamyelocytes, myelocytes, and basophils as well.

All of the following are likely to be true EXCEPT:
A) The patient has an underlying infection with leukemoid reaction
B) The patient has a balanced translocation between chromosomes 9 and 22
C) The patient will likely develop progressive leukocytosis, fevers, anemia, and thrombocytopenia if untreated
D) This condition may be treated with oral tyrosine kinase inhibitors

The correct answer (and exception) is "A." Although a leukemoid reaction is a possibility, it would be unusual to see a full range of maturation of myeloid cells (e.g., metamyelocytes and myelocytes) in the peripheral blood along with increased basophils and a palpable spleen. Rather, this patient likely has chronic myelogenous leukemia (CML), which is a clonal myeloproliferative disorder, characterized by the "Philadelphia chromosome" (translocation between chromosomes 9 and 22), which encodes for an abnormal tyrosine kinase protein. This protein is the target for the tyrosine kinase inhibitors, such as imatinib (Gleevec), which have resulted in significant improvement in survival. Patients with CML typically present between the ages of 40 and 60. Up to 40% of patients are asymptomatic at presentation. Others complain of weight loss, fatigue, abdominal pain, night sweats, and fever. Five-year overall survival can be up to 85% depending on the age at diagnosis.

 QUICK QUIZ: ACUTE LEUKEMIA

You have a febrile 37-year-old male with a very high WBC count, most of which are blasts. Most likely, he has an acute leukemia. A bone marrow has not yet been done, and it is unknown if this is an acute myeloid leukemia or an acute lymphoblastic leukemia.

Which of the following statements is INCORRECT?
A) The patient's fever is likely due to the leukemic cells, and antibiotics should be started only if you identify a specific infection
B) The patient is at risk for tumor lysis syndrome and should be started on allopurinol
C) Aggressive inpatient chemotherapy is required for both the treatment of acute myeloid leukemia and acute lymphoblastic leukemia
D) You should consult a hematologist/oncologist as soon as possible

The correct (or rather incorrect) answer is "A." Patients with acute leukemia and fever should be cultured, **and antibiotics should be started as soon as possible** since a fever is often the result of a concurrent infection. These patients should be kept well hydrated and given allopurinol ("B") to prevent tumor lysis syndrome, which can occur even without chemotherapy if the tumor burden is high enough. Treatment of acute leukemias requires intensive chemotherapy and should be started as soon as possible, so prompt evaluation by a hematologist/oncologist is imperative ("C" and "D").

▶ **CASE 6.21**

A 65-year-old male who is on quinine for leg cramps (a non–FDA-approved indication) is brought into the ED. Last night he was complaining of a headache, fever, and numbness on the right side of his face. This morning, he was acting erratically.

His physical examination demonstrates a confused male, with a temperature of 39°C, pulse 110 bpm, BP 180/94 mm Hg, and respirations 14 bpm. He has a few petechiae on his palate. He is tachycardic and lungs are clear to auscultation bilaterally. His abdomen is soft, without organomegaly. His neurologic examination is difficult to complete due to his inability to cooperate.

Laboratory findings include WBC 6,000/mm³, Hgb 8.4 g/dL, and platelet count 50,000/mm³. Schistocytes are noted on a peripheral blood smear.

Question 6.21.1 **All of the following may be expected in this patient EXCEPT:**
A) Creatinine of 3.2 mg/dL
B) LDH of 640 IU/L
C) Elevated haptoglobin
D) Elevated indirect bilirubin
E) Negative direct antiglobulin test (direct Coombs)

Answer 6.21.1 **The correct answer is "C."** An elevated haptoglobin would suggest the absence of active hemolysis. The presence of schistocytes suggests ongoing microangiopathic hemolysis, in this case due to thrombotic thrombocytopenic purpura (TTP). TTP is due to the lack of activity of the ADAMTS13 enzyme either via inheritance of a faulty enzyme (inherited) or via antibodies produced against the enzyme (acquired). It is classically described by a pentad of findings: microangiopathic hemolytic anemia (suggested by schistocytes on peripheral smear), thrombocytopenia, fever, renal insufficiency, and mental status changes. Not all five features need to be present for the diagnosis, but your patient seems to have the pentad. An otherwise unexplained microangiopathic hemolytic anemia in the presence of thrombocytopenia is enough to trigger treatment for TTP; fever, renal insufficiency, and mental status changes are not necessary to make the presumptive diagnosis of TTP. The negative direct antiglobulin test (direct Coombs), "E," suggests that the hemolytic anemia is not due to an autoimmune process. Note that the patient is on quinine, one of the drugs that can cause TTP. Clopidogrel (Plavix) and ticlopidine (Ticlid) can also cause TTP, although it is less common with clopidogrel.

 HELPFUL TIP:
Schistocytes are the result of intravascular trauma to RBCs. Any microangiopathic hemolytic anemia can result in schistocytes as can other intravascular trauma such as that secondary to artificial heart valves, HELLP syndrome, malignant hypertension, some malignancies, transjugular intrahepatic portosystemic shunts (TIPS), eclampsia, etc.

Question 6.21.2 **Which of the following laboratory findings would you expect to see in this patient with TTP?**
A) Normal PT/INR
B) Elevated PTT
C) Elevated fibrin degradation products
D) Low level of fibrinogen

Answer 6.21.2 **The correct answer is "A."** Patients with TTP should have a normal PT/INR. This is important because TTP can be confused with DIC, in which the PT/INR should be elevated and fibrinogen should be low.

Your patient is started on plasma exchange. You note that he has not had any change in his hemoglobin or platelet count, and his renal function is worsening.

Question 6.21.3 Which of the following may mimic TTP and should be considered in a poorly responsive patient?
A) Rocky Mountain spotted fever
B) Disseminated aspergillosis
C) Disseminated malignancy
D) Malignant hypertension
E) All of the above

Answer 6.21.3 **The correct answer is "E."** When patients are poorly responsive to therapy, an alternative diagnosis should be sought. In pregnant patients, preeclampsia or HELLP syndrome can mimic TTP. Autoimmune disease (e.g., systemic lupus erythematosus and scleroderma), malignant hypertension, and disseminated malignancy may also mimic TTP. Infections that can be confused with TTP include Rocky Mountain spotted fever, disseminated aspergillosis, as well as any other disease that can cause mental status changes and a low platelet count such as Ehrlichiosis, Anaplasmosis, West Nile virus, etc.

HELPFUL TIP:
Therapy with plasma exchange has reduced the mortality rate for TTP from 90% to less than 25%. Other treatments may include glucocorticoids, rituximab (*Transfusion*. 2012 Dec;52(12):2525–2532), and splenectomy in refractory cases. Platelet transfusion should be avoided as it can worsen the patient's condition.

▶ **Objectives: Did you learn to …**
· Recognize the clinical presentation of TTP?
· Treat a patient with TTP?
· Develop a differential diagnosis for a patient with microangiopathic anemia?

▶ CASE 6.22

A 23-year-old G1 P0 term female goes to emergency cesarean section after she is noted to have placental abruption. She has no other significant medical history. After the delivery, you note that she is having brisk vaginal bleeding and oozing from her venipuncture sites. You obtain laboratories: WBC 9,000/mm³, Hgb 8.2 g/dL, platelet count 80,000/mm³, INR 2.4, PTT 22 seconds, and fibrinogen 80 mg/dL (normal 190–420 mg/dL). Fibrin degradation products are elevated. A CBC at admission was normal.

Question 6.22.1 **Which of the following statements is INCORRECT?**
A) The patient may benefit from platelet transfusion
B) The patient may benefit from cryoprecipitate transfusion
C) The patient may benefit from FFP transfusion
D) The patient may benefit from crystalloid infusion

Answer 6.22.1 **The correct answer (and what not to do) is "A."** This patient is exhibiting signs of disseminated intravascular coagulation (DIC), which is characterized by the disordered

regulation of coagulation. It can be precipitated by a sepsis, malignancy, CNS trauma with release of tissue plasminogen activator, obstetrical problems (preeclampsia, retained products of conception, amniotic fluid embolism), ABO incompatibility with hemolysis, extensive burns, snake bites, etc. Thrombin also activates platelets, causing platelet aggregation and consumption. Antithrombin, previously known as antithrombin III, is consumed in this process as well. Treatment is directed at correcting the underlying cause of DIC whenever possible. *Don't treat the numbers; patients may have a low-grade DIC and be relatively asymptomatic.* If this is the case, reversing the underlying process is enough. If the patient is bleeding, she may benefit from platelet transfusion to maintain a platelet count above 20,000/mm³, but transfusion at higher levels can worsen platelet aggregation. Transfusion of FFP will replace consumed factors. Patients with low fibrinogen levels will benefit from transfusion of cryoprecipitate. The use of heparin is generally limited to those with low grade, chronic DIC with thrombotic complications. It may also be considered acutely if there are prominent thrombotic complications.

HELPFUL TIP:
Laboratory findings in DIC include low platelets, prolonged PT/INR, normal or prolonged PTT, low fibrinogen, and increased fibrin degradation products. Further, D-dimer and thrombin time are also increased, antithrombin may be low, and peripheral blood smear will reveal schistocytes. An elevated D-dimer in isolation is not helpful since D-dimer is elevated in many states, including DVT/PE.

▶ **Objectives: Did you learn to …**
· Distinguish DIC from TTP?

▶ CASE 6.23

A 22-year-old female college student presents to your office with complaints of an enlarged cervical lymph node and sore throat. She has felt feverish on and off for several weeks, but never measured her temperature. She is afebrile today, a rapid strep test is negative, and there is no evidence of lymphadenitis; you treat her symptomatically. You ask her to return if her symptoms do not resolve within 2 to 4 weeks.

She returns 4 weeks later. The sore throat has resolved; however, she now complains of intense pruritus and sweats at night. The cervical lymph node now measures 3 cm. The remainder of her physical examination is negative.

Question 6.23.1 **What is the most appropriate next step?**
A) Direct laryngoscopy
B) Empiric antibiotic trial
C) Lymph node biopsy
D) MRI of the neck
E) Observation for another 4 weeks

Answer 6.23.1 The correct answer is "C." The prolonged (>1 month) presence of a large (>1 cm) lymph node deserves a biopsy. MRI of the neck and laryngoscopy may be indicated depending on the biopsy results. Empiric antibiotic therapy ("B") is inappropriate and unlikely to be helpful, as you have no source of primary infection. At this point in time, observation ("E") will just delay the diagnosis. Note that delaying the biopsy for 1 month after initial presentation does not change outcomes even if the node is malignant.

You obtain a lymph node biopsy that is consistent with nodular sclerosing Hodgkin lymphoma.

Question 6.23.2 Which of the following statements is INCORRECT?
A) The patient has B symptoms
B) Further staging is necessary
C) Chemotherapy is palliative only in this patient
D) Treatment includes both radiation and chemotherapy

Answer 6.23.2 The correct (and untrue) answer is "C." Chemotherapy regimens for Hodgkin lymphoma have resulted in response rates of more than 90%, with fewer long-term complications than prior regimens. Despite the fact that it is well-known, Hodgkin lymphoma is an uncommon disease, with about 8,000 cases occurring each year in the United States. It is a disease of young people, occurring typically in patients in their 20s. Patients often present with lymphadenopathy. Symptoms, known as "B symptoms," include weight loss, fever, and drenching night sweats. The presence of "B symptoms" correlates with more advanced disease. Other symptoms may include pruritus, diffuse pain after consuming alcoholic beverages, and symptoms related to the development of a mediastinal mass. After a diagnostic lymph node biopsy, further staging includes CT scans, bone marrow biopsy, and routine laboratory tests.

HELPFUL TIP:
Non-Hodgkin lymphoma (NHL) is increasing in incidence and is more common than Hodgkin lymphoma. Risk factors for NHL include HIV infection and advancing age.

HELPFUL TIP:
The differential diagnosis of generalized lymphadenopathy is broad, and a good history is imperative. The initial evaluation should include a CBC and CXR. If these are negative and lymphadenopathy persists, consider obtaining syphilis testing and ANA and testing for TB and HIV. Also, consider testing for Epstein–Barr virus (antibody test or heterophile) as appropriate. Some medications can cause generalized lymphadenopathy secondary to serum sickness.

▶ **Objectives: Did you learn to …**
· Recognize presentation of a patient with Hodgkin lymphoma?
· Describe "B symptoms"?

▶ **CASE 6.24**

A 34-year-old woman presents to your office with calf pain and swelling. She denies trauma to the leg. She has no other significant medical history and takes only oral contraceptives. She smokes half a pack of cigarettes daily but does not drink alcohol. Her physical examination is also unremarkable, with the exception of swelling and tenderness of the left calf. A lower extremity Doppler study demonstrates a new thrombus occluding the common femoral vein.

Question 6.24.1 Which of the following would NOT be appropriate in this patient?
A) Start the patient on heparin or a heparinoid and warfarin to maintain an INR of 2 to 3 or start a factor Xa inhibitor (e.g., rivaroxaban) or a direct fibrin inhibitor (e.g., dabigatran)
B) Have the patient scheduled for placement of an inferior vena cava filter
C) Discontinue hormonal contraceptives
D) Encourage the patient to stop smoking
E) Obtain further history regarding her family

Answer 6.24.1 The correct (and inappropriate) answer is "B." This patient has an acute DVT and risk factors for developing a DVT, including smoking and hormonal contraceptive use. You should start her on heparin (or low–molecular-weight heparin) and warfarin with a goal INR of 2 to 3. Heparin should be used for **at least** 5 days and overlapped with therapeutic doses of warfarin that have reached the target INR for **at least** 48 hours. Alternatively, you can start rivaroxaban (Xarelto), apixaban (Eliquis), or dabigatran (Pradaxa). Dabigatran requires an overlap with low–molecular-weight heparin; rivaroxaban and apixaban do not. Dabigatran has a reversal agent (idarucizumab, "Praxbind") available as do the factor Xa inhibitors (andexanet alfa, "AndexXa"). Avoid edoxaban (Savaysa) as it is less effective and more problematic when adjusting for renal disease. She should be anticoagulated for at least 3 months. Encourage her to stop smoking and to find an alternative form of birth control. "B" deserves special mention. There is no evidence that vena caval filters are of benefit in patients that can be anticoagulated except as a temporary measure for inpatients where the vena caval filter will be removed prior to discharge. There is **no** reduction in PE risk with vena caval filters in those who can be anticoagulated, and there is likely an increased risk of DVT. The role in those who cannot be anticoagulated is unclear; there is scant data.

HELPFUL TIP:
Homan sign is neither sensitive nor specific enough to allow it to be used to rule in or rule out DVT. Don't bother. However, use of a clinical prediction tool (e.g., Well's criteria) can reduce unnecessary testing.

The patient returns 3 months later. She has been relatively easy to anticoagulate (somebody has to be, right?), maintaining a stable INR. She stopped smoking and knows to avoid hormonal contraception. She has learned that her mother had a DVT and her maternal aunt died of a pulmonary embolus. Now, the patient wants to know how this new information will affect her long-term care. You decide to screen her for thrombophilia.

Question 6.24.2 **Which of the following sets of tests should NOT be performed while she remains on warfarin?**
A) Factor V Leiden mutation
B) Antiphospholipid antibodies
C) Protein C
D) Prothrombin gene mutation

Answer 6.24.2 **The correct answer is "C."** There are several types of thrombophilia for which you might initially test: factor V Leiden mutation, antithrombin (previously antithrombin III) deficiency, prothrombin gene mutation, protein C deficiency, protein S deficiency, and antiphospholipid antibody syndrome. Not all causes of thrombophilia can be tested for while on anticoagulant therapy. Factor V Leiden gene mutation, prothrombin gene mutation, and antiphospholipid antibodies are not affected by warfarin. However, warfarin can reduce protein C and S levels (giving false-positive test results) and increase antithrombin levels (giving a false-negative result). Also, proteins C

and S are depleted during the acute phase of thrombosis, so the levels should not be measured when a patient is experiencing a VTE event.

Factor V Leiden mutation is the most common cause of inherited thrombophilia, being found in 3% to 6% of non-Black blood donors. Antithrombin deficiency is less common, occurring in 1/1,000 to 1/5,000 individuals. The homozygous condition is fatal in utero. Heterozygotes have a 30% chance of developing a thromboembolic event by the age of 30 years. Protein C deficiency occurs in 1/200 to 1/300 people; however, fewer than 1/1,000 heterozygotes develop venous thromboses. Protein S deficiency is estimated to occur in 1/750 to 1/3,000 of persons and has a clinical presentation similar to protein C deficiency. The prevalence of prothrombin gene mutation varies widely and occurs most commonly in persons of southern European descent. Unlike the other thrombophilias discussed antiphospholipid antibody syndrome is an acquired disorder that is associated with arterial as well as venous thromboembolic events.

Importantly, bridging atrial fibrillation patients on warfarin with heparin increases the bleeding risk while doing nothing to prevent stroke, PE, etc. Be selective in whom you bridge. Bridge patients with a CH2ADS2-VASC score of >5 (see cardiology chapter for more on the CH2ADS2-VASC score), those with a prosthetic mitral valve or metal aortic valve, those with a history of thromboembolic events while off anticoagulation, etc. For "average" risk patients bridging with heparin adds nothing and has significant downsides (see *N Engl J Med.* 2015;373:823–833 and *Circulation.* 2015;131:488–494). *Note that it isn't necessary to bridge patients who are on dabigatran, rivaroxaban, apixaban, etc.* They are short acting enough that just holding one dose prior to surgery is adequate; there is a minimal window for clot formation. See below for further discussion of heparin bridging in those who have had a recent thromboembolic event.

▶ **Objectives: Did you learn to …**
  * Obtain an appropriate history in a patient with clotting problems?
  * Recognize common inherited and acquired hypercoagulable risk factors?

▶ **CASE 6.25**

A 19-year-old gravid female presents during her second trimester and complains of left calf swelling. With the help of Doppler studies, you diagnose her with a DVT.

Question 6.25.1 Which of the following statements is correct?
A) DVT occurs most commonly in the right lower extremity in pregnant women
B) DVT is common in pregnancy due to increased venous stasis and increased levels of fibrinogen, factor VIII, and vWF
C) Anticoagulation with heparin introduces no risk to the fetus or mother
D) DVT is most common in the third trimester

Answer 6.25.1 **The correct answer is "B."** DVT, and the broader category of venous thromboembolism (VTE), occurs two to four times more often in pregnant women compared to nonpregnant controls. Increased risk is found with cesarean delivery versus vaginal delivery. The majority of DVTs occur in the **left** lower extremity of pregnant women, likely due to the compression of the left iliac vein by the right iliac artery as they cross. The increased incidence of VTE is multifactorial, including the presence of all three components of Virchow's triad: venous stasis, endothelial injury (increased venous distension secondary to increased estrogen), and a hypercoagulable state (increased levels of fibrinogen, factor VIII, and vWF).

VTE occurs equally during all three trimesters, **but the highest risk is postpartum (2–5 times the risk during pregnancy).**

Warfarin crosses the placenta and has teratogenic effects in addition to increased risk of fetal bleeding. Heparin and danaparoid (available in Canada) do not cross the placenta but are associated with a 2% risk of maternal bleeding. Heparin also carries the risks of heparin-induced thrombocytopenia with thrombosis, osteoporosis, and bleeding at the uteroplacental junction. Dosing of unfractionated heparin is difficult during pregnancy, and low–molecular-weight heparin (e.g., enoxaparin) is probably the best choice for anticoagulation. There is increased use of enoxaparin in the immediate postpartum for DVT prophylaxis for higher risk mothers, so don't be surprised if your patient is discharged home after her delivery with a few more days or weeks of enoxaparin. Heparin and warfarin are safe for lactating mothers.

▶ **Objectives: Did you learn to …**
  * Recognize the risks of VTE in the pregnant patient?

▶ **CASE 6.26**

A 52-year-old woman presents to the ED with shortness of breath and pleuritic chest pain. She has been on warfarin for atrial fibrillation. Despite her anticoagulation, you suspect pulmonary embolism (PE) and obtain a spiral CT scan, which shows a thrombus in the right pulmonary artery. Prior to the initiation of any therapy, her coagulation studies return and show INR of 2.8 (normal = 1) and PTT 49 seconds (prolonged).

Question 6.26.1 Which of the following is the most appropriate next step?
A) Test the patient for antiphospholipid antibodies
B) Place an inferior vena cava filter
C) Repeat the INR and PTT since the patient's sample was probably contaminated with heparin
D) Confront the patient about her noncompliance with warfarin
E) Throw up your hands in disgust. Aren't they done with the hematology chapter yet?

Answer 6.26.1 **The correct answer is "A."** Patients who have a new VTE while on appropriate anticoagulation therapy should be evaluated for antiphospholipid antibody syndrome. This patient has a prolonged PTT, which is also suspicious for an antiphospholipid antibody. Remember that warfarin prolongs the PT, not the PTT. She was an outpatient prior to having her blood drawn and was not taking heparin, so contamination with heparin is unlikely (although heparin definitely causes an increase in the PTT). The increased INR suggests that the patient has been compliant with her warfarin. As to "B," see the note above about vena caval filters.

 HELPFUL TIP:
Previously, retrospective studies resulted in the recommendation that patients with an antiphospholipid antibody and VTE be maintained at an INR of 3 to 4. This

recommendation has changed with newly available prospective data, and these patients should have a target INR of 2 to 3. Some patients with antiphospholipid antibody syndrome may have marked INR fluctuations that make monitoring anticoagulation difficult.

HELPFUL TIP:
Genetic testing is now available for warfarin sensitivity that can help predict which patients will need higher (or lower) doses of warfarin to maintain adequate anticoagulation. However, these tests are very expensive and contribute little to the care of most patients.

▶ **Objectives: Did you learn to …**
  · Identify a patient presenting with antiphospholipid antibodies and understand the management of such patients?

▶ CASE 6.27

A 50-year-old male is admitted to the hospital with a fractured tibia after a motor vehicle collision. You are asked to assist in his perioperative management. The patient is generally healthy but is taking warfarin for a DVT that he developed after a total knee arthroplasty 3 weeks ago. His INR is 1.8, and he is scheduled for open reduction/internal fixation tomorrow.

Question 6.27.1 **Which of the following statements is INCORRECT?**
A) The patient has an approximate 50% risk of recurrent VTE without appropriate therapy
B) Heparin should be started preoperatively
C) Heparin should be continued postoperatively
D) Resumption of warfarin alone postoperatively is adequate anticoagulation

Answer 6.27.1 **The correct answer is "D."** Perioperative management of a patient with recent VTE is complicated. While there are established guidelines for VTE prophylaxis depending on the type of surgery planned, this patient already has an active thrombotic event. Discontinuing warfarin may result in a rebound hypercoagulable state, and surgery creates a prothrombotic state.

Patients who have a VTE within 1 month of surgery have a 50% risk of a second VTE if not treated aggressively with anticoagulation. These recurrent events carry a mortality rate of approximately 6%. Such patients should be placed on heparin before and after surgery if they are on warfarin. If they are on one of the newer anticoagulants, hold a dose of dabigatran, apixaban, or rivaroxaban and then restart the drug postoperatively.

Patients with a VTE within 1 to 3 months before a scheduled surgery should be considered for *postoperative* heparin/warfarin *or* dabigatran, apixaban, or rivaroxaban. A VTE > 3 months before the scheduled surgery should not pose significant additional risk, and established prophylaxis guidelines should be followed. See above for a discussion of heparin bridging in atrial fibrillation and heart valves.

▶ **Objectives: Did you learn to …**
  · Describe anticoagulation approaches in perioperative care?

We will leave you with a quick primer on the direct oral anticoagulants ("DOACs"). All of these now carry indications for nonvalvular atrial fibrillation and venous thromboembolism. None are approved for use with mechanical heart valves. Transitioning between warfarin and DOACs (and vice versa) is dependent on the DOAC. Refer to FDA labeling. For VTE treatment, dabigatran (Pradaxa) and edoxaban (Savaysa) require initial therapy with a parenteral anticoagulant, such as heparin or enoxaparin.

Dabigatran (Pradaxa): A direct thrombin inhibitor. Contributes to less bleeding overall than warfarin, but prevents fewer myocardial infarctions and causes more GI bleeds. May also increase dyspepsia. The dose must be decreased in those with renal disease. May be reversed with idarucizumab (Praxbind).

Rivaroxaban (Xarelto): An oral factor Xa inhibitor (similar to enoxaparin). Does not require heparin at initiation. There are multiple drug interactions (though fewer than with warfarin). Not indicated in those with severe renal disease and those with moderate liver disease.

Apixaban (Eliquis): An oral direct factor Xa inhibitor. Does not require heparin at initiation. Not recommended for patients with moderate hepatic impairment. Dose must be decreased in renal impairment. May cause hypercoagulable state when stopped, increasing the risk of stroke if stopped without adequate continuous anticoagulation.

Other oral direct factor Xa inhibitors: *Betrixaban (Bevyxxa), Edoxaban (Lixiana, Savaysa)*

Annexa (Andexanet alfa, Portola Phamaceuticals): A new recombinant modified factor Xa to work as an antidote for patients receiving Xa inhibitors.

Clinical Pearls

○ A platelet count of >20,000/mL is adequate for hemostasis.

○ Do not perform an exhaustive hypercoagulability workup in patients with VTE who have a major risk factor (e.g., systemic estrogen, surgery, trauma, prolonged immobility).

○ Do not use plasma or a prothrombin complex concentrate to reverse anticoagulation unless there is significant bleeding (e.g., intracranial bleed).

○ Do not use venocaval filters to prevent a second PE in a patient with a prior history of DVT. They do not work.

○ If a patient is on warfarin and the INR is 10 or less and the patient is asymptomatic, do not treat with vitamin K; simply hold the warfarin. If the INR is >10, give 1 to 5 mg of PO vitamin K.

○ It is not necessary to anticoagulate patients with a first DVT *that can be explained by a reversible cause* (e.g., estrogen, surgery, and immobilization) for more than 3 months.

○ The PTT is the most useful single test when screening for coagulopathy.

○ Transfuse stable patients to a hemoglobin of 7 to 8 mg/dL. A higher target can worsen outcomes.

○ Transfusing platelets will not work in ITP. The platelets will just get destroyed.

○ With iron deficiency anemia, the reticulocyte count should go up within 10 days when appropriately treated with iron. If this doesn't happen, reconsider your diagnosis.

BIBLIOGRAPHY

Abramson N, Melton B. Leukocytosis: basics of clinical assessment. *Am Fam Physician*. 2000;62(9):2053–2060.

Adkinson NF, et al. Comparative efficacy of intravenous ferumoxytol vs. ferric carboxymaltose in iron deficiency anemia: a randomized trial. *Am J Hematol*. 2018;93(5):683–690.

Allen GA, Glader B. Approach to the bleeding child. *Pediatr Clin North Am*. 2002;49(6):1239–1256.

Bain BJ. Diagnosis from the blood smear. *N Engl J Med*. 2005;353:498–507.

Booth KK, et al. Systemic infections mimicking thrombotic thrombocytopenic purpura. *Am J Hematol*. 2011;86(9):743–751.

Brandhagen DJ, et al. Recognition and management of hereditary hemochromatosis. *Am Fam Physician*. 2002; 65(5):853.

Carson JL, et al. Red blood cell transfusion: a clinical practice guideline from the AABB. *Ann Intern Med*. 2012;157(1):49–58.

Crownover BK, Covey CJ. Hereditary hemochromatosis. *Am Fam Physician*. 2013;87(3):183–190.

Douketis JD, et al. Perioperative bridging anticoagulation in patients with atrial fibrillation. *N Engl J Med*. 2015;373:823–833.

Freifeld AG, Bow EJ, Sepkowiz KA. Clinical practice guideline for the use of antimicrobial agents in neutropenic patients with cancer: 2010 update by the Infectious Diseases Society of America. *Clin Infect Dis*. 2011;52(4):e56–e93.

Ganetsky M, et al. Dabigatran: review of pharmacology and management of bleeding complications of this novel oral anticoagulant. *J Med Toxicol*. 2011;7(4):281–287.

Guyatt GH, et al., for the American College of Chest Physicians Antithrombotic Therapy and Prevention of Thrombosis Panel. Executive summary: antithrombotic therapy and prevention of thrombosis, 9th ed: American College of Chest Physicians Evidence-Based Clinical Practice Guidelines. *Chest*. 2012;141(2)(suppl):7S–47S.

Kearon C, et al. D-dimer testing to select patients with a first unprovoked venous thromboembolism who can stop anticoagulant therapy: a cohort study. *Ann Intern Med*. 2015;162:27.

Kearon C, et al. Antithrombotic therapy for VTE disease. *Chest*. 2016;149(2):315–352.

Killip S, Bennett JM, Chambers MD. Iron deficiency anemia. *Am Fam Physician*. 2007;75(5):671–678.

Landgren O. Monoclonal gammopathy of undetermined significance and smoldering myeloma: new insights into pathophysiology and epidemiology. *Hematology Am Soc Hematol Educ Program*. 2010;2010:295–302.

Moake J. Thrombotic thrombocytopenia purpura (TTP) and other thrombotic microangiopathies. *Best Pract Res Clin Haematol*. 2009;22(4):567–576.

National Institutes of Health. What causes thrombotic thrombocytopenic purpura? Available at https://www. nhlbi.nih.gov/health/health-topics/topics/ttp/causes. Accessed April 1, 2019.

O'Connell TX, Horita TJ, Kasravi B. Understanding and interpreting serum protein electrophoresis. *Am Fam Physician*. 2005;71(1):105–112.

Prandoni P, et al. Recurrent venous thromboembolism and bleeding complications during anticoagulant treatment in patients with cancer and venous thrombosis. *Blood*. 2002;100:3484–8.

Short MW, Domagalski JE. Iron deficiency anemia: evaluation and treatment. *Am Fam Physician*. 2013;87(2):98–104.

Som S, et al. Decreasing frequency of plasma exchange complications in patients treated for thrombotic thrombocytopenia purpura-hemolytic uremic syndrome, 1996 to 2001. *Transfusion*. 2012;52(12):2525-2532.

Steinberg BA, et al. Use and outcomes associated with bridging during anticoagulation interruptions in patients with atrial fibrillation: findings from the Outcomes Registry for Better Informed Treatment of Atrial Fibrillation (ORBIT-AF). *Circulation*. 2015;131:488–494.

Stoffel NU, et al. Iron absorption from oral iron supplements given on consecutive versus alternate days and as single morning doses versus twice-daily split dosing in iron-depleted women: two open label, randomized controlled trials. *Lancet Haematol*. 2017;4(11):e524–e533.

Wigle P, et al. Updated guidelines on outpatient anticoagulation. *Am Fam Physician*. 2013;87(8):556–566.

Wilbur J. Surveillance of the adult cancer survivor. *Am Fam Physician*. 2015;91(1):29–36.

Other helpful office resource links:

American Society of Clinical Oncology. www.asco.org.

American Society of Clinical Oncology. www.plwc.org. (Website for patients living with cancer.)

American Society of Hematology. www.hematology.org. (Links to many blood disease websites.)

American Association for Clinical Chemistry. www. labtestsonline.org. (Information on general hematology/ oncology subjects and laboratory testing.)

Multiple Myeloma Research Foundation. www.themmrf.org. (Everything about myeloma.)

Gastroenterology

7

Jason Kruse and Mark A. Graber

▶ CASE 7.1

A 43-year-old woman complains of a burning pain in the retrosternal area. Her symptoms started about 2 years ago and initially responded to self-medication with antacids or histamine-2 receptor antagonists (H₂ blockers). However, within the last 4 months, she has had nearly daily problems. She frequently wakes up in the middle of the night with retrosternal, burning pain radiating to her neck. She also frequently notices an acidic taste in her mouth. While antacids help somewhat, they only provide transient relief. She has otherwise been healthy. She currently takes up to 150 mg of ranitidine twice daily plus the antacids. She denies tobacco or alcohol use. Her physical examination is normal.

Question 7.1.1 Which of the following is NOT considered a "red flag" when it comes to patients with acid reflux/ dyspepsia?
A) Weight loss
B) Trouble swallowing liquids
C) Trouble swallowing solids
D) A craving for doughnuts

Answer 7.1.1 The correct answer is "D." OK, we will give you this one. One of the most critical parts of patient assessment is to make sure there are no "red flag" symptoms that may indicate more than simple gastroesophageal reflux disease (GERD). "Red flag" symptoms include: dysphagia, weight loss, anemia, aspiration, early satiety or vomiting, and cough. Dysphagia for solids progressing to dysphagia for liquids is especially problematic. A craving for doughnuts is benign (although eating them is not) and may be seen among the book editors, police, college students, and others.

Question 7.1.2 Which of the following statements is true?
A) All patients with GERD need endoscopy
B) Routine endoscopy in patients with GERD markedly reduces the risk of esophageal cancer

C) The diagnostic sensitivity and specificity of typical symptoms of GERD is >90%
D) Patients over the age of 45 with new onset symptoms are considered to be at high risk
E) C and D

Answer 7.1.2 The correct answer is "E." Because of the high sensitivity and specificity of symptoms (>90%), most patients do not need endoscopy or any other procedure or test to make the diagnosis of GERD. Patients with refractory GERD or those with new symptoms over the age of 45 years (50 by some sources) warrant endoscopy. "B" is incorrect. Screening for the presence of Barrett esophagus in patients with GERD is low yield. Targeted, not routine, endoscopy may be beneficial.

HELPFUL TIP:
The link between *Helicobacter pylori* and GERD is poorly defined. There is no good evidence to support eradication of *H. pylori* for the treatment of GERD. The thinking in dyspepsia has evolved (more on this later).

The patient denies any "red flags." Based on the history, you assume that this patient has GERD.

Question 7.1.3 You recommend:
A) Barium swallow study
B) Esophageal manometry
C) Esophagogastroduodenoscopy (EGD)
D) Ambulatory pH study of the esophagus
E) Trial of omeprazole and life style modifications

Answer 7.1.3 The correct answer is "E." As noted above, the sensitivity and specificity of classical symptoms allows for the diagnosis of GERD without additional studies. Testing is actually less sensitive than symptoms for GERD with the sensitivity of tests varying between 50% and 70%. Many patients have a false-negative EGD. H₂ blockers can be used as the first-line treatment in patients with GERD, but this patient has already failed ranitidine. Starting a proton pump inhibitor (PPI) like omeprazole is the next step and is preferred as the first-line therapy in patients with severe symptoms. Lifestyle modifications should be made including weight loss (if overweight); avoidance of carbonated beverages, caffeine, excessive alcohol, and large or late evening meals; avoidance of anticholinergics, calcium channel blockers, NSAIDs, and sedative drugs; smoking cessation; and elevation of the head of the bed using 6-in blocks.

HELPFUL TIP:
Most patients with GERD will have negative endoscopic findings (termed nonerosive reflux disease [NERD]— really, we didn't make this one up). Symptoms do not correlate well with the presence or degree of esophageal inflammation or erosion.

Your patient is willing to try the PPI you prescribe, but she also wants to know about surgery that a friend had.

Question 7.1.4 Regarding surgery for GERD, you can tell her:
A) Bloating and inability to belch do not occur with antireflux surgery
B) Antireflux surgery should be thought of as the first-line because it is vastly superior to medical therapy
C) Years after antireflux surgery, many patients will require medication for GERD symptoms
D) Laparoscopic fundoplication will ruin her fabulous bikini body by leaving a large midline scar

Answer 7.1.4 The correct answer is "C." Surgery may be an option in select patients with reflux disease. The usual indications for antireflux surgery include failure of medical therapy to control symptoms and failure of medical therapy to prevent complications (e.g., stricture and pneumonia). The most commonly performed surgery is fundoplication, in which the lower esophageal sphincter is "wrapped" to enhance its competency. While fundoplication will alleviate symptoms in 80% to 95% of patients, there is progressive loss of effectiveness over time (only 40% are without medication after 10 years). Adverse effects of surgery include persistent dysphagia (requiring additional interventions in 3–7%), gas, bloating, and inability to belch. "D" is incorrect because a laparoscopic procedure should result in just a few small scars.

After making lifestyle changes and a trial of your favorite PPI (that her insurance will cover after you play "Guess What's on Our Formulary"), the patient feels markedly better. She is so pleased with your care, she refers her brother to you. He just turned 52 and has been struggling with heartburn for many years. He smokes 1 ppd and has a BMI of 35 kg/ m². He was hoping for a prescription of PPI and a quick exit. You inform him that he has multiple risk factors and needs screening for Barrett esophagus. You refer him for EGD. The

esophageal biopsy is consistent with the visual report, which shows Barrett esophagus.

Question 7.1.5 All of the following are true regarding Barrett esophagus EXCEPT:
A) Males are more likely to have Barrett esophagus than females
B) Barrett esophagus is due to a change in the esophageal mucosa from columnar to squamous
C) Barrett esophagus occurs in 10% to 15% of patients with erosive esophagitis
D) Barrett esophagus increases the risk of adenocarcinoma by up to 30-fold
E) Patients with Barrett esophagus should undergo periodic screening EGD

Answer 7.1.5 The correct answer is "B." Barrett esophagus is diagnosed histologically when esophageal mucosal metaplasia has occurred **and the usual squamous epithelial cells have changed to columnar epithelium. Targeted screening for Barrett's in males with >1 additional risk factors is recommended.** Risk factors for Barrett include long-standing reflux (>5 years of weekly symptoms), male gender (6:1 male:female preponderance), advancing age (>50 years old), central adiposity, tobacco use, and white race. Barrett esophagus occurs in 10% to 15% of patients with erosive esophagitis, and it dramatically increases the risk of esophageal adenocarcinoma by up to 30-fold (*N Engl J Med.* 2011;365:1375). However, the absolute risk of adenocarcinoma is still small, about 0.2% to 0.5% annually. Surveillance for Barrett depends on the level of dysplasia found on initial examination, and guidelines exist that dictate the frequency with which repeat EGD should be performed.

Question 7.1.6 The patient returns to you alarmed by his new diagnosis of Barrett esophagus. He quit smoking and is working to lose weight. He admits to a glass of wine nightly with dinner. His symptoms are well controlled on daily PPI. He will follow up as directed for surveillance endoscopy. Which of the following regarding management of this patient's Barrett's esophagus is true?
A) The patient should increase to twice daily PPI to prevent progression
B) The patient should be on aspirin or NSAID prophylaxis to prevent progression to cancer
C) The patient should consider antireflux surgery to prevent further damage
D) The patient should quit drinking alcohol, his nightly glass of wine is accelerating his progression to malignancy
E) None of the above are true

Answer 7.1.6 The correct answer is "E." In patients with good symptom control there is no additional benefit to twice daily PPI and patient should remain on his daily dose. Current ACG guidelines *recommend against* aspirin or NSAID as an antineoplastic strategy. While antireflux surgery should be considered in patients with poor control on optimized medical therapy, it is not recommended for management of Barrett's in a patient with good symptom control. Alcohol consumption is not associated with progression of Barrett's (though there is an association of hard liquor with squamous cell cancer of the esophagus). The patient's wine may in fact be protective.

HELPFUL TIP:
Prokinetic agents, like metoclopramide (Reglan), can be useful in the treatment of GERD. In addition to promoting stomach emptying, metoclopramide increases gastroesophageal sphincter tone. Remember that metoclopramide can cause extrapyramidal side effects with chronic use.

HELPFUL TIP:
Complications of chronic GERD include erosive esophagitis, peptic stricture, and adenocarcinoma of the esophagus. However, the absence of heartburn symptoms does not rule out reflux-related complications since approximately one-fourth of patients with peptic stricture (a stricture of the esophagus, which results from the healing of ulcerative esophagitis) and one-third of those with adenocarcinoma of the esophagus had no heartburn prior to diagnosis. Barrett esophagus can regress with the adequate treatment of GERD.

▶ **Objectives: Did you learn to …**
  · Describe the diagnosis and management of GERD?
  · Use H₂ blockers and PPIs in the management of GERD?
  · Recognize complications of GERD and risk factors for Barrett esophagus?

▶ **CASE 7.2**

A 53-year-old woman comes to your office complaining of chest pain and problems swallowing. She says food seems to hang up in the retrosternal area. This started several years ago, has gradually worsened, and now occurs at least twice per week. Generally, only solid foods cause problems. She has become very careful, only taking small bites and chewing them well before swallowing. Should she experience problems, she has found that drinking additional liquids alleviates her symptoms within minutes. She does not regurgitate food and has not lost weight.

Question 7.2.1 What is the symptom this patient is complaining of?
A) Dysphagia
B) Globus sensation
C) Odynophagia
D) Aerophagia
E) Phagophobia

Answer 7.2.1 The correct answer is "A." Dysphagia, from the Greek *dys* (meaning "with difficulty" … as opposed to "*Dis*,"

which is a city in Dantes's Hell in addition to being a neologism) and *phagia* (meaning "to eat"), refers to the sensation that food is being hindered in its passage from the mouth to the stomach. Odynophagia refers to pain upon swallowing, aerophagia to swallowing of air, and globus sensation to a perception of a lump or fullness in the throat that is temporarily relieved by swallowing. Phagophobia is just what you think it is: fear of eating or swallowing.

HELPFUL TIP:
Aerophagia is a common and underdiagnosed cause of abdominal symptoms. Generally, patients will complain of belching associated with abdominal bloating, especially after meals. It is not uncommon for patients to mention that they have to loosen their belt after meals. Aerophagia is exacerbated by gum chewing (which causes frequent swallowing of air), eating quickly, drinking carbonated beverages, and smoking. Aerophagia can be mitigated by eating more slowly, avoiding carbonated beverages, etc.

Question 7.2.2 Given the above patient's description of symptoms and the location of her discomfort (food sticking in the retrosternal esophagus), what type of dysphagia is she most likely to suffer from?
A) Oropharyngeal dysphagia
B) Esophageal dysphagia
C) Functional dysphagia
D) Aberrant dysphagia

Answer 7.2.2 The correct answer is "B." Dysphagia can be differentiated by where the symptoms seem to occur. Oropharyngeal dysphagia, also known as "transfer dysphagia," arises from difficulty in the upper esophagus and pharynx. Patients complain of food getting stuck immediately upon swallowing, and when asked to point to the location, patients frequently identify the cervical region. Patients with oropharyngeal dysphagia often have more problems with liquids than solids and may complain that liquid comes out of their nose when they try to swallow. The best initial test for oropharyngeal dysphagia is a modified barium swallow (video fluoroscopic swallow exam) with a liquid phase and a solid phase. Esophageal dysphagia is usually described as beginning several seconds after swallowing, and patients frequently point to the suprasternal notch or retrosternally when trying to localize the area causing symptoms. Patients in whom no cause can be found after detailed investigation are often categorized as having functional dysphagia. There is no such thing as aberrant dysphagia.

A complete review of systems and physical examination is unrevealing. She is not taking pills that can cause erosive esophagitis such as doxycycline or bisphosphonates, she is not HIV positive making candidal and HSV esophagitis unlikely, and she again notes progressive dysphagia, initially to solids and now to liquids.

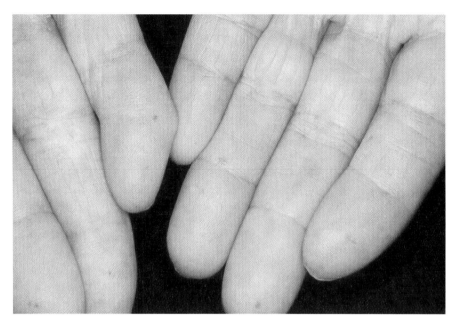

FIGURE 7-1. Telangiectasias in a patient with Raynaud's.

Question 7.2.3 Which of the following is the single best test to arrive at a diagnosis in this patient?
A) Barium swallow
B) Esophageal manometry
C) Esophagogastroduodenoscopy (EGD)
D) Ambulatory pH study of the esophagus
E) Diagnostic trial of a high-dose PPI

Answer 7.2.3 The correct answer is "C." Visualization of the esophagus is critical in patients with esophageal dysphagia. Our patient presents with esophageal dysphagia for solids, which is most consistent with a structural problem, such as a stricture, web, or neoplasm. Endoscopy is the best diagnostic study to evaluate the esophageal mucosa as it allows one to obtain biopsies and perform endoscopic interventions such as dilations, if indicated. Barium swallows are second best and have fallen out of favor when endoscopy is available. That said, barium swallow is inexpensive, noninvasive, and does not require sedation. Barium swallow can help map the esophagus and assess for lesions posing a high risk of perforation (*Cleve Clin J Med.* 2009;76(2):105–111). Should the endoscopy come back negative, esophageal manometry ("B") may be useful as it will help determine if a motility disorder is the cause of symptoms. While a "diagnostic" trial with a PPI ("E") is an appropriate strategy in patients with typical GERD, the presence of an alarm symptom, such as dysphagia, requires further testing. "D," an ambulatory pH study, does not help in defining the etiology of the dysphagia.

HELPFUL TIP:
Many patients have breakthrough pain at night even when on a PPI. The reason for this is that PPIs only act on cells that have been activated (such as by a meal). PPIs should be taken 30 minutes before eating. Try adding an H₂ blocker at nighttime for patients having breakthrough pain.

HELPFUL TIP:
Rebound acid hypersecretion can lead to symptom recurrence if potent antisecretory agents, such as PPIs, are stopped abruptly. Many experts recommend stepping down to H₂ blockers prior to cessation. However, even H₂ blockers can also cause a lesser degree of rebound acid hypersecretion. So, consider tapering these drugs as well.

The patient returns from her endoscopy. According to the report, she had severe esophagitis with confluent erosions in the distal esophagus. During your physical examination, you find the skin changes shown in Figure 7-1. When you ask about these, the patient reports a history of bluish fingertip discoloration with cold temperatures. She also complains that her fingers feel "tight" at times.

Question 7.2.4 With this new information, which of the following diagnoses are you considering?
A) CREST syndrome
B) Esophageal adenocarcinoma
C) Metastatic colonic adenocarcinoma
D) Sicca syndrome
E) Peptic ulcer disease (PUD)

Answer 7.2.4 The correct answer is "A." Note the telangiectasia on the finger pads in Figure 7-1. CREST is an acronym for a syndrome that includes **C**alcinosis cutis, **R**aynaud phenomenon, **E**sophageal dysmotility, **S**clerodactyly, and **T**elangiectasias. Up to 60% of patients with CREST have erosive esophagitis. Dysphagia is common and is due to esophageal stricture and/or dysmotility.

Question 7.2.5 Given her endoscopic findings and the fact that she likely has CREST syndrome, what treatment do you suggest?
A) H₂ blocker
B) PPI
C) High-dose corticosteroids
D) *H. pylori* eradication
E) Laparoscopic fundoplication

Answer 7.2.5 The correct answer is "B." Severe reflux and dysphagia are hallmarks of CREST syndrome. The esophagus has poor motility with impaired function of the lower esophageal sphincter allowing reflux while poor motility reduces esophageal clearance. Chronic and potent acid suppressive medications, such as PPIs, are indicated. Fundoplication is **relatively contraindicated**, as the poor contractile function of the esophagus may not generate enough force to overcome the barrier created by fundoplication. *H. pylori* treatment has no role in the management of this illness. Steroids could certainly worsen the gastrointestinal (GI) symptoms by irritating the gastric mucosa. Other causes of esophageal dysphagia are listed in Table 7-1.

HELPFUL (AND IMPORTANT) TIP:
It would not surprise us to see this one on the board examination. An increasingly recognized cause of dysphagia is **eosinophilic esophagitis**. The classic adult patient presents with dysphagia, "GERD symptoms" and upper abdominal pain unresponsive to PPIs, and possibly food impaction. Children often present with feeding problems (age 2), recurrent vomiting (age 8), and chronic abdominal pain (age 12), or food impaction (teenage years). Association with childhood asthma is strong and dietary elimination therapy may be helpful in children. This entity is found especially in those who are atopic and requires both symptoms and an esophageal biopsy result showing an increased number of eosinophils. Treatment in adults (and often children) involves swallowing inhaled corticosteroids (e.g., fluticasone or budesonide), and, in severe cases, systemic steroids. Systemic eosinophilia is rare; montelukast has a checkered record when it comes to treating eosinophilic esophagitis and appears less effective than steroids.

HELPFUL TIP:
Dysphagia that progresses from solids and then to liquids is a classic symptom of esophageal cancer and cannot be ignored.

▶ **Objectives: Did you learn to …**
- Differentiate dysphagia from other GI symptoms?
- Take an adequate history to evaluate the etiology of dysphagia?

TABLE 7-1 CAUSES OF ESOPHAGEAL DYSPHAGIA

Mechanical Lesions	
Intrinsic	**Extrinsic**
Benign tumors	Aberrant subclavian artery
Caustic esophagitis/stricture	Cervical osteophytes
Radiation esophagitis/stricture	Enlarged aorta
Peptic esophagitis/stricture	Enlarged left atrium
Eosinophilic esophagitis	Mediastinal mass
Diverticula	Postspinal surgery
Malignancy	
Post-GI surgery	
Rings and webs	
Foreign bodies	

Motility Disorders
Achalasia
Chagas disease (*Trypanosoma cruzi*)
Diffuse esophageal spasm
Hypertensive lower esophageal sphincter
Nonspecific esophageal motility disorder
Nutcracker esophagus
Scleroderma

- Describe different types of dysphagia and identify various causes of dysphagia?
- Recognize that CREST syndrome as a cause of dysphagia?

 QUICK QUIZ: REGURGITATION

You see a 61-year-old woman in your office complaining of halitosis, heartburn, and regurgitation of undigested food 4 hours after eating. She also feels that the food is sticking in her throat.

What is the most likely cause of her symptoms?
A) Schatzki ring
B) Zenker diverticulum
C) Achalasia
D) Foreign body
E) Esophageal web

The correct answer is "B." Late regurgitation of undigested food is pathognomonic for Zenker diverticulum. A Zenker diverticulum is an acquired out-pouching of esophageal mucosa, which typically becomes symptomatic in middle age or later in life. The diagnosis is confirmed by lateral view of a barium swallow or by visual confirmation with EGD. The other diagnoses listed can cause dysphagia and regurgitation but are less likely. "A," Schatzki ring, is a lower esophageal mucosal ring that can "catch" food and cause dysphagia. "C," achalasia, results from a loss of innervation of the lower esophagus with impaired esophageal motility and generally occurs in young and middle-aged adults. Patients with achalasia typically have dysphagia with solids and liquids. "D," foreign body, should be diagnosable by history. Elderly adults, children, and patients with psychiatric disease are most at risk for foreign body in the esophagus. "E," esophageal web, is caused by a thin layer of mucosa across the esophageal lumen and presents much like a Schatzki ring.

▶ CASE 7.3

A 48-year-old woman presents with 3 years of intermittent GI complaints after eating. She describes epigastric pain and bloating after food intake. Pain is described as pressure, mild-to-moderate in intensity, and nonradiating. Her weight is stable. She denies heartburn, dysphagia, vomiting, diarrhea, constipation, or blood in her stools. She only takes a multivitamin and she has not tried any specific remedies. The physical examination is normal. CMP and CBC are benign.

Question 7.3.1 What is the most likely diagnosis given the information above?
A) Pyrosis
B) Peptic ulcer disease (PUD)
C) Functional dyspepsia
D) Stomach cancer

Answer 7.3.1 **The correct answer is "C"** functional dyspepsia. "A," pyrosis, is just another name for heartburn. "B," PUD, is relatively unlikely, given the lack of risk factors and mild nature of illness. "D" is unlikely for similar reasons.

There have been significant shifts in evaluation and management of dyspepsia. ACG/CAG 2017 guidelines define dyspepsia as "predominant epigastric pain lasting at least one month." Associated symptoms often include epigastric fullness, vomiting, and heartburn. Conventional wisdom has been upended with the most recent evidence-based guidance, so let's review…

Question 7.3.2 What is the most appropriate next step in this 48-year-old female patient?
A) Obtain *H. pylori* serum antibodies
B) Obtain an abdominal ultrasound examination of liver, biliary tree, and pancreas
C) Obtain a detailed dietary history
D) Obtain an upper GI x-ray series
E) Refer for gastroscopy

Answer 7.3.2 **The correct answer is "C."** A good history and physical is always a good starting point! While food intolerance does not cause functional dyspepsia, the symptoms of the two types of disorders overlap to some degree. Considering the prevalence of selective carbohydrate malabsorption syndromes, high intake of lactose- and fructose-containing foods and beverages may contribute to GI symptoms in a significant number of patients. Therefore, the history should always contain a detailed assessment of dietary habits and symptoms in relation to food intake.

You obtain a detailed dietary history, suggesting a potential contribution of fructose intolerance and excessive carbonated beverage intake (it's those five Giant Gulp soft drinks a day). After appropriate dietary modification, her symptoms of postprandial pain and bloating are unchanged.

Question 7.3.3 Now what is the most appropriate next step in this patient?
A) Obtain *H. pylori* stool antigen
B) Obtain an abdominal ultrasound examination of liver, biliary tree, and pancreas
C) Run a trial of PPI
D) Obtain an upper GI x-ray series
E) Refer for gastroscopy

Answer 7.3.3 **The correct answer is "A."** Patients under the age of 60 with dyspepsia should have noninvasive testing for *H. pylori*, with plans to treat if positive. Preferred noninvasive testing includes stool antigen and 13C urea breath test. Treat for *H. pylori* if positive. If symptoms persist despite treatment, or if *H. pylori* testing is negative, it's appropriate to proceed to PPI trial. If symptoms persist with PPI, addition of a tricyclic antidepressant or prokinetic agent is reasonable. When all else fails, consider psychotherapy to help your patient cope with ongoing symptoms. Without focal symptoms or lab abnormalities, there is no indication for ultrasound at this point. Endoscopy is not indicated for dyspepsia in patients <60 years old unless they are high risk (e.g., family history, growing up in South East Asia or South America). Note that even an isolated alarm feature (including weight loss, anemia, vomiting) in the **absence** of refractory or new onset GERD > age 45–50 years of age is no longer considered reason for endoscopy!

HELPFUL TIP:
The shift away from endoscopy is uncomfortable for this author and flies in the face of traditional practice. In the end, remember these are guidelines and not standards of care. A move away from unnecessary invasive testing is good for patient safety and cost management. Patients with progressive symptoms, progressive weight loss, risk factors for malignancy, and ***all patients greater than age 60 with dyspepsia warrant EGD***.

Question 7.3.4 Which of the following is true of the natural history of functional dyspepsia?
A) Most patients will not have symptom-free periods, instead having constant dyspepsia
B) Most patients improve with placebo treatment
C) Most patients will go on to develop ulcers
D) Spontaneous resolution of symptoms is rare

Answer 7.3.4 **The correct answer is "B."** Up to 60% of patients in placebo-controlled trials respond to placebo, making it difficult to prove the efficacy of medications. As the above number suggests, spontaneous resolution of symptoms is common, while many patients will have a chronic, intermittent course characterized by symptom-free periods. Most patients will not develop serious pathology.

HELPFUL TIP:
For functional dyspepsia, general management principles call for reassurance by the physician and the avoidance of repeated diagnostic testing. Patients should make appropriate life style modifications (avoid tobacco, caffeine products, and alcohol) and limit or avoid aggravating medications (NSAIDs). Patients should chew their foods slowly and eat more frequent, smaller meals. Finally, if there is underlying psychiatric morbidity, relaxation training, or treatment of specific diseases can be helpful.

Back to our 48-year-old. *H. pylori* **testing is negative. You continue to avoid invasive testing and start the patient on a PPI with modest benefit. One week later, your nurse receives a call from your patient about abdominal cramping and diarrhea. She has not noticed blood in her stool.**

Question 7.3.5 What is the best next step?
A) She is having withdrawal from the five Giant Gulp sodas. Add back the fructose and the 2,000 kcal
B) Check fasting gastrin level
C) Add antibiotic therapy for bacterial overgrowth
D) Discontinue the PPI
E) Add an antidiarrheal

Answer 7.3.5 **The correct answer is "D."** Diarrhea, including from *Clostridium difficile*, is a common adverse effect of PPIs that occurs in at least 5% to 7% of patients. Discontinuation of the PPI generally leads to a rapid resolution in the majority of cases (although maybe not in *C. difficile*-related diarrhea). While reduced stomach acidity from PPIs or H₂ blockers may result in bacterial colonization of the proximal GI tract, the early onset and severity of symptoms described argue against bacterial overgrowth as the etiology of this patient's symptoms ("C"). While PPIs can elevate gastrin levels, the hypergastrinemia seen is not comparable to levels seen in Zollinger–Ellison syndrome, which can also cause diarrhea. Stool studies and empiric therapy with antidiarrheals may be considered if discontinuing the PPI does not improve symptoms.

HELPFUL TIP:
For dyspepsia, prokinetic agents may be helpful, and in the United States this means metoclopramide or erythromycin. Cisapride (Propulsid) has been removed from the market secondary to cardiac arrhythmias (QT prolongation with torsades de pointes). Metoclopramide (Reglan), of course, is associated with tardive dyskinesia and extrapyramidal reactions. Erythromycin causes GI side effects and QT prolongation.

HELPFUL TIP:
PPIs are not benign drugs and have been associated with (1) increased risk of osteoporosis and hip fracture in the elderly, (2) increased risk of pneumonia, (3) increased risk of *C. difficile* colitis, (4) interference with vitamin and mineral absorption (B vitamins, iron, calcium), and (5) diarrhea as noted previously. Initially, data suggested that PPIs were associated with dementia. This association has not held up (*J Am Geriatr Soc.* 2018 Feb;66(2): 247–253, etc.) and the association with pneumonia has been questioned (*BMJ.* 2016 Nov 15;355:i5813). Nonetheless, stop PPIs after the treatment is completed (if you can . . . . GERD is a chronic disease and stopping a PPI is associated with rebound acid secretion) and aim for the lowest effective dose.

▶ **Objectives: Did you learn to …**
· Diagnose and manage nonulcer dyspepsia?
· Appreciate the natural history of nonulcer dyspepsia?
· Recognize important side effects of PPIs?

▶ **CASE 7.4**

A 56-year-old woman comes to the emergency department after a sudden episode of hematemesis. Yesterday, she had two bowel movements that were dark, sticky, and foul-smelling. She woke up nauseated and has since twice vomited a small amount of bright red blood. She also feels dizzy. Because of knee pain related to skydiving 1 week ago, she started taking five tablets of naproxen (1,100 mg) twice daily. She takes no other medicines and denies any significant past medical history.

On physical examination, you find a pale, uncomfortable, but alert patient. She is tachycardic (pulse of 115 bpm) and has a blood pressure drop from 116/72 mm Hg supine to 93/65 mm Hg standing. Her abdomen is flat with hyperactive bowel sounds. You note epigastric tenderness but no rebound or guarding. There is melena on rectal examination.

Question 7.4.1 Which of the following steps will be LEAST helpful at this point in time?
A) Admission to the hospital
B) Immediate treatment with an intravenous (IV) H₂ blocker
C) Referral for emergent endoscopy
D) IV access and fluid resuscitation
E) Laboratory tests including hemoglobin, coagulation studies, and blood type and cross-match

Answer 7.4.1 **The correct answer is "B."** The patient has symptoms and clinical findings of a hemodynamically significant upper GI tract bleed. Although she is "walking and talking" just fine, fluid administration and hospital admission with close monitoring in an intensive care environment are indicated. A baseline hemoglobin and hematocrit should be obtained. **However, a normal hemoglobin concentration does not** exclude a significant acute bleed, as hemodilution (in the absence of IV fluids) requires several hours. Two large-bore IVs should be placed. Given the presentation, a blood transfusion may become necessary in the future; therefore, blood should be sent for type and cross-match. Early endoscopy (ideally within 24 hours) should be performed to identify the cause of her bleeding, and endoscopic therapy should be undertaken if appropriate. Treatment with H_2 blockers does not affect the rate of bleeding; however, IV PPI therapy **does** decrease the risk of rebleeding in high-risk patients by increasing gastric pH to enhance coagulation. **PPI therapy and endoscopy are standard of care for upper GI bleeding.**

HELPFUL TIP:
Orthostatic vital signs are not that useful in determining a patient's volume status. Many hypovolemic patients are **not** orthostatic and many patients who are euvolemic **have** orthostatic changes (e.g., patients on antihypertensives and the elderly). So, use orthostatic vital signs to confirm your clinical suspicion, but do not use them as an absolute guide to the patient's volume status (*JAMA.* 1999;281:1022–1029).

HELPFUL TIP:
Nasogastric aspirate may be heme (e.g., Gastroccult®) negative in up to 72% of upper GI bleeds. A positive test is confirmatory, but a negative test is fairly meaningless. NG tubes are not routinely recommended.

Question 7.4.2 What is the risk of suffering a clinically significant GI event on NSAIDs?
A) Up to 4% per year
B) Up to 10% per year
C) Up to 25% per year
D) Up to 50% per year
E) Nearly 99% per year

Answer 7.4.2 The correct answer is "A." The risk of a clinically significant NSAID-related GI event, including GI bleeding, perforation, or obstruction, is about 1% to 4% per year.

The patient undergoes endoscopy, which shows a small duodenal ulcer in the bulb with a visible vessel in the ulcer base. Biopsies show chemical gastropathy and no evidence of *H. pylori.* After endoscopic treatment, the patient recovers nicely. Then, 3 months later, she returns to your office for a follow-up evaluation. She is asymptomatic and continues taking a PPI. Her physical examination is normal. Laboratory tests show normal hemoglobin.

Question 7.4.3 What is the best next step?
A) Repeat endoscopy to document healing and rule out malignancy
B) Perform upper GI x-ray series to document healing

C) Switch to a H_2 blocker
D) Discontinue acid-suppressive medication
E) Obtain serum *H. pylori* antibody test

Answer 7.4.3 The correct answer is "D." While nonhealing ulcers may be due to a neoplasm, the vast majority of **duodenal** ulcers are benign. Therefore, neither endoscopic nor radiologic documentation of healing is necessary. See Table 7-2 for more on risk factors for malignancy in gastric ulcers. "C" is incorrect. Patients with uncomplicated and small (<1 cm) duodenal or gastric ulcers who have received adequate treatment of *H. pylori* or NSAID-induced ulcer do not need long-term therapy directed at ulcer healing as long as they are asymptomatic following therapy. Antisecretory drugs can be discontinued after 4 to 6 weeks in these patients. "E" is incorrect. Serology for *H. pylori* will not be helpful in this patient. First, histology is as sensitive as other tests for *H. pylori* infection and the patient's biopsies were negative for *H. pylori.* Second, **serologic testing does not tell us if the patient is currently infected**, as many patients maintain antibody positivity even a year after treatment.

HELPFUL TIP:
Sensitivity of serologic testing for *H. pylori* is 90% to 100%. But this does not indicate current infection and may reflect prior infection. Breath testing is 88% to 95% sensitive with most false negatives the result of the use of antibiotics and antacids, including H_2 blockers and PPIs. Thus, make sure that the patient has been off antibiotics for at least a month prior to testing and has not taken acid suppressors for 2 weeks prior to testing. This also holds true for CLO testing. Stool antigen testing (94% sensitive, 92% specific) is also available to help with the noninvasive documentation of *H. pylori* infection or eradication. False-negative stool antigen assays may be due to recent (within 2 weeks) use of antibiotics or antacids.

Question 7.4.4 If your patient had come back *H. pylori* positive, which of the following combinations IS NOT indicated in the treatment of *H. pylori?*
A) Omeprazole, clarithromycin, metronidazole
B) Cephalexin, omeprazole, amoxicillin

TABLE 7-2 RISK FACTORS FOR MALIGNANCY IN GASTRIC ULCERS

- Occurrence in ethnic groups raised in endemic areas (Asians, Latinos, etc.)
- *Helicobacter pylori* infection
- Absence of recent NSAID use
- Absence of concomitant duodenal ulcer or a prior history of duodenal ulcer (duodenal ulcers require higher acid secretion, which is incompatible with the pangastritis typical of most gastric cancers)
- Giant ulcers (>2–3 cm)
- Absence of a protracted ulcer history—in general, the longer the ulcer history, the lower the risk that a gastric ulcer is cancer. Gastric ulcers require acid and gastric cancer usually develops in the setting of atrophic pangastritis

C) Metronidazole, amoxicillin, omeprazole
D) Bismuth subsalicylate, metronidazole, tetracycline, lansoprazole
E) Omeprazole, clarithromycin, amoxicillin

Answer 7.4.4 The correct answer (and the regimen you would not want to use) is "B." All of the other regimens can be used to treat *H. pylori* infection. Of note are regimens "A" and "D." There is resistance to metronidazole, so it should only be used when the patient is penicillin allergic or taking quadruple therapy. Triple therapy with PPI should be used where clarithromycin resistance is low. Quadruple therapy should be used in patients with recent or repeated exposure to clarithromycin or metronidazole or areas with high clarithromycin resistance (>15%).

Question 7.4.5 Which of the following IS NOT useful for testing for *H. pylori* eradication after treatment?
A) Serum IgG antibody titers
B) CLO test
C) Breath urea test
D) Radioactive CO_2 blood test
E) Stool antigen test

Answer 7.4.5 The correct answer is "A." Remember the helpful tip mentioned previously? Only 57% of patients are antibody negative to *H. pylori* a year after successful treatment. Thus, antibody titers cannot document eradication. All of the other tests mentioned are functional tests for the presence of *H. pylori*. The CLO test is done on biopsy specimens and documents the presence of urea splitting. The same is true for the breath urea test and the radioactive CO_2 blood test. In both of these tests, urea is ingested. If *H. pylori* is present, radioactive CO_2 is generated that can be measured in the blood or breath. Confirmation of eradication should be considered for all patients receiving *H. pylori* treatment 1 month after treatment and at least 1 to 2 weeks off of PPI, but definitely should be performed in the following: (1) patients with persistent symptoms of dyspepsia despite *H. pylori* treatment; (2) patients with *H. pylori* associated ulcer; (3) patients with gastric mucosa–associated lymphoid tissue–type lymphoma; (4) patients who had resection for early gastric cancer (*N Engl J Med*. 2010;362:1597–1604).

 HELPFUL TIP:
NSAID-induced ulcers can occur in the stomach, duodenum, and occasionally in the small bowel and colon. However, NSAIDs are more frequently found to be the cause of gastric ulcers (up to 30%) than the cause of duodenal ulcers (up to 20%). Remember that NSAIDS (except for aspirin) can precipitate acute coronary syndrome.

▶ **Objectives: Did you learn to …**
• Appreciate the role of NSAID use in peptic ulcer disease (PUD)?
• Manage an acute GI bleed?
• Identify patients at high risk for gastric malignancy?
• Diagnose and treat *H. pylori*?

 QUICK QUIZ: PILL PROBLEMS

Which of these medications would be the LEAST likely cause of esophagitis if caught in the esophagus?
A) Potassium chloride
B) Ferrous sulfate
C) Alendronate
D) Loratadine
E) Tetracycline

The correct answer is "D." Many medications can cause "pill esophagitis," including potassium chloride, ferrous sulfate, alendronate, tetracycline antibiotics, and ascorbic acid. Aspirin and other NSAIDs can also cause esophagitis. Smaller pills are less likely to cause problems. In addition to not being irritating, loratadine is tiny.

 QUICK QUIZ: THE CASE OF THE HOLY STOMACH

One of your patients presents complaining of diarrhea and epigastric pain unresponsive to H_2 blockers or PPIs. He denies smoking tobacco, taking NSAIDs, or drinking alcohol. Endoscopy reveals several ulcers. Biopsy for *H. pylori* is negative and there is no malignancy.

Which of the following would be the most appropriate laboratory test to obtain in order to discover an etiology for the *multiple* ulcers (and diarrhea)?
A) Vasoactive intestinal peptide (VIP)
B) Gastrin
C) Glucagon
D) Somatostatin

The correct answer is "B." Some sort of screening test for gastrinoma is warranted in a patient who has recurrent or refractory ulcers and who is *H. pylori* negative and does not use NSAIDs. Zollinger–Ellison syndrome is the name given to the state in which there is acid hypersecretion secondary to increased gastrin production, usually from a gastrin-producing tumor (gastrinoma). Up to 1% of patients with PUD have a gastrinoma. Serum gastrin levels should be obtained with the patient fasting **and off PPIs, as PPIs will increase gastrin levels.** If the serum gastrin is elevated (>10 times upper normal limit), further investigations will need to be performed. Other reasons to consider obtaining a serum gastrin level include ulcers in unusual locations (distal duodenal and jejunum), family history of ulcers, and ulcers associated with severe esophagitis. "A" is incorrect. VIP actually works to suppress acid secretion. VIPomas do occur, but VIPomas are associated with watery diarrhea and hypokalemia—not ulcers. "C," glucagon, will not be of much help here. Glucagon over secretion results in hyperglycemia and anemia. "D," somatostatin, is a hormone that inhibits the secretion of gastrin and thus would be protective vis-à-vis ulcers. Somatostatin secreting tumors are very rare.

 QUICK QUIZ: GI BLEEDING

Isolated bright red hematemesis (e.g., no tachycardia and no fever), which occurs after several bouts of vomiting or dry heaves, is referred to as:
A) Boerhaave syndrome
B) Mallory–Weiss tear
C) Cameron lesion
D) None of the above

The correct answer is "B." A Mallory–Weiss tear occurs after repeated trauma to the lower esophageal and gastric mucosa from forceful retching. This can be differentiated from a Boerhaave tear by the (generally) self-limited nature of the bleeding and the absence of other symptoms. Boerhaave syndrome ("A") is a perforation of the esophagus resulting from a sudden increase in intraesophageal pressure, caused by vomiting, retching, less frequently by coughing, childbirth, or weight lifting. It occurs higher in the esophagus and is associated with mediastinitis, fever, shock, and death if intervention is not forthcoming. Cameron lesions ("C") are small ulcers in patients with a hiatal hernia, are usually an incidental finding, and are likely caused by rubbing of the stomach against the diaphragm as the hernia slides. They can bleed, but the history given above is classic for a Mallory–Weiss tear.

 QUICK QUIZ: ABDOMINAL PAIN

A 35-year-old female presents to your clinic complaining of onset of severe mid-epigastric pain, weight loss, and vomiting following meals. Between meals she is asymptomatic. This has been going on for the past 2 years ever since she purposefully lost 25 lb to attain a healthy weight for her height. Unfortunately, she has continued to lose weight because of the postprandial pain and vomiting. On her examination you notice a mid-epigastric bruit.

The most likely diagnosis is:
A) Aortic aneurysm
B) Atherosclerotic disease of the celiac trunk
C) Superior mesenteric artery (SMA) syndrome
D) Chronic pancreatitis
E) None of the above

The correct answer is "C." This is a typical history and physical examination for SMA syndrome. SMA syndrome is more likely to occur in a patient who has lost significant weight, resulting in thinning of the mesenteric fat pad. Here's the pathophysiology: the SMA runs above the duodenum and becomes stretched and partially occluded in response to meals (as the stomach and duodenum expand), leading to mesenteric ischemia and

food aversion; the fat pad is protective. SMA syndrome can be diagnosed using Doppler ultrasound to demonstrate increased velocity of blood in the SMA or by a CT-angiogram. "A" and "B" are unlikely in a young patient, and "D" should not be associated with a bruit. Celiac artery syndrome may have a similar presentation to SMA syndrome but, obviously, involves the celiac trunk.

▶ **CASE 7.5**

A 54-year-old man comes to your office for his annual physical. He is taking naproxen for a recent ankle injury. Based on your recommendation last year, he started taking one aspirin (81 mg) daily. He does not take any other medications. He exercises regularly, does not smoke, and drinks one glass of wine every day. Your examination is completely normal, except that a test for occult fecal blood is positive.

Question 7.5.1 What is the next best step?
A) Upper endoscopy
B) CBC
C) Colonoscopy
D) A and B
E) B and C

Answer 7.5.1 **The correct answer is "E."** This patient has heme positive stools and needs a colonoscopy. See below for details of colon cancer screening. Since the patient currently has no symptoms referable to upper GI pathology, evaluation of the upper GI tract should only be considered if the colonoscopy is negative.

 HELPFUL TIP:
Iron supplements may cause stool to darken but they DO NOT cause false-positive guaiac tests. Guaiac tests rely on the presence of hemoglobin in the stool, not iron. Don't blame a positive guaiac on an iron supplement.

Question 7.5.2 Regarding colon cancer, what is the most likely type of cancer you will find?
A) Squamous cell carcinoma
B) Adenocarcinoma
C) Clear cell carcinoma
D) Lymphoma

Answer 7.5.2 **The correct answer is "B."** Adenocarcinoma represents the overwhelming majority of colon cancers. Other histologic types of colon cancer include adenosquamous, poorly differentiated cancers with neuroendocrine aspects, small cell carcinomas (of neuroendocrine origin), and others.

Your patient asks the perennial question that theologians are usually better qualified to answer: "Why me?" In this case, however, we can provide some insight.

Question 7.5.3 Which of the following is NOT considered a risk factor for colon cancer?
A) Familial polyposis
B) Alcohol use
C) Obesity
D) Inflammatory bowel disease
E) Chronic constipation

Answer 7.5.3 **The correct answer is "E."** Chronic constipation is not a risk factor for colon cancer. Aside from those listed above, risk factors include: acromegaly, diabetes mellitus, African-American race, immunosuppression, and tobacco use, among others. African Americans have the highest risk for colon cancer of any ethnic group, as well as a higher mortality (20% higher compared to white Americans). Screening for colon cancer in African Americans should begin at age 45 (see the following).

Review of his records shows that he underwent a colonoscopy 3 years ago. Three small adenomatous polyps were found. He also had scattered diverticula in the sigmoid.

Question 7.5.4 Based on this new information, which strategy do you now recommend?
A) Colonoscopy now
B) Colonoscopy in 5 years
C) Yearly tests for fecal occult blood
D) Yearly tests for fecal occult blood and colonoscopy in 7 years
E) Colonoscopy in 7 years

Answer 7.5.4 **The correct answer is "A."** Adenomatous polyps are considered precancerous. Recommended follow-up of an adenomatous polyp is by colonoscopy every 3 to 5 years. So, he did not truly have a "negative" colonoscopy 3 years ago. Plus, we are not doing the colonoscopy in this case for screening purposes; it is diagnostic. We may find another source of his bleeding. If his previous colonoscopy was completely normal (no adenomatous polyps), you could argue for stopping the aspirin and NSAIDs and following up with serial fecal occult blood tests (FOBTs). In this alternative scenario, persistently positive tests for occult blood would lead to colonoscopy as well.

HELPFUL TIP:
Adenomatous colon polyps, either pedunculated or sessile, are associated with transformation to cancer. Hyperplastic polyps are considered benign.

HELPFUL TIP:
US Preventive Services Task Force recommends routine screening for colorectal cancer, starting at the age of 50 to 75 years for average-risk patients (earlier in high-risk patients—positive family history, known adenomatous polyps, etc.). Any of the following modalities is

acceptable. The USPSTF does not favor one screening method above others:
1) **Annual FOBT alone** (fecal immunochemical test [FIT] or high sensitivity guaiac [e.g., SENSA] ... other guaiac tests are less sensitive). **Fecal immunochemical test** (FIT) detects human hemoglobin by immunologic means and is more sensitive and specific than guaiac. It also circumvents many of the weaknesses of the old guaiac test (e.g., false positive with rare meat), but will still give a false positive secondary to bleeding from NSAIDs
2) **FOBT every 3 years with sigmoidoscopy every 5 years**
3) **Colonoscopy every 10 years (without annual FOBT)**
4) **FIT + DNA** is more sensitive but less specific than FIT alone
5) **Other options** include fecal DNA testing (Cologuard), computed tomography colonography

In general, the FIT and guaiac-based FOBT have lower sensitivity for proximal neoplasm. Also, FIT does not detect serrated polyps that are the progenitors of 20% to 30% of malignancies. Between the ages of 75 and 85 years, *routine screening* is not recommended but select patients should be counseled on screening. After the age of 85, no screening should be done.

HELPFUL TIP:
US Multi-Society Task Force on Colon Cancer (includes the American College of Gastroenterology, the American Gastroenterological Association, and The American Society for Gastrointestinal Endoscopy) published recommendations in 2017 to start screening African Americans of average risk at age 45. First-tier options include annual fecal immunochemical testing or colonoscopy every 10 years. Second-tier screening options include CT colonography every 5 years, FIT testing every 3 years, or flexible sigmoidoscopy every 10 years. Third-tier option was capsule colonoscopy every 5 years. Guaiac-based FOBT was dropped from their screening recommendations.

You refer the patient for a colonoscopy. The report from the endoscopist shows one small tubular adenomatous polyp in the sigmoid colon that was completely removed. The patient wants to know when he needs another colonoscopy.

Question 7.5.5 **Your answer is:**
A) In 3 months
B) In 1 year
C) In 5 years
D) In 10 years
E) Any of the above is an equally valid recommendation

Answer 7.5.5 The correct answer is "C." The current surveillance guidelines recommend the following intervals for screening:

1. No polyps or only rectal hyperplastic polyps, repeat in 10 years.
2. One to two tubular adenomas less than 1 cm in size with only low-grade dysplasia should have repeat colonoscopy in 5 years.
3. Three to ten tubular adenomas, or villous features or high-grade dysplasia should have surveillance in 3 years.
4. Patients with >10 adenomas should be screened more frequently, and familial colon cancer syndromes should be considered.
5. If a large sessile polyp is removed in piecemeal fashion, then a repeat examination in 3 months is appropriate to assure complete removal.
6. If the prep is not good, repeat colonoscopy at earliest convenience is indicated.

. . . .

Whoops, the pathologist calls back and it turns out your patient has a colon cancer. He is justifiably worried about the possibility of colon cancer in his offspring. Unfortunately, none of his kids exercise (which reduces colon cancer risk) and they are avowed carnivores, eschewing fruit, vegetables, and anything with fiber (which may reduce colon cancer risk, although the data is conflicting).

Question 7.5.6 Which of the following has been shown to reduce cancer risk and takes so little effort that even your patient's slothful offspring may partake?
A) Metformin
B) Aspirin
C) Antioxidants
D) Vitamin B6 but no other antioxidants
E) B and C

Answer 7.5.6 The correct answer is "B." Aspirin does have a slight protective effect on colon cancer (USPSTF found 40% relative risk reduction in incident colon cancer with aspirin use) but not heart disease. Unfortunately, the rest of the answers are incorrect and none have been found to reduce the risk of colon cancer.

Question 7.5.7 Patients presenting with hereditary nonpolyposis colorectal cancer (HNPCC), or "Lynch syndrome," are more likely than patients with sporadic colon cancer to have which of the following findings?
A) Left-sided colon cancers
B) Late age onset of colon cancer
C) Multiple colon cancers diagnosed simultaneously
D) An unusual desire to visit Lynchburg, Tennessee, and a dedication to all things Jack Daniels

Answer 7.5.7 The correct answer is "C." Patients with HNPCC (Lynch syndrome) are at increased risk of developing colon cancer. About 5% of colon cancers occur in patients with Lynch syndrome. Transformation from an adenoma to cancer is faster in patients with Lynch syndrome. In addition, many of the neoplasms are located in the right colon, so "A" is incorrect.

Compared to sporadic colon cancer patients, those with Lynch syndrome are younger at the time of diagnosis, more frequently present with multiple colon tumors, and are more likely to have extracolonic tumors—especially endometrial cancer. This is a genetic disorder, and the occurrence of colorectal and/or **endometrial** cancer in three relatives before the age of 50 should suggest HNPCC. The current recommendation is to perform surveillance colonoscopies at least every 3 years in these patients.

. . . .

It is time to stage your patient's cancer. The Duke's classification system is no longer used for colon cancer and has been replaced with the more standardized TMN system.

Question 7.5.8 Which of the following is the most common first site of metastasis of colon cancer?
A) Lungs
B) Liver
C) Bone
D) Brain

Answer 7.5.8 The correct answer is "B." The liver is the most common first site of colon cancer metastases, which arrive via the portal system. Colon cancer can also metastasize to the lungs, bone, lymph nodes, and brain (uncommon). Intraperitoneal spread may also occur.

. . . .

Your patient wonders if blood tests can predict his death (and the direction of the stock market … and if the Cubs will ever again win the world series).

Question 7.5.9 While tumor markers for colon cancer are not used in staging disease, the presence of which of these markers suggests a poor prognosis if it remains elevated after surgical resection of the tumor?
A) Carcinoembryonic antigen (CEA)
B) β-hCG
C) CA-125
D) Vasoactive intestinal peptide (VIP)
E) α-Fetoprotein (AFP)

Answer 7.5.9 The correct answer is "A." The presence of CEA after resection of a colon cancer is a poor prognostic factor. This should be obvious: there is still tumor present. β-hCG is elevated in some testicular cancers. CA-125 is a marker for ovarian cancer (although it is also expressed by colon cancer cells and is *not* to be used as a screening test for ovarian cancer). VIP is either the patient who everyone swarms over and nobody can please *or* vasoactive intestinal peptide, which is found with some pancreatic adenocarcinomas and carcinoid tumors. AFP is elevated in germ-cell tumors, such as testicular and ovarian cancer, and liver cancer.

. . . .

HELPFUL TIP:
Flushing? Diarrhea? Elevated heart rate? While 5-HIAA sounds like an acronym for some new government initiative, it is a marker of carcinoid tumor activity.

John undergoes surgery and ends up with a total colectomy and ileostomy.

Question 7.5.10 Which of the following is NOT true of ileostomy care?
A) Fluid output tends to be relatively high with an ileostomy requiring increased fluid intake to prevent dehydration
B) Since the diameter of the ileostomy is limited, avoiding large amounts of nondigestible fiber helps to prevent bezoar formation
C) Extended-release drugs are usually well absorbed
D) Proteolytic enzymes are present in the effluent and may lead to skin breakdown

Answer 7.5.10 **The correct answer is "C."** Extended-release medications should be used with caution. Many extended-release medications are absorbed through the entire length of the bowel. Have your patient notify you if they are finding undigested pills in their ostomy bag. All of the rest are correct.

HELPFUL TIP:
Loperamide can be used to reduce output in short bowel syndrome (including in those with an ostomy) as long as bacterial overgrowth is not an issue.

Your patient does well and has a happy and long life, although his children remain slugs and he supports them well into their forties.

▶ **Objectives: Did you learn to …**
• Describe the limitations of FOBT?
• Choose the appropriate tests and screening and surveillance intervals for colorectal neoplasia?
• Learn how family and personal history of colorectal neoplasia affects screening and surveillance strategy?

▶ **CASE 7.6**

A 28-year-old graduate student comes to your office complaining of diarrhea. About 6 months ago, she noted a sudden onset of loose stools. While she initially attributed these symptoms to "stomach flu," her problem has persisted. She currently has about four to six loose bowel movements per day with nighttime defecations. She has not seen blood in her stool. In addition, she complains of cramps located in the left and occasionally right lower abdomen. The cramps are made worse with food intake and often are associated with a need to defecate. She has lost about 8 kg unintentionally within the last 3 to 4 months. She denies any travel or antibiotic use. On physical examination, you notice some tenderness in the right lower quadrant. You see a painless anal fissure in the anterior commissure, and by the appearance, you judge that the fissure is probably chronic in nature.

Question 7.6.1 What do you recommend as the next step in the evaluation and management of this patient?
A) Trial of loperamide on a scheduled basis
B) Referral to a holistic clinic for a coffee colonic cleansing regimen (using fair trade, shade grown organic coffee only, of course)
C) Titers for atypical antineutrophil cytoplasmic antibodies (ANCA)
D) Colonoscopy
E) Botulinum toxin injection into the area of the anal fissure

Answer 7.6.1 **The correct answer is "D."** The patient's history and physical findings with a painless, anteriorly located anal fissure and diarrhea are consistent with Crohn disease. The best next step in her evaluation is colonoscopy with inspection of the terminal ileum. You may want to do some stool testing before colonoscopy. Testing for *Giardia*, *C. difficile* toxin, and other pathogens is appropriate. CRP can be helpful to track response to therapy if elevated but is normal in 40% of patients with active flare so cannot be used to "rule out" Crohn disease. But of the choices presented, colonoscopy is the best option. "A" is inappropriate since this is long-standing with weight loss; symptomatic control is fine, but we need to figure out what is going on with this patient. "B" is incorrect, coffee is better PO. "C," serologic testing, is a reasonable choice but not ANCA, and here's why: Crohn disease is associated with antibodies against saccharomyces (ASCA), while ulcerative colitis (UC) patients are more often positive for ANCA. However, the sensitivity of these tests is only about 60%. Moreover, there is about a 20% overlap (e.g., ANCA positive in Crohn disease), raising further questions about the overall usefulness of these tests. ASCA can also be positive in celiac disease. "E" is also incorrect. Fissures are one of the anal manifestations of Crohn disease and should be approached by treating the underlying disease rather than using surgical techniques, botulinum injection, etc. Botulinum injections, nitroglycerin ointment, and nifedipine have all been used for anal fissures with success, but we need to diagnose this patient and address the underlying disease. Botulinum injections also get rid of those embarrassing anal wrinkles.

HELPFUL TIP:
Fecal calprotectin levels are helpful in distinguishing irritable bowel syndrome (IBS) from inflammatory bowel disease (IBD) in adults. Calprotectin is produced by granulocytes, and its presence in the stool indicates active inflammation and suggests IBD. Sensitivity 93% and specificity 96% (*BMJ*. 2010;341:c3369). Despite being markers of white cells, neither fecal leukocytes nor fecal lactoferrin are helpful.

HELPFUL TIP:
In Crohn disease, about 25% of patients have disease confined to the colon. Another 40% have disease in the ileum and cecum, and 30% have disease confined to the small bowel. The remainder have more diffuse disease and/or disease in the proximal GI tract.

Question 7.6.2 Which of the following is true regarding the pathophysiology and natural history of Crohn disease?
A) Crohn disease is a genetic disorder, transmitted in an auto-somal-dominant fashion
B) Crohn disease is a relapsing/remitting disease, and 30% of patients will improve spontaneously
C) Patients with Crohn disease rarely progress to disease requiring surgery
D) Maintenance therapy with glucocorticoids will reduce the rate of recurrence of Crohn disease
E) GI fistulae and abscesses are rare complications of Crohn disease

Answer 7.6.2 The correct answer is "B." Crohn disease and UC are both relapsing/remitting diseases. Up to 30% of initial exacerbations of Crohn disease will remit without any intervention. While there is a genetic component to inflammatory bowel disease (up to a 100-fold increase in risk among first-degree relatives with IBD), no single, autosomal-dominant gene has been identified. "C" is incorrect because half or more of patients with Crohn disease will ultimately require some sort of surgery. "D" is incorrect. Unfortunately, chronic glucocorticoid administration does not lower the rate of relapse. There are many complications of IBD (see next question), and GI abscesses and fistulae occur with a relatively high frequency (20–40%) in Crohn disease.

HELPFUL TIP:
Although considered a disease of young adults, there is a bimodal distribution of IBD with a second peak in older adults in their seventies.

Question 7.6.3 Extraintestinal features of IBD include all of the following EXCEPT:
A) Alopecia
B) Arthritis
C) Sclerosing cholangitis
D) Uveitis
E) Cholelithiasis

Answer 7.6.3 The correct answer is "A." Alopecia is not an extraintestinal manifestation of IBD. Arthritis ("B") related to IBD (enteropathic arthritis) is fairly common and usually migratory in nature, involving the large joints. Spondyloarthropathy may also be seen. Sclerosing cholangitis ("C") and autoimmune hepatitis can occur and may be fatal. Eye disease may include uveitis ("D") and episcleritis. Importantly, the main treatment of extraintestinal manifestations is to treat the IBD. IBD spondyloarthropathy and pyoderma gangrenosum are important exceptions, as these do not always improve with the treatment of the underlying IBD.

HELPFUL TIP:
Toxic megacolon is a potentially deadly complication of IBD that should be suspected in a patient with IBD who presents with fever, abdominal pain, and shock. Even in

nontoxic patients a transverse colon diameter >5.5 cm or sigmoid colon diameter >10 cm should prompt evaluation for obstruction or impending disaster.

....

Returning to your patient, you next see her in the emergency department, where she presents with fever, abdominal pain, and bloody diarrhea. She is tachycardic and slightly hypotensive but alert and oriented. You suspect a relapse of her Crohn disease.

Question 7.6.4 All of the following are important aspects of her management at this time EXCEPT:
A) Surgical consultation
B) IV access and fluid administration
C) Glucocorticoids
D) NSAIDs
E) Metronidazole and ciprofloxacin

Answer 7.6.4 The correct answer is "D." What's in a name? NSAIDs are contraindicated and in spite of being "anti-inflammatory" can actually exacerbate IBD. Acetaminophen or narcotics can be used for pain control if necessary. The patient should be stabilized, and this includes IV access and fluid resuscitation. An exacerbation (or relapse) of IBD can be treated with glucocorticoids in the acute setting. Metronidazole and ciprofloxacin are no longer used to induce remission of Crohn disease and occupy a niche role in preventing recurrence after bowel resection. However, antibiotics are often used in unstable patients. In this patient, who may have an abscess or obstruction, antibiotics and further evaluation (e.g., labs and abdominal CT) and surgical consultation are necessary. Finally, thalidomide has been used for Crohn disease but is not standard of care.

Question 7.6.5 Which of the following is indicated in the long-term treatment of Crohn disease?
A) Azathioprine
B) Methotrexate
C) 5-ASA moieties
D) Loperamide
E) All of the above

Answer 7.6.5 The correct answer is "E." All the options are indicated for the treatment of IBD. Systemic steroids (e.g., prednisone) are useful acutely to induce remission but should be tapered and stopped as soon as possible. Use of steroids for greater than 4 months is discouraged.

Methotrexate and thiopurines (azathioprine, 6-mercaptopurine) are mainstays of oral therapy. Advanced therapy options continue to grow and include TNF inhibitors (e.g., infliximab [Remicade], Etanercept [Enbrel], Adalimumab [Humira]), interlukin 12 and 23 inhibitors (e.g., ustekinumab [Stelara]), alpha-4 integrin binders (e.g., natalizumab [Tysabri] and vedolizumab [Entyvio]), and Janus kinase inhibiters. Mesalamine is a mainstay of ulcerative colitis treatment, but is not used to treat active Crohn disease. Antidiarrheal drugs such as loperamide are useful to control symptoms. However, be sure to avoid antidiarrheal drugs in patients who may have impending toxic megacolon. Probiotics and lactose avoidance may also be useful (although there is less evidence for these).

HELPFUL TIP:
Test for thiopurine methyltransferase (TPMT) enzyme prior to starting thiopurines. Around 10% of the population is deficient and are at higher risk of toxicity with these medications.

After discussions with your patient about ongoing therapy at discharge, you find that cost is a major consideration for her. Therefore, you consider discharging her on sulfasalazine.

Question 7.6.6 Which of the following is an absolute contraindication to the use of sulfasalazine?
A) Sulfa allergy
B) Aspirin allergy
C) Anemia
D) A and B
E) B and C

Answer 7.6.6 **The correct answer is "D."** Sulfasalazine contains both sulfa and salicylate moieties and thus is contraindicated in patients with sulfa or aspirin allergy.

Question 7.6.7 Which of the following is LEAST likely to be a complication of anti-tumor necrosis factor (TNF)-alpha antibody therapy (e.g., infliximab [Remicade®]) for IBD?
A) Sepsis
B) Headache
C) Abdominal pain
D) Diarrhea
E) Anemia

Answer 7.6.7 **The correct answer is "E."** Anemia will generally improve with the treatment of IBD. Anemia in IBD is often due to a combination of iron deficiency and anemia of chronic disease, but IBD can cause an autoimmune hemolytic anemia as well. All of the rest are common complications of infliximab. Infection deserves special mention. Patients on anti-TNF drugs are more prone to sepsis. In fact, ongoing infection is an absolute contraindication to the use of anti-TNF drugs. Take any complaints attributable to infection (e.g., fever) very seriously in patients on anti-TNF drugs (not that you don't take them seriously in all patients ... just more seriously in these). Tuberculosis and active hepatitis B are contraindications to the use of anti-TNF drugs and patients need to be screened for these before prescribing these drugs.

Question 7.6.8 All of the following characteristics differentiate ulcerative colitis (UC) from Crohn disease EXCEPT:
A) The risk of colon cancer is greater in UC than in Crohn disease
B) Histologically, UC appears as transmural disease, whereas Crohn disease involves only the mucosal and submucosal layers
C) UC almost always involves the rectum, whereas Crohn disease may or may not
D) In UC, the diseased segments are continuous, while "skip" areas of healthy bowel are seen in Crohn disease

Answer 7.6.8 **The correct answer (and exception) is "B."** Histologically, UC involves only the mucosa and submucosal tissue, while Crohn disease is transmural. All of the other statements are true. UC involves the rectum in 95% of cases and advances proximally.

HELPFUL TIP:
Patients with long-standing UC with frequent relapses are candidates for colectomy.

HELPFUL TIP:
IBD increases the risk of colon cancer, so more frequent and earlier colonoscopies are recommended. Recommendations vary, but most expert guidelines recommend colonoscopy every 1 to 2 years in patients with UC after 8 years with disease. Screening parameters in those with Crohn disease are less well established.

HELPFUL TIP:
Sclerosing cholangitis is an inflammatory process that causes strictures of the intrahepatic and/or extrahepatic ducts. Biochemically, there is evidence of cholestasis manifested by an elevated alkaline phosphatase. This progresses to fibrosis, cirrhosis, and hepatic failure with a median survival of 10 years without a transplant. The rate of cholangiocarcinoma is also elevated in these patients. The diagnosis of sclerosing cholangitis is made by cholangiography, which demonstrates strictures and dilatation (beaded appearance) of intrahepatic and/or extrahepatic ducts. The majority of cases are related to inflammatory bowel disease, particularly UC.

▶ Objectives: Did you learn to ...
· Diagnose IBD?
· Differentiate Crohn disease from UC?
· Manage a patient with IBD?
· Recognize extraintestinal manifestations and complications of IBD?

▶ CASE 7.7

A 52-year-old woman complains of abdominal pain, bloating, and constipation. Her symptoms started about 5 years ago and became more bothersome within the last 6 months. She describes a dull pain in the left lower abdomen occurring 2 to 3 days a week. This pain is alleviated by passing gas or having a bowel movement, which she does with excessive straining. The pain is generally related to eating, and she has had intermittent diarrhea and constipation, with constipation predominating. Two years ago, she underwent a screening colonoscopy, which was completely normal. Her review of systems is notable for a weight gain of about 5 lb within the last 3 years. She is taking only a multivitamin daily. Her physical examination is normal.

Question 7.7.1 Which is the best next step?
A) Defecogram
B) Barium enema
C) Anorectal manometry
D) TSH level
E) Colonoscopy

Answer 7.7.1 **The correct answer is "D."** The patient's presentation with pain and constipation meets criteria for constipation-predominant IBS. Of note, irritable bowel is not an uncommon complication of GI infections including *E. coli*, *Campylobacter*, viral infections, and *Giardia* (*Gut*. 2010;59:605). There is also a relationship between anxiety and the presence of irritable bowel. This patient underwent colonoscopy for screening 2 years prior to presentation, so further evaluation for colon cancer ("B" and "E") can be delayed unless there is another indication. Secondary causes of constipation, such as hypothyroidism, medication side effects, or hypercalcemia, should be ruled out. Therefore, a TSH level should be obtained prior to deciding on additional diagnostic or therapeutic steps. At this point in time, anorectal manometry ("C") and defecogram ("A") are

unnecessarily invasive procedures, and neither will help you to determine if this patient has IBS. New Rome IV criteria provide an algorithm (see Figure 7-2).

The patient is euthyroid. Hypercalcemia and other electrolyte abnormalities have been ruled out. Since she does not use medications other than the multivitamin, you decide to initiate the treatment of IBS. Based on available evidence, you suggest using fiber supplements such as psyllium.

Question 7.7.2 What do you tell your patient to expect?
A) Complete resolution of her symptoms
B) Increase in stool frequency and stool volume with less need for straining
C) Not much. Fiber supplementation doesn't work very well for IBS
D) Decrease in abdominal pain and bloating
E) Enlightenment and absolute bliss

Answer 7.7.2 **The correct (and unfortunate) answer is "C."** Although it has been one of the mainstays of irritable bowel therapy, the efficacy of fiber for IBS has always been in question. A meta-analysis (*Am J Gastroenterol*. 2014;109(9):1367–1374) suggests an NNT of 7 with psyllium to benefit one patient. Perhaps surprisingly, there are only 14 randomized trials of only 906 patients. While bowel habits can be successfully changed with bulking agents for constipation or loperamide for diarrhea-predominant IBS, pain is generally not affected by

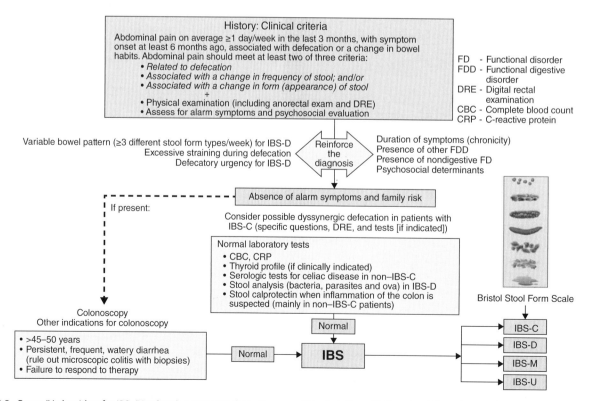

FIGURE 7-2. Rome IV algorithm for IBS. (Used with permission from Drossman DA, et al. *Rome IV: Functional Gastrointestinal Disorders for Primary Care and Non-GI Clinicians*. Raleigh, NC: The Rome Foundation; 2016.) Copyright © 2016 Rome Foundation, Inc. All rights reserved.

these measures. In fact, increased fiber intake may transiently worsen some symptoms due to fermentation and generation of gas, potentially resulting in flatulence or bloating. "E" requires special mention. Bliss and enlightenment can only occur with proper colon purging procedures provided at a very expensive resort!

Question 7.7.3 Which of the following has the best record in treating IBS?
A) Eliminating FODMAPs from the diet
B) Probiotics
C) Rifaximin
D) St. John's wort
E) Eliminating the use of GOOGLEMAPS

Answer 7.7.3 The correct answer is "A." First, you need to know what FODMAPs are. **FODMAP** stands for "**F**ermentable, **O**ligo-, **D**i-, **M**onosaccharides, **A**nd **P**olyols" (say that five times fast). These are poorly absorbed carbohydrates that can cause fermentation and gas in the colon. Some FODMAPs include fructose, lactose, fructans (from wheat … think this is why everyone believes they have gluten intolerance?), and others. Eliminating FODMAPs from the diet seems to have the best NNT of any of the irritable bowel treatments. Of the others, probiotics ("B") have an NNT of 7 to 11 (*Am J Gastroenterol.* 2014;109:1547), rifaximin ("C") (at $1,200/month) has an NNT of 11 and a marginal benefit at best (*N Engl J Med.* 2011;364:22–32), and St. John's wort ("D") actually increases the symptoms of IBS and should be avoided. Use of GOOGLEMAPS ("E") has not been shown to have any effect on IBS symptoms that we know of. Remember that a strong patient–physician relationship is key to treatment. Acknowledge the patient's disease experience without ordering unnecessary testing or providing unnecessary medications.

HELPFUL TIP:
About 4% of *children* diagnosed with IBS *who are referred to an academic GI clinic* have celiac disease. The number will be less in the general patient population (*JAMA Pediatr.* 2014;168(6):514–515).

HELPFUL TIP:
IBS has a relatively good prognosis. Up to 60% of patients improve with placebo treatment in trials, making it hard to show benefit with any treatment. There is no increase in mortality with IBS, and symptoms usually improve over time.

HELPFUL TIP:
TCAs, SSRIs, may be beneficial in IBS. Psychologic management including CBT can be helpful in managing symptoms.

▶ **Objectives: Did you learn to …**
• Diagnose and manage IBS?
• Describe the role of FODMAPs in irritable bowel?
• Realize that both you and your patient will be frustrated with the treatments for IBS?

▶ **CASE 7.8**

A 32-year-old male complains about fatigue and episodic abdominal pain. His pain is located in the periumbilical region and the left lower quadrant. It is cramp-like in nature and is associated with flatulence and diarrhea. Passing gas alleviates his symptoms. He notes that milk and other dairy products worsen his symptoms. His weight has remained stable. His prior medical history, family and social history, and physical examination are unremarkable. Laboratory tests reveal hemoglobin of 11.5 g/dL and a normal glucose and TSH.

Question 7.8.1 What is the most appropriate next step in your evaluation?
A) Lactose breath test
B) Dietary trial of strict lactose avoidance
C) Enteroclysis
D) Colonoscopy
E) Tissue transglutaminase antibody titer

Answer 7.8.1 The correct answer is "B." The patient's symptoms are consistent with lactose intolerance. He may have malabsorption secondary to lactose intolerance, which may be partially responsible for his anemia. If his symptoms resolve with a trial of a lactose-free diet, you have your diagnosis. Follow-up should include re-checking his CBC and perhaps other studies, such as stool for occult blood. If these symptoms are new, he could have a secondary form of lactase deficiency (e.g., Crohn disease or bacterial overgrowth) or a coincidental problem with the absorption of this carbohydrate. Colon cancer is not common at this age, but endoscopy should also be considered if anemia does not resolve.

The patient tries a lactose-free diet, but this is of no benefit and his abdominal cramping and diarrhea continue. At this point, you are considering additional diagnoses.

Question 7.8.2 Which of the following is LEAST likely in this patient?
A) Bacterial overgrowth syndrome
B) Gluten-sensitive enteropathy
C) *Giardia lamblia*
D) *C. difficile*
E) Whipple disease

Answer 7.8.2 The correct answer is "E." It is unlikely that this patient has Whipple disease, which is a result of an infection with *Tropheryma whippelii*. Whipple disease is associated with nondeforming arthritis, weight loss, fever, diarrhea, etc. All of the others are possibilities in this patient. "A," bacterial overgrowth syndrome, presents with bloating, diarrhea, dyspepsia, and possible malabsorption and weight loss. It can occur as a result of bowel dysmotility, bowel redundancy or diverticula, chronic pancreatitis, etc. "B," gluten-sensitive enteropathy (nontropical or celiac sprue), presents with symptoms similar to those in our patient including malabsorption. "C," *Giardia* infection, can be chronic and presents with gas, diarrhea, and occasionally constipation. Finally, *C. difficile* infection (pseudomembranous colitis) can also be chronic in nature with chronic diarrhea and blood loss.

HELPFUL TIP:
Giardia is a common pathogen that may be contracted in the day care setting. Symptoms may consist of diarrhea, malaise, and nausea. The treatment of choice is metronidazole.

You continue to work up this patient's diarrhea with stool cultures, stool for *C. difficile* toxin, direct immunofluorescence analysis for *Giardia* and *Cryptosporidium*, and three stools for ova and parasites. All of the studies are negative. You now turn your attention to possible bacterial overgrowth syndrome.

Question 7.8.3 The best test(s) for bacterial overgrowth syndrome is (are):
A) Quantitative stool culture
B) Stool leukocytes
C) 72-hour fecal fat
D) [14-C] d-xylose breath test
E) B and D

Answer 7.8.3 **The correct answer is "D."** The d-xylose breath test takes advantage of the fact that the bacteria responsible for bacterial overgrowth syndrome (Gram-negative aerobes) catabolize d-xylose. The breath test measures radioactive CO_2 that is formed as a result of bacterial breakdown of radioactive d-xylose (you too, like Godzilla, can have radioactive breath). The glucose breath test, in which glucose is administered to the patient and breath hydrogen is measured, is also helpful and commonly used. However, it is less sensitive and specific than the d-xylose test and has a 30% to 40% false-negative rate. Workup of bacterial overgrowth syndrome should also include an upper GI endoscopy and possible small bowel biopsy. GI hypomotility, small bowel dilatation, or small bowel diverticula support the diagnosis of bacterial overgrowth syndrome. Of the others, "B," stool leukocytes are pretty useless in general and do not have a good correlation with infectious causes of diarrhea (high false-positive and false-negative rates). "C," fecal fat collection, is useful in documenting fat malabsorption syndromes, including those secondary to severe pancreatic insufficiency (e.g., cystic fibrosis with >90% pancreatic dysfunction) and short bowel syndrome.

HELPFUL TIP:
Another option to diagnose bacterial overgrowth is empiric treatment for 7 to 10 days with medications to cover aerobes and anaerobes (cephalexin plus metronidazole, TMP/SMX plus metronidazole, amoxicillin/clavulanate). Rifaximin can be used but is expensive. Definitive treatment may require surgical intervention to shorten the bowel, resect diverticula, etc.

This patient's d-xylose test is negative, and you consider the possibility of gluten-sensitive enteropathy (celiac disease).

Question 7.8.4 Of the following, the BEST test for the diagnosis of gluten-sensitive enteropathy is:
A) Antiendomysial antibodies
B) Tissue transglutaminase antibodies
C) Antigliadin antibodies
D) Radiolabeled wheat flour absorption test
E) All of the above are equally accurate for detecting celiac disease

Answer 7.8.4 **The correct answer is "B."** Tissue transglutaminase antibodies are sensitive and specific for severe gluten-sensitive enteropathy, but may be falsely negative in mild-to-moderate cases. Antiendomysial IgA antibodies are less sensitive than tissue transglutaminase antibodies for gluten-sensitive enteropathy, but very specific for gluten-sensitive enteropathy. Antigliadin antibodies are less sensitive and specific and have fallen out of favor. The definitive test ("gold standard") is a small bowel biopsy and should be considered if your clinical suspicion is high and the patient has negative antibodies. Patients with positive antibodies should also have an endoscopy; the diagnosis should be confirmed by endoscopy and biopsy before committing the patient to a gluten-free diet for life.

HELPFUL TIP:
Up to 1:200 Caucasians living in the United States may be affected with gluten-sensitive enteropathy (while 1:20 grocery store aisles appear to be devoted to gluten-free products).

HELPFUL TIP:
Remember FODMAPs from earlier? Studies of patients who believe that they have gluten-sensitive enteropathy show that eliminating FODMAPs will improve the symptoms of many of these patients (*Gastroenterology*. 2013;145(2):320-8.e1-3). The culprit here is not the whole wheat bread but the seven Big-Gulp-Fructose-Laden pops the patient drinks each day. To be fair, wheat has FODMAPs, so wheat, but not gluten sensitivity, may make symptoms worse in these patients. **Differentiating gluten-sensitive enteropathy from FODMAP-induced symptoms is important. Keep reading…**

Eureka! The results of his tissue transglutaminase test are positive. You educate him about gluten-sensitive enteropathy (celiac disease) and have an endoscopy performed. A small bowel biopsy demonstrates blunted villi with a significant increase in intraepithelial lymphocytes, consistent with gluten-sensitive enteropathy. With a gluten-free diet, the patient experiences a significant increase in his energy level. Two years later he comes for a routine visit. He has gradually reintroduced some wheat products into his diet and tolerates these very well.

Question 7.8.5 What do you recommend?
A) Resume gluten-free diet
B) Continue dietary challenge and repeat examination in 6 months
C) Repeat small bowel biopsy
D) Check tissue transglutaminase antibody titer
E) Completely liberalize diet and return to a typical American diet

Answer 7.8.5 **The correct answer is "A."** While there is no good data on the benefit of a long-term gluten-free diet in patients who can tolerate small amounts of gluten, several factors argue for continuing a gluten-free diet. The first is that many patients will have subclinical nutrient deficiencies if they reintroduce gluten. For this reason, patients with gluten-sensitive enteropathy should be screened for osteoporosis and take a multivitamin. This is especially true in pediatric patients where deficiencies may lead to stunted growth. The second is that there is some data that patients who reintroduce gluten may have increased mortality from GI lymphoma despite the fact that they are tolerating the gluten well (*Ann Intern Med.* 2013;159(3):169–175).

Question 7.8.6 All of the following are gluten-free grains EXCEPT:
A) Oats
B) Corn
C) Sticky (glutinous) rice
D) Rice
E) Rye

Answer 7.8.6 **The correct answer is "E."** Rye contains gluten (as does barley). Despite its name, glutinous rice contains no gluten. The rest are gluten-free. Other gluten-free grains/starches include: buckwheat, flax, quinoa, teff, millet, amaranth, and tapioca. Oats have a gliadin peptide that can activate celiac disease in *some* patients. Generally, oats are fine in small quantities as long as they are not contaminated with wheat in the processing.

HELPFUL TIP:
With a gluten-free diet, antibodies (tissue transglutaminase, antigliadin, antiendomysial) often return to normal levels.

HELPFUL TIP:
Patients with gluten-sensitive enteropathy must be compulsive about their diet. Rice, corn, and soybean-based flours are safe to consume.

▶ **Objectives: Did you learn to …**
- Evaluate a patient with chronic diarrhea?
- Recognize clinical manifestations of gluten-sensitive enteropathy?
- Manage a patient with gluten-sensitive enteropathy?

▶ CASE 7.9

A 22-year-old previously healthy male reports a 3-day history of explosive and watery diarrhea. He is having up to six bowel movements per day. He recalls eating at a new Mexican restaurant 5 days ago. His head sinks a little low as he recalls drinking a "fish bowl-sized" margarita … or at least he thinks he remembers drinking it. He denies fever, blood in his stool, or recent travel. Multiple people ate the same food but he is the only one who is sick. His vital signs are normal (including supine and standing blood pressures), and the remainder of the physical examination is remarkable only for mild, diffuse abdominal tenderness.

Question 7.9.1 What is the most likely diagnosis?
A) Celiac sprue
B) Viral gastroenteritis
C) Lactose intolerance
D) Small bowel bacterial overgrowth
E) *C. difficile* colitis

Answer 7.9.1 **The correct answer is "B."** This is always a dilemma. It can be difficult to differentiate acute gastroenteritis from food poisoning. What makes gastroenteritis more likely is that there is no clustering of cases among people who ate the same food. With only 3 days of symptoms, it would be premature to diagnose "A," "C," or "D." Without recent antibiotic exposure, "E" would be unlikely in an otherwise healthy male. See Table 7-3 for a differential diagnosis for diarrhea.

Question 7.9.2 What is the MOST appropriate next step in the care of this patient at this point?
A) Order a CBC
B) Order electrolytes
C) Order stool examination for ova and parasites
D) Recommend oral hydration and antidiarrheals as needed
E) Order an abdominal film

Answer 7.9.2 **The correct answer is "D."** No workup is needed for a mild case of acute diarrhea, since such cases are usually self-limited. Generally, the history and physical examination should provide the diagnosis and indicate need for further workup. Further workup and treatment are indicated if the patient has severe or bloody diarrhea, dehydration, systemic toxicity, or severe pain.

TABLE 7-3 DIFFERENTIAL DIAGNOSIS FOR DIARRHEA

Acute Diarrhea

- Bacteria (e.g., *Campylobacter*, *Salmonella*, and *Clostridium*)
- Viruses (e.g., Norwalk and rotavirus)
- Parasites (e.g., *Giardia*)
- Protozoa (especially in HIV-infected patients)
- Medications
- Anything that causes chronic diarrhea

Chronic Diarrhea

- Inflammatory (e.g., IBD and radiation enteritis)
- Osmotic (e.g., gluten-sensitive enteropathy and lactase deficiency)
- Secretory (e.g., Zollinger–Ellison syndrome and villous adenoma)
- Disordered motility (e.g., irritable bowel syndrome and overflow from fecal impaction)

HELPFUL TIP:
Patients with severe, bloody diarrhea, and fever (T >101°F, >6 stools per day) should be treated with a single dose or 3-day course of a fluoroquinolone while awaiting stool culture results. **Bloody diarrhea in an afebrile patient should suggest *Escherichia coli* 0157:H7.** These patients should **NOT** get antibiotics because of an increased risk of hemolytic–uremic syndrome. As always, there is an "except." Patients who have been traveling to areas with resistant organisms should be treated with azithromycin 1,000 mg once or 500 mg daily for 3 days. This includes most of Asia.

You treat the patient with oral rehydration and prochlorperazine for nausea and he does well. He returns to see you a few weeks later after a trip to Mexico. He liked that fish bowl-sized margarita so much that he decided to go for an original. He has diarrhea that began a couple of days after his arrival in Cancun and has now been present for 5 days. He has had frequent, watery diarrhea with nausea but no vomiting. He has noticed no blood in the stool. He was very careful to avoid salads and water, but did have some ice in a soft drink and his margarita was "on the rocks."

Question 7.9.3 The most likely organism causing illness in this patient is:

A) *Salmonella*
B) *Shigella*
C) Enterotoxigenic *E. coli*
D) Enterohemorrhagic *E. coli*
E) *Campylobacter*

Answer 7.9.3 The correct answer is "C." Enterotoxigenic *E. coli* is the most common cause of traveler diarrhea in patients traveling to Mexico. **Enterohemorrhagic** *E. coli* is less likely and should be associated with bloody diarrhea. The others are much less likely to be causes of travelers' diarrhea.

HELPFUL TIP:
Many physicians would not treat a patient with *Shigella* unless that patient is clinically ill (e.g., fever). Treatment with antibiotics is **relatively** contraindicated in *Salmonella* because it prolongs the carrier state. However, use judgment in the patient who is particularly ill.

HELPFUL TIP:
A variety of PCR panels are now available to help identify the pathogen causing GI distress. These panels are superior to traditional evaluation in both sensitivity and timeliness (results in hours). These tests are useful in determining treatment (or nontreatment for viral infections), but are unnecessary in mild disease as they will not change management. Note these tests are so sensitive they can detect nonpathogenic levels of potential pathogens, yielding a false-positive result.

Question 7.9.4 Which of the following is/are appropriate for the treatment of this patient's travelers' diarrhea (remember, he has no vomiting)?

A) Oral rehydration
B) Antidiarrheals
C) Eat any food (e.g., no need for a bland diet with slow advancement)
D) All of the above
E) None of the above

Answer 7.9.4 The correct answer is "D." This patient has non-bloody diarrhea and no systemic signs, so it should be safe to treat him with antidiarrheal agents (e.g., loperamide) and avoid antibiotics. Oral rehydration is the rule unless a patient is too nauseated or has some other reason that he cannot take adequate fluids by mouth. *Patients (including children) should eat anything they can tolerate.* The concept of "gut rest" is a misnomer and actually leads to increased bowel permeability and more persistent diarrhea. **Lactose deserves special mention.** The American Academy of Pediatrics has changed its recommendation about lactose in diarrhea, recommending caregivers withhold lactose **only** in children less than 3 months of age. This seems to be the group in which transient lactase deficiency occurs.

▶ **Objectives: Did you learn to …**

- Evaluate a patient with acute diarrhea?
- Treat acute diarrhea?
- Recognize different bacterial causes of diarrhea?

▶ CASE 7.10

A 49-year-old man comes to your office, requesting testing for hepatitis C. He recently attended his 25-year college reunion where an old friend he had "partied" with during experimentation with injectable drugs related that he has cirrhosis due to hepatitis C. The patient is otherwise healthy and denies any symptoms except for occasional fatigue after a long day at work. Physical examination of the patient is unremarkable. There are no stigmata of chronic liver disease.

Question 7.10.1 Which of the following is the most appropriate course of action?
A) Check a quantitative Hepatitis C virus (HCV) PCR ("viral load")
B) Order a recombinant immunoblot assay (RIBA)
C) Order HCV antibody test (enzyme immunoassay)
D) Order a qualitative HCV PCR
E) Order ALT and AST

Answer 7.10.1 **The correct answer is "C."** The sensitivity and specificity of the present-day HCV antibody test are excellent; thus, this is the best initial test to perform to diagnose HCV infection. Rarely, patients with immunologic impairment, such as HIV infection, have HCV viremia without detectable antibody, but this would not be a concern in this otherwise healthy patient. Quantitative HCV PCR is not a reliable means for diagnosing HCV infection because currently used methods are insensitive at low levels of viremia; thus, infection cannot be ruled out if the level of HCV viremia is below the lower limit of detection of the test. RIBA is an old test that is no longer used. **Qualitative** HCV PCR is the most sensitive test for the presence of HCV RNA, with a limit of detection that is lower than that of quantitative PCR. It is useful to establish the presence of viremia, but is more expensive than antibody testing and thus not a first-line test. Many patients with chronic HCV infection (including patients with cirrhosis) have normal liver enzymes and can still have progressive disease; therefore, in a high-risk patient, ALT and AST are not appropriate for screening for HCV.

HELPFUL TIP:
Hepatitis C antibody can remain positive lifelong even in patients who have cleared their infection. Unlike HAV and HBV antibodies, HCV antibodies are not protective. Just because a patient cleared HCV once does not mean they cannot be reinfected. If these patients have ongoing high-risk behaviors, consider periodic evaluation with qualitative PCR to assess for reinfection.

The patient returns several weeks later to discuss his test results. His HCV antibody test is positive. A liver panel obtained that day shows an ALT of 48 IU/L (reference range, 0–20) and an AST of 39 IU/L (0–31). His albumin and total bilirubin are within normal limits. Subsequent HCV PCR confirms active disease. He is extremely anxious about his liver.

Question 7.10.2 To most accurately assess the degree of liver disease, your next step is to:
A) Obtain a liver–spleen scan to assess for evidence of cirrhosis
B) Order a right upper quadrant ultrasound with Doppler to assess for evidence of cirrhosis
C) Order elastography for evidence of cirrhosis
D) Obtain an abdominal CT to assess for evidence of cirrhosis
E) Reassure the patient that his mild liver test abnormalities rule out cirrhosis

Answer 7.10.2 **The correct answer is "C."** Having established that the patient has hepatitis C with elevated liver enzymes, the next step is to determine the severity of his liver disease. Although his liver function tests are reassuring, this does not exclude the possibility of advanced fibrosis or even well-compensated cirrhosis. While biopsy has been the definitive test for liver fibrosis in the past (and you would not be wrong to order a biopsy if it were an option in this question), ultrasound elastography, a noninvasive technique of determining liver fibrosis, is being used more and more. The idea is that a fibrotic liver is a stiff liver, and that stiffness can be determined by imaging modalities, including ultrasound. The sensitivity of elastography for detecting cirrhosis ranges from 70% to 87% and specificity of 84% to 91% (with better accuracy at higher stages of cirrhosis). The "F" score, discussed below, should allow you to make decisions about your hepatitis C patients. You would not be incorrect to order ultrasound imaging as well, but it would not be the best modality for determining degree of cirrhosis.

HELPFUL TIP:
Fibrosis is scored from F0 to F4, with F0 representing no fibrosis and F4 representing cirrhosis. In addition to elastography, another noninvasive method of determining the degree of fibrosis is the AST/platelet ratio index, abbreviated APRI. This is calculated as follows:

APRI = [(patient AST / upper normal of lab AST) / platelet count] × 100. Platelet count should be given as $\times 10^9/L$ (e.g., if the count is 100,000/µL, use 100).

Significant fibrosis (F2–F4) is present if the APRI is 0.7 or greater (77% sensitivity, specificity 72%), although some sources use 0.5 as the lower limit for "significant fibrosis." An APRI of 1 or greater represents cirrhosis. Finally, the FibroSure, Fibrotest, and ActiTest are proprietary methods of determining liver fibrosis—all of which have separate scoring systems for fibrosis. Note that a biopsy is not necessary for making a decision about who to treat: more on this below.

After a few phone calls, you find that elastography is not available anywhere nearby. The patient agrees to a liver biopsy to diagnose cirrhosis and you make the referral. He is still very concerned about his situation and asks what you think the chances are that he already has cirrhosis.

Question 7.10.3 Regarding the development of progressive liver disease in hepatitis C, all of the following are true EXCEPT:
A) Approximately 20% of patients with chronic HCV infection will develop serious liver disease
B) Heavy alcohol use is a risk factor for development of serious liver disease

C) Acquisition of HCV infection after the age of 40 is associated with increased risk of developing serious liver disease

D) HCV genotype affects the probability of developing end-stage liver disease

E) Males are more likely than females to develop serious liver disease

Answer 7.10.3 **The correct answer is "D."** While only a minority of persons *infected* with HCV develop serious liver disease (about 20%), the likelihood of progression is difficult to predict in an individual patient. Of the rest of those infected, 80% will not clear the virus and have a chronic infection that *does not* progress to end-stage liver disease. Nonetheless, male gender, heavy alcohol use, and acquisition of HCV infection after the age of 40 are associated with increased risk of progressive liver disease, while genotype is not. In addition, Japanese ancestry, smoking (both cigarettes and marijuana), and acquiring hepatitis C from a blood transfusion have been associated with an increased risk of progression. The genotype of the hepatitis C certainly makes a difference when it comes to treatment but not with progression to cirrhosis.

HELPFUL TIP:
Screen for hepatitis C at least once in all U.S. adults aged 18-79 years (per USPSTF draft recommendation published for public comment in 2019). Other populations deserving of screening include those with HIV, dialysis patients, and incarcerated patients.

The patient is concerned that he may transmit the virus to his wife or children. They are tested and are found to be negative for HCV antibody. He is relieved but asks for advice to prevent infecting them.

Question 7.10.4 **You advise all of the following EXCEPT:**

A) No change in sexual practices is recommended for couples in a long-term monogamous relationship in which one partner is HCV+ and the other HCV−

B) The use of condoms is recommended for couples in a long-term monogamous relationship in which one partner is HCV+ and the other HCV−

C) Hepatitis C is not spread by hugging, sneezing, or sharing a drinking glass

D) Household members of persons infected with HCV should not share items that might be contaminated with small amounts of blood, such as razors or nail clippers

E) Parenteral exposure to infected blood is a major route of transmission of HCV

Answer 7.10.4 **The correct answer is "B."** HCV is spread by parenteral contact with infected blood. In contrast to hepatitis B, sexual transmission of HCV is inefficient and appears to be a minor route of spread. In addition, the efficacy of latex condoms in preventing disease is not known. The NIH and the US Public Health Service do not recommend condom use for patients in a stable, long-term, and monogamous relationship. That said,

using condoms will likely reduce an already low risk even further (0.1% per year without condoms).

The patient's liver biopsy shows mild-to-moderate inflammatory activity and portal and periportal fibrosis (stage 2). He is relieved to find out that he does not have cirrhosis, but remains very concerned about his hepatitis and wants to do everything possible to "get rid of" hepatitis C. He asks about the treatment of his HCV.

Question 7.10.5 **At what stage of fibrosis should treatment be considered?**

A) F2 or higher

B) F3 or higher

C) F4, no need to treat until cirrhosis sets in

D) Any stage

Answer 7.10.5 **The correct answer is "D."** Current recommendation is to treat everybody. Unless the patient has a short life expectancy, they should be treated regardless of fibrosis score. F-score still matters, as duration of therapy is determined in part by severity of disease but there is not a minimal level of disease to qualify for treatment. The current regimens of antivirals are effective and well tolerated. Unfortunately, the cost of these new drugs—at least, in the United States—remains immorally high, in some cases over $100,000 for a complete 12-week treatment depending on the drug. Public and private insurers have been forced into outright rationing. If the United States treated all of the approximately 3 million HCV-infected persons with the new drugs, it would cost our country about $300 billion. Because of the pharmaceutical companies setting prices differently in different markets, at least one of these new HCV drugs costs about 1% of the US price in Egypt. So … one option is to send your HCV patients to Egypt for the treatment and put them up in a nice hotel—it would be significantly cheaper.

Question 7.10.6 **You tell him which of the following?**

A) Combination therapy with interferon and ribavirin results in sustained virologic responses (SVR) in 40% to 70% of patients treated

B) Combination therapy with interferon and ribavirin can cause numerous side effects including pancytopenia, flu-like symptoms, worsening of autoimmune conditions, depression, and hemolytic anemia

C) The HCV genotype is a strong predictor of response to the treatment

D) Newer treatment regimens including ledipasvir/sofosbuvir are much more effective than the traditional combination of interferon/ribavirin

E) All of the above

Answer 7.10.6 **The correct answer is "E."** Combination therapy with interferon and ribavirin is the traditional treatment of HCV and it is clearly not as effective at achieving an SVR as the newer drugs. In fact, it is no longer part of the recommended treatment algorithm. Similarly, the protease inhibitors (telaprevir and boceprevir) have also come and gone. Current treatments are based on genotype, fibrosis score, whether or not a cirrhotic patient is compensated or decompensated, and prior treatment status. Higher baseline viral levels also tend to predict poorer response to the treatment. There are currently safe, effective oral regimens for all 6 genotypes. While there is a higher rate of success in the treatment of naïve patients, the new regimens are useful even in patients with prior treatment failure.

Question 7.10.7 Overall, the new oral "direct acting antiviral" drugs for hepatitis C have a cure rate of approximately:

A) 50%
B) 70%
C) 80%
D) 90%

Answer: 7.10.7 The correct answer is "D." The direct acting antivirals have a cure rate of over 90% (and some up to 99%). Some of these drugs include: Harvoni, Viekira, and Technivie. Epclusa (sofosbuvir and velpatasvir) is effective in all genotypes. However, knowing and targeting the genotype is crucial. Patients should be tested 12 weeks after treatment is completed. About 1% will relapse between 12 and 24 weeks post-treatment, so some practitioners recheck viral levels at 24 weeks.

HELPFUL (AND CRUCIAL) TIP:
HCV treatment is rapidly changing. In order to keep pace, the Infectious Disease Society of America (IDSA) and American Association for the Study of Liver Disease (AASLD) maintain current guidelines at www.hcvguidelines.org.

▶ **Objectives: Did you learn to …**
- Evaluate a patient at risk for hepatitis C?
- Understand the natural history of the disease process in hepatitis C?
- Describe the transmission of hepatitis C?
- Discuss the treatment issues for a patient with hepatitis C?

▶ CASE 7.11

A 24-year-old female graduate student from China comes to your office complaining of fatigue for the past month. She has also had a poor appetite and has lost about 3 lb over this period. She reports that she was told that she had "hepatitis" when she was about 10 years old, but does not recall what type. She is otherwise healthy and takes no medications. She has no history or percutaneous exposures or blood transfusion. Her grandfather died of liver cancer.

Physical examination reveals a thin, tired-appearing woman. The liver edge is palpable 2 cm below the right costal margin and is slightly tender. There is no ascites, splenomegaly, or cutaneous stigmata of chronic liver disease.

Laboratory studies are remarkable for anemia (hemoglobin 9.1 g/dL). Liver tests reveal elevated aminotransferases (ALT 289 IU/L, AST 158 IU/L), albumin 3.2 g/dL, and total bilirubin 1.5 mg/dL (normal 0.2–1.0 mg/dL).

Question 7.11.1 Diagnostic possibilities at this point include:

A) Hepatitis A
B) Hepatitis B
C) Hepatitis C
D) Autoimmune hepatitis
E) All of the above

Answer 7.11.1 The correct answer is "E." Constitutional symptoms such as fatigue and anorexia can be seen with any form of acute or chronic liver disease; thus, they are not helpful in establishing a specific diagnosis. The first priority is to rule out infectious hepatitis including hepatitis A, B, and acute hepatitis C. Autoimmune hepatitis deserves consideration, particularly in female patients. While HCV infection is a worldwide problem, HBV infection is endemic in Asia and Africa, and the possibility of chronic hepatitis B also warrants special attention in this patient.

Question 7.11.2 Appropriate laboratory studies at this point include which of the following?

A) Quantitative HCV PCR
B) Hepatitis B surface antigen (HBsAg)
C) Antihepatitis A antibodies (IgG and IgM)
D) B and C
E) All of the above

Answer 7.11.2 The correct answer is "D." As discussed previously, the quantitative HCV PCR is not a useful test for diagnosing HCV infection. HCV antibody testing would be a better choice. Both HBsAg and anti-HAV are useful tests in this patient. HBsAg identifies active infection (but does not distinguish between acute and chronic). HBsAb IgM indicates acute infection but usually gives way to HBsAb IgG within 6 months of infection. Anti-HAV antibodies will rule out acute hepatitis A infection. A positive total anti-HAV (positive IgG) with a negative IgM would indicate past infection, while a positive IgM would suggest acute HAV infection. In this scenario, you might also consider testing for Epstein–Barr virus (mononucleosis), CMV virus, and other viral infections. Interpreting the HBV antigens (Ag) and antibodies (Ab) can be confusing, and Table 7-4 may help.

The patient's results show a positive HBsAg, indicating ongoing hepatitis B infection. She is immune to hepatitis A and is hepatitis C negative.

After being out of contact for 4 months, she returns for a follow-up visit. She tells you that she took an herbal medicine her mother sent from China and has been feeling much better recently. Her HBsAg remains positive, but her liver enzymes, albumin, and total bilirubin are now completely normal.

Question 7.11.3 Appropriate actions at this time include:

A) Treatment with interferon-alpha 5 million units daily for 16 weeks
B) Order hepatitis Be antigen, anti-HBe, and HBV DNA level

TABLE 7-4 HEPATITIS B VIRAL SEROLOGIES FOR DIFFERENT PHASES OF INFECTION

Antigen/Antibody	Acute	Chronic	Recovered	Vaccinated/Immune
HBsAg	+	+	−	−
HBeAg	+	+	−	−
Anti-HBsAb	−	−	+	+
Anti-HBcAb	+ (IgM)	+ (IgG)	+ (IgG)	−
Anti-HBeAb	−	+/−	+	−
HBV DNA	+	+/−	+/−	−

Ab, antibody; Ag, antigen; HBc, core antigen or antibody; HBe, "e" antigen or antibody; HBs, surface antigen or antibody.

C) Begin periodic screening for hepatocellular carcinoma (HCC) with ultrasound and alpha-fetoprotein (AFP)
D) A and C
E) B and C

Answer 7.11.3 The correct answer is "E." The HBe antigen reflects viral replication. Loss of HBeAg indicates decreased viral replication and less of a risk of progression to cirrhosis. Loss of HBeAg may occur spontaneously; it is also the therapeutic endpoint of the antiviral treatments of HBV infection (interferon, lamivudine, entecavir). If she is negative for HBeAg and is anti-HBe antibody positive (anti-HBe +) or has low or undetectable levels of HBV DNA, she has a low level of viral replication and will not benefit further from the antiviral treatment.

Her liver panel should be monitored periodically as should AFP and liver ultrasound. Ultrasound is recommended every 6 months with or without AFP. An AFP alone should not be done because of the poor sensitivity and specificity. Even asymptomatic HBV carriers with minimal liver disease are at risk for HCC. Screening for HCC in those who are carriers of hepatitis B is indicated in: Asians (men >40 years old, women >50 years old); those with a family history of HCC; cirrhotic patients; and those of African ancestry >20 years of age. Our patient had positive family history of HCC, so monitoring for HCC is indicated.

....

The patient returns to discuss the results of her tests. Laboratory results show that she is positive for HBsAg and is anti-HBeAb positive. Her HBV DNA is undetectable using an unamplified assay, making her a carrier without evidence of viral replication (no chronic, active, hepatitis B). AFP is within limits and abdominal ultrasound is unremarkable. She continues to feel well. She also tells you that she will be getting married in 2 months. She asks you what can be done to prevent her fiancé and future children from becoming infected with HBV.

Question 7.11.4 All of the following are accurate responses to her question EXCEPT:
A) No special precautions need to be taken because she has undetectable HBV and is therefore not infectious

B) If her fiancé has not been immunized against HBV, he should be tested and vaccinated if not immune
C) If her fiancé is not immune to HBV, they should use barrier contraceptives (e.g., condoms) until he has completed his HBV vaccination series
D) She should cover any open cuts or scratches with a bandage and clean up any blood spills with bleach
E) Administration of hepatitis B immune globulin (HBIG) and HBV vaccination begun immediately after birth is 95% effective in preventing perinatal transmission of HBV

Answer 7.11.4 The correct answer is "A." Although patients with higher levels of HBV DNA are more infectious than those with lower levels of viral DNA, the risk of transmission in the latter case is not zero. In the case of this patient, having "undetectable" HBV DNA simply indicates a level of HBV DNA that falls below the limit of detection of an unamplified assay (on the order of 10^5 copies/mL). Also, the positive HbsAg means she is still a carrier. Thus, precautions should be taken to prevent sexual or household transmission to her fiancé (use of condoms, immunization if required, etc.) and to her future children (HBIG and HBV vaccination).

VERY HELPFUL (IF LONG) TIP
ALT and AST can be elevated secondary to:
- **Viral agents:** Hepatitis (A, B, C, D, E), CMV, Epstein–Barr virus, and other viruses.
- **Drugs and chemicals:** Acetaminophen overdose, the "glitazones," HMG-CoA reductase inhibitors, INH, griseofulvin, anticonvulsants, NSAIDs, chemicals (carbon tetrachloride, etc.), alcohol, and many other agents.
- **Primary liver diseases:** Primary sclerosing cholangitis, primary biliary cirrhosis (positive antimitochondrial antibody [AMA]).
- **Metabolic diseases:** Wilson disease (decreased ceruloplasmin), hemochromatosis, alpha-1 antitrypsin deficiency, and cystic fibrosis.
- **Mechanical difficulties:** Ductal obstruction secondary to common duct stone or carcinoma (especially pancreatic, hepatoma, metastatic), Budd–Chiari syndrome (thrombosis of the hepatic vein).

- **Cholestasis** from central venous nutrition (CVN), pregnancy, or ceftriaxone therapy.
- **Infiltrative processes:** Fatty liver (especially those with diabetes, hypothyroidism, obesity; determine by U/S), amyloid, granulomatous hepatitis, liver abscess (including amebic or echinococcal; diagnosis by U/S or CT; may have eosinophilia), AIDS-related lymphoma, or other neoplasm.
- **Other:** Congestive heart failure, celiac sprue, muscle diseases (e.g., polymyositis).

Alkaline phosphatase may be elevated secondary to:

- Pregnancy, after a fatty meal in persons with type O or B blood.
- **Liver:** Cholestasis, partial obstruction of the biliary ducts, primary sclerosing cholangitis, adult bile ductopenia, primary biliary cirrhosis, sarcoidosis, and other granulomatous disease.
- **Bone diseases** such as Paget disease and metastatic disease.

For elevated liver tests, workup should include (in approximate order, which may vary depending on patient presentation):

- Rule out toxin exposure (alcohol, drugs).
- Hepatitis A, B, and C serology.
- Serum ferritin, iron, TIBC, transferrin saturation (hemochromatosis).
- Ultrasound or CT imaging (ultrasound first).
- ANA and antismooth muscle antibody (autoimmune hepatitis but only 28–40% sensitive).
- Serum alpha-1 antitrypsin.
- Serum protein electrophoresis (elevated levels in autoimmune hepatitis, 80% sensitive).
- Antiendomysial antibodies or tissue transglutaminase (gluten-sensitive sprue).
- Serum ceruloplasmin (Wilson disease).

(What a long strange tip it's been!)

▶ **Objectives: Did you learn to …**

- Generate a differential diagnosis for patients with abnormal liver enzymes?
- Identify patients at risk for hepatitis B?
- Use the various hepatitis B antigens and antibodies to determine a patient's infection status?
- Describe the route of transmission of hepatitis B?
- Workup elevated liver tests in a stepwise fashion?

▶ **CASE 7.12**

A 73-year-old man comes to your office, complaining of abdominal and ankle swelling, decreased energy, and poor appetite for the past 2 months. He dates the onset of his symptoms to a "reaction" to penicillin given for dental work. He says that before taking the penicillin, he was in excellent health and walked 3 miles per day. Now he is too weak and tired to even care for his own yard.

His past medical history is remarkable for coronary artery bypass surgery done 6 years ago. He also recalls having "yellow jaundice" (as opposed to the purple kind?) when he was stationed in Vietnam decades ago. He has no significant family history. He "drank a bit" on the weekends when he was in the service but has drunk very little alcohol in the past 50 years. He also quit smoking about 50 years ago. His medications are aspirin 81 mg daily and ibuprofen 600 mg as needed for knee pain due to degenerative joint disease.

Question 7.12.1 **Diagnostic considerations suggested by the history should include which of the following?**
A) Adverse drug reaction to penicillin
B) Malignancy
C) Cirrhosis
D) Heart failure
E) All of the above

Answer 7.12.1 **The correct answer is "E."** The patient's history of abdominal and lower extremity swelling suggests fluid overload. Penicillin is known to cause interstitial nephritis and secondary nephrotic syndrome, which can lead to fluid retention. Sources of fluid overload besides the kidneys should be considered in this patient, including liver and heart disease. Malignancy, especially with liver involvement, can cause ascites. He is on an NSAID, which can cause fluid retention, although rarely to this degree.

Physical examination reveals a fragile-appearing elderly man with temporal wasting. There is no JVD. The lungs are clear to auscultation. The heart sounds are regular, with no murmurs or gallops. The abdomen is protuberant with bulging flanks. Shifting dullness is present. There is 2+ ankle edema bilaterally and scattered telangiectasias on skin examination. He has no asterixis.

Question 7.12.2 **Which of the following findings would you expect on laboratory examination?**
A) Elevated hemoglobin and HCT (17.5 g/dL and 55%)
B) Decreased platelet count of 80,000/mm^3
C) Elevated serum albumin
D) BUN/Cr ratio <20
E) All of the above

Answer 7.12.2 **The correct answer is "B."** This patient likely has portal hypertension given his ascites and stigmata of liver disease (spider angiomata/telangiectasias). Blood flow is shifted toward the spleen because of the increased portal pressure (the blood, like the rest of us, takes the path of least resistance). Shunting of blood through the spleen results in thrombocytopenia through increased platelet destruction. Spider telangiectasias and palmar erythema develop due to excess circulating estrogens. Along with this, gynecomastia and testicular atrophy can be an issue in men. "A" is wrong since liver patients often have anemia. "C" is incorrect because liver patients frequently have a low albumin. And, "D," a BUN/Cr ratio <20 is associated with intrinsic kidney disease (see Chapter 5).

Diagnostic paracentesis is performed and approximately 50 mL of clear light yellow fluid are obtained.

Question 7.12.3 Appropriate laboratory studies on the ascitic fluid include which of the following?
A) pH
B) Albumin
C) Lactate
D) Triglycerides
E) All of the above

Answer 7.12.3 **The correct answer is "B."** The ascitic fluid albumin is needed to calculate the serum-ascites albumin gradient (SAAG), which is helpful in distinguishing between ascites resulting from portal hypertension and ascites due to other causes. Lactate ("C") and pH ("A") have been proposed as markers for spontaneous bacterial peritonitis (SBP) but have proven unreliable. Measurement of triglycerides ("D") is useful to confirm chylous ascites; however, in the absence of grossly milky-appearing fluid, there is no need to perform this test.

> **HELPFUL TIP:**
> In addition to albumin, all ascitic fluid should be sent for total protein, cell count, and cultures. A cell count showing ≥250 polymorphonuclear leukocytes/mm³ is presumptive evidence of SBP and mandates treatment for such. Gram stain is nearly useless since ascitic fluid bacterial counts are typically so low that bacteria are rarely seen on Gram stain. Serum albumin and total protein should be obtained within an hour before or after the tap.

Your patient's laboratory tests reveal an ascitic fluid total protein of 2.2 g/dL with an ascitic fluid albumin of 1.9 g/dL. A liver panel reveals normal aminotransferases, normal bilirubin, serum albumin 3.3 g/dL, and alkaline phosphatase 147 IU/L. Electrolytes, BUN, and creatinine are within normal limits.

Question 7.12.4 Which of the following is the most accurate interpretation of these results?
A) The SAAG is 1.7, which is consistent with portal hypertension as its cause
B) The SAAG is 1.7, which rules out portal hypertension as its cause
C) The SAAG is 1.4, which is consistent with portal hypertension as its cause
D) The SAAG is 1.4, which rules out portal hypertension as its cause
E) The SAAG confuses me, so I don't want to do it

Answer 7.12.4 **The correct answer is "C."** The SAAG can tell us whether the fluid is a transudate or exudate. The SAAG is simply the difference between the serum albumin and the ascitic fluid albumin, or 3.3 − 1.9 = 1.4, in this case. **A SAAG of ≥1.1**

indicates portal hypertension with 97% accuracy. Remember this by remembering that a high SAAG means high pressure in the portal system.

> **HELPFUL TIP:**
> **Ascites from any cause of portal hypertension will have a high SAAG.** Aside from cirrhosis, portal hypertension also may result from schistosomiasis, sarcoidosis, portal vein thrombosis (Budd–Chiari syndrome), congenital hepatic fibrosis, heart failure, myxedema, etc. **Causes of a low SAAG include:** serositis from connective tissue disorders, nephrotic syndrome, pancreatic-related ascites, and peritoneal carcinomatosis, among others.

> **HELPFUL TIP:**
> SAAG >1.1 and ascites total protein >2.5 suggests a cardiac process with congestive hepatopathy (e.g., heart failure or constrictive pericarditis). This should prompt further evaluation if cause of the ascites is not already known.

Question 7.12.5 In addition to a complete evaluation to determine the cause of his portal hypertension, which of the following is/are appropriate action(s) at this time?
A) Refer the patient to a nutritionist for instruction on a low-sodium diet
B) Discontinue ibuprofen and prescribe a COX-2-selective inhibitor for arthritis
C) Prescribe spironolactone 100 mg daily and furosemide 40 mg daily
D) A and C
E) A, B, and C

Answer 7.12.5 **The correct answer is "D."** The initial approach to the management of ascites due to portal hypertension is sodium restriction and diuretics. The goal is a 2-g sodium diet (which is very difficult to follow—just look at a can of soup!). The majority of patients will **not** have an adequate response to sodium restriction alone, so it is reasonable to begin diuretics at the outset. Typically, diuretics are *started* at furosemide 40 mg and spironolactone 100 mg (or ½ this in patients <50 kg). They are escalated by 40 mg and 100 mg increments to max of furosemide 160 mg daily and spironolactone 400 mg daily. The ratio is dictated largely by potassium levels. **Remember the focus is on sodium balance, and if the patient is nonadherent to their diet, max dose diuretics will remain ineffective.** NSAIDs should be avoided, due to sodium retention and GI bleeding. COX-2-selective inhibitors have no advantage over nonselective NSAIDs in this regard. Other approaches to the patient's knee pain should be considered, including intra-articular injections, acetaminophen (up to 2 g daily is likely safe in cirrhosis), and narcotics, provided encephalopathy is not a problem.

HELPFUL TIP (AND PET PEEVE):
Don't use NSAIDS in liver disease. The patient may already have a coagulopathy and a low platelet count. They may have varices prone to bleeding. NSAIDS can also cause GI bleeding and are **NOT** a safe alternative to acetaminophen.

HELPFUL TIP:
In the author's experience it is not uncommon for cardiologists and hepatologists to express concern about each other's spironolactone regimen. Hypertension and heart failure doses range from 25 to 100 mg. Be sure you know WHY your patient is on the medication they are on so you can communicate effectively with your consultants.

The patient does relatively well and abstains from alcohol. He is now taking spironolactone and furosemide and following a low-salt diet. He seems to be following your instructions well but returns to the clinic because of increasing dyspnea, abdominal distention, and pain. He admits to eating his way through the state fair including the Giant Pork Tenderloin and just about anything fried on a stick (he insists he removed the pickles). On examination, he has no peritoneal signs but obviously has massive ascites. You are considering a large-volume paracentesis in your office.

Question 7.12.6 Which of the following statements best reflects the current thinking on large-volume paracentesis?
A) A patient who has over 4 L of fluid removed should receive IV albumin
B) There is no consistent data with regard to the use of albumin in large-volume paracentesis
C) Under no circumstance should more than 5 L of ascites be removed at one time
D) Given this patient's dyspnea, large-volume paracentesis is contraindicated
E) If more than 10 L of ascites fluid is removed, an equal volume of normal saline should be replaced intravenously

Answer 7.12.6 The correct answer is "B." It is unclear what patient factors indicate albumin replacement. "A" is incorrect. Unless the patient has had prior issues with renal insufficiency or hypotension with paracentesis, there is no need for albumin in patients who have less than 5 L of fluid removed. However, for patients who have more than 5 L of fluid removed, the standard of care is replacement with albumin although the data are limited. "C" is incorrect. Large-volume paracentesis can be done with even the removal of >10 L. "D" is incorrect. In fact, respiratory compromise is one reason to do a large-volume paracentesis. Removal of fluid will help with diaphragmatic excursion and may help with the resolution of pleural effusions. "E" is wrong as albumin replacement is

recommended instead of normal saline. Giving normal saline will further induce fluid shifting and increase sodium load. And, it just sounds wrong, don't you agree? That's a lot of fluid shifting.

HELPFUL TIP:
A meta-analysis of albumin replacement following paracentesis suggests that 6 to 8 g of albumin be given per liter of ascites removed in those patients having more than 5 L of ascitic fluid removed (*Hepatology*. 2012;55:1172–1181). Be sure to use the 25% concentrated version; more dilute versions result in a higher sodium load and the rapid re-accumulation of ascites.

A few months later, your patient comes to the emergency department "feeling sick." He complains of diffuse abdominal pain and swelling, stating that his abdomen feels "tense." On examination, you find a pale, uncomfortable male with a temperature of 38.3°C. His other vital signs are normal. His abdomen is tense, distended, and diffusely tender with hypoactive bowel sounds. You perform a paracentesis that shows 400 polymorphonuclear leukocytes/mm^3.

Question 7.12.7 What is the most appropriate next step in the evaluation and treatment of this patient?
A) Discharge to home with increased doses of spironolactone and furosemide
B) Discharge to home with amoxicillin and the same doses of diuretics
C) Perform a large-volume paracentesis for symptomatic relief and discharge to home
D) Admit to the hospital and start IV ceftriaxone
E) Admit to the hospital and place a peritoneal tube for drainage

Answer 7.12.7 The correct answer is "D." This patient meets criteria for spontaneous bacterial peritonitis (SBP), which is diagnosed when the peritoneal fluid contains ≥250 polymorphonuclear leukocytes/mm^3 and clinical findings suggest infection. This patient could become unstable quickly, so discharge from the emergency department is not recommended. Increasing doses of diuretics and/or large-volume paracentesis may be required, but these interventions should only be considered in the setting of hospital admission once the patient is stabilized. Beta-blockers, which may be used for portal hypertension, should be stopped; mortality is increased in SBP with continued use. Broad-spectrum antibiotics are the standard of care for SBP, and IV third-generation cephalosporins (e.g., ceftriaxone, cefotaxime) are typically the first-line agents in hospitalized patients. Levofloxacin is a good second-line agent, *but should not be used in those on levofloxacin prophylaxis as resistance is likely.* Amoxicillin ("B") is not sufficient.

In addition, albumin in the dose of 1.5 g/kg on day 1 followed by 1 g/kg on day 3 reduces the chance of renal failure, which occurs in 30% to 40% of patients with SBP. Albumin also improves mortality and should be given to all patients with SBP. Also, send the ascitic fluid for culture. Blood cultures, CBC, serum chemistries, and PT/PTT should be obtained as well. Consider imaging the abdomen with ultrasound or CT. Further tests should be ordered as indicated.

HELPFUL TIP:
The most common organisms in SBP include *Streptococcus pneumoniae*, *E. coli*, and *Klebsiella*.

HELPFUL TIP:
Fluoroquinolones and TMP/SMX have been used prophylactically to decrease the frequency of SBP episodes. Prophylaxis is indicated in anyone with cirrhosis and either (1) an episode of SBP **or** (2) an ascitic fluid protein of <1.0 **or** (3) an active GI bleed. *For active GI bleeding in those with ascites, ceftriaxone or norfloxacin for 7 days has been shown to reduce SBP and mortality.* Consider SBP prophylaxis in those with an ascites protein of <1.5 g/dL, if the Cr >1.2 mg/dL or Na is <130 mg/dL, or the BUN >25 mg/dL or the bilirubin is >3 mg/dL.

▶ **Objectives: Did you learn to …**
- Generate a differential diagnosis for ascites?
- Analyze ascitic fluid to determine potential causes of ascites?
- Initiate appropriate treatment for a patient with ascites?
- Diagnose and manage SBP?

▶ **CASE 7.13**

A 42-year-old male with known hepatitis C who is also a heavy drinker presents to your office because of increasing confusion. He hasn't noticed much of anything (hey, most of his life has been like this …), but his family states that he is somewhat confused and on occasion difficult to wake up. He has a known history of end-stage liver disease. He recently decided to start a running regimen and has been "carb loading" on boxed mac and cheese.

Question 7.13.1 Which of the following is NOT a common cause of hepatic encephalopathy?
A) GI bleeding
B) Constipation
C) High-carbohydrate diet
D) Sepsis
E) Alteration in gut flora

Answer 7.13.1 **The correct answer is "C."** High-carbohydrate diets are not associated with hepatic encephalopathy, but a high-protein diet is. Similarly, a GI bleed ("A") delivers a large protein load to the GI tract. **Thus, any patient with hepatic encephalopathy should be evaluated for a GI bleed.** Other causes of acute hepatic encephalopathy include constipation,

sedative use (e.g., benzodiazepines), and hypokalemic metabolic alkalosis.

HELPFUL TIP:
An elevated ammonia level is associated with hepatic encephalopathy, although there is not a direct linear correlation between serum ammonia level and mental status.

HELPFUL TIP:
While it's true a high protein diet *does* result in increased ammonia production in the gut, **DO NOT put your patient on a low protein diet.** Protein malnutrition is a predictor of mortality in patients with cirrhosis. The current recommendation is actually for a robust 1 to 1.5 gram per kg of dry weight (nonedematous, nonascitic state). Don't trade a short-term decrease in encephalopathy for a higher mortality rate.

You decide to admit the patient to the hospital for treatment of his hepatic encephalopathy.

Question 7.13.2 Which of the following IS NOT part of the standard treatment of hepatic encephalopathy?
A) Oral lactulose
B) Polyethylene glycol (e.g., GoLytely and Mira-Lax)
C) Oral antibiotics
D) Fluid and electrolyte management

Answer 7.13.2 **The correct answer is "B."** Polyethylene glycol does have some evidence for efficacy (*JAMA Intern Med.* 2014;174(11):1727–1733), but it is not currently the standard for treatment of hepatic encephalopathy and requires more study. There are concerns about excess volume depletion and electrolyte shifts. While polyethylene glycol and lactulose both increase bowel movements, the action of the drugs in the bowel differs. The mechanism of action of lactulose is dependent on bacterial metabolism of lactulose into lactic and acetic acids. This reduces the pH of the colon leading to precipitation of nonabsorbable ammonia in the colon, which reduces serum ammonia levels. **Enemas (soap suds, etc.), on the other hand, may help acutely** by removing colonic contents. "C" is of particular note. Oral antibiotics like rifaximin, metronidazole, or neomycin can be used when patients do not respond to lactulose or when lactulose is contraindicated (e.g., severe diarrhea). Rifaximin (though expensive) has become the standard in treating hepatic encephalopathy acutely and for chronic management. Neomycin is inexpensive (but also likely ineffective) and is only approved for episodic use. Metronidazole comes with risk of peripheral and central neurotoxicity.

The patient recovers his mental status on a regimen of lactulose and oral rifaximin.

Question 7.13.3 Which of the following problems do you need to worry about in this patient?
A) Prolonged bleeding time
B) Elevated PT/INR
C) Thrombocytopenia
D) A and B
E) All of the above

Answer 7.13.3 **The correct answer is "E."** Patients with end-stage liver disease tend to have a lack of vitamin K-dependent clotting factors (and thus elevated PT/INR and prolonged bleeding times) and have thrombocytopenia due to shunting of blood from the liver to the splanchnic bed because of elevated portal pressures. However, a platelet count of 50,000 is generally considered adequate for clotting. In addition, it is likely that there is platelet dysfunction in cirrhosis, although the clinical significance is not clear.

HELPFUL TIP:
The INR is not a great measure of coagulation in liver disease. Even when the INR is elevated, the patient may be hypercoagulable due to low levels of Protein C and Protein S, both synthesized in the liver. Thromboelastography (TEG), a measure of clot formation, or a fibrinogen level (which should be >120mg/dl) are better markers for whether the patient needs anticoagulation for an appropriate indication or is "autoanticoagulated" (data are limited). Unfractionated heparin can be used for DVT/PE, portal vein thrombosis in those with stable cirrhosis. This can be followed by a DOAC, LMWH or warfarin. Cirrhosis without varices does not increase bleeding risk. (Get the article free online: Gastroenterology July 2019 Volume 157, Issue 1, Pages 34–43.e1)

Several months after the index hospitalization, the patient returns with severe ascites and recurrent encephalopathy. Patient and family are adamant he is sober and adherent to diet and medication regimens.

Question 7.13.4 What evaluation needs to be done at this time?
A) Diagnostic paracentesis
B) Vascular ultrasound of the liver
C) ETOH level
D) All of the above

Answer 7.13.4 **The correct answer is "D."** While nonadherence is a major concern, it is important to rule out SBP and evaluate for portal vein thrombosis (PVT). Patients with cirrhosis are at elevated risk for bleeding AND clotting. PVT is surprisingly common in those with cirrhosis (11% over 5 years). It can present as acute decompensation of chronic liver failure. Anticoagulation for *acute* PVT (fever, chills, abdominal pain, tender liver, acute decompensation) is indicated.

The benefit of anticoagulation in long-standing PVT, such as that found incidentally on ultrasound, is not defined. However, in the non-cirrhotic patient portal thrombosis should prompt an evaluation for a hypercoagulable state (e.g., cancer). Long-term treatment with non-warfarin anticoagulants can be undertaken but increases bleeding episodes and has an uncertain benefit. There is a high risk of re-thrombosis when anticoagulation is stopped (39% in 6 weeks [*Clin Gastroenterol Hepatol.* 2012;10(7):776–783]).

After a few bowel movements the patient admits he has been skipping his lactulose ("Doc, even my dog won't touch the stuff!"). During hospitalization, he underwent EGD which revealed him to have large esophageal varices. He is ready for discharge.

Question 7.13.5 Which of the options is/are indicated for this patient at the time of discharge, assuming he is hemodynamically stable?
A) Nadolol
B) Propranolol
C) Carvedilol
D) A or B
E) Any of A, B, or C

Answer 7.13.5 **The correct answer is "E."** All of the above are indicated in the further treatment of this patient. It should go without saying (but we'll say it) that only one beta-blocker should be prescribed, not three. Nonselective beta-blockers ("A" and "B") will reduce portal pressures, decreasing the risk of variceal bleeding. Recently, low-dose carvedilol, 3.125 to 6.25 mg PO BID, has been shown to be effective. Other selective beta-blockers should NOT be used in patients with varices.

Primary prophylaxis is indicated for medium or large varices or small varices with red wale sign (evidence of a recent bleed) on EGD or Child Pugh Class C. In patients *without* prior variceal bleed, primary prevention with one of the above beta-blockers is noninferior to *recurrent banding*. Patients who start beta-blockers do not need a follow-up EGD unless they have a bleed. Note that beta-blockers may need to be stopped or reduced if patient has renal insufficiency, systolic pressures <90 mm Hg, or other side effects like fatigue. Also note that nitrates for reducing portal pressures are out. They do reduce portal pressures but do not reduce bleeds.

HELPFUL TIP:
Prednisolone (40 mg/day) for 28 days then tapered over 2 to 4 weeks may have some benefit in severe alcoholic hepatitis. This is controversial as steroids can increase risk of sepsis and most of alcoholic hepatitis patients die of sepsis. In order to determine which patients with alcoholic hepatitis are candidates for corticosteroids, calculate the **discriminant function (DF)**. Simply measure prothrombin time and total bilirubin and plug the numbers into an online calculator (Qxmd.com). If the DF ≥32, the patient may benefit from corticosteroid therapy.

Unfortunately, between hospital admissions, the patient continues to drink. You next admit him when he presents vomiting blood. There is clear concern for a variceal bleed in spite of adherence to his beta-blocker regimen. Two large-bore IVs are placed and aggressive volume resuscitation is initiated.

Question 7.13.6 Which of the following medications should be started in this patient?
A) Octreotide
B) IV Proton pump inhibitor
C) Ceftriaxone
D) A and B
E) All of the above

Answer 7.13.6 **The correct answer is "E," all of the above.** Octreotide is a somatostatin analog and will decrease the amount of blood going to the intestinal (splanchnic) circulation. This means less blood to go to the portal vein and up the collaterals to the bleeding vessels. A PPI should be started to cover for possible ulcer disease in this briskly bleeding patient. Start ceftriaxone for SBP prophylaxis (which will also reduce rebleeding).

HELPFUL TIP:
The goal hemoglobin in patients with acute variceal bleed is 7 to 9 g/dL. Higher transfusion targets result in higher rates of rebleeding.

The patient survives the initial bleed and appears to be recovering. Guidelines suggest placing a transjugular intrahepatic portosystemic shunt (TIPS) within 72 hours to help reduce portal pressures, prevent the re-accumulation of ascites, and hopefully prevent further bleeding (*Hepatology.* 2017;65(1):31–35).

Question 7.13.7 Which of the following statements best reflects the status of TIPS?
A) TIPS unequivocally worsens survival from end-stage liver disease
B) TIPS is associated with an increased risk of hepatic encephalopathy
C) Once placed, TIPS remains effective for at least 3 years
D) TIPS is only indicated for waiters, bar tenders, baristas, and cab drivers

Answer 7.13.7 **The correct answer is "B."** TIPS **is effective** in controlling variceal bleeding and may help ascites by reducing portal pressures. It is clearly indicated in this patient, but is not an entirely benign procedure. TIPS is clearly associated with an increased risk of hepatic encephalopathy; the effect on mortality in patients **after** a bleed when compared to a beta-blocker is still not well-studied. "A" is incorrect. In fact, there may be some survival **advantage** to TIPS in those who are at high risk but have never had a variceal bleed (not standard of care but you may see it done [*Hepatology* 2019;69(1):282–293]). "C" is incorrect

because TIPS shunts tend to clot and may need to be evaluated for patency by Doppler if ascites re-accumulates or other symptoms occur. Newer devices, however, tend to clot off less often.

HELPFUL TIP:
Over-diuresis can lead to hepatorenal syndrome, which is characterized by oliguric renal failure. Sepsis, GI bleeding, etc., can also lead to hepatorenal syndrome. The mechanism has more to do with altered circulation to the kidneys from hepatic disease than with the diuresis itself.

▶ **Objectives: Did you learn to …**
· Recognize causes of hepatic encephalopathy and identify patients at risk?
· Manage a patient with hepatic encephalopathy?
· Discuss risks and benefits of TIPS and large-volume paracentesis?

 QUICK QUIZ: AUTOIMMUNE LIVER DISEASE

Which of the following is a marker for primary biliary cirrhosis?
A) Antimitochondrial antibodies (AMA)
B) Antismooth muscle antibodies
C) Alpha-1 antitrypsin
D) Polyclonal antibodies on serum protein electrophoresis

The correct answer is "A." Antimitochondrial antibodies are found in primary biliary cirrhosis (95% sensitive and 98% specific). "B," antismooth muscle antibodies, are found in autoimmune hepatitis. "C," **reduced levels** of alpha-1 antitrypsin, are found in hepatitis from alpha-1 antitrypsin deficiency (surprise!). "D," polyclonal antibodies, are found in autoimmune hepatitis.

Autoimmune liver disease encompasses multiple etiologies including primary biliary cirrhosis, primary sclerosing cholangitis, and autoimmune hepatitis. Immune infiltrates feature prominently on biopsy in drug-induced liver injury. Other causes of liver disease, including NASH and alcohol abuse, can be associated with positive ANA and antismooth muscle antibodies leading to diagnostic uncertainty. In these cases, biopsy is reasonable.

▶ **CASE 7.14**

A 31-year-old man comes to your office for evaluation of "abnormal liver tests." He had labs for disability insurance and the following was noted: elevated total bilirubin (2.1 mg/dL) with normal direct bilirubin. AST, ALT, GGT, albumin, and alkaline phosphatase are normal. A CBC obtained at that time was unremarkable.

The patient feels generally well. When you ask about jaundice, he recalls that once when he was sick with the "flu" while in college, his roommate told him that he "looked a little yellow." He went to the student health service a few days later when he felt better and was told there was nothing to be concerned about. He drinks 6 to 8 beers/week and takes ibuprofen once or twice a month for knee pain.

Physical examination is unremarkable. A repeat liver panel shows a total bilirubin of 2.4 mg/dL with normal conjugated (direct) bilirubin, an elevated unconjugated (indirect) bilirubin, and normal AST, ALT, and alkaline phosphatase. CBC and reticulocyte count are also normal. A blood smear, LDH, and haptoglobin are normal.

Question 7.14.1 The most likely diagnosis is:
A) Crigler–Najjar syndrome type I
B) Choledocholithiasis
C) Gilbert syndrome
D) Hemolytic anemia
E) Occult acetaminophen abuse

Answer 7.14.1 **The correct answer is "C."** Gilbert syndrome is the most common inherited disorder of bilirubin metabolism, affecting up to 5% of Caucasians. It is characterized by isolated mild unconjugated (indirect) hyperbilirubinemia, with serum bilirubin levels usually less than 3 mg/dL. However, bilirubin levels in patients affected with Gilbert syndrome can increase with fasting or during febrile illnesses, though rarely exceeding 6 mg/dL. Crigler–Najjar syndrome type I is a rare disorder leading to severe unconjugated neonatal jaundice and neurologic impairment due to kernicterus. Both choledocholithiasis and acetaminophen hepatotoxicity would be unlikely to cause an isolated increase in unconjugated bilirubin; the LFTs should be elevated with these. The normal blood smear, reticulocyte count, normal LDH, and normal haptoglobin make significant hemolysis unlikely. Thus, this presentation is most consistent with Gilbert syndrome.

Several months later, the patient's older sister comes to see you. She had gone to a local health fair where screening liver tests were found to be abnormal. She recalled her brother mentioning something about a familial problem causing liver test abnormalities and wonders if she has the same thing.

She is 39 years old with good general health, although she wishes she could lose weight. She says she has been 30 to 40 lb overweight for at least 10 years and is now at her heaviest weight ever. She is a nonsmoker, who takes no medications and drinks no alcohol. She denies any risk factors for viral hepatitis.

Physical examination reveals an obese woman. Blood pressure is 138/88 mm Hg; BMI is 35 kg/m². There is no scleral icterus or other cutaneous stigmata of chronic liver disease. The abdomen is protuberant with the liver edge palpable about 3 to 4 cm below the right costal margin and is slightly tender to palpation. There is no splenomegaly and no evident ascites.

Her liver panel from the health fair 3 months ago shows the following: ALT 87 IU/L (normal range, 0–20), AST 53 IU/L (0–31), alkaline phosphatase 110 IU/L (30–115), total

protein 7.8 g/dL (6.0–8.0), albumin 4.2 g/dL (3.3–5.0), total bilirubin 0.9 mg/dL (0.2–1.0), and conjugated (direct) bilirubin 0.1 mg/dL (<0.2).

Question 7.14.2 Appropriate steps at this time include all of the following EXCEPT:
A) Repeat the liver panel
B) Counsel the patient that her labs suggest Gilbert syndrome
C) Counsel the patient regarding weight loss
D) Recommend a serologic evaluation to assess for chronic viral and autoimmune hepatitis if the liver test abnormalities persist
E) Right upper quadrant ultrasound

Answer 7.14.2 **The correct answer is "B."** As discussed above, Gilbert syndrome is defined by *isolated* unconjugated hyperbilirubinemia. This patient's pattern of liver test abnormalities with aminotransferase elevations clearly indicates a different type of problem. If these abnormalities persist, an evaluation for causes of chronic aminotransferase elevations is warranted (see differential earlier in this chapter of elevated liver enzymes). Chronic viral hepatitis and autoimmune hepatitis would be among the diagnostic considerations. Given the apparent hepatomegaly and tenderness on physical examination, an imaging study of the liver is also indicated.

The repeat liver panel is remarkable for ALT 129 IU/L and AST 76 IU/L. The other tests are normal. HBsAg and HCV antibody are negative. Antinuclear and antismooth muscle antibodies are <1:40 (normal). The ultrasound examination shows an enlarged liver with increased echogenicity, suggestive of diffuse fatty infiltration.

Question 7.14.3 Regarding nonalcoholic fatty liver disease (NAFLD), or nonalcoholic steatohepatitis (NASH), all of the following are true EXCEPT:
A) It is frequently associated with one or more features of the metabolic or insulin resistance syndrome
B) It is more common in women than men
C) The histologic features can closely mimic those of alcoholic hepatitis
D) It may cause cirrhosis in a minority of patients

Answer 7.14.3 **The correct answer is "B."** NAFLD prevalence is two times higher in men than in women and is among the most common causes of elevated liver enzymes. NAFLD refers to a spectrum of histologic findings that range from simple steatosis to an aggressive injury pattern. NAFLD often occurs in association with obesity, dyslipidemia, and/or glucose intolerance, hypothyroidism, and occurs more commonly in men than women. While most patients with NAFLD will not develop progressive liver disease, a minority are at risk to develop cirrhosis. However, due to its high prevalence in our population (thank you, fast food nation!), NAFLD/NASH is now the most common cause of cirrhosis and second only to hepatitis C for liver transplant.

Question 7.14.4 In this patient with NAFLD, all of the following are appropriate actions EXCEPT:
A) Obtain a fasting lipid panel
B) Obtain fasting serum glucose
C) Recommend weight loss to get her BMI to the normal range
D) Start ursodeoxycholic acid

Answer 7.14.4 **The correct answer is "D."** Weight loss, including from gastric surgery, can improve NAFLD. However, too rapid weight loss may be counterproductive in the setting of NAFLD, as mobilization of peripheral fat stores may worsen hepatic steatosis. Also, addressing underlying metabolic illnesses (e.g., diabetes and hypothyroidism) would be important elements in the treatment. Treating hyperlipidemia and diabetes can also improve NAFLD. Ursodeoxycholic acid has been shown to be ineffective in NAFLD as has metformin. Evidence for statin use to treat NASH is mixed, but many patients with NASH warrant statin therapy (see the following).

Question 7.14.5 Which of the following are acceptable options for assessing fibrosis score in NAFLD?
A) NAFLD fibrosis score (NFS)
B) Elastography
C) Liver biopsy
D) FIB-4
E) All of the above

Answer 7.14.5 **The correct answer is "E."** While liver biopsy is the gold standard, it is generally not required. The role of liver biopsy is primarily in patients with possible alternative diagnosis (very elevated iron studies, positive antismooth muscle or ANA, etc.). "A" and "D" are both noninvasive scores using easily obtained labs and patient data. The NAFLD fibrosis score (NFS) takes into account the patient's age, BMI, glucose, platelet count, albumin, and transaminase levels. The Fibrosis-4 (FIB-4) includes transaminase levels, platelet count, and age. Both NFS and FIB-4 are useful to categorize patients as low-to-moderate fibrosis (F1-2) or near cirrhosis and cirrhosis (F3-4) (see mdcalc.com). "B," elastography, was discussed previously and is useful in determining fibrosis levels in NAFLD as well as HCV infection. Higher fibrosis scores require additional management including surveillance for HCC and esophageal varices.

▶ **Objectives: Did you learn to …**
- Evaluate a patient with abnormal liver tests?
- Recognize the clinical and laboratory presentation of Gilbert syndrome?
- Describe findings of nonalcoholic liver disease?
- Manage a patient with fatty liver disease?

▶ CASE 7.15

A 70-year-old female presents to the emergency department complaining of mid-epigastric pain associated with vomiting. This started approximately 12 hours ago and now she notes vomiting, fever, and myalgia. Her vital signs are blood pressure 110/70 mm Hg, pulse 115 bpm, and temperature 38.5°C. On examination, the patient is quite tender in the mid-epigastric region with guarding and some rebound. Her past history is significant for lone atrial fibrillation and a seizure disorder. Her only medication is phenytoin.

Question 7.15.1 Your next steps in the diagnosis of this patient should include all of the following EXCEPT:
A) Chest radiograph
B) CBC
C) Liver enzymes
D) Abdominal CT with contrast
E) Amylase

Answer 7.15.1 **The correct answer is "D."** An abdominal CT is not indicated in this patient as part of the initial workup. "A," an upright chest radiograph, is the single best *plain* radiograph for finding free abdominal air and is indicated for this reason. In addition, the etiology of abdominal pain may also include pneumonia (especially consider this in the elderly) and other thoracic pathology that may be evident on a chest radiograph. Liver enzymes, amylase, and CBC are indicated since mid-epigastric pain with fever can be related to pancreatitis, acute cholecystitis, etc.

Her chest x-ray is normal and her laboratory results are as follows: elevated AST and ALT (both mild), normal amylase, mildly elevated white count (13.5×10^3 cells/mm³), and elevated GGT.

Question 7.15.2 The correct interpretation of these results is:
A) The patient does not have pancreatitis
B) The elevated GGT is specific for biliary outlet obstruction
C) The elevated AST and ALT may indicate biliary outlet obstruction
D) None of the above

Answer 7.15.2 The correct answer is "C." Early in the course of biliary outlet obstruction (e.g., biliary colic and common duct stone), AST and ALT may be mildly elevated. "A" is incorrect because amylase is only 80% sensitive for pancreatitis, meaning 20% of patients with pancreatitis have a normal amylase—a false-negative test. "B" is incorrect because GGT is nonspecific. GGT helps differentiate biliary tract disease from bony disease, but is an inducible enzyme and can be elevated in response to alcohol and various medications including phenytoin.

HELPFUL TIP:
In alcohol-related liver disease, AST is generally twice the level of the ALT. Part of this is due to decreased breakdown of AST, and part of this is from mitochondrial toxicity and AST leak from skeletal muscle. Rhabdomyolysis will also present with elevated AST-to-ALT ratio. When you encounter an elevated AST-to-ALT ratio, consider checking CK—in the right clinical scenario, of course.

We still don't know what is causing this patient's pain. You consider your differential. The patient has a history of atrial fibrillation and is not on anticoagulation (appropriately, given her CHA2-DS2-VASc score). You are concerned that there may be bowel ischemia from an embolism.

Question 7.15.3 Which of the following is true of mesenteric thrombosis and bowel ischemia?
A) Patients generally have guarding and rebound early in the course
B) The pain is out of proportion to the examination and patients may have a normal initial examination
C) A serum lactate level is helpful and specific for the diagnosis of bowel ischemia
D) The best study to diagnose this disease entity is CT with contrast

Answer 7.15.3 The correct answer is "B." Patients with small bowel ischemia from either embolism or mesenteric thrombosis will generally present with severe abdominal pain and an examination that is unremarkable. Late in the course there will be guarding, rebound, and other peritoneal signs as the bowel perforates. However, early in the course of the illness, severe pain with a relatively benign examination is consistent with the presentation of bowel ischemia. "A" is incorrect for the reasons stated above. "C" is incorrect because the serum lactate can be elevated in a number of states, not just bowel ischemia. However, abdominal pain plus lactic acidosis should raise the suspicion that there may be bowel ischemia. "D" is incorrect because radiographic findings on CT scan are present in only about 65% of patients with mesenteric thrombosis/embolism. The **best** study remains angiography or CT angiography, which has largely replaced traditional angiography.

Since the patient's examination includes guarding and rebound that is not out of proportion to your exam, you put the diagnosis of bowel ischemia lower in your list of possibilities. Based on the elevated white count, ALT and AST, you order an ultrasound of the right upper quadrant, which shows evidence of a common duct stone. There is thickening of the gallbladder wall but no pericolic fluid noted. You decide that there is a mild cholecystitis and want to admit the patient to the hospital. Clearly, this patient needs to be started on antibiotics.

Question 7.15.4 Which antibiotic is the most appropriate choice for this patient?
A) IV clindamycin
B) IV vancomycin
C) IV gentamicin
D) IV ampicillin/sulbactam

Answer 7.15.4 The correct answer is "D." The most appropriate antibiotic choice of those provided is ampicillin/sulbactam (Unasyn). The main organisms that need to be covered are Gram-negative organisms and anaerobes (*E. coli*, *Enterococcus*, *Klebsiella*, and *Enterobacter*). Ampicillin/sulbactam will cover all of these organisms. You might also choose piperacillin/tazobactam (Zosyn), which includes pseudomonal coverage, or metronidazole with either ceftriaxone or levofloxacin. "A" is incorrect because clindamycin covers Gram-positive organisms and anaerobes, but does not cover most Gram-negative organisms. In addition, many enterococci are resistant to clindamycin. "B" is incorrect because vancomycin only covers Gram-positive organisms and even then it is a relatively weak antibiotic for such (e.g., mortality is higher for MSSA than with nafcillin). "C" is incorrect because gentamicin does not cover anaerobic organisms. Other antibiotic options for treating this patient include cefotetan and cefoxitin, among others.

The patient is admitted to the hospital. She is treated with ampicillin/sulbactam, IV fluids, and pain medication.

Question 7.15.5 The next step for this patient is:
A) Percutaneous "T" tube placement to drain the gallbladder
B) 2 weeks of IV antibiotics followed by cholecystectomy
C) Endoscopic retrograde cholangiopancreatography (ERCP) with sphincterotomy
D) Lithotripsy

Answer 7.15.5 The correct answer is "C." The patient should have an ERCP with sphincterotomy in an attempt to retrieve the stone in her common bile duct. "A" is incorrect because in this healthy patient, percutaneous drainage would certainly be a third-line procedure. "B" is incorrect because the patient essentially has a closed abscess (the gallbladder blocked by a stone), which requires drainage. If the patient had cholecystitis **without** obstruction, prolonged antibiotics followed by cholecystectomy would be an option—but not the best one. In patients with cholecystitis without obstruction, outcomes are overall better with an early cholecystectomy. "D" is also incorrect and would be a less desirable approach than is ERCP with sphincterotomy.

HELPFUL TIP:
Studies have shown improved outcome in patients with severe gallstone pancreatitis and/or cholangitis that receive early (within 72 hours after admission) ERCP with biliary sphincterotomy.

The ERCP is successful but the patient develops worsening pain in the mid-epigastric region.

Question 7.15.6 **Which of the following is the most common adverse consequence of ERCP?**
A) Pancreatitis
B) Contrast allergy
C) Perforation
D) Bleeding
E) Sepsis

Answer 7.15.6 **The correct answer is "A."** Of the complications listed, pancreatitis is the most common, with an incidence of about 5% of patients after ERCP. In fact, elevations in pancreatic enzymes (mostly not significant) occur in up to 75% of patients post-ERCP. The others are less common and in order of descending incidence are bleeding, perforation, sepsis, and contrast allergy (rare).

Although you suspect that this patient has pancreatitis secondary to the ERCP, you also consider other potential causes of pancreatitis.

Question 7.15.7 **All of the following are causes of pancreatitis EXCEPT:**
A) Viral infection
B) HMG-Co A reductase inhibitors (statins)
C) Alcohol
D) Indinavir
E) Bee stings

Answer 7.15.7 **The correct answer is "E."** The most common causes of acute pancreatitis in the United States are ethanol ingestion, biliary tract disease, and endoscopic procedures with biliary tract disease. "A" is true. Common viruses that can cause pancreatitis include HIV, hepatitis viruses, EBV, and Coxsackieviruses. "B" and "D" are true. Many other drugs can also cause pancreatitis: of note are didanosine, some diuretics, some NSAIDs, some antibiotics, etc. See Table 7-5 for more on drugs that cause pancreatitis. The venom of a scorpion sting can result in pancreatitis, as can brown recluse spider bites but not bee stings (OK, there are one or two cases with wasps).

TABLE 7-5 DRUGS ASSOCIATED WITH PANCREATITIS

Drugs with Definitive Association	Drugs with Probable Association
Thiazide diuretics	Acetaminophen
Sulfonamides	Salicylates
Azathioprine	Metronidazole
6-Mercaptopurine	Nitrofurantoin
Furosemide	Erythromycin
Estrogens	NSAIDs
Tetracycline	ACE inhibitors
Valproic acid	Methyldopa
Pentamidine	Steroids
Valproic acid	
Dideoxyinosine	

The patient unfortunately develops worsening pancreatitis from the ERCP. You have the patient's pain well managed with morphine. However, over the next couple of days, her condition worsens. The patient begins to vomit and have increased pain as well as tachycardia and fever. Repeat labs are pending.

Question 7.15.8 **Which of the following are helpful in assessing prognosis?**
A) Hematocrit
B) BUN
C) SIRS criteria
D) All of the above

Answer 7.15.8 **The correct answer is "D."** Scores including the Ranson (no longer used), APACHE II, and newer scores like the Bedside Index of Severity in Acute Pancreatitis are not particularly helpful as early prognostic tools. They basically tell you that sick patients are sick after they are sick! Markers of severity include elevated or rising BUN, creatinine and/or hematocrit, and SIRS criteria and help identify who is sick without the cumbersome scoring of the Ranson criteria. Evidence of organ dysfunction, pleural effusions, pulmonary infiltrates, and altered mental status all suggest a more severe disease state. Patients with persistent tachycardia or tachypnea warrant close monitoring in the ICU including vitals, I's and O's, and serial evaluation for other organ system failure.

Baseline characteristics including advanced age (>55 years old), elevated BMI, and multiple comorbidities are associated with worse outcomes, and clinicians should remain vigilant in these patients.

HELPFUL TIP:
Fluid resuscitation in acute pancreatitis is important. Aggressive fluid resuscitation in the first 24 hours has been associated with reduced morbidity and mortality. Some experts recommend up to 5 to 10 mL/kg/hour with either normal saline or lactated ringers. In such patients—as with all patients with acute

pancreatitis—fluid status must be monitored frequently, and fluids adjusted as the clinical scenario dictates.

There are concerns about the patient's nutrition status. A spirited debate erupts on rounds regarding route, type, and timing of nutrition with a rather gray-haired doctor droning on about central venous nutrition (CVN).

Question 7.15.9 Which of the following IS NOT a complication of CVN?
A) Infection
B) Cholestasis
C) Hypoglycemia
D) Ileus

Answer 7.15.9 **The correct answer is "D."** Infection, cholestasis, and hypoglycemia can all be a result of CVN. Hypoglycemia generally occurs when stopping CVN because of increased levels of circulating insulin. This can be mitigated by tapering CVN or administering IV dextrose.

HELPFUL TIP:
In acute pancreatitis, enteral nutrition is preferred. CVN is now discouraged unless absolutely necessary. Increasingly, early feeding in the first 24 hours with a low-fat diet is gaining traction over waiting 24 hours and advancing from a clear liquid diet. Refeed patients early who are free of nausea/vomiting (and other signs of ileus) and have decreasing pain and improving inflammatory markers (*Curr Opin Gastroenterol.* 2018;34(5):330–335). Early refeeding is not harmful and decreases bowel permeability and bacterial translocation to the circulation.

Since the patient has continued to do poorly, you order a CT scan of the abdomen that shows evidence of a pseudocyst.

Question 7.15.10 Which of the following IS NOT true about a pancreatic pseudocyst?
A) Pseudocysts occur in 10% of patients with pancreatitis
B) Pseudocysts can be drained by forming a fistula with the stomach endoscopically
C) Pseudocysts can lead to the formation of arterial pseudoaneurysms that can cause severe bleeding
D) Open drainage is the preferred method of treatment
E) Not all pseudocysts require drainage

Answer 7.15.10 **The correct (and untrue) answer is "D."** The formation of a fistula with the stomach using an endoscope ("B") is actually the preferred method of drainage. The one major contraindication to endoscopic treatment is a pseudoaneurysm ("C"). Injury to an artery can cause significant bleeding that is difficult to control. Not all pseudocysts may require drainage ("E") and can be observed.

HELPFUL TIP:
CT scan can be used to look for a pseudoaneurysm before endoscopic drainage. An aneurysm should also be suspected in these circumstances: evidence of an upper GI bleed, a drop in the HCT, or a sudden expansion of the pseudocyst. Uncomplicated pseudocysts can be observed with serial imaging. Indications for drainage include infection, a rapidly enlarging cyst, or patients who are symptomatic from the pseudocyst. It is best to let the pseudocyst "mature" to have a well-defined "wall" for several weeks before drainage.

▶ **Objectives: Did you learn to …**
- Recognize and diagnose mesenteric thrombosis?
- Identify causes of acute pancreatitis?
- Diagnose and manage a patient with acute pancreatitis?
- Manage the complications of pancreatitis?
- Describe some side effects of parenteral nutrition in a hospitalized patient?
- Describe the principles of narcotic choice in patients with pancreatitis?

 QUICK QUIZ: GALLSTONES

A 40-year-old female presents to you with gallstones found on a "full body CT scan" performed at Live4Ever Imaging Technologies, Inc. She is anxious that she will become sick like her sister who had an emergent cholecystectomy for her gallstone pancreatitis. She asks you if she should have her gallbladder removed. She is asymptomatic and her liver enzymes are normal.

Which of the following should you recommend?
A) Laparoscopic cholecystectomy because of family history of severe gallstone pancreatitis
B) Ultrasound to confirm gallstones and to check for common bile duct stones
C) No treatment or follow-up is needed unless she develops symptoms
D) ERCP with sphincterotomy to allow stones to pass without obstructing common bile duct or compressing pancreatic duct
E) Recheck liver enzymes and if elevated recommend cholecystectomy

The correct answer is "C." Asymptomatic gallstones do not need special attention since 70% to 80% remain asymptomatic. Only 2% to 3% of patients will present with acute cholecystitis or other complications and therefore prophylactic cholecystectomy is not indicated. American-Indian populations have high risk of stone-associated gallbladder cancer and are an exception to this rule. Diabetics or sickle cell disease patients have higher risk of complications from gallstones but still **should not** have their gallbladder removed if asymptomatic. Family history of complication from gallstones is not an indication for prophylactic cholecystectomy.

▶ CASE 7.16

A 58-year-old woman with type 2 diabetes mellitus comes to your clinic with nausea, vague epigastric abdominal pain, bloating, early satiety, and intermittent vomiting for 3 weeks. Her past medical history is significant for hypertension and hyperlipidemia and her diabetes is complicated by retinopathy and neuropathy. She is on metformin, glyburide, lisinopril, aspirin, and atorvastatin.

She is afebrile and not ill appearing on examination. She has gained 5 kg in the last year. She has mild epigastric tenderness without rebound or guarding. Bowel sounds are normal and there is no abdominal distention. Laboratory results show normal CBC and differential with HbA1c of 9.4%. You suspect diabetic gastroparesis.

Question 7.16.1 Which statement is FALSE regarding diagnosis of gastroparesis?
A) On scintigraphy (gastric emptying study) >60% of the standard meal present in stomach at 2 hours suggests gastroparesis
B) On scintigraphy >10% of the standard meal present in the stomach at 4 hours suggests gastroparesis
C) EGD looking for evidence of food after an uncontrolled restaurant meal is a good test for diagnosing gastroparesis
D) Gastroparesis can be diagnosed by exhaled radiolabeled CO_2 measurement

Answer 7.16.1 The correct answer (the false statement) is "C." Simply looking for retained gastric contents at an unspecified time after an unspecified ingestion is not the way to diagnose gastroparesis. The most widely used test for diagnosing gastroparesis is radionucleotide scan. The patient is given standardized meal containing 99m technetium sulfur colloid in low-fat eggs, and nuclear activity is measured at 2 and 4 hours, respectively. If radioactivity in the stomach is >60% at 2 hours or >10% at 4 hours, the patient is considered to have delayed gastric emptying. You can do a liquid phase gastric emptying study if you suspect dumping syndrome, but it is not a test for gastroparesis. "D," radiolabeled CO_2 breath test, correlates well with nuclear scintigraphy and is easier to perform in the community setting. However, a radiolabeled CO_2 breath test requires normal small bowel, pancreas, liver, and lung function.

You order a radionucleotide gastric emptying study, and it shows that 75% of the meal was present in the stomach at 2 hours and 20% at 4 hours. You diagnose gastroparesis.

Question 7.16.2 The best long-term treatment option for her is:
A) Cisapride
B) Domperidone
C) Erythromycin
D) Metoclopramide
E) Improved glucose control

Answer 7.16.2 The correct answer is "E." The treatment of diabetic gastroparesis is often difficult and frustrating for patients and clinicians. Although not proven in prospective trials, most experts believe improved glucose control with dietary and lifestyle modification is the key to long-term success in diabetic gastroparesis. All of the above medications ("A"–"D") have shown benefit in the *short term* to reduce symptoms associated with diabetic gastroparesis. Cisapride was removed from the market because of prolongation of the QT interval. Domperidone is not available in the United States and causes a prolonged QT interval but is used in other countries for gastroparesis. Erythromycin and metoclopramide are effective and available. However, both can cause cramps, and erythromycin can cause nausea, prolonged QT interval, and often rapidly becomes ineffective (tachyphylaxis), while metoclopramide may cause tardive dyskinesia, dystonia, and a prolonged QT. Other macrolides are not effective. Liquid metoclopramide is suggested for gastroparesis and seems to work better than tablets (leaves the stomach faster and is better absorbed).

You add insulin to the diabetic regimen in an attempt to tighten glucose control and prescribe metoclopramide 5 mg, 30 minutes before meals.

Question 7.16.3 In addition to this you recommend all of the following dietary and life style modifications EXCEPT:
A) Increase dietary fiber
B) Change from four large to six small meals daily
C) Moderate exercise
D) Decrease dietary fat
E) ADA 1,800 kcal diet

Answer 7.16.3 The correct answer is "A." Fiber and raw vegetables can form gastric bezoars (phytobezoar) in gastroparesis and this is often seen on endoscopy. Bezoars cause early satiety and bloating and add to the symptom burden of gastroparesis. If a bezoar is found, it can be dissolved using cellulase (Kanalase®) or mechanically broken up. More frequent, smaller meals help with symptoms; and moderate exercise can be helpful but excessive exercise may slow gastric emptying. Your patient is gaining weight, so it is important to reinforce the ADA diet. Fat slows gastric emptying; therefore, dietary fat should be reduced to less than 40 g/day.

Question 7.16.4 Which of the following medications can exacerbate preexisting gastroparesis?
A) Fluoxetine
B) Oxycodone
C) Angiotensin converting enzyme (ACE) inhibitors
D) Metformin
E) Insulin

Answer 7.16.4 The correct answer is "B." Oxycodone and all narcotics reduce GI motility and are rarely tolerated by patients with gastroparesis. This can be clinically challenging, and attention to the cause of pain and alternative management options should be explored. Fluoxetine does not have significant effects on gastric motility, but tricyclic antidepressants and other drugs with anticholinergic activity do and are not good options for pain syndromes in gastroparesis. ACE inhibitors do not affect GI motility. Although metformin is associated with GI side effects, it does not affect GI motility. Insulin has no adverse effect on GI motility. Other medications that reduce gastric emptying are dopaminergic agents, antiadrenergic antihypertensives, calcium channel blockers, and anticholinergic agents. All drugs known to affect gastric motility should be stopped prior to obtaining a gastric emptying study.

HELPFUL TIP:
There are multiple causes of gastroparesis other than diabetes. Some of these include: postviral syndrome after gastroenteritis (may persist for >1 year), thyroid disease, neurologic diseases, and autoimmune diseases. Forty percent of gastroparesis is idiopathic. So, consider this in your differential of the patient with any of the following: postprandial fullness, upper abdominal pain, nausea, vomiting, early satiety, and regurgitation of food hours after intake (yum!).

▶ **Objectives: Did you learn to …**
- Diagnose gastroparesis?
- Identify medications that can exacerbate gastroparesis?
- Manage gastroparesis?

 QUICK QUIZ: GI BLEED

You admit a 65-year-old woman with end-stage renal disease on hemodialysis. She is being admitted because of recurrent episodes of melena requiring transfusions. She is anemic with low ferritin, iron, and iron saturation. The gastroenterologist performs an upper and lower endoscopy without any bleeding source found. Subsequently, a capsule enteroscopy shows multiple small angiodysplasias throughout the small bowel, without any large, endoscopically treatable lesions.

Your patient is discharged after a blood transfusion. Her hemoglobin is 11 g/dL. At follow-up 1 month later, her hemoglobin is 9 g/dL. The patient is on maximum doses of erythropoietin with dialysis and is still having guaiac positive stools. She refuses to take oral iron because of constipation.

Which of the following is the next best step in the management of this case?
A) Prescribe iron dextran or sucrose IV with dialysis to maintain her iron stores
B) Try to convince the gastroenterologist to repeat the endoscopy and treat any angiodysplasia lesions that can be reached

C) Prescribe octreotide
D) Order a Meckel scan
E) Prescribe estrogen–progesterone

The correct answer is "A." This is an appropriate situation for the administration of IV iron. It is safer than blood transfusions and can be given on an outpatient basis during hemodialysis. There are rare occurrences of anaphylaxis with iron dextran, and a test dose should be given. Some reports suggest iron sucrose is safer. "B," repeat endoscopies with treatments of angiodysplasias, may help but should be adjunctive therapy to maintenance of iron stores. The scope only reaches the proximal jejunum and the patient has lesions throughout the small bowel. "C," octreotide, has been reported in case series to have a beneficial effect, but no randomized trials have been performed and it cannot be recommended at this time. "D," a Meckel scan (done to look for Meckel diverticula), would be redundant as another cause has been found and the patient does not fit the most likely age group. "E," hormone replacement therapies initially seemed effective at reducing bleeding from angiodysplasia but randomized trials failed to show benefit.

HELPFUL TIP:
Angiodysplasias are commonly missed and are associated with increasing age, end-stage renal disease, aortic stenosis, hereditary telangiectasias (autosomal dominant), and are more likely to bleed in patients on long-term anticoagulation and antiplatelet therapies. Other commonly missed lesions include Cameron lesions (small ulcers caused by rubbing of hiatal hernia sac against diaphragm) and peptic ulcer disease.

HELPFUL TIP:
Capsule endoscopy of the small bowel using a small camera can be helpful if a small bowel follow-through does not show a source of bleeding. Other possible studies include tagged red blood cell (RBC) scan and angiography, but these are only really useful in overt bleeding. The tagged RBC scan needs 0.1 mL/min bleeding rate and angiography requires 0.5 mL/min bleeding rate to detect bleeding sites. Finally, double balloon enteroscopy can allow visualization and treatment of small bowel lesions.

 QUICK QUIZ: HEMATOCHEZIA

A 30-year-old female comes to your clinic with the complaint of intermittent blood on toilet paper for 3 years. She says she always has been constipated and takes polyethylene glycol (MiraLax) on regular basis. She has no family history of colorectal cancer and is asymptomatic and has no weight loss. On examination, she does not appear anemic and abdominal examination is normal. Rectal examination is normal and nontender. Anoscopy is normal.

What is the most appropriate action?

A) Reassurance

B) Hydrocortisone suppositories three times/week for 6 weeks; follow up as needed

C) Flexible sigmoidoscopy

D) Colonoscopy

E) Anorectal manometry

The correct answer is "C." The message is that everybody reporting persistent blood in stools without lesions seen on anoscopy warrants endoscopic evaluation. Colon cancer is rare in this age group but can happen. The symptom of red blood per rectum suggests that the cause could be found distal to descending colon and likely in the rectum. If there is only a single episode of bleeding, some would argue for a more conservative approach in patients less than 50 years of age without other alarm symptoms (constitutional symptoms or change in bowel habits). In this young patient, a full colonoscopy is not necessary unless there is a strong family history of colorectal cancer or other symptoms suggestive of colitis such as urgency, weight loss, or diarrhea. Anorectal manometry is not useful in the evaluation of rectal bleeding. Hydrocortisone suppositories can be helpful in reducing pain associated with hemorrhoids, but if bleeding is the only symptom, fiber supplements and stool softeners are sufficient. If the patient is older than 50 years with rectal bleeding, full colonoscopy is indicated.

▶ CASE 7.17

A 73-year-old male comes to your office with a 3-day history of left lower quadrant abdominal pain. He has felt cold and clammy at times but has not checked his temperature. He has had no nausea, vomiting, or diarrhea. The pain does not worsen after meals, but his appetite has been poor since this started. On review of systems, he reports increased urinary frequency and urgency for the same amount of time. He has had no abdominal surgeries. He has diabetes mellitus type 2 and is on metformin. He also takes aspirin 81 mg/day. He has always declined screening colonoscopy, stating, "If it ain't broke, don't fix it"—apparently, his family motto. On examination, he is in no distress with blood pressure 125/75 mm Hg, pulse 90 bpm, respirations 15, and temperature 38.5°C. His heart sounds are normal, and his chest is clear bilaterally. He has moderate left lower quadrant tenderness without rebound tenderness or guarding. There is no abdominal distention or organomegaly. Bowel sounds are normal, and the rectal examination is normal without stool in the rectal vault. Urinalysis is normal.

Question 7.17.1 What is the most likely diagnosis?

A) Ischemic colitis

B) Colon cancer with large bowel obstruction

C) Irritable bowel syndrome (IBS)

D) Pyelonephritis

E) Diverticulitis

Answer 7.17.1 The correct answer is "E." Diverticulitis is the most likely cause of the patient's pain. Fever associated with acute onset abdominal pain located in left lower quadrant makes this pain more likely to be due to diverticulitis. Diverticulitis can, however, occur in any part of the colon. Ischemic colitis ("A") can present with disproportionate abdominal pain in this location, but is usually associated with bloody diarrhea, so it is less likely. IBS ("C") almost never initially presents in this age group, is not associated with fevers unless there is a fistula or megacolon, and is a chronic condition, not acute. Pyelonephritis ("D") was a good thought until the urine dipstick returned normal. Urinary symptoms are common in diverticulitis because of bladder irritation. Colon cancer with large bowel obstruction ("B") would present with severe abdominal pain and distention. In obstruction, bowel sounds are typically hyperactive with intermittent rushing.

Question 7.17.2 The most appropriate next step in the workup of the patient is:

A) CT scan of abdomen and pelvis

B) Surgical consult

C) Gastroenterology consult

D) Abdominal ultrasound

E) Colonoscopy

Answer 7.17.2 The correct answer is "A." CT scan is very sensitive and specific for diverticulitis and can simultaneously evaluate for other causes of abdominal pain. Radiocontrast (oral or IV) does not add to the diagnostic accuracy for diverticulitis *or* appendicitis (*Ann Emerg Med.* 2010;55(1):51–59), but try telling that to your radiologist. Compromise with them and use IV contrast alone if they insist. In general, CT scan is indicated if the patient has peritoneal signs or mass suggesting diverticular abscess formation. In a patient who has had previously documented attacks and who has none of the above symptoms, empiric treatment is appropriate. Surgical and/or GI consults may be indicated but are premature at this point. Abdominal ultrasound can diagnose diverticulitis and/or abscess, but it is less sensitive than a CT scan. Colonoscopy is only indicated in the acute setting if obstruction is present or if colitis is thought to be more likely. In the setting of acute diverticulitis, the risk of perforation during colonoscopy is increased, and colonoscopy is preferably delayed until inflammation has subsided. Note that you specifically do not want to use rectal contrast if there is a question of a perforation (or that you may cause a perforation).

You get the CT scan the same day (with only IV contrast … you partially win this round with the radiologist) and have the patient return to your office to discuss the results. The CT scan shows inflammation in the sigmoid colon with some outpouching structures suggesting diverticulosis. There is a 1.5 cm fluid collection posterior to the sigmoid colon suggesting pericolonic abscess. No other findings were noted, and the colon above sigmoid appeared normal. No free air was seen.

Question 7.17.3 Which of the following is the most appropriate next step in management?

A) CT-guided drainage of the abscess

B) Surgical consult for immediate diverting colostomy and abscess drainage

C) Admission to the hospital for IV antibiotics and serial abdominal examinations

D) Discharge to home on levofloxacin and metronidazole

E) GI consult for endoscopic ultrasound guided transcolonic drainage of abscess

Answer 7.17.3 **The correct answer is "C."** This patient should be admitted for IV antibiotics. Mild attacks of diverticulitis can be managed on an outpatient basis. Our patient has small abscess that requires inpatient therapy. In addition, he is immunosuppressed by his diabetes, and all immunosuppressed patients with diverticulitis should be admitted for IV antibiotics since they are more likely to develop complications and need surgery. "A" is not the best choice. It is reasonable to ask the radiologist if this abscess can be drained, but the likely answer is no, because it is very small and is posterior to colon. "B" is also incorrect. The patient does not have peritoneal signs, and the abscess likely will respond to IV antibiotics. Thus, immediate surgery is not indicated. As discussed above, colonoscopy (and by extension endoscopic ultrasound) is relatively contraindicated in the setting of acute diverticulitis. Additionally, no gastroenterologist has been found crazy enough to try to drain abscesses by a transcolonic approach to our (and Pubmed's) knowledge. However, maybe the emerging Natural Orifice Transluminal Endoscopic Surgeons (NOTES) will attempt this in the future but not on our patient today. (Editor's note: we didn't make this one up either …. They have been doing cholecystectomies via a transvaginal approach … don't ask us why …)

HELPFUL TIP:
Antibiotic regimens for diverticulitis must include both Gram-negative and anaerobic coverage. Some common regimens include ciprofloxacin + metronidazole, ampicillin/sulbactam, amoxicillin/clavulanate, ampicillin + gentamicin + clindamycin, and ceftriaxone + metronidazole.

Question 7.17.4 Which of the following is true of diverticulosis?

A) The majority of patients with this disease will develop symptoms at some time

B) The condition is associated with a high malignant potential

C) The condition has peak incidence of occurrence in sixth, seventh, and eighth decades of life

D) The condition primarily affects the ascending colon

Answer 7.17.4 **The correct answer is "C."** Diverticu**losis** is an acquired disease that peaks in the sixth, seventh, and eighth decades with about 50% of octogenarians having the condition. "A" is incorrect. Most are **asymptomatic** with only 10%

to 20% going on to develop symptomatic diverticu**litis**. Acute diverticulitis has a variety of presentations. Peri-diverticular inflammation occurs when a fecalith becomes entrapped in a diverticular wall resulting in a localized, contained, microperforation. Pain is typically acute and located in the left lower quadrant. Examination may reveal only a mildly tender abdomen without any masses. A peri-diverticular abscess and phlegmon will typically result in worsening left lower quadrant abdominal pain, and *may* have an associated palpable mass.

HELPFUL TIP:
Epiploic appendagitis (not appendicitis, yes, it is spelled correctly) can mimic both appendicitis and diverticulitis. It generally will present similarly to appendicitis but on the left. It occurs mostly in people in their thirties. It occurs when there is torsion or infarction of an epiploic appendage on the peritoneal aspect ("outside") of the colon. Diagnosis is by CT scan and it generally resolves on its own without surgical intervention.

The patient is admitted and he responds to IV antibiotics and supportive measures. A repeat CT scan 2 weeks later shows resolution of the abscess. The local gastroenterologist performs colonoscopy 2 months after the attack and confirms left-sided diverticulosis with otherwise normal colonoscopy.

Question 7.17.5 Which of the following statements is true about this patient's prognosis?

A) When the patient has his second attack of uncomplicated diverticulitis, a resection of the diseased segment is always indicated (sigmoid colectomy)

B) 50% of patients will have a repeat attack within 5 years

C) He has 20% to 30% chance of diverticular perforation in the next 2 years

D) He has 30% chance of diverticular bleeding in the next 2 years

E) 33% of patients will have a second attack

Answer 7.17.5 **The correct answer is "E."** Only 33% of patients with an episode of diverticulitis will have a second episode. There is no set rule for the number of attacks needed before partial colectomy is indicated. The commonly used rule of three attacks is not based on prospective evidence. The decision has to be individualized, but the tendency is to operate on healthy young people with frequent attacks while opting for observation of elderly patients with comorbidities (even if they have more than three attacks). Diverticular perforation is rare and occurs in only 5% to 10% of patients within 2 years of the initial event. Diverticular bleeding happens in 3% to 5% of patients with diverticulosis and the risk is not increased with diverticulitis; if GI bleeding occurs during an episode of presumed diverticulitis, other diagnoses should be strongly considered.

On a weekend call 6 months later, your patient presents to the emergency department after experiencing sudden onset of bright red blood per rectum mixed within stools. He has passed five stools in last 3 hours and the last one had blood clots. He feels dizzy but has not passed out. He stopped taking his aspirin after his last illness, but otherwise his health and medications are unchanged. His abdomen is nontender and bowel sounds are normoactive. Rectal examination reveals fresh blood on the glove but no masses in rectum. Hemoglobin is 10 g/dL, and you place two large-bore IVs and admit him to the hospital. He has no more bowel movements overnight, his hemoglobin is 8.2 g/dL the next morning, and he is feeling well. You assume that the bleeding was diverticular.

Question 7.17.6 Which of the following statements is true?
A) Urgent colonoscopy is needed to localize and treat the lesion
B) Colonoscopy is needed but can be done on an outpatient basis
C) Tagged RBC scan followed by angiography is indicated to prevent rebleeding
D) No further workup is indicated at this point
E) Sigmoid colon resection is indicated because of the dynamic diverticular duo (diverticular bleed and diverticulitis)

Answer 7.17.6 **The correct answer is "D."** The patient has classic presentation of diverticular bleeding with rapid onset and spontaneous resolution of bleeding (75% stop spontaneously). The patient underwent colonoscopy recently and the only finding was diverticulosis. Since the patient has stopped bleeding, colonoscopy is unlikely to help in the management of his condition. For the same reason, colonoscopy does not need to be done as an outpatient. If the patient had continued to bleed, there would be two options for managing this patient, and both are acceptable. One approach is to perform rapid colonic lavage by placing an NG tube and giving 6 L (1.5 gallons) of polyethylene glycol (GoLytely) over 4 hours and perform colonoscopy to try to find the bleeding site and treat it. Often multiple blood-filled diverticuli are seen, and the source of the bleed cannot be identified. The second approach is to perform a tagged RBC scan to confirm active bleeding, followed by selective angiography to identify the bleeding vessel and embolize it. The approach taken depends on the local expertise available. Without treatment, 25% of patients eventually rebleed and of those who rebleed, 50% will have a third bleed.

HELPFUL TIP:
The whole thing about avoiding seeds and nuts in those with diverticular disease is—pun intended—nuts. In fact, patients who eat popcorn, nuts, seeds, etc., have a *lower* incidence of recurrent diverticular disease (*JAMA*. 2008;300(8):907–914). Good thing, too, popcorn has helped fuel our book editing!

▶ **Objectives: Did you learn to …**
· Identify signs and symptoms of diverticulitis?
· Appreciate the natural history of diverticular disease?
· Manage complications of diverticular disease?

 QUICK QUIZ: CAN'T STOP PUKING

Mary Jane is a 27-year-old female who presents to your clinic complaining of recurrent abdominal pain and vomiting daily for the last 6 months. The only way that she can relieve the symptoms is to either sit in a hot bath or take a hot shower. She does this compulsively and is the cleanest patient you have ever seen; she literally shines. In this case, though, cleanliness may not be next to godliness. Social history is remarkable for daily use of marijuana, tobacco use of ½ pack per day, and about 1 to 2 alcoholic drinks per day. When her back hurts, she will take her boyfriend's oxycodone—about once per week.

This behavior is typical for which of the following disorders?
A) Cyclic vomiting syndrome
B) Cannabis hyperemesis syndrome
C) Opioid bowel syndrome
D) Catamenial cyclic vomiting syndrome
E) Vomit-shower-vomit syndrome

The correct answer is "B." This history is typical of cannabis hyperemesis syndrome. This occurs in patients who are frequent marijuana users. Cannabis hyperemesis syndrome is resistant to typical antiemetics, but patients will have an abatement of their symptoms while they are in a hot bath or shower (why is unknown). The syndrome resolves once they stop using marijuana. "A," cyclic vomiting syndrome, **occurs in a stereotypical pattern**; for example, a patient may have onset at 3:00 AM (2:00 to 7:00 AM is the most common time) with preceding nausea, pallor, abdominal pain, and anorexia. Children usually have 12 cycles per year as compared to 4 in adults. Each cycle may last several days or more and the patient has normal health in between episodes. Cyclic vomiting syndrome may be a migraine variant, and antimigraine medications are worth trying. "C", opioid bowel syndrome, refers to bloating, pain, distension, and vomiting found in opioid users (not just due to constipation). It is probably a hyperalgesia syndrome and resolves when opioids are stopped (good luck with that!). "D," catamenial cyclic vomiting syndrome, is cyclic vomiting related to menses, which is not described in this case since it is occurring daily. "E" sounds silly and fictional—which it is.

 QUICK QUIZ: ALL BOUND-UP

A 64-year-old male who is a long-time patient with a history of constipation-predominant irritable bowel disease (at least that is the diagnosis he came to you with) presents to your office complaining of worsening constipation. He tells you that he is taking psyllium (Metamucil), senna (a stimulant laxative), and polyethylene glycol (MiraLax). His regimen is not working quite as well as it had in the past. He is once again having to strain.

Which of the following is/are FALSE?

A) You should review his medicine list with an eye toward eliminating anticholinergic drugs
B) He has become resistant to senna since resistance develops to stimulant laxatives
C) Increasing exercise may help regulate his bowel movements
D) Opioid-induced constipation is best treated with an antiopioid such as naldemedine as first line
E) Both B and D are false

The correct (and false) answer is "E." "A" is true. You should try to eliminate constipating medications if possible, including anticholinergics and opioids. "B" is false. Despite what we have been taught, there is no tolerance developed to stimulant laxatives (*J Clin Gastroenterol*. 2003;36(5):386–389). "C" is true. Exercise will help. Finally, "D" is false. The initial treatment of opioid-induced constipation should be a "traditional" laxative (especially an osmotic laxative such as polyethylene glycol). If the patient fails usual laxatives, peripheral mu-opioid receptor antagonists such as naldemedine (Symproic), methylnaltrexone (Relistor), and naloxegol (Movantik) can be used (*Gastroenterology*. 2019;156(1):218–226). As an aside, did you notice that we didn't mention docusate (Colace)? It tends to be ineffective long-term (*Gastroenterology*. 2013 Jan;144(1):218–238).

> **HELPFUL TIP:**
> The definition of constipation requires two of the following: straining to pass stools >25% of the time, lumpy or hard stools >25% of the time, sensation of incomplete evacuation >25% of the time, relying on manual maneuvers to promote defecation, and having fewer than three unassisted bowel movements per week. Prior criteria were difficulty passing stools, incomplete passage of stool, or fewer than three bowel movements per week.

Clinical Pearls

- All patients 50 years old or older with at least a 10-year life expectancy should undergo routine colon cancer screening; various methods are acceptable.
- Do not refer patients for cholecystectomy if they have asymptomatic cholelithiasis.
- Do not refer patients for upper endoscopy (EGD) if they have typical heartburn and no alarm symptoms (e.g., dysphagia, weight loss).
- Feed patients with pancreatitis once their nausea begins to subside. Early feeding is associated with better outcomes. There is no need for a jejunal tube if they tolerate oral feedings.
- Gastroparesis can be caused by diabetes and also by viral GI infections, thyroid disease, and autoimmune disease. Postviral gastroparesis can last for up to a year.
- If a screening colonoscopy is completely negative, do not repeat colon cancer *screening* of any kind for 10 years.
- Most pancreatitis is caused by gallstones or alcohol; other causes (viral, drug induced, elevated triglycerides, scorpion stings, etc.) are much less common.
- Screen for hepatitis C at least once in all U.S. adults aged 18-79 years (per USPSTF draft recommendation published for public comment in 2019).
- There is no absolute number of episodes of diverticulitis that mandates surgery. Tailor the treatment to the patient.
- Titrate proton pump inhibitor therapy to the lowest tolerable dose—or discontinue, if possible—after initial therapy for GERD. Remember that there is rebound hyperacidity when stopping PPIs or H_2 blockers.

BIBLIOGRAPHY

Allen BC, et al. Role of barium esophagography in evaluating dysphagia. *Cleve Clin J Med*. 2009;76(2):105–111.

American Association for the Study of Liver Disease and Infectious Disease Society of America. Recommendations for testing, managing, and treating hepatitis C. HCVguidelines.org. Accessed September 1, 2018.

Bernardi M, et al. Albumin infusion in patients undergoing large-volume paracentesis: a meta-analysis of randomized trials. *Hepatology*. 2012;55:1172–1181.

Bharucha AE, et al. American Gastroenterological Association technical review on constipation. *Gastroenterology*. 2013;144(1):218–238.

Biesiekierski JR, et al. No effects of gluten in patients with self-reported non-celiac gluten sensitivity after dietary reduction of fermentable, poorly absorbed, short-chain carbohydrates. *Gastroenterology*. 2013;145(2): 320–328. e1–3.

Crockett SD, et al. American Gastroenterological Association Institute guideline on the medical management of opioid-induced constipation. *Gastroenterology* 2019;156(1):218–226.

Delgado MG, et al. Efficacy of anticoagulation on patients with cirrhosis and portal vein thrombosis. *Clin Gastroenterol Hepatol*. 2012;10(7):776–783.

Drossman DA. Functional gastrointestinal disorders: history, pathophysiology, clinical features, and Rome IV. *Gastroenterology*. 2016;150(6):1262–1279.

Drossman DA, et al. *Rome IV: Functional Gastrointestinal Disorders for Primary Care and Non-GI Clinicians*. Raleigh, NC: The Rome Foundation; 2016.

Eisenberg JM. Managing chronic gastroesophageal reflux disease: AHRQ comparative effectiveness reviews. Available at: www.effectivehealthcare.ahrq.gov/gerdupdate.cfm. Accessed January 16, 2012.

Ford AC, et al. Efficacy of prebiotics, probiotics, and synbiotics in irritable bowel syndrome and chronic idiopathic constipation: systematic review and meta-analysis. *Am J Gastroenterol*. 2014;109:1547–1561.

Garcia-Tsao G, et al. Portal-hypertensive bleeding in cirrhosis: risk stratification, diagnosis, and management: 2016 practice guideline by the American Association for the Study of Liver Diseases. *Hepatology*. 2017;65(1):31–335.

Gray SL, et al. Proton pump inhibitor use and dementia risk: prospective population-based study. *J Am Geriatr Soc*. 2018;66(2):247–253.

Havid-Jensen F, et al. Incidence of adenocarcinoma among patients with Barrett's esophagus. *N Engl J Med*. 2011;365:1375.

Hernandez-Gea V, et al. Preemptive-TIPS improves outcome in high-risk variceal bleeding: an observational study. *Hepatology*. 2019;69(1):282–293.

Hlibczuk V, et al. Diagnostic accuracy of noncontrast computed tomography for appendicitis in adults: a systematic review. *Ann Emerg Med*. 2010;55(1):51–59.

Jacobs DO. Clinical practice: diverticulitis. *N Engl J Med*. 2007;357:2057–2066.

James TW, Crockett SD. Management of acute pancreatitis in the first 72 hours. *Curr Opin Gastroenterol*. 2018;34(5):330–335.

Jiang D. Care of chronic liver disease. *Prim Care*. 2011;38:483–498; viii–ix.

Kwo PY, et al. ACG clinical guideline: evaluation of abnormal liver chemistries. *Am J Gastroenterol*. 2017;112(1):18–35.

Laine L, Jensen DM. Management of patients with ulcer bleeding. *Am J Gastroenterol*. 2012;107(3):345–360.

Lanza FL, et al. Practice Parameters Committee of the American College of Gastroenterology. Guidelines for prevention of NSAID-related ulcer complications. *Am J Gastroenterol*. 2009;104:728–738.

Lebwohl B, et al. Mucosal healing and risk for lymphoproliferative malignancy in celiac disease: a population-based cohort study. *Ann Intern Med*. 2013;159(3):169–175.

Lichtenstein GR, et al. ACG clinical guideline: management of Crohn's disease in adults. *Am J Gastroenterol*. 2018;113(4):481–517.

Malfertheiner P, et al. Peptic ulcer disease. *Lancet*. 2009; 374(9699):1449–1461.

Marshall JK, et al. Eight year prognosis of postinfectious irritable bowel syndrome following waterborne bacterial dysentery. *Gut*. 2010;59:605.

McColl KEL. *Helicobacter pylori* infection. *N Engl J Med*. 2010;362:1597–1604.

McGee S, et al. The rational clinical examination: is this patient hypovolemic? *JAMA*. 1999;281:1022–1029.

Moayyedi PM, et al. The effect of fiber supplementation on irritable bowel syndrome: a systematic review and meta-analysis. *Am J Gastroenterol*. 2014;109(9):1367–1374.

Moayyedi PM, et al. ACG and CAG clinical guideline: management of dyspepsia. *Am J Gastroenterol*. 2017;112(7):988–1013.

Nery F, et al. Causes and consequences of portal vein thrombosis in 1,243 patients with cirrhosis: results of a longitudinal study. *Hepatology*. 2015;61:660–667.

Othman F, et al. Community acquired pneumonia incidence before and after proton pump inhibitor prescription: population based study. *BMJ*. 2016;355:i5813.

Pimentel M, et al. Rifaximin therapy for patients with irritable bowel syndrome without constipation. *N Engl J Med*. 2011;364:22–32.

Rahimi RS, et al. Lactulose vs. polyethylene glycol 3350-electrolyte solution for treatment of overt hepatic encephalopathy: the HELP randomized-clinical trial. *JAMA Intern Med*. 2014;174(11):1727–1733.

Rex DK, et al. Colorectal cancer screening: recommendations for physicians and patients from the society task force on colorectal cancer. *Gastroenterology*. 2017;153(1):307–323.

Riddle MS, et al. ACG clinical guideline: diagnosis, treatment, and prevention of acute diarrheal infections in adults. *Am J Gastroenterol*. 2016;111(5):602–622.

Sanyal AJ, et al. Pioglitazone, vitamin E, or placebo for nonalcoholic steatohepatitis. *N Engl J Med*. 2010;362:1675.

Shaheen NJ, et al. ACG clinical guideline: diagnosis and management of Barrett's esophagus. *Am J Gastroenterol*. 2016;111(1):30–50.

Squires JE, et al. Role of celiac disease screening for children with functional gastrointestinal disorders. *JAMA Pediatr*. 2014;168(6):514–515.

Strate LL, et al. Nut, corn, and popcorn consumption and the incidence of diverticular disease. *JAMA*. 2008;300(8):907–914.

Swaroop VS, et al. Severe acute pancreatitis. *JAMA*. 2004;291:2865–2868.

United States Preventive Services Task Force. Screening for colorectal cancer: US Preventive Services Task Force recommendations statement. *JAMA*. 2016;315(23):2564–2575.

van Rheenen PF, et al. Faecal calprotectin for screening of patients with suspected inflammatory bowel disease: diagnostic meta-analysis. *BMJ*. 2010;341:c3369.

Vilstrup H, et al. Hepatic encephalopathy in chronic liver disease: 2014 Practice Guideline by the American Association for the Study of Liver Diseases and the European Association for the Study of the Liver. *Hepatology*. 2014;60(2):715–735.

Wald A. Is chronic use of stimulant laxatives harmful to the colon? *J Clin Gastroenterol*. 2003;36(5):386–389.

Infectious Diseases

A. Ben Appenheimer

8

Flu season is right around the corner and you are preparing your clinic for the onslaught. First things first ... you need to know how much vaccine to order and who will be receiving it. The Centers for Disease Control and Prevention (CDC) annually publishes recommendations for administering influenza vaccine to the American public.

Question 8.1.1 The CDC recommends vaccination for all of the following groups EXCEPT:

A) Health care workers
B) Nursing home residents
C) Febrile neonates
D) Diabetics
E) The elderly

Answer 8.1.1 The correct answer is "C." We start this chapter with an easy one. Patients 6 months of age or younger should not be vaccinated nor should children who are febrile. *Egg allergy is no longer a contraindication to any influenza vaccine product.* Also, patients with egg allergies no longer need to be observed for 30 minutes. Those who have more than hives as an egg allergy should be given the vaccine in a health care facility able to treat anaphylaxis, which seems prudent (CDC 2018).

HELPFUL TIP:
Vaccinate all persons older than 6 months annually. There are **several types** of vaccine available: trivalent and quadrivalent inactivated influenza vaccines (the old-fashioned flu shot, e.g., Fluzone) for patients 18 to 64 years of age, high-dose intramuscular vaccine for the elderly, and the intranasal live attenuated influenza vaccine (e.g., FluMist). However, the intranasal live attenuated influenza vaccine was not recommended for the 2017–2018 influenza season due to concerns about efficacy against the circulating strains. It was once again recommended for the 2018–2019 season. Check annually.

Oh, no! The virus has struck. Like a zombie apocalypse, it started with just a few cases, but now it's out of control. (For fun, google "zombie apocalypse CDC"—it's a real thing, an educational tool for patients.) Every other patient who calls complains of influenza-like illness and there have been a few cases noted in the local nursing home.

Question 8.1.2 During this outbreak, what intervention(s) is/are most appropriate for all your unvaccinated, frail nursing home patients who have no symptoms of febrile respiratory illness?

A) Antiviral prophylaxis with oseltamivir
B) Antiviral prophylaxis with amantadine
C) Influenza immunization
D) A and C given together
E) B and C given together

Answer 8.1.2 The correct answer is "D." Persons at high risk for complications of influenza can still be vaccinated after an outbreak of influenza has begun in the community, but development of antibodies in adults can take up to 2 weeks. Thus, for those patients who have not been vaccinated but are at high risk for complications, chemoprophylaxis should be considered. These include children <5 years old, adults > 65 years old, pregnant or recently postpartum women, immunosuppressed patients, those with significant comorbidities, etc. In an outbreak setting, oseltamivir prophylaxis is recommended for all nursing home residents *regardless of their immunization status.* "A" alone might be appropriate for individuals who have a contraindication to vaccination and wish to protect themselves from influenza. "B" is not correct because influenza A is increasingly resistant to M2 drugs (e.g., amantadine, rimantadine) and influenza B has never been sensitive to them. Vaccination alone ("C") can be used in individuals **without** known high-risk conditions such as asthma, diabetes, renal dysfunction, immunodeficiency, or cardiovascular disease. But, as noted above, vaccine alone is inadequate for those who are institutionalized or have significant comorbidities. These higher risk patients also need to be covered by oseltamivir until immunity has developed (2 weeks).

HELPFUL TIP:
Sensitivity of rapid antigen tests for influenza is low, estimated at 62%. Therefore, a negative rapid antigen test should not preclude treatment in those patients in which a high clinical suspicion is maintained. However, newer PCR testing has a much higher sensitivity of around 92%. Both tests have relatively high specificity.

HELPFUL TIP:
For a specific patient, tests of the virus for susceptibility to specific antivirals are not clinically useful due to the time required to get results. However, trends in the community guide empiric therapy. Resistance varies by year. Resistance of influenza A H1N1 to oseltamivir was 99% in 2009. However, in 2013 to 2014 98.2% of influenza A H1N1 isolates tested were **susceptible** to oseltamivir. The CDC monitors and reports annual influenza antiviral sensitivity results on their website, https://www.cdc.gov/flu/.

Question 8.1.3 Which of these patients would qualify for antiviral therapy during an influenza outbreak?
A) A healthy 29-year-old male who presents 72 hours after onset of symptom **and** has a positive rapid test for influenza
B) A 70-year-old patient hospitalized with influenza who presents 72 hours after onset of symptoms
C) A pregnant women who presents within 48 hours of symptom onset and has a positive rapid test for influenza
D) B and C
E) All of the above

Answer 8.1.3 The correct answer is "D." In outpatients, antiviral drugs are reserved for high-risk groups including pregnancy, age >65 years, significant underlying medical illness (DM, immunosuppression, morbid obesity, asthma, etc.), nursing home residents, and children age <2 years. Normal risk outpatients should be prioritized lower on the treatment ladder. However, the CDC does recommend that antiviral drugs be considered for otherwise healthy outpatients with confirmed influenza who can start medication *within 48 hours* of symptom onset. All hospitalized patients should be treated even if it is >48 hours after onset of symptoms.

The director of nursing at your community nursing home calls about an outbreak of febrile respiratory infections. In the last 24 hours, three patients have become ill on the dementia care unit. All residents of the home were vaccinated with the current year's influenza vaccine 2 months ago in November. Several of the aides have not been vaccinated and two recently left work after complaining of feeling tired, feverish, and achy.

Question 8.1.4 You suspect an influenza outbreak and take the following actions EXCEPT:
A) Quarantine the nursing home and restrict access for visitors, new admissions, and ill staff
B) Hospitalize all patients suspected of having influenza
C) Limit the interaction of ill residents with non-ill residents
D) Administer antiviral prophylaxis to all well residents
E) Provide influenza vaccine to any unvaccinated residents and staff

Answer 8.1.4 The correct answer is "B." Moving sick patients only risks spreading the infection to the hospital. In addition to measures above, employees should be assigned to one work area only to prevent spread via the staff. Activities, visits, and gatherings in central common areas should be curtailed during the outbreak.

HELPFUL TIP:
Influenza vaccine is only about 50% effective in nursing home patients (thus the admonition to treat with prophylaxis during an outbreak in the nursing home regardless of vaccination status). Still, there is some herd immunity, and vaccination is recommended as the primary way to prevent an influenza outbreak. Considering all the options, vaccinating staff may be the most effective method to prevent nursing home outbreaks.

QUICK QUIZ: THE NEW KID ON THE BLOCK

Baloxavir (Xofluza®) has the advantage of:
A) Being effective even 72 hours after the onset of influenza symptoms
B) Influenza viruses having very little resistance *and* very little chance of developing resistance
C) Being recommended for treatment of all inpatients with influenza
D) Being available in an IV form
E) None of the above

The correct answer is "E", "none of the above." Baloxavir is a single-dose agent active against influenza A and B that is equivalently effective to oseltamivir and should be started within the first 48 hours of symptoms to be effective. It is given orally only (not IV), and there is about a 10% rate of resistance development *after a single dose*. Although it is not clear, this may also reduce communicability (so *that* is a plus). Its role in therapy is not currently well-defined and it is not necessary for inpatients with influenza. There seems to be no role at this point in using it in combination with oseltamivir. As to "D," you are thinking of peramivir (Rapivab®). It also has no well-defined role but may be used IV for hospitalized patients who cannot take PO; it reduces symptoms by 4 hours when compared to oral oseltamivir at several times the cost (close to $1,000).

Question 8.1.5 Time to update the pneumococcal vaccine protocol at your nursing home! In accordance with 2015 CDC recommendations for older adults, you institute the following schedule for all patients at age 65 who have not yet received a pneumococcal vaccination:

A) 23-valent pneumococcal polysaccharide vaccine (PPSV23) once only

B) 13-valent pneumococcal conjugate vaccine (PCV13) once only

C) PPSV23 followed by PCV13 one year later

D) PCV13 followed by PPSV23 one year later

E) Cowpox … lots and lots of cowpox

Answer 8.1.5 **The correct answer is "D."** Indications for pneumococcal vaccination include patients with chronic illness at high risk for invasive pneumococcal disease (e.g., diabetes, chronic pulmonary disease, and cardiovascular disease), institutionalization, age 65 or older, immunocompromised state, and **tobacco use**. Note that the tobacco use applies to all patients age 19 to 64 years old. There are two pneumococcal vaccinations, the 23-valent pneumococcal polysaccharide vaccine (PPSV23 or Pneumovax) and 13-valent pneumococcal polysaccharide conjugate vaccine (PCV13 or Prevnar-13). While the PPSV23 covers more serotypes than the PCV13 (23 vs. 13), the PCV13 induces a stronger immune response. Therefore, all adults aged 65 or older should receive both vaccines. PCV13 should be administered before PPSV23 when practical. PCV13 is also recommended for patients with end-stage renal disease, asplenia, HIV, and many other conditions. As opposed to PPSV23, **PCV13** vaccine is **NOT** indicated for those <age 65 only on the basis of smoking or the presence of lung disease (as of 2019).

HELPFUL TIP (AND BREAKING NEWS):
It turns out that Prevnar-13 is not needed in most adults: Adults are protected by herd immunity secondary to children getting vaccinated. Thus, by the time you read this, the CDC will recommend shared decision making when deciding whether or not to give Prevnar-13 in adults over 65 without an immunocompromising condition. Continue to suggest both Prevnar-13 and Pneumovax 23 to those >65 or with chronic disease that might effect immunity (DM, CKD, etc.). We don't know what the answer on the exam will be.

HELPFUL TIP:
The most common cause of bacterial pneumonia complicating influenza is *S. pneumoniae*. However, *Staphylococcus aureus* pneumonia (usually uncommon in the community) is an important entity during influenza outbreaks and generally presents with more severe symptoms.

▶ **Objectives:** Did you learn to …
- Describe who should receive influenza and pneumococcal vaccines?
- Identify appropriate interventions to halt the transmission of influenza in community and care facility outbreaks?
- Lead a successful influenza prevention program in a health care setting?
- Prescribe influenza antivirals appropriately?

 QUICK QUIZ: THE COMING PLAGUE

The clinic triage nurse comes to you with a concern about a patient who has just walked into clinic and is at the front desk. She is a 28-year-old Peace Corps worker who returned 10 days ago from a western African country in the midst of an Ebola epidemic. She is otherwise healthy but started having a fever suddenly last night. She describes fatigue, night sweats, myalgia, and temperature of 38.5°C. This morning she notes vomiting and diarrhea with blood in the stool. The patient thinks that she has a benign viral illness ("everyone was coughing on the plane") and does not recall any contacts with persons with Ebola.

You tell the nurse:

A) "We will work her in. Just have her hang out in the waiting room."

B) "Give her any mask you can find and send her to the ER. Pronto."

C) "Isolate the patient immediately in an examination room (preferably negative laminar flow if available) and call the health department."

D) "Shut down the whole clinic! We're on lockdown!"

The correct answer is "C." This patient has been in an area of Ebola epidemic, has the classic symptoms of Ebola (fever, diarrhea, vomiting, bleeding [in this case in her stools]). Other symptoms include meningoencephalitis, diffuse rash, and a relative bradycardia for the degree of fever (similar to that seen with typhoid). Treat her as though she has Ebola until proven otherwise. Ebola is highly contagious and is spread by contaminated body fluids, including aerosolized droplets. You should endeavor to limit exposure of others to the ill patient, so "A" and "B" are incorrect, as both options expose more persons. The health department in your area should be involved immediately, and they would be in contact with the CDC. The CDC recommends symptomatic patients at risk for Ebola exposure be isolated (a private examination room with doors closed is likely sufficient) and treated at the direction of public health authorities. "D" is incorrect. Despite its contagious nature, casual exposure to a patient with Ebola (e.g., sitting 10 ft away in the reception area as she walks by) is unlikely to result in transmission. Remember that the persons at highest risk during the 2014–2015 Ebola outbreak in West Africa were health care workers and caregivers of the Ebola patients. The incubation period of Ebola is 2 to 21 days. The virus can persist in the sperm, eye, breast milk, and CNS for months after symptoms have resolved (so quit eating eyeballs and you will be fine).

▶ CASE 8.2

An 80-year-old female fell, broke her hip, and underwent intraoperative repair with pinning of the fracture. She developed a local infection at the site of the repair and was treated with a 10-day course of oral clindamycin. She was transferred to the nursing home for rehabilitation and has developed loose, watery stools. Today when you visit her, she reports feeling diffuse abdominal discomfort and has had 10 bowel movements. She is very concerned because she cannot work with the therapist and risks losing her Medicare benefit for skilled nursing.

Question 8.2.1 **You plan to do the following:**
A) Begin loperamide (Imodium) as needed to prevent diarrhea during the therapy sessions
B) Obtain stool specimens for *Clostridium difficile*
C) Obtain an abdominal CT scan looking for evidence of obstruction
D) Ask your favorite gastrointestinal (GI) doctor to perform emergency endoscopy for evaluation of lower GI bleed
E) Obtain stool specimens for ova and parasites

Answer 8.2.1 **The correct answer is "B."** *C. difficile* is the most common **bacterial** cause of infectious diarrhea in **hospitalized** patients in the United States (*Campylobacter jejuni* is the most common bacterial cause overall). Multistep diagnostic algorithms using polymerase chain reaction (PCR) for the toxin gene(s) have the best test performance characteristics (sensitivity 68–100% and specificity 92–100%). Testing should be performed on only symptomatic patients. There is no benefit from testing more than one stool specimen or for checking for test of cure. Although symptomatic therapy is important, "A" is incorrect because antiperistaltic agents should be avoided in patients with *C. difficile*. Although other causes of diarrhea are possible, the most cost-effective approach in this patient would be laboratory testing for *C. difficile* according to local laboratory protocol prior to any other more invasive procedure. As an aside, ***Clostridium difficile is no more.*** The new nomenclature is "*Clostridioides difficile.*" We are using the old nomenclature in this book due to the general familiarity with it among physicians—either way, "*C diff*" still works!

HELPFUL TIP:
Testing for *C. difficile* infection has become more complicated. Therefore, the specifics of testing are not likely to be on the boards. However, the following information could be clinically useful depending on your lab's testing algorithm for *C. difficile*. Different labs test for *C. difficile* using different assays (see Table 8-1). The simplest approach (and one used by many labs) is to use PCR to test for the presence of the gene encoding the toxin responsible for *C. difficile* disease. However, this is not specific as not all *C. difficile* with this gene are actively producing toxin. Other labs have recently started utilizing an algorithm that incorporates three different assays. These include the GDH antigen (present on all *C. difficile*) which picks up all *C. difficile*, even the nontoxigenic strains that cannot cause disease. This is coupled with an assay that looks directly for the toxin responsible for *C. difficile* disease. If GDH and the toxin assay are both positive, the patient has *C. difficile* **infection**. If both are negative, the patient does not have *C. difficile*. If the patient has a positive GDH but **negative** toxin assay, then the PCR for the toxin gene is used to see if the patient's *C. difficile* is capable of producing toxin (see Table 8-2). The gold standard test for detecting *C. difficile* in the stool is the tissue culture cytotoxicity assay, but it is not commonly performed because it takes up to 2 days to perform and is more costly.

TABLE 8-1 *CLOSTRIDIUM DIFFICILE* DIAGNOSTIC TESTS

Test Name	What It Tests For	Comments
GDH assay	Presence of *any Clostridium difficile* bacteria	This test does not differentiate between toxigenic strains (that are capable of causing disease) and nontoxigenic strains that are asymptomatic. If negative, the patient does not have *Clostridium difficile*. Only used in conjunction with other tests
Toxin PCR	Presence of the gene responsible for producing toxin	This test identifies infection with *C. difficile* that has the gene to produce toxin (i.e., it is capable of causing disease). It does not detect the toxin itself. Many labs use this as the sole diagnostic test for *C. difficile*. It has a high sensitivity at detecting disease but its specificity is questionable
Toxin assay	Detects presence of the toxin itself	This test confirms the diagnosis of *C. difficile* disease as it directly detects the toxin. The specificity of this test is high but it is not highly sensitive

A stool specimen reveals the presence of *C. difficile* toxin A gene. The patient is nontoxic with a normal complete blood count (CBC) and creatinine.

Question 8.2.2 **The preferred, first-line, treatment of this patient should include:**
A) Fecal microbiota transplantation (i.e., stool transplant)
B) Lactose restriction and acidophilus milk products
C) Metronidazole 500 mg PO TID for 10 days
D) Vancomycin 125 mg PO QID for 10 days
E) B and C

TABLE 8-2 INTERPRETING *CLOSTRIDIUM DIFFICILE* MULTISTEP TESTING

Initial Result	Follow-Up Testing	Interpretation
GDH assay – Toxin assay –	None	Negative for *C. difficile* disease
GDH assay + Toxin assay +	None	Definitive positive for *C. difficile* disease
GDH assay + Toxin assay –	Toxin PCR –	Negative for *C. difficile* disease. Patient is colonized with nontoxigenic *C. difficile*
GDH assay + Toxin assay –	Toxin PCR +	Interpret based on clinical scenario[a]

[a]There are two potential interpretations of this scenario. Presuming all testing is accurate, this represents colonization with a strain of *C. difficile* that has the gene to produce toxin but is not actively producing the toxin (as indicated by the negative toxin assay). Interpreted literally, this is a negative test. However, the toxin assay has variable sensitivity and is therefore prone to false-negative tests. Therefore, the alternative possibility with this testing result is that the patient has true *C. difficile* disease but the toxin assay was a false negative. In the correct clinical scenario, these patients should be treated, but other causes of diarrhea should be considered if they do not respond to therapy.

Answer 8.2.2 The correct answer is "D." Treatment of *C. difficile* infection (CDI) includes supportive care, discontinuation of the offending antimicrobial agent, and initiation of an oral antibiotic. The previous recommendation in this setting was metronidazole. However, the Infectious Disease Society of America (IDSA) guidelines were updated in 2018 and removed metronidazole as a preferred option for initial, nonsevere *C. difficile*. There are currently two favored choices for an initial episode of *C. difficile* disease: oral vancomycin at 125 mg every 6 hours for 10 days or fidaxomicin (Dificid) 200 mg twice daily for 10 days. Randomized studies demonstrate similar cure rates between fidaxomicin and oral vancomycin, with fewer recurrences with fidaxomicin. However, fidaxomicin has a much higher cost (potentially over $3,000 for a course), and therefore vancomycin is used more often as first-line therapy. Fecal microbiota transplantation is associated with resolution of recurrent CDI, but its role in primary and severe CDI has not been established. There is limited evidence that use of probiotics is effective in the treatment of *C. difficile* infection and prevention of recurrence. See helpful tip below.

Question 8.2.3 Risk factors for *C. difficile* infection in nursing home patients include:
A) Advanced age
B) Recent acute hospitalization
C) Proton pump inhibitor (PPI) use
D) Long-term residence in a chronic care facility
E) All of the above

Answer 8.2.3 The correct answer is "E." Risk factors for acquisition of CDI in nursing home patients are similar to that of hospitalized patients and include hospitalization, advanced age, GI surgery/procedures, antibiotic exposure, and importantly **PPI use**. H_2 blockers are much less likely to contribute to *C. difficile* colitis.

HELPFUL TIP:
C. difficile diarrhea and colitis can be caused by **any** antibiotic, including metronidazole and vancomycin. The probability of diarrhea seems highest with clindamycin. Fluoroquinolones and broad-spectrum cephalosporins are increasingly associated with *C. difficile* infection, including a highly toxigenic strain. Simply stopping the antibiotic can lead to resolution in 25% of the mild cases.

Recurrence of *C. difficile*-associated diarrhea after a 10-day course of antibiotic therapy is common. Guess what? Your patient's diarrhea has recurred shortly after discontinuation of her vancomycin.

Question 8.2.4 The most reasonable treatment approach is to:
A) Repeat a course of oral vancomycin
B) Treat with a prolonged vancomycin pulse-taper regimen
C) Treat with a course of intravenous (IV) vancomycin
D) Treat with a course of fidaxomicin
E) B or D

Answer 8.2.4 The correct answer is "E." Relapse and/or recurrence are very common. Typically, about 20% of patients have a recurrence of symptoms, often within about 1 week of completing therapy. These patients usually respond to retreatment. The new IDSA guidelines have changed the recommendations for how to treat an initial recurrence. Previous recommendations included either metronidazole or oral vancomycin. However, the new guidelines suggest treating an initial recurrence with a "step-up" in therapy. If metronidazole was used initially (despite the new guidelines), a 10-day course of vancomycin is recommended. If oral vancomycin was used, recommendations include either a prolonged vancomycin pulse-taper or fidaxomicin. For additional recurrences, guidelines suggest either fidaxomicin, vancomycin pulse-taper, vancomycin followed by rifaximin, or fecal microbiota transplantation. IV vancomycin is **ineffective** treatment of *C. difficile* since vancomycin does not enter into the GI tract from the vascular space.

HELPFUL TIP:
Klebsiella oxytoca and *Clostridium innocuum* can produce an antibiotic-related diarrhea that is indistinguishable from *C. difficile*. In those with a negative stool for *C. difficile* antigen, consider (1) false-negative test (some of the newer strains of *Clostridium* toxin are not detected by traditional stool antigen), (2) *K. oxytoca* or *C. innocuum*, (3) inappropriate care of the stool sample; since *C. difficile* toxin degenerates rapidly at room temperature (no toxin may be detectable after 2 hours of exposure to room temperatures) or (4) ELISA tests generally only test for Type A antigen. The patient

may have an antigen Type B producing strain **or** there may be a mutation of antigen Type A. Know the type of test your laboratory does: enzyme immunoassay (EIA) may miss type B toxin; glutamate dehydrogenase (GDH) assay is sensitive *for the organism*, but does not prove it is causing disease; and nucleic acid amplification test (NAAT) is prone to overdiagnosis.

HELPFUL TIP:
Although frequently used in the prevention and treatment of CDI, the effectiveness of probiotics is uncertain. Gut flora is amazing (about 10^{14} bacteria from 1,200 different species live in symbiosis with you—we are actually about 50% bacteria), and adding a little acidophilus might not cut it. In particularly recalcitrant cases, fecal microbiota (stool, basically) transplantation can be performed. Patients are given "healthy" stool via NG tube or colonoscopy to reestablish normal GI flora. Yum. Although it sounds a little yucky, it appears quite safe and effective (and tastes fine with a little ketchup). Finally, bezlotoxumab is a monoclonal antibody against *C. difficille* toxin that can reduce recurrences. Added to antibiotics it reduces recurrence rate (17% vs. 28% for placebo). May be worth a try if you have a patient with recurrent disease.

▶ **Objectives: Did you learn to …**
  · Recognize the presentation of *C. difficile* infection?
  · Identify risk factors for the development of *C. difficile* diarrhea and colitis?
  · Treat patients with initial and recurrent *C. difficile* infections?

▶ **CASE 8.3**

You are called to the emergency department (ED) to examine a 40-year-old man with fever (temperature of 39°C) and headache. His past history is remarkable only for a splenectomy secondary to trauma at age 10. He is not allergic to any antibiotics. Upon examination you note that he has meningeal signs. Nondilated fundal examination shows sharp disc margins, and he is neurologically intact with a nonfocal examination.

Question 8.3.1 **The most appropriate action is:**
A) Obtain a head CT so that you can safely proceed with lumbar puncture (LP)
B) Order IV penicillin as you prepare to perform LP
C) Perform an LP immediately and begin antibiotic therapy empirically
D) Order IV erythromycin as you prepare to perform LP
E) Order IV vancomycin and IV ceftriaxone as you wait for the CBC. If the CBC is abnormal, you will do the LP

Answer 8.3.1 **The correct answer is "C."** Once you suspect bacterial meningitis, rapid diagnostic evaluation and emergent treatment are imperative, including LP and blood cultures. **If LP is going to be delayed, then appropriate empiric antimicrobial and adjunctive therapy should be given without delay.** Head CT is necessary only in those who are immunocompromised (HIV/AIDS, those receiving immunosuppressive drugs, transplant recipients), have a history of CNS disease (brain tumor and stroke), develop new-onset seizures, display papilledema on examination, or who have an abnormal/focal neurologic deficit or abnormal level of consciousness. Antibiotics for a 40-year-old male should cover *Neisseria meningitidis* and *S. pneumoniae* and would include vancomycin and ceftriaxone with pneumococcus predominating in this age group ("E"). However, "E" is not the best choice. Never wait for a CBC to determine if an adult needs an LP. The decision to do an LP is a clinical one.

HELPFUL TIP:
If the preponderance of initial clinical and laboratory data indicate that bacterial meningitis is likely and the LP cannot be done immediately, draw blood cultures and administer dexamethasone and appropriate antibiotics. You won't change the CSF culture results (in most cases) if you give a single dose of antibiotics before the LP. However, it is considered prudent to do the LP within 2 hours of administering IV antibiotics. Although *not* used routinely, PCR and immunochromotographic studies of the CSF can be used to diagnose bacterial meningitis if needed. The standard of care for suspected meningitis is to administer antibiotics within 30 minutes of the patient presenting to the ED.

Results of the cerebrospinal fluid (CSF) obtained after LP are as follows: cloudy, WBC count 5,000 cells/mm³, 95% neutrophils, glucose 20 mg/dL, and Gram-positive cocci in pairs (see Figure 8-1).

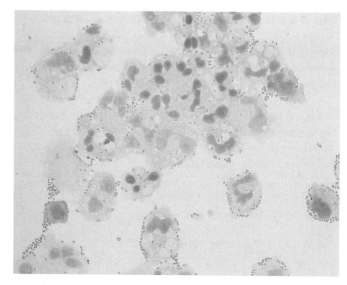

FIGURE 8-1. Gram positive bacteria with polymorphonucleocytes. Courtesy of Dr. Bradley Ford.

Question 8.3.2 **The most likely pathogen is:**

A) *S. pneumoniae*
B) *Listeria monocytogenes*
C) *S. aureus*
D) *N. meningitidis*
E) *Pseudomonas* species

Answer 8.3.2 **The correct answer is "A."** Gram stain examination of CSF may permit rapid identification of the causative organism in bacterial meningitis with a sensitivity of 60% to 90%. Prior antibiotic therapy (e.g., a partially treated meningitis ... not a single dose of antibiotics in the ED) may reduce the sensitivity by 20%. The likelihood of a positive Gram stain is highest in cases of *S. pneumoniae* (a Gram-positive diplococcus). Only about one-third of *L. monocytogenes* meningitis cases demonstrate a positive Gram stain. "D" requires special mention. *N. meningitidis* is a diplococcus but is Gram negative. As you can see in Figure 8-1, there are numerous dark blue (Gram positive) organisms in pairs and chains among the polymorphonucleocytes.

Question 8.3.3 **An adjunctive therapy that has been shown to improve neurologic outcomes in pneumococcal meningitis is:**

A) Dexamethasone
B) Activated protein C
C) Vasopressors
D) CSF shunt implantation
E) Monoclonal antibody directed against the capsule antigen of the bacterium.

Answer 8.3.3 **The correct answer is "A."** The IDSA guideline recommends adjunctive dexamethasone to be administered to all adult patients with pneumococcal meningitis. No other adjunctive therapy has proven benefit. However, benefit is only proven if given with (or just prior to) the first dose of antibiotics. Since the organism is not usually known at the time of initiation of therapy, dexamethasone should be given empirically until the causative organism is identified. If the meningitis is not due to *S. pneumoniae*, dexamethasone should be discontinued. Additionally, patients should receive standard supportive therapies in an intensive care setting. Complications, when they occur, usually develop within the first 2 to 3 days of therapy. Complications include sepsis, mental status changes, neurologic complications, and electrolyte abnormalities.

Question 8.3.4 **Highly resistant *S. pneumoniae* infections of the CNS should be treated with:**

A) Third-generation cephalosporin
B) Vancomycin and a third-generation cephalosporin
C) High-dose penicillin G
D) Ampicillin
E) Vancomycin, gentamycin, and rifampin

Answer 8.3.4 **The correct answer is "B."** Vancomycin should be combined with a third-generation cephalosporin (e.g., ceftriaxone and cefotaxime) for highly resistant pneumococcus. It

is important to understand that the use of empiric vancomycin in community-acquired meningitis is to cover for highly resistant *S. pneumoniae* as opposed to MRSA (which doesn't generally cause community-acquired meningitis). Therefore, even when *S. pneumoniae* meningitis is definitively diagnosed, you should continue vancomycin until susceptibilities are available. If it is highly resistant to beta-lactams, both vancomycin and ceftriaxone should be continued. Do not use vancomycin alone. The newer generation fluoroquinolones have enhanced in vitro activity against *S. pneumoniae* and may be used as alternative agents in very specific situations but should not be used routinely in this setting. Fluoroquinolones are not recommended unless the patient cannot tolerate or is allergic to standard drugs. In general, empiric coverage for community-acquired meningitis in adults includes vancomycin and ceftriaxone. Ampicillin is added for certain patient groups where *Listeria* is more common (infants, age > 50, or immunocompromising condition).

HELPFUL TIP:
You may be asking yourself why we need to add vancomycin to cover for highly resistant *S. pneumoniae* in the setting of meningitis, but not when covering for community-acquired pneumonia. The answer has to do with drug penetration. Ceftriaxone reaches high enough levels in the lungs to overcome this resistance. However, levels of ceftriaxone in the CSF are not high enough for this, even when used with the standard CNS dosing of 2 g every 12 hours.

HELPFUL TIP:
The combination of Kernig and Brudzinski signs carries a sensitivity and specificity of 5% and 95%, respectively. Thus, the great majority of patients do not manifest these signs when they have meningitis, and they are useless to rule out meningitis. The sensitivity and specificity of nuchal rigidity (stiff neck) is 30% and 68%, respectively. In adults, the classic triad of fever, nuchal rigidity, and altered mental status was found in only 46%, with 85% having fever, 70% having neck stiffness, and 67% having mental status changes. If they have **none** of these, you have effectively ruled out meningitis.

▶ **Objectives: Did you learn to ...**
- Diagnose meningitis?
- Identify the most likely causative organism based on epidemiology and patient characteristics?
- Describe proper use of empiric antibiotics and steroid therapy for bacterial meningitis?

 QUICK QUIZ: BIG MENINGITIS ON CAMPUS

What is the most common bacterial cause of meningitis in college-aged patients who live in dormitories?

A) *N. meningitidis*
B) *S. pneumococcus*
C) *L. monocytogenes*
D) *Haemophilus influenzae*
E) *Escherichia coli*

The correct answer is "A." Although *S. pneumococcus* is the most common cause of bacterial meningitis in the adult population in the United States, *N. meningitidis* remains the leading cause in adolescents despite vaccination and is particularly prevalent in the setting of dormitory living (e.g., college or military). The presence of petechial (or purpuric) rash in the lower extremities and pressure points is typical of *N. meningitidis*. The advent of vaccination has made *H. influenzae* a less common cause. *L. monocytogenes* is more prevalent in those over age 50, infants, and the immunocompromised. *E. coli* is a common cause for meningitis in neonates and infants, but is very uncommon in adolescents and adults (see Table 8-3).

 QUICK QUIZ: SPLEENLESS IN SEATTLE

Patients undergoing elective splenectomy should receive all of the following EXCEPT:
A) PCV13 followed by PPSV23 at least 8 weeks later
B) *H. influenzae* type B conjugate vaccine
C) Influenza vaccine
D) Meningococcal vaccine
E) Oral polio vaccine

TABLE 8-3 RECOMMENDED EMPIRICAL ANTIBIOTIC THERAPY FOR PURULENT MENINGITIS BASED ON PATIENT AGE

Age	Most Likely Bacterial Pathogens	Recommended Antibiotics
<1 month	*Streptococcus agalactiae* *Escherichia coli* *Listeria monocytogenes* *Klebsiella*	Ampicillin + Cefotaxime or Ampicillin + Aminoglycoside
1–23 months	*Streptococcus pneumoniae* *Neisseria meningitidis* *Streptococcus agalactiae* *Haemophilus influenzae* *Escherichia coli*	Vancomycin + Ceftriaxone[a]
2–50 years	*Neisseria meningitidis* *Streptococcus pneumonia*	Vancomycin + Ceftriaxone[a]
>50 years	*Streptococcus pneumoniae* *Neisseria meningitidis* *Listeria monocytogenes* Aerobic Gram-negative rods	Vancomycin + Ceftriaxone[a] + Ampicillin

[a]Or cefotaxime.
Adapted from Tunkel AR, et al. Practice guidelines for the management of bacterial meningitis. *Clin infect Dis.* 2004;39:1267–1284.

The correct answer is "E." Oral polio vaccine is no longer recommended in the United States for anyone. The risk of developing polio from the live vaccine outweighs the benefit of oral administration. All patients undergoing elective splenectomy should receive preoperative vaccination against encapsulated organisms at least 14 days prior to splenectomy; this includes vaccines against *S. pneumoniae*, meningococcus, and *H. influenzae* type B (all encapsulated bacteria). New recommendations for all pneumococcal vaccine-naive immunosuppressed adults, including those with asplenia, advise vaccination with a dose of PCV13 first, followed by a dose of PPSV23 at least 8 weeks later. Splenectomized individuals should be re-immunized against pneumococcus in 5 years with a second PPSV23. Patients who have undergone splenectomy need to be educated about seeking prompt medical attention for fever.

▶ CASE 8.4

A 74-year-old woman is in your office for a complete physical. As part of her routine labs, you obtain a urinalysis (although why is beyond us … there is no recommendation for a screening urinalysis for any nonpregnant patients). On further questioning, she has actually had stress urinary incontinence for a number of years, which is unchanged. She reports no fevers, hematuria, dysuria, flank pain, or other symptoms. The urinalysis shows 10 to 20 WBC/hpf and is nitrite positive on dipstick. A culture of the urine shows 100,000 cfu/mL of *E. coli*.

Question 8.4.1 How should you treat this patient?
A) Trimethoprim–sulfamethoxazole DS 1 tab PO BID for 10 days
B) Erythromycin 500 mg PO q 6 hours for 14 days
C) Ampicillin 250 mg PO q 6 hours for 10 days
D) Ceftriaxone 1 g IM every day for 3 days
E) With courtesy and respect, but not with antibiotics

Answer 8.4.1 **The correct answer is "E."** A positive urine culture in an asymptomatic patient (i.e., asymptomatic bacteriuria) should not be treated with antibiotics except during pregnancy. Asymptomatic bacteriuria is a very common finding, especially in elderly females, persons with indwelling catheters, and institutionalized persons. Treatment does not reduce the incidence of symptomatic infection or sequelae. Treatment also does not reduce mortality in frail elderly patients and does not improve chronic urinary incontinence symptoms. Persistent asymptomatic bacteriuria does not result in renal insufficiency or the development of hypertension.

Question 8.4.2 Which statement is true of asymptomatic bacteriuria?
A) The finding of pyuria in a urinalysis distinguishes urinary tract infection (UTI) from asymptomatic bacteriuria and guides treatment decisions
B) The prevalence of asymptomatic bacteriuria in women is unrelated to age, function, or hormonal status

C) Asymptomatic bacteriuria need not be treated in the pregnant patient

D) None of the above

Answer 8.4.2 The correct answer is "D." None of the statements are true. "A" is incorrect because the finding of pyuria with low numbers of WBCs in a urinalysis specimen is nonspecific, common, and frequently unrelated to infection. "B" is incorrect. The prevalence of asymptomatic bacteriuria in women increases with age, declining functional capabilities, and institutionalization. More than 10% of community-dwelling women over the age of 65 and up to 50% of elderly women in nursing homes will have asymptomatic bacteriuria. "C" is incorrect. Pregnancy is one state in which treating asymptomatic pyuria/bacteriuria is indicated. The risk of infection from asymptomatic bacteriuria is high in pregnant patients.

HELPFUL TIP:
Treat asymptomatic bacteriuria in the following patients: those with urinary tract obstruction (functional or anatomic), pregnancy, transplanted kidney (only within the first 3 months after transplant … though we always call the transplant surgeon), or planned urinary instrumentation. In the past, **men** with asymptomatic bacteriuria were considered candidates for treatment. This is no longer the case. **Men** *with asymptomatic bacteriuria should not be treated;* it does not improve outcomes and leads to resistant organisms (see http://www.choosingwisely.org/societies/infectious-diseases-society-of-america/).

HELPFUL TIP:
Not all pyuria is from UTI. Other pathologic causes of pyuria include vaginitis (infectious and atrophic), urethritis (*Chlamydia trachomatis*, *Neisseria gonorrhoeae*), and genital herpes infections.

A few years later, the same patient is now 80 years old (you're still paying off your med school loans and will probably work until you're 80), and she is admitted to a nursing home. Her initial tuberculin skin test (TST) with 5-tuberculin unit injection of purified protein derivative was interpreted as 0 mm diameter of induration after 48 hours.

Question 8.4.3 What is your next step?
A) Repeat a TST now
B) Repeat a TST in 2 weeks
C) Repeat a TST in 1 year
D) Declare the patient free of TB
E) Obtain a chest x-ray

Answer 8.4.3 The correct answer is "B." This is called a two-step TST test. If many years have passed since a patient became infected with latent TB, they can have an initial false-negative due to immune senescence. However, the initial TST stimulates

their ability to react to the test, prompting a positive second test. This type of testing is recommended at the time of *initial* testing for individuals who will thereafter be tested periodically (e.g., persons living in nursing homes CDC recommendations have changed for health care workers). If the first TST is negative, a second test should be performed approximately 2 weeks later in order to detect this "booster phenomenon." Without this two-step approach in this setting, the patient might react in their 1-year routine screen and may be incorrectly labeled as a recent converter (as opposed to long-standing, latent TB).

HELPFUL TIP:
False-positive TSTs can be due to Bacille Calmette–Guerin (BCG) vaccine and infection with other mycobacteria. However, most patients who had the BCG vaccine will experience a decline in immunity (a maximum of 20% will have a positive TST due to BCG 10 years after the vaccine was given). Therefore, the CDC recommends interpreting a positive skin test as a true positive, even in the presence of a prior BCG, saying, "TST reactions should be interpreted based on risk stratification regardless of BCG vaccination history." To remove this variable from the equation, Interferon Gamma Release Assays (IGRAs) are considered the preferred testing in patients who have received the BCG vaccine previously (see the following).

HELPFUL TIP:
In general, once the decision is made to test with either the TST or IGRA, the result should be trusted. An IGRA test should not be viewed as a "confirmatory" test for a positive TST (or vice versa) as they have similar test characteristics. More information on the exceptions to this rule is available at https://www.cdc.gov/tb/publications/ltbi/appendixd.htm.

The TST is repeated 2 weeks later and is interpreted again as 0 mm diameter of induration after 48 hours. You reassure the patient that her tuberculin test is negative.

Question 8.4.4 What would most accurately represent a positive TST in *THIS* patient?
A) Erythema 5 mm in diameter
B) Induration 5 to 10 mm in diameter
C) Erythema of 10 mm in diameter
D) Induration 10 mm in diameter
E) Erythematous induration of any size

Answer 8.4.4 The correct answer is "D." Here is the bottom line. Routine screening is not recommended for low-risk patients (e.g., community dwelling individuals from a low-risk country) unless they are at high risk for reactivation (such as with initiation of TNF-inhibitor). Screen only the following: close contacts of those with TB, HIV-infected patients, IV drug users, those with predisposing factors to TB infection (diabetes, immunosuppressive drugs, lung

TABLE 8-4 INTERPRETATION OF TUBERCULIN SKIN TESTS

Diameter of Induration	Positive in These Situations
>5 mm	Chest x-ray consistent with past TB infection HIV positive Recent close contact of person with active TB Organ transplant recipients Other immunosuppressed conditions (>15 mg/day prednisone, TNF inhibitor, etc.)
>10 mm	Employees or residents of high-risk congregate settings (hospitals, nursing homes, etc.) IV drug users Recent immigrants (<5 years) from high-prevalence countries Children <5 y/o or those exposed to high-risk adults TB lab personnel
≥15 mm	Persons without risk factors. These are people who probably should not have been tested in the first place (e.g., the general public without any exposure to TB)

cancer, etc.), foreign-born individuals arriving in the United States within the last 5 years, nursing home and other institutionalized individuals, and the homeless. Measure the **induration** and not the erythema. The definition of a positive TST changes with the population tested. A general rule is that the cutoff for immunosuppressed people or those with very high-risk exposures (e.g., known close contact with known case of active pulmonary TB) is 5 mm. For other people at risk the cutoff is 10 mm. For people who shouldn't have been tested in the first place the cutoff is 15 mm. See Table 8-4 for specific details. A note about health care workers: As of 2019 the CDC no longer recommends annual screening for health care workers unless they are at high risk (pulmonologists, respiratory therapists, some emergency department staff, etc.). (https://www.cdc.gov/tb/topic/testing/healthcareworkers.htm)

HELPFUL TIP:
Whole blood interferon-gamma release assays, or IGRAs (e.g., QuantiFERON-TB Gold test, T-SPOT) are Food and Drug Administration (FDA)-approved for use in any situation in which the TST is currently employed. IGRAs are more expensive and should not be the front-line screening test, but may help in certain situations such as with prior BCG vaccination or in someone who may not reliably return for their TST read. Similar to TSTs, IGRAs are **not 100% sensitive and should not** be used in patients who are symptomatic to attempt to confirm a diagnosis of active TB; they are for asymptomatic screening only and cannot differentiate latent from active infection.

A year later, the nursing home calls about her annual TST. You examine the patient and find the diameter of induration is 12 mm. The patient denies cough, weight loss, fever, or chills.

Question 8.4.5 The most appropriate next step in this case is to:
A) Obtain a chest radiograph and, if *normal*, initiate isoniazid 300 mg and pyridoxine for 9 months
B) Obtain a chest radiograph and, if *normal*, observe the patient annually for signs of active TB (weight loss, cough, fever, etc.)
C) Obtain a chest radiograph and, if *abnormal*, initiate isoniazid 300 mg and pyridoxine for 9 months
D) Obtain sputum specimens for acid-fast bacilli (AFB) stains and mycobacterial culture and sensitivity testing, and initiate therapy with isoniazid, pyridoxine, pyrazinamide, and rifampin for 6 months
E) Obtain an interferon-gamma release assay, and if negative, observe the patient annually for signs of active TB (weight loss, cough, fever, etc.)

Answer 8.4.5 The correct answer is "A." The patient lives in a high-risk setting (nursing home). The results of her TST 1 year ago suggest that she was not infected with *Mycobacterium tuberculosis* at that time. She has newly converted—probably due to exposure to an active case of TB in the facility. The risk of developing active disease following TB infection is greatest in the first 2 years following infection. The risk/benefit ratio favors prophylactic therapy with isoniazid (INH) for the patient who has converted within the last 2 years, regardless of age, as long as there is no sign of active disease and the chest x-ray is negative. Pyridoxine should also be given to prevent peripheral neuropathy from isoniazid. A negative chest x-ray does not mean that you can forego prophylactic therapy, and thus "B" is incorrect. "C" is incorrect because an **abnormal** chest radiograph must be followed with collection of sputum specimens for AFB staining and culture. "D" is incorrect because a chest radiograph is necessary to evaluate all patients with a positive TST to evaluate for active TB. Sputum specimens should be collected and multiple drug regimens initiated only in patients with signs and symptoms of active disease based on clinical history, examination, and radiographic findings. "E" is incorrect. Since this patient has converted from 0 to 12 mm induration in 1 year, her pretest probability is high enough that performing an IGRA adds nothing.

HELPFUL TIP:
It is extremely important to understand the difference between latent TB and active TB. People with latent TB are **asymptomatic** and without any imaging findings concerning for TB disease. They are infected with TB but their immune system has the infection contained. These people **are not infectious** and cannot transmit TB. Treating them for latent TB will lower the risk of converting to active TB in the future. In contrast, in people with active TB, the infection has overcome the patient's immune system. These people are symptomatic and usually have radiographic findings. People with untreated active pulmonary TB are infectious and should be isolated.

HELPFUL TIP:

A directly observed 3-month course of isoniazid (INH) plus rifapentine (RIF) once weekly may be an equal alternative to a 9-month course of daily self-supervised INH in otherwise healthy patients of at least 12 years of age. Contraindications to this regimen include persons <2 years of age, people with HIV, women who are pregnant or who may become pregnant, or those with presumed INH- or RIF-resistant TB.

HELPFUL TIP:

If active disease is diagnosed, appropriate therapy should be initiated with a four-drug regimen for 6 to 8 weeks followed by a simpler regimen for 4 to 7 months once sensitivities are known (average 6 months total). A number of regimens are available, and all include isoniazid (INH) and rifampin. INH alone is never appropriate for active TB because of resistance. First-line drugs used for active TB include isoniazid, rifampin, pyrazinamide, and ethambutol. Ethambutol may be dropped if the organism is sensitive to isoniazid, rifampin, and pyrazinamide. Second-line drugs include levofloxacin, streptomycin, and others. Regimens vary by location and local resistance patterns. Contact your local health department.

The patient's son is somewhat distraught that his mother has TB. He asks if she should have received a vaccine before coming into the nursing home.

Question 8.4.6 Regarding the BCG vaccine, which of the following statements is true?
A) Foreign-born persons who received the BCG vaccine should never have a TST administered
B) The BCG vaccine is most efficacious for older adults, and children benefit much less from the vaccine
C) A TST in an individual with a remote history of BCG vaccine should be interpreted as if the BCG had not been given
D) The BCG vaccine is made from killed *M. tuberculosis*
E) People who have received the BCG vaccine are not at risk for developing active TB

Answer 8.4.6 The correct answer is "C." Of course, you have been paying attention and know that the TST should be interpreted exactly the same way whether or not the patient has received the BCG. "B" is incorrect. BCG is most efficacious in children but protection from the vaccine wanes over a few years. Even in children, it is a poor vaccine, protecting children from TB only about 50% of the time, making "E" incorrect. Persons vaccinated with BCG should still be evaluated by TST when appropriate and an induration of >10 mm (age <35 years) or >15 mm (age ≥35 years) is considered positive. "D" is incorrect. The BCG vaccine is made from attenuated *Mycobacterium bovis*.

Prior to starting INH, you measured the patient's aminotransferase levels, which were normal. Now, 3 months into treatment, her alanine aminotransferase (ALT) is 42 IU/L (about twice the upper limit of normal).

Question 8.4.7 Your next step is to:
A) Stop her INH since she has had a few months of treatment
B) Continue the INH as scheduled and follow up with clinical and laboratory monitoring
C) Switch to rifampin and pyrazinamide
D) Refer her to a hepatologist for liver biopsy
E) Start her on milk thistle

Answer 8.4.7 The correct answer is "B." While liver injury is a significant problem with INH, the drug need not be stopped unless the liver enzymes rise to more than three times the upper limit of normal in the presence of associated symptoms or five times the upper limit of normal if asymptomatic. "A" is incorrect because she should have 9 months of prophylactic therapy. "C" is incorrect because rifampin and pyrazinamide have potentially more hepatotoxicity than INH. Finally, "D" and "E" are incorrect. Neither liver biopsy nor milk thistle (touted for its benefit in liver disease) is likely to be useful.

HELPFUL TIP:

Unfortunately, TB has developed resistance to numerous first-line agents. There is drug-resistant TB, multidrug-resistant TB (MDR-TB), and extensively drug-resistant TB (XDR-TB). The differences:
- Drug-resistant TB is resistant to one of the first-line drugs (INH, rifampin, ethambutol, streptomycin, pyrazinamide).
- MDR-TB is resistant to at least INH and rifampin and possibly more drugs.
- XDR-TB is resistant to at least INH, rifampin, fluoroquinolones, and aminoglycosides or capreomycin or both. A new drug for XDR-TB, pretomanid (2019), is approved for use with bedaquiline (approved 2012) and linezolid for highly resistant TB with about a 90% response rate.

▶ **Objectives: Did you learn to …**
- Determine who needs to be treated for asymptomatic bacteriuria?
- Interpret TST results?
- Describe the BCG vaccine and how patients who receive it should be approached?
- Recommend appropriate treatment of a positive TST?
- Recognize complications of isoniazid therapy?
- Define and recognize the importance of drug-resistant TB?

▶ **CASE 8.5**

A 37-year-old woman with a history of mitral valve prolapse and mitral regurgitation presents for evaluation. She reports no symptoms of shortness of breath or exercise intolerance.

She plans to undergo health-screening procedures, including dental exams for routine cleaning and filling of several caries, pelvic examination with removal of an intrauterine device (IUD), and colonoscopy in the next year (for a family history of polyps and early colon cancer).

Question 8.5.1 According to the American Heart Association (AHA) 2007 guidelines (and focused update in 2017) on prevention of infective endocarditis, what should she receive prior to these procedures?
A) Amoxicillin 2 g orally
B) Azithromycin 500 mg orally
C) Clindamycin 600 mg orally
D) Nothing

Answer 8.5.1 **The correct answer is "D."** Even now it seems the news has not made it to every corner of the world. In 2007 there were major changes to the AHA guidelines on infective endocarditis prevention which were affirmed in 2017. The one change that would seem to affect the greatest number of patients in primary care practices is the "downgrading" of mitral valve prolapse with regurgitation, which is no longer considered a high-risk condition. If the patient had a condition for which prophylaxis was warranted, all of the other regimens ("A," "B," "C") are options depending on the patient's allergies and other medications, conditions, etc.

Question 8.5.2 According to the AHA 2007 guidelines on the prevention of infective endocarditis, which of the following conditions is NOT a high-risk condition for the adverse outcome of infective endocarditis?
A) Bioprosthetic aortic valve
B) Mechanical aortic valve
C) Congenital heart disease completely repaired with prosthetic material
D) Bicuspid aortic valve
E) Previous history of infective endocarditis

Answer 8.5.2 **The correct answer is "D."** The guidelines recommend antibiotic prophylaxis for conditions considered to be high risk for adverse outcomes of infective endocarditis. High-risk conditions include prosthetic valves (bioprosthetic homograft and allograft valves and mechanical valves), previous infective endocarditis, and complex cyanotic congenital heart disease.

HELPFUL TIP:
Moderate-risk conditions, **for which prophylaxis is *not* indicated**, include acquired valvular dysfunction, such as rheumatic heart disease, hypertrophic cardiomyopathy, bicuspid aortic valve, and mitral valve prolapse with auscultatory evidence of valvular regurgitation and/or thickened leaflets. **Joint replacement is also not a reason for routine dental prophylaxis** (but that doesn't stop orthopedists from prescribing antibiotics).

HELPFUL TIP:
Infective endocarditis is much more likely to result from transient bacteremia that occurs with routine dental care at home, like brushing and flossing, than from dental, GI, and GU procedures. Accordingly, good oral hygiene to lower the risk of bacteremia is more important than prophylactic antibiotics.

Question 8.5.3 If your patient had a mechanical aortic valve, appropriate endocarditis prophylaxis might include:
A) Ampicillin IV 2 hours prior to colonoscopy if biopsy of lesions is anticipated
B) Ampicillin IV 2 hours prior to pelvic examination and IUD removal
C) Amoxicillin PO 2 hours prior to routine dental cleaning
D) Amoxicillin PO 2 hours prior to any injection of local anesthesia and filling of caries
E) All of the above

Answer 8.5.3 **The correct answer is "C."** For high-risk conditions (e.g., mechanical aortic valve), antibiotic prophylaxis is recommended by the AHA prior to cleaning of teeth and removal of plaque. The risk of endocarditis is highest for dental procedures that might traumatize the oral mucosa and periapical tissue, such as tooth extractions, periodontal procedures, and cleaning of teeth with removal of adherent plaque. "A," "B," and "D" are incorrect. Prophylaxis is not recommended prior to these procedures. The risk of endocarditis is low for procedures such as upper endoscopy, colonoscopy, and pelvic examination with IUD removal, because the microorganisms likely to cause transient bacteremia following these interventions are not capable of adhering to cardiac valve tissues. Antibiotic prophylaxis is NOT recommended for restorative dental procedures (e.g., fillings). Other procedures where prophylaxis *may* be indicated include procedures involving the respiratory tract with incision or biopsy of mucosa (e.g., tonsillectomy or adenoidectomy, incision and drainage of peritonsillar abscess) or other procedures including *actively infected* areas (e.g., skin, musculoskeletal, gastrointestinal, or genitourinary tracts) in those individuals at highest risk of infectious endocarditis as per above.

HEPFUL TIP:
Catheter-based cardiac valve prostheses (e.g., TAVR/TAVI, annuloplasty rings) should be treated like any other prosthetic valve from the standpoint of endocarditis prophylaxis, according to the AHA 2017 update.

All of the evaluations, including the dental examination, seem to go well. However, 1 month later, she returns to see you for gradually (perhaps even subacutely?) worsening fever, malaise, and night sweats. You are concerned that she may have developed infective endocarditis.

Question 8.5.4 The evaluation of a patient suspected of having subacute bacterial endocarditis (SBE) should include all of the following EXCEPT:

A) Three sets of blood cultures before starting antibiotics
B) Auscultation of chest for evidence of new or changing murmur
C) Transthoracic or transesophageal echocardiogram
D) Spiral chest CT
E) Electrocardiogram

Answer 8.5.4 The correct answer is "D." Endocarditis is on the rise because of the opioid epidemic. Spiral chest CT is NOT indicated in the diagnosis of SBE. History is important: onset of infection can sometimes be related to a recent dental extraction, IV drug abuse, or invasive medical procedure. Symptoms generally begin insidiously and may include weakness, fatigue, fever, night sweats, arthralgia/myalgia, and hematuria. "C," echocardiography, is indicated. The yield for visualization of vegetations for transthoracic echocardiography is 60% to 77% and increases to 96% with transesophageal echocardiography. A prolongation of the PR interval on an electrocardiogram, "E," may suggest involvement of the cardiac conduction system while a new or changing heart murmur, "B," may be suggestive of newly turbulent flow over a vegetation.

....

You carefully examine the patient and find that she is febrile and slightly tachycardic.

Question 8.5.5 You look for signs of infective endocarditis, paying particular attention to all of the following EXCEPT:

A) Osler nodes
B) Painless erythematous macules on the palms and soles
C) Splinter hemorrhages
D) Painless nodules over bony prominences
E) Roth spots

Answer 8.5.5 The correct answer is "D." Classical physical examination findings of SBE include: intermittent fever; petechiae; conjunctival hemorrhage; splinter hemorrhages under the nails; erythematous painful nodules on the pads of fingers, and toes (Osler nodes); fundic hemorrhages (Roth spots); painless erythematous macules on the palms and soles (Janeway lesions); and a new diastolic murmur. "D" is not a physical examination finding in SBE. Painless nodules over bony prominences are observed in *rheumatic fever* and are a Jones criterion. Remember that in a modern medical practice, most patients with SBE will not present with these findings, and you must maintain a high degree of suspicion for SBE in the appropriate clinical scenario.

HELPFUL TIP:
Laboratory evaluation in endocarditis may be remarkable for anemia, leukocytosis, elevated erythrocyte sedimentation rate (ESR), and microscopic hematuria.

TABLE 8-5 DUKE CRITERIA FOR BACTERIAL ENDOCARDITIS

Definite endocarditis is established by the presence of two major criteria, OR one major and three minor criteria, OR five minor criteria. Probable endocarditis is established by the presence of one major and one minor criterion, or three minor criteria.

Major Duke criteria	• New valvular regurgitation • Echocardiographic evidence of vegetations • Two positive blood cultures of a typical organism known to cause endocarditis (*Streptococci viridans, Staphylococcus aureus, Streptococci bovis, Enterococcus,* HACEK organism) • Persistently positive blood cultures with other, nontypical, organisms drawn at least 12 hours apart • Single blood culture or antibody evidence of *Coxiella burnetii* (Q fever)
Minor Duke criteria (not an exhaustive list but these are the most common manifestations)	• Fever >38°C • Vascular phenomena (e.g., Janeway lesions, splinter or conjunctival hemorrhages, and septic emboli) • History of predisposing illness (e.g., IV drug abuse, heart lesion, and artificial valve) • Immunologic phenomena (e.g., glomerulonephritis and Osler nodes) • Microbiologic finding not meeting major criteria

Question 8.5.6 Which of the following is/are included in the major criteria of the modified Duke criteria for endocarditis?

A) Positive blood cultures
B) Janeway lesions (painless macules on palms and soles)
C) Echocardiographic evidence of valvular vegetation
D) A and B
E) A and C

Answer 8.5.6 The correct answer is "E." The modified Duke criteria were developed to provide clinicians with standardized criteria for the diagnosis of endocarditis. They have been validated by pathologic examination and are more sensitive than other endocarditis criteria systems. See Table 8-5.

....

You draw a CBC, which shows leukocytosis with a "left shift" (e.g., a high percentage of bands and other immature neutrophils). Chest x-ray and urinalysis are unrevealing. You draw blood cultures and admit her to the hospital and start antibiotics (vancomycin). The next morning two blood cultures are reported to grow Gram-positive cocci in clusters. You order a transesophageal echocardiogram. Indeed, the echocardiogram shows a small vegetation on her mitral valve. Blood cultures return (wow—that was fast!) showing methicillin-sensitive *S. aureus*.

Question 8.5.7 What is the most appropriate treatment of this patient now?

A) Nafcillin IV for 4 to 6 weeks
B) Penicillin G IV for 4 to 6 weeks
C) Vancomycin IV for 4 to 6 weeks

D) Ceftriaxone IV for 2 weeks
E) Levofloxacin 500 mg IV for 4 to 6 weeks

Answer 8.5.7 The correct answer is "A." Nafcillin is the drug of choice for the treatment of methicillin-sensitive *S. aureus* endocarditis. The next best agent for severe MSSA infections would be cefazolin. Vancomycin should be reserved for patients with a penicillin allergy or patients with methicillin-resistant *S. aureus* (MRSA) as *it has been shown to be inferior to both nafcillin and cefazolin for severe MSSA infections.* Neither ceftriaxone nor levofloxacin would be considered appropriate first-line therapy for staphylococcal endocarditis.

> **HELPFUL (AND IMPORTANT) TIP:**
> **Patients who have a sensitive organism (MSSA) actually have better outcomes (fewer deaths, etc.) with nafcillin or cefazolin than with vancomycin.** While providing broad coverage for Gram-positive organisms, vancomycin is actually a relatively weak antibiotic, so save vancomycin for MRSA or other resistant organisms. Other options for hospital-acquired MRSA include linezolid and daptomycin.

While hospitalized, the patient develops symptoms of heart failure and worsening mitral regurgitation by echocardiogram. The heart failure is managed medically, but the regurgitation is now categorized as "severe." She has had 3 days of antibiotics and is currently hemodynamically stable.

Question 8.5.8 Which of the following is the most appropriate course of action?
A) Complete 6 weeks of antibiotics and manage her heart failure medically for the foreseeable future
B) Complete 6 weeks of antibiotics and manage her heart failure medically, if possible; plan for valve replacement after 6 weeks of antibiotics
C) Refer her for emergent valve replacement surgery, while being treated with the course of antibiotics
D) Refer her for heart transplant

Answer 8.5.8 The correct answer is "C." Progressive heart failure due to moderate-to-severe valvular dysfunction is an indication for surgery. There is evidence that early surgery reduces mortality and embolic complications especially in patients who have left-sided endocarditis associated with large vegetations and severe valvular dysfunction. This is true even in the absence of congestive heart failure and in the presence of less virulent pathogens. Thus, "B" is incorrect. Also, "A" is incorrect, as the patient should have surgery. "D" is incorrect, as there is no indication for heart transplant at this time.

> **HELPFUL TIP:**
> Other indications for surgery in cases of endocarditis include multiple embolic events, infections that are

difficult or impossible to treat adequately with medications (e.g., fungal infections), cardiac conduction abnormalities due to infection, persistent bacteremia, partially dehisced prosthetic valve, and perivalvular infection (e.g., cardiac abscess and fistula).

Question 8.5.9 Which of the following organisms is most often responsible for causing infective endocarditis?
A) *E. coli*
B) *Streptococcus viridans*
C) *Proteus mirabilis*
D) None of the above

Answer 8.5.9 The correct answer is "B." Of all these choices, *S. viridans* is the most likely organism to cause endocarditis. Gram-negative organisms, such as *E. coli* and *P. mirabilis*, are infrequent causes of infective endocarditis. Other organisms that cause endocarditis include the HACEK organisms (*Haemophilus* species, *Actinobacillus actinomyces comitantes*, *Cardiobacterium hominis*, *Eikenella* species, and *Kingella kingae*). In summary, organisms typically found causing endocarditis are *S. aureus*, *S. viridans*, enterococci (aerobic, Gram-positive organisms in chains that are GI or vaginal flora), *Streptococcus bovis*, and HACEK organisms.

▸ **Objectives: Did you learn to …**
· Determine who is an appropriate candidate for infective endocarditis prophylaxis?
· Recognize signs and symptoms of infective endocarditis?
· Diagnose infective endocarditis?
· Prescribe appropriate treatment for infective endocarditis?

 QUICK QUIZ: DRUG INTERACTIONS

Which of the following medications is/are contraindicated in patients taking linezolid?
A) MAOIs
B) SSRIs
C) Gentamicin
D) Vancomycin
E) A and B

The correct answer is "E." Linezolid can cause serotonin syndrome when combined with SSRIs, lithium, MAOIs, and other serotonergic drugs.

▸ **CASE 8.6**

A 10-year-old boy presents with his mother, complaining of intense itching, worse at night, since the first week of school. He has numerous excoriations in the interdigital web spaces, wrists, and anterior axillary folds (see Figure 8-2). His infant sister (10 kg) has recently developed intensely pruritic linear lesions on her palms, soles, face, and scalp. Their mother

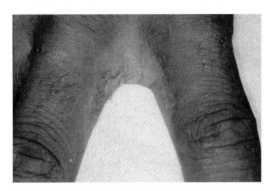

FIGURE 8-2. Scabies rash often occurs between the fingers. Used with permission from Taylor SC, et al. *Taylor and Kelly's Dermatology for Skin of Color*, 2nd ed. Copyright © McGraw-Hill Education. All rights reserved.

works in a nursing home and has developed pruritus and reddish-brown nodular lesions in her axillae and perineum that have persisted several months after she treated herself with a lotion that was provided at her place of work. As you examine the patient, your skin begins to itch—you need to solve this puzzle quickly.

Question 8.6.1 **The most likely ectoparasite affecting this family is:**
A) Head lice (pediculosis)
B) Chiggers (mites)
C) Ticks
D) Fleas
E) Scabies

Answer 8.6.1 **The correct answer is "E."** Scabies' mites (*Sarcoptes scabiei*) burrow into the epidermis, lay eggs, and hatch larvae in cycles of 3 to 4 days. The most notable clinical symptom is intense pruritus that is worse at night. The typical lesion is small, erythematous, and papular and may resemble eczema in quality and distribution. About 7% of individuals develop a nodular variant (like the mother in this case). Transmission is typically by direct contact and infestations may appear as epidemics in institutions like nursing homes. The organism may be spread by fomites as well, although to a lesser extent. Young children and infants often have involvement of palms, soles, face, and scalp. A clinical diagnosis may be made in the setting of pruritic rash, typical distribution, and multiple family members affected.

Question 8.6.2 **What is the next best step in this case (remember that one child weighs 10 kg)?**
A) Removal of the individual organisms
B) Tetracycline 10 mg/kg divided TID for all affected family members
C) Single-dose oral ivermectin 200 µg/kg, repeated in 2 weeks for all affected family members
D) Symptomatic treatment with topical steroids and oral antihistamines

E) Single-dose oral ivermectin 200 µg/kg repeated in 2 weeks for the mother; one application of 5% permethrin cream for all family members for 8 to 14 hours, followed by bathing

Answer 8.6.2 **The correct answer is "E."** Permethrin 5% cream is the topical medication of choice. Ivermectin, an antihelmintic medication, is indicated for adults with nodular disease (like the mother in this case), in epidemic settings and for treatment of scabies crustosa. "B" is incorrect because tetracycline is not helpful in this situation and should be avoided in children. "C" is incorrect because oral ivermectin should be avoided in infants weighing <15 kg due to concerns about increased penetration of the blood–brain barrier. Finally, "D" is incorrect because scabies should be treated with specific therapy rather than simply symptomatic therapy. Oh, and "A" is just insane—how could you do that? Is there even a CPT code for that?

HELPFUL TIP:
All household members should be treated, regardless of the presence or lack of symptoms. Microscopic examination of a skin scraping may identify the mite but has **poor sensitivity (46–90%).** Other viable treatment alternatives include crotamiton 10% solution precipitated sulfur in petroleum and lindane but avoid lindane in children <10 years old per the FDA. Additionally, lindane hasn't been manufactured in the United States for several years. Launder or isolate any worn/suspect bedding, clothing, etc. for 1 week (although scabies mites generally die within 3 days away from human skin). You can instruct patients to put bedding into a garbage bag outside for a week and then wash it. Patients will continue to itch for 2 to 4 weeks after treatment. This does not mean you have failed (although some providers routinely retreat at 1–2 weeks).

You successfully treated the whole family. They are now comfortable, happy, and totally confident in your abilities. The mother returns with her girl, who is now 3 years old, with a new complaint. Apparently, the girl's "bottom" is hurting, a symptom that her mother has interpreted to mean perineal pain. The pain is worse at night, even waking her at night with vaginal pain. The mother thinks that she may have a bladder infection, but there are no urinary symptoms. In the office, the patient complains only of "itchy butt" and her examination is normal.

Question 8.6.3 **What is the next best step in diagnosis of this problem?**
A) Reassurance that this is "just a stage"
B) Vaginal speculum examination with cultures
C) "Scotch tape" test
D) Stool collection for ova and parasites
E) Psychiatry consultation for the mother who obviously has Munchausen by proxy syndrome

Answer 8.6.3 The correct answer is "C." The presentation is consistent with pinworm (*Enterobius vermicularis*) infection. Clinical manifestations of pinworm infection are related to the life cycle of the parasite, in which the adult worm resides in the colon, exits the anus at night, lays eggs in the perianal skin, and may also infest the female genitourinary tract. Typical symptoms include pruritus ani, vulvitis, vaginal pain, poor sleep, and—rarely—abdominal pain (pinworms can migrate and cause appendicitis and other intra-abdominal illness). The diagnostic test of choice is the "Scotch tape" test. Clear cellophane tape is wrapped around a tongue depressor, sticky side up, and used to sample the perianal area first thing in the morning before bathing. Multiple specimens should be obtained and stored in a refrigerator (it's a good thing OSHA has no jurisdiction in the home). The tape is then examined microscopically for the characteristic ova.

Your "Scotch tape" test is a success, proving your clinical suspicions.

Question 8.6.4 The best intervention is to:
A) Treat the patient with mebendazole 100 mg orally once, repeat in 2 weeks, and encourage good hand washing for the whole family
B) Treat the patient and the entire family with mebendazole 100 mg orally daily for 14 days
C) Treat the patient and the entire family with mebendazole 100 mg orally once, and repeat in 2 weeks
D) Treat the patient with metronidazole 500 mg orally once, and repeat in 2 weeks

Answer 8.6.4 The correct answer is "C." As with scabies, the entire family should be treated. Mebendazole is the agent of choice, although other antiparasitic agents (e.g., albendazole, pyrantel pamoate) may also be used. Pyrantel pamoate is second-line and only has a 90% response rate. "D," metronidazole, is not used for helminthic infections but is effective against protozoal infections, including amebiasis and trichomoniasis. Make sure to wash all of the bed linens and clothing: eggs can stay viable for 20 days (although 3 days is more typical).

▶ **Objectives: Did you learn to …**
  • Diagnose and treat scabies infestations?
  • Diagnose and treat pinworm infections?

⧗ **QUICK QUIZ:** SWEATING IN SAVANNAH

A 54-year-old construction worker with no significant travel history presents with a fever. He developed the fever 4 weeks ago and has been febrile daily since. He saw another doctor recently. He was evaluated but received no antibiotics or other treatment. His evaluation, including history, physical examination, CBC

with differential, urinalysis, serum chemistries, and chest x-ray, has been unrevealing. Today his temperature is 38.5°C.

Which of the following is the most appropriate next step in the evaluation and management of this patient?
A) ESR and/or CRP
B) PET CT
C) Bone scan
D) PSA
E) Vancomycin IV daily and ceftriaxone IV daily for 2 weeks

The correct answer is "A." This patient has a fever of unknown origin (FUO). FUO in adults is defined as fever greater than 38.3°C of at least 3 weeks duration with no obvious cause despite extensive evaluation. Infections are the most common source of FUO in children and young adults. The most common infections worldwide include tuberculosis and abscesses. In older adults (sorry to say that this patient's age of 54 counts!), collagen-vascular diseases, such as giant cell arteritis and rheumatoid arthritis, are more likely sources of FUO. Therefore, tests for inflammatory markers, like ESR and CRP, are indicated. Other tests to consider at this point include ANA, rheumatoid factor, creatine kinase (CK), and blood and urine cultures. Although malignancy is a consideration, PSA ("D") should not be ordered without other symptoms associated with underlying prostate disease. A bone scan ("C") would be indicated to look for osteomyelitis, which is an unlikely occult source of fever in this patient with no other reason to believe he has a bone infection. PET CT can be part of the workup for FUO, but is usually reserved until after a broad initial workup has returned as negative. There is no indication for antibiotics ("E") at this point—wait until you have something to treat.

HELPFUL TIP:
The most common malignancies that present with an FUO are lymphoma, leukemia, renal cell carcinoma, and hepatoma. A CT scan of the abdomen should pick all of these up, except leukemia, of course. However, the diagnostic yield of a CT scan is lower than the yield of FDG-PET/CT, which may detect active inflammation prior to any specific anatomic change. See Table 8-6 for a partial list of causes of FUO.

▶ **CASE 8.7**

A 45-year-old physician who has recently returned from an early summer fishing vacation (in reality he mostly studied for his upcoming board examination) in rural North Carolina presents for a febrile illness. He reports a 5-day history of fever, malaise, headache, and vomiting. Today, he has developed a nonpruritic rash that began on his extremities and has spread to his body. On examination he has a fever of 38.3°C with a pulse of 120 bpm and otherwise normal

TABLE 8-6 PARTIAL LIST OF ETIOLOGIES OF FEVER OF UNKNOWN ORIGIN

Infections
- Tuberculosis
- Lyme disease
- HIV
- Endocarditis
- Dental abscess
- Abdominal/pelvic abscess
- CMV
- Epstein–Barr virus

Malignancies
- Metastatic cancer
- Lymphoma
- Leukemias
- Renal cell carcinoma

Autoimmune Conditions
- Polymyalgia rheumatica/giant cell arteritis
- Rheumatoid arthritis
- Inflammatory bowel disease
- Lupus
- Vasculitides

Drug-induced Fever

Factitious fever

Venous thrombosis

Sarcoidosis

vitals. **The rash is maculopapular and generalized, involving his palms and soles. Oral mucosa is dry but intact, and the examination is otherwise nonspecific.**

Question 8.7.1 **What is the most appropriate next step?**
A) Reassurance and symptomatic treatment
B) CBC, electrolytes, BUN, creatinine
C) Dermatology referral
D) Punch biopsy of leading edge of rash
E) Admission to the ICU

Answer 8.7.1 **The correct answer is "B."** This gentleman is sick (febrile, pulse of 120 bpm, dry oral mucosa, headache, vomiting). We would be amiss to simply reassure ("A") or refer ("C") this patient. A CBC and electrolytes may give us an indication of the degree of dehydration and help us narrow the differential (bacterial, viral, etc.). Blood cultures would also be indicated at this time. While he is febrile and tachycardic, his other vital signs are stable and he does not appear to be ill enough to warrant ICU admission ("E") given the information provided. "D," punch biopsy of the rash may be warranted as part of the evaluation but would not provide timely diagnosis or treatment; therefore, this would not be the most appropriate next step.

The test results return quickly. **CBC shows mild thrombocytopenia and leukopenia but is otherwise normal. BUN and creatinine are at the upper limits of normal, and the electrolytes are normal aside from mild hyponatremia.**

Question 8.7.2 **The most likely diagnosis is:**
A) Chicken pox
B) Syphilis
C) Parvovirus B19
D) Rocky Mountain spotted fever (RMSF)
E) Human monocytic ehrlichiosis

Answer 8.7.2 **The correct answer is "D."** RMSF is a tick-borne (dog or wood tick) disease caused by *Rickettsia rickettsii*. It presents with a prodrome of fever and headache several days before the onset of the characteristic rash—a maculopapular eruption that begins at the wrists and ankles and spreads centrally. Eventually, the rash becomes petechial. While the rash is characteristic, most patients present to medical care before the development of the rash and up to 10% of patients never develop a rash. Therefore, the lack of a rash does not rule out RMSF. Despite its name, RMSF is endemic in the southeastern United States, the Atlantic states, and the northern Rocky Mountains. Laboratory manifestations of RMSF are generally nonspecific: mild thrombocytopenia (rarely becoming severe), hyponatremia, azotemia, elevated transaminases, and prolonged PTT and PT. WBC count is variable and can be low, normal, or elevated.

"B" is incorrect because the secondary stage of syphilis is characterized by a generalized maculopapular rash (including the palms and soles) and is **not** associated with systemic symptoms.

"E" is also incorrect. Human monocytic ehrlichiosis is caused by *Ehrlichia chaffeensis*, and other related bacteria, and presents with a fever and nonspecific "flu-like" symptoms (headache, fever, myalgias, chills, cough). Rarely a rash, maculopapular or petechial, is seen. Thus, it may be easily confused with RMSF (and in fact some physicians refer to ehrlichiosis as "Rocky Mountain *Spotless* Fever"). Patients are often leukopenic and thrombocytopenic. The disease is tick-borne and endemic to midwestern, south central, and southeastern states. So, if you think you have a case of RMSF but there is no rash, consider human monocytic ehrlichiosis.

Regarding distribution, a quick general rule (albeit an oversimplification) is that Lyme, Babesiosis, and Anaplasmosis cover similar geographic areas including the Atlantic states and upper Midwest. Likewise, Ehrlichiosis and RMSF cover similar geographic areas, focused on the southeastern US and southern Midwest. Outside of Babesiosis, all others should respond to doxycycline. See Table 8-7 for more details on tick-borne illnesses. Yeah … we know … *everything* presents with fever, headache, and myalgias. They all sound the same to us too …

Question 8.7.3 **What is the appropriate next step for this patient?**
A) Obtain serologic studies and await results while treating symptomatically
B) Obtain skin biopsy and await results while treating symptomatically

TABLE 8-7 TICK-BORNE ILLNESSES

Disease	Etiologic Agent	Geographic Distribution	Clinical Findings
Babesiosis	*Babesia species*	New England, upper Midwest, California	Fever, sweats, myalgias, arthralgias, red urine, hemolytic anemia (most severe cases occur in splenectomized patients). **Similar to malaria,** in that there are periodic fever spikes. Diagnosis is by Giemsa stain
Human monocytic ehrlichiosis	*Ehrlichia chaffeensis* and *ewingii*	South, Midwest	Fever, headache, myalgias (similar to RMSF but rarely a rash). Diagnosis is by buffy coat examination, clinical presentation, PCR
Human granulocytic anaplasmosis	*Anaplasma phagocytophilum*	Atlantic states, upper Midwest	Fever, headache, myalgias. Similar to Ehrlichia but often milder presentation. Diagnosis is by buffy coat examination, clinical presentation, PCR
Lyme disease	*Borrelia burgdorferi*	Northeast, upper Midwest	Erythema migrans, myalgias, arthralgias, arthritis, fever, headache. Diagnosis is by serology
Rocky Mountain Spotted Fever (RMSF)	*Rickettsia rickettsii*	Southeast, Atlantic coast states	Fever, headache, GI symptoms, maculopapular rash that may involve wrists, ankles, palms, and soles of feet→petechiae, myalgias. Diagnosis: clinical, serology (but not + early)
Tularemia	*Francisella tularensis*	South, Midwest	Fever, headache, cough, myalgias, GI symptoms, tender lymphadenopathy with rare skin ulceration. Diagnoses by agglutination or ELISA. Exposure history (rabbits, ticks, flies)

C) Obtain serologic studies and start doxycycline 100 mg orally BID

D) Obtain skin biopsy and start levofloxacin 500 mg orally daily

E) Hospitalize and start ceftriaxone 1 g IV daily until fever has resolved

Answer 8.7.3 The answer is "C." Early treatment for RMSF is essential. Individuals treated after 5 days of symptoms have worse outcomes than those treated earlier. Awaiting serologic studies is inappropriate and treatment should not be delayed. The drug of choice in the treatment of RMSF is doxycycline 100 mg PO BID for 14 days. **This is true for children as well!** Despite prior concerns, doxycycline does not stain the teeth of children (per FDA). Pregnant women should be treated with chloramphenicol. Agents such as penicillin, fluoroquinolones, and cephalosporins are inappropriate in this situation.

The following year the patient returns from another fishing trip, this time in Northern Wisconsin. Three weeks after returning, he notices an erythematous rash behind his knee with central clearing. He then develops low-grade fevers and eventually becomes short of breath and fatigued. An EKG is notable for third-degree heart block.

Question 8.7.4 In addition to ordering further testing, what should be your next step in management?

A) Start IV ceftriaxone

B) Start oral doxycycline

C) Emergent permanent pacemaker placement

D) Start an anti-arrhythmic

Answer 8.7.4 The answer is "A." This patient likely has Lyme carditis with AV block. His prior rash was likely erythema migrans. In this setting, IV therapy is indicated, at least until the heart block resolves. Therefore, "B" is incorrect. While hospitalized patients with Lyme-related heart block occasionally require a *temporary pacemaker*, the heart block resolves with effective therapy and it would be premature to place a permanent pacemaker ("C") at this time.

Your patient is started on ceftriaxone and improves significantly. His Lyme disease titers (you need BOTH a positive ELISA and Western Blot) come back as positive. His fever resolves and his heart block disappears. He completes a full course of therapy targeting his Lyme disease. However, his fatigue persists. He comes back to see you 7 months after completing his therapy and is asking about additional antibiotics.

Question 8.7.5 What should you do at this visit?

A) Send additional studies to look for co-infection with other tick-borne diseases

B) Re-prescribe a course of doxycycline

C) Consider noninfectious causes of his symptoms

D) A and C

E) All of the above

Answer 8.7.5 The correct answer is "D." Occasionally someone with a prior diagnosis (or presumed diagnosis) of Lyme disease will develop chronic symptoms which is referred to as post-Lyme disease syndrome. This syndrome is **not** related to active infection and patients **do not** respond to re-treatment with doxycycline ("B"). However, other explanations for his symptoms are possible and should be investigated. Babesia is carried in the same species of tick as Lyme disease and co-infection can occur. Unlike the other tick-borne infections, Babesia does not respond to doxycycline (or ceftriaxone in this case), and therefore infection can persist despite treatment for Lyme disease. While much is not currently known about post-Lyme disease syndrome, the IDSA guidelines state, "There is no convincing biologic evidence for the existence of symptomatic chronic *B. burgdorferi* infection among patients after receipt of recommended treatment regimens for Lyme disease [and] antibiotic therapy has NOT proven to be useful and is NOT recommended for patients with chronic (> 6 months) subjective symptoms after administration of recommended treatment regimens for Lyme disease."

HELPFUL TIPS:
The CDC has approved doing TWO ELISAs (AKA EIA) either at the same time or sequentially to diagnose Lyme Disease. Use an FDA approved test. See: https://www.cdc.gov/mmwr/volumes/68/wr/mm6832a4.htmn.

HELPFUL TIPS ABOUT LYME:
- Prophylaxis after a bite requires ALL of the following be true:
  - Attached tick identified as an adult or nymphal *I. scapularis* tick (deer tick now known as the "black legged tick").
  - Tick is estimated to have been attached for ≥36 hours (by degree of engorgement or time of exposure).
  - Prophylaxis is begun within 72 hours of tick removal.
  - Local rate of infection of ticks with *B. burgdorferi* is ≥20 percent—basically, only New England, parts of the mid-Atlantic States, and parts of Minnesota and Wisconsin.
  - Use a single, 200 mg dose of doxycycline for those 8 years of age and older.
- Only 20–40% of patients will have positive serology for Lyme at the time of the rash (erythema migrans); so, labs cannot be used to rule out infection in these patients.
- Lyme symptoms can include: Rash, neuropathy (Bell's palsy, others), arthritis, heart block. But there is *no* chronic Lyme disease, only untreated disease, which progresses to include the above manifestations. There is "Post-Lyme Syndrome" which is subjective aches, fatigue, etc. There is no evidence that this is related to persistent infection.

▶ Objectives: Did you learn to ...
- Identify and diagnose RMSF?
- Initiate treatment of RMSF?
- Identify complications of Lyme disease?
- Recognize other tick-borne illnesses?

 QUICK QUIZ: FLUCTUANCE IN FLINT

A 27-year-old male carpenter presents with pain, redness, and swelling of the distal aspect of the right index finger. He reports getting a splinter in the site 2 days ago while working. The pain is now so severe that he cannot work. On examination, the patient is afebrile, the right index fingertip is extremely tender, and there is an area of fluctuance at the palmar aspect of the finger. All of the redness and warmth are distal to the proximal interphalangeal joint.

What is the most appropriate diagnosis?
A) Paronychia
B) Felon
C) Whitlow lesion
D) Tenosynovitis
E) Achy-breaky-finger

The correct answer is "B." A felon is an abscess of the distal fingertip (not the person convicted of grand theft auto), and it most commonly occurs in the index finger and thumb. It can be distinguished from paronychia ("A") because a felon is located in the fat pad of the finger and not the tissue around the nail. Often, an area of fluctuance is palpable. A felon can spread quickly and can involve the tendon sheath, periosteum, and bone. Appropriate management includes x-ray of the finger (to rule out osteomyelitis), antibiotics, and incision and drainage. "C" is incorrect because a whitlow lesion results from inoculation of broken skin of the hand with type 1 or 2 herpes simplex virus. The whitlow lesion is often typical of herpes (vesicles on erythematous papules), but can also be confused with paronychia or felon if at the distal finger. "D" is incorrect as well. Tenosynovitis should involve the tendon sheath. "E" is just silly but could be another big country hit!

▶ CASE 8.8

The Smith family presents to your office in December seeking travel vaccines for a trip to Nigeria. John (34) and Jane (35) Smith have two children, Jack (7) and Jill (5). They will be in Nigeria for a month and will be living in a suburb of Lagos, Nigeria's largest city (Boko Haram not withstanding). They expect to take sightseeing trips into less developed areas. John has no previous medical problems. Jane is currently taking venlafaxine (Effexor) for depression and is known to have a sulfa allergy. Jack has had occasional bouts of reactive airway disease and also has a sulfa allergy. Jill is healthy. Everyone in the family is up-to-date on all routine North American vaccines.

Question 8.8.1 Regarding pathogens they might encounter in Africa, which of the following is caused by a virus?
A) *Plasmodium ovale*
B) *Plasmodium falciparum*
C) Dengue fever
D) *Entamoeba histolytica*
E) All of the above

Answer 8.8.1 **The correct answer is "C."** Dengue fever (aka "break bone" fever) is a viral infection caused by *Flavivirus* (more later). "A" and "B," *P. falciparum* and *P. ovale*, are two species of malaria parasites. *P. falciparum* tends to produce more severe infections that can be rapidly fatal in malaria naïve patients. "D," *E. histolytica*, is the intestinal protozoan parasite responsible for amebiasis.

Question 8.8.2 Mr. Smith asks for advice on the use of insect repellent. What do you recommend?

A) Any repellent will do, they're all the same. Just use the cheapest
B) Pleasant-smelling repellents, such as Avon Skin So-Soft™, are just as effective as any DEET-containing formulation
C) Use repellent with DEET concentrations of at least 50% for the children, since their protection is so vital
D) Apply permethrin insecticide to the skin to enhance any other repellent's efficacy
E) Use DEET or picaridin-containing repellents, as they are the most efficacious insect repellents available, but avoid DEET concentrations greater than 30% in children

Answer 8.8.2 The correct answer is "E." Repeated experiments clearly show DEET- and picaridin-containing repellents to be the most effective for deterring bites and these are the two recommended by the CDC. Picaridin-containing insect repellents do not cause neurotoxicity. The American Academy of Pediatrics recommends not exceeding 30% DEET concentration in repellants for children, due to a slight risk of toxicity seen in frequent applications over a long period of time. Applying DEET to clothing rather than skin reduces the risk of toxicity. Adults can theoretically use any concentration, but 30% is usually sufficient for most situations and you do not get more "bang for your buck" with concentrations above 50%. Often, more cosmetically pleasing products ("B") are less effective and last a mere fraction of the duration of DEET compounds. Permethrin insecticide, *when applied to clothes, tents, and bed nets,* is synergistic with insect repellent, but permethrin itself is not formulated for use as an insect repellent on skin. Even if permethrin does not kill a tick or mosquito, it makes them incapable of biting. Of note, many countries have a combination DEET–Permethrin product available for use on clothes.

....

Mrs. Smith reports that her friends get sick with diarrhea every time they travel abroad. She would like to avoid this.

Question 8.8.3 Which of the following is (are) true about traveler's diarrhea?

A) Enterotoxigenic *E. coli* (ETEC) is the most common cause of this condition
B) Even carefully avoiding the consumption of tap water or unwashed vegetables may not be sufficient to prevent the disease
C) Fluoroquinolones can help to rapidly cure this condition but are contraindicated in pregnancy and young children
D) The use of loperamide is effective in reducing the duration of symptoms but is contraindicated in children <2 years of age
E) All of the above are true

Answer 8.8.3 The correct answer is "E." In most parts of the world, including Africa, ETEC is the most common cause of travelers' diarrhea followed by other pathogens such as *Campylobacter*, *Salmonella*, and *Shigella*. Although it is advisable to avoid tap water, unwashed foods, and raw foods, these measures are usually insufficient to completely eliminate the risk of contracting the disease. A traveler may drink only bottled liquids but might not realize that the ice in the glass is made from tap water. Although the disease is self-limited, a single dose of ciprofloxacin 750 mg **(see following note)** may shorten the course of symptoms: use ciprofloxacin 500mg BID for 2-3 days for more severe disease. A patient's symptoms can be further shortened by adding loperamide, which is safe in the absence of bloody stools and fever. Loperamide is potentially toxic to infants and toddlers.

HELPFUL (AND VERY IMPORTANT) TIP:
The CDC no longer recommends fluoroquinolones for travelers' diarrhea acquired in Southeast Asia because of resistance, seen in *Campylobacter* and increasingly in *Shigella* and *Salmonella*. The current recommendation is to use azithromycin for travelers' diarrhea in Southeast Asia.

HELPFUL TIP:
The FDA has continued to issue new warnings regarding potentially serious side effects of fluoroquinolones to include: increased risk of tendinopathies, development of *C. difficile* infection, CNS side effects, mental health side effects, and aortic dissection that may cause more risk than benefits with their use. However, the very short duration of fluoroquinolone use for traveler's diarrhea is not felt to pose significant risk. Moral of the story: use fluoroquinolones sparingly and stay tuned for emerging recommendations.

HELPFUL TIP:
The CDC maintains a user-friendly and up-to-date travel website at https://wwwnc.cdc.gov/travel. Always check here first to assure you are giving the right vaccines and advice.

....

Finally, you discuss the medication options for malaria prophylaxis.

Question 8.8.4 Which of the following is TRUE?

A) Mefloquine (Lariam) is relatively contraindicated for Jane due to her history of psychiatric illness
B) Doxycycline would be a safe and effective option for the whole family
C) Although malaria is resistant to chloroquine in many parts of the world, it can still be used for prophylaxis in West Africa

D) Atovaquone/proguanil (Malarone) is contraindicated for Jane and Jack due to their sulfa allergy

E) A month is too long a time to use malaria prophylaxis safely; recommend against it

Answer 8.8.4 The correct answer is "A." Mefloquine is an effective, once-a-week prophylaxis for malaria. However, it carries a significant risk of CNS side effects including vivid or disturbing dreams. There have been case reports of the medication inducing psychosis, so the drug is relatively contraindicated for patients with a history of psychiatric illness (such as Jane Smith ...careful with that axe, Jane). "B," doxycycline, may be a good option for the parents, but is not recommended for children < 8 years. "C" is incorrect. Malaria throughout Africa, India, Southeast Asia, and South America is now assumed to be resistant to chloroquine. Finally, "D" atovaquone/proguanil is relatively contraindicated in patients with G6PD deficiency due to a risk of hemolysis, but it does not contain sulfa. Of particular note is answer "E." Medications used to provide malarial chemoprophylaxis have been shown to be well-tolerated for at least a year or more (http://www.cdc.gov/malaria/about/faqs.html). Therefore, 1 month is not too long to use malaria prophylaxis safely, and it should be recommended to the family for their travel. The main cause of long-term travelers getting malaria is poor compliance with antimalarials.

Weeks pass, and you hear nothing more until you are called to the acute care clinic, where Jack Smith has been brought in by his parents for fever and lethargy. Jack's father had been treated in Lagos, Nigeria, for malaria with an unknown medication, and he subsequently recovered. Jack was apparently well until 10 days after returning home, when he developed rapid onset of a fever and shaking chills. He also complained to his parents of generalized abdominal pain and watery, nonbloody diarrhea. The parents treated him at home for a day with ibuprofen and acetaminophen, but he seemed to worsen. He became lethargic, stopped drinking and eating, and the fever continued.

Jack appears drowsy and listless but is arousable. He does not respond to questions about current symptoms but cooperates with an examination. Findings are temperature 39.1°C, pulse 136 bpm, blood pressure 100/50 mm Hg, and respiratory rate 24. His neck is supple with mild lymphadenopathy. He is tachycardic with a mild flow murmur. His abdomen is nontender with a palpable spleen. No rash or petechiae are noted. The rest of the examination is unremarkable. Malaria is suspected.

Question 8.8.5 What is the best method for confirming this diagnosis?

A) Blood culture

B) Malaria serology

C) Malaria PCR

D) Thin and thick blood smears

E) Stool ova and parasite

Answer 8.8.5 The correct answer is "D." Malaria is usually diagnosed by blood smear. The thick blood smear is the more sensitive screening test, and the thin blood smear is used to identify the species of parasite. There are rapid antigen tests that are often important in resource-limited settings but should be ***used in conjunction*** with the thin and thick smears. While many rapid antigen tests can distinguish *P. falciparum* from other species, they do not allow specific identification of the other species. If one suspects malaria and the rapid test is negative, thick and thin smears are still indicated and remain the gold standard. Malaria will not grow in blood cultures ("A"), and malaria serologies ("B") are used only in research experiments and are not clinically helpful for diagnosis of an individual patient. The PCR-based testing ("C") has excellent sensitivity and specificity but is expensive and not widely available. The malaria parasite cannot be identified in stool ("D").

HELPFUL TIP:
It is important to determine the species of malaria for a few reasons. First, *P. falciparum* is the most aggressive species of malaria and has a higher mortality rate than the other species. These patients often require closer monitoring. Second, there are two species of malaria that have hypnozoite forms that can remain dormant in the liver, *ovale* and *vivax*. In addition to routine therapy for malaria, these species require an additional agent, primaquine, to clear the dormant parasites in the liver. Because of this dormant stage, infection with these species can cause relapses of malaria weeks, months, or even years after travel if left untreated.

You begin IV fluids and arrange hospital admission. The relevant laboratory tests are drawn and sent, including CBC, blood cultures, tests for malaria, chemistry profile, blood type and screen, and urinalysis. LP is performed and the CSF is normal. In the meantime, the laboratory calls with the report that *P. falciparum* has been identified.

Question 8.8.6 What antimicrobial should be chosen as initial therapy?

A) Oral hydroxychloroquine (Plaquenil), since many hospitals do not stock chloroquine

B) Oral mefloquine (Lariam)

C) Oral quinine

D) IV quinidine, since IV quinine is not generally available in the United States

E) IV atovaquone/proguanil (Malarone)

Answer 8.8.6 The correct answer is "D." This is a difficult question. For severe malaria such as this, IV therapy is generally indicated. In the US, quinidine is the best option available but is sometimes used in conjunction with other therapy. For uncomplicated or outpatient treatment of malaria, atovaquone/proguanil is an option along with artemether-lumefantrine (Coartem) which works well but may prolong the QT interval. In patients from chloroquine-sensitive zones (currently Central America and the Middle East), treatment with chloroquine is acceptable. Hydroxychloroquine is an option if chloroquine is not available.

> **HELPFUL TIP:**
> Artesunate, another antimalarial, clears parasitemia faster than quinidine but is not approved by the FDA. It is available from the CDC on protocol. The CDC maintains a 24-hour hotline for malaria advice that will connect you directly to a real, live clinician for assistance in managing patients with malaria.

Despite a frightening hospital course that included generalized seizures, hypoglycemia, hematuria, renal insufficiency, and an exchange transfusion, Jack eventually recovers completely. The Smith family thanks you for your help and hopes you'll accompany them on their next trip to Africa.

▶ Objectives: Did you learn to …
- Identify important elements of a patient's travel plans and unique risks when providing counseling for overseas travel?
- Identify preventative measures for malaria, including chemoprophylaxis and insect bite avoidance?
- Diagnose travelers' diarrhea and describe its prevention and treatment?
- Recognize the signs and symptoms of malaria, describe methods of diagnosis, and initiate therapy?

 QUICK QUIZ: CRITTERS IN CLEVELAND

A family comes to see you because the two children, ages 7 and 4, have developed itchy scalps. The parents seem unaffected. So far, they have not tried any treatments. On examination of both children, you find erythematous papules on the occiput and small white eggs firmly attached to the hair shaft about 1 cm from the scalp. Upon leaving the room, you head straight for the shower and scrub your scalp for 5 minutes.

The most appropriate treatment for the suspected diagnosis is:
A) Application of 1% permethrin cream to all family members for 10 minutes followed by rinsing, combing out all nits with a special louse comb, and decontaminating affected garments and bed linens. Repeat in 7 days
B) Elimination of animal or fomite sources of infestation and use of insect repellents
C) Removal of any adherent organisms and oral doxycycline for 14 days
D) Application of 5% permethrin cream to all family members for 8 to 14 hours, followed by showering
E) Shave everyone's head

The correct answer is "A." These are head lice. Pediculosis infestations of the hair and scalp are usually asymptomatic but can present with itching. The diagnosis is made by demonstration

of the louse or nits, which fluoresce a pale blue under a Wood's light. Treatment with topical agents such as permethrin cream for two applications and wet combing to remove nits is recommended by the CDC. Ivermectin may be effective in cases of resistant organisms. It is reasonable to recommend washing clothing and bedclothes of an infested person, but head lice do not survive off the scalp longer than 48 hours. "B" is appropriate for chiggers (mites) or fleas. "C" is appropriate for ticks (see above for management of Lyme). "D" is a treatment of scabies (note the difference in strength of permethrin). Of note, *there is no benefit to keeping children with head lice out of school.* Avoid sharing hats, etc. But just try to get this one past the school nurse.

▶ **CASE 8.9**

A 19-year-old female college student presents to student health services with "the flu." She has noted a fever of 38.9°C and myalgia. She is treated with symptomatic care and discharged back to her dormitory. Three hours later her roommate finds her lethargic and difficult to arouse, so she calls 911. On examination, her blood pressure is 70/30 mmHg with a pulse of 145 bpm. Her neck is supple, but she is lethargic and complaining of severe muscle aches. She denies headache. There is a fine macular rash over her abdomen.

Question 8.9.1 **You need to obtain a little more history. The *most* important historical factor in this case is:**
A) History of splenectomy
B) Previous history of acetaminophen overdose
C) History of tobacco use
D) History of alcohol abuse

Answer 8.9.1 **The correct answer is "A."** "A" is important since patients with a splenectomy can get sick rather rapidly from pneumococci and other encapsulated bacteria. The rest are much less important. Shock is not a prominent feature of acetaminophen overdose ("B")—if it occurs at all. In addition, acetaminophen overdose is not associated with a rash. "C" and "D" are incorrect. These elements of social history, while important to her overall care, will not aid you in the diagnosis and immediate management. Another very pertinent historical feature would be tampon use, which is important because this patient may have toxic shock syndrome.

The patient is able to give you the additional history that she does not use tampons and has not taken any medication except for occasional acetaminophen and ibuprofen in recommended doses. She has her spleen … in a jar in her dorm room—no, wait, we mean in her left upper quadrant.

Question 8.9.2 **On the basis of this information you decide that:**
A) It is unlikely that this is toxic shock syndrome given that she does not use tampons

B) The combination of acetaminophen and ibuprofen in this patient with the flu has led to hypotension

C) Given that she is immunocompetent and has her spleen intact, this cannot be sepsis since it started so quickly

D) Toxic shock, which was a big problem in the 1980s and early 1990s, no longer occurs since the advent of less absorbent tampons

E) None of the above

Answer 8.9.2 The correct answer is "E." "A" is incorrect because up to 50% of cases of toxic shock occur as the result of staphylococcal infections unrelated to tampons. These may be ingrown toenails, infected abrasions, etc. "B" is incorrect. Acetaminophen and ibuprofen are frequently combined without difficulty (but likely no benefit either). "C" is also incorrect. Splenectomized patients are more prone to sepsis from encapsulated organisms, but the fact that the patient has a spleen does not grant invincibility. Sepsis obviously occurs in the normal host as well. Finally, "D" is incorrect. While absorbent tampons are a major culprit in toxic shock syndrome, as noted earlier, there are other causes. Thus, toxic shock syndrome is not going away anytime soon.

Question 8.9.3 The organism(s) responsible for toxic shock syndrome is (are):

A) *Staphylococcus*

B) *H. influenzae*

C) *Streptococcus*

D) A and B

E) A and C

Answer 8.9.3 The correct answer is "E." There are two major types of toxic shock syndrome, one caused by *Staphylococcus* and the other by *Streptococcus*. There are certain subtypes of these bacteria that make the toxin responsible for toxic shock syndrome and only certain hosts are thought to be susceptible. Of note, most patients with streptococcal toxic shock are bacteremic, whereas those with staphylococcal toxic shock are not.

Question 8.9.4 Which of the following lab abnormalities is NOT part of the criteria for suspected toxic shock syndrome?

A) Creatinine of 2 mg/dL (normal 1 mg/dL)

B) Elevated ALT/AST

C) Platelets of 900,000/mm^3

D) Elevated CPK

Answer 8.9.4 The correct answer is "C." By the definition of toxic shock syndrome, the platelet count should be <100,000/mm^3 in staphylococcal-related toxic shock. All of the other findings are representative of the multisystem dysfunction that categorizes toxic shock syndrome. Since Staphylococcal Toxic Shock Syndrome is a clinical diagnosis, the clinical criteria are as follows: fever (temperature > 38.9°C), rash, desquamation, hypotension, and three or more of the following: vomiting or diarrhea, severe myalgia or CPK > 2x upper limit of normal (ULN), mucous membrane involvement, Cr > 2x ULN or pyuria in the absence of UTI, LFTs > 2x ULN, platelets < 100,000/mm^3, or altered mental status (AMS).

Your patient is a little more alert, most likely NOT due to your charming wit. A second set of vitals shows: blood pressure 72/44 mm Hg, pulse 140 bpm, respirations 24, temperature 39°C. Labs are pending.

Question 8.9.5 What is the single best next step in the care of this patient?

A) Start IV nafcillin

B) Place two large-bore IV lines and start aggressive fluid replacement

C) Start IV norepinephrine

D) Give a single dose of IV dexamethasone

E) Transfuse two units of packed red cells

Answer 8.9.5 The correct answer is "B." Treatment is mainly supportive. She's in shock. Two large-bore IV lines should be placed with fluids running wide open, and norepinephrine (or other pressor) should be available if her blood pressure does not improve rapidly. "A" is of special note. Patients with classic toxic shock syndrome (staphylococcal) are not bacteremic. They are suffering from the effects of a localized infection that has produced a toxin that is the causative agent in their illness. Therefore, while an anti-staphylococcal drug is important (as is locally treating the site of infection with incision and drainage, toenail removal, etc.), the anti-staphylococcal drug is not to treat bacteremia. However, the patient should receive empiric antibiotics (IV clindamycin and vancomycin) to treat a suspected localized infection, with narrowing of the spectrum when more data (e.g., cultures and susceptibilities) become available. Since we have not ruled out sepsis you might consider broader spectrum antibiotics including piperacillin/tazobactam (Zosyn). "A", nafcillin alone, would be inappropriate, however. Of note, the clindamycin in this setting is used more to *limit toxin production* than as an anti-staphylococcal agent. "D" and "E" are incorrect since neither steroids nor blood products are currently indicated.

HELPFUL TIP:
Norepinephrine is the initial pressor of choice in most shock situations. It has superior survival when compared to dopamine in sepsis and is clearly better in cardiogenic shock.

▶ **Objectives: Did you learn to …**
- Identify signs and symptoms of toxic shock syndrome?
- Describe the pathophysiology of toxic shock syndrome?
- Initiate management for a patient with sepsis and toxic shock syndrome?

 QUICK QUIZ: BOILS IN BOSTON

A 15-year-old male presents with his mother who had to drag him in to your clinic. He won't look up from his iPhone as his mother gives an exasperated history. He's had "boils" several times on his buttocks and legs that he prefers to "pop" rather than to have treated by a medical professional. ("Darn," you think, "I'd really like to pop those.") Today he has a large red lump on his anterior left thigh. On examination, you find a healthy-looking male with normal vital signs and a 3 cm area of erythema with central pustule and fluctuance. You incise the lesion, obtain a sample for culture and drain it completely (just in time for lunch).

If the culture returns with MRSA as you suspect it will, you must treat with:
A) Good local wound care
B) Packing the wound daily
C) Chlorhexidine baths and mupirocin to nares daily
D) Cephalexin orally for 2 weeks
E) Oritavancin (Orbactiv°) 1,200 mg IV, single dose

The correct answer, and the only thing you must do for this patient, is "A." You have already treated the local infection, the abscess on his skin, with incision and drainage. Packing a small abscess after incision and drainage ("B") is a time-honored method of inflicting mild torture on patients. This practice is grounded in tradition and perceived benefits of packing large, deep soft tissue wounds. However, wound packing has not been shown to benefit small skin abscesses (e.g., less than 5 cm), but it has been shown to increase pain, prolong healing, and result in greater health care utilization. "C" sounds good for a patient who has a history of skin abscesses and is probably worth a try in patients with recurrent MRSA skin infections; but the benefits are minimal at best. Even after clearing MRSA, the little bugger has a tendency to recur; re-colonization rates are as high as 75% several months after decolonization. "Bleach baths" have also been tried, and these seem to be marginally effective if they are effective at all (*Clin Infect Dis.* 2014;58:679).

As to "D", cephalexin does not cover MRSA, and this patient is not systemically ill so IV antibiotics are not necessary. Antibiotics do seem to improve cure rates after drainage of an abscess of 2 cm or greater (NNT 14, NNH 23) (*Ann Emerg Med.* 2018 Mar 9). For abscesses >2 cm, antibiotics are not unreasonable especially if there is surrounding cellulitis. Other factors may push your hand including indwelling medical devices/lines, prior history of endocarditis, immunosuppression, multiple lesions, etc.

If treating a MRSA cellulitis, many options are available. Antibiotic therapy should be dictated by culture and susceptibility when available. Empiric oral antimicrobials that are generally regarded as effective against MRSA include trimethoprim–sulfamethoxazole, tetracyclines (e.g., doxycycline), and linezolid. Clindamycin can be effective as well, but resistance rates are much higher than for the other agents and this should not be used unless susceptibility data is known and resistance is less than 10–15%. For more serious MRSA infections and those failing to respond to empiric oral antibiotics, vancomycin is still first-line IV therapy. Other options include daptomycin and cefraroline. For isolated skin infections, the newer lipoglycopeptides (e.g. oritavancin and dalbavancin) are long-acting antimicrobials that have the advantage of infrequent administration-- in fact, oritavancin

is given as a single dose. The lipoglyopeptides are expensive and have no medical advantage over less expensive options. Remember that they they are only approved for skin infections, not systemic infections.

▶ CASE 8.10

One of your patients has recently been in Indonesia for a prolonged period of time. Upon return to the United States, he develops a febrile illness 5 days after landing in Iowa (yes, we have airports). When he presents to the ED, he recalls being bitten by a particularly large and persistent mosquito just before boarding the airplane. On arrival to the ED, he complains of severe, diffuse body pain, headache, and eye pain and eye redness. Vitals show a temperature of 38.5°C, pulse 145 bpm. After taking his blood pressure, you note a few petechiae under the location of the blood pressure cuff (the so-called "tourniquet test"). Labs show a low white count and thrombocytopenia. He does NOT report cyclic fevers. His eosinophil count is normal. A Giemsa stain of the blood shows no organisms.

Question 8.10.1 The most likely cause of this illness is:
A) Pneumococcal sepsis
B) Dengue fever
C) Malaria
D) Filariasis
E) Kuru

Answer 8.10.1 **The correct answer is "B."** This patient likely has Dengue fever. Dengue fever is most common in Asia but also occurs in Africa, South and Central America, and the Caribbean (and may eventually occur in the southern United States if global temperatures continue to rise). Patients typically present with fever, conjunctivitis, headache, retro-orbital pain, leukopenia, and thrombocytopenia. The *sine-qua-non* of Dengue fever is severe myalgia and arthralgia, hence the moniker "break bone fever." More mild forms do occur, however. "A" is incorrect since patients with pneumococcal sepsis will *generally* not have thrombocytopenia and a low WBC count (yes, we know there are exceptions). "C" is incorrect because the patient does not have cyclic fevers and a blood smear is negative (plus, we've already had our malaria case—why would we repeat it?). Filariasis, "D," presents with eosinophilia and microfilaria in the bloodstream. Again, this should be evident on the blood smear. "E," kuru, is a prion-driven degenerative neurological disease found in Papua, New Guinea associated with eating brains and ritual cannibalism (another reason not to eat your family). This patient does not have any evidence of neurological disease, aside from a headache, which also makes this option less likely.

....

With supportive care, the patient recovers. However, not having learned his lesson he returns to Indonesia. When he comes home to Iowa again, he presents again to the ED, suspecting that he has another episode of Dengue fever.

Question 8.10.2 Signs and symptoms of a second occurrence of Dengue fever include all of the following EXCEPT:
A) Capillary leak with hypovolemia and hemoconcentration
B) Hemorrhagic complications including capillary fragility
C) Onset of symptoms >14 days after exposure
D) Severe thrombocytopenia

Answer 8.10.2 The correct answer is "C." If a returning traveler presents more than 14 days after returning home, Dengue fever can be effectively ruled out. In this case, think of other infectious diseases including malaria. The incubation period of Dengue fever is 3 to 7 days. The rest are correct. Patients with their *second or subsequent* episode of Dengue fever can present with capillary leak syndrome, marked thrombocytopenia, and severe hemorrhage. It is usually the second or subsequent infection that leads to mortality.

HELPFUL TIP:
The treatment of Dengue fever is supportive care. In many countries, treatment is begun with albumin to replace the circulating volume (given the capillary leak syndrome). However, saline is just as good and a lot less expensive.

▶ **Objectives: Did you learn to …**
- Describe the presentation of Dengue fever?
- Distinguish between the first and subsequent episodes of Dengue fever?

▶ CASE 8.11

Ahh… Spring Break…beaches in Mexico, palm trees, and margaritas (drug cartels be damned!). However, on return, a 20-year-old female patient presents to your clinic with a low-grade fever (37.8°C [100.4°F]), a pruritic rash on the body, face, hands, and feet, small joint arthralgia, and conjunctivitis (but no eye drainage). Her mother is on the phone demanding she be checked for STIs (spring break, you know).

Question 8.11.1 The most likely diagnosis is:
A) Dengue
B) Chikungunya
C) Typhoid
D) Zika
E) MERS-CoV (Middle East Respiratory Syndrome-Corona Virus)

Answer 8.11.1 The correct answer is "D." This is Zika. Consider Zika in a patient who has two of these and an appropriate travel history: often **pruritic** rash ("micro" papular) involving hands, feet, face, body; low-grade fever (generally <38.5°C); arthralgia, especially in the small joints of the hands and feet; conjunctivitis without evidence of drainage. Patients with two or more of these have a disease *consistent* with Zika. **Only 20–25% of infected individuals are *symptomatic*.** And

that comment about STIs? Zika can be transmitted both by mosquito (*Aedes* species) as well as sexually (male to male, male to female, and female to male). Zika can persist in semen for 6 months. "A," Dengue, is discussed earlier. "B," Chikungunya, which is also mosquito borne, presents similarly to Dengue with abrupt fever and malaise. Only 15% of Chikungunya cases are *asymptomatic*. Fever is often >39°C and patients have arthralgia (bilateral, symmetrical) in often >10 joints and edema (including facial edema). Rash is common as well as about every other nonspecific symptom: myalgia, headache, GI symptoms, adenopathy. Chikungunya is associated with lymphopenia and thrombocytopenia. Patients can have elevated transaminases and organ failure. *Thinking Dengue? Think also Chikungunya.* "C," typhoid, caused by *Salmonella typhi*, is water borne and presents with fever, myalgias, and abdominal pain. Diarrhea is actually variable and often there is constipation. There is often pulse-temperature disassociation (low pulse, high temperature). It can go on to GI bleeding, bowel perforation, shock, and death. Diagnosis is by culture of *Salmonella typhi* (now called *Salmonella enterica* [thus the moniker "enteric fever"]) from blood or bone marrow (marrow has the best sensitivity at 90%). But bone marrow culture is not fun. We can say this from personal experience. Treatment for typhoid is with antibiotics (start with ceftriaxone while sensitivities are being obtained). The Widal test that you learned about in medical school is fairly useless with a high false-positive rate. Finally, "E," MERS-CoV, is a coronavirus that presents with URI symptoms and may proceed to an influenza-like illness progressing to respiratory distress and renal failure. Avoid snogging with camels and other people with the illness.

Question 8.11.2 Your patient has an illness consistent with Zika. Which of the following *is not* associated with the Zika virus?
A) Guillain–Barre like illness
B) Microcephaly in newborns
C) Acute tubular necrosis
D) Increased risk of miscarriage

Answer 8.11.2 The correct answer (and what you don't generally see with Zika) is "C," acute tubular necrosis. All of the others are associated with the Zika virus.

Question 8.11.3 Which of the following is FALSE about diagnosing this patient with an illness consistent with Zika?
A) You need do nothing else. She meets the case definition so that is enough
B) You can perform PCR on the blood or urine collected within 14 days of symptom onset
C) You can perform serum IgM but not IgG within first 14 days of symptom onset
D) You can perform a PRNT (plaque reduction neutralization test)
E) All of the above

Answer 8.11.3 The correct answer, and false statement, is "A." You SHOULD do some further evaluation. Let's look at them each. Generally, you want to do some testing to confirm, especially if the patient is considering pregnancy—the results could have a huge impact on her life in the near-term. A PCR of blood and urine may be positive for the virus and clinches the diagnosis. However, a negative test does not rule out disease since the virus may be cleared. The next step might be an IgM which is often detectable within 3 days of the onset of symptoms. IgG is not generally recommended. If the IgM is anything but clearly positive (intermediate, etc.), do PRNT (plaque reduction neutralization test). This looks for neutralizing antibodies. Fourteen days after the onset of symptoms, typical testing with IgM and IgG is reliable.

Her tests for Zika come back positive. Her boyfriend, who is asymptomatic, was in Cancun with her on spring break. They are getting married in the next month and would like to start a family. Unfortunately, he is needle phobic and refuses to pee in a cup, saying, "I don't think so, doc. What happened in Cancun might stay in Cancun, but the pee doesn't lie."

Question 8.11.4 **What do you recommend?**
A) Avoid conception for the next month
B) Avoid conception for the next 3 months
C) Avoid conception for at least 6 months
D) Test the female partner for Zika before conception using a nucleic acid test of urine and serum as well as IgM testing.
E) C and D

Answer 8.11.4 **The correct answer is "E."** This is for a couple of reasons. First, the virus is transmissible for up to 6 months in the semen. Since most infections are asymptomatic (remember that only 20% or so are symptomatic), we need to know the serostatus of the boyfriend. He is refusing testing. Thus, the best course of action is to wait 6 months before trying to conceive (unless she wants to get a new potential mate who isn't such a whiner about getting tested). "D" is also correct. Viremia may persist in the female partner so checking her viral status before conception is prudent. Thus, testing for the presence of the virus with a nucleic acid test will help assure there is no active virus persisting.

▶ **Objectives: Did you learn to …**
· Describe the presentation of Zika?
· Distinguish between Zika and some other tropical infections?
· Counsel a patient and partner exposed to Zika?

▶ **CASE 8.12**

A 50-year-old male presents to your clinic in summer. He has noticed a relatively abrupt onset of fever, myalgia, back pain, and anorexia. In the past 4 days he has noticed progressive weakness and headache along with fever. He was visiting Minnesota 1 week ago with his 30-year-old son on vacation doing a slow paddle through the Boundary Waters (very pretty). His son was bitten just as much by mosquitoes yet is asymptomatic. You are wondering what the problem might be.

Question 8.12.1 **Highest on your differential is which of the following?**
A) West Nile Virus (WNV)
B) Lead poisoning from drinking water in a polluted stream
C) Poliomyelitis
D) Zika Virus
E) Bacterial meningitis

Answer 8.12.1 **The correct answer is "A."** Summer, when adventure and mosquitos are in the air, is WNV season. You can rule out lead poisoning, "B"; this is an ID chapter after all. Plus, lead poisoning generally presents with a radial neuropathy (wrist drop) and should not have fever and systemic symptoms more commonly associated with infection. "C" is unlikely given his age and the fact he likely had immunizations, and, lest we forget, polio has been eradicated in North America. "D" is wrong; the *Aedes* mosquito does not live that far north—yet. Finally, you would expect him to be sicker with bacterial meningitis ("E").

Question 8.12.2 **Factors associated with an increased expression of systemic symptoms with WNV include which of the following?**
A) Advanced age
B) Hematologic malignancies
C) Genetic factors
D) Female gender
E) All of the above

Answer 8.12.2 **The correct answer is "E."** All of the above increase the risk of systemic symptoms. *Male gender* may increase the risk of encephalitis, however. Large viral load, immunosuppression, and organ transplant round out the list. Only 20–40% of those infected with WNV become symptomatic.

Question 8.12.3 **The symptoms of WNV include all of the following EXCEPT:**
A) A "Dengue-like" syndrome of sudden onset of headache, body aches, fever (+/−), nausea, vomiting
B) Confusion perhaps progressing to loss of consciousness
C) A "polio-like" syndrome with symmetric (or asymmetric) extremity weakness **with** reflexes preserved
D) A "Guillain–Barre like" syndrome **with loss of** reflexes
E) Hematuria

Answer 8.12.3 **The correct answer is "E."** Hematuria is generally NOT seen in WNV. The symptoms of WNV are protean, necessitating a high index of suspicion among clinicians. WNV presentations may include a "Dengue-like" illness, encephalitis with meningeal signs and mental status changes, neurologic symptoms including Guillain–Barre, a poliomyelitis-type syndrome, neuropathies, meningitis, a rash, and rarely cranial nerve involvement, including a "Bell's-like" illness. Of those with encephalitis only 30% recover entirely, with 50% having prolonged fatigue, memory issues, or parkinsonian-like syndrome. If you are thinking, "This could be Dengue, but they haven't left the U.S.," then you need to think of WNV. Treatment is supportive.

HELPFUL TIP(S):

* You may choose not to test for WNV in mild disease (bit of an ache, low-grade fever, etc.). To diagnose WNV: check an IgM which will be 90% positive at 4 to 10 days. This does NOT mean acute infection since the IgM can persist >12 months. If IgM is negative, consider repeating at a later date. IgG doesn't help rule out acute infection; the patient may have had an asymptomatic infection in the past, as IgG persists for years after infection.

* For those with neurological manifestations (encephalitis, weakness, etc.) a firm diagnosis should be made requiring an LP. With WNV encephalitis/meningitis, LP will show a pleocytosis with lymphocytes and, early on, perhaps PMNs will predominate. CSF IgM (MAC-ELISA) should be done. **IgM does not normally cross into the CSF.** Thus, if the CSF is positive for IgM, it is evidence of acute encephalitis (the IgM can cross the blood–brain barrier because of inflammation). If positive, this should be followed up by neutralizing antibodies (acute and convalescent).

HELPFUL TIP:

WNV is tracked by dead crows and sentinel chickens. Crows and blue jays seem susceptible to dying from WNV. Sentinel chickens (a real thing) have their blood drawn regularly to check for WNV antibodies in an attempt to track the distribution of WNV. Think of these sentinel chickens standing guard like brave heroes—it makes a great mental picture.

▶ **Objectives: Did you learn to …**

* Differentiate WNV from similar illnesses?
* Describe symptoms of WNV, including the protean neurological manifestations?
* Recognize the long-term sequelae of WNV infection?
* List patient-specific factors that increase the potential for symptoms development in WNV?

Clinical Pearls

○ Do not delay antibiotics in a suspected case of meningitis. If the lumbar puncture is going to be delayed, administer antibiotics first.

○ Do not rely on Kernig and Brudzinski signs to rule out meningitis. The sensitivity is as low as 9%.

○ Do not treat asymptomatic bacteriuria in most patients; it is not helpful and only leads to resistance. Pregnant females are one of the important exceptions to this rule.

○ Do not treat Lyme disease with prolonged courses of antibiotics. Postinfectious complications are not due to persistent infection.

○ Do not treat viral upper respiratory infections with antibiotics.

○ Do not use pre-procedural prophylactic antibiotics for most valvular heart disease. Exceptions include: prosthetic valves,

previous infectious endocarditis, and some congenital heart diseases.

○ Do not use vancomycin in patients who prove to have methicillin-sensitive *Staphylococcus aureus*; outcomes are worse with vancomycin than with targeted coverage such as nafcillin.

○ Start fluids and antibiotics as soon as possible in cases of presumed sepsis. It may take 3 L or more of crystalloid to stabilize the septic patient.

○ There is no need to exclude patients with head lice from school. Avoid sharing hats and head-to-head contact, however.

○ Treat patients with a positive PPD who have had the BCG vaccine just the same as any other patient with a positive PPD. Age is not a limitation to treating with isoniazid.

BIBLIOGRAPHY

Angus DC, van der Poll T. Severe sepsis and septic shock. *N Engl J Med.* 2013;369:840–851.

Bagdasarian N, et al. Diagnosis and treatment of *Clostridium difficile* in adults: a systematic review. *JAMA.* 2015;13(4):398–408.

Bratton RL, Corey R. Tick-borne disease. *Am Fam Physician.* 2005;71(12):2323–2330.

Centers for Disease Control and Prevention. Section on influenza. Available at: http://www.cdc.gov/flu/professionals/index.htm. Accessed July 13, 2018.

Center for Disease Control and Prevention. Section on latent tuberculosis infection. Available at: https://www.cdc.gov/tb/publications/ltbi/diagnosis.htm#TST. Accessed August 23, 2018.

Centers for Disease Control and Prevention. Section on traveler's health. Available at: https://wwwnc.cdc.gov/travel. Accessed January 21, 2019.

Centers for Disease Control and Prevention. Vaccine recommendations and guidelines of the ACIP. Available at: https://www.cdc.gov/vaccines/hcp/acip-recs/index.html. Accessed January 19, 2019.

Connor BA. The pre-travel consultation: Traveler's diarrhea. In: Centers for Disease Control and Prevention. *CDC Yellow Book 2018: Health Information for International Travel.* New York: Oxford University Press; 2017:chap. 2. Available at: https://wwwnc.cdc.gov/travel/yellowbook/2018/the-pre-travel-consultation/travelers-diarrhea. Accessed January 19, 2019.

Harper SA, Bradley JS, Englund JA, et al. Seasonal influenza in adults and children—diagnosis, treatment, chemoprophylaxis, and institutional outbreak management: clinical practice guidelines of the Infectious Diseases Society of America. *Clin Infect Dis.* 2009;48(8):1003–1032.

Kang DH, Kim YJ, Kim SH, et al. Early surgery versus conventional treatment for infective endocarditis. *N Engl J Med.* 2012;366:2466–2473.

Lawn SD, Zumla AI. Tuberculosis. *Lancet.* 2011;378:57–72.

MacDonald JR. Acute infective endocarditis. *Infect Dis Clin North Am.* 2009;23(3):643–664.

Mcdonald LC, Gerding DN, Johnson S, et al. Clinical practice guidelines for *Clostridium difficile* infection in adults and children: 2017 update by the Infectious Diseases Society of America (IDSA) and Society for Healthcare Epidemiology of America (SHEA). *Clin Infect Dis.* 2018;66(7):e1–e48.

Merckx J, Wali R, Schiller I, et al. Diagnostic accuracy of novel and traditional rapid tests for Influenza infection compared with reverse transcriptase polymerase chain reaction: a systematic review and meta-analysis. *Ann Intern Med.* 2017;167(6):394–409.

Nichol KL, Nordin JD, Nelson DB, et al. Effectiveness of influenza vaccine in community-dwelling elderly. *N Engl J Med.* 2007;357:1373–1381.

Sterling TR, Villarino ME, Borisov AS, et al. Three months of rifapentine and isoniazid for latent tuberculosis infection. *N Engl J Med.* 2011;365(23):2155–2166.

Tal S, Guller V, Gurevich A. Fever of unknown origin in older adults. *Clin Geriatr Med.* 2007;23(3):649–668, viii.

Talan DA, Mower WR, Krishnadasan A, et al. Trimethoprim–sulfamethoxazole versus placebo for uncomplicated skin abscess. *N Engl J Med.* 2016;374:823–832.

Tolan RW Jr. Fever of unknown origin: a diagnostic approach to this vexing problem. *Clin Pediatr.* 2010;49(43):207–213.

Tunkel AR, Hartman BJ, Kaplan SL, et al. Practice guidelines for the management of bacterial meningitis. *Clin infect Dis.* 2004;39(9):1267–1284.

U.S. Food and Drug Administration. FDA drug safety communication: FDA updates warnings for oral and injectable fluoroquinolone antibiotics due to disabling side effects. Updated December 20, 2018. Available at: https://www.fda.gov/Drugs/DrugSafety/ucm511530.htm. Accessed January 21, 2019.

Wendel K, Rompalo A. Scabies and pediculosis pubis: an update of treatment regimens and general review. *Clin Infect Dis.* 2002;35(suppl 2):S146–S151.

Wilson W, Taubert KA, Gewitz M, et al. Prevention of infective endocarditis: guideline from the American Heart Association. *Circulation.* 2007;116(15):1736–1754. Focused update 2017. Available at: https://www.ahajournals.org/doi/10.1161/JAHA.117.007596. Accessed March 31, 2019.

Wormser GP, Dattwyler RJ, Shapiro ED, et al. The clinical assessment, treatment, and prevention of Lyme disease, human granulocytic anaplasmosis, and babesiosis: clinical practice guidelines by the Infectious Diseases Society of America. *Clin Infect Dis.* 2006;43(9):1089–1134.

HIV/AIDS

9

A. Ben Appenheimer

Note: The antiretroviral treatment of HIV/AIDS (HAART) continues to evolve, and guidelines for use are regularly updated (https://aidsinfo.nih.gov/guidelines). This chapter focuses on the primary care aspects of HIV/AIDS including initial evaluation, drug side effects, and infectious disease prophylaxis.

▶ CASE 9.1

A 23-year-old female presents to your clinic complaining of sore throat, fever, and body aches. She reports that the illness began about a week ago and has persisted despite therapy with NSAIDs, acetaminophen, and throat lozenges. She denies cough, abdominal pain, nausea, or vomiting, but reports a persistent headache. Her past medical and surgical history is unremarkable. The patient smokes about one pack of cigarettes a week, drinks occasional alcohol, and denies other drugs, including intravenous (IV) use. She is heterosexual and has had eight male sexual partners in the past year. She takes oral contraceptives, and her partners usually do not use condoms.

On examination, her vital signs are T 38.9°C, P 112 bpm, BP 115/68 mm Hg, R 20 bpm. She has pharyngitis and enlarged tonsils with exudates. There is diffuse cervical lymphadenopathy, but the neck is supple. There are enlarged lymph nodes in her axillae and inguinal areas as well. The spleen is palpable and nontender. The rest of the examination is unremarkable. You obtain a throat culture, CBC with differential, and heterophile antibody (Monospot) test. Given her history of unprotected intercourse with eight new partners within the last year, you also consider testing for HIV.

Question 9.1.1 The most appropriate laboratory test(s) to rule out the acute retroviral syndrome would be:
A) HIV-1/2 antibody by ELISA followed by a confirmatory Western blot
B) HIV-1/2 antibody by rapid detection method
C) CD4 T lymphocyte count
D) Combined HIV-1/2 antibody and antigen test by ELISA

Answer 9.1.1 **The correct answer is "D."** This presentation is consistent with an acute retroviral syndrome, which occurs very early in the infection and is characterized by a mononucleosis-like illness that can last several weeks. Current HIV diagnostic ELISA methods include the option for both antibody and antigen detection. Since the antibody to HIV will not develop for at least 2 to 8 weeks after infection and the retroviral syndrome typically occurs before seroconversion, HIV antibody tests, including rapid detection methods ("B"), may well be negative. During the acute HIV infection, HIV viral loads are very high, and patients are more infectious compared to other times during their HIV infection. Consequently, the HIV antigen assay, which measures HIV p24 protein, is typically positive during this period. Not all laboratories have adopted the combined HIV antibody–antigen ELISA. If this option is not available, the alternative approach would be to measure the HIV **RNA** by PCR. However, the PCR test is more expensive and has a longer turnaround time, thus the antibody–antigen ELISA is preferred as the initial screen. The CD4 count ("C") is not a reliable way of diagnosing HIV infection; it can become depressed with any acute illness or may be normal in early HIV disease.

 HELPFUL TIP:
If your clinical suspicion is high and the antibody–antigen combination ELISA test is *negative*, the next step would be an HIV **RNA** PCR. This can be detected approximately 10 days after infection and is typically positive 5 to 7 days prior to the HIV p24 antigen, but this timing can vary (see Figure 9-1).

The ELISA returns positive for HIV-1 antigen and negative for antibody and confirmatory testing comes back positive. After appropriate counseling about her test results, blood is also sent for CD4 count, HIV RNA viral load testing, and drug-resistance (genotype) testing. Follow-up is arranged for the patient, and she returns in 4 weeks with no complaints or symptoms. A complete history and physical examination are performed. The patient has mild cervical lymphadenopathy

281

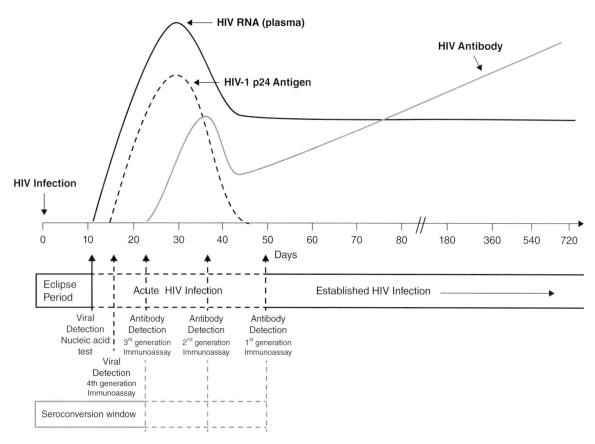

FIGURE 9-1. Sequence of appearance of laboratory markers for HIV-1 infection. Taken from Centers for Disease Control and Prevention and Association of Public Health Laboratories. Laboratory testing for the diagnosis of HIV infection: updated recommendations. Available at: http://stacks.cdc.gov/view/cdc/23447. Published June 27, 2014. Accessed August 22, 2018.

and no other findings. Laboratory studies are ordered and show:

> WBC 3,200 cells/mm^3
> HCT 42%
> Platelets 185,000 cells/mm^3
> Chemistry panel (normal)
> Liver enzymes (normal)
> CD-4 lymphocytes 645 cells/mm^3
> HIV viral load 5,000 copies/mL
> HIV genotype has K103 N mutation

Question 9.1.2 At her next visit, what baseline studies should be ordered?
A) PPD or Quantiferon Gold testing
B) Syphilis IgG
C) Repeat HIV ELISA
D) Hepatitis B and C antibody
E) All of the above

Answer 9.1.2 **The correct answer is "E."** During the initial assessment of an HIV-infected person, all of these studies are important. A positive PPD (>5 mm induration in a person infected with HIV) warrants treatment for latent tuberculosis (TB) if the

patient is found to not have active disease. Since patients with any sexually transmitted infection (STI) are at risk for another STI, screening for syphilis with syphilis IgG (RPR, VDRL) testing is recommended. The same rationale applies for hepatitis B and C, which can be acquired via the same routes as HIV. The patient has documented HIV by virtue of the positive HIV antigen test and positive HIV RNA; however, documentation of seroconversion is important, and a repeat HIV antibody ELISA should be sent at 12 weeks with positives confirmed by HIV-1/HIV-2 antibody differentiation immunoassay. Genotype testing should also be done at this time. The K103 N mutation suggests that the virus will be resistant to efavirenz and nevirapine, two of the most commonly used non-nucleoside reverse transcriptase inhibitors (NNRTIs).

HELPFUL TIP:
Genotype testing for resistance against certain medications should be performed at baseline diagnosis regardless of whether antiretroviral (ARV) therapy will be initiated or deferred. See this Stanford University website at https://hivdb.stanford.edu/ for a mutation-resistance database.

The patient is counseled appropriately about all her results.

Question 9.1.3 What is the most important factor in determining when to start highly active antiretroviral therapy (HAART)?
A) A rising viral load
B) A decrease in CD4 count
C) The development of an opportunistic infection
D) The patient's willingness and ability to maintain strict adherence to an antiviral regimen
E) An undetectable viral load (<50 copies/mL)

Answer 9.1.3 The correct answer is "D." The decision to start HAART must be done on an individual basis. The most important consideration by far, however, is the willingness of the patient to strictly adhere to complicated medical regimens. Poor compliance puts the patient at risk for the development of resistance, hampers treatment of the patient in later stages, and risks the spread of resistant strains to other patients. The current recommendations are to start all HIV-infected individuals on HAART therapy regardless of CD4 count, although the strength of these recommendations varies depending on the CD4 count. Early HAART therapy helps prevent disease progression for HIV-infected individuals and is also an important step in helping prevent transmission of HIV. Evidence does not support using the viral load ("E") as an independent determinant of initiating therapy.

HELPFUL TIP:
HAART regimens have become increasingly complex with the addition of many new drugs, classes, and combination pills. However, the basics can be broken down and simplified. The backbone usually consists of two nucleoside reverse transcriptase inhibitors (NRTIs). There are a few popular combination pills used for this backbone, but the two often used are Truvada (tenofovir/emtricitabine) and Epzicom (abacavir/lamivudine). These are popular because they are both once daily and are combined with an additional medication for relatively simple regimens. To complete a regimen, an additional medication is added from a different class, usually either an NNRTI (e.g., efavirenz), protease inhibitor (e.g., darunavir/ritonavir), or integrase inhibitor (e.g., dolutegravir, raltegravir, bictegravir, or elvitegravir). Current guidelines favor using integrase inhibitors over the other classes. The three current one-pill once-daily recommended regimens combine an NRTI backbone with an integrase inhibitor. These are Triumeq (abacavir/lamivudine + dolutegravir), Stribild (tenofovir/emtricitabine + elvitegravir/cobicistat), and Biktarvy (tenofovir/emtricitabine + bictegravir). Common adverse effects of common antiretroviral drugs are listed in Table 9-1.

HELPFUL TIP:
Current guidelines recommend treatment immediately for pregnant women at any stage of HIV infection to prevent transmission to the fetus, including during the acute retroviral syndrome. HIV medications suitable for use during pregnancy must be used. Although HIV itself is not associated with birth defects, it can be transmitted to the fetus during pregnancy, delivery, and breastfeeding. Use of antiretroviral drugs lowers the risk of transmission to the fetus from as high as 70% to 1–2%.

Question 9.1.4 Aside from considering HAART and stressing the importance of partner notification, what other intervention should be offered at this stage?
A) 13-valent conjugated pneumococcal (Prevnar) and hepatitis B vaccines (Engerix-B)
B) Trimethoprim/sulfamethoxazole (TMP/SMX) DS one tablet per day for the prevention of *P. jiroveci* pneumonia (PCP)
C) Azithromycin 1,200 mg per week for the prevention of *Mycobacterium avium* complex (MAC)
D) Fluconazole 100 mg per day for the prevention of cryptococcal meningitis

Answer 9.1.4 The correct answer is "A." Adequate immunizations at a clinical stage when the patient is likely to benefit from the vaccines (i.e., CD4 > 200 cells/mm³) are important. Live vaccines, such as the MMR, Zostavax, and *intranasal* influenza should be avoided in immunocompromised persons, generally considered those HIV-infected persons with a CD4 count <200 cells/mm³. Pneumococcal vaccines are indicated for HIV-positive patients. While the polysaccharide 23-valent vaccine (Pneumovax) covers more serotypes, the 13-valent conjugate vaccine (Prevnar) elicits a more robust immune response. If previously unvaccinated, the recommendation is to start with the 13-valent conjugate vaccine followed by the 23-valent polysaccharide pneumococcal vaccine after at least 8 weeks. After 5 years, boost with the 23-valent pneumococcal vaccine. The CDC makes no specific recommendation regarding the live shingles vaccine (Zostavax) in HIV patients with CD4 count > 200 cells/mm³ but does state that it is *contraindicated* in patients with CD4 count < 200 cells/mm³; and CDC states that the use of the recombinant vaccine (Shingrix) is "under review" as of 2019.

TMP/SMX ("B") for PCP prevention is indicated when the CD4 drops below 200 cells/mm³, and azithromycin ("C") is indicated for MAC prophylaxis when the CD4 count drops

TABLE 9-1 COMMON ADVERSE EFFECTS OF ANTIRETROVIRAL AGENTS

Medication	Adverse Effects
Tenofovir (component of Truvada)	Renal failure, decreased bone mineral density
Abacavir (component of Epzicom)	Hypersensitivity reaction
Efavirenz	CNS effects including increased suicidality, depression, vivid dreams
Atazanavir	Asymptomatic hyperbilirubinemia

below 50 cells/mm^3. If the patient is started on HAART immediately, MAC prophylaxis can be deferred. Fluconazole ("D") is used for chronic suppression after the treatment of cryptococcal meningitis or for the treatment of esophageal candidiasis; but it is **NOT currently used as primary prophylaxis**. There is no survival benefit to prophylaxis for cryptococcal meningitis. See Table 9-2 for recommended prophylaxis in patients with HIV.

HELPFUL (BUT CONFUSING) TIP:
PCP is no longer *P. carinii*. It is now *Pneumocystis jiroveci*. We didn't do it, honest. It was some microbiologist-taxonomist who wanted to confuse us all. Just to add to the confusion, *P. jiroveci* pneumonia is still often abbreviated "PCP" as in **P**neumo **C**ystis jiroveci **P**neumonia.

HELPFUL TIP:
Partner notification is **VERY** important. State laws vary considerably regarding partner notification, and state health departments are usually very helpful in facilitating this. Some states have criminal transmission statutes for having sex without telling the partner of one's HIV status. Prosecution may not require actual transmission.

After consultation with an HIV specialist, the patient elects not to start therapy at this time and is scheduled for follow-up with regular checks of her viral load and CD4 count. After 1 year, the patient's lab values have changed: CD-4 lymphocytes

TABLE 9-2 RECOMMENDED PROPHYLAXIS IN HIV PATIENTS

CD4± Count	Organism	Recommended Prophylaxis
<200	*Pneumocystis jiroveci*	TMP/SMX, atovaquone, or dapsone (should make sure patient is not G6PD deficient)
<100	Toxoplasmosis[a]	TMP/SMX, combination of dapsone + pyrimethamine + leucovorin, or atovaquone
<50	*Mycobacterium avium* complex (MAC)[b]	Azithromycin, clarithromycin, or rifabutin

[a]Toxoplasmosis prophylaxis is only indicated if patient has documented positive toxoplasma IgG.
[b]MAC prophylaxis is not needed if patient is already on ART or starting ART at that visit.
Adapted from Panel on Opportunistic Infections in HIV-Infected Adults and Adolescents. Guidelines for the prevention and treatment of opportunistic infections in HIV-infected adults and adolescents: recommendations from the Centers for Disease Control and Prevention, the National Institutes of Health, and the HIV Medicine Association of the Infectious Diseases Society of America. Available at: http://aidsinfo.nih.gov/contentfiles/lvguidelines/adult_oi.pdf. Accessed August 22, 2018. Table 1.

280 cells/mm^3 and HIV viral load 75,000 copies/mL. In the past year, she has been treated three times for lobar pneumonia and once for oral candidiasis (without esophageal disease).

Question 9.1.5 Does this patient meet the CDC case definition for the acquired immune deficiency syndrome (AIDS)?
A) No, because she has not had an AIDS-defining illness
B) No, because her CD4 count is >200 cells/mm^3
C) No, because she has only been diagnosed with HIV infection for 1 year
D) Yes, because she has had recurrent (two or more episodes) of lobar pneumonia
E) Yes, because her viral load is >10,000 copies/mL

Answer 9.1.5 The correct answer is "D." The CDC HIV classification system requires that a case of HIV infection be reported as AIDS if the CD4 count is less than 200 cells/mm^3 **or** the patient develops an AIDS-defining illness. These AIDS-defining illnesses include esophageal (not oral) candidiasis, cryptococcal infection, disseminated histoplasmosis, invasive cervical cancer, tuberculosis, HIV wasting disease, and recurrent pneumonia (more than one episode per year). Other infections, Kaposi sarcoma, and certain lymphomas may also define AIDS in an HIV-infected person. Duration of infection and viral load are not currently criteria.

The patient is started on one of the current first-line regimens, a combination pill of tenofovir/emtricitabine/elvitegravir/cobicistat (Stribild). She does well with the treatment and tolerates the medications. Her laboratory results over several visits are listed in Table 9-3.

Question 9.1.6 Most HIV regimens include three active drugs. What is the benefit of the fourth medication (cobicistat) in the patient's regimen?
A) Adds a fourth active antiretroviral to increase efficacy of the regimen
B) Counteracts a potential adverse effect of her regimen
C) Inhibits metabolism of some of her regimen, allowing for once-daily dosing
D) Increases the rate of CD4 increase

Answer 9.1.6 The correct answer is "C." Most HAART regimens for HIV consist of three medications active against HIV. In this case, the active agents are tenofovir, emtricitabine, and elvitegravir. For specific regimens a fourth "boosting" agent is added to decrease metabolism of an active drug, allowing for easier dosing schedules. The two boosting agents that are

TABLE 9-3 CASE 1, LABORATORY RESULTS

	January	March	May
CD4 count	204 cells/mm^3	178 cells/mm^3	244 cells/mm^3
Viral load	5,500 copies/mL	<50 copies/mL	<50 copies/mL

used include cobicistat and ritonavir. Since these affect drug metabolism by design, they also have several important drug interactions. If you have someone on a boosted regimen, it is important to check for interactions with any new medications.

HELPFUL TIP:
If the virus is undetectable, HIV is NOT transmissible sexually (*Lancet HIV* 2018 Jul 16); While this is good news, both partners need to have undetectable virus levels (to prevent sharing of different strains), and there are always other STIs to worry about.

The patient comes at her 4-week follow-up and has been taking her tenofovir/emtricitabine/elvitegravir/cobicistat faithfully and not having any notable side effects. Her viral load is checked and is undetectable. However, she is complaining of headaches and nasal congestion thought to be secondary to uncontrolled allergies. She has tried over-the-counter oral antihistamines without effect. Every year she has required inhaled intranasal corticosteroids for several months to control her symptoms.

Question 9.1.7 What inhaled intranasal corticosteroid would be the safest for her to use chronically?
A) Fluticasone
B) Triamcinolone
C) Mometasone
D) Beclomethasone

Answer 9.1.7 The correct answer is "D." One of the major drug interactions with the boosting agents is with intranasal (or inhaled) corticosteroids. Systemic exposure with these is increased significantly when combined with ritonavir or cobicistat to the point where there are well-established reports of Cushing syndrome with use (as little as 7 days) as well as reports of adrenal insufficiency after withdrawal of the intranasal corticosteroid. Concurrent use of these medications leads to >100x increased systemic exposure to the intranasal steroid. Therefore, these are category X drug interactions with these "boosting" agents. The **ONE** inhaled corticosteroid that seems to be exempt from this interaction is beclomethasone (but good luck with that prior authorization!). Other important interactions to always keep in mind in patients on HIV medications include acid suppressants (which can decrease absorption of some common HIV medications), statins (interactions can either increase or decrease statin levels significantly), and polyvalent cations like calcium and iron (which can decrease absorption of some HAART).

The patient misses her next two appointments and returns to clinic 6 months later. She reports missing several doses of her medications and complains of a 10-lb unintended weight loss. She also notes increased frequency of night sweats but no fevers. A physical examination is unremarkable except for a gaunt appearance and temporal muscle wasting.

Her laboratory results show:

CD4 count: 78 cells/mm^3
Viral load: 6,400 copies/mL
WBC: 2,400 cells/mm^3
Hgb: 11.3 g/dL
Platelets: 145,000 cells/mm^3

After that visit, she starts taking her HAART faithfully. Repeat CD4 count and viral load 4 weeks later shows:

CD4 count: 32 cells/mm^3
Viral load: 7,100 copies/mL

Question 9.1.8 At this point, what changes, if any, should be made to the patient's regimen?
A) The patient has failed HAART treatment and her ARV regimen should be adjusted
B) The viral load is not over 50,000 copies/mL, so the current regimen should be continued
C) The patient is doing well and her regimen should be continued
D) None of the above

Answer 9.1.8 The correct answer is "A." The patient has failed HAART based on several criteria, including the reemergence of detectable viral RNA after it had been completely suppressed. Her ARV regimen should be changed once the results of the repeat genotype testing are known.

HELPFUL TIP:
When changing drug regimens for virologic failure, it is important to repeat genotype testing while on their current regimen to determine whether the patient's virus has now developed resistance to their current regimen. This is most helpful if the patient is still taking the medication as it maintains the selective pressure for the resistance mutations.

Based on the genotype results, a new ARV therapy regimen is recommended, along with PCP prophylaxis with TMP/SMX. Because you are starting therapy, MAC prophylaxis with azithromycin can be deferred. Two weeks later, the patient's CD4 count rises to 210 cells/mm^3 and she has more energy. However, she returns to clinic 3 weeks later (5 weeks after starting her new ARV regimen) and is complaining of severe shortness of breath. She says that she had been taking her HIV medications but that she lost her PCP prophylaxis prescription (TMP/SMX) and had forgotten to get a new one. Her current illness began 6 days ago as a fever and mild cough. She developed significant dyspnea with minimal exertion, and now is even short of breath at rest. Her chest hurts bilaterally, worse with inspiration. She has drenching night sweats. She denies hemoptysis, sputum production, nausea, vomiting, or abdominal pain.

Physical examination reveals the following vital signs: T 39°C, BP 90/60 mm Hg, P 135 bpm, RR 38 bpm, and SpO$_2$ 78% on room air. The patient is in severe respiratory distress and in the tripod position. The lung examination shows diffuse rales and tachypnea. You call the ambulance because she looks like she needs help! You place oxygen to help improve her oxygen saturation and her respiratory rate. She does not respond to oxygen and becomes unresponsive.

Question 9.1.9 Aside from respiratory isolation, what should be done immediately?
A) Sputum culture to evaluate for any lung organisms that may be causing her respiratory distress
B) Bronchoalveolar lavage (BAL) for PCP via direct immuno-fluorescence (DFA)
C) Bag mask the patient and have your nurse place an IV in order to prepare for rapid sequence intubation and IV fluids
D) Oxygen, furosemide, and nitroglycerin. She clearly is volume overloaded
E) Chest x-ray (CXR), blood count, CD4 count, and viral load to assess for underlying infection

Answer 9.1.9 The correct answer is "C." The patient presented in severe respiratory distress and now has impending respiratory failure. She is also hypotensive and tachycardic and must be stabilized before any further workup is done. Remember those ABCs (Airway, Breathing, Circulation) from all those certification classes you had to take? "D," oxygen, furosemide, and nitrates are useful treatments of congestive heart failure, but this is unlikely in this young woman. *P. jiroveci* pneumonia (PCP) is the most likely diagnosis that explains her findings; however, community-acquired pneumonia remains on the differential. Further workup including sputum culture, PCP direct immunofluorescence, CXR, and blood count are all indicated but only after the patient is stabilized. Given the timing of the onset of symptoms in the setting of a rapid CD4 response to ARV therapy, this is likely complicated by immune reconstitution inflammatory syndrome (IRIS).

HELPFUL TIP:
Immune reconstitution inflammatory syndrome (IRIS—as opposed to ISIS the terrorist organization) is well named. It is identified by a paradoxical **symptomatic** worsening of a preexisting infectious process as the immune system reconstitutes with ARV therapy. Basically, the body's immune response wreaks havoc at the sites of infection (e.g., CMV retinitis, tuberculosis, cryptococcal meningitis, and obviously, PCP). The infection may be under treatment or subclinical and becomes symptomatically worse when IRIS develops. Common findings are fever, increased fatigue and malaise, unexplained weight loss, worsening respiratory and neurological status. IRIS usually occurs within the first 4 to 8 weeks after initiation of therapy, but it can be delayed several months in some cases.

After appropriate resuscitation and transportation to a higher level of care at the local emergency room, laboratories and a CXR are obtained. The x-ray is shown in Figure 9-2.
Laboratory results are:

WBC 3,400 cells/mm^3
Hgb 11 g/dL
Platelets 180,000 cells/mm^3
Creatinine 2.4 mg/Dl (high)
LDH 1,280 IU/L (high)
PT 12.4 seconds, PTT 27 seconds
Liver enzymes normal
ABG: pH 7.56, PaCO$_2$ 23 mm Hg, PaO$_2$ 68 mm Hg (on 100% FiO$_2$)
Sputum and blood cultures are pending

Question 9.1.10 What should be the *initial* antibiotic therapy?
A) Four drug anti-tuberculosis regimen
B) Doxycycline
C) IV TMP–SMX
D) IV corticosteroids followed by IV TMP–SMX
E) No antibiotics initially—just wait for the culture results

Answer 9.1.10 The correct answer is "D." The patient is acutely ill, and likely has PCP. Steroids decrease the mortality in patients with severe PCP (PaO$_2$ <70 on room air or arterial–alveolar O$_2$ gradient >35 mm Hg). The best antibiotic for PCP is TMP–SMX. IV Pentamidine may be used in cases of sulfa allergy, but it has been associated with hypotension and hypoglycemia. Although the classic CXR appearance for PCP is bilateral interstitial infiltrates, it can present differently (as in this case, showing more centrally located patchy infiltrates). Approximately 10% of people diagnosed with PCP have a normal CXR on presentation. Since the infecting organism is not known with certainty, it would be prudent to secondarily add empiric therapy for bacterial pneumonia with ceftriaxone and azithromycin or

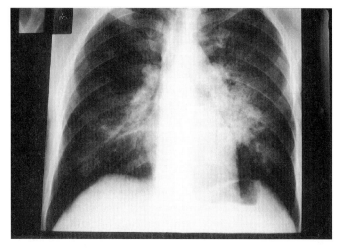

FIGURE 9-2. Chest radiograph.

respiratory fluoroquinolone pending bronchoscopy results. Of note, PCP does not grow in standard cultures, but it can be visualized by silver staining or direct immunofluorescence assays (DFA) on BAL specimens. The yield of the PCP DFA testing is much higher with BAL than sputum. Detection of PCP is not reduced during the first 48 hours after starting therapy, and cysts may be seen for much longer in people responding to therapy, despite effective treatment.

The patient is admitted to the ICU and given antibiotics. Her condition stabilizes until 4 hours into her ICU stay. At that time, her respiratory rate on assisted-control ventilation dramatically increases from 18 to 42. Peak airway pressures according to the ventilator are greater than 60 cm of water, when they were less than 30 cm water previously. Breath sounds are absent on the right side of her chest, and her trachea is deviated to the left. Heart sounds are audible, but tachycardic. Neck veins are distended bilaterally.

Question 9.1.11 **What is the next appropriate step, BEFORE a repeat CXR is taken?**
A) Give Versed 2 mg IV for sedation, the patient must be very anxious
B) Pull the ET tube back 1 to 2 cm, as it is likely in the right main stem bronchus
C) Perform a blind pericardiocentesis, as the patient is developing tamponade
D) Insert a large Angiocath into the left second intercostal space to relieve the tension pneumothorax on the left
E) Insert a large Angiocath into the right second intercostal space to relieve the tension pneumothorax on the right

Answer 9.1.11 **The correct answer is "E."** The patient has developed a dreaded complication of PCP, a pneumothorax. The organism, *Pneumocystis*, has a propensity to cause blebs (cysts) in the lung tissue. Since the patient was receiving positive pressure ventilation, a tension pneumothorax developed that requires immediate needle decompression. This should be done without waiting for a portable CXR. When the pneumothorax is later confirmed, a tube thoracostomy may be performed under controlled conditions.

HELPFUL TIP:
Over the past several years, the placement location of an angiocath for relief of tension pneumothorax has changed. The current preferred placement is in the mid-axillary line, fourth or fifth interspace (similar to where you would place a chest tube).

Following a protracted ICU admission, the patient improves and is re-started on HAART based on her drug resistance testing. She is discharged, and in response to this life-threatening complication, she is highly motivated and becomes very adherent with her medications. Two years

later her CD4 is 385 cells/mm³, her HIV RNA concentration is <20 copies/mL (nondetectable), and she recently started a job that she enjoys.

▶ **Objectives: Did you learn to …**
- Identify the signs and symptoms of the acute retroviral syndrome?
- Use appropriate tests for the diagnosis of HIV infection?
- Evaluate a patient with HIV and monitor that patient's progress?
- Review the preventative health measures and vaccinations important in patients with HIV infection?
- Define acquired immune deficiency syndrome?
- Understand the guidelines for initiating and changing HAART?
- Recognize some of the more common medications used to treat HIV and their side effects?
- Recognize some of the more common opportunistic infections in patients with HIV and how to prevent them?
- Describe IRIS?

▶ CASE 9.2

A 32-year-old female presents to the office seeking prenatal care. Her last menstrual period was 2-and-1/2 months prior to her visit. She believes that she is pregnant and has tested positive with a home pregnancy test. She has been pregnant twice before, with one living child and one spontaneous abortion (G₃P₁). She is married to the father of her children. She has no health problems but does smoke 1/2 pack of cigarettes per day. She also admits to occasional alcohol use (one drink every 2 weeks). She denies illicit drug use, including IV drug use.

Question 9.2.1 **Besides prenatal vitamins with iron and folate, you recommend:**
A) Smoking cessation
B) Confirming the home pregnancy test with a serum HCG in your laboratory
C) HIV testing and counseling
D) A and C
E) All of the above

Answer 9.2.1 **The correct answer is "D."** Smoking during pregnancy is associated with lower birth weight and preeclampsia, and smoking in the house with a young child is associated with respiratory diseases, especially asthma. Although confirming pregnancy by examination (uterine size or fetal heart tones) and/or urine HCG is appropriate, serum HCG is unnecessary and expensive. In addition, when used correctly, home pregnancy tests are highly sensitive and specific. But really, this is the HIV chapter, and we want you to know that HIV screening should be included in the routine panel of prenatal tests for **all women** seeking prenatal care. Routine testing for HIV in expectant females has dramatically reduced the HIV prevalence in children in developed countries. Vertical transmission of HIV is still a tremendous problem in Africa and other developing regions of the world.

HELPFUL TIP:
Special consent is not needed prior to testing for HIV. However, the patient **must** be notified and given the opportunity to opt-out.

HELPFUL TIP:
Partners of pregnant women should be encouraged to undergo HIV testing if their HIV status is unknown.

You explain that HIV testing is routine, but that the patient can "opt out," and the patient agrees to HIV testing. Her pregnancy is confirmed. Her HIV Ab/Ag combination test is positive.

Question 9.2.2 What is the next step in confirming the diagnosis of HIV?
A) HIV viral load
B) HIV-1/HIV-2 multispot test
C) HIV Western blot
D) HIV genotype
E) CD4 count

Answer 9.2.2 **The correct answer is "B."** The recommended testing algorithm has recently changed. Previously an HIV antibody ELISA "screening" test was done initially, followed by a "confirmatory" Western blot. However, the current recommendation (based on CDC guidelines) starts with the HIV antigen/antibody combination immunoassay. This combines the p24 antigen test (which is positive before seroconversion) with an antibody test for IgM and IgG. This will diagnose any HIV infection 2 to 3 weeks after infection (including HIV-2). If the antigen–antibody test is positive, it is followed by an HIV-1/HIV-2 antibody differentiation immunoassay. If positive, HIV diagnosis is confirmed. If negative, an HIV RNA viral load should be sent to determine whether the patient truly has HIV (see Figure 9-3).

Your patient is understandably shaken by the news of this test result. Being an empathetic physician, you say something like, "I can see that you are shaken by the news of this test result." She is most concerned about her unborn child.

Question 9.2.3 What should you tell her?
A) Her child is almost certainly also infected
B) A therapeutic abortion at this point is the only humane thing to do
C) With effective therapy, the risk of transmission to the child can be lowered to less than 2%
D) With effective therapy, the risk of transmission to the child can be lowered to 15%
E) Despite effective therapy, the risk of transmission remains at 25%

Answer 9.2.3 **The correct answer is "C."** Although it is possible for HIV to infect the fetus in utero, the large majority

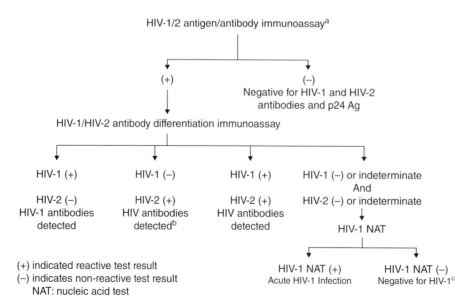

Recommended Laboratory HIV Testing Algorithm for Serum or Plasma Specimens

HIV-1/2 antigen/antibody immunoassay[a]

(+) → HIV-1/HIV-2 antibody differentiation immunoassay

(−) → Negative for HIV-1 and HIV-2 antibodies and p24 Ag

HIV-1 (+)
HIV-2 (−)
HIV-1 antibodies detected

HIV-1 (−)
HIV-2 (+)
HIV antibodies detected[b]

HIV-1 (+)
HIV-2 (+)
HIV antibodies detected

HIV-1 (−) or indeterminate
And
HIV-2 (−) or indeterminate
HIV-1 NAT

HIV-1 NAT (+)
Acute HIV-1 Infection

HIV-1 NAT (−)
Negative for HIV-1[c]

(+) indicated reactive test result
(−) indicates non-reactive test result
NAT: nucleic acid test

FIGURE 9-3. Algorithm for HIV Testing. Taken from Centers for Disease Control and Prevention and Association of Public Health Laboratories. Laboratory testing for the diagnosis of HIV infection: updated recommendations. Available at: http://stacks.cdc.gov/view/cdc/23447. Published June 27, 2014. Accessed August 22, 2018.

of mother-to-child HIV transmission occurs vertically (due to exposure to maternal genital-tract virus during delivery). The most important variable for transmission is the HIV viral load (HIV RNA concentration in plasma) in the mother. ARV drugs reduce perinatal transmission by several mechanisms, including lowering maternal antepartum viral load and providing infant pre- and postexposure prophylaxis. Therefore, combined antepartum, intrapartum, and infant ARV prophylaxis is recommended to prevent perinatal transmission of HIV.

Your patient is somewhat relieved that her baby can be protected and wants to know what can be done to treat her. She feels fine, is now in the second trimester, and would rather not take medications unless she had to.
Some additional laboratory tests are ordered:

CD4 count: 756/mm^3
HIV viral load: 80,000 copies/mL
Hgb: 11.2 g/dL
BUN: 11 mg/dL
Cr: 0.7 mg/dL

Question 9.2.4 **What should you tell her about HAART in pregnancy?**
A) To minimize the risk of transmission to her child, she should start HAART as soon as possible
B) ARV medications are teratogenic and should be avoided at all costs during pregnancy, except just before delivery
C) Since her CD4 count is normal and she feels well with no sign of opportunistic infections, starting HAART is not indicated
D) Her renal function makes HAART relatively contraindicated
E) Her hemoglobin level makes HAART relatively contraindicated

Answer 9.2.4 **The correct answer is "A."** ARV therapy is recommended for all pregnant women regardless of their viral load to prevent transmission to the child. Factors that increase risk of transmission of HIV include high maternal viral load, low maternal CD4 count, advanced clinical stage of her HIV, and lack of maternal use of ARV therapy. Vaginal delivery is also a risk factor—but only if the mother did not receive antepartum ARV therapy. Although the patient's hemoglobin is low, it does not preclude her from taking therapy. Her renal function is normal, so it should not be an issue.

Ideally, the mother should be initiated on ARV as soon as her HIV is diagnosed and have her HIV suppressed (undetectable viral load) on combination antiretroviral therapy (HAART) prior to delivery. If the HIV viral load (HIV RNA concentration in plasma) is nondetectable at 36 weeks, the transmission risk is <2%.

If the mother's viral load is unknown or >1,000 copies/mL, current guidelines recommend also adding continuous infusion of zidovudine (ZDV) to the mother *during labor* as well as scheduled cesarean delivery. Postpartum prophylactic medications for the newborn should be given for 4 to 6 weeks regardless of maternal viral load. Women who present in labor without HIV testing during pregnancy, should be tested by rapid HIV ELISA. If this is positive, continuous infusion ZDV should be started. Current guidelines do not recommend additional intrapartum drugs in this setting, **including nevirapine, which has been shown to cause rapid resistance when used in this setting.**

The patient is started on HAART (Truvada plus raltegravir) and tolerates her regimen well. Repeat laboratory results at a return visit 4 weeks later are as follows:

CD4 count: 692/mm^3
HIV viral load: 5,500 copies/mL
Hgb: 10.9 g/dL

Her HAART seems to be effective. Her viral load has decreased by >10-fold (one $\log_{10}$). You remember from your last patient how sick patients can get with *P. jiroveci* pneumonia.

Question 9.2.5 **What do you recommend to this patient regarding PCP prophylaxis?**
A) She should start prophylaxis with TMP–SMX immediately, because PCP in pregnancy can be particularly severe
B) She should start PCP prophylaxis with inhaled pentamidine, because TMP–SMX is contraindicated in pregnancy
C) PCP prophylaxis is not indicated since her CD4 count is >200/mm^3
D) PCP prophylaxis is not a major concern for pregnant patients

Answer 9.2.5 **The correct answer is "C."** PCP is particularly severe in pregnant patients, but prophylaxis is not generally indicated for CD4 counts >200 cells/mm^3. TMP–SMX is associated with hyperbilirubinemia in newborns but is still indicated for PCP prophylaxis. Oral dapsone is another option, as is inhaled pentamidine.

She continues her HAART, but at 36 weeks, her viral load is still detectable (2,500 copies/mL). You recommend changing the ARV, but at the next appointment (37.5 weeks), the patient tells you that she did not fill the new prescriptions, and admits that she has not been adherent with her medications. At this visit, you renew discussions about adherence, and about delivery plans with the patient.

Question 9.2.6 **Which of the following is/are true regarding the delivery?**
A) A cesarean section (C-section) is likely to reduce the risk of transmission to her infant
B) A C-section is indicated because this patient's viral load remains greater than 1,000 copies/mL despite HAART
C) A C-section should be performed at 38 weeks gestation, prior to the onset of labor
D) Postpartum ARV therapy should be given to the mother and infant
E) All of the above

Answer 9.2.6 **The correct answer is "E."** If a patient achieves effective suppression with ARV therapy (undetectable viral load), the risk of transmission is minimal, and the mode of delivery should depend on the preferences of the mother and the other usual obstetric factors. Vaginal delivery is not contraindicated if the mother's viral load is suppressed. If, as in this patient's case, the viral load is >1,000 copies/mL, current guidelines recommend delivery by C-section at 38 weeks. When performed at 38 weeks, prior to the onset of labor, the relative risk of transmission is reduced by 50%. Intrapartum ZDV, as discussed previously, may also help reduce the risk of transmission. Also, the premature rupture of membranes should be addressed promptly in HIV-infected mothers. Children born to mothers more than 4 hours after rupture are **twice** as likely to acquire HIV. After birth, infants born to any HIV-positive mothers regardless of viral load should receive prophylactic ARV therapy. If the maternal viral load is >1000 copies/mL, the infant should receive combination therapy with two to three drugs, such as zidovudine plus lamivudine plus raltegravir.

....

The patient delivers a healthy, 3-kg male infant via C-section. The postpartum course is uneventful. Blood is taken from the infant at day 1 and at 2 weeks, and both test positive for HIV antibodies.

Question 9.2.7 **What does this mean?**
A) The infant is infected with HIV
B) The infant's infection status is unclear from the information given
C) Maternal HIV antibodies are expected to be circulating in the infant, but it can be assumed that no transmission of infection took place
D) A positive test at day 1 is expected due to maternal antibodies, but a repeat positive at 2 weeks indicates infant antibody production and is evidence of infection

Answer 9.2.7 **The correct answer is "B."** Because the antibodies cross the placenta, children born to HIV-positive mothers will test positive for HIV antibodies for up to 6 moths post-partum. Therefore, it requires 2 negative serologic tests at >= 6 months OR two or more negative virologic tests at >=1 and 4 months to rule out HIV infection.

Question 9.2.8 **How should the HIV status of the infant be determined?**
A) Serial HIV antibody tests: a fourfold drop in titer can be considered negative
B) p24 antigen testing in the first 48 hours of life
C) Viral load by PCR in the first 48 hours of life
D) Viral load by PCR at 14 to 21 days, 1 to 2 months, and 4 to 6 months
E) p24 antigen and PCR viral load on cord blood samples

Answer 9.2.8 **The correct answer is "D."** The best test to assist with diagnosis of HIV infection is viral load by PCR, and a positive test (by DNA PCR or RNA assays) indicates

likely HIV infection. Confirmation of HIV infection is provided by two positive virologic tests obtained from separate blood samples. Overall, the sensitivity of virologic testing increases rapidly by 2 weeks. One can consider obtaining virologic testing within the first 48 hours in newborns who are at high risk for HIV infection, such as infants born to HIV-infected mothers who did not receive prenatal ARV therapy or who had HIV viral loads >1,000 copies/mL close to the time of delivery. If this returns positive, this would be indicative of an intrauterine infection rather than intrapartum infection, which is normally acquired during delivery. "A" is incorrect. HIV antibody testing is useless in infants, and quantified titers are not typically generated. "B" is incorrect because the p24 antigen is less sensitive and specific than the viral load in this setting. "E" is incorrect. Tests done on the cord blood may be contaminated with maternal blood and do not give an accurate assessment of the infant's status.

HELPFUL TIP:
Serial testing of neonates at risk is indicated. Test at age 2 to 3 weeks, 4 to 8 weeks, and 4 to 6 months. If the child is high risk (no prenatal care, known HIV+ mother, known elevated viral load, etc.), consider testing at birth as well.

Question 9.2.9 **What should you advise your patient about breastfeeding her son?**
A) HIV is not transmitted by breast milk
B) HIV is transmitted by breast milk, but the benefits of breastfeeding outweigh the risk of transmission in this setting
C) HIV is transmitted by breast milk, but her son will be protected from serious infection due to maternal antibodies in the breast milk
D) HIV is transmitted by breast milk, and breastfeeding should be avoided if possible

Answer 9.2.9 **The correct answer is "D."** Postpartum transmission of HIV from mother to child occurs in 10% to 14% of breastfeeding mothers. This is not a major problem in developed nations, where there is reliable access to formula. HIV-positive mothers should be discouraged from breastfeeding in the developed world, including the United States. The recommendations may be different in developing areas of the world, where the mother's milk may be the only clean source of nutrition available to the infant. In fact, in many developing nations, the benefit of breastfeeding outweighs the risk of HIV transmission; formula feeding can increase mortality due to inadequate access to good nutrition, lack of clean water source with which to mix the formula, and risk of diarrheal illnesses. The World Health Organization (WHO) suggests that "when replacement feeding is an acceptable, feasible, affordable, sustainable and safe, bottle-feeding is the best option."

Despite the best efforts of your patient and all the physicians and nurses participating in her care, her child tests positive by PCR for HIV at 4 weeks and 4 months. Now, you need to think about how to treat this child with HIV.

Question 9.2.10 Which of the following is true about the use of ARV therapy in children?
A) Treatment should be initiated immediately for all children as soon as HIV infection is diagnosed
B) Since they are just little adults with relatively big heads compared to their torsos, treatment indications for children and adults are the same
C) HAART is highly toxic in children and treatment should be reserved until the child's life is in immediate danger from HIV-related complications
D) Single-drug ARV therapy is recommended in children rather than HAART

Answer 9.2.10 The correct answer is "A." As of May 2018, the Panel on Antiretroviral Therapy and Medical Management of Children Living with HIV now recommends that **all** children receive antiretroviral therapy, regardless of symptoms or CD4 count, as soon as possible after diagnosis. HAART regimens are more difficult to choose and adjust in children because of a limited number of pediatric (non-pill) formulations and a lack of data about long-term efficacy and safety. However, combination therapy can effectively and safely suppress viral load and stimulate immunologic reconstitution. Monotherapy is NOT recommended.

Question 9.2.11 Which of the following statements regarding the natural history of HIV complications in children is true?
A) Hepatobiliary complications, such as AIDS cholangiopathy, are more common in children than adults
B) Kaposi sarcoma is more common in children than adults
C) Focal brain lesions in children are almost always due to toxoplasmosis
D) Many children show cognitive and motor deficits, but frank AIDS dementia is uncommon
E) Lymphocytic interstitial pneumonitis (LIP) is more common in adults than in children

Answer 9.2.11 The correct answer is "D." Twenty-five percent of children with HIV infection demonstrate some cognitive and motor deficits. They face problems with verbal expression, attention deficits, hyperactivity, and hyperreflexia. LIP is characterized by diffuse reticulonodular infiltrates and hilar lymphadenopathy and occurs in up to 40% of children with perinatally acquired HIV. **LIP is very rare in adults**. Kaposi sarcoma is associated with a herpes virus infection and is very rare in children. Toxoplasmosis, usually presenting as focal mass brain lesions, is a reactivation of previous infection, and is therefore also very rare in children. **Hepatobiliary complications are more common in adults** than in children, but the reason for this is unclear.

Question 9.2.12 What should you recommend for this infant regarding PCP prophylaxis?
A) Prophylaxis is unnecessary because children do not get PCP
B) Prophylaxis is unnecessary if the child's CD4 count is >200 cells/mm^3
C) Prophylaxis is unnecessary until the child reaches 1 year of age
D) Prophylaxis with TMP–SMX is contraindicated in infants less than 6 months of age due to the risk of hyperbilirubinemia
E) Prophylaxis with TMP–SMX as the first-line agent should be initiated at 4 weeks of age because the highest risk for PCP in children is at 3 to 6 months of age

Answer 9.2.12 The correct answer is "E." The highest incidence of PCP occurs in the first year of life with peak onset at 3 to 6 months of age. TMP/SMX is still considered first-line therapy for prophylaxis and should be started at 4 to 6 weeks of age. CD4 counts are naturally higher in children and decrease to adult levels by the age of 6 years. PCP prophylaxis is recommended for all HIV-infected infants <12 months regardless of CD4 count or percentage. It should be continued until the infant is determined to be HIV uninfected or presumptively uninfected. If this drug is not tolerated, dapsone or aerosolized pentamidine are acceptable alternatives. Remember that TMP/SMX can cause kernicterus.

The child tolerates the HAART very well and demonstrates a consistently suppressed viral load. He has further follow-up by a pediatric infectious disease specialist. The mother returns to you for further care. She had been taking the previously prescribed HAART, but quit all her medications 3 months ago because she was having trouble remembering doses causing her to miss several doses per week.

Her latest laboratory results show the following:

CD4 count: 254 cells/mm^3
HIV viral load: 50,000 copies/mL
(Previously CD4 count: 692/mm^3; HIV viral load: 5,000 copies/mL)

Question 9.2.13 In addition to encouraging her to contact your office immediately when she stops or changes medication, which of the following is the most appropriate advice to provide her now?
A) She should have continued to take the medications because now the HIV has a "foothold" and it will be much harder to treat
B) It would not have mattered if she took the medications or not. Her disease is progressing as expected
C) With the degree of drop seen in her CD4 count, the virus must be resistant, and further HAART is futile
D) She should have continued the medications, even if she was missing doses. A little of ARV activity is better than nothing

E) She did the right thing by stopping the medications. If a patient is not able to comply fully, it is often better to not take any HAART at all

Answer 9.2.13 The correct answer is "E." Starting HAART is a very difficult and serious decision and should be made after careful and complete counseling. If taken intermittently, her virus could potentially develop resistance to the medications she is taking, making them ineffective. Patients missing doses of HAART frequently are more likely to have their HIV disease progress. Once multidrug resistance develops, it is more difficult to find an effective regimen to slow disease progression.

....

After the drug resistance genotype testing did not identify any mutations associated with drug resistance, she agrees to try a new regimen of Truvada (tenofovir/emtricitabine) and dolutegravir. She does not want to have any more children and is using effective contraception, which is important as the dolutegravir is potentially teratogenic.

At her follow-up visit, laboratory results are repeated and show an improvement in her viral load:

CD4 count: 261 cells/mm^3
HIV viral load: 7,000 copies/mL.

You explain that if her viral load continues to fall and becomes undetectable, she can expect an improvement in her CD4 count over the next 1 to 2 years. You take this office visit as an opportunity to catch up on preventative medicine. On one prior occasion, 6 years ago, she had an abnormal Pap smear result that returned to normal after a repeat examination and colposcopy. Prior to her diagnosis of HIV, she had never been diagnosed with an STI. A pelvic examination today reveals a normal appearing cervix. A sample for Pap smear is collected and sent to pathology.

Question 9.2.14 How often should this patient get screened for cervical cancer with Pap smear?
A) Cervical cancer is inevitable, so you should recommend prophylactic radical resection
B) She must be tested every 6 months, regardless of results of this Pap smear
C) She may be screened with pap test and HPV co-testing. If both are negative, she may be screened at 3-year intervals
D) She may be screened per the usual guidelines for HIV-negative women
E) She has almost no chance of developing cervical cancer and screening may be discontinued

Answer 9.2.14 The correct answer is "C." Women with HIV are at significant risk of cervical cancer with adolescent women at particularly higher risk due to the higher likelihood of contracting the human papilloma virus (HPV), implicated as the leading cause of cervical cancer. The increased risk of cervical cancer is regardless of how the HIV virus was acquired (e.g., vertical transmission at birth or horizontal contraction through sexual activity). Prior pap smear screening recommendations for women with HIV were to perform screening at 6 to 12 month intervals pending her CD4 count. However, newer recommendations are more in line with those for women without HIV and do not utilize CD4 counts as part of the screening criteria. For women <30, it is now recommended to START pap smear screening **within 1 year of sexual activity** or age 21, whichever is first. Note, this is a variation from screening recommendations in women without HIV, who should start pap smears at age 21 *regardless* of sexual activity status. For women aged 21 to 29 with new diagnosis of HIV, pap smear should be performed at the time of initial diagnosis. If pap smear is NEGATIVE, a follow-up pap smear should be performed at 12-month intervals until three negative pap smears and then may lengthen out to 3-year intervals.

For those women with HIV infection and > age 30, a pap test can be performed at 12-month intervals until three negative paps and then may lengthen out to 3-year intervals. Another very effective, and preferred, option is to obtain a pap smear with HPV co-testing at baseline and then at every 3-year intervals (*NOTE: this is different than the guidelines for non-HIV-infected women*). Any detection of cervical intraepithelial neoplasia is treated the same as with HIV-negative women. HPV testing alone is NOT recommended for screening or follow-up of an abnormal pap smear in HIV-infected women as there is a high prevalence of oncogenic HPV and results may be suboptimal.

Screening in HIV-infected women should continue even beyond age 65 years due to the higher risk of cervical cancer in this population (**another variation from recommendations for non-HIV-infected women**). However, clinicians should take patient factors such as comorbidities and life expectancy into account and use shared decision-making when determining if continued screening is warranted.

HELPFUL TIP:
Any STI causing genital ulcers (e.g., herpes) increases the risk of transmission of HIV.

Question 9.2.15 Aside from an increased risk of aggressive HPV and a high rate of menstrual disorders, how does the natural history of HIV infection in women differ from that in men?
A) Women have a lower rate of progressive multifocal leukoencephalopathy (PML) and bacterial pneumonia
B) Women are more likely to present with oral thrush and recurrent genital candidiasis
C) Women with the same level of medical care as men have significantly shortened survival
D) HAART is more effective and better tolerated in women
E) Most women in the United States acquire HIV from same-sex partners

Answer 9.2.15 The correct answer is "B." The natural history of HIV infection in women and men is very similar. Women with the same level of access to medical care have similar survival rates to men, and HAART is equally effective in both sexes. Women are more likely to present with recurrent, refractory vaginal candidiasis, oral thrush, PML, and bacterial pneumonias. The majority of women in the United States with HIV have acquired it from heterosexual contact. The second largest route of exposure for US women is IV drug use. Females who have sex with other women are at low risk of contracting HIV; the opposite is true for men who have sex with other men. Worldwide, heterosexual contact is by far the most common means of transmission.

▶ **Objectives: Did you learn to …**
- Interpret HIV antibody and viral load tests?
- Evaluate the risk of vertical transmission of HIV?
- Reduce the risk of vertical transmission of HIV?
- Interpret HIV tests in the neonatal period?
- Initiate HAART in children?
- Identify some difference in the clinical manifestations of HIV in women and children?
- Recommend appropriate pap smear screening for HIV-infected women?

▶ CASE 9.3

A 39-year-old female working as a nursing assistant in your hospital comes into the emergency department looking quite upset. About 30 minutes earlier, she was helping to move a patient with known HIV when his IV was pulled out and he bled. Several drops of blood got on her hands, but she washed them immediately and thoroughly. On examination, she has intact skin on the hands, no signs of trauma, and no residual blood on her.

Question 9.3.1 The most appropriate action to take is:
A) Reassure her that her risk of contracting HIV for this event is almost zero
B) Obtain HIV antibody testing
C) Start her on HAART for prophylaxis
D) Have her return in 6 weeks for HIV antibody testing
E) B and D

Answer 9.3.1 The correct answer is "A." Fortunately, HIV is not the most efficient virus when it comes to spreading itself. Health care workers are at risk of contracting HIV when working with HIV-infected patients, but exposure to infected bodily fluid must occur through a percutaneous route or contact with a mucous membrane or nonintact skin. Even percutaneous exposure (e.g., open bore needle) with HIV-infected blood carries a transmission rate of only about 0.3%, and the mucous membrane exposure to HIV-infected blood carries a 0.09% risk. Therefore, contracting HIV through contact with an infected patient's blood with intact skin is very low risk.

The patient is reassured that her risk of contracting HIV is negligible. She looks a little sheepish when she tells you, "In all the commotion I knocked over the urinal and spilled the patient's urine on my leg." She changed clothes and washed her leg. You inspect her and find some eczema in the area where the urine was spilled.

Question 9.3.2 Now, you recommend that she:
A) Not worry, as the risk of transmission from this event is also negligible
B) Start ZDV for 4 weeks for prophylaxis
C) Be tested for HIV by viral load
D) Start HAART

Answer 9.3.2 The correct answer is "A." Your patient now has an area of nonintact skin, which is a concern. However, urine is not considered infectious unless it is grossly bloody. Other bodily fluids **NOT** considered infectious: feces, vomitus, sputum, tears, sweat, nasal secretions, and saliva (things you don't want contact with anyway). Any visibly bloody fluids, blood, semen, and vaginal secretions are all considered infectious. Other bodily fluids not already mentioned (e.g., CSF and amniotic fluid) should be considered potentially infectious.

HELPFUL TIP:
HIV post-exposure prophylaxis (PEP) should be considered for contact of nonintact skin or oral or genital mucosa (though how this would happen in a health care environment is somewhat sketchy) with potentially infected body fluid (see above) from a source that is HIV positive or has an unknown HIV status. PEP should be started with a three-drug regimen as soon as possible and continued for 4 weeks. There are many options for prophylaxis with various advantages and disadvantages. The Public Health Service currently recommends tenofovir and emtricitabine (Truvada) in addition to raltegravir. A single dose can be given while awaiting rapid HIV testing from the source patient (if known). Note that most institutions have a set of guidelines that may vary from what is discussed here (including "mandatory" baseline testing).

You see the patient back in your clinic 6 months later for routine follow-up.

Question 9.3.3 Given that you did not screen her initially, and she has never been screened, should she be screened for HIV at this time?
A) No, both of these events were low risk for transmission and there are no recommendations for routine screening
B) No, both of these events were low risk for transmission, and she does not meet the criteria for risk factor-based testing
C) Yes, she meets the recommendations for risk factor-based testing
D) Yes, everyone should be routinely screened for HIV

Answer 9.3.3 The correct answer is "D." In 2013, the United States Preventive Services Task Force (USPSTF) updated its screening recommendation for HIV, recommending universal HIV testing for all individuals between the age of 15 and 65 who present to any health care setting. The screening interval is not currently well-defined. Repeated screening should be considered in patients known to be at risk for HIV infection, those engaged in risky behaviors, and those who live or receive medical care in high-prevalence settings (i.e., HIV seroprevalence of at least 1%). Depending on their risk, this could be either yearly or every 3 to 5 years. According to the CDC, universal screening may be discontinued if the prevalence of HIV in a population has been documented to be less than 0.1% (1/1,000).

▶ **Objective: Did you learn to …**
- Identify when a health care worker is at risk for contracting HIV?
- Apply the USPSTF recommendations for routine HIV screening?

▶ CASE 9.4

A 32-year-old male patient comes in to establish care. He does not have any significant past medical history and is not currently taking any medications. However, his male partner is known to be HIV positive and is currently on HAART. He is not sure what his partner's viral load is but thinks he is well-controlled. They use protection "most of the time." He is wondering what he can do to decrease his risk of acquiring HIV.

Question 9.4.1 What should you tell him?
A) Recommend condom use
B) Discuss prophylaxis with ARV medications
C) Discuss sexual risk-reduction counseling
D) A and C
E) All of the above

Answer 9.4.1 The answer in this case is "E." Since he is in a relationship with a known HIV-positive man, it would be reasonable to consider pre-exposure prophylaxis (PrEP). Indications for PrEP go beyond men who have sex with men (MSM) and also encompass high-risk heterosexual adults and IV drug users. To be eligible for PrEP, the patient must be an adult, not have acute or established HIV infection, and not be in a monogamous relationship with a known HIV-negative person. For MSM, it is indicated for anyone with any male sex partner in the past 6 months AND one of the following: any anal sex without condoms in the past 6 months, any sexually transmitted infections in the past 6 months, or in an ongoing sexual relationship with an HIV-positive male partner (current recommendations do not take into account the viral suppression of the HIV-positive partner although studies in IV drug users and heterosexual adults show negligent of transmission if the partner's viral load is undetectable). For heterosexual adults, PrEP is recommended if condoms are infrequently used with a partner who is known to be at substantial risk for HIV infection or if

the patient is in an ongoing relationship with an HIV-positive partner. For IV drug users, PrEP should be considered if the patient has shared injection or drug preparation equipment in the past 6 months.

You decide to start the patient on PrEP based on his risk of acquiring HIV through his infected partner.

Question 9.4.2 What medications should be used?
A) Tenofovir
B) Tenofovir/Emtricitabine (Truvada)
C) Efavirenz (Sustiva)
D) Tenofovir/Emtricitabine/Efavirenz (Atripla)
E) None of the above

Answer 9.4.2 The correct answer is "B." The combination pill of tenofovir and emtricitabine (Truvada) is the only current FDA-approved regimen for PrEP. In trials in IV drug users or heterosexually active adults, tenofovir alone has shown efficacy but is not FDA-approved and has not been adequately studied in MSM. Any PrEP regimen should be taken daily with strict adherence. Coitally timed or other noncontinuous use is not recommended at this point. Pharmacologic PrEP should be done in combination with repeated condom provision, counseling on sexual risk reduction, and evaluation and treatment for other sexually transmitted infections. While the combination pill of Atripla ("D") would be effective, it would unnecessarily subject the patient to an additional medication (efavirenz) and its associated adverse effects.

When initiating PrEP, discussions regarding an appropriate follow-up plan are imperative.

Question 9.4.3 Which of the following is NOT necessary for monitoring a patient prior to starting and while continuing PrEP?
A) HIV testing at baseline and again every 3 months
B) Baseline assessment of creatinine and repeat levels every 6 months
C) Hepatitis B serologies at baseline
D) Liver function tests at baseline and at 3 months
E) Assessment of adherence at each visit

Answer 9.4.3 The correct answer is "D." LFTs need not be monitored every 3 months. Prior to initiating PrEP, it is important to rule out HIV infection as the two-drug therapy of Truvada would be inadequate in treating HIV and could lead to resistance. In addition, HIV testing should be repeated every 3 months **prior to refilling the prescription**. If signs or symptoms of acute HIV occur, an HIV viral load should be considered. Tenofovir, one of the components of Truvada, has been associated with renal failure and Fanconi's syndrome. In the trials, only patients whose CrCl was >60 mL/min were included, and therefore the current recommendation is to not prescribe PrEP with Truvada for any patient with a CrCl of <60 mL/min. Once PrEP is initiated, creatinine clearance should be rechecked every 6 months. In addition, hepatitis B serologies should be checked prior to initiating PrEP with Truvada. Both components of Truvada have activity against hepatitis B and, if stopped in a patient with active hepatitis B, can lead to reactivation and severe hepatic damage.

▶ **Objective: Did you learn to …**
- Recognize the effectiveness of PrEP?
- Determine when PrEP is indicated?

Clinical Pearls

○ A positive PPD in patients with HIV is considered to be 5 mm of induration.

○ All pregnant women should be tested for HIV.

○ Daily tenofovir/emtricitabine (Truvada) can be used as pre-exposure HIV prophylaxis in high-risk patients such as IV drug abusers and those who engage in risky sexual behavior.

○ Do not treat patients with highly active antiretroviral therapy (HAART) if they are unable to comply with the treatment regimen. Missing doses of HAART can lead to resistant strains of the virus and more difficulty treating the patient later in the disease course.

○ HIV does not seem to cause birth defects, and HAART should be continued during pregnancy to reduce vertical transmission risk.

○ HIV genotype testing for drug resistance should be done when starting or changing a HAART regimen.

○ Neonates suspected of exposure to HIV should be screened with a PCR for viral load.

○ Screening for HIV (not in the neonate) should be done using a P24 antigen and with an evaluation of IgM and IgG antibodies. This will detect HIV as soon as 2 weeks after initial infection.

○ Start HAART early. In general, the earlier the better.

○ The USPSTF suggests that *all* patients age 15 to 65 be screened for HIV.

○ Use steroids in patients with pneumocystis pneumonia if the PaO_2 is <70 or the A-A gradient is >35.

○ Pap smear screening is important in HIV-infected women due to increased risk of cervical cancer. It is recommended to screen with pap smears more frequently and longer (even past age 65) compared to the general population.

BIBLIOGRAPHY

Boyd SD, Hadigan C, McManus M, et al. Influence of low-dose ritonavir with and without darunavir on the pharmacokinetics and pharmacodynamics of inhaled beclomethasone. *J Acquir Immune Defic Syndr.* 2013;63(3):355–361.

Centers for Disease Control and Prevention and Association of Public Health Laboratories. Laboratory testing for the diagnosis of HIV infection: updated recommendations. Available at: http://dx.doi.org/10.15620/cdc.23447. Published June 27, 2014. Accessed August 22, 2018.

Khalsa AM. Preventive counseling, screening, and therapy in the patient with newly diagnosed HIV infection. *Am Fam Physician.* 2006;73(2):271–280.

Mofenson LM, Brady MT, Danner SP, et al. Guidelines for the prevention and treatment of opportunistic infections among HIV-exposed and HIV-infected children: recommendations from CDC, the National Institutes of Health, the HIV Medicine Association of the Infectious Diseases Society of America, the Pediatric Infectious Diseases Society, and the American Academy of Pediatrics. *MMWR Recomm Rep.* 2009;58(RR-11):1–166.

Moyer VA, U.S. Preventative Services Task Force. Screening for HIV: U.S. Preventative Services Task Force recommendation statement. *Ann Intern Med.* 2013;159(1):51–60.

Panel on Antiretroviral Guidelines for Adults and Adolescents. Guidelines for the use of anti-retroviral agents in adults and adolescents living with HIV. Department of Health and Human Services. Updated October 2018. Available at: http://www.aidsinfo.nih.gov/ContentFiles/AdultandAdolescentGL.pdf. Accessed August 22, 2018.

Panel on Antiretroviral Therapy and Medical Management of HIV-Infected Children. Guidelines for the use of antiretroviral agents in pediatric HIV infection. Updated December 2018. Available at: https://aidsinfo.nih.gov/contentfiles/lvguidelines/pediatricguidelines.pdf. Accessed January 21, 2019.

Panel on Treatment of HIV-Infected Pregnant Women and Prevention of Perinatal Transmission. Recommendations for use of antiretroviral drugs in pregnant HIV-1-infected women for maternal health and interventions to reduce perinatal HIV transmission in the United States. Updated March 2018. Available at: https://aidsinfo.nih.gov/contentfiles/lvguidelines/PerinatalGL.pdf. Accessed January 21, 2019.

Panlilio AL, Cardo DM, Grohskopf LA, et al. Updated U.S. Public Health Service guidelines for the management of occupational exposures to HIV and recommendations for postexposure prophylaxis. *MMWR Recomm Rep.* 2005;54(RR-9):1–17.

Saberi P, Pehngrasamy T, Nguyen DP. Inhaled corticosteroid use in HIV-positive individuals taking protease inhibitors: a review of pharmacokinetics, case reports and clinical management. *HIV Med.* 2013;14(9):519–529.

U.S. Department of Health and Human Services. AIDSInfo: Guidelines for prevention and treatment of opportunistic infections in HIV-infected adults and adolescents. Updated November 29, 2018. Available at: https://aidsinfo.nih.gov/contentfiles/lvguidelines/glchunk/glchunk_343.pdf. Accessed January 21, 2019.

Endocrinology 10

Emad Abou-Arab

▶ CASE 10.1

A 27-year-old female presents to the office with the chief complaint of fatigue for 4 months. She has gained 17 lb in that same time, despite a decreased appetite. She also complains of depression, increased sleepiness, lack of energy, hair loss, and cold intolerance. Her past medical history is unremarkable, and she takes no medications. She has never had any surgeries. She did a little Internet research, and according to Dr. Oz, she might have a thyroid problem.

Question 10.1.1 Which of the following physical examination findings would be expected?
A) Tachycardia
B) Exophthalmos
C) Fine tremor
D) Peripheral sensory loss
E) Delayed relaxation in reflexes

Answer 10.1.1 **The correct answer is "E."** The history given is consistent with a hypothyroid state. Symptoms of hypothyroidism include thinning hair, dry skin, a hoarse and deep voice, bradycardia, and a prolonged relaxation in the reflexes. Tachycardia and a fine tremor are more typical of hyperthyroidism, and exophthalmos is characteristic of Graves' disease (one specific cause of hyperthyroidism). Proximal muscle weakness may occur in hypothyroidism, but sensory loss is not typical (although hypothyroidism, diabetes, gout, rheumatoid arthritis, obesity, and connective tissue disorders can contribute to carpal tunnel syndrome, and carpal tunnel syndrome may be the initial presenting symptom of these diseases).

Question 10.1.2 How can the diagnosis of hypothyroidism best be confirmed?
A) Elevated thyroid-stimulating hormone (TSH) level
B) Low TSH level
C) Thyroid biopsy
D) Radionuclide scan
E) Serum thyroglobulin

Answer 10.1.2 **The correct answer is "A."** The TSH is the most sensitive test for both hypo- and hyperthyroidism, and changes in the TSH can precede abnormalities in serum thyroxine (best measured as free T4) level. An elevated TSH occurs when the pituitary detects insufficient thyroid hormone production (low free thyroxine), and TSH production is shut off when the pituitary detects an excess of thyroid hormone circulating (elevated free thyroxine). With pituitary dysfunction, there is insufficient TSH production resulting in a low TSH *and* decreased free thyroxine (T4). Since pituitary disorders are rare, and often suggested by other clues in the history and physical (lack of gonadotropins [amenorrhea, hypogonadism], impaired vision from mass effect), TSH alone is sufficient for initial screening for thyroid disease. "C," a biopsy, is used to evaluate thyroid masses and nodules as is "D," a radionuclide scan. A radionuclide scan ("D") can also be used in the evaluation of thyroid masses. "E," the serum thyroglobulin measurement, is used to monitor thyroid carcinoma and is not a screening test.

Her laboratory results are normal except for glucose 115 mg/dL, TSH 22.3 μIU/mL (normal 0.27–4.20), free T4 0.56 ng/dL (normal 0.93–1.70).

Question 10.1.3 Based on prevalence, labs, and presentation, what is the MOST likely cause of this patient's disease?
A) Autoimmune hypothyroidism
B) Iatrogenic hypothyroidism
C) Tuberculosis infiltration of the thyroid gland
D) Nonfunctioning pituitary adenoma
E) Congenital hypothyroidism

Answer 10.1.3 **The correct answer is "A."** Autoimmune hypothyroidism (Hashimoto thyroiditis) is the most common cause of hypothyroidism in areas where there is adequate iodine. If this patient had a pituitary adenoma causing hypothyroidism, the TSH (as well as the free T4) would be low. Congenital hypothyroidism causes severe developmental delay and a constellation of other signs termed "cretinism"; screening for hypothyroidism is generally part of neonatal screening.

Tuberculosis is a rare cause of hypothyroidism but is the most common cause of **adrenal** failure worldwide.

> **HELPFUL TIP:**
> Outside the United States, iodine deficiency is the most common cause of hypothyroidism, with an estimated 2 billion persons being iodine deficient although not all being hypothyroid.

Question 10.1.4 How should this patient be managed?
A) I^{131} administration
B) Surgical excision of thyroid gland
C) Start synthetic thyroxine hormone at 25 micrograms (µg) PO daily, and re-check symptoms and TSH in 2 months
D) Start synthetic thyroxine hormone at 200 µg PO daily, and re-check symptoms and TSH in 2 months
E) Start synthetic thyroxine hormone at 25 µg PO daily, and double every week until the patient experiences weight loss, tremor, and poor sleep (and the desire to find a new doctor)

Answer 10.1.4 The correct answer is "C." The patient is deficient in thyroid hormone and needs supplementation. Two strategies may be used: (1) start with 25 µg daily and titrate up every 1 to 2 months until the TSH is in the normal range or (2) start with full-dose therapy based on weight (1.6 µg/kg daily) and adjust based on TSH in 1 to 2 months. Either option is appropriate in young, otherwise healthy adults. **However, older patients (>65 years old) or those with cardiac disease or multiple comorbidities should be started at a low dose (25 µg daily) due to increased cardiac risks associated with being overly replaced (see helpful tip below).** If the patient is titrated up to 200 µg of levothyroxine and does not seem to be responding, the diagnosis needs to be reconsidered or the patient's adherence needs to be carefully assessed. Iron and food will decrease the absorption of levothyroxine by as much as 40%. Thyroid medication should be taken under similar circumstances each day, and ideally it should be taken on an empty stomach. If it is taken with a meal, it should always be taken with a meal to prevent variable absorption. Peak serum levels occur 2 to 4 hours after an oral dose, but the half-life is 7 days, so day-to-day levels can be misleading. It usually takes 6 to 8 weeks for the body's endocrine response and TSH to reach a steady state. The goal of therapy is a euthyroid state with the patient experiencing neither hyper- nor hypothyroid symptoms. "A" and "B" are treatments of **hyper**thyroidism. Surgical excision and radioablation with I^{131} are approaches to the treatment of Graves' disease. Both can result in iatrogenic hypothyroidism that requires lifelong thyroid hormone therapy.

You start the patient on 25 µg levothyroxine (Synthroid) and schedule a return appointment in 2 months. At follow-up, she reports a general improvement in symptoms but is not "back to normal." She reports continued constipation, a lack of energy, and feeling depressed. Though she initially lost weight in the first month, she has not lost any further weight and reports a thickening of her hair. Laboratory results are as follows: TSH 11.8 µIU/mL (0.27–4.20) and free T4 0.75 ng/dL (0.93–1.70).

Question 10.1.5 What adjustments, if any, should be made to her regimen?
A) None, she will continue to improve at the current dose
B) Increase the dose to 50 µg/day, and re-check in 2 months
C) Increase the dose to 200 µg/day, and re-check in 2 months
D) She is becoming hyperthyroid, so cut the dose to 12.5 µg/day, and re-check in 2 months
E) Levothyroxine is ineffective in this patient. Change her to desiccated thyroid tissue (e.g., Armour Thyroid) or triiodothyronine (T3)

Answer 10.1.5 The correct answer is "B." This patient has improved from her initial presentation, but she is clinically and chemically (elevated TSH) still hypothyroid. Since 2 months have elapsed, she is now at steady state. It is doubtful that her thyroid levels will change much if you wait, so now is a good time to increase her dose. Since you started with a low dose, doubling of the dose is a reasonable increase that is unlikely to make her hyperthyroid. The goals of therapy are amelioration of symptoms and normalization of TSH secretion by maintaining the TSH within the normal reference range—except in the elderly or during pregnancy. There is evidence of better outcomes if the TSH is kept at the *high normal* end in the elderly and the *low normal* end during pregnancy. "E" deserves special mention. Desiccated thyroid is generally avoided due to variability in concentration of thyroid hormone content. T3 has nothing to offer over levothyroxine (T4) despite what the Internet "experts" (and your patients' grandmothers) say.

> **HELPFUL TIP:**
> Poor adherence is the most common reason for failure of medical therapy. Other causes include malabsorption, drug interactions (e.g., rifampin and amiodarone), drug–food interactions, or drugs that reduce absorption (e.g., phosphate binders, PPIs, iron, and sucralfate).

Your patient worries about taking too much thyroid hormone.

Question 10.1.6 Which of the following can result from oversuppression of the TSH (iatrogenic hyperthyroidism)?
A) Renal failure
B) Pulmonary fibrosis
C) Hirsutism
D) Osteoporosis
E) Loss of secondary sex characteristics

Answer 10.1.6 The correct answer is "D." Hyperthyroidism, either iatrogenic or endogenous, causes osteoporosis. For this reason, it is important to monitor the TSH and assure that the patient is not over-replaced.

The patient has been doing great for a couple of years when she returns to see you for a routine follow-up. Both her TSH and her free T4 are within the normal range. She then informs you that she had no menses for 5 weeks. You check a urine pregnancy test in the clinic and it is positive. The patient is excited about the pregnancy.

Question 10.1.7 What is the most appropriate management for the patent's hypothyroidism?
A) Continue the current levothyroxine dosage without any change
B) Increase the levothyroxine dose by 10% now
C) Increase the levothyroxine dose by 30% now
D) No change of the levothyroxine dose, but have the thyroid function re-checked in 6 weeks
E) Refer her to an endocrinologist (wait time is currently 6 months)

Answer 10.1.7 **The correct answer is "C."** Women with preexisting hypothyroidism who are planning to become pregnant should optimize their thyroid hormone dose preconception if possible. The majority of women with preexisting hypothyroidism require a higher dose of levothyroxine during pregnancy to maintain goal TSH levels. The increase in levothyroxine requirements occurs as early as the fifth week of gestation and plateaus by 16 to 20 weeks. It is generally recommended that the levothyroxine dose be increased by 30% to 50% at the time of the positive pregnancy test through the first trimester. Note that there are trimester-specific goals that differ from the goal in the usual patient. The goal TSH level for the first trimester is 0.1 to 2.5 μIU/mL, second trimester 0.2 to 3.0 μIU/mL, and third trimester 0.3 to 3.0 μIU/mL (*Am Fam Physician.* 2014;89,4:273–278). Thyroid function should be assessed every 4 weeks. If the TSH values are above goal, the dose of levothyroxine is increased and thyroid function is re-checked in 2 to 4 weeks. "A," "B," and "D" are incorrect because of the reasons mentioned above. Also, "E" is incorrect. If you do not feel comfortable managing the patient's hypothyroidism during her pregnancy, you may still need to increase her levothyroxine first, then refer her to an endocrinologist. Good care transition is critical: assure that the patient's hypothyroidism is managed until she is under the care of the consultant.

HELPFUL TIP:
Hashimoto thyroiditis is associated with primary thyroid lymphoma, which typically presents with an enlarged neck mass and may be associated with local compression symptoms and "B-symptoms" such as fever, weight loss, and night sweats. If lymphoma is suspected, a core needle or excisional biopsy is indicated.

▶ **Objectives: Did you learn to …**
- Recognize the presentation of hypothyroidism and its most common causes?
- Identify common physical examination findings consistent with hypothyroidism?
- Describe the basic medical and laboratory management of patients with hypothyroidism?
- Manage hypothyroidism during pregnancy?

▶ **CASE 10.2**

A 32-year-old male presents complaining of severe anxiety. For the last 4 months, he has had difficulty sleeping, progressively worsening anxiety, a 25-lb weight loss, and constantly feels "too warm." He feels "shaky" and has difficulty concentrating. He denies diarrhea, but reports having normally shaped stools four to five times per day—more than usual for him. The patient denies neck or eye discomfort and has not noticed any neck swelling. He has no other significant medical history. His mother, who died 3 years ago from coronary artery disease (CAD), had a "thyroid problem," but he doesn't know any details.

Physical examination reveals an anxious young adult male. He has a noticeable resting tremor. You note mild exophthalmos, conjunctival injection, and lid lag. His thyroid is diffusely, mildly enlarged, is non-tender, and a bruit is audible over the gland. The cardiac examination reveals tachycardia with a flow murmur. The rest of the examination is unremarkable.

Question 10.2.1 What is the most likely diagnosis?
A) Viral thyroiditis
B) Graves' disease
C) Anaplastic thyroid carcinoma
D) Hyperactive thyroid adenoma
E) Surreptitious thyroid hormone ingestion

Answer 10.2.1 **The correct answer is "B."** This is a classic presentation of Graves' disease. The family history, the symptoms and signs of hyperthyroidism (especially the diffusely enlarged goiter with a bruit), and the exophthalmos are typical; conjunctival injection is also frequently noted. "A" is unlikely. Viral thyroiditis can cause hyperthyroidism and a goiter, but the thyroid gland is usually tender. Also, viral thyroiditis will likely not last 4 months, but is usually self-limited to less than 6 weeks. Anaplastic carcinoma ("C") is a devastating disease with a dismal prognosis: the thyroid gets very large very quickly, but the disease does not present with hyperthyroid symptoms. A hyperactive adenoma ("D") and surreptitious ingestion of thyroid hormone ("E") would not cause a goiter or exophthalmos.

HELPFUL TIP:
75% of patients with viral thyroiditis will progress from 2 weeks of self-limited hyperthyroidism to 3 to 6 months

of hypothyroidism that is also self-limited. About 15% of patients go on to a permanent hypothyroid state requiring thyroid replacement. The hyperthyroid phase is best treated with NSAIDs, beta-blockers, and prednisone if needed.

Question 10.2.2 **Which of the following tests is most specific for Graves' disease?**
A) Anti-thyrotropin receptor (anti-TSH receptor) antibody
B) Anti-thyroglobulin antibody
C) Antithyroid peroxidase antibody
D) Markedly suppressed TSH

Answer 10.2.2 **The correct answer is "A."** Graves' disease is an autoimmune process, and lymphocytes in the thyroid gland itself are responsible for a large amount of the thyroid autoantibodies produced. Although several types of antibodies can be assayed, anti-thyrotropin receptor antibody is the most specific. Here is a breakdown of selected thyroid serum assays and where you may see them elevated:

- **Anti-thyrotropin receptor antibody (anti-TSH receptor antibody)** ("A") is found in 80% to 95% of patients with Graves' disease, but also in 10% to 20% of those with other forms of autoimmune thyroiditis.
- **Anti-thyroglobulin antibodies** ("B") are found in Graves' disease, autoimmune thyroiditis, some patients with type 1 diabetes, and in up to 20% of the general population.
- **Antithyroid peroxidase antibody** ("C") is elevated in Graves' disease, autoimmune thyroiditis, type 1 diabetes, and some pregnant patients, etc.
- **Serum thyroglobulin:** A form of T3/T4 produced by follicular cells. Used to monitor thyroid cancer.

You obtain labs and find that the CBC is normal and TSH is undetectable. He is tachycardic at 130 bpm.

Question 10.2.3 **How should the patient be treated acutely?**
A) Propranolol and methimazole started immediately
B) Control the patient's symptoms with propranolol now, then start propylthiouracil (PTU) when the patient feels better
C) Iodine (Lugol solution)
D) Radioablation with I^{131}
E) Thyroidectomy

Answer 10.2.3 **The correct answer is "A."** There is no need to wait before starting methimazole (Tapazole), which blocks production of thyroid hormone. PTU can also be used, but methimazole is preferred because (1) it affords better control and (2) PTU is associated with more liver toxicity and bone marrow suppression (although these adverse effects can occur with both drugs). PTU is preferred during the **first trimester** of pregnancy due to the risk of birth defects (aplasia cutis and choanal and esophageal atresia) associated

with methimazole. Current guidelines recommend switching from PTU to methimazole for the second and third trimesters because the risk of liver toxicity for the mother (with PTU) is greater than the risk of congenital defects in the fetus; however, some experts still prefer PTU throughout pregnancy.

Propranolol is helpful for controlling the symptoms of hyperthyroidism (tachycardia, tremor, etc.) and prevents the conversion of T4 to active T3. Metoprolol is an alternative. "C" is incorrect, as iodine will provide further substrate for the body in the production of thyroid hormone and should not be given until a thyroid-blocking agent has been started. Iodine is useful during thyroid storm to prevent the release of stored thyroid hormone, but it is given 1 hour after PTU or methimazole. Radioablation is used for patients who prove refractory to medicine or have poor compliance. Thyroidectomy is rarely used for Graves' disease in current medical practice because of the ease and efficacy of radioactive iodine administration (except in the case of pregnancy and few other unusual cases).

Question 10.2.4 **Which of the following is/are possible side effects of PTU and methimazole therapy?**
A) Granulocytopenia
B) Aplastic anemia
C) Elevated liver transaminases
D) Inhibition of fetal thyroid gland
E) All of the above

Answer 10.2.4 **The correct answer is "E."** All of the above are known side effects of antithyroid drugs (thionamides). Granulocytopenia occurs in about 0.5% of patients and is a sudden, idiosyncratic reaction. **Classically, patients present with a severe sore throat. If you have a patient on PTU or methimazole with a sore throat or fever, check a CBC.** Aplastic anemia may occur but is rare. For these reasons, patients starting these medications should have a baseline CBC. Mild, transient elevation of the liver transaminases is common, and the drug should be discontinued only if the transaminases increase to greater than three times the upper limit of the reference range. Both PTU and methimazole cross the placenta and will inhibit the fetal thyroid, increasing the risk for congenital hypothyroidism. The risk to a fetus posed by the drugs is less than the danger posed by a mother with accelerating hyperthyroidism, so the medications should be used even during pregnancy if indicated. The smallest doses possible should be used. If a pregnant patient is not controlled medically, consider thyroidectomy. Finally, PTU and methimazole can cause an ANCA-positive vasculitis.

HELPFUL TIP:
When treating *hyperthyroidism* in pregnancy, aim for a serum-free T4 level in the upper one-third of the reference range. Avoid radioactive iodine treatment during pregnancy since it will affect the fetus as well.

The patient is interested in treating the ophthalmopathy.

Question 10.2.5 What is the *primary* method for treating Graves' ophthalmopathy?
A) Orbital radiation
B) Glucocorticoids
C) Rituximab
D) Thyroidectomy
E) Radioactive iodine therapy

Answer 10.2.5 The correct answer is "B." Approximately 5% to 10% of patients with Graves' disease develop clinically significant ophthalmopathy. Graves' ophthalmopathy manifests as inflamed, red eyes and diplopia/proptosis. The treatment of Graves' ophthalmopathy includes establishing a euthyroid state. PTU and methimazole are preferred since radioactive iodine may worsen Graves' ophthalmopathy. Other measures include reducing eye irritation (e.g., artificial tears/methylcellulose eye drops) followed by a trial of corticosteroids. Glucocorticoids have been shown to be effective in treating Graves' ophthalmopathy. Intravenous (IV) steroids are more effective than oral steroids, but either can be used. Orbital radiation has been used but with little success. Rituximab (C") is another option that seems to be effective, but it is not first line. Radioactive iodine treatment ("E") has been associated with *worsening* of Graves' ophthalmopathy. Thyroidectomy ("D") is usually reserved for patients who fail antithyroid drugs, have large or obstructive goiters, or who have coexisting hyperparathyroidism requiring parathyroidectomy.

Your patient complies with the recommended regimen and improves. He is not symptomatic at a return visit in 2 months, and his eye pathology has not progressed. After 6 months of good control, the patient elects to have cosmetic eye surgery for his exophthalmos, which has not responded well to glucocorticoids. A preoperative physical is unremarkable. Laboratory studies prior to surgery are normal except TSH 0.21 μIU/mL (0.27–4.20) and free T4 3.01 ng/dL (0.93–1.70).

After an uneventful surgery, you are called to the postanesthesia room by the oculoplastic surgeon. She reports that the patient has become very anxious and tachycardic. A quick review of the chart reveals no known allergies, no personal or family history of reactions to anesthesia, and the only medication that the patient takes regularly is methimazole (propranolol had been discontinued 2 months earlier due to lack of symptoms).

Physical examination shows T 39.8°C, BP 98/25 mm Hg, RR 34, and P 166 bpm. The patient is agitated but alert and in acute distress. He is tachypneic and tremulous and is unable to carry on a conversation. He seems confused and distracted. The skin is diaphoretic and flushed. His mucous membranes are dry, and his surface veins are flat. There is no JVD and the vena cava looks normally filled on ultrasound. Pulmonary examination reveals diffuse rales. Reflexes are brisk.

Question 10.2.6 What is the likely cause of this patient's symptoms and signs?
A) The patient became fluid overloaded during the surgery due to excessive hydration
B) The patient has neuroleptic malignant syndrome (NMS)
C) The patient has thyroid storm induced by the stress of surgery
D) The patient has endocarditis and suffered a valve rupture
E) The patient has euthyroid sick syndrome (AKA nonthyroidal illness syndrome)

Answer 10.2.6 The correct answer is "C." The syndrome of thyroid storm is characterized by fever, tachyarrhythmias, altered mental status, and high-output cardiac failure. It is induced by a major stress (infection, surgery, myocardial infarction, etc.) in a patient with underlying hyperthyroidism (usually undiagnosed). This patient, although **clinically** well-controlled, had a **low TSH and high free T4 prior to surgery**, suggesting he may have suffered a recurrence of disease or had stopped taking his medications. The patient is not fluid overloaded, as evidenced by his clinically dry status (dry mucous membranes, flat neck veins, normal vena caval filling); thus "A" is incorrect. His pulmonary edema (rales) is due to high-output failure rather than fluid overload. NMS presents with altered mental status and hyperthermia (due to increased metabolic activity). But the patient is not currently taking neuroleptics. A ruptured valve due to endocarditis would fit the patient's clinical picture, but he had no fever preceding the surgery or other evidence of endocarditis. Euthyroid sick syndrome (now termed "nonthyroidal illness syndrome") ("E") is used to define a state in critically ill patients with laboratory findings of low free T3, low free T4, and/or low TSH (a central hypothyroidism in response to illness). It is an adaptation which lowers tissue energy requirements in the face of systemic illness. He could have malignant hyperthermia secondary to anesthesia, but this isn't a choice.

HELPFUL TIP:
Thyroid storm is a clinical diagnosis consisting of hyperthermia, tachycardia, CNS dysfunction, and signs and symptoms of peripheral hyperthyroidism. While most patients will have an elevated T3 and free T4, there is no laboratory level of these hormones that defines thyroid storm. Thyroid storm may cause right upper quadrant pain due to liver congestion secondary to high-output congestive heart failure.

HELPFUL TIP:
A pheochromocytoma can be confused with hyperthyroidism. Both include tachycardia and possible hypertension. Interestingly, serum catecholamines **are normal** (often high normal—but normal) in thyroid storm. But catecholamine sensitivity seems to play a role in thyroid storm. Catecholamines will be elevated in patients with a pheochromocytoma.

Question 10.2.7 How should this patient now be treated?

A) Administer aggressive fluid hydration, cooling measures, benzodiazepines, and dantrolene

B) Administer fluid hydration, cooling measures, IV propranolol, IV corticosteroids, methimazole or PTU, then iodine 1 hour later

C) Administer fluid hydration, dopamine drip for his hypotension, and antibiotics; consult cardiovascular surgery immediately

D) Hold fluids; administer nitroglycerin drip and furosemide for his heart failure; consider an intra-aortic balloon pump

E) Administer fluid hydration (even 3 L or more) and antibiotics; consider norepinephrine drip if patient becomes more hypotensive

Answer 10.2.7 The correct answer is "B." This is the appropriate management for thyroid storm and the correct sequence of therapies. This patient is in distress (hypotensive and tachycardic) and needs fluid hydration, despite his pulmonary edema (but be judicious and use clinical judgment). Cooling measures address his hyperthermia, and beta-blockade (propranolol) will improve his high-output failure (and reduce the pulmonary edema). Corticosteroids help block release of thyroid hormone and decreases peripheral conversion of T4 to T3. In addition, corticosteroids will treat any underlying adrenal insufficiency. Methimazole prevents thyroxine synthesis. This must be given before iodine. The iodine blocks any further release of thyroid hormone. Some experts recommend using PTU instead of methimazole for the patient with life-threatening thyroid storm admitted to an ICU because PTU blocks T4 to T3 conversion and results in lower serum T3 level. "A" is the appropriate management of NMS. "C" is an appropriate approach for valve rupture from endocarditis. "D" describes the management of severe heart failure. "E" describes essential steps in the treatment of sepsis.

HELPFUL TIP:
In patients with hyperthyroidism, diarrhea is a sign that can presage thyroid storm.

HELPFUL TIP:
Surgery or radioactive iodine can be used to treat Graves' disease. Radioactive iodine can take months to work. Otherwise, hyperthyroid patients are treated for 1 to 2 years followed by a taper of their medications. A taper can be tried earlier in the course (at 6 months) if desired by the patient.

Your patient is treated appropriately and eventually recovers. He continues on methimazole and propranolol and remains in good control. You can try tapering the medications in 6 months to see how he does.

▶ **Objectives: Did you learn to …**
- Identify the more common causes of hyperthyroidism?
- Recognize the presentation of Graves' disease?
- Manage hyperthyroidism and describe the indications and risks of each treatment option?
- Recognize and treat thyroid storm?

▶ **CASE 10.3**

You are seeing a 45-year-old female who is a nursing assistant at a local nursing home. As part of a life insurance mandated blood panel, the patient's TSH is noted to be elevated at 7.2 µIU/mL (0.27–4.20 µIU/mL). She has a normal free T4 and is asymptomatic. You repeat the labs, with very similar results.

Question 10.3.1 The best option is to:
A) Start levothyroxine at a low dose to normalize the TSH
B) Begin T3 at a low dose
C) Reassure the patient and have her follow-up for repeat thyroid studies
D) Begin a workup for central hypothyroidism
E) Begin methimazole

Answer 10.3.1 The correct answer is "C." This patient has subclinical hypothyroidism (asymptomatic, TSH between 5 and 10, and normal free T4). There is convincing evidence that **asymptomatic** patients with a mildly elevated TSH (generally <10 µIU/mL) and normal free T4 do not benefit from treatment in terms of quality of life, etc. In fact, treated patients tend to have more symptomatic anxiety, atrial fibrillation, etc. Follow-up thyroid studies are indicated, although the interval may differ depending on the clinician's judgment. Of note, many patients will have transient changes in their thyroid hormone levels due to comorbid illness, viral thyroiditis, etc. Generally, the best thing to do is re-check rather than start treatment except in those patients with high risk for progression to overt hypothyroidism (TSH level >10 µIU/mL, positive family history, goiter, presence of antithyroid peroxidase antibodies, or desire to become pregnant; see *Clin Endocrinol (Oxf)*. 2015 May 23. doi: 10.1111/cen.12824 for hypothyroidism clinical guidelines).

HELPFUL TIP:
Among patients with hyperlipidemia, overt and subclinical hypothyroidism is common. Thus, patients with hypercholesterolemia and hypertriglyceridemia should be screened for hypothyroidism.

HELPFUL TIP:
T3 tends to have rapid gastrointestinal (GI) absorption and relatively short half-life leading to erratic T3 serum levels. It is best to avoid T3 in the vast majority of patients with hypothyroidism.

▶ **Objectives: Did you learn to …**
- Describe subclinical hypothyroidism?

 QUICK QUIZ: SOMETHING SUBACUTE

A 32-year-old white female without significant past medical history except an upper respiratory tract infection 4 weeks ago presents to the clinic for a 1-week history of dull anterior neck pain, palpitations, anxiety, poor sleep, and chills. Physical examination is unremarkable except tachycardia (100 bpm). with anterior neck tenderness, but no mass appreciated. Laboratory results: C-reactive protein 5 mg/dL (high), TSH <0.01 μIU/mL (low), and free T4 5 ng/dL (high). A bedside ultrasound shows an enlarged thyroid gland.

What is the most appropriate next step in management?
A) Fine needle aspiration for biopsy
B) Antithyroid medications like methimazole or PTU
C) 24-hour radioactive iodine uptake test
D) Neck soft tissue computer tomography (CT)

The correct answer is "C." Considering her recent viral infection, tender thyroid gland, elevated inflammatory marker, and the low TSH and high T4, this is most likely subacute thyroiditis. The 24-hour radioactive iodine uptake (RAIU) test measures thyroid gland iodine uptake over 24 hours. We need to determine the etiology of this patient's thyroiditis. In patients with destructive thyroiditis like subacute thyroiditis, the RAIU will be low, usually less than 5% over 24 hours. In contrast, Graves' disease will have an elevated or normal RAIU. Fine needle aspiration ("A") is used for evaluation of thyroid nodule but the patient does not have one. Antithyroid agents ("B") have no role in the treatment of subacute thyroiditis since it is usually a self-limiting disease after transient (2–8 weeks) hyperthyroidism. The primary treatment focus is symptom relief and includes NSAIDs, nonselective beta-blockers, and/or corticosteroids (prednisone) if patient has severe pain or no improvement is seen after 2 to 3 days of more conservative treatment. Ultrasound is an excellent imaging modality to evaluate the thyroid gland, whereas CT scan ("D") offers little value in this case.

 QUICK QUIZ: THYROID TESTS

A 52-year-old male is being seen in your clinic for weight loss, tachycardia, and anxiety. You suspect hyperthyroidism and decide to check blood work. The patient has a low TSH suggestive of hyperthyroidism but has a normal free T4.

The most likely explanation of this patient's symptoms and laboratory findings is:
A) He has pituitary dysfunction with a pending central hypothyroidism
B) He has an isolated T3 hyperthyroidism
C) He has Addison disease
D) He is taking aspirin that interferes with the assay for free T4
E) He is taking aspirin that interferes with the assay for TSH

The correct answer is "B." Five percent of patients with hyperthyroidism have an isolated T3-toxicosis. Thus, if you suspect hyperthyroidism and the patient has a low TSH but a normal free T4, check a T3. Of note, "D" and "E" are incorrect. However, many drugs can interfere with thyroid-binding globulin and cause changes in the measurable amounts of **total** T4 (not free) and T3 in the serum. In most cases, the free T4 and free T3 (unbound thyroid hormones) are not affected by the changes in thyroid-binding globulin levels.

 QUICK QUIZ: HYPERTHYROIDISM

Which of the following cause(s) *hyper*thyroidism?
A) Lithium
B) Amiodarone
C) Peginterferon alfa-2 a
D) Phenytoin
E) B and C

The correct answer is "E." Amiodarone (see Helpful Tip) and peginterferon alfa-2 a can cause both hypothyroidism and hyperthyroidism. Amiodarone causes hypothyroidism in approximately 10% of patients who take it chronically and hyperthyroidism in approximately 1%. "A" and "D," lithium and phenytoin, respectively, cause hypothyroidism. Phenytoin reduces TSH secretion so patients may have a low TSH and a low T4.

▶ **CASE 10.4**

A 45-year-old female presents to the office complaining of a "ball in my neck." She noticed a lump in her anterior neck approximately 1 month ago. She is not sure if it has increased in size. She has not noticed any other lumps or masses. She denies dysphagia, odynophagia, neck pain, cough, weight loss, fever, chills, sweats, or a change in bowel habits. She also denies any hyperthyroid or hypothyroid symptoms. In 1993, she immigrated to the United States from Kiev (still in the Ukraine at the time of this writing … at least until Putin takes it), where she had grown-up and lived—including all of the 80s (you remember—Madonna, leg warmers, Chernobyl). She has no family history of thyroid or other endocrine disorders, but several relatives in Kiev have been diagnosed with various cancers.

Question 10.4.1 Which of the following factors from history INCREASES the likelihood that the nodule is malignant?
A) Nodule **not** increasing in size
B) **No** regional adenopathy
C) Age >40 years
D) Male gender
E) History of radiation exposure

Answer 10.4.1 **The correct answer is "E."** This patient lived in Kiev, near the Chernobyl nuclear power plant, during and after the reactor accident in 1986. She was exposed to radiation and, like her family members, is at significantly increased risk for cancer, especially thyroid malignancies. Other clinical factors that suggest a malignant etiology include (in general, not necessarily in this patient): a nodule >2 cm or increasing in size, dysphagia, hoarseness, regional lymphadenopathy, a fixation to the surrounding tissues, female gender, age <40, and family history.

 HELPFUL TIP:
There are a lot of cancer survivors walking around who received radiation to the neck (e.g., mantle radiation for Hodgkin lymphoma). These patients are at increased risk of developing thyroid cancers.

Physical examination reveals an obese female in no acute distress. Her head, eye, nose, and oral examinations are normal. She has a 2-cm firm nodule on the right pole of the thyroid. The nodule moves along with the other subcutaneous structures upon swallowing. She has no lymphadenopathy. The rest of the examination is normal.

Question 10.4.2 Which of the following next steps would be most likely to yield a *definitive* diagnosis?
A) Thyroid ultrasound
B) Fine needle aspiration (FNA)
C) Thyroid scan (Tc^{99})
D) Serum thyroglobulin level
E) Serum calcitonin level and CEA level

Answer 10.4.2 **The correct answer is "B."** FNA can conclusively prove or disprove the presence of neoplasm and should be considered for all thyroid nodules and cysts. That is the bottom line; the rest are interesting—but do the FNA.

Ultrasound can be used if there is low malignant potential in order to look for worrisome sonographic features, but it cannot definitively differentiate a benign nodule from a malignant one. Besides, *any thyroid nodule with diameter greater than 1 cm should be evaluated with FNA.* Thus, no ultrasound is needed in this case except to guide the FNA.

A thyroid scan ("C") will identify if a nodule is actively processing thyroid hormone ("functional" or "hot") or is not metabolically active ("nonfunctional" or "cold"). A "hot" nodule may cause hyperthyroidism, is usually benign ("hot is not" malignancy), and can be treated with I^{131}. A cold nodule is either an adenoma or a malignancy, and a biopsy is mandated.

A serum thyroglobulin ("D") is the tumor marker for thyroid carcinoma and should be drawn before thyroidectomy. It has no value as a diagnostic test in the initial evaluation before malignancy is diagnosed but can be followed as a marker. Anti-thyroglobulin antibodies may interfere with the assay, however.

Serum calcitonin and CEA levels ("E") are elevated in the case of medullary carcinoma, but would have low yield in the initial evaluation. Refer to the American Thyroid Association guidelines for management of thyroid nodules (*Thyroid* 2016;26(1):1–132) for additional details on the evaluation of thyroid nodules.

Fine needle aspiration is consistent with papillary carcinoma. A serum thyroglobulin level, TSH, basic chemistries, a blood count, and a blood type are ordered.

Question 10.4.3 What should be done next?
A) Observe the nodule for 1 month
B) Computerized tomography (CT) of the head and neck with contrast
C) Radiation therapy with I^{131}
D) Radiation therapy with external beam radiation
E) Suppression of TSH levels with levothyroxine

Answer 10.4.3 **The correct answer is "B."** Surgery for removal of the tumor is the most appropriate next step, but a CT scan is indicated to delineate the extent of the neoplasm. Radiotherapy with I^{131} is used after surgery for metastatic disease, but external beam radiation is not used for thyroid cancers except for palliative therapy of anaplastic carcinoma. Because these tumors are TSH responsive, suppression of TSH level **following surgery** for papillary carcinoma is achieved with levothyroxine (usually 2.2–2.5 µg/kg—fairly high dose to completely suppress TSH production).

 HELPFUL TIP:
The most common thyroid cancer is papillary carcinoma. Medullary carcinoma may be associated with an elevated calcitonin and other endocrine malignancies (e.g., multiple endocrine neoplasia II [MEN II]).

 HELPFUL TIP:
There's a caveat to the emphatic endorsement of FNA (which has a deservedly good reputation for diagnosis). Here it is: thyroid follicular lesions. When an FNA returns material from a thyroid follicular neoplasm, 15% to 25% of these may be harboring cancer. Follicular thyroid cancer cannot be ruled out on the basis of an FNA due to inability to differentiate a malignancy from a benign adenoma. Usually, a thyroid lobectomy or total thyroidectomy is recommended to further evaluate a follicular neoplasm so that a pathologic examination can be completed.

▶ **Objectives: Did you learn to …**
· Recognize the major risk factors influencing the development and prognosis of thyroid carcinomas?
· Evaluate a thyroid nodule?
· Describe the management of papillary carcinoma, the most common of the thyroid cancers?

A 78-year-old female is brought to the emergency department (ED) for strange behavior. According to her family, she has been more sleepy and weak throughout the last week. She is acting more withdrawn and depressed and seems to respond to nonexistent external stimuli. When asked about her depression, she reports she is sad because a man in a clown suit who trains poodles keeps telling her she is going to die (or maybe she just has bad flashbacks to the circus when she was younger). She complains of abdominal cramps and blames it on "being plugged up," and her family reports no bowel movement for 2 days. She also notes chronic bone pain in her hips and back. That's about all you can get before the bad news clown returns.

A physical examination is notable only for a 3 cm irregular mass in her right breast (we're very impressed that you did a breast examination in the ED). The family thinks that the mass is new. Her neurological examination is normal, except for her apparent confusion.

Question 10.5.1 What finding would you expect from an ECG?
A) Peaked T-waves
B) Long QT interval
C) Short QT interval
D) Torsades de pointes

Answer 10.5.1 The correct answer is "C." This patient is likely to have hypercalcemia, probably from an undiagnosed metastatic breast cancer. The ECG in a patient with significant hypercalcemia will show a short QT interval with possibly J-waves (aka Osborne waves, more frequently seen in hypothermia); rarely there is diffuse ST elevation (which is more commonly seen in pericarditis). **Hypo**calcemia is associated with a long QT interval, which can occasionally lead to arrhythmias due to an R on T phenomenon (an R-wave of a PVC fuses with the previous T-wave predisposing to torsades de pointes). **Hyper**calcemia produces symptoms in the CNS (confusion, psychosis, depression), GI system (abdominal pain, cramps, constipation), kidneys (nephrolithiasis, polyuria, renal insufficiency), and musculoskeletal system (weakness, myopathy, osteoporosis). To help you remember the symptoms of hypercalcemia, use the phrase "stones, bones, moans, groans, and psychiatric overtones." "A," peaked T-waves, are associated with hyper**kalemia**.

Your patient's total serum calcium level is reported as 15.3 mg/dL (upper limit 10.4 mg/dL).

Question 10.5.2 What is the NEXT step in her treatment?
A) Moderately aggressive normal saline hydration
B) IV chlorthalidone administration
C) IV calcitonin administration
D) PO bisphosphonate
E) IV glucocorticoids

Answer 10.5.2 The correct answer is "A." Although "C" and "D" may be indicated, adequate hydration and establishing urine output is critical to the treatment of hypercalcemia and should be the next step. A normal saline infusion will increase urinary calcium excretion by inhibiting proximal tubular sodium and calcium reabsorption. **Note that IV furosemide (and diuretics in general) are falling out of favor and should not be used. Hydration is the most important goal.** An IV bisphosphonate infusion (not PO, "D"), such as zoledronic acid, should be started concurrently and will lower the calcium level over 2 to 4 days. Calcitonin has a limited duration of action and can be used in emergencies where saline is ineffective. Glucocorticoids are generally useful in hypercalcemia secondary to granulomatous diseases and some lymphomas neither of which our patient has. "B" is of special note. Chlorthalidone and other thiazide diuretics **increase** calcium levels and are contraindicated. In addition to the above, dialysis can be used in a hypercalcemic emergency (generally in patients with unresponsive severe hypercalcemia [e.g., those with renal failure]).

⋯⋯⋯⋯⋯⋯⋯⋯⋯⋯⋯⋯⋯⋯⋯⋯⋯⋯⋯⋯⋯⋯⋯⋯⋯⋯⋯⋯⋯⋯

The patient is treated appropriately for her hypercalcemia and her mental status improves. A biopsy of her breast mass is done and reveals an infiltrating ductal carcinoma. A bone scan reveals diffuse metastatic disease.

Question 10.5.3 Which of the following statements about the mechanism for malignancy-associated hypercalcemia is/are TRUE?
A) Decreased bone reabsorption increases the serum calcium
B) Secretion of osteoclast-inhibiting factors increases the serum calcium
C) Secretion of parathyroid hormone (PTH)-like substances increases the serum calcium
D) Direct erosion of bone by tumor cells does not cause hypercalcemia
E) All of the above

Answer 10.5.3 The correct answer is "C." This is a case of humoral hypercalcemia of malignancy (HHM). Secretion of PTH-like substances causes retention of calcium by the kidneys, which elevates the serum calcium. Tumors can also produce osteoclast-**activating** (not inhibiting as in answer "B") factors leading to increased bone resorption and elevation of the serum calcium (remember that osteoblasts deposit bone and osteoclasts reabsorb bone). Finally, direct erosion of bone by tumor cells also contributes to the release of calcium from the bones (and predisposes the patient to fractures). The neoplasms most commonly associated with hypercalcemia are cancers of the breast, lung, prostate, and kidney as well as multiple myeloma and a few other hematologic cancers.

Question 10.5.4 Your patient's cancer cannot be cured. How can her chronically elevated calcium level be managed?
A) Oral glucocorticoids
B) Oral phosphates
C) Oral bisphosphonates
D) All of the above

Answer 10.5.4 The correct answer is "D." Glucocorticoids (e.g., prednisone 20–40 mg/day) *decrease intestinal calcium absorption*, but in and of themselves can lead to bone density loss and an increased risk for fractures. Oral phosphates can decrease intestinal calcium absorption and bone reabsorption of calcium. Bisphosphonates, as previously discussed, decrease the serum calcium and increase bone density.

HELPFUL TIP:
Granulomatous diseases like tuberculosis, sarcoidosis, Crohn disease, and leprosy are associated with hypercalcemia because of increased levels of active vitamin D.

▸ **Objectives: Did you learn to …**
- Recognize neoplastic causes of hypercalcemia?
- Identify presenting symptoms of hypercalcemia?
- Understand the mechanisms underlying hypercalcemia in malignancy?
- Initiate emergency treatment for symptomatic hypercalcemia?

▶ CASE 10.6

A 42-year-old male presents to the office for routine follow-up of his hypertension. He denies any complaints. He has primary hypertension, for which he takes benazepril 20 mg PO daily and hydrochlorothiazide 25 mg PO daily. The patient takes no other medications. His vital signs are as follows: BP 135/70 mm Hg, P 72 bpm, R 18, and T 98.6°F. The physical examination is completely normal. His calcium is elevated at 12.8 mg/dL (upper limit normal 10.4 mg/dL). The rest of his electrolytes, BUN, and creatinine are normal as is a CBC and ECG. "Hmm …" you think. "This calcium level could be falsely elevated."

Question 10.6.1 Which of the following is/are responsible for spuriously elevated serum calcium?
A) High phosphate diet
B) Fever and active metabolic state
C) Use of alendronate or risedronate
D) Prolonged application of the tourniquet while drawing blood
E) All of the above

Answer 10.6.1 The correct answer is "D." Prolonged application of the tourniquet or a high calcium meal before a blood draw can cause a spuriously elevated serum calcium. In fact, up to 50% of patients with hypercalcemia have a normal calcium when it is checked a second time. So, the next step after finding elevated calcium is to repeat the test. "A" and "C" will cause a low calcium level.

Question 10.6.2 Assuming you repeat the laboratory value and the calcium remains elevated, your next step is:
A) A bone scan for occult cancer
B) Immediate dialysis
C) Nothing, since the patient is asymptomatic
D) Discontinue the hydrochlorothiazide and re-check calcium in 2 weeks
E) Discontinue the benazepril and re-check potassium in 2 weeks

Answer 10.6.2 The correct answer is "D." This patient has hypercalcemia. Asymptomatic hypercalcemia is not uncommon on routine screening examinations. It should be addressed because it is always abnormal and can be treated early before any symptoms develop. In this patient, the most likely cause is hydrochlorothiazide. Thiazide drugs increase the renal reabsorption of calcium. Angiotensin-converting enzyme (ACE) inhibitors may cause hyperkalemia but are usually not associated with hypercalcemia. An investigation for occult cancer may be in this patient's future, but it is reasonable to address the potential adverse drug effect first. Dialysis is not indicated.

Being the smart practitioner that you are, you think that the hypercalcemia could be related to his hydrochlorothiazide use, so you ask him to stop it. He returns for a laboratory draw 2 weeks later. The calcium level is now 12.9 mg/dL. "Rats," you say. "Where's my thinking cap—I mean iPad?"

Question 10.6.3 What should you do next?
A) Wait another month and re-check before taking any other action
B) Order a 24-hour bisphosphonate infusion
C) Perform prostate and testicular examination for masses, chest x-ray, and serum assay for intact PTH (iPTH)
D) Perform prostate and testicular examination for masses, chest/abdomen/pelvis CT, and bone scan
E) Perform prostate and testicular examination for masses, chest x-ray, then reassure patient if normal

Answer 10.6.3 The correct answer is "C." In this patient, it is reasonable to rule out primary hyperparathyroidism while also checking for other potential causes. A chest x-ray will rule out significant lung masses and sarcoidosis. A testicular and prostate examination for masses is important so that **large** tumors in these organs do not go unnoticed (remembering that a digital rectal examination is neither sensitive nor specific as a screening test for prostate cancer, but it may be useful in conjunction with prostate-specific antigen testing if prostate cancer is on your differential). An elevated or high normal iPTH in the presence of hypercalcemia confirms the diagnosis of hyperparathyroidism after ruling out familial hypocalciuric hypercalcemia. *The test for iPTH will not significantly cross-react with the PTH-like hormone produced by neoplasms.* Unless the history or physical is suspicious for lymphoma, or some other occult neoplasm, a pan-body scan is a waste of money and exposes the patient to unnecessary radiation. At this point, it is not necessary to acutely lower the calcium level because the cause has not been identified and the patient is asymptomatic. See Table 10-1 for more causes of hypercalcemia.

TABLE 10-1 CAUSES OF HYPERCALCEMIA

Pseudohypercalcemia (from elevated albumin or rarely in multiple myeloma....an ionized calcium will be normal).
Excessive calcium intake
Hypervitaminosis D
Hyperparathyroidism (primary and secondary)
Hyperthyroidism
Malignancy
Hypervitaminosis A
Adrenal insufficiency
Pheochromocytoma
Rhabdomyolysis
Familial hypocalciuria
Immobilization
Medications
- Lithium
- Megestrol
- Methyltestosterone
- Mycophenolate
- Tacrolimus
- Tamoxifen
- Theophylline (toxicity)
- Thiazides

The patient's complete examination is normal as is the chest x-ray. The iPTH level is twice the upper limit of normal and his urinary calcium scores, which should be done as part of the workup of hypercalcemia (24-hour urinary calcium excretion and his calcium-to-creatinine clearance rate) are *not* suggestive of familial hypocalciuric hypercalcemia (a discussion of which is outside the scope of this book).

Question 10.6.4 **How should this patient be treated?**
A) Immediate CT of the chest, abdomen, and pelvis
B) IV bisphosphonate infusion
C) Daily dialysis until the calcium level is normal
D) Referral for parathyroidectomy
E) Referral for thyroidectomy

Answer 10.6.4 **The correct answer is "D."** This patient has primary hyperparathyroidism. Patients with symptomatic primary hyperparathyroidism (e.g., nephrolithiasis, symptomatic hypercalcemia) should have parathyroid surgery, which is the only definitive therapy. In asymptomatic patients, surgical indications also include a serum calcium level greater than 1.0 mg/dL over the upper limit of the reference range, a creatinine clearance less than 60 mL/min, a 24-hour urinary calcium >400 mg/day, nephrolithiasis or nephrocalcinosis by imaging, bone density T-scores less than −2.5 in any area, a previous osteoporotic fracture, and age less than 50 years. In elderly patients with mild hyperparathyroidism and asymptomatic hypercalcemia, medical management is an option. If the iPTH is low, then measuring the parathyroid hormone-related peptide (PTHrp, which is made by malignancies) and vitamin D metabolites is needed to further work up the cause. If PTHrp is elevated, a bone scan or body CT may be warranted. Although bisphosphonates will lower the serum calcium and may be used in an emergency, a parathyroidectomy is curative. Dialysis is not indicated in this patient.

Your patient undergoes a parathyroidectomy and is discharged from the hospital. The pathology report on the removed tissue confirms the presence of a parathyroid adenoma and no malignancy. He returns for his first postoperative appointment 1 week later, and he is complaining of weakness. He says that the day after the surgery he felt fine but has progressively gotten weaker since that time. Last night, he was kept awake by recurrent muscle spasms in his legs and arms. He denies fever, chills, nausea, or vomiting. He says he is eating, drinking, and passing urine normally. He has had no hematuria or dysuria. His vital signs are normal.

On physical examination, he appears anxious. Just after taking the patient's vital signs, his left arm develops a muscle spasm and an involuntary flexion of the wrist that lasts for about 20 to 30 seconds. Tapping the cheek just anterior to the tragus causes the ipsilateral face to twitch (to your great delight … it is just like in the books!). The rest of cranial nerve examination is normal. His neck wound is healing well, with minimal erythema and no tenderness. The rest of the physical examination is unremarkable.

Question 10.6.5 **What is causing this patient's symptoms?**
A) He suffers from vitamin D deficiency
B) This patient has MEN II and also has a pheochromocytoma
C) Too much parathyroid tissue was removed during the surgery
D) The stress of the surgery precipitated thyrotoxicosis
E) The stress of the surgery precipitated the onset of multiple sclerosis

Answer 10.6.5 **The correct answer is "C."** This patient likely has **hypo**calcemia due to excessive removal of parathyroid gland tissue—a rare and unfortunate complication of parathyroidectomy. It is usually detected in the immediate postoperative course. The patient's physical examination demonstrates Chvostek sign (tapping over the facial nerve elicits a twitch) and Trousseau signs (carpopedal spasm after placement of a blood pressure cuff). Vitamin D deficiency, although a cause of hypocalcemia, is unlikely to develop so quickly. The usual causes of vitamin D deficiency are malabsorption or inadequate intake. There is nothing to suggest MEN II (hyperparathyroidism, medullary thyroid carcinoma, and pheochromocytoma). There is also nothing here to suggest pheochromocytoma (episodic diaphoresis, labile blood pressure, recurrent palpitations, and near-syncope). There is no clinical evidence of thyrotoxicosis (tachycardia, tremor, etc.).

HELPFUL TIP:
Another consideration for a patient who had a recent parathyroidectomy for primary hyperparathyroidism: "hungry bone syndrome" (great name, right?), in which the unmineralized bone matrix produced during the period of hyperparathyroidism begins to mineralize after the PTH has normalized. This results in hypocalcemia and hypophosphatemia.

HELPFUL TIP:
It is always difficult to remember the MEN types. Here is a tip for you by Dr. Mark Yoffe (who wanted to see his name in print … and a shout-out to his mom!).
MEN 1: the number "1" in MEN1 should remind you of **p**rimary or **p**rime number. MEN1 involves things that start with the letter **P**:

- **P**ituitary adenoma
- **P**arathyroid hyperplasia
- **P**ancreatic islet cell tumors (gastrinoma, insulinoma, glucagonoma)

MEN 2A: happens to involve the letter **C** (This is MEN **2**A, so there are two C's in each item!):

- **C**al**c**itonin (medullary **c**arcinoma of the thyroid with elevated **c**alcitonin level)
- **C**al**c**ium (parathyroid hyperplasia, which causes elevated **c**alcium levels)
- **C**ate**c**holamines which are made in the **c**hromo**c**ytes (as in pheo**c**hromo**c**ytoma)

MEN 2B: **B** is for **b**ig (marfanoid habitus) and for **b**elly problems (mucosal neuromas)

. . . .

A calcium and albumin level is sent, as well as a CBC and routine chemistry panel including magnesium. Everything is normal except: calcium 5.1 mg/dL (8.8–10.4 mg/dL) and albumin 3.0 g/dL (3.4–5.0 g/dL). His phosphate level is 4.2 mg/dL (2.5–4.5 mg/dL).

Question 10.6.6 Does this patient have hypocalcemia?
A) No, the serum calcium level is normal
B) No, the serum calcium level when corrected for the albumin is normal
C) Yes, because the serum calcium-phosphate product is >20
D) Yes, because the serum calcium level is still low when corrected for albumin
E) Not enough information given to determine

Answer 10.6.6 **The correct answer is "D."** The patient's calcium level is low, even after correcting for hypoalbuminemia. To correct for albumin, add 0.8 mg/dL to the serum calcium level for each 1 g/dL the albumin is <4 g/dL. In other words, corrected serum calcium = [(4 – albumin) × 0.8] + measured serum calcium. In this case the equation is [(4 – 3) × 0.8] + 5.1 = 5.9 mg/dL. When evaluating hypocalcemia, it is prudent to check a BUN and creatinine to rule out renal failure as a cause (from renal osteodystrophy … see Chapter 5 for more information).

HELPFUL TIP:
If you want to take the easy route and avoid the math, check an ionized calcium. The ionized calcium need not be corrected for albumin. An ionized calcium will also be useful in patients with monoclonal gammopathy or multiple myeloma. Occasionally, these proteins can also bind calcium.

Question 10.6.7 How should this patient now be treated?
A) Calcium gluconate 1 g by rapid IV push
B) Correct his hypomagnesemia with IV MgSO₄
C) Administer IV normal saline 1 L bolus
D) Initiate calcium carbonate 1 to 4 g with vitamin D orally divided in two to three doses daily
E) No therapy, as the calcium level will correct itself

Answer 10.6.7 **The correct answer is "D."** The patient now requires oral calcium supplementation, usually given with vitamin D to stimulate absorption. He will likely require vitamin D and calcium supplementation for the rest of his life. This patient has neither hypomagnesemia nor hyperphosphatemia, nor any other electrolyte abnormalities. If he had, correcting either would also raise the serum calcium. "A" deserves special mention. IV calcium gluconate or calcium chloride is usually indicated for severe hypocalcemia with signs and symptoms (e.g., tetany, seizures, or prolonged QT), but they should not be given by rapid IV push but rather by slow push over a couple of minutes.

▸ **Objectives: Did you learn to …**
- Describe the evaluation and treatment of primary hyperparathyroidism?
- Recognize the signs and symptoms of hypocalcemia and hypercalcemia?
- Recognize the causes of hypercalcemia and hypocalcemia?
- Evaluate and treat hypocalcemia?

▶ CASE 10.7

A 36-year-old female presents to the office complaining of difficulty losing weight for 2 years. She seeks a prescription drug to aid in these efforts. She has tried every fad diet she comes across (grapefruit, banana, alkaline diet, blood-type diet, etc.), but nothing seems to help. She tries to exercise regularly but manages only walking a couple of miles each week. A nutritional history reveals that she is eating a sensible low-fat diet (how often do you see that!). Her past medical history includes hypertension treated with medications for the last 3 years and type 2 diabetes mellitus (DM2) treated for 1 year. She also has been seeing a psychiatrist over the last 6 months for emotional lability, which she blames on anxiety over her inability to get pregnant. The patient takes glyburide 5 mg PO daily and chlorthalidone 25 mg PO daily. A review of systems reveals thinning hair, irregular menses, delayed wound healing, and infertility (she's been trying to get pregnant for over 1 year).

Question 10.7.1 What advice do you offer this patient now?
A) She is eating right; she just needs to exercise more
B) Low-fat diets are ineffective; she needs to reduce her carbohydrate intake
C) She has failed lifestyle modifications, and appetite suppressant medications are indicated

D) She is likely depressed and needs to continue psychiatric therapy and probably should start treatment with a selective serotonin-reuptake inhibitor (SSRI)

E) Reserve any dietary advice at this time, as she first needs a medical workup

Answer 10.7.1 The correct answer is "E." The patient's symptoms of weight gain and associated findings on review of systems (emotionally labile, thinning hair, infertility, irregular menses, and delayed wound healing) suggest a secondary cause, most likely an endocrine abnormality. (What else would you expect? This is the endocrine chapter after all ….)

Her vitals in the office: P 88 bpm, BP 155/94 mm Hg, R 20, and T 37.7°C. On physical examination, you note an obese female with truncal obesity and thin extremities. She has thinning hair, round facies, hirsutism, and a buffalo hump at her upper back. Her skin is hyperpigmented with abdominal striae. The rest of the examination is unremarkable.

Question 10.7.2 Based on this patient's history and physical examination, what diagnosis is most likely?
A) Hypothyroidism
B) Hyperthyroidism
C) Cortisol excess secondary to chronic steroid therapy
D) Cortisol excess secondary to an endogenous process
E) Cortisol deficiency secondary to autoimmune adrenal insufficiency

Answer 10.7.2 The correct answer is "D." This patient has the classic symptoms and signs of Cushing *syndrome*, or cortisol excess. This may be due to corticosteroid therapy (the most common cause), ectopic ACTH production from neoplasms (lung, pancreas, kidney, etc.), adrenal neoplasms producing cortisol, or ACTH-production from a pituitary neoplasm (termed Cushing *disease*). Her condition is unlikely due to steroid therapy, as this should have been revealed in her medical history. At this point in the evaluation, it is not clear what the source of the ACTH is, just that there is excess ACTH being produced. Note that the hyperpigmentation of this patient's skin indicates an ACTH excess. ACTH stimulates melanocytes causing the hyperpigmentation. Hyperpigmentation will not be seen with exogenous steroid use. The same mechanism is in play in Addison's secondary to adrenal destruction; the pituitary is pumping out ACTH in an attempt to flog the adrenals into producing cortisol. Other skin findings may include easy bruisability, purplish striae, and skin atrophy.

Labs are sent, most of which are normal except for an elevated glucose of 210 mg/dL and an elevated 24-hour urinary free cortisol of 115 μg (normal <100 μg). Based on these findings, a dexamethasone suppression test is ordered. The patient is given huge (gargantuan, way big), supratherapeutic dexamethasone doses for 2 days, and then serum ACTH is drawn, and another 24-hour urine collection is done. The

repeat serum ACTH is still *slightly* elevated and 24-hour urinary free cortisol is 78 μg (normal).

Question 10.7.3 What is the source of this patient's cortisol excess?
A) An ACTH-producing tumor
B) A cortisol-producing adrenal tumor
C) Surreptitious use of oral steroids
D) Not enough information to determine

Answer 10.7.3 The correct answer is "A." When the patient was given exogenous steroids during the test, there was a partial suppression of cortisol production (a decrease in 24-hour urinary free cortisol). But more importantly, the serum ACTH level remained above normal despite the high steroid load. The ACTH level should have been low in the presence of dexamethasone, or any exogenous steroid, which would act to shut off ACTH production in the normal patient. If ACTH is still being produced despite a high steroid load, then there must be an ACTH-producing neoplasm somewhere in the body (either ectopic production from a lung, renal, or pancreatic cancer, or an ACTH-producing pituitary tumor that has escaped normal regulatory feedback mechanisms).

On physical examination, the patient has a visual field cut.

Question 10.7.4 What is the best next step in this patient's evaluation?
A) Ultrasound of kidneys to assess for masses and adrenal flow
B) CT scan of the brain to rule out metastatic lesions and assess pituitary size
C) CT scan of the adrenals to evaluate for adrenal neoplasms
D) MRI of the pancreas to evaluate for neoplasms
E) MRI of the pituitary gland to evaluate for a neoplasm

Answer 10.7.4 The correct answer is "E." The previous studies strongly suggest Cushing syndrome and the visual field cut suggests a pituitary source of excess ACTH (e.g., ACTH-producing tumor of the pituitary gland). An MRI of the pituitary is the best means to confirm this. CT scan may suggest enlargement of the sella turcica (where the pituitary gland sits), but it is insensitive for detecting abnormalities in the pituitary, especially microadenomas.

HELPFUL TIP:
If the MRI is negative, then the rarer case of ectopic ACTH production from occult cancer must be considered, and a body CT scan is indicated.

▶ **Objectives: Did you learn to …**
- Recognize the common presenting signs and symptoms of Cushing syndrome?
- Differentiate Cushing syndrome from Cushing disease?
- Identify the causes of cortisol excess and how they are best evaluated?

▶ CASE 10.8

JFK is a 38-year-old male presenting to the office with the chief complaint of weakness. He reports that he lacks the energy to complete his previously busy work schedule (such as invading Cuba) and has cut his hours back the last 2 to 3 weeks, which has recently become a financial hardship. He also reports poor appetite and a 20-lb weight loss over the last month. He has had alternating periods of diarrhea and constipation. He is often feeling faint and has come near to passing out after standing up quickly a few times; this is different for him from baseline. He used to rescue sailors at sea. He has no previous medical or surgical history. He denies medications or allergies. He reports that several of his relatives on his mother's side have had thyroid problems. "I can't go on like this," he complains in an accent that betrays his Boston roots.

On physical examination, his vitals reveal BP 85/38 mm Hg, P 85 bpm, R 20, and T 37°C. The examination shows hyperpigmentation of buccal mucosa and weakness in the proximal musculature (4+/5 strength in both upper and lower extremities) but with normal reflexes and sensation in all extremities. His skin is hyperpigmented at the elbows, knuckles, knees, and the palmar creases. There is no edema.

Question 10.8.1 What is the most likely cause of this patient's symptoms?
A) Hyperthyroidism
B) Hypothyroidism
C) Adrenal gland hyperactivity
D) Adrenal insufficiency
E) Depression

Answer 10.8.1 **The correct answer is "D."** Several clues point you in this direction, aside from the patient's name. First, the hyperpigmentation found at stress/crease points on the skin suggests the diagnosis of adrenal insufficiency. The low blood pressure and orthostasis is also more likely to be seen in adrenal insufficiency.

This patient has a number of symptoms consistent with both depression and hypothyroidism ("B" and "E"), but his physical examination suggests another diagnosis. A patient with depression and no underlying medical cause would have a normal physical examination. A patient with hypothyroidism may have a slightly low blood pressure, but not markedly low as in this patient. The heart rate in symptomatic hypothyroidism is usually low. Hypothyroidism may also cause changes in the hair, skin, and thyroid gland that are not seen here. Finally, the patient's reflexes are normal, rather than delayed. There is nothing in this case to suggest hyperthyroidism or cortisol excess ("A" or "C").

Laboratory results show a low sodium (129 mg/dL), low glucose (69 mg/dL), and high potassium (5.4 mg/dL) along with a normal TSH and a mildly low hemoglobin.

Question 10.8.2 Based on the information provided thus far, what is the best test to diagnose this patient's condition?
A) Cosyntropin stimulation test
B) Random serum cortisol
C) Bone marrow biopsy
D) Plasma renin
E) Ultrasound of kidneys to measure their size

Answer 10.8.2 **The correct answer is "A."** The laboratory chemistry results (hyperkalemia, hyponatremia, and hypoglycemia), combined with the history and physical examination, strongly suggest a mineralocorticoid deficiency. A cosyntropin stimulation test uses synthetic ACTH to try to induce a burst of cortisol secretion. No adequate increase in the serum cortisol in response to the cosyntropin suggests that the adrenal glands are unable to respond to the body's mineralocorticoid and glucocorticoid needs. A positive cosyntropin test makes the diagnosis of adrenal insufficiency. A random serum cortisol is definitely second best, as cortisol levels normally fluctuate widely throughout the diurnal cycle. Plasma renin is used in the evaluation of mineralocorticoid *excess* (hyperaldosteronism) and should be **low in adrenal insufficiency secondary to adrenal dysfunction** (aldosterone causes sodium reabsorption and potassium excretion, the exact opposite seen in this patient whose adrenals don't make aldosterone). "E" is not likely to be helpful. Even in the case of adrenal insufficiency, the kidneys are unlikely to change in size. Although an ultrasound may show small, shrunken adrenals that have been destroyed by tuberculosis, a CT scan is a better tool for assessing the adrenals. "C" is way off base. This patient has no indication for a bone marrow biopsy.

HELPFUL TIP:
An early morning serum cortisol level is often low in patients with adrenal insufficiency. However, this test alone is insufficient for screening, as it has a high false-negative rate. But a low (<5 μg/dL) early morning serum cortisol is likely to be due to adrenal insufficiency.

HELPFUL TIP:
Interpreting the cosyntropin stimulation test is not always straightforward. The current criteria used to indicate normal adrenal function are a minimum serum cortisol concentration ≥18 to 20 mcg/dL (500–550 nmol/L) BEFORE OR AFTER corticotropin injection. An algorithm is available at http://www.arupconsult.com/Algorithms/AdrenalInsufficiency.pdf

Further laboratory results are as follows:
Random serum cortisol: 4 μg/dL (normal >/= 20 μg/dL)
Serum cortisol 1 hour after 0.25 mg cosyntropin IV: 4.5 μg/dL (low)

Question 10.8.3 Based on the prevalence in the United States, what is the most likely underlying cause of this patient's condition?
A) Autoimmune disease
B) Invasive carcinoma
C) Meningococcal septicemia
D) Sarcoidosis
E) Tuberculosis

Answer 10.8.3 The correct answer is "A." All the conditions listed are known causes of *primary* adrenal insufficiency, and all cause this disorder by destruction of the adrenal glands. However, in the United States the most common cause is autoimmune destruction of the adrenal glands; tuberculosis is the most common cause worldwide. Adrenal destruction will result in a lack of adrenal hormone secretion and a blunted response of the adrenals to ACTH—hence, the minimal rise of cortisol despite administration of synthetic ACTH (cosyntropin). Cortisol level after cosyntropin stimulation test should be higher than 18 to 20 mcg/dL (500 to 550 nmol/L) in patients with normal adrenal function.

....

Without measuring the serum ACTH or 24-hour urine ACTH level, it is still possible to tell the difference between primary (lack of adrenal response to ACTH) and secondary (pituitary lack of ACTH) adrenal insufficiency.

Question 10.8.4 Which of the following suggests primary adrenal insufficiency (e.g., adrenal destruction) rather than secondary?
A) Baseline serum cortisol level >7 μg/dL
B) Presence of hyperpigmentation on physical examination
C) Presence of neuropathy on physical examination
D) Predominant symptoms of depression

Answer 10.8.4 The correct answer is "B." Hyperpigmentation at skin creases occurs in primary adrenal insufficiency (but not secondary adrenal insufficiency). This is because in primary adrenal insufficiency, the **pituitary** is intact. As a result, the ACTH level is high, as is the level of melanocyte-stimulating hormone. It is this melanocyte-stimulating hormone that causes hyperpigmentation. An early morning baseline serum cortisol level of 5 mcg/dL or above ("A") would suggest primary adrenal insufficiency **unlikely** (the adrenals are still making cortisol). Hypoglycemia and depression ("D") are symptoms common to all causes of adrenal insufficiency so don't differentiate between primary adrenal failure and secondary causes of adrenal insufficiency. Neuropathy ("C") is not a common finding in adrenal insufficiency.

HELPFUL TIP:
Patients with primary adrenal insufficiency **may** present with low serum sodium and high serum potassium (although many will have normal electrolytes). This is primarily because of loss of the aldosterone

system. Patients with secondary adrenal insufficiency (e.g., pituitary cause) have intact adrenal glands and therefore intact aldosterone production. Thus, they will generally have normal electrolytes and less dehydration, hypotension, etc.

Question 10.8.5 How should this patient now be treated?
A) Prednisone 60 mg PO for 5 days, then slowly tapered over 2 weeks
B) Cosyntropin 0.5 mg SC daily indefinitely
C) Corticosteroids (prednisone 5 mg or hydrocortisone 15 mg) daily indefinitely
D) Corticosteroids (prednisone 5 mg or hydrocortisone 15 mg) daily plus mineralocorticoid (fludrocortisone 0.1 mg) daily indefinitely
E) Adrenal transplant

Answer 10.8.5 The correct answer is "D." This patient requires chronic corticosteroid supplementation, and because he has primary adrenal insufficiency, he also requires mineralocorticoid supplementation. Usually, mineralocorticoid administration is not necessary in the acute setting, like adrenal crisis, but the vast majority of patients with primary adrenal insufficiency eventually require mineralocorticoid replacement with fludrocortisone. Cosyntropin treatment ("B") would have no effect since the adrenals are not functioning. A short burst of prednisone ("A") is important if this patient experiences a sudden stressor, such as an infection, but it is not the primary therapy. Medical therapy is fairly effective, so adrenal (or renal) transplant ("E") is not a usual treatment option.

....

JFK is treated appropriately and, after 4 weeks, is feeling much better, has regained most of his lost weight, and feels well enough to take on both Castro *and* Khrushchev (local competitors to his dry-cleaning business). He no longer suffers spells of lightheadedness or depression. To celebrate his new good health, he and a blond starlet go out for a lavish seafood dinner, including fresh oysters. Within 8 hours of the meal, JFK develops severe cramping abdominal pain and profuse watery diarrhea (so much for the date …). He tries to treat himself at home with Pepto–Bismol and oral fluids but becomes progressively weaker. After 12 hours of intestinal symptoms, he calls for an ambulance because he is too weak to stand.

Upon presentation in the ED, his vital signs are: P 130 bpm, BP 70/20 mm Hg, R 30, and T 38°C. He is diaphoretic, ill-appearing, and in severe distress.

Question 10.8.6 After establishing adequate IV access, what should be done next?
A) Order a chest x-ray
B) Start "renal-dose" dopamine through a peripheral line
C) Give 2 L normal saline by bolus
D) Start normal saline at 125 cc/hr
E) Give levofloxacin 500 mg IV

Answer 10.8.6 The correct answer is "C." This patient is severely volume depleted and needs crystalloid immediately. All other treatment concerns, although they may eventually be done, are secondary.

Despite fluid boluses, he remains hypotensive. You scratch your head and ponder what you may have forgotten.

Question 10.8.7 What should have been done simultaneously for this patient when the fluids were started?
A) Intubation by rapid sequence and mechanical ventilation
B) Administration of a phenylephrine drip
C) Administration of 4 mg dexamethasone IV
D) Administration of 100 mg hydrocortisone IV
E) C or D.

Answer 10.8.7 The correct answer is "E." This patient has adrenal insufficiency and requires additional "stress doses" of steroids in times of severe physical stress (e.g., infection, trauma, myocardial ischemia). The steroids he regularly takes for his disease may not be sufficient during these periods, precipitating addisonian crisis. Without this additional treatment, the patient may experience intractable hypotension and possibly death. In a less acute situation in which the patient has a minor illness, two to three times the usual maintenance glucocorticoid dose for 3 days (known as the "3 × 3 rule") may benefit the patient.

HELPFUL TIP:
If you suspect adrenal insufficiency crisis (addisonian crisis), start steroids immediately even if you do not have laboratory confirmation. Dexamethasone is an option for treatment, and it will not interfere with the cortisol assay when doing a cosyntropin stimulation test. **But note that dexamethasone does not have mineralocorticoid activity and should be replaced by hydrocortisone succinate just as soon as the cosyntropin stimulation test is done.**

The next day when you are doing your inpatient rounding, you meet your patient's cousin Kenneth, who is a 59-year-old white male with a past medical history of hypertension, COPD, alcohol abuse, and osteoarthritis in his shoulders and knees; he is an enthusiastic, if not clumsy, tennis player. A particularly enthusiastic colleague injected 80 mg of triamcinolone in both of the patient's knees and shoulders several months ago (total dose of 320 mg). He had just gone to a joint injection workshop and figured, what the heck, let's practice! The patient notes weakness, lightheadedness, nausea, and decreased appetite recently. His home medications are lisinopril and inhaled albuterol. Vitals are BP 70/44 mm Hg, HR 60 bpm, T 35.6°C, oxygen saturation 98%. Physical examination shows a mildly distressed patient with mild expiratory wheezing on auscultation and unsteady gait when he tries to stand up.

Lab results: sodium 123 mEq/L (low), K 3.8 mEq/L (normal), BUN 30 mg/dL (normal range <20 mg/dL), creatinine 2.1 mg/dL (patient's baseline is 0.6 mg/dL), Cl 84 mEq/L (low), and CO_2 26 mEq/L. CBC, LFTs, total protein, and albumin are normal. A troponin, TSH, urine drug screen, alcohol level, and urinalysis are also normal.

He receives a couple of liters of normal saline, and his blood pressure normalizes. A repeat lab shows sodium 130 mEq/dL and creatinine 1.1 mg/dL. One of your resident physicians decides to further workup the hyponatremia and checks the cortisol level, which returns 1.5 μg/dL (low) with ACTH at 18 pg/mL (normal 7–63 pg/mL). A cosyntropin stimulation test is done and the serum cortisol level goes up to 14.9 μg/dL.

Question 10.8.8 What is the most likely cause of the patient's hyponatremia?
A) Secondary adrenal insufficiency due to panhypopituitarism
B) Secondary adrenal insufficiency due to exogenous steroid use
C) COPD exacerbation
D) Hypothyroidism

Answer 10.8.8 The correct answer is "B." The patient received ridiculous doses of intra-articular triamcinolone several months ago causing adrenal suppression. "A" is incorrect because the initial ACTH is normal, which is not the typical finding for central causes of adrenal insufficiency. "C," COPD exacerbation, is not consistent with the adrenal function tests. "D," hypothyroidism, can cause fatigue and hyponatremia, but the patient's TSH is within the normal limits.

▶ **Objectives: Did you learn to …**
· Recognize the presentation of adrenal insufficiency?
· Evaluate a patient with adrenal insufficiency?
· Treat a patient chronically for adrenal insufficiency and when in adrenal crisis?
· Understand secondary adrenal insufficiency due to exogenous steroid use?

 QUICK QUIZ: DIABETES DIAGNOSIS

Which of the following can be used to diagnose diabetes mellitus (DM)?
A) Fasting blood glucose on one occasion
B) Glycosylated hemoglobin (HbA1C) on one occasion
C) A random blood sugar of >160 mg/dL
D) None of the above

The correct answer is "D." Here is why: The diagnosis of DM requires **two** elevated fasting blood sugars of ≥126 mg/dL or **two** HbA1c levels of ≥6.5%. It can also be diagnosed if the patient has a **single** random blood sugar of >200 mg/dL with typical signs and symptoms of DM (polyuria, polydipsia, weight loss, and blurred vision). To be complete, a 2-hour postprandial glucose tolerance test result of >200 after 1.75 g/kg of glucose (max dose 75 g) is diagnostic of DM. However, this is rarely used in the United States.

 QUICK QUIZ: A1c IN SPECIAL CONDITIONS

Which of the following conditions artificially *raises* the value of hemoglobin A1c (HbA1c)?
A) Iron deficiency anemia
B) Sickle cell disease
C) Chronic liver disease
D) Acute blood loss anemia
E) All of the above

The correct answer is "A." Iron deficiency may **falsely elevate** the HbA1c. Several other conditions can cause a **falsely low** HbA1c including sickle cell disease, malaria, acute blood loss, and hemolysis (see a pattern developing here?). This makes sense: in all these conditions the bone marrow is pumping out new cells that have not been exposed to the elevated glucose levels. Conversely, iron deficiency and vitamin B12 and folate deficiencies may be associated with falsely high HbA1c levels, which is due to the proportion of older red cells (and therefore more glycosylated cells) in the blood being high compared to the normal individual. Chronic kidney disease may cause either a falsely elevated or falsely low HbA1c.

▶ **CASE 10.9**

You are called to the ED to see a 17-year-old man brought in by his parents who found him in his room at home. He is lethargic, but not unconscious or comatose. He is unable to give a coherent history. His parents state that they have been concerned because the patient has been losing weight in the last 2 months and acting more tired than usual. They are worried that he might be abusing drugs, but have not found any drugs or drug paraphernalia in the home. They have observed no other signs of illness. The family history is positive for hypertension in multiple family members, and the patient's mother has hyperlipidemia. There is no family history of kidney or liver disease, heart attacks, strokes, diabetes, or cancer. His vitals are: T 36.9°C, P 125 bpm, BP 98/54 mm Hg, respirations are deep with a rate of 28, SpO2 95% on room air. He is lethargic and nonverbal but arouses to pain. His mucous membranes are dry with a fissured tongue. You smell a fruity aroma on his breath that reminds you of that bowl of fruity cereal you left at home. His breathing is fast and he is tachycardic. His abdominal examination reveals a soft abdomen with mild, generalized tenderness. No rebound or guarding.

EKG shows sinus tachycardia. CBC shows an Hgb 17.9 g/dL, WBC 16,200 cells/mm³ with neutrophil predominance, and platelets 650,000 cells/mm³. Electrolytes show sodium 131 mEq/L (slightly low), potassium 5.7 mEq/L (high), chloride 97 mEq/L, bicarbonate 10 mEq/L (low), BUN 63 mg/dL

(high), creatinine 1.8 mg/dL (baseline 0.7 mg/dL), and glucose 635 mg/dL (high). Serum ketones are positive. You are concerned about his respiratory status so you obtain a venous blood gas (just as good as an ABG in almost every circumstance and it hurts less ... and you can get the oxygen saturation off a monitor) on room air with pH 7.20, PaCO₂ 27 mm Hg, PaO₂ 101 mm Hg, and bicarbonate 10 mEq/L.

You diagnose diabetic ketoacidosis (DKA) with dehydration >10% and admit the patient to the intensive care unit. As the first stage of therapy you wish to replace the lost fluid volume.

Question 10.9.1 Which of the following regimens is the most appropriate initial intervention?
A) 5% dextrose in 0.45% (half-normal) saline to run at 150 cc/hr
B) 0.45% (half-normal) saline with 20 mEq potassium/L, to run at 150 cc/hr
C) 0.9% (normal) saline 1 L to infuse as quickly as possible
D) 0.9% (normal) saline with 20 mEq potassium/L to run at 1,000 cc/hr
E) 5% dextrose in 0.225% (quarter-normal) saline with 20 mEq potassium/L to run at 1,000 cc/hr

Answer 10.9.1 The correct answer is "C." Initial volume replacement should be with isotonic saline infused at a rapid rate until the volume deficit is corrected. "D" is of special note. In general, potassium should be added to the fluid later (often the second bag) unless the patient is already hypokalemic on the initial blood work (getting a potassium, glucose, and sodium on the first blood gas is good policy). Potassium replacement may be essential even in the hyperkalemic patient, as correction of the ketoacidosis leads to a rapid shift of potassium into the intracellular compartment. Remember that an acidosis artificially increases the serum potassium by shifting potassium extracellularly. The potassium increases by approximately 1 mEq/L for every pH point of 0.1 below 7.4 (so, a pH of 7.3 will increase the potassium from 4 to 5 mEq/L). See Chapter 5 for more on acidosis, alkalosis, and the effects on potassium. "D" is incorrect because you would like the first liter to infuse as quickly as possible in DKA and not over an hour. Besides, 20 mEq of potassium IV in 1 hour should not be routine and only given if the patient has continuous cardiac monitoring.

 HELPFUL TIP:
Patients with severe hyperglycemia (like this guy) will have hyponatremia secondary to the osmotic effect of glucose pulling water into the intravascular space, increasing the plasma water content. What is the corrected sodium for this patient? It is approximately 140 mEq/dL based on the formula: **corrected sodium = measured sodium + [1.6 (glucose − 100)/100]**. This is very approximate. If the glucose is >400 mg/dL, use "2" rather than 1.6 for the correction. As an aside, the bowl of fruity cereal the provider left at home? All of the colors of Fruit Loops taste exactly the same. Another bubble broken ...

HELPFUL TIP:
Urine ketones are >99% sensitive for DKA in the right circumstance. Thus, checking serum ketones is superfluous in most cases.

HELPFUL TIP:
When should you start insulin? When should you start potassium? The American Diabetes Association gives us guidance. (1) DO NOT start insulin if the potassium is LESS THAN 3.3 mEq/L. Give fluid and potassium replacement first. The risk of hypokalemia and arrhythmias is too great. (2) Start potassium in the patient with DKA if their potassium is <5.3 mEq/L; give 20 to 40 mEq/hr IV (cardiac monitored). Once you correct the acidosis the potassium will drop, of course.

Question 10.9.2 What is the most appropriate initial insulin regimen for this patient?
A) Subcutaneous NPH insulin, 1 unit/kg; repeat as necessary
B) IV regular insulin, 5 unit IV bolus, followed by constant infusion at 0.05 to 0.1 unit/kg/hr; adjusted as needed
C) Subcutaneous regular insulin, 0.5 to 1 unit/kg; adjust dose by fingerstick blood glucose results
D) Intramuscular regular insulin, 5 to 10 units hourly; adjust dose by fingerstick blood glucose results
E) Insulin glargine 10 units daily adjusted based on fasting glucose levels

Answer 10.9.2 The correct answer is "B." A bolus of IV regular insulin, followed by a constant infusion, adjusted to reduce the blood glucose level by 50 to 75 mg/dL/hr, is the appropriate therapy. This may frequently require >0.1 unit/hr, but 0.05 to 0.1 unit/kg/hr is a good place to start. Intramuscular insulin administration is an alternative, but absorption is unreliable, especially in hypotensive patients. Long-acting insulins and subcutaneous insulin administration have no place in the initial management of DKA.

HELPFUL TIP:
Although tradition, the bolus of regular insulin is unnecessary and does not change outcomes. Starting a drip of regular insulin is the critical step here.

Question 10.9.3 Which of the following types of insulin can be administered IV?
A) NPH insulin
B) Glargine insulin (e.g., Lantus)
C) Lente insulin
D) Ultralente insulin
E) None of the above

Answer 10.9.3 The correct answer is "E." The only insulin that can be administered IV is regular insulin. As an aside, some insulins are incompatible when mixed together in the same syringe. For example, insulin glargine should not be mixed with any other forms of insulin due to the low pH of its diluent. Further, phosphate-buffered insulins (e.g., NPH) should not be mixed with Lente insulins.

The patient's status improves, and you re-check his blood sugar. His glucose is now 200 mg/dL and his insulin drip is running at 5 units per hour. His pH is 7.30 with a bicarbonate level of 14 mEq/L.

Question 10.9.4 Given that his glucose has almost normalized, your reaction at this point is to:
A) Administer bicarbonate in order to finish correcting the pH
B) Decrease the rate of the insulin infusion to 2 units per hour
C) Add 5% to 10% dextrose to his IV fluids
D) Consider the addition of an oral hypoglycemic agent
E) Discontinue IV fluids and switch to oral rehydration

Answer 10.9.4 The correct answer is "C." This patient is still acidotic and will need continued insulin to reverse his catabolic state. Thus, the appropriate treatment is to increase the amount of sugar he is getting—add some dextrose to his IV fluids. Remember, DKA is not primarily a result of too much sugar but rather of too little insulin. "A" is incorrect. **Bicarbonate plays no role in the treatment of DKA no matter what the pH.** In fact, the administration of bicarbonate actually prolongs acidosis and ketosis and produces a paradoxical CNS acidosis. In addition, it shifts the oxygen disassociation curve to reduce oxygen delivery to the tissue. Finally, **the only predictor of cerebral edema in children treated for DKA is the administration of bicarbonate.** So, there is no need to restrict fluids in children being treated for DKA (although this does NOT mean you should over-hydrate them).

HELPFUL TIP:
The common causes of DKA: "the 5 I's" mnemonic.
    Insulin or medication noncompliance; Infection; myocardial Infarction; Incision (surgery); Incidental (new diagnosis of DM presenting with DKA). (Not by Dr. Mark Yofee … but still a shout out to his mom.)

Question 10.9.5 Which of the following statements is FALSE?
A) The Somogyi phenomenon occurs when a patient's blood sugar becomes elevated and there is a reactive hypoglycemia
B) Patients who are being treated appropriately for DKA may have an increase in serum ketones during treatment
C) An elevated WBC count is not a strong predictor of infection in patients with DKA
D) Glucagon is an inappropriate treatment of patients with alcoholic **hypo**glycemia

Answer 10.9.5 The correct answer (and false statement) is "A." Consensus is that **the Somogyi phenomenon does not exist regardless of what we were taught** (*N Engl J Med.* 1987;317(25):1552). **But just for the record,** it was thought to occur when a patient becomes **hypoglycemic** (often in the middle of the night) and experiences a reactive hyperglycemia from adrenergic outpouring. Actually, quite a different phenomenon appears to occur: nocturnal **hyper**glycemia is strongly associated with elevated morning glucose levels. All of the rest are true statements. "B" is correct because beta-hydroxybutyrate is metabolized to acetoacetic acid that will increase serum ketone measurements. "C" is true since DKA is a pro-inflammatory state and the WBC count is often elevated due to DKA and not infection. "D" is a true statement. Patients with alcoholic hypoglycemia have exhausted their glycogen stores and are also generally NAD deficient and thus have impaired gluconeogenesis. Thus, glucagon will not work. Another group on which glucagon will not work is the infant or child who becomes hypoglycemic overnight and has a seizure in the morning. They have already depleted their stores of glycogen.

HELPFUL TIP:
Consider the possibility of a silent myocardial infarction in a diabetic patient who is generally well-controlled but suddenly has elevated blood sugars.

HELPFUL TIP:
Twenty percent of patients with DKA have relatively "normoglycemic" DKA and present with a blood sugar under 300 mg/dL.

It is time to transition this patient to a home-going insulin regimen.

Question 10.9.6 Which of the following statements is FALSE regarding the use of insulin in this patient?
A) Insulin detemir and insulin glargine are both long-acting, essentially equivalent, and can (almost always) be used once a day as basal insulin
B) If you use NPH, start with 0.1 to 0.2 units/kg/day and give 2/3 in the AM and 1/3 HS
C) Regular insulin should be given with meals to cover blood sugars and generally requires 0.1 to 0.2 units/kg/day as a start
D) Metformin can markedly reduce the need for insulin in this patient
E) This patient's insulin need may markedly diminish over the next 2 weeks

Answer 10.9.6 The correct answer (which is false) is "D." Metformin is used only in DM2. By virtue of the fact that he's presenting with DKA, our patient almost assuredly has type 1 diabetes mellitus (DM1). The rest are true statements. Insulin detemir and glargine can both be used once a day in most patients (although not always). The starting dose of both regular and NPH insulin is about 0.1 to 0.2 units/kg/day for a total initial insulin dose of 0.2 to 0.4 units/kg/day to start. "E" refers to the "honeymoon period." Patients usually present with DM in relation to some metabolic stress. Once this stress resolves, the need for insulin may decrease markedly. Thus, close monitoring is required. (Editor's note: Yes, metformin has been studied in DM1 but seems to not lead to changes in the HbA1c [although it can reduce the insulin dose needed]).

HELPFUL TIP:
There is no outcome advantage to brand name insulins versus generic insulins (*JAMA* 2018 Jul 3; 320:53). Cost and convenience should be the main considerations in choosing one versus the other. Lantus, Novolog, and Humalog cost up to $250/bottle with generic NPH costing as little as $25/bottle.

HELPFUL TIP:
DKA often presents as an acute abdomen with abdominal pain, nausea and vomiting and can be mistaken for appendicitis, etc.

▶ **Objectives: Did you learn to …**
- Diagnose a patient with DKA?
- Initiate therapy in DKA?
- Identify causes of DKA?
- Realize that the Somogyi phenomenon is scary but not real (like Godzilla)?

 QUICK QUIZ: DIABETES PREVENTION

Which intervention has been shown to have the *greatest effect* in preventing or delaying the onset of DM2 in patients with impaired fasting glucose or impaired glucose tolerance?
A) Dietary modifications and increased activity
B) Early glipizide treatment
C) Early metformin treatment
D) Intensive fitness training
E) Weight loss >25% of baseline

The correct answer is "A." Metformin has been shown to have some benefit in delaying progression to diabetes but is less effective than diet and activity modifications. The studies showing benefit from lifestyle modifications used much less aggressive targets for weight loss and activity level than the 25% listed in answer "E." Thus, "E" is incorrect. Other medications that have been used (successfully) to reduce progression to diabetes include the thiazolidinediones ("glitazones") and acarbose. However, exercise and diet are superior to drugs. The benefit of drugs is marginal. In addition, the thiazolidinediones have significant downsides including edema and possibly increased cardiac events.

HELPFUL TIP:
Nonpharmacologic therapies that can reduce insulin resistance include engaging in 30 minutes of modest aerobic exercise 5 days per week (tell patients to aim for 150 minutes of exercise per week—how it's divided is not important), having high fiber in the diet, decreasing caloric intake (small portions), and losing weight. Magic pill? We're still waiting … However, weight loss surgery has been shown to "cure" diabetes in those with Type 2 DM and reverse hypertension and dyslipidemia in substantial minorities—up to 30% for diabetes, 50% for hypertension (*JAMA* 2018 Jan 16; 319:291 and *JAMA* 2018 Jan 16; 319:266).

QUICK QUIZ: DIABETIC RETINOPATHY

Which of the following interventions has NOT been shown to prevent loss of vision in patients with retinopathy due to type 2 diabetes?
A) Laser photocoagulation therapy
B) Aspirin
C) Tight glycemic control
D) Tight blood pressure control

The correct answer is "B." Aspirin has not been shown to be of any benefit in the Early Treatment Diabetic Retinopathy Study. All the other options have been shown to be useful in delaying the development of diabetic retinopathy or preventing its progression to visual loss.

▶ CASE 10.10

You are seeing a new patient in your office. He is a 47-year-old man with a presenting complaint of fatigue for several months. He denies fever, rigors, cough, nausea, or diarrhea. He has lost about 10 lb. Upon questioning him you discover that he is also having nocturia and is thirsty all the time. He has asthma, for which he uses an albuterol-metered dose inhaler occasionally. He has no other chronic medical problems and takes no other medications on a regular basis. He has a family history of diabetes, hypertension, and heart disease. He smokes about one pack per day, and he works as a teacher at the local high school. He is aware of no occupational exposure to toxins.

Physical examination reveals the following: T 37°C, BP 135/83 mm Hg, P 72 bpm, BMI 38 kg/m². Aside from obesity, the remainder of the examination is normal.

Laboratory test results reveal the following: normal CBC, BUN/creatinine, and electrolytes. You ask him to return to the office the next day for fasting laboratory tests, which reveal a fasting glucose of 123 mg/dL and an HbA1c of 7.5%.

Question 10.10.1 Does this patient have diabetes?
A) Yes; he has an elevated fasting glucose
B) Probably; he needs a second fasting glucose to confirm the diagnosis
C) Probably; he needs a second HbA1c to confirm the diagnosis
D) Yes; he has the classic symptoms of diabetes: fatigue, weight loss, and thirst, associated with an elevated glucose
E) Probably not; his HbA1c is not >8%

Answer 10.10.1 The correct answer is "C." If results of two different diagnostic tests for DM are discordant, the test that is diagnostic of diabetes should be repeated. "A" and "B" are incorrect because the fasting glucose is <126 mg/dL (the threshold for diabetes). "D" is incorrect because we do not have his random glucose value that is ≥200 mg/dL. "E" is incorrect because the A1c cutoff for diabetes diagnosis is ≥6.5%.

HELPFUL TIP:
The 2018 ADA guidelines recommend screening *all* asymptomatic adults every 3 years starting at age 45; earlier screening is recommended for adults at high risk of type 2 diabetes (BMI ≥25 kg/m²; first-degree relative with DM; history of CVD; habitual physical inactivity; high-risk race/ethnicity [African Americans, Asian Americans, Mexican Americans, Native Americans, Pacific Islanders, and Native Hawaiians]; previously identified impaired glucose tolerance; hypertension; dyslipidemia [HDL<35 or triglycerides >250]; history of gestational diabetes or delivery of a baby weighing >9 lb; and polycystic ovary syndrome). Pre-diabetics should be tested yearly. Of note, the USPSTF recommendations on *who* to screen for diabetes are similar, but include the age ranges of 40 to 70 years and do not specify a screening frequency.

Question 10.10.2 Assuming another A1c is above 6.5%, what further study must be done to complete the diagnosis of diabetes and determine whether the patient has type 1 or type 2 diabetes?
A) C-peptide level
B) Anti-islet cell antibodies
C) Anti-insulin antibodies
D) None of the above

Answer 10.10.2 The correct answer is "D." This patient's age, history, examination (BMI 38), and laboratory findings are consistent with the diagnosis of DM2. None of the other studies listed needs to be performed. However, if questions remain regarding the type of diabetes (which will then affect therapy, prognosis, follow-up, etc.), you may choose to perform further studies. In DM1, the C-peptide level (a marker of endogenous insulin production) is low. If it is equivocal, give a glucose load (e.g., large meal) and see if it goes up. If it goes up, the diagnosis is likely DM2. Anti-islet cell antibodies are present in 80% of type

1 diabetics and, if found in the patient with criteria for diabetes, are essentially diagnostic of type 1 diabetes. "C" is incorrect because anti-insulin antibodies have a low sensitivity for DM1 and may be elevated secondary to the use of exogenous insulin.

 HELPFUL TIP:
To be complete, anti-glutamic acid decarboxylase (anti-GAD) antibodies are present in 70% of patients with DM1 at the time of diagnosis.

Question 10.10.3 The pathologic factors involved in type 2 diabetes in adults include:
A) Pancreatic beta-cell destruction through a yet undetermined infectious process
B) The production of anti-insulin antibodies that cause precipitation of insulin/antibody complexes
C) Resistance to the effects of insulin at peripheral tissues and *a* relative insulin deficiency that is progressive over time
D) An autosomal-dominant process, with the diabetes gene located on the long arm of chromosome 18
E) Too much exercise and a complete lack of a "beer gut"

Answer 10.10.3 **The correct answer is "C."** DM2 is the result of the development of insulin resistance at the peripheral tissues (e.g., fat and muscle cells) and a relative lack of insulin compared to the increasing amount that the body requires. "A" is incorrect. Autoimmune destruction of beta-cells in the pancreas is responsible for causing DM1. "B" is incorrect, although there are anti-insulin antibodies found in **DM1**. "D" is incorrect as well, but there is a strong genetic component to DM2. The exact genetic factors that cause DM2 in adults have not been completely elucidated, but no single responsible gene is transmitted in an autosomal dominant fashion. "E" is incorrect because lack of exercise, weight gain, dietary factors, and truncal obesity (the "beer gut") predispose persons to the development of DM2.

You meet with the patient and his husband to go over the test results and explain the diagnosis of diabetes. Given his age, body habitus, and lack of exercise, you feel certain that this patient has type 2 diabetes. You provide some basic education on the nature of diabetes, its natural history, and what can be done to manage it.

Question 10.10.4 What is the *most* important next step for this patient?
A) Initiation of insulin therapy
B) Initiation of an ACE inhibitor
C) Referral to an endocrinologist
D) Diabetic education classes
E) Initiation of glyburide or other sulfonylurea

Answer 10.10.4 **The correct answer is "D."** A general education program that includes information on diet, disease management, and the family's role in successful diabetes care is the most important intervention listed. While specialist consultation may be useful in complex diabetic patients or in those who are not responding to treatment, primary care physicians provide care to the majority of patients with diabetes. Insulin therapy is not indicated at this point, and an ACE inhibitor may or may not be helpful depending on the patient's blood pressure and urine protein. "E" is also incorrect (keep reading to learn why).

Upon his return, you find that the patient's blood pressure is elevated. On three separate occasions, he has systolic pressure ≥140 and diastolic pressure ≥90 mm Hg.

Question 10.10.5 Which class of medications is the best choice for initial therapy of hypertension in diabetics?
A) ACE inhibitors
B) Calcium-channel blockers
C) Loop diuretics
D) Vasodilators
E) Beta-blockers

Answer 10.10.5 **The correct answer is "A."** ACE inhibitors have been shown to provide renal protection in patients with diabetes (types 1 and 2). Patients with albuminuria and hypertension will certainly benefit from an ACE inhibitor. Loop diuretics (e.g., furosemide) are not indicated for the **primary** treatment of hypertension in diabetics (or, really, anyone else). Angiotensin receptor blockers (ARBs) are a reasonable alternative in the hypertensive patient with albuminuria if an ACE inhibitor is not tolerated. Vasodilators and calcium-channel blockers are not optimal choices in this patient although *non-dihydropyridine* calcium channel blockers (verapamil, diltiazem) are an option for renal protection in patients with worsening albuminuria especially in those who cannot tolerate an ACE inhibitor or ARB. "E," beta-blockers, should not be used first line for treating hypertension in patients without cardiac disease.

Question 10.10.6 Which of the following is NOT a side effect of ACE inhibitors?
A) Acute renal failure
B) Hyperkalemia
C) Dry cough
D) Angioedema
E) Cooties

Answer 10.10.6 **The correct answer is "E."** All of those listed—except cooties—are side effects of ACE inhibitors. Cooties are airborne parasites for which obnoxious fourth-grade boys serve the main host. Hope you got your "cooties shot" when you were younger. If so, you should be fine.

Adverse effects of ACE inhibitors are due to either reduced angiotensin II formation or to increased kinin formation. Those related to reduced angiotensin II formation include hypotension, acute renal failure, hyperkalemia, and problems during pregnancy. Side effects thought to be related, at least in part, to increased kinins include cough, angioedema, and anaphylactoid reactions. Termination of the ACE inhibitor should be considered if hyperkalemia cannot be controlled or the serum creatinine concentration increases more than 30% above the baseline value within the first 6 to 8 weeks when blood pressure is reduced. Also, both ACE inhibitors and ARBs are contraindicated in pregnancy.

HELPFUL TIP:
Guidelines published by JNC8 (2014) and the ADA (2018) endorse higher blood pressure goals for hypertensive diabetics than was the case in prior guidelines. The blood pressure target for most diabetic patients is now <140/90 mm Hg. A lower target (e.g., 130/80) may be appropriate for certain individuals, such as younger patients, if it can be achieved without undue treatment burden.

After 3 months of dietary therapy and lifestyle modifications, the patient returns to see you with his husband. While he has been adherent to the recommendations given by you and the diabetes education staff, his HbA1c remains elevated at 7.9%. You decide to begin pharmacologic therapy.

Question 10.10.7 Which medication is the most appropriate *first-line* therapy for an obese patient with type 2 diabetes?
A) A thiazolidinedione ("glitazone" [e.g., Actos])
B) A sulfonylurea (e.g., glipizide)
C) Insulin
D) Metformin
E) A dipeptidyl peptidase-4 inhibitor (DPP-4 or "gliptin" [e.g., Januvia])

Answer 10.10.7 The correct answer is "D." Too easy? Well, every once in a while, you deserve a break, right? Metformin does not cause weight gain (unlike many other treatments for diabetes), has evidence for reducing the complications of diabetes, and is generally well-tolerated and inexpensive. Thus, it is the drug of choice in most DM2 patients. In addition, it carries very little risk of hypoglycemia. GI side effects are common, however (nausea, diarrhea). Some patients will lose weight from use of metformin. Thiazolidinediones known as "glitazones" ("A") are not first-line for several reasons, chief among these being the possibility of increased cardiovascular events (rosiglitazone and pioglitazone can exacerbate CHF). The track record of rosiglitazone is somewhat spotty: it was removed from the market due to an increase in cardiovascular events and then was reintroduced even though there was no additional safety data; avoid it if you can. Sulfonylureas ("B") are also effective and well-tolerated, but have a significant risk for hypoglycemia and are associated with weight gain. Studies comparing effects on end-organ disease show better outcomes with metformin than with sulfonylureas. All other oral drugs are best considered second-line agents. "E" is of special note. DPP-4 inhibitors, also known as "gliptins," block the degradation of the body's endogenous incretin, which helps to lower blood sugar. DPP-4 acts as a "glucagon-like peptide-1" (GLP-1). DPP-4 inhibitors (sitagliptin [Januvia], saxagliptin [Onglyza], alogliptin [Nesina] … see below for a caution) can be used as an "add-on" therapy if traditional hypoglycemic agents are not effective and have the benefit of some weight loss. In a patient with very poor control (e.g., A1c >9%) at diagnosis, insulin ("C") would be a potential first-line agent, but not in this patient whose is partially controlled.

HELPFUL TIP:
New data suggests an association (or maybe causality) of congestive heart failure with saxagliptin (Onglyza) and alogliptin (Nesina). This does not seem to be a problem with sitagliptin (Januvia). These drugs only reduce HbA1c by about 0.5% and have no data demonstrating cardiovascular benefit. Other reported side effects include headache, nasopharyngitis, and upper respiratory tract infections. Also, acute pancreatitis has been reported in association with DPP-4 inhibitors, but currently there is insufficient evidence to determine a causal relationship.

HELPFUL TIP:
Another class of "glucagon-like peptide-1" (GLP-1) drugs act as receptor agonists (e.g., exenatide [Byetta or Bydureon], liraglutide [Victoza], albiglutide [Tanzeum], etc.) which bind to the GLP-1 receptor. They are resistant to breakdown by the body and thus provide sustained glucose control. These are given by subcutaneous injection and are fairly costly, but have the advantage of being more potent than the gliptins and may even cause weight loss in type 2 diabetics.

HELPFUL TIP:
Good glucose control can cost an arm and a leg (or at least a leg). Can't they leave well enough alone? Just what we need, more abbreviations. The last new(ish) class of drugs for DM2 are the "flozins" properly known as **"SGLT2 inhibitors"** (sodium-glucose cotransporter-2). Examples are canagliflozin (Invokana), empagliflozin (Jardiance), etc. They promote the renal excretion of glucose (literally peeing out the sugar) and thereby lowering A1c levels by 0.5% to 0.7%. The overall benefits of SGLT2 inhibitors include a decrease in blood pressure and weight and a low incidence of hypoglycemia. There is some evidence that they improve cardiac and renal outcomes (although marginally). Invokana (one of Trump's daughters?) and the other flozins are associated with an increased risk of amputations (*BMJ* 2018;363:k4365). The other side

effects are exactly what you would think, given that the mechanism of action increases sugar content of urine: vulvovaginal candidiasis, urinary frequency, hypovolemia/dehydration, and (serious) urinary tract infection. LDL goes **up** 4% to 8%. Also, the FDA has issued a warning regarding Fournier's gangrene, keto-acidosis, and fractures. There is also some concern about an association with bladder cancer that requires further post-market monitoring.

Question 10.10.8 **Which of the following is NOT a side effect of GLP-1 receptor agonists (exenatide, liraglutide, albiglutide)?**
A) Weight gain
B) Pancreatitis
C) Hypoglycemia
D) GI upset
E) Thyroid tumor

Answer 10.10.8 **The correct answer is "A."** Actually, GLP-1 agonists may cause weight loss of 1.5 to 2.5 kg over 30 weeks. These drugs are associated with pancreatitis although rarely, and the association is tenuous. Due to an association with thyroid cancer, their use is contraindicated in patients with a personal or family history of medullary thyroid carcinoma or MEN 2A or 2B. The risk of hypoglycemia is small—but not zero—with GLP-1 agonists. Somewhere between 10% and 50% of patients may develop GI symptoms.

Question 10.10.9 **Metformin should NOT be used in which class of patients?**
A) Patients with COPD
B) Patients with a GFR<30 mL/min
C) Patients with leukemias or lymphomas
D) Postmyocardial infarction patients with normal systolic function
E) Patients with insufficient fat stores

Answer 10.10.9 **The correct answer is "B."** Patients with renal disease are at a higher risk of lactic acidosis, the most severe complication of metformin therapy, although it is exceedingly rare (3 cases per 100,000 vs. 2 cases per 100,000 with other hypoglycemic agents). Current manufacturer recommendations state that metformin should be avoided if the serum creatinine ≥1.5 mg/dL in males and ≥1.4 mg/dL in females. However, metformin is safe to start as long as the GFR is >45 mL/min and can be used until the GFR is 30 mL/min (max dose 1,000 mg/day for those with a GFR between 30 and 60 mL/min, per FDA Package Labeling 2016). Outcomes in patients with mild CHF and renal failure (GFR>30 mL/min) **are actually better** with metformin than without (*Ann Intern Med.* 2017;166(3):191–200). Patients with pulmonary or neo-plastic diseases may take metformin unless they also have severe hepatic or renal failure. **Metformin should be held for 48 hours after contrast studies.** Please refer to the general

recommendations regarding anti-hyperglycemic therapy in type 2 diabetes by the ADA (Figure 10-1).

 HELPFUL TIP:
Metformin is associated with vitamin B12 deficiency, and periodic testing of vitamin B12 should be considered in metformin-treated patients, especially in those with anemia or peripheral neuropathy.

Question 10.10.10 **Which one of the following is NOT a risk factor or prognostic marker for lower-extremity amputation in patients with diabetes?**
A) Diabetic retinopathy
B) Bony deformity of the feet or ankles
C) C-reactive protein (CRP) level
D) Abnormal monofilament testing for sensory function
E) Severe nail pathology

Answer 10.10.10 **The correct answer is "C."** The risk of ulcers or amputations is increased in patients who have had diabetes for 10 years or more, are male, have a history of poor glucose control, have evidence of microvascular complications of diabetes (e.g., retinopathy), or are on Invokana. Bony deformities, loss of protective sensation, and severely dystrophic toenails are also risk factors for amputation. The Semmes–Weinstein 10-gram monofilament sensory examination is the most sensitive neurologic test for predicting the future occurrence of a diabetic foot ulcer. An elevated CRP in and of itself is not a known risk factor for amputation, but CRP may be elevated if there is lower extremity infection present.

....

At the next visit, you review the patient's medical record and try to assure that he is up to date on his preventive health care.

Question 10.10.11 **Which of the following is NOT true regarding preventive services in diabetics?**
A) Patients diagnosed with type 2 diabetes should have a dilated eye examination at the time of diagnosis
B) Patients with type 1 diabetes should have a dilated eye examination at the time of diagnosis if they are over age 12
C) Check TSH annually in type 1 diabetes, in patients with dyslipidemia, or diabetic women over age 50 years
D) A urine microalbumin should be checked at least yearly in all type 2 diabetics
E) A foot examination using a 10-g nylon microfilament should be done annually for all diabetics

Answer 10.10.11 **The correct answer is "B."** Patients with diabetes type 1 should have an eye examination **3 to 5 years** after the diagnosis and then yearly. Age at the time of diagnosis is not a factor in determining when an eye examination should be done. See Table 10-2 for components of recommended diabetes follow-up.

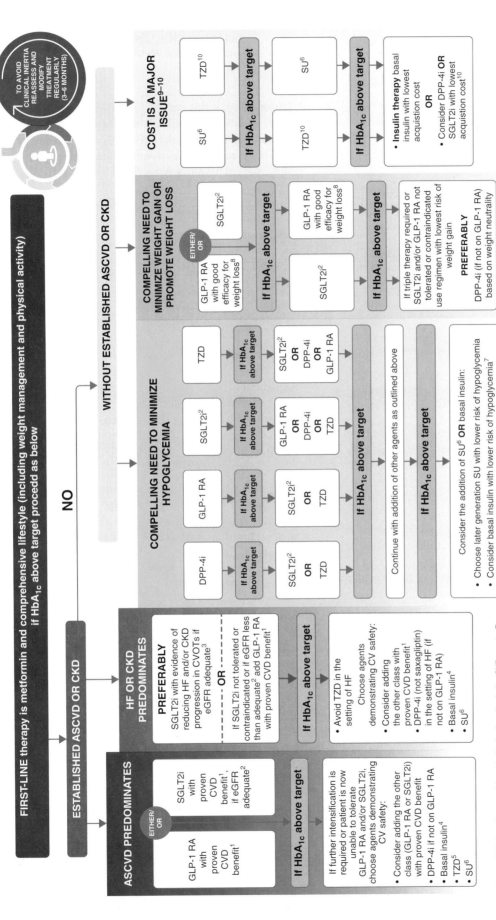

FIGURE 10-1. Recommendations for medical treatment of diabetes mellitus type 2.
From American Diabetes Association. Standards of Medical Care in Diabetes 2019. *Diabetes Care.* 2019;42:S90–S102.

1. Proven CVD benefit means it has label indication of reducing CVD events. For GLP-1 RA strongest evidence for liraglutide > semaglutide > exenatide extended release. For SGLT2i evidence modestly stronger for empagliflozin > canagliflozin.
2. Be aware that SGLT2i vary by region and individual agent with regard to indicated level of eGFR for initiation and continued use
3. Both empagliflozin and canagliflozin have shown reduction in HF and reduction in CKD progression in CVOTs
4. Degludec or U100 glargine have demonstrated CVD safety
5. Low dose may be better tolerated though less well studied for CVD effects

6. Choose later generation SU with lower risk of hypoglycemia
7. Degludec / glargine U300 < glargine U100 / detemir < NPH insulin
8. Semaglutide > liraglutide > dulaglutide > exenatide > lixisenatide
9. If no specific comorbidities (i.e., no established CVD, low risk of hypoglycemia, and lower priority to avoid weight gain or no weight-related comorbidities)
10. Consider country- and region-specific cost of drugs. In some countries TZDs relatively more expensive and DPP-4i relatively cheaper

TABLE 10-2 SUMMARY OF SCREENING RECOMMENDATIONS

Diabetes mellitus type 1:

- Urine microalbumin starting at age 12 and then every 6 to 12 months
- Dilated eye examination within 5 years of diagnosis and then annually
- HbA1c every 6 months for stable patients achieving glycemic goals, every 3 months for patients changing therapy or not meeting glycemic goals
- Blood pressure screening at every visit
- Foot examination and screening for polyneuropathy at diagnosis and annually
- If not performed/available within past year
- Fasting lipid profile, including total, LDL, and HDL cholesterol and triglycerides, as needed
- Serum creatinine and calculated glomerular filtration rate
- TSH in type 1 diabetes, dyslipidemia, or women over age 50 years

Diabetes mellitus type 2:

Same as DM1 above, except:

- Eye examination at time of diagnosis and then yearly
- Urine microalbumin at the time of diagnosis and then every 6–12 months

American Diabetes Association. Comprehensive medical evaluation and assessment of comorbidities. *Diabetes Care.* 2019;42(S1):S34–S45.

Question 10.10.12 Speaking of prevention, your patient, now 48 years old with his diabetes controlled, asks if he should be taking an aspirin daily to protect his heart. You respond:
A) "Take aspirin 325 mg daily because it will lower your risk of myocardial infarction"
B) "Diabetes does not automatically qualify you for aspirin therapy. Let's check your atherosclerotic cardiovascular disease (ASCVD) score"
C) "The risks and benefits of aspirin in your case are unknown"
D) "Take it by the truckload. I've got a lot of stock in Bayer"

Answer 10.10.12 **The correct answer is "B."** The ADA recommends considering aspirin therapy (75–162 mg/day) as a primary prevention strategy in those with type 1 or type 2 diabetes at increased cardiovascular risk (10-year risk ≥10%). Who would be in this category of risk? Diabetic men AND women aged >=50 years who have at least one additional major risk factor (family history of cardiovascular disease, hypertension, smoking, dyslipidemia, or microalbuminuria). ADA recommends AGAINST aspirin use for CVD prevention for adults with diabetes at low ASCVD risk, since the potential adverse effects from bleeding likely offset the potential benefits. If you decide to prescribe aspirin for primary CVD prevention in a diabetic, use 81 mg daily.

HELPFUL TIP:
As diabetes itself confers increased risk of ASCVD, a moderate to high intensity statin is recommended as primary prevention for those patients 40 years or older.

Moderate intensity is recommended for patients without known ASCVD and high intensity for those patients with known ASCVD. See Chapter 2 (Cardiology) for more information.

Unfortunately, this patient follows the "rule" of type 2 diabetes and ends up on multiple medications. When he returns to your clinic a few months later, he is complaining of shortness of breath and lower extremity edema. You decide to follow the "rule" of blaming drugs first …

Question 10.10.13 Which of the following drugs (by itself—not in combination with other drugs) is the most likely cause of this patient's edema, shortness of breath, and possible heart failure?
A) Metformin
B) Glyburide
C) Pioglitazone
D) Lisinopril
E) Insulin

Answer 10.10.13 **The correct answer is "C."** The thiazolidinediones ("glitazones") tend to cause fluid retention as one of their major side effects. Thus, they are contraindicated in patients with a history of heart failure. Some drug combinations can cause edema, including the combination of glimepiride and metformin.

Because of the problem with edema, you decide to change this patient to a sulfonylurea, and you choose to start glyburide. The patient does well on this for several weeks but is then found unconscious in his home with a blood sugar of 20 mg/dL. Strike two, doc! He is rapidly revived by the paramedics with an amp of D50. You are called to see the patient in the ED. He is currently awake, conversant, and eating ("a great excuse for a couple of cookies!"). He would like to go home since he is back to his baseline.

Question 10.10.14 Which of the following is the best next step in the management of this patient's hypoglycemic episode?
A) Discharge the patient from the ED and have him continue his regimen, including glyburide
B) Discharge the patient from the ED and have him stop his glyburide and start insulin
C) Admit the patient and start him on IV dextrose 5% infusion
D) Admit the patient and observe him for 24 hours
E) Give him a gift card to local casino buffet, and tell him, "Pretend it's your birthday!"

Answer 10.10.14 **The correct answer is "D."** Patients on an oral hypoglycemic agent—especially longer-acting agents like glyburide—should be admitted for observation. It would be reasonable to let him eat, check his glucose periodically, and hold his diabetic medications. He is currently stable and does not appear to need IV dextrose ("C"), but the patient should have IV access, and a half- or full-ampule of D50 can be given if necessary. The absorption of oral hypoglycemic agents is somewhat erratic, and their effect can be prolonged. The patient may have an additional episode of hypoglycemia for up to 36 to 48 hours after the initial episode. This is not true of patients on insulins (NPH or short-acting insulin [e.g., regular, lispro]), who may be discharged from the ED after a few hours. But for this patient, discharge from the ED ("A," "B," and "E") would be unwise.

HELPFUL TIP:
Fifteen to 20 g of fast-acting carbohydrates such as glucose tablets, honey, corn syrup, nonfat or 1% milk, jellybeans, gumdrops, gel tube, raisins, hard candy, regular soda, and sweetened fruit juice can be used to treat symptomatic hypoglycemia. For severe hypoglycemia, glucagon injection may be needed. Glucagon, 1 mg IM or IV, is another option.

HELPFUL TIP:
The following medications generally do not cause hypoglycemia: metformin, acarbose, dipeptidyl peptidase (DPP-4) inhibitors, and glucagon-like peptide-1 (GLP-1) receptor agonists. Hypoglycemia is rare with the SGLT2 inhibitors.

It turns out that one of your partners has started this patient on a beta-blocker for its cardioprotective and antihypertensive effects while you were on vacation. The patient wants to know if this may have prevented him from noticing the signs and symptoms of hypoglycemia.

Question 10.10.15 Your response is:
A) "Beta-blockers reduce your ability to recognize hypoglycemia and the drug should be stopped"
B) "Beta-blockers reduce your ability to recognize hypoglycemia but the benefits are worth it"
C) "Beta-blockers do not decrease your ability to recognize hypoglycemia to any great degree. Don't worry about it"
D) "ACE inhibitors are better drugs because they do not contribute to hypoglycemia in diabetics"

Answer 10.10.15 **The correct answer is "C."** Beta-blockers do not significantly interfere with patient ability to recognize hypoglycemia, but they have been associated with hypoglycemia (mechanism is purported to be impairment in gluconeogenesis). The main thing that contributes to unawareness of hypoglycemia in diabetics is the rate of glucose drop (a slow drop is less likely to be noticed) and autonomic insufficiency (patients cannot respond with tachycardia, sweating, etc., to the outpouring of adrenergics). "D" is incorrect. ACE inhibitors, like beta-blockers, have been associated with hypoglycemia in diabetics. Other nondiabetic drugs that have been associated with hypoglycemia include quinolones, salicylates, and pentamidine.

HELPFUL TIP:
The ADA recommends the target A1c in nonpregnant adults with diabetes be <7%. However, it also advises more or less stringent glycemic goals may be appropriate for individual patients and goals should be individualized on the basis of duration of diabetes, age/life expectancy, comorbid conditions, known CVD or advanced microvascular complications, hypoglycemia unawareness, and individual patient considerations. For patients with multiple comorbidities and higher risks for hypoglycemia and other drug adverse effects, a higher A1c, even up to 8.5%, may be acceptable (but try telling that to the insurance companies). **It is recommended to perform A1c twice yearly in those patients who are meeting treatment goals, and quarterly in patients with poor glycemic control.**

You admit the patient and advise him to carry a source of glucose with him at all times and everybody has a happy outcome until …

The patient has developed persistent hyperglycemia despite being on maximal doses of metformin and glyburide. He is willing to begin insulin therapy but wants to give himself as few injections as possible.

Question 10.10.16 Which of the following regimens would be best for him?
A) A single injection of insulin glargine (Lantus™) or NPH insulin at bedtime
B) A single injection of 70/30 NPH/regular insulin at bedtime
C) A baseline bedtime injection of insulin glargine and up to three injections of short-acting insulin with meals
D) Regular insulin with meals to control postprandial blood sugars.

Answer 10.10.16 **The correct answer is "A."** Because of its slow release, insulin glargine provides a steady-state insulin level throughout 24 hours; insulin detemir and NPH are alternatives. In fact, NPH likely causes *less* hypoglycemia than do insulin glargine and insulin detemir, and the outcomes are the same (and glargine and detemir cost 10× as much as NPH; see *JAMA* 2018;320:53). Regular insulin (as found in 70/30) is generally not the place to start with type 2 diabetics ("B"). Multiple daily insulin injections may be necessary for type 1 diabetics, but this is not true for type 2 patients. For type 2 diabetes, long-acting insulin is usually started first and bolus mealtime insulin added later, so "C" would not be the first choice. As noted above, regular insulin ("D") isn't the place to start in DM2. If you are trying to start with the simplest possible regimen, choose something like "A."

HELPFUL TIP:
Sulfonylureas and insulin work in the same manner: they both increase circulating insulin levels. For this reason, some choose not to use these two drugs together and will taper the sulfonylurea after the patient is on a stable dose of insulin.

Your patient is hospitalized for acute diverticulitis and requires urgent partial colectomy.

Question 10.10.17 Which of the following statements regarding the management of diabetes in hospitalized patients is TRUE?
A) Hyperglycemia in the hospital has minimal, if any, effect on outcomes of myocardial infarction.
B) A standardized sliding-scale insulin regimen is adequate to control hyperglycemia in all hospitalized diabetic patients.
C) Insulin requirements will be lower for acutely ill, hospitalized diabetic patients.
D) Metformin should be discontinued in seriously ill, hospitalized patients.

Answer 10.10.17 The correct answer is "D." In general, one should consider discontinuation of metformin in severely ill, hospitalized patients due to the possible need for contrast studies, changes in fluid balance, changes in glomerular filtration rate, uncertainty about oral intake (e.g., NPO status), etc. "A" is incorrect. Hyperglycemia is associated with worse outcomes in hospitalized patients with cardiac disease and those who are in an intensive care unit for most reasons. But this may be because elevated blood sugars suggest they are under greater metabolic stress and sicker to begin with. "B" is also incorrect. Sliding-scale regimens, if used at all, should be individualized to each patient, rather than prescribed as a standardized regimen. It has become clear that a sliding scale is not the best way to control blood sugars in hospitalized patients. Continuing some type of basal insulin (or basal-bolus) regimen is best, using correctional insulin as needed. In hospitalized patients, it is generally recommended to discontinue oral antidiabetic agents and control the glucose using insulin only, provided in a combination form including basal long-acting insulin plus pre-meal short-acting insulin if on diet and correctional insulin (aka basal/bolus insulin). The stress of acute illness and surgery will likely increase insulin requirements in most diabetics, not decrease them.

> **HELPFUL TIP:**
> Chasing the glucose in an attempt to maintain tight control in the hospital is counterproductive and does not improve outcomes! *Even though patients with hyperglycemia may do worse, it is clear that the elevated glucose is a marker for metabolic stress which is why outcomes might be worse … they are sicker to begin with.* Thus, for sicker patients, aim for a blood sugar of between 120 and 180 mg/dL. This has been found to be superior to more intensive glycemic control. Some studies suggest a goal of as high as 250 mg/dL (*Crit Care Med* 2018;46:935). For now, 180 mg/dL seems reasonable.

He does well and is ready for discharge. He asks about self-monitoring of blood glucose.

Question 10.10.18 How often should a type 2 diabetic on oral hypoglycemic agents measure his or her blood glucose?
A) Once or twice a week, at varying times during the day
B) Four times daily—before meals and at bedtime
C) Twice daily—fasting and 2 hours after a meal
D) Once or twice daily—fasting and before a meal
E) Routine blood sugars are not indicated on a daily basis for type 2 diabetics

Answer 10.10.18 The correct answer is "E." Daily measurements of finger stick sugars in patients on oral hypoglycemic agents do nothing to improve glycemic control (*BMJ*. 2012;344:e486). In these patients, we are not reacting to daily fluctuations in glucose control but rather making changes in response to long-term trends, and typically HbA1c is used. Occasional random sugars are not unreasonable to get a general idea about glycemic control. Type 2 diabetics on insulin (and all type 1 diabetics) should measure their blood glucose at least daily, and ideally two or three times per day, regardless of the presence or absence of symptoms.

The patient has come back to your clinic several times for follow-up, and his current medications are adjusted to their maximum doses. The patient is not interested in injectable medication—he changed his tune from earlier after reading online how he might get addicted to insulin. You discuss adding a third oral agent (to his metformin and glyburide), and muster an expression that you hope conveys enthusiasm. However, the patient's diabetes is not optimally controlled, and he develops diabetic neuropathy years later.

Question 10.10.19 Which of the following agents is LEAST effective in treatment of diabetic neuropathic pain?
A) Tricyclic antidepressants
B) SSRIs
C) Duloxetine (Cymbalta)
D) Pregabalin (Lyrica) or gabapentin
E) Venlafaxine (Effexor XR)

Answer 10.10.19 The correct answer is "B." SSRIs are generally ineffective in treating neuropathic pain. Several drugs have been approved specifically for relief of diabetic peripheral neuropathic pain in the United States (pregabalin, duloxetine, and tapentadol), but none affords complete relief, even when used in combination. **Low-dose tricyclic antidepressants are the most effective of this group (e.g., nortriptyline or amitriptyline 25 mg qhs), but also have anticholinergic side effects** (*Lancet Neurol.* 2015 Feb; 14:162). Pregabalin, gabapentin, amitriptyline (except in older adults), or duloxetine should be used as first-line treatment for painful diabetic neuropathy. Venlafaxine and opioid-like medications (tramadol, tapentadol) may be considered second- or third-line. Remember that gabapentin is ONLY FDA approved for post-herpetic neuralgia. It is overused and causes weight gain, mental slowing, sleepiness, and is abusable.

▶ **Objectives: Did you learn to …**

- Recognize diagnostic criteria for diabetes?
- Differentiate diabetes type 1 from type 2?
- Evaluate a patient with new-onset type 2 diabetes?
- Identify risk factors for complications of diabetes?
- Initiate and manage oral therapy in type 2 diabetes?
- Start a type 2 diabetic patient on insulin?
- Manage diabetes in the hospital setting?
- Treat painful diabetic peripheral neuropathy?

▶ CASE 10.11

A 32-year-old female presents to your office complaining of "hypoglycemia." She notices that about 2 to 3 hours after a meal she gets nauseated, shaky, and irritable. When she wakes up in the morning, she generally feels well even though she eats dinner at about 5:00 PM and does not eat any snacks afterward and generally does not have breakfast until 8:00 AM.

Question 10.11.1 **You can tell her that:**
A) She likely has an insulinoma
B) She likely will have normal blood sugars when she feels shaky
C) Hypoglycemia does not exist as an entity in this form and she likely has anxiety
D) She likely has "fasting" hypoglycemia
E) Hypoglycemia is an uncommon problem in nondiabetics but it could explain her symptoms

Answer 10.11.1 **The correct answer is "E."** "A" is incorrect because a patient with an insulinoma should be hypoglycemic after a 15-hour fast (when she's not eating between 5:00 PM and 8:00 AM). "B" is incorrect. This patient may have postprandial hypoglycemia that occurs 2 to 4 hours after eating. The process leading to postprandial hypoglycemia is as follows: the patient has a large meal with simple carbohydrates, the serum insulin level increases in response but overshoots, and the patient becomes transiently hypoglycemic for 15 to 20 minutes usually 2 to 4 hours after eating. This is associated with adrenergic outpouring in an attempt to correct the problem. It is the adrenergic outpouring

that causes the symptoms of tremor, nausea, etc. "C" is incorrect because hypoglycemia does exist. "D" is incorrect. The patient does not have symptoms of fasting hypoglycemia, which occur 4 to 6 hours (or longer) after the last meal.

Question 10.11.2 **All of the following are associated with postprandial hypoglycemia EXCEPT:**
A) Diuretics
B) Alcohol intake
C) Postgastrectomy syndrome
D) Beta-blockers

Answer 10.11.2 **The correct answer is "A."** Diuretics tend to **increase** the blood sugar a bit. Aspirin, indomethacin, ACE inhibitors, pentamidine, and renal failure may be associated with postprandial **hypo**glycemia. Other medications that are associated with **hyper**glycemia include quinolones, atypical antipsychotics, corticosteroids, calcineurin inhibitors, protease inhibitors, and some lipid-lowering agents like niacin and atorvastatin. It is worth noting that carvedilol and nebivolol are not associated with the development of **hyper**glycemia, and that quinolones (especially gatifloxacin) are associated with both hyper- and hypoglycemia. It turns out that the kidneys are responsible for about 50% of gluconeogenesis. If the kidneys aren't working, the ability to respond to hypoglycemia is blunted.

Question 10.11.3 **You advise this patient to do all of the following EXCEPT:**
A) Increase the amount of simple carbohydrates with her meals
B) Increase the amount of complex carbohydrates with her meals
C) Increase the amount of protein with her meals
D) Increase the amount of fat with her meals
E) Eat smaller, more frequent meals

Answer 10.11.3 **The correct answer (and what you would not want to do) is "A."** Her problem is caused at least in part by a high intake of simple carbohydrates, leading to a rapid and high peak in her blood sugar followed by an excessive release of insulin. Thus, one would want to decrease the amount of simple carbohydrates in the diet and add protein, fat, and complex carbohydrates. There is little data suggesting that any of these is particularly effective, however. Delaying gastric emptying (using an agent like propantheline, an anticholinergic/antispasmodic) does **not** seem to make a difference (but might make the patient sleepy enough that she doesn't notice the symptoms!). Reducing the spike in carbohydrate absorption using alpha-glucosidase inhibitors (e.g., acarbose) makes sense but also does not have any good supporting data for this indication.

INTERESTING (BUT MAYBE NOT SO HELPFUL) TIP:
Gin and tonic and ackee fruit (from Caribbean islands) are known causes of hypoglycemia. In "gin and tonic hypoglycemia" (the actual name of the syndrome), alcohol prevents effective counter-regulatory measures to the hypoglycemia produced by the quinine. Ackee fruit, common in the Jamaican diet, contains "hypoglycin" that prevents gluconeogenesis. And, no, you cannot use gin and tonic to control your diabetes!

HELPFUL TIP:
For insulinoma, watch the patient during a **controlled** fast during which the patient is observed and can be treated for hypoglycemia if necessary. If you are considering self-induced hypoglycemia with insulin (e.g., factitious hypoglycemia), measure the c-peptide. This will be **low** if the patient is being administered exogenous insulin because pancreatic insulin production will be shut off in response to hypoglycemia (remember, however, that it will also be low in type 1 diabetes).

▶ Objectives: Did you learn to ...
- Evaluate a patient with possible hypoglycemia?
- Treat a patient with postprandial hypoglycemia?
- Identify causes of hypoglycemia?

 QUICK QUIZ: CARBOHYDRATES AND CALORIES

Which of the following statements is FALSE?
A) The use of the glycemic index (GI) and load may help diabetic patients improve their carbohydrate-containing food selection
B) Diabetics should avoid sucrose-containing foods because they worsen glycemic control more than a comparable amount of starch
C) For weight loss, either low-carbohydrate or low-fat calorie-restricted diets may be effective in the short term (up to 1 year)
D) Moderate alcohol intake may reduce the risk of developing diabetes
E) Carbohydrates have fewer calories per gram than alcohol

The correct (and false) answer is "B." Several studies demonstrate that dietary sucrose does not increase glycemia more than isocaloric amounts of starch. For example, the glycemic index (GI) of sucrose is 84 while that of a banana is 88 (higher GI being worse). GI represents how much the serum glucose will increase after the ingestion of 50 g of the carbohydrate in the food when compared to a standard (often oral glucose). It typically ranges between 50 and 100, where 100 represents the standard blood sugar response to an equivalent amount of pure glucose. GI < 55 is considered low, 56 to 69 medium, and 70 or over high.

A related measure, the glycemic load (GL), uses white bread as the standard of comparison. It takes into account not only the carbohydrates in a food but also the fiber and other nutrients and *how much* carbohydrate is in the food. For example, the carbohydrate in whole grains may be absorbed more slowly so the glucose will not rise as much for a given amount of carbohydrate in the food (when compared to white bread).

Both GI and GL are helpful in medical nutritional therapy for diabetes. For "C," although low-fat diets have traditionally been promoted for weight loss, studies found that subjects on low-carbohydrate diets lost more weight. Nonetheless, either low-carbohydrate or low-fat calorie-restricted diets are effective for weight loss. Regarding "D," observational studies report that moderate alcohol intake may reduce the risk for diabetes, but the data do not support recommending alcohol consumption to individuals at risk of diabetes. Did you know that 1 g of alcohol has 7 calories while 1 g of carbohydrates has only 4? Now you do!

▶ **CASE 10.12**

A 24-year-old female presents to the office complaining of amenorrhea. Six months ago, her menses became irregular and light. For the last 4 months, she has not had a period at all. This is causing her great distress, as she constantly worries about being pregnant. She does desire to have children "some day," but not now. She has run multiple home pregnancy tests, all of which have been negative. Last week, she developed clear leakage from her nipples, and the patient is now convinced she is pregnant and that the home pregnancy tests must be faulty. She requests that you perform "a real pregnancy test."

Question 10.12.1 **Which of the following may cause her amenorrhea?**
A) Emotional stress
B) Pregnancy, despite multiple negative tests
C) Thyroid dysfunction
D) Pituitary tumor
E) All of the above

Answer 10.12.1 **The correct answer is "E."** The differential diagnosis for amenorrhea is rather broad but includes all of the above diagnoses and more. The most common cause in a woman of childbearing age is, of course, pregnancy. Although urine-based pregnancy tests have become very sensitive (able to detect as little as 20 IU/mL of β-hCG), the patient may have been using the tests incorrectly and thus was getting false-negative results. Other causes of amenorrhea include hypothyroidism, strenuous exercise or anorexia, emotional stress, pituitary tumor, certain medications (e.g., phenothiazines, dopaminergic agents, chemotherapy, and estrogens), and ovarian failure or agenesis. See Chapter 15 for a more thorough discussion of amenorrhea.

Further history from the patient reveals menarche at age 12, no pregnancies, and no previous history of menstrual irregularities. She participates in low-impact exercise regularly and

does not engage in long-distance running or other demanding endurance sports. Review of systems reveals frequent mild headaches, but no visual disturbances or symptoms of hypothyroidism.

Physical examination demonstrates a well-developed, well-nourished (neither obese nor excessively thin) adult female. She has appropriate secondary sex characteristics, no hirsutism, and a normal thyroid gland to palpation. Galactorrhea is noted on breast examination. The pelvic examination is normal, with appropriately developed external genitalia, vagina, and cervix. The uterus is palpable and small, and the ovaries are neither palpable nor tender.

Question 10.12.2 In addition to a serum β-hCG and a TSH, what other test(s) should be ordered?

A) Karyotype, to evaluate for testicular feminization (now called "complete androgen insensitivity syndrome") and Turner syndrome
B) Adrenal MRI, to evaluate for adrenal hyperplasia
C) Prolactin level
D) All of the above
E) None of the above

Answer 10.12.2 **The correct answer is "C."** A prolactin level is an essential component of this evaluation. A prolactinoma is the most common form of pituitary adenoma, and it can cause secondary amenorrhea, galactorrhea (as in this patient), and infertility (or erectile dysfunction and hypogonadism in men). Expansion of the mass in the sella turcica may cause headaches or visual field defects (bitemporal hemianopsia), but the tumors are more often too small to have any local effects. Adrenal hyperplasia is unlikely in the patient because of a lack of virilizing characteristics from androgen excess (such as hirsutism). Also, adrenal imaging is not usually the first step in the diagnosis of this disorder (24-hour urine collection for cortisol and 17-OHS is indicated if adrenal hyperplasia is suspected). A karyotype is not indicated in this patient because she has secondary amenorrhea, or amenorrhea that has developed after a period of time of normal menses. Patients who complain of never having a menstrual cycle are considered to have primary amenorrhea, which may be evidence of either Turner syndrome (XO genotype) or complete androgen insensitivity (aka testicular feminization, which has an XY genotype with end-organ resistance to testosterone, resulting in a female phenotype). Both cases result in ovarian agenesis and, therefore, no menstrual cycles.

You obtain laboratory tests, and the results are as follows: TSH 3.1 IU/mL (0.27–4.20), β-hCG undetectable, prolactin 150 ng/mL (3.4–24.1).

Question 10.12.3 What is the best next step in this patient's evaluation?

A) Reassure patient that stress is causing her amenorrhea and she will improve when she learns to deal with her life
B) No additional tests at this time but return in 2 weeks for a repeat prolactin level

C) Admit the patient to the hospital and start bromocriptine therapy STAT
D) MRI brain to evaluate for pituitary mass
E) Refer patient for neurosurgical intervention

Answer 10.12.3 **The correct answer is "D."** This patient has a high prolactin level and symptoms of prolactin excess. In the absence of medications causing an elevated prolactin (phenothiazines, narcotics, estrogens, etc.) and a normal TSH, this prolactin result is virtually diagnostic for a prolactinoma. Imaging is indicated regardless of visual symptoms. A visual field examination by confrontation is insensitive for a minor visual field loss. If she had a mild elevation in prolactin (up to two times the upper limit of normal), and no other symptoms/signs, then repeating the level over several visits may be appropriate. If the level remains elevated, imaging and medical therapy should then be considered. Neurosurgical intervention is not immediately indicated, since a trial of medical therapy is usually the first step in treatment.

This patient undergoes a brain MRI, which shows a 1.3-cm pituitary mass.

Question 10.12.4 How should this finding be interpreted and managed?

A) This is a microadenoma, and the result can be ignored
B) This is a microadenoma, and medical therapy with a dopamine agonist is indicated
C) This is a macroadenoma, so medical therapy is futile, and the patient should be referred for surgery
D) This is a macroadenoma, but medical therapy with a dopamine agonist should still be attempted
E) This is a macroadenoma, which tends to be self-limited, so therapy can be held for 6 months when a repeat scan will be done

Answer 10.12.4 **The correct answer is "D."** A pituitary tumor <1 cm in size is considered a microadenoma, and tumors 1 cm or greater in size are considered macroadenomas. The treatment implications are slightly different. In both cases, medical therapy with a dopamine agonist (e.g., bromocriptine, cabergoline) is indicated. Successful shrinkage of even macroadenomas is possible with this therapy. Remember that the secretion of prolactin is under a negative feedback loop. As CNS dopamine levels go up, prolactin levels go down. When dopamine levels go down, prolactin levels go up.

HELPFUL TIP:
Many psychoactive medications inhibit dopamine and can result in hyperprolactinemia. Resist the knee-jerk reaction of stopping a psychoactive medication in a patient found to have hyperprolactinemia. High prolactin levels do not kill patients, but untreated mental illness does. Risks, benefits, and likelihood that the drug is to blame must all be considered.

The patient is started on bromocriptine and is scheduled for follow-up in 3 weeks. She returns earlier than scheduled due to severe nausea and lightheadedness. No other new symptoms have occurred. The patient's vital signs are normal, but the systolic blood pressure decreases by 20 mm Hg and the pulse increases by 20 beats/minute upon standing.

Question 10.12.5 Aside from a bolus of IV fluids, how should you address this problem?
A) This is a common side effect from bromocriptine. Decrease or stop the bromocriptine, and consider another type of dopamine agonist, such as cabergoline
B) Admit her to the hospital and arrange for a STAT head CT scan to rule out bleeding from the pituitary adenoma
C) Repeat the pregnancy test
D) She is having an anaphylactic allergic reaction. Administer epinephrine and diphenhydramine immediately
E) She has failed medical therapy and must be referred for neurosurgical intervention

Answer 10.12.5 **The correct answer is "A."** The most common side effects of dopamine agonists are nausea, postural hypotension, and difficulty concentrating. These symptoms tend to be lessened when lower doses are used, and the dose is increased very slowly. Cabergoline tends to be better tolerated than bromocriptine.

The patient is able to tolerate cabergoline and continues the medication for 6 months. During this time, the prolactin level decreases slowly. She has had resumption of her menses. A repeat MRI is done after 6 months and shows a marked decrease in size of the adenoma. The patient has reached that magical inflection point in life where she recognizes that her own mortality is inevitable, and she desires to get pregnant "as soon as possible." She wants to know if she should have surgery to remove the adenoma.

Question 10.12.6 What is/are the indication(s) for transsphenoidal pituitary surgery?
A) Failure to respond to dopamine agonists
B) Failure to tolerate dopamine agonists
C) Treatment of giant adenoma (>3 cm) in a patient who desires pregnancy, despite efficacy of medical therapy
D) A and B
E) All of the above

Answer 10.12.6 **The correct answer is "E."** Surgery should be reserved for those patients who fail to respond to or cannot tolerate medical therapy. Note that visual field defects are not a specific indication for surgery, since medical therapy can be effective in decreasing the size and related local effects of the tumor. If a patient desires pregnancy and has a large mass (>3 cm), surgery may be considered as an adjunct to medical therapy. During pregnancy, there is a physiological increase in the size of the prolactinoma. If such a patient becomes pregnant

(without a prior reduction in tumor size) and discontinues the dopamine agonist for the duration of pregnancy, the adenoma may increase to a clinically important size before delivery.

HELPFUL TIP:
Bromocriptine and cabergoline are classified as category B for pregnancy risk (in other words, they are generally considered safe). These medications can be continued during pregnancy, but a careful risk–benefit analysis and discussion between patient and physician must occur before making treatment decisions.

The patient wants to know how long she should be on cabergoline or bromocriptine and when a trial off of the medication is indicated.

Question 10.12.7 You tell her which of the following?
A) Patients with a pituitary adenoma have to be on medication "forever" to suppress the tumor
B) A trial off of a dopamine agonist should be done at 6 months
C) Prolactin levels can be allowed to rise after menopause without problem unless visual symptoms or other local symptoms develop. So, she should continue the medication until menopause
D) None of the above

Answer 10.12.7 **The correct answer is "C."** Dopamine agonists can be stopped at menopause. Follow-up can be done using blood levels of prolactin. If prolactin levels rise, an MRI can be done to see if the adenoma is becoming larger. If not, there is no reason to treat the adenoma in postmenopausal patients. "A" is incorrect because "C" is correct—a simple test taking skill! If you see "forever" on a test it is probably wrong. (Also, never answer "never" and never answer "always.") "B" is incorrect. **If there is no adenoma noted on MRI at baseline,** and the prolactin in normal, a trial off of dopamine agonists can be tried at 1 year. Taper the drug and follow the prolactin. **In those with an adenoma on MRI at baseline,** a trial off of medications at 2 years is *reasonable*, provided the prolactin level has fallen to normal and there is no evidence of adenoma by MRI in the past 2 years. If prolactin levels remain under control, there is no need to continue medication.

▶ **Objectives: Did you learn to …**
- Generate a list of potential causes of secondary amenorrhea?
- Evaluate a patient with secondary amenorrhea?
- Diagnose and treat hyperprolactinemia secondary to a pituitary prolactinoma?

▶ **CASE 10.13**

A 39-year-old female presents to the office complaining of amenorrhea. She has had normal menses until 8 months ago, when they became infrequent and then stopped. She insists she cannot be pregnant, because she has not been sexually active "in years." She believes she is going through "the change" but wants to know why she is reaching menopause at a much earlier age than other women she knows. On review of systems, she complains of headaches "for years" and recent onset of weakness and fatigue. She also complains of arthritis in the hip and knees, something she attributes to "getting old." She reports that her hands are swollen, and her rings do not fit any more. She denies other complaints.

On physical examination, vitals are normal. The patient is an adult female of average height, with a noticeably large jaw and hands. Her hair is thick and coarse, and hirsutism is present. Her thyroid gland is slightly enlarged, but regular in shape. No bruit or tenderness is present. The point of maximal impulse is displaced laterally, but the heart rhythm is regular and without murmur. The rest of the examination is normal.

Question 10.13.1 What is the most appropriate next step?

A) Reassure the patient that menopause is a normal process and offer estrogen replacement therapy for symptomatic relief (but warn the patient about risks of long-term use)
B) Tell the patient you suspect depression and offer a regimen of counseling combined with SSRI therapy
C) Tell the patient she may suffer from growth hormone (GH) excess and recommend sending a serum insulin-like growth factor-I (IGF-I) level
D) Tell the patient to quit being a hypochondriac and that her Internet search is not equivalent to your medical degree

Answer 10.13.1 **The correct answer is "C."** This patient represents a classic presentation of acromegaly due to GH excess, and the best single test for this is the IGF-I level. Although GH levels will often be elevated, the IGF-I does not vary from hour to hour and is not dependent on food intake, as is the case with GH. An elevated GH after a glucose load is also very suggestive of GH excess. Acromegaly of adult onset (after fusion of the long bones) does NOT result in increased height, but does cause coarsening of facial features, prognathism, and thickening of the feet and hands. These changes can be very subtle, and there is generally a lag of **12 years** before diagnosis. Comparing older photographs of the patient to their current appearance may be a clue (a driver's license photograph may be a convenient source … although nobody looks good in their driver's license photo). Patients with acromegaly also develop hypertrophy of certain organs (such as the thyroid and heart) and may present with heart failure due to cardiomyopathy. Eighty-five percent of females with acromegaly have at least some menstrual dysfunction and 60% are amenorrheic. Finally, arthropathy is common in acromegaly and may be the overriding symptom that prompts a patient to be evaluated.

HELPFUL TIP:
Premature ovarian failure is defined as menopause at age 40 or younger (two standard deviations below the mean).

The patient's IGF-I is elevated, and her TSH is normal. An MRI is performed that reveals a pituitary mass slightly <1 cm in diameter.

Question 10.13.2 What is the most effective therapy for this condition?

A) Weekly anti-IGF-I antibody infusions
B) Bromocriptine therapy
C) Transsphenoidal pituitary resection
D) Somatostatin analogs (such as octreotide)
E) Pegvisomant (GH receptor antagonist)

Answer 10.13.2 **The correct answer is "C."** Acromegaly is caused by a GH-secreting pituitary tumor. Surgery is the treatment of choice for patients with a microadenoma (1 cm or less in diameter) or for patients with a macroadenoma that appears to be fully resectable. Somatostatin analogs and pegvisomant (Somavert®) may be useful adjuncts to surgery and are an option for patients who are not surgical candidates. Bromocriptine is not very effective, and only about 10% of acromegaly patients will achieve normal IGF-I levels with bromocriptine; however, cabergoline seems to work in about half of patients. Cabergoline has an advantage over somatostatin analogs, in that it can be taken orally. Radiation is also an option for therapy, especially for those patients who are not surgical candidates and do not tolerate or do not respond to medical therapy. "A," anti-IGF-I antibody (if it existed as a medication), would not have an effect on a GH-secreting tumor. But it does not exist. It's a made-up answer, so it's wrong. By the way, there's no made-up stuff on the real examination … we think.

▶ **Objectives: Did you learn to …**
  • Recognize signs and symptoms of GH excess?
  • Evaluate and manage a patient with GH excess?

 QUICK QUIZ: GROWTH HORMONE

A 6-year-old boy is brought into the office by his concerned mother due to "growing too slowly." She has noticed that he is significantly shorter than his classmates at school, and she wants something done about it. She heard a report on the nightly news about a medication that makes children grow taller and insists on getting it for her son. Both parents are deluded and expect their son to play in the NBA or NFL and believe he will not make it unless he "gets a lot taller really soon." She informs you in no uncertain terms that if you don't prescribe this "growing pill," she will just find someone that will.

You believe this mother is in need of some education about GH deficiency.

What are the *approved* indications in children and adolescents for GH replacement therapy?

A) Growth hormone deficiency
B) Growth failure due to chronic renal insufficiency, intrauterine growth retardation with lack of "catch-up" growth by age 2, Turner syndrome, and Prader–Willi syndrome

C) An adolescent male who wishes to play college or pro basketball but is only 5 feet 9 inches on a good day

D) A and B

E) All of the above

The correct answer is "D." GH replacement is specifically approved for GH deficiency and growth failure due to chronic renal insufficiency, intrauterine growth retardation and no "catch-up" growth by age 2, Turner syndrome, and Prader–Willi syndrome. It has been approved for use in "idiopathic short stature" (more than two standard deviations below the mean height for age). Not all patients with GH deficiency require GH replacement, because not all will suffer the negative end-organ effects, such as marked short stature, growth failure, hypoglycemia in infancy, and central distribution of body fat.

HELPFUL TIP:
As with acromegaly, IGF-I should be checked when considering short stature secondary to pituitary failure. It is also important to check IGF-binding protein-3 levels. Low levels of IGF-binding protein-3 may cause problems with binding of IGF to the proper receptors.

HELPFUL TIP:
Even when used appropriately, GH only leads to a couple of inches increase in adult height. Poof … there go the NBA dreams.

Clinical Pearls

- Do not order a thyroid ultrasound to routinely evaluate abnormal thyroid function tests.
- Do not prescribe/recommend multiple daily blood glucose monitoring in patients on oral hypoglycemic regimens.
- Do not use bicarbonate to help correct the acidosis of DKA. The main intent is to provide IV fluid hydration and insulin to help bring down the sugars and correct the acidosis.
- Do not use diuretics to treat acute hypercalcemia. The important point is to aggressively hydrate the patient.
- Do not use T3 for hypothyroidism as its rapid gastrointestinal absorption and relatively short half-life lead to erratic T3 serum levels.
- Initiate thyroid replacement at a low dose (e.g., 25 mcg levothyroxine) in the elderly (>65 years old) or those with cardiac disease, and slowly titrate upward every 4 to 8 weeks.
- Rely primarily on the TSH to screen for thyroid disease in symptomatic individuals and as part of monitoring thyroid function in thyroid disease.
- Screen all obese adults from ages 40 to 70 for diabetes.

- Start steroids immediately if you suspect an adrenal insufficiency (addisonian) crisis.
- Start with an ACE inhibitor (or an ARB if ACEI is contraindicated or has side effects) in the treatment of proteinuria and hypertension in patients with diabetes.

BIBLIOGRAPHY

American Diabetes Association. Standards of medical care in diabetes—2018. *Diabetes Care.* 2018;41:S1–S144.

Betterle C, Morlin L. Autoimmune Addison's disease. *Endocr Dev.* 2011;20:161-172.

Bonora E, Tuomilehto J. The pros and cons of diagnosing diabetes with A1C. *Diabetes Care.* 2011;34(Suppl 2):S184–S190.

Carroll MF. A practical approach to hypercalcemia. *Am Fam Physician.* 2003;67:1959.

Findling JW. Diagnosis and differential diagnosis of Cushing's syndrome. *Endocrinol Metab Clin North Am.* 2001;30:729.

Finklestein BS. Effect of growth hormone therapy on height in children with idiopathic short stature: a meta-analysis. *Arch Pediatr Adolesc Med.* 2002;156:230.

Fraser WD. Hyperthyroidism. *Lancet.* 2009;374:145-158.

Grozinsky-Glasberg S, et al. Thyroxine-triiodothyronine combination therapy versus thyroxine monotherapy for clinical hypothyroidism: meta-analysis of randomized controlled trials. *J Clin Endocrinol Metab.* 2006;91:2592.

Habib G, et al. Intra-articular methylprednisolone acetate injection at the knee joint and the hypothalamic-pituitary-adrenal axis: a randomized controlled study. *Clin Rheumatol.* 2014;1:99–103.

Herrick B. Subclinical hypothyroidism. *Am Fam Physician.* 2008;77:953.

Kearns AE. Medical and surgical management of hyperparathyroidism. *Mayo Clin Proc.* 2002;77:87.

Knox MA. Thyroid nodules. *Am Fam Physician.* 2013;88(3):193-196.

Moghissi ES, et al. American Association of Clinical Endocrinologists and American Diabetes Association consensus statement on inpatient glycemic control. *Diabetes Care.* 2009;32:1119–1136.

Norris SL, et al. Effectiveness of self-management training in type 2 diabetes: a systematic review of randomized controlled trials. *Diabetes Care.* 2001;24:561–587.

Rao G. Insulin resistance syndrome. *Am Fam Physician.* 2001;63(6):1159-1163, 1165-1166.

Sherlock M, et al. Medical therapy in acromegaly. *Nat Rev Endocrinol.* 2011;7:291–300.

Siu AL et al. for Screening for U.S. Preventive Services Task Force. Abnormal blood glucose and type 2 diabetes mellitus: U.S. Preventive Services Task Force recommendation statement. *Ann Intern Med.* 2015;163:861.

Snyder M, et al. Treating painful diabetic peripheral neuropathy: an update. *Am Fam Physician.* 2016;94(3):227–234.

Tritos NA, et al. Medscape: management of Cushing disease. *Nat Rev Endocrinol.* 2011;7:279-289.

U.S. Preventive Services Task Force. Screening for gestational diabetes mellitus: U.S. Preventive Services Task Force recommendation statement. *Ann Intern Med.* 2014;160(6):414.

Unger J. Latent autoimmune diabetes in adults. *Am Fam Physician.* 2010;81:843.

Yassa L, Marqusee E, Fawcett R, Alexander EK. Thyroid hormone early adjustment in pregnancy (the THERAPY) trial. *J Clin Endocrinol Metab.* 2010;7:3234–3241.

Rheumatology

Priyanka Iyer, Sanjeev Patil, and Bharat Kumar

11

A few words on "rheumatology panels." Doing a "rheumatology panel" will never be the right answer. *The diagnosis of rheumatologic disease is clinical with specific clinical criteria for each illness.* While antinuclear antibody (ANA), rheumatoid factor (RF), erythrocyte sedimentation rate (ESR), C-reactive protein (CRP), and other tests may be useful in supporting a clinical diagnosis and assessing disease activity, these tests have **poor specificity** and may be positive in a variety of disease states. A positive ANA without a clinical diagnosis is meaningless. Likewise, RF helps to gauge prognosis (seropositive vs. seronegative) in rheumatoid arthritis (RA) but has limited value as a diagnostic test. RF may also be positive in sarcoidosis, viral infections (especially hepatitis C), and autoimmune diseases such as granulomatosis with polyangiitis (formerly known as Wegener granulomatosis), as well as a variety of primary lung and liver diseases. ESR and CRP may support the clinical impression of inflammatory disease but are again nonspecific.

▶ CASE 11.1

A 43-year-old female presents with body aches and stiffness, which are worse in the morning. She further describes a low-grade fever and pain in her hands, feet, and left knee. She feels that her grip strength is diminished. These symptoms started rather abruptly 2 weeks ago and have not responded to acetaminophen.

She frequently camps with her family. She remembers that 1 week they could not go because her 8-year-old daughter had a fever, mild diarrhea, abdominal pain, and a skin rash ("legs, arms, and especially face were red and warm, and she seemed 'flushed' all the time"). Her daughter's symptoms resolved in a few days, she did not see a doctor, and no one else was sick. She has no other illnesses, and review of systems is otherwise negative.

On physical examination, her vitals are normal. She is unable to close her hands completely. Although the physical examination is somewhat limited by pain, there appears to be swelling of all metacarpophalangeal (MCP) and

proximal interphalangeal (PIP) joints, as well as mild erythema over the MCP joints bilaterally. In addition, upon examination of the left knee, the bulge sign (indicating effusion) is detected.

Question 11.1.1 If found on physical examination, which of the following would be LEAST useful in helping you in *narrowing* your diagnosis?
A) Bilateral metatarsophalangeal (MTP) joint swelling and tenderness
B) Painless oral ulcerations, with clean edges
C) Firm, slightly tender subcutaneous nodules at the olecranon bursae
D) A "bull's eye" rash in the right axilla
E) Icterus and tender hepatomegaly

Answer 11.1.1 The correct answer is "A." This patient presents with polyarticular inflammatory arthritis of unclear etiology. While important to note, MTP joint swelling would not add much to the picture of subacute, symmetrical, small joint polyarthritis that you have already found on examination. The differential diagnosis includes acute viral arthritis, specifically parvovirus B19 (due to the daughter's history of acute illness resembling erythema infectiosum), coxsackievirus, hepatitis B (hinted at in "E"), and HIV. Also on the differential will be Lyme disease ("D," although small joint symmetrical arthritis would be atypical), RA ("C," the presence of rheumatoid nodules would be helpful although these would be unlikely in early disease), and other inflammatory disorders. "B," *painless* ulcerations, are classically associated with SLE (systemic lupus erythematosus), but it ought to be noted that lupus aphthae (ulcers) may be painful as well.

After you sneak off to do a little reading, you examine her again. She has no rash. You detect bilateral pain and swelling of the third and fourth MTP joints. There are no oral ulcerations and no lymphadenopathy. She is not icteric, and her abdomen is diffusely, mildly tender. There is no hepatomegaly. You decide to order some blood tests.

Question 11.1.2 If positive, which of the following tests would be MOST helpful in ruling *in* a *specific* diagnosis?
A) Positive ANA
B) Elevated white count
C) Positive parvovirus B19 IgM
D) Positive urinalysis for white blood cells (WBCs)
E) Elevated ESR and CRP

Answer 11.1.2 **The correct answer is "C."** The presence of IgM antibodies to parvovirus B19—or rising titers of IgG antibodies—indicates acute viral infection, which may present with symptoms and signs seen in this patient. "A," positive ANA, will not help you rule in a diagnosis at this point. While the ANA is a highly sensitive test, it is not specific and has a low positive predictive value in the absence of the appropriate clinical symptoms and signs (just hammering this home). "B," "D," and "E" are all important findings, but would not lead you toward a specific diagnosis. "D," WBC in the urine could be from interstitial nephritis, a UTI, a nephritic urine from other causes, etc. Table 11-1 presents a framework for who should be tested for and diagnosed with RA.

HELPFUL TIP:
Note that the diagnosis of RA no longer requires 6 weeks of symptoms, although a longer duration of polyarthritis makes RA more likely. Similarly, it would be unusual for parvovirus B19 to cause symptoms for 6 weeks. However, the virus can cause prolonged joint pain in 10% of affected adults.

TABLE 11-1 AMERICAN COLLEGE OF RHEUMATOLOGY 2010 CLASSIFICATION CRITERIA FOR RHEUMATOID ARTHRITIS

Patients:

1. Who have at least 1 joint with definite clinical synovitis with the synovitis not better explained by another disease. 6 points makes the diagnosis of RA:

A. Joint involvement	
1 large joint	0
2–10 large joints	1
1–3 small joints (with or without involvement of large joints)	2
4–10 small joints (with or without involvement of large joints)	3
>10 joints (at least 1 small joint)	5
B. Serology (at least 1 test result is needed for classification)	
Negative RF and negative ACPA	0
Low-positive RF or low-positive ACPA	2
High-positive RF or high-positive ACPA	3
C. Acute-phase reactants (at least 1 test result is needed for classification)	
Normal CRP and normal ESR	0
Abnormal CRP or abnormal ESR	1
D. Duration of symptoms	
<6 weeks	0
>6 weeks	1

ACPA, anti-citrullinated peptide antibodies; RF, rheumatoid factor; CRP, c-reactive protein; ESR, erythrocyte sedimentation rate.

Diagnose rheumatoid arthritis if: Score of categories A–D is at least 6/10.

Used with permission from Aletaha D. Rheumatoid arthritis classification criteria: An American College of Rheumatology/European League Against Rheumatism collaborative initiative. *Arthritis Rheum.* 2010;62:2569–2581.

Her laboratory results return as follows:
- **Hepatitis B: Surface antibody positive, surface antigen negative**
- **CMV: IgG positive, IgM negative**
- **Parvovirus: IgG positive, IgM negative**
- **RF: 200 (normal: <14 units)**
- **Anti-citrullinated peptide antibodies (ACPA) 64 units (strong positive >60 units)**
- **ANA: Negative**
- **ESR: 58 mm/hr**

Note that based on results so far and according to Table 11-1, she has 7 points (4–10 joints involved, high titers of RF and ACPA, and elevated ESR.

Question 11.1.3 Which of the following is the most appropriate next step?
A) Bilateral hand x-rays
B) CT of the chest
C) Smith antibody, double-stranded DNA (dsDNA), complement levels

D) Start methotrexate 15 mg weekly by mouth and daily folic acid, with or without low-dose prednisone and follow-up in 4 to 5 weeks
E) Start prednisone 60 mg daily by mouth and follow up in 4 to 5 weeks

Answer 11.1.3 **The correct answer is "D."** This patient most likely has seropositive RA (see criteria in Table 11-1). The patient should be started on a disease-modifying anti-rheumatic drug (DMARD), such as weekly methotrexate at a moderate dose, along with folic acid 1 mg daily and prednisone 10 to 20 mg daily. Evidence suggests that there is a "window of opportunity" when treating early RA and that an early remission *may* lead to sustained remission.

Note that investigating for any evidence of other systemic involvement should be included as part of the initial evaluation. It is appropriate to obtain CBC, liver function tests, electrolytes, BUN, creatinine, and urinalysis (to rule out glomerulonephritis). "A" is incorrect. She is presenting fairly early after the onset of symptoms, so it is unlikely that hand x-rays will provide any significant findings. "B" is also incorrect. Without further symptoms or signs of lung involvement (e.g., pulmonary osteoarthropathy and respiratory symptoms), a CT scan would be inappropriate. As to "C," she has no other symptoms of lupus and also had a negative ANA, so further testing for lupus (Smith antibody, dsDNA [also known as anti-native DNA antibodies], complement levels) is not appropriate. "E" is incorrect. Although steroids are indicated, *low doses* are fine; higher doses are rarely necessary and are associated with greater side effects. Therefore, early institution of a DMARD would be preferable.

HELPFUL TIP:
Anti-citrullinated protein antibodies (ACPA), also known as anti-CCP (anti-cyclic citrullinated peptides), are very *specific* for RA; however, their *sensitivity* is 67% and therefore may be negative in RA.

HELPFUL (IF LONG) TIP:
In all cases of RA, and especially in those with a poorer prognosis, DMARDs should be instituted promptly, and escalated fairly rapidly, with goal being disease remission. Methotrexate (MTX) is the most commonly used DMARD in the United States, but combination therapy (methotrexate plus hydroxychloroquine or sulfasalazine) or triple therapy (methotrexate, hydroxychloroquine, and sulfasalazine) improves outcomes over methotrexate alone. *Low-dose* prednisone is indicated for immediate symptomatic relief. Recent data suggests that *low-dose* prednisone in the first 6 months up to 2 years after diagnosis is associated with better prognosis and more sustained remission. Occupational therapy referral is helpful in identifying and treating functional impairment due to RA. Vitamin D 800 IU/day and calcium 600 to 800 mg BID should be initiated with prednisone therapy to help prevent corticosteroid-induced osteoporosis. Evaluation of bone density (DEXA scan) and a bisphosphonate (e.g., alendronate) should be considered if >5 mg of prednisone is to be used for >3 months.

HELPFUL TIP:
RA typically has an insidious onset with a fluctuating course; however, a significant minority of patients (perhaps one-third) will experience rapid onset, over days to weeks.

She returns in 4 weeks and is now about 7 weeks into her illness. She reports a moderate response to your intervention (you started methotrexate 15 mg weekly with 1 mg folic acid daily and prednisone 20 mg daily), but now she has 1 to 2 hours of morning stiffness. She continues to complain of pain in her hands and feet, with poor grip. In fact, she had to take time off from work during the last week. On examination, she has persistent swelling of MCPs 2 to 5 bilaterally and

MTPs 3 and 4 bilaterally. You also note swelling in the left wrist and both knees, but tenderness is reduced and there is no erythema. You are now reconsidering your diagnosis. Did you miss something?

Question 11.1.4 What examination finding is so general that it would NOT help you support/reconsider your diagnosis?
A) Pleural rub auscultated on lung examination
B) Firm, slightly tender subcutaneous nodules at the olecranon bursae
C) Faint pink rash over chest, which is not visible 15 minutes later
D) Reduced passive flexion in left knee
E) Left foot drop

Answer 11.1.4 **The correct answer is "D."** While important to note, limitation of passive movements of the knees is indicative only of knee effusion (or pain), which you have already observed, and is not specific for any particular etiology. She responded modestly to methotrexate and prednisone but clearly still has active arthritis. What can you use to expand or limit your differential diagnosis? Pleural friction rub ("A") is indicative of possible lupus. Diagnostic criteria for lupus include serositis, which may be detectable as a pleural rub on auscultation of the lungs (also, look for malar rash, discoid lesions, alopecia, and oral ulcerations). Although not part of the diagnostic criteria for the disease, RA may also present with pleuritis or pericarditis. Rheumatoid nodules ("B") are found in RA. A salmon-colored, evanescent macular rash ("C") would lead you to consider adult-onset Still disease. Still disease, also known as juvenile idiopathic arthritis (JIA, discussed in Chapter 13), presents with an evanescent rash, intermittent fever, and arthritis. "Adult onset" Still disease is Still disease with onset after age 16. In addition, RF and CCP antibodies are typically negative in adult-onset Still disease. A finding of isolated foot drop ("E") may be the result of mononeuritis multiplex, a feature of vasculitides, and paraneoplastic syndromes. In fact, foot drop is the most common weakness with mononeuritis multiplex followed by wrist drop. Mononeuritis multiplex is defined as injury of two or more *named* nerves secondary to a vasculitis (e.g., ANCA-associated vasculitis, polyarteritis nodosum, cryoglobulin-associated vasculitis, lupus, RA, Sjogren syndrome, etc.).

Question 11.1.5 Since your patient is taking methotrexate, you caution her to avoid which of the following?
A) Aspirin
B) Sulfonamide antibiotics
C) Ibuprofen
D) Folate
E) Penicillin antibiotics

Answer 11.1.5 **The correct answer is "B."** Methotrexate is a folate antagonist. Antifolate medications, such as sulfonamide antibiotics, must be avoided in patients taking methotrexate because the combination may result in pancytopenia. Supplemental folate, 1 mg daily, reduces the adverse effects of methotrexate. Patients with RA are often treated with aspirin or NSAIDs in combination with methotrexate. Penicillin antibiotics can be administered safely with methotrexate, although methotrexate levels may increase by 8% or so.

HELPFUL TIP:
Drug interaction programs often warn about concomitant use of NSAIDs and methotrexate, as well as aspirin and methotrexate. These warnings are most relevant to high-dose methotrexate used to treat cancer, not the lower doses used for inflammatory arthritis.

At her first return visit, she had only mild improvement so you (rightly) added hydroxychloroquine (good job!). Initial hand x-rays demonstrate mild periarticular osteopenia. Liver function tests, urinalysis, CBC, BUN, and creatinine are normal. She returns 6 weeks after starting the hydroxychloroquine and is much improved, having returned to work full-time. She tells you that she still has problems with opening jars and about 45 minutes of morning stiffness, "But nothing like it was."

Question 11.1.6 What is the BEST course of action to follow now?
A) Continue her current therapy and follow up in 6 to 12 months with transaminases, RF, and hand x-rays
B) Continue her current therapy and follow up in 3 to 4 months with transaminases, RF, and hand x-rays
C) Continue current therapy and follow up in 3 to 4 months; arrange for monthly BUN, creatinine and CBC; and schedule for an annual ophthalmology examination
D) Begin prednisone taper, continue other medications, and arrange for monthly transaminases and CBC; schedule for baseline ophthalmology exam; and schedule follow-up in another 2 to 3 months
E) Instruct her to discontinue methotrexate, taper the prednisone dose, and continue hydroxychloroquine; arrange for follow-up in 1 year

Answer 11.1.6 The correct answer is "D." She seems to be responding to therapy, and a 3-month trial on her current medications (during which the methotrexate dose may be increased) is indicated. A slow prednisone taper should be initiated to minimize the cumulative dose of corticosteroids. Close follow-up is critical; she should contact you, should symptoms return during the steroid taper. Guidelines for monitoring her DMARD regimen recommend measurement of transaminases and CBC every 8 to 12 weeks for methotrexate and routine eye examination to assess for hydroxychloroquine-related retinal toxicity. A baseline eye examination is necessary when starting hydroxychloroquine; annual screening should begin after 5 years, unless the patient is at high risk for complications. Hand x-rays are recommended at 2-year intervals. "E" is incorrect: DMARD therapy reduces her risk of joint destruction and disease progression and should not be discontinued.

At her next visit 3 months later, she feels better. Although she still has difficulty opening jars, she now has <30 minutes of morning stiffness and almost no pain. On examination, she has no rash, nodules, or evidence of serositis. She now has swelling over MCPs 2 to 4 on the right and 2 to 3 on the left. Her grip is still somewhat weak but improved. Laboratory data shows an ESR of 28 mm/hr, CRP 0.7 mg/dL, and normal transaminases and CBC. Her symptoms increased when she tapered prednisone to less than 10 mg/day, so she is taking 20 mg/day once again.

Question 11.1.7 Which of the following is the most appropriate next step?
A) Increase methotrexate to 25 mg weekly, continue hydroxychloroquine, and refer to rheumatology
B) Stop methotrexate and switch to leflunomide 20 mg/day
C) Increase prednisone to 60 mg daily
D) Discontinue all medications except methotrexate
E) Discontinue methotrexate, taper prednisone, and continue hydroxychloroquine

Answer 11.1.7 The correct answer is "A." Despite her initial response, she has evidence of ongoing inflammatory activity by history and examination. Discontinuing or reducing medication is inappropriate. According to published guidelines, consultation with a rheumatologist is now indicated—if it had not been sought sooner. She has had a fair initial response to methotrexate, prednisone, and hydroxychloroquine. Further benefit may be gained with increasing the methotrexate dose. Addition of sulfasalazine would also be appropriate. If "triple therapy" with methotrexate, hydroxychloroquine, and sulfasalazine fails, she will need a biological agent. "B" is incorrect: since she had an initial response to methotrexate, and may show further efficacy at a higher dose, it would be wise to further increase the methotrexate dose, rather than substituting another agent, such as leflunomide. Leflunomide is a nonbiologic immunosuppressant that can cause liver injury. Its place in therapy is in patients who cannot tolerate or have a contraindication to a biologic agent (see below). "C" is incorrect: doses of prednisone this high are not indicated for RA.

Question 11.1.8 This patient wants to become pregnant. You can tell her that:
A) Symptoms remit in 70% of women during pregnancy
B) She should avoid pregnancy while taking methotrexate
C) RA is a contraindication to pregnancy
D) Prednisone cannot be taken during pregnancy
E) A and B

Answer 11.1.8 The correct answer is "E," both "A" and "B" are correct. RA is an autoimmune disease, and it tends to remit during pregnancy when a woman is relatively immunosuppressed. Methotrexate is class X for pregnancy and is actually used in ectopic pregnancy to arrest fetal growth. Women taking methotrexate should use an effective form of contraception and continue contraception for 3 months after stopping methotrexate. "D" is incorrect since prednisone is often used to control RA during pregnancy, when methotrexate is contraindicated. Prednisone does not cross the placenta, but use during pregnancy is associated with higher risk for gestational diabetes.

....

The patient is an avid runner and, prior to her diagnosis, participated in numerous outdoor activities. She is concerned about whether she will eventually become disabled.

Question 11.1.9 **You can let her know that:**
A) RA tends to progress without any remissions to involve almost all joints in all patients
B) Prednisone-free disease remission has become the goal of treatment
C) Patients with RA have the same life expectancy as the general public
D) Renal involvement is common with RA and is a major source of morbidity and mortality
E) She won't need to worry about having a life after she gets pregnant and has a child. All her energy will be absorbed by that little parasite … er, child.

Answer 11.1.9 **The correct answer is "B."** With the advent of new potent disease-modifying agents, it is now possible for RA patients to achieve remission, defined as the absence or near absence of joint pain and swelling. "A" is incorrect. Untreated RA may progress to involve further joints, but not all joints are affected by RA. Classically, the distal interphalangeal joints are spared and, if there is DIP involvement, should prompt reassessment of the diagnosis. Moreover, treatment with DMARDs can, and frequently does, induce remission. "C" is incorrect. RA reduces the life expectancy by up to 10 years (due to earlier cardiac disease, infections, lymphoma). "D" is incorrect. Renal disease is a rare complication of RA; however, it can be a result of some of the medications used to treat RA. Finally, "E." If she wants a life after becoming a parent, she can borrow a life from us—we're chained to this book. Or, she can buy one at Costco wholesale.

....

She has an exacerbation of her disease despite triple therapy. You refer to a rheumatologist who recommends the use of a biologic agent for RA.

Question 11.1.10 **Which of the following screenings are required before beginning a biological agent to treat rheumatoid arthritis?**
A) CMV
B) TB
C) Heart failure
D) Mucosal candidiasis
E) B and C

Answer 11.1.10 **The correct answer is "E."** There are a number of biologics for treating rheumatoid arthritis that are TNF inhibitors. Etanercept (Enbrel) is a soluble TNF receptor antagonist. Infliximab (Remicade) and adalimumab (Humira) are monoclonal antibodies that bind TNF both at the cell and when it is in its soluble form. These drugs can also reduce the resistance to infection and promote malignancies. *All of the TNF inhibitors essentially have the same efficacy.* Any one of these agents can be added to MTX. Things to watch for with TNF inhibitors include serious infections (e.g., TB, fungal infections) and malignancies. Rule out TB and hepatitis B before starting TNF inhibitors. There is also a concern for worsening congestive heart failure in those with preexisting disease. Thus, "E" is the correct answer. Mucocutaneous candidiasis is not a contraindication to TNF inhibitors, and routine testing for CMV is not recommended.

HELPFUL TIP:
Does joint replacement work in RA? Yes. Remember, however, that the maximum life span of an artificial joint is about 15 years with current technology. Thus, replacement should not be undertaken lightly in a young patient—or any patient for that matter.

▶ **Objectives: Did you learn to …**
· Describe an appropriate diagnostic strategy for polyarthritis?
· Recognize the diagnostic criteria for RA?
· Develop a management strategy for RA?
· Recognize the importance of early DMARD therapy for RA?
· Identify the uses and adverse effects of medications used to treat RA?

 QUICK QUIZ: AN ILL CHILD

A concerned mother brings in her 2-year-old son with a 1-week history of fever. She is worried because she had expected the fever to resolve by now. According to his mother, the patient also has a rash, poor appetite, and lethargy. On examination, he looks ill and his temperature is 39.0°C. There is a diffuse, erythematous, macular rash, and peeling skin on the fingertips. The oropharynx is injected and the tongue is bright red with white papillae. Cervical lymph nodes are enlarged and tender.

Based on the available information, what is your leading diagnosis?
A) Rheumatic fever
B) Parvovirus B19 infection
C) Kawasaki syndrome
D) Juvenile idiopathic arthritis (JIA)
E) Varicella infection

The correct answer is "C." Kawasaki syndrome is an acute vasculitis of unknown etiology, which is most often seen in children. Kawasaki syndrome presents *with at least 5 days of fever* (required fever duration for the diagnosis of Kawasaki disease), polymorphous rash, conjunctival injection, mucous membrane involvement (e.g., "strawberry" tongue), cervical lymphadenopathy, and extremity findings of erythema and desquamation. The usual treatment is aspirin and IVIG. Corticosteroid therapy is controversial and does not seem to improve outcomes. There may be cardiac involvement with the formation of coronary artery aneurysms.

"A," rheumatic fever, which is rare in developed countries, is recognized by the Jones criteria. The major Jones criteria consist of polyarthritis, carditis, Sydenham chorea, erythema marginatum, and subcutaneous nodules. Here's a fun mnemonic: "JONES" with a heart shape in place of the "O," so that J = joints, O = carditis, N = nodules, E = erythema marginatum, and S = Sydenham chorea. "B" is incorrect. Generally, children do not appear this ill with parvovirus B19 infection (fifth disease). "D," JIA, would be unusual at such a young age, and is discussed in Chapter 13. "E" is incorrect, as this is obviously not varicella.

▶ CASE 11.2

A 62-year-old male who you have followed for hypertension for several years presents with complaints of worsening fatigue and aching in his back, shoulders, and neck. He notes 3 months of symptoms unresponsive to acetaminophen.

Further history reveals that your patient has experienced stiffness of the neck and shoulders each morning for over 30 minutes. He occasionally has difficulty getting out of bed due to pain. Vital signs are within normal limits. There is no evidence of synovitis of the hands, wrists, or elbows. Active range of motion in the neck and shoulders is slow but full. There is tenderness to palpation of the shoulders, upper back, and neck, but no apparent muscle atrophy.

Question 11.2.1 **Which of the following is the most appropriate next step in the diagnosis of this illness?**
A) Obtain an ESR and CRP
B) Obtain a urinalysis
C) Prescribe a diagnostic trial of corticosteroids
D) Order a rheumatology panel, including ANA, uric acid, ESR, CRP, and RF
E) Perform shoulder radiograph

Answer 11.2.1 **The correct answer is "A."** This patient's presentation is consistent with the diagnosis of polymyalgia rheumatica (PMR). Elevations of ESR and/or CRP contribute further evidence to such a diagnosis and are useful in following the treatment of PMR. While a urinalysis ("B") may be important in some rheumatologic illnesses (e.g., lupus, Behçet syndrome), PMR is not likely to be associated with renal disease.

A trial of corticosteroid therapy ("C"), may be appropriate, but an ESR should be obtained first to more conclusively establish the diagnosis. At this point all we know is that he has bilateral shoulder and neck pain, which could be mechanical from the cervical spine, etc. As you already know from earlier discussion, "D" is incorrect; a "rheumatology panel" will typically include tests that are not indicated, and positive results can be misleading. In the absence of small joint symptoms or examination findings, an RF is not indicated in this case. Likewise, there is no history to suggest an ANA-related

TABLE 11-2 EUROPEAN LEAGUE AGAINST RHEUMATISM AND AMERICAN COLLEGE OF RHEUMATOLOGY CLASSIFICATION CRITERIA FOR POLYMYALGIA RHEUMATICA

Required Criteria	
Age > 50 years	
Bilateral shoulder pain	
Elevated ESR and/or CRP	
Clinical Criteria	
Morning stiffness lasting over 45 minutes	2 points
Hip pain or restricted range of motion	1 point
Negative RF and ACPA	2 points
Absence of other joint involvement	1 point
Ultrasound Criteria	
>1 shoulder with subdeltoid bursitis, biceps tenosynovitis, or glenohumeral synovitis, AND >1 hip with synovitis or trochanteric bursitis	1 point
Both shoulders with subdeltoid bursitis, biceps tenosynovitis, or glenohumeral synovitis	1 point

ACPA, anti-citrullinated peptide antibodies; CRP, c-reactive protein; ESR, erythrocyte sedimentation rate; RF, rheumatoid factor.

A score ≥4 points without ultrasonography, or >5 with ultrasonography, in addition to fulfillment of the required criteria, is categorized as polymyalgia rheumatica.

Adapted from Dasgupta B, et al. 2012 provisional classification criteria for polymyalgia rheumatica. *Arthritis Rheum.* 2012;64(4):943–954.

disorder. "E" is incorrect. This patient does not need shoulder radiographs. In a patient with bilateral shoulder pain and neck pain, a neck radiograph may be more useful than shoulder imaging. Neck radiographs help to evaluate for cervical canal narrowing and degenerative disc disease, which may result in pain and neurologic findings in the upper extremities. An MRI of the neck might be useful if cervical spine disc disease or a syrinx were suspected. Diagnostic criteria for PMR are given in Table 11-2. Small joint synovitis, or puffy swelling of hands and feet, will occur in 20% of patients with PMR; and in these cases, it is appropriate to check RF and ACPA during your initial evaluation.

HELPFUL TIP:
Physical examination findings of PMR are subtle. Active ROM in the affected areas is often limited by pain, but passive ROM should be full. Strength is intact. In general, PMR affects shoulders to a greater degree than hips, and the hips more than the neck. The essential pathology is inflammation of the synovia, and muscles are not directly involved.

Question 11.2.2 The sensitivity of an elevated ESR in the diagnosis of PMR and giant cell arteritis (GCA) is:
A) 100%
B) 85%
C) 50%
D) 25%

Answer 11.2.2 **The correct answer is "B."** Up to 15% of patients with PMR or GCA (a closely related disorder—keep reading) have a false-negative ESR. Using ESR and CRP together is 97% to 99% sensitive for GCA. Double false negatives of ESR and CRP are uncommon but do occur. Thus, in the patient in whom GCA is suspected but in whom there is a normal ESR and/or CRP, biopsy is still recommended. In those suspected of PMR with normal ESR and/or CRP, a trial of empiric therapy is warranted.

HELPFUL TIP:
Patients with PMR often have a low-grade fever and a normocytic anemia.

HELPFUL TIP:
PMR is uncommon in non-white populations. The mean age of onset is approximately 70 years. Women are affected twice as often as men.

You order radiographs of the neck, which demonstrate mild degenerative disease. A CBC is unremarkable, except for a mild thrombocytosis. The ESR is 80 mm/hr. You relate these findings to the patient and tell him that your presumptive diagnosis is PMR.

Question 11.2.3 Which of the following is the most appropriate initial treatment in this case?
A) Naproxen 500 mg twice daily
B) Prednisone 15 mg daily
C) Aspirin 650 mg twice daily
D) Prednisone 50 mg daily
E) Referral to physical therapy

Answer 11.2.3 **The correct answer is "B."** Prednisone is the treatment of choice in PMR. Doses of prednisone ranging from 10 to 20 mg daily are usually sufficient to control the disease. Higher doses (up to 30 mg/day) should be tried if there is no response in 1 to 2 weeks. If the patient fails to respond to 30 mg or less of prednisone, the diagnosis of PMR should be reconsidered. "A" is incorrect. NSAIDs may provide some symptomatic relief, but are not the treatment for PMR. It remains controversial whether low-dose aspirin 81 mg/day may decrease the risk of vision loss in giant cell arteritis. In general, use it only in patients in whom it is indicated for another diagnosis. However, high-dose aspirin therapy ("C") without corticosteroids is not recommended. "E" is incorrect.

Since patients usually respond quickly to corticosteroids, physical therapy is not necessary—although you could hardly be faulted for employing physical therapy as part of your overall treatment approach.

HELPFUL TIP:
Looking at the long-term outcomes, initial low-dose therapy prednisone for PMR works better than high-dose therapy. Patients have fewer relapses and are spared some of the adverse effects of high-dose corticosteroids.

You prescribe prednisone 15 mg daily, aspirin 81 mg daily, and calcium and vitamin D supplementation. Your patient presents for follow-up 4 weeks later, reporting marked improvement. On examination, there is no joint inflammation, or muscle tenderness with a range of motion exercises. His ESR is 20 mm/hr. You believe that the patient's disease is now in remission.

Question 11.2.4 Which of the following is the most appropriate next step in his management?
A) Discontinue prednisone and initiate naproxen
B) Continue the current dose of prednisone for the next 12 months
C) Continue the current dose of prednisone for the next 6 months
D) Taper prednisone by 1 to 2 mg every 2 weeks to reach the minimum effective dose
E) Taper prednisone by 5 mg over 2 weeks and then discontinue the drug

Answer 11.2.4 **The correct answer is "D."** Relapse of PMR occurs more frequently when corticosteroids are abruptly discontinued or tapered too quickly. However, due to complications associated with corticosteroid therapy, the dose should be reduced as soon as possible; therefore, maintaining prednisone 15 mg daily for 6 to 12 months is inappropriate. The usual recommendation is to reduce the dose of prednisone by 10% every 1 to 2 weeks until the minimum effective dose is reached. While tapering prednisone, the patient should be monitored with an ESR and/or CRP every 2 to 4 weeks. If symptoms worsen, prednisone should be increased slightly to achieve symptomatic control. If the ESR increases to 40 mm/hr or greater and the patient is asymptomatic, consider continuing the same dose of prednisone until the ESR normalizes, then continue the taper. *However, an isolated elevation in ESR without symptoms is not a reason to increase prednisone.*

Question 11.2.5 Which of the following is true regarding the prognosis of PMR?
A) PMR is associated with an increased risk of mortality
B) Most patients with PMR will require corticosteroid therapy for life

C) Up to 50% of patients who initially have a successful remission will experience a relapse while tapering prednisone

D) A relapse of PMR requires high-dose corticosteroids (prednisone 50 mg daily) for successful treatment

Answer 11.2.5 The correct answer is "C." Relapses occur in 30% to 50% of patients after induction of remission and should be treated by resuming or increasing prednisone. Usually, successful treatment of a relapse requires increasing the prednisone dose by a few milligrams. "A" is incorrect. Although the pathogenesis of PMR is incompletely understood, it has features in common with vasculitides, including potential vascular complications of GCA. However, PMR is not associated with an increase in mortality. "B" is incorrect because PMR is a self-limited disease, and most patients recover within a few months to a few years. Thus, patients require prednisone for 6 months to 2 years, but prednisone therapy is typically not lifelong. Remote relapses of PMR after prednisone has been successfully stopped are seen in about 20% of cases and can occur up to years later.

....

Your patient does well and is able to taper off prednisone over a year. Twelve months after stopping corticosteroids, he presents to the ED one weekend. His shoulder and neck pain and stiffness have returned, as well as severe fatigue and subjective fevers. He has lost 5 pounds over 2 weeks. He is now experiencing frequent left-sided headaches. Finally, he is most concerned about a new visual disturbance starting today. He notes that he has a "hole" in his vision. On physical examination, there is a prominent, tender vessel palpable at the left temporal area. Funduscopic examination of the left eye shows a pale disc with blurred margins. The remainder of the neurologic examination is normal. The ESR is 70 mm/hr.

Question 11.2.6 Which of the following is the most likely diagnosis for the visual symptoms?
A) Polymyalgia rheumatica (PMR)
B) Stroke (CVA)
C) Giant cell arteritis (GCA)
D) Multiple sclerosis (MS)
E) Acute angle-closure glaucoma

Answer 11.2.6 The correct answer is "C." Many of the patient's symptoms can be explained by PMR ("A"), but visual symptoms do not occur with this disease. GCA (aka temporal arteritis) is a related diagnosis that is commonly seen in conjunction with PMR. Most experts now agree that PMR and GCA are different presentations of the same disease process. With the new symptoms of localized headache and tenderness of the temporal artery and the previously known findings consistent with PMR, this patient now meets diagnostic criteria for GCA (see Table 11-3). The visual symptoms described are typical of GCA and can occur acutely or chronically. As to the other answers, vision loss in multiple sclerosis is attributable to optic neuritis, which is associated with pain and presents initially in a younger population. Acute angle-closure glaucoma is associated with eye pain and redness. The lack of other neurological symptoms makes stroke less likely.

TABLE 11-3 AMERICAN COLLEGE OF RHEUMATOLOGY CLASSIFICATION CRITERIA FOR GIANT CELL ARTERITIS

A patient with vasculitis may be classified as having giant cell arteritis if she or he fulfills three of the following five criteria:
- Age ≥ 50 years at onset of symptoms
- New localized headache, jaw claudication, visual symptoms
- Temporal artery tenderness or decreased pulsation
- ESR ≥ 50 mm/hr
- Abnormal temporal artery biopsy findings

HELPFUL TIP:
The initial visual loss in GCA is peripheral, while the vision loss in macular degeneration is initially central. If you think about it, this makes sense. GCA basically causes an anterior ischemic optic neuropathy (AION) secondary to involvement of the retinal artery by vasculitis. Areas further from the artery will have poorer perfusion.

Question 11.2.7 Which of the following is the most appropriate initial management of this patient?
A) Withhold treatment for now and arrange for temporal artery biopsy within 48 hours
B) Withhold treatment for now and arrange for an ultrasound of his temporal artery next week
C) Refer to an ophthalmologist as soon as possible
D) Initiate prednisone 20 mg daily and refer for temporal artery biopsy
E) Admit and administer methylprednisolone 1 g intravenously (IV) and arrange for temporal artery biopsy

Answer 11.2.7 The correct answer is "E." When symptoms of vision loss occur, IV methylprednisolone 15 mg/kg/day (up to 1 g) daily for 3 days, followed by prednisone 40 to 60 mg daily is the standard of care. Compared to PMR, higher doses of corticosteroids are necessary to treat GCA. In the absence of vision loss, prednisone doses of 40 to 60 mg daily are usually required to relieve symptoms. Consultation with ophthalmology is also necessary in providing proper care to the patient. "A" is incorrect. You do not want to withhold treatment from this patient whose vision is at risk (see "Helpful Tip" below). Ultrasonography for the "Halo Sign" is being actively investigated. It has a high specificity (94%) but low sensitivity (42%) and so should not be used to rule out cases of GCA. "B" and "C" are incorrect for the same reason. "D" is incorrect because a dose of 20 mg of prednisone is too low to be effective in GCA.

HELPFUL TIP:
Temporal artery biopsy is the gold standard test for the accurate diagnosis of GCA. Characteristic giant cell inflammation pathology can be seen for up to 4 weeks after initiating high-dose corticosteroids. However, corticosteroid therapy should never be delayed for fear of reducing the inflammatory findings on the temporal artery biopsy.

Six years after his diagnosis of GCA, your patient has experienced several remissions and relapses. Although he has been able to discontinue prednisone on occasion, he is now taking 5 mg daily with good symptomatic control. He asks about whether there are other treatments that may help him to wean off prednisone.

Question 11.2.8 **Which of the following medications may be used as a part of a steroid-sparing regimen for the treatment of GCA?**
A) Hydroxychloroquine
B) Adalimumab
C) Tocilizumab
D) Azathioprine
E) All of the above

Answer 11.2.8 **The correct answer is "C."** It is believed that in patients with GCA, elevated serum levels of interleukin-6 correlate with disease activity. Tocilizumab, an interleukin-6 receptor alpha inhibitor, allows for reductions in glucocorticoid doses that are used to control GCA and to maintain remission. It is currently FDA approved for subcutaneous use in the treatment of GCA. Hydroxychloroquine ("A"), TNF inhibitors (including adalimumab, "B"), and azathioprine ("C") are incorrect. There have been no studies supporting their use in GCA.

One dark and stormy night, 3 AM in the ED—the weather is cold and the coffee is colder—your patient presents with tearing substernal chest pain radiating to his back. He is alert but anxious and diaphoretic. His left radial pulse is diminished compared to the right. His heart rate is 120 bpm, and his blood pressure is 92/56 mm Hg.

Question 11.2.9 **Which of the following studies will confirm the most likely diagnosis?**
A) Chest radiograph
B) Chest CT
C) ECG
D) Venous blood gas
E) Troponin-T

Answer 11.2.9 **The correct answer is "B."** Your patient's symptoms are classic for a dissecting thoracic aortic aneurysm, which is often mistaken for a myocardial infarction. Thoracic aortic aneurysm is a late complication of GCA; aortic aneurysms generally occur an average of 6 to 7 years after the initial diagnosis of GCA. Thoracic aortic aneurysms occur 17 times more often in patients with GCA when compared to the general population. The diagnosis of thoracic aortic aneurysm is confirmed by CT scan of the chest, transesophageal echocardiogram, or angiogram. While the other studies listed should be done, none of them are going to make the diagnosis of a dissecting aneurysm for you.

HELPFUL TIP:
With the initiation of corticosteroids in PMR or GCA, start calcium 1,200 to 1,500 mg daily and vitamin D 400 to 800 IU daily for osteoporosis prevention. Once the diagnosis is confirmed (and prednisone will be continued for an extended period), bone mineral density should be measured with a DEXA scan and bisphosphonates instituted on the basis of FRAX calculated risk of fracture or DEXA results (do you see a pattern here of prophylaxis for osteoporosis when starting corticosteroids?).

▶ **Objectives: Did you learn to …**
- Describe the appropriate evaluation, including physical examination and laboratory tests, of diffuse pain in the older patient?
- Recognize the diagnostic criteria for PMR and GCA?
- Describe the appropriate management, including medical therapy, of PMR and GCA?
- Identify complications of PMR and GCA?

▶ **CASE 11.3**

A 22-year-old graduate student presents to the ED on a Monday night with an acutely swollen left knee. He admits to "wild partying" over the weekend but only had "a couple of beers" (that is the "college couple"… so, 6 or 7). His knee was OK then. However, when he woke up this morning, he noticed the knee was swollen and painful (so was his head, but that's another matter). By early afternoon, he had difficulty bearing weight. He denies fever, but feels tired.

He reports a history of JIA (juvenile idiopathic arthritis) and has had ankle and knee swelling previously, but not to this degree. He took prednisone intermittently, as well as hydroxychloroquine and methotrexate, for his JIA until age 18. He then continued on hydroxychloroquine until 8 months ago, when he stopped it because he felt fine. He denies any other medical problems. He smokes only when drinking—which happens way too often.

Question 11.3.1 **What other information from the history would be most helpful in establishing the diagnosis?**
A) Sexual history, including sexual orientation, practices, and last contact
B) Personal or family history of gout or kidney stones
C) History of IV drug use
D) Family history of pseudogout
E) A, B, and C

Answer 11.3.1 **The correct answer is "E."** While all of these points are important in the history, this patient is too young to have pseudogout. While gout is unusual in young adults, there are uncommon syndromes of familial hyperuricemia and early gout. Although there are several possible etiologies for this patient's presentation, septic arthritis should be considered first and foremost due to its high morbidity and mortality. As such, the history and examination should focus on those clues that point toward an infectious etiology and its source. The clinician must also consider noninfectious inflammatory arthropathies. IV drug abuse can lead to a septic joint as can gonorrhea. Thus "A" and "B" are important parts of the history.

Your patient is heterosexual and *thinks* he had intercourse Saturday night (2 nights ago), but admits that his memory is somewhat blurry (maybe he had more than the "couple" of beers he claims). He denies a history of gout and IV drug use. He complains of poor sleep and feeling stiff in the mornings and evenings lately.

Question 11.3.2 What findings on physical examination would be LEAST helpful in determining the diagnosis?
A) A few vesiculopustular lesions on the back, arms, and legs
B) Swollen, tender, nonerythematous MCP joints
C) Nontender hepatomegaly
D) Diastolic murmur at the right sternal border
E) Whitish discharge from the tip of penis

Answer 11.3.2 **The correct answer is "C."** Although nontender hepatomegaly may indicate presence of liver disease, it is unlikely to help identify the etiology of this patient's arthritis. Hepatitis B arthritis usually presents as a symmetric polyarthritis, although it can be migratory or additive (sequential joints becoming involved without resolution in the initial joints). Our patient has a single swollen, hot joint, which is unlikely to occur as a result of hepatitis. "A" is helpful: a vesiculopustular rash occurs in disseminated gonococcal infections. "B" is also helpful: the presence of other swollen joints should prompt consideration of noninfectious inflammatory arthritis, and the swelling of the MCPs in particular may be a clue for active RA. The detection of a diastolic murmur ("D") is significant, since diastolic murmurs are almost always pathologic in adults, and may represent infective endocarditis. Finally, "E," penile discharge, can result from acute gonorrheal infections.

On examination, vital signs are significant only for tachycardia and fever (pulse 112 bpm, temperature 38.2°C). He has no other swollen joints, rashes, heart murmurs, or penile discharge. You palpate a smooth, nontender liver edge 2 cm below the costal margin; it percusses to 15 cm. You note mild cervical lymphadenopathy and whitish pharyngeal exudates.

Question 11.3.3 Which of the following is the most appropriate next step in the management of this patient?
A) Order hepatitis serologies
B) Order blood cultures, urine PCR for chlamydia and gonorrhea, and abdominal ultrasound
C) Administer ceftriaxone 1 g IV and inject the knee with triamcinolone

D) Perform knee aspiration
E) Prescribe prednisone 20 mg PO QD and arrange consultation with a rheumatologist

Answer 11.3.3 **The correct answer is "D."** Did you get distracted by a big liver? If so, redirect your attention to the knee. The single most important step in evaluating acute monoarthritis is joint aspiration, which will allow differentiation between inflammatory and noninflammatory disease. Although blood cultures and urine PCR for chlamydia and gonorrhea should also be sent in this case, obtaining these studies must not delay joint aspiration. Without determining whether the arthritis is infectious, it would be inappropriate—and potentially hazardous to the patient—to start treatment with corticosteroids. "C" and "E" are incorrect because you would **not** want to give corticosteroids—especially intra-articular corticosteroids—to a patient with an infected joint. Analysis of the synovial fluid will aid in determining the appropriateness of treating with antibiotics or anti-inflammatory medications. Joint aspiration will also provide a specimen for crystal examination. While you would probably use empiric antibiotics (treat as septic until proven otherwise), you will need to first obtain cultures (from the knee aspiration and blood).

HELPFUL TIP:
CBC, ESR, and CRP are not useful in diagnosing a septic joint. While they may be somewhat sensitive, they are hopelessly nonspecific. You have to tap the joint if they are normal or if they are abnormal. There's just no getting around it. Just do it!

You have obtained blood cultures and urine PCR for chlamydia and gonorrhea. A metabolic profile, CBC, and hepatitis B and C serologies are pending. Knee aspiration yields 45 cc of turbid, blood-tinged fluid.

Question 11.3.4 You send the synovial fluid for all of the following studies EXCEPT:
A) Cell count and differential
B) Crystal analysis
C) Culture
D) Glucose and protein
E) Gram stain

Answer 11.3.4 **The correct answer is "D."** In contrast to analysis of some other bodily fluids (e.g., cerebrospinal fluid [CSF], pleural fluid, and ascitic fluid), chemistry analysis on synovial fluid is of little diagnostic value. Low glucose levels in synovial fluid are associated with the degree of inflammation but do not help to determine its cause. Likewise, synovial protein levels do not help differentiate between types of arthritis. Cell count with differential, Gram stain, and cultures should be routine when suspecting infection; crystal analysis is also part of the standard examination, but positive crystal analysis does not rule out concomitant infection.

The synovial fluid analysis reveals the following findings: 50,000 WBC/mm³, 95% polymorphonuclear cells, and no crystals. Gram stain shows Gram-negative diplococci. Cultures are pending. Gonorrhea and chlamydia PCR tests are also pending.

Question 11.3.5 What is the sensitivity of a synovial fluid white count of 100,000/mm³ for infection?
A) 30%
B) 40%
C) 50%
D) 60%
E) 75%

Answer 11.3.5 The correct answer is "A." Unfortunately, a synovial white count of 100,000/mm³ is only 30% sensitive for a septic joint but is 99% specific. 50,000 WBC/mm³ is 62% sensitive and 92% specific while a WBC count of 25,000/mm³ is 75% sensitive and 73% specific. The point is that what we were taught in school about the synovial WBC count being >100,000/mm³ in a septic joint is wrong.

Question 11.3.6 Which of the following studies will be most important to the OVERALL care of this patient?
A) HIV testing and RPR
B) Chest x-ray
C) ANA and RF
D) Uric acid
E) ESR and CRP

Answer 11.3.6 The correct answer is "A." His presentation is very suggestive of disseminated gonococcal infection with acute arthritis, and the presence of diplococci is virtually diagnostic. Therefore, the clinician must also consider the presence of other sexually transmitted diseases and screen the patient appropriately. Assays for hepatitis B and C and chlamydia have been sent, and tests for HIV and syphilis should now be performed. Also, the patient must be counseled regarding safe sexual practices (e.g., condom use, reduced alcohol use, become a monk…). In this setting, the other studies are less relevant to his overall health.

HELPFUL TIP:
Gonococcus is cultured from the joint fluid only about 50% of the time in patients with gonococcal arthritis. Thus, urine and joint fluid PCR should be done even if the Gram stain is negative.

Question 11.3.7 Which of the following is the most appropriate treatment plan for this patient's septic arthritis?
A) Ceftriaxone 1 g IV once, followed by cefixime 400 mg twice daily by mouth for 14 days; follow-up in 7 days
B) Admit to hospital, administer ceftriaxone 1 g IV daily, and perform repeat knee aspirations

C) Admit to the hospital and administer IV and intra-articular ceftriaxone 1 g daily
D) Ciprofloxacin 500 mg by mouth twice daily for 14 days; follow-up in 7 days
E) Penicillin G 4 million units IV once, followed by amoxicillin 500 mg PO three times daily for 14 days; follow-up with a rheumatologist

Answer 11.3.7 The correct answer is "B." In order to ensure the best outcome, this patient should be admitted for monitoring and repeated joint aspiration. Purulent fluid tends to collect rapidly in the joint spaces in patients with septic arthritis, necessitating frequent drainage until antibiotics work and inflammation begins to subside. Most cases of gonococcal arthritis respond to needle aspiration plus antibiotics, but arthroscopic or open debridement is occasionally necessary. Because IV antibiotics have good penetration into synovial fluid, intra-articular antibiotics are not recommended. When culture, PCR, and sensitivity results become available, antibiotic therapy should be tailored to the particular infectious agent and its susceptibilities.

HELPFUL TIP:
The initial antibiotic of choice in gonococcal arthritis is ceftriaxone, administered IV. Spectinomycin IV is an acceptable alternative when ceftriaxone is contraindicated. Remember that there is now fluoroquinolone-resistant gonococcus. Because of this, fluoroquinolones are no longer recommended as treatment of gonorrhea.

Within 48 hours, your patient shows signs of improvement. His knee appears much better, there is no recurrent effusion, and he is afebrile. He wants to leave the hospital. By the way, his chlamydia PCR turned up positive.

Question 11.3.8 Which of the following management strategies do you recommend?
A) Continue the hospital admission and ceftriaxone 1 g IV daily
B) Discharge with ciprofloxacin 500 mg by mouth twice daily
C) Discharge with penicillin V 500 mg by mouth three times daily
D) Discharge with cefixime 400 mg by mouth twice daily, and doxycycline 100 mg by mouth twice daily

Answer 11.3.8 The correct answer is "D." Since the patient is improving, continued hospitalization and IV antibiotics are not needed. Thus, "A" is incorrect. Without knowing the antibiotic sensitivities of the gonococcus, you should assume that it is penicillin-resistant, making "C" a poor choice. Once local and systemic signs are resolving, you can safely discharge the patient with oral antibiotic therapy, using cefixime 400 mg twice daily (or an acceptable alternative based on culture and susceptibilities) to complete a 7- to 14-day course. In cases of gonococcal infection, you should *always* presumptively treat for concurrent chlamydia infection.

Question 11.3.9 What is the mortality rate of septic arthritis?
A) 0.5%
B) 5%
C) 10%
D) >15%

Answer 11.3.9 **The correct answer is "C."** The mortality rate of septic arthritis is 10%, with up to one-third of survivors having persistent joint problems, such as limited range of motion, pain, and swelling. Note that the mortality is probably not due to the infection alone but rather due to a combination of the underlying illness (e.g., immunosuppression) and the infection.

▸ **Objectives: Did you learn to …**
- Describe the appropriate evaluation of monoarthritis?
- Appropriately manage a patient with septic arthritis?
- Identify risk factors for septic arthritis?
- Recognize the prognosis of septic arthritis?

▶ CASE 11.4

A 55-year-old male presents to your office complaining of severe left knee pain of 2 days duration. Although he was also out partying over the weekend (is there a pattern here to the patients in our practice?), he went home early (say, 2 or 3 o'clock). He denies any previous history of knee pain or arthritis. He has felt feverish over the last 2 days. He recalls a similar episode of pain in his right great toe 2 years before, but the pain resolved in a few days and he did not seek medical attention. He has hypertension treated with chlorthalidone but is otherwise healthy. He drinks about a case of beer per week—unless he's been partying, in which case he doubles his effort. His family history is remarkable for osteoarthritis.

Physical examination reveals an uncomfortable-appearing obese male in no acute distress. His temperature is 37.9°C, blood pressure 168/98 mm Hg, and pulse 84 bpm. The left knee is red, warm, and diffusely tender with a palpable effusion. There are no visible or palpable subcutaneous nodules on the fingers, toes, or at the elbows.

Question 11.4.1 Which of the following is the most appropriate next step to accurately diagnose this condition?
A) Radiograph of the affected knee
B) CBC
C) Serum uric acid level

D) Knee aspiration and synovial fluid analysis
E) Diagnostic corticosteroid injection

Answer 11.4.1 **The correct answer is "D."** We don't mean to sound like a broken record, but the diagnostic study of choice in a monoarthritis is synovial fluid analysis. Synovial fluid analysis allows the clinician to determine whether there is an inflammatory, infectious, or crystalline cause of the arthritis. "A" is incorrect. Radiographs are typically not helpful acutely in inflammatory arthritis (but would be indicated if there was trauma or suspicion of tumor). "B" and "C," a CBC is nonspecific and uric acid may be normal during an acute attack of gout. Neither of these laboratory results will be diagnostic. Finally, corticosteroid injection must be avoided in monoarthritis until the possibility of infection is eliminated.

You successfully aspirate 5 cc of slightly cloudy yellow synovial fluid from the left knee. While the patient is waiting, the laboratory reports the following findings: 5,000 WBC/mm^3, Gram stain negative for bacteria, and many needle-shaped negatively birefringent crystals.

Question 11.4.2 These synovial fluid findings are most consistent with which of the following diagnoses?
A) Osteoarthritis
B) Septic arthritis
C) CPPD ("pseudogout")
D) Gout

Answer 11.4.2 **The correct answer is "D."** Monosodium urate crystals of gout are needle-shaped as seen in this patient's synovial fluid (a good way to remember this is that being stuck with a needle hurts and so does gout). Calcium pyrophosphate dihydrate crystals are rod-, square-, or rhomboid-shaped and positively birefringent in polarized light. Thus, the synovial fluid findings given above are most consistent with gout. "A" and "B" are incorrect. Normally, synovial fluid contains <180 WBC/mm^3, but it is generally considered noninflammatory if the WBC count is still <2,000/mm^3. Low WBC counts are seen in the synovial fluid of osteoarthritic joints. Synovial fluid containing ≥2,000 WBC/mm^3 is consistent with an inflammatory process. When there are >100,000 WBC/mm^3, the monoarthritis is considered septic until proven otherwise (although as noted above this is only 30% sensitive for septic arthritis). See Table 11-4 for the diagnostic criteria for gout. Note that up to 20% of patients with a crystalline arthritis will have a coexisting septic arthritis (*J Rheumatol.* 2012; 39:157) so be sure to do the gram stain and culture.

TABLE 11-4 CLASSIFICATION CRITERIA FOR ACUTE GOUT

The presence of characteristic urate crystals in the joint fluid or tophus proved to contain urate crystals by chemical means or polarized light microscopy or the presence of 6 of the following 12 phenomena:

1. More than 1 attack of acute arthritis
2. Maximal inflammation developed within 1 day
3. Attack of monoarticular arthritis
4. Joint redness observed
5. First MTP joint painful or swollen
6. Unilateral attack involving first MTP joint
7. Unilateral attack involving tarsal joint
8. Suspected tophus
9. Hyperuricemia
10. Asymmetric swelling within a joint (radiograph)
11. Subcortical cysts without erosion (radiograph)
12. Negative joint fluid culture for microorganisms during attack of joint inflammation

Used with permission from Wallace SL, Robinson H, Masi AT, Decker JL, McCarty DJ, Yu TF. Preliminary criteria for the classification of the acute arthritis of primary gout. *Arthritis Rheum.* 1977;20(3):895–900.

Question 11.4.3 Which of the following may be used as a noninvasive imaging modality to diagnose gout at joints that are inaccessible to an arthrocentesis?
A) Bone scan
B) Dual energy CT
C) MRI
D) X-rays

Answer 11.4.3 The correct answer is "B." A diagnosis of gout is usually reached by evaluating clinical, laboratory, and radiologic findings. In uncertain cases, dual energy CT scan may be useful (sensitivity 90% and specificity 82% in one literature review [*Ann Rheum Dis.* 2015;74(6):1072–1077]). It may also identify subclinical tophi and quantify burden of disease. While a bone scan ("A"), MRI ("C"), and x-rays ("D") may help to identify joint/bony abnormalities commonly seen in gout, findings may not be specific for gout.

Question 11.4.4 In general, all of the following are risk factors for gout EXCEPT:
A) Tobacco use
B) Alcohol use
C) Obesity
D) Diuretic use
E) Family history

Answer 11.4.4 The correct answer is "A." Your patient exhibits many of the risk factors for gout, which include male sex, obesity, high-protein diet, use of diuretics (either loop or thiazide), alcohol, and family history. However, tobacco use is not associated with gout.

   HELPFUL TIP:
Many patients with hyperuricemia do **not** develop gout or nephrolithiasis; it is unclear whether asymptomatic hyperuricemia should be treated with uric

acid-lowering agents, and research is ongoing to answer this question. What is the risk at 5 years? Risk is 0.33% if the uric acid is <6 mg/dL, and 26% if the baseline level is >10 mg/dL. At 15 years, it is 49% for the highest risk group (baseline uric acid > 10 mg/dL). Let the uric acid level guide you when deciding whether to treat otherwise asymptomatic hyperuricemia (*Ann Rheum Dis.* 2018;77:1048).

Question 11.4.5 Which of the following is the *next step* in the management of this patient?
A) Prescribe allopurinol
B) Prescribe acetaminophen
C) Discontinue chlorthalidone
D) Prescribe naproxen at a full anti-inflammatory dose
E) Perform a therapeutic joint aspiration

Answer 11.4.5 The correct answer is "D." An acute attack of gout should first be treated with NSAIDs, such as naproxen or indomethacin. The doses prescribed should be at the upper limit for the particular NSAID (e.g., naproxen 500 mg three times daily). Earlier treatment is associated with greater relief of symptoms and shorter duration of the acute event. Other potential first-line agents are colchicine and corticosteroids. The effectiveness of colchicine is best if started within 36 hours of onset of symptoms. Colchicine is typically prescribed as one dose of 1.2 mg, followed by 0.6 mg twice daily for 1 to 2 weeks, and then 0.6 mg daily for 2 to 6 months. Note that this is a much lower dose than we have prescribed in the past! Due to significant toxicity at high doses, it is no longer recommended to "titrate to diarrhea." Oral or intra-articular corticosteroid administrations are also options for patients who have contraindications to NSAIDs, who have failed NSAID therapy, or who have more severe attacks. Corticosteroids are just as efficacious as NSAIDs and may be more appropriate for patients with heart failure, ulcers, or kidney disease. Prednisone, 30 mg/day for five days is a reasonable dose (this is the authors' choice). Narcotic pain medication may be needed as an adjunct to your anti-inflammatory but will do nothing to shorten the duration of an attack.

"A" is incorrect. Allopurinol is indicated to treat hyperuricemia and prevent the next gout attack in patients *who have had more than one attack in the last year, when tophi are present, or, when a single gout attack occurs with chronic kidney disease grade 2 or higher.* Some will treat those with a particularly bad attack (e.g., polyarticular gout, disabling pain resistant to treatment) without regard to the frequency of attacks. "B" is incorrect because acetaminophen lacks the anti-inflammatory properties of NSAIDs and is less effective. Discontinuing chlorthalidone, "C" (a thiazide diuretic), and switching to a nondiuretic antihypertensive is probably appropriate but will not treat this gout attack. Joint aspiration is not therapeutic in gout but may be helpful in pseudogout.

HELPFUL TIP:
Other drugs that increase the risk of gout include ACEIs, ARBs, and beta-blockers. Calcium-channel blockers do not increase the risk of gout (*BMJ.* 2012;344:d8190).

You start an NSAID. He returns in a few days to discuss his labs and x-rays. A radiograph of the left knee demonstrates an effusion but is otherwise unremarkable. His knee pain is much improved, and knee effusion is nearly resolved. His uric acid level is 10.1 mg/dL (the upper limit of normal for your lab is 7.2 mg/dL). CBC, creatinine, sodium, and potassium are normal. You instruct the patient to reduce his alcohol intake (especially beer) and try to lose weight to decrease his risk of gout attacks and for overall health. You schedule a follow-up visit, but he is a no-show and you don't see him again for more than a year (was it something you said?). When the patient returns 18 months later, he reports frequent use of naproxen, and at least five more acute attacks of gout. He continues to consume alcohol. His examination reveals no swollen or tender joints today, but there is a small whitish subcutaneous nodule overlying a toe PIP joint. Creatinine is 1.1 mg/dL, serum uric acid 10.5 (normal < 7.2 mg/dL); liver enzymes and CBC are normal.

Question 11.4.6 Which is the most appropriate regimen to start now in this patient to reduce the frequency of gout attacks?
A) Twice daily colchicine
B) Daily allopurinol 300 to 600 mg
C) Daily probenecid
D) Daily allopurinol 100 mg, with once or twice daily colchicine
E) Daily probenecid and allopurinol

Answer 11.4.6 The correct answer is "D." The presence of a tophus and the history of more than one attack in the last year are both indications for starting long-term urate-lowering therapy. Colchicine administered once or twice daily has been shown to reduce the frequency of gout attacks 75% to 85% and is especially useful as prophylaxis (prevention of the next gout attack) during the first 6 to 12 months of urate-lowering therapy. But "A," colchicine alone, is incorrect in this case because the patient now has tophaceous gout and allopurinol is indicated.

Starting allopurinol at a low dose of 100 mg daily and then increasing the dose every few weeks is less likely to provoke new gout attacks than starting at a larger dose. "B" is incorrect because it is a higher dose of allopurinol, given without prophylaxis, and could induce new gout attacks (which will make this patient think that your treatment is not very good, and that you are not a very good doctor). Probenecid ("C" and "E") is a uricosuric agent that also reduces the frequency and severity of acute gout attacks but has multiple drug interactions (including with allopurinol) and contraindications (e.g., decreased renal function, kidney stones, or presence of tophi). Another option for a uricosuric drug is lesinurad (Zurampic). It is more expensive than probenecid,

and can lead to increased creatinine, an influenza-like syndrome, etc. It should *only be used in combination* with allopurinol or febuxostat; otherwise it increases the risk of renal failure and kidney stones. It may not add anything to maximize allopurinol or febuxostat. In combination, it is less effective than probenecid. Bottom line: just say no to lesinurad.

You prescribe allopurinol 100 mg daily and once daily colchicine and schedule the patient to return every 2 to 4 weeks to re-check his uric acid level and make further allopurinol dose adjustments.

Question 11.4.7 The target for uric acid lowering in this patient is:
A) Less than 7.2 mg/dL, because this is the upper limit of normal for a man his age
B) Less than 6.0 mg/dL
C) Less than 5.0 mg/dL
D) Less than 3.14159 mg/dL, because precision counts
E) As low as possible

Answer 11.4.7 The correct answer is "C." This patient has a tophus; in order to resolve tophi, and minimize the risk for further attacks, allopurinol should be increased in 100-mg steps until his uric acid level is consistently less than 5.0 mg/dL. Uric acid crystals start to form at serum levels >6.7 mg/dL, which is within the 95% confidence range in the adult population, so within the "normal"—but not necessarily "harmless"—range. "A" is not correct, as levels higher than 6.7 mg/dL would continue to cause gout attacks and will not resolve tophaceous deposits. "B" is the correct target for patients without evidence of tophi, but <6.0 mg/dL is not sufficient in this patient. "D" is the first few digits of the mathematical constant pi. We know you didn't fall for "D." In fact, in this patient with gout, we should encourage him to avoid pie (but not pi). Please also note that these are guidelines from the American College of Rheumatology. Like the name suggests, these are meant to guide practitioners. Depending on the patient, the target can be modified to account for individual risks and benefits. Uric acid is a normal product of purine metabolism. There have been some studies that show it may have some role in neuroprotection as well as fighting infection. Too much is bad, but too little ("E") could be a problem as well, so we do not target uric acid to zero.

HELPFUL TIP:
Febuxostat (Uloric) is an alternative to allopurinol. However, it is rather expensive (10× the cost of allopurinol), and the FDA now states that there is a higher incidence of cardiovascular events in those on febuxostat when compared to allopurinol and a *higher risk of death.* Febuxostat should be reserved for use in patients who fail allopurinol. Febuxostat can be started low and titrated up, like allopurinol. It well may be off the market some time during the life of this publication because of the increased cardiac mortality.

HELPFUL TIP:
Although colchicine is recommended as prophylaxis when allopurinol is initiated, it should be discontinued within 6 months (if possible) due to the potential side effects of GI irritation, diarrhea, and myopathy.

Question 11.4.8 All of the following are side effects of allopurinol EXCEPT:
A) Aseptic meningitis
B) Rash
C) Leukopenia
D) Fever
E) GI disturbance

Answer 11.4.8 The correct answer is "A." Additional side effects include elevated liver enzymes, glomerulonephritis, aplastic anemia, and vasculitis. Hypersensitivity reactions are especially common—with incidence rates as high as 15%—in some Asian populations (e.g., Chinese, Koreans, Thais). Consider checking for HLA-B*5801 in these groups before starting allopurinol. Not a pretty drug, but look on the bright side… it's not associated with meningitis!

HELPFUL TIP:
Probenecid should be avoided in patients with a creatinine of clearance <50 mL/min, as it is ineffective and there may be an increased risk of toxicity.

....

It is 9 years later. Congress has passed a law banning the Kardashians from being on TV (the sad part is that we have had this same joke in multiple editions and the Kardashians *still* haven't gone away!). Your favorite gout patient is back. He's had 9 years of acute intermittent gout attacks ("Of course I took my medication, Doc, but it didn't work so I stopped taking it"). He presents complaining of pain in his knees and feet that has been present for several months. He has also developed swelling and pain in his hands. The pain is less intense than his attacks of gout, but occurs in the same areas and never completely resolves between attacks. He has no morning stiffness, no muscle complaints, and no other systemic complaints. You find diffuse edema of both hands and palpable hard nodules on the knees, fingers, toes, and in the olecranon bursa.

Question 11.4.9 Which of the following is the most likely cause of his current symptoms?
A) RA
B) Osteoarthritis
C) Tophaceous gout
D) PMR

Answer 11.4.9 The correct answer is "C." This patient has a long history of acute intermittent gout. After years of acute attacks, patients with gout may develop a form of the disease called chronic tophaceous gout (the nodules are deposits of uric

acid called tophi; tophus for a single nodule), in which the intercritical periods are no longer free of pain. There are no clinical associations between gout and the other rheumatic conditions mentioned and, therefore, no reason to suspect that another rheumatic disorder is causing the chronic pain.

HELPFUL TIP:
Hyperlipidemia occurs in 80% of patients with gout—check lipids. Recall also that there can be renal injury with longstanding gout as well as an increased risk of urate stones.

HELPFUL TIP:
In addition to being a fun word, podagra (from the Greek meaning "foot seizure") is a useful diagnostic tool. The first MTP joint is affected in 90% of patients with gout, and the initial attack involves the first MTP joint in 50%.

▶ **Objectives: Did you learn to …**
· Evaluate recurrent monoarthritis?
· Describe the diagnostic synovial fluid findings in gout?
· Define diagnostic criteria for gout?
· Manage a patient with gout and describe adverse effects of the medications used to treat gout?
· Identify the appropriate target uric acid level for urate-lowering therapy?

▶ **CASE 11.5**

Citing your characteristic compassion and attention to detail, your "gout guy" (as he now calls himself) refers a friend he met at a meeting of his favorite club, Gouty Retirees in Love with Life ("GRILL"). This friend of his is a 65-year-old female who reports a history of joint swelling, pain, and redness, usually involving her knees, wrists, and hands; she has never had first MTP joint involvement. Although she has never had a joint aspiration performed, she has been treated for gout for 5 years. She faithfully takes her medication but has found allopurinol unhelpful. She is currently asymptomatic but uses ibuprofen for acute attacks. The joint examination is notable only for some knee crepitus and reduced wrist range of motion—but, again, she is currently asymptomatic.

Question 11.5.1 Which of the following studies is most appropriate for this patient?
A) Diagnostic knee injection with corticosteroids
B) CBC
C) RF
D) Radiographs of the knees and wrists

Answer 11.5.1 The correct answer is "D." The initial evaluation should include radiographs of the affected joints, which may lend clues to the diagnosis. Radiographs may reveal osteophyte formation typical of osteoarthritis, subchondral cysts, chondrocalcinosis typical of CPPD (calcium pyrophosphate dehydrate crystal deposition disease), or erosions with an overhanging edge typical of gout. Chondrocalcinosis is most often seen in the knees and triangular fibrocartilage of the wrists. "A," an injection of corticosteroids, might help relieve symptoms, but it will not be diagnostic. "B," CBC, is nonspecific and will not be helpful. "C," RF, is also unlikely to be helpful, given this patient's symptoms, which are not suggestive of RA. Also, RF may be elevated in inflammatory arthritides other than RA.

HELPFUL TIP:
The crystals of gout (uric acid) and pseudogout (calcium pyrophosphate) can be seen in synovial fluid during intercritical periods. If there is an effusion even in the absence of acute symptoms and you are thinking gout or pseudogout, tap that joint!

HELPFUL TIP:
The diagnosis of pseudogout (CPPD) is not as straightforward as gout. To confuse the clinician all the more, CPPD tends to travel with other types of arthritis (e.g., osteoarthritis, gout). Patients with CPPD are more likely older than 65 and have knee arthritis, but clinical criteria alone are insufficient for the diagnosis, which requires demonstration of crystals in the joint fluid.

Your patient's knee radiographs demonstrate chondrocalcinosis (see Fig. 11-1). Examination of synovial fluid from the knee shows positively birefringent, rhomboid crystals consistent with CPPD (pseudogout). Maybe this is why her gout medicine wasn't working….

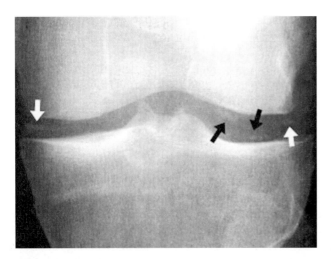

FIGURE 11-1. Chondrocalcinosis of the knee joint. (Note arrows highlighting calcification.)

Question 11.5.2 Which of the following do you recommend to decrease her risk of recurrent acute attacks of pseudogout?
A) Serial joint aspiration
B) Daily allopurinol
C) Twice daily colchicine
D) Serial intra-articular corticosteroid injections
E) Chondroitin sulfate

Answer 11.5.2 **The correct answer is "C."** Pseudogout is diagnosed by the presence of CPPD crystals (as described) in synovial fluid and/or typical x-ray findings (basically, chondrocalcinosis). Although prophylaxis is more predictably successful in gout, colchicine 0.6 mg BID has been shown to reduce the frequency of pseudogout attacks in CPPD. NSAIDs or colchicine may be used in acute attacks with prednisone/steroids as third line (whereas they can be used as first line in gout). "A" and "D" are incorrect. While joint aspiration and corticosteroid injection may be helpful during acute attacks, they have no role in prophylaxis. "B" is also incorrect. Since CPPD is not caused by abnormalities in uric acid metabolism, allopurinol has no role in the management of pseudogout. Finally, chondroitin sulfate ("E") is not useful in pseudogout (or much of anything else, for that matter).

HELPFUL TIP:
Gout is more likely to occur during middle age and is more common in men. Pseudogout has a peak incidence later in life and is about equally prevalent in both males and females.

Question 11.5.3 CPPD (pseudogout) is associated with which of the following?
A) Hypothyroidism
B) Hyperparathyroidism
C) Amyloidosis
D) Hemochromatosis
E) All of the above

Answer 11.5.3 **The correct answer is "E."** All of the above are associated with pseudogout. Additional associated conditions include hypophosphatemia and hypomagnesemia. For this reason, order the following studies in patients newly diagnosed with CPPD: thyroid-stimulating hormone (TSH), calcium, phosphate, magnesium, transferrin saturation, and alkaline phosphatase.

HELPFUL TIP:
Precipitants of acute attack of gout and pseudogout (CPPD) include trauma, surgery, severe medical illness, and alcohol overindulgence.

▶ **Objectives: Did you learn to …**
 · Identify clinical and diagnostic characteristics of CPPD?
 · Implement appropriate therapy for CPPD?

QUICK QUIZ: CRYOGLOBULINEMIA

Cryoglobulinemia, a vasculitic disease caused by antibodies that precipitate in cold temperatures, is most often caused by which of the following viral infections?

A) HIV
B) Hepatitis B
C) Hepatitis C
D) Parvovirus B19

The correct answer is "C." Hepatitis C is found in 80% of vasculitis cases associated with mixed cryoglobulinemia. Although up to 50% of patients with hepatitis C will eventually express cryoglobulins, only a minority of patients have clinical vasculitis. As to the other options, hepatitis B and parvovirus B19 infection may cause a symmetric polyarthritis. HIV is less commonly a cause of cryoglobulinemia and is associated with reactive arthritis. The symptoms of mixed cryoglobulinemia associated with HCV infection typically include arthralgias, fever, renal disease, palpable purpura, and neuropathy.

▶ CASE 11.6

A 13-year-old male presents to your office with his father. The patient complains of pain in his wrists, elbows, and knees bilaterally. He has felt fatigued and has been unable to work his usual summer job as a busboy at his father's restaurant (what happened to child labor laws?). He complains of intermittent fevers and an evanescent rash that appears during febrile episodes but which is short-lived. All of these symptoms have emerged in the last 6 weeks, after a week-long backpacking trip in the tick-infested woods of Minnesota. He has no significant past medical history. His only medication is acetaminophen daily for joint pain. He denies tobacco use, alcohol use, and sexual activity.

Question 11.6.1 The differential diagnosis should include all of the following EXCEPT:

A) Lyme disease
B) JIA
C) PMR
D) Viral illness

Answer 11.6.1 **The correct answer is "C," of course.** From earlier in the chapter, you will recall that the diagnosis of PMR is highly unusual in adults under the age of 50. JIA is a chronic arthritis of childhood that can present in a variety of ways, but must include arthritis of one or more joints, lasting 6 weeks or more, with symptom onset before age 16 years. Likewise, Lyme disease has several presentations, presenting with arthritis early or late in the course. Many viral illnesses can result in arthralgia and/or arthritis. Any of the diseases listed may have associated

symptoms of fatigue, malaise, headache, and myalgia. One factor that makes Lyme disease a more likely diagnosis is the history of being outdoors in an endemic area (90% of Lyme disease in the United States occurs in New York, New Jersey, Connecticut, Rhode Island, Massachusetts, Pennsylvania, Wisconsin, and Minnesota—although the geographic distribution is widening slightly).

Question 11.6.2 Which of the following findings on physical examination would be more consistent with Lyme disease than JIA?

A) Bell palsy
B) Temperature ≥38°C
C) Rash
D) Lymphadenopathy
E) A and C

Answer 11.6.2 **The correct answer is "A."** All of the other findings are seen in both Lyme disease and JIA. Neurologic symptoms, including Bell palsy ("A") and even meningitis, may occur with Lyme disease but not JIA. Rash ("C") is present in both diseases but differs substantially. The characteristic rash of Lyme disease is erythema migrans. The rash of systemic-onset JIA (also known as Still disease) is macular, salmon-pink, and brought on by heat. Erythema migrans occurs in about 80% of patients with acute Lyme disease. The lesion is often described as "targetoid," meant to convey a red circular rash with central clearing. However, most patients do not have the classic lesion. Instead, most patients present with a mildly to brightly erythematous patch in the axilla or belt line, where the tick bite occurs. The tick itself is rarely seen. Erythema migrans is usually not painful or pruritic. Both Lyme disease and JIA may have associated systemic findings, including fever and lymphadenopathy, so neither "B" nor "D" is a good discriminator.

HELPFUL TIP:
There is a "new" form of Lyme disease in the upper Midwest caused by *Borrelia mayonii* (why does this have to happen to Iowa?). Rather than the typical bull's eye rash, it can present with a diffuse rash, perhaps neurologic symptoms, nausea, vomiting, and a spirochetemia often visible on dark-field examination. So far it is uncommon and limited to the upper Midwest (see https://www.cdc.gov/ticks/mayonii.html).

Physical examination reveals a thin male in no acute distress. His temperature is 37.3°C, pulse 100 bpm, and blood pressure 120/70 mm Hg. Small, nontender, mobile lymph nodes are palpable in the neck and axillae. There is a large, warm, erythematous patch with central clearing at the patient's left axilla. There is limited range of motion in his right wrist and left elbow. An effusion is palpable at the left knee, which is diffusely tender.

Question 11.6.3 **If you were to aspirate the patient's knee—so often the right answer in this chapter—which of the following would you expect to find in the synovial fluid?**
A) Greater than 100,000 WBC/mm^3
B) Predominance of eosinophils
C) Monosodium urate crystals
D) Spirochetes
E) Predominance of polymorphonuclear cells

Answer 11.6.3 **The correct answer is "E."** This patient is presenting now with classic features of Lyme disease. If synovial fluid is obtained in a patient with Lyme arthritis, analysis of the fluid reveals leukocytes, most commonly polymorphonuclear cells. "A" is incorrect. If the synovial fluid has >100,000 WBC/mm^3, you should consider septic arthritis (arthritis in Lyme disease is mostly an immunological phenomenon rather than true septic arthritis. But remember that more often patients with a septic joint have <100,000 WBC/mm^3). "B" is incorrect because eosinophils are not the predominant cell in synovial fluid of Lyme arthritis. "C" is wrong since monosodium urate crystals are observed in gout—an unlikely cause of this patient's joint complaints. Finally, "D" is wrong. In general, *Borrelia burgdorferi* spirochetes, the causative organism in Lyme disease, are not observed in the synovial fluid.

You strongly suspect Lyme disease. Because it is so swollen, you aspirate the joint and find slightly cloudy yellow fluid, with cell count 10,000/mm^3, and 95% polymorphonuclear cells. Gram stain is negative, and culture was subsequently found to be negative.

Question 11.6.4 **Which of the following is true regarding laboratory tests for Lyme disease?**
A) Serologic tests are reliable within 1 week of the tick bite
B) Serologic tests are useful in screening for Lyme disease
C) Blood cultures remain positive for *B. burgdorferi* for months after the tick bite
D) Serologic tests remain positive for up to 10 years after antibiotic treatment
E) The diagnosis of Lyme disease is based on serologic tests

Answer 11.6.4 **The correct answer is "D."** Serologic tests for Lyme disease can remain positive for up to 10, and in some cases 20, years after exposure. *Thus, serologic tests alone are not diagnostic of active Lyme disease.* "E" is incorrect: the diagnosis of Lyme disease is clinical with laboratory tests used to confirm the diagnosis. A positive ELISA test is not adequate to make the diagnosis of Lyme disease. Positive or equivocal ELISA tests should be confirmed with Western blot analysis. "A" is incorrect: serologic assays may be falsely negative early in infection. Only 20% to 40% will have a positive serology at the time of presentation (e.g., when the rash is present). Serology is more likely to be positive if they present with Lyme carditis or CNS *Borrelia*. "B" is incorrect. Lyme serology is set to be a very sensitive test: there are few false negatives assuming enough time has elapsed since *Borrelia* exposure, but it is not highly specific and there are many false positives. Because of the high false-positive rate, serologic assays should not be used as a screening tool in the general population but are a good step when Lyme disease is suspected. Most laboratories will automatically do a Lyme Western Blot study to confirm positive Lyme serology. "C" is incorrect: positive blood cultures for *B. burgdorferi* are rarely obtained. When cultures do grow *B. burgdorferi*, it is only early in the disease. Cultures of skin biopsied from the erythema migrans lesion are more likely to be positive. **The CDC now also endorses doing two FDA approved ELISA (EIA) tests either simultaneously or serially instead of a Western Blot. (see: MMWR** August 16, 2019 / 68(32);703).

Question 11.6.5 **For this 13-year-old patient, whose weight is 50 kg and who has no known allergies, which course of therapy is safest and most efficacious?**
A) Amoxicillin 500 mg by mouth three times daily for 1 week
B) Ceftriaxone 2 g IM, single dose
C) Doxycycline 100 mg by mouth twice daily for 4 weeks
D) Levofloxacin 250 mg by mouth daily for 2 weeks
E) Erythromycin 250 mg by mouth four times daily for 4 weeks

Answer 11.6.5 **The correct answer is "C."** Recommended therapy for Lyme arthritis (without neurologic disease) is **4 weeks** of either amoxicillin 500 mg **three** times daily, doxycycline 100 mg twice daily, or cefuroxime axetil 500 mg twice daily. The old chestnut that *doxycycline* causes tooth staining has been disproven (https://www.cdc.gov/rmsf/doxycycline/index.html). So, doxycycline can be used in younger patients (even children <5 year olds) if needed (e.g., Rocky Mountain Spotted Fever). *The same thing is not true for tetracycline which does stain the teeth.* The duration of amoxicillin prescribed here is too short, so "A" is wrong. Ceftriaxone is prescribed when neurologic abnormalities are present (such as Bell palsy or meningitis), and it must be dosed daily for 2 to 4 weeks. Levofloxacin is not indicated for Lyme disease. Treatment with erythromycin for 4 weeks, while an acceptable alternative, appears to be less efficacious.

HELPFUL TIP:
There is no known resistance of *B. burgdorferi* to standard antibiotic regimens. One round of treatment is enough.

Several hours after starting antibiotics, the patient's father calls to report worsening symptoms of fever, shaking, and dizziness. You hear his lawyer talking in the background…

Question 11.6.6 **You recognize this condition as which of the following?**
A) An allergic reaction to the antibiotic
B) *B. burgdorferi* sepsis
C) Secondary bacterial infection
D) A cytokine-mediated reaction to the antibiotic-mediated killing of spirochetes (Jarisch–Herxheimer reaction)
E) The expected, natural course of Lyme disease

Answer 11.6.6 The correct answer is "D." A Jarisch–Herxheimer reaction occurs in 5% to 15% of patients treated with antibiotics for Lyme disease. (Remember syphilis? Lyme is also a spirochete disease.) The reaction is mediated by the release of cytokines and occurs within hours of initial administration of antibiotics. In Lyme disease, the reaction is self-limited and usually resolves within a day. Only supportive treatment is necessary, and antibiotics should be continued (but hey, you know you got the diagnosis right!). "A" is incorrect because this reaction is not typical of a drug allergy. "B" is incorrect because *B. burgdorferi* does not cause sepsis. "C" is incorrect because it is unlikely that a secondary bacterial infection has occurred so quickly. Finally, this does not represent the natural history of Lyme disease ("E"). See Table 11-5 for more on the natural history of Lyme disease.

HELPFUL TIP:
Lyme disease symptoms typically improve a few days after starting antibiotics.

....

Since he spends much of his free time hunting deer in Minnesota (trying to shoot Bambi), your patient's father is worried about contracting Lyme disease himself.

Question 11.6.7 What do you recommend for primary prevention of Lyme disease?
A) Weekly tick checks
B) *N,N*-diethyl-m-toluamide (DEET) application prior to hunting
C) Daily doxycycline when in endemic areas
D) Lyme vaccine
E) Kill as many deers as possible in order to reduce the risk of Lyme disease transmission to humans

Answer 11.6.7 The correct answer is "B." Primary prevention is best accomplished with the use of insect repellents when in endemic areas. Also, when in endemic areas, tick checks should be performed daily (not weekly as in answer "A"). A tick that has been attached for <24 hours is not likely to transmit

B. burgdorferi. Unfortunately, the species that transmit Lyme disease (ticks of the *Ixodes ricinus* complex) are very small and difficult to see. "C" is incorrect. There is no role for routine prophylactic antibiotics. However, if a tick bite from the appropriate species is noticed, a single dose of doxycycline 200 mg administered orally reduces the risk of erythema migrans (see "Helpful Tip" below for prophylaxis criteria). The dose should be administered within 72 hours of a known *I. ricinus* tick bite. "D" is not an option for this patient. In 2002, the vaccine was removed from the U.S. market due to low demand. When it was available, antibody titers tended to wane quickly and protection was not complete. After the administration of three vaccinations, the efficacy of the vaccine to prevent Lyme disease was 76% at best. "E" is just plain wrong … what with Bambi and all … And furthermore, the white-footed field mouse, not the white-tailed deer, is the major reservoir of *B. burgdorferi* bacteria.

HELPFUL TIP:
Who should get prophylactic doxycycline for a tick bite? According to the CDC **ALL of the following need to be present** (https://www.cdc.gov/ticks/tickbornediseases/tick-bite-prophylaxis.html).
Prophylaxis is doxycycline 200 mg as a single dose.
1. Doxycycline is not contraindicated.
2. The attached tick can be identified as an adult or nymphal *I. scapularis* tick.
3. The estimated time of attachment is ≥36 hours based on the degree of tick engorgement with blood or likely time of exposure to the tick.
4. Prophylaxis can be started within 72 hours of tick removal.
5. Lyme disease is common in the county or state where the patient lives or has recently traveled to (i.e., CT, DE, MA, MD, ME, MN, NH, NJ, NY, PA, RI, VA, VT, WI).

HELPFUL TIP:
Repeat after us: there is no such thing as "chronic Lyme disease" requiring months-to-years of antibiotics. The CDC does recognize an entity called "post-Lyme disease syndrome" that may include fatigue, myalgia, cognitive slowing, and numbness. However, post-Lyme disease syndrome does NOT improve with prolonged antibiotics. Focus on looking for other causes (e.g., depression, fibromyalgia, hypothyroidism) in these patients, as most of them do not have post-Lyme disease syndrome, and work to alleviate symptoms. However, avoid the temptation to prescribe antibiotics that do not work.

HELPFUL TIP:
If Lyme meningitis is suspected, confirm by analysis of CSF. Lyme meningitis must be treated with IV ceftriaxone or penicillin G.

TABLE 11-5 STAGES OF LYME DISEASE

Early localized disease (Stage I): Occurs days to a month after the tick bite and includes erythema migrans, fatigue, fever, malaise, myalgias, arthralgia, arthritis, headache, and lymphadenopathy. Except for erythema migrans, it can be confused with a viral illness.
Early disseminated disease (Stage II): Occurs weeks to months after the tick bite; 5–10% have cardiac manifestations (atrioventricular block of any degree, myocarditis/pericarditis, and heart failure); and 10–15% have neurologic manifestations (see below).
Late disease (Stage III): Occurs months to years after the tick bite and includes myalgias, arthralgias, fatigue, polyarthritis, and neurologic symptoms (encephalopathy, cognitive dysfunction, and peripheral neuropathy)

Adapted from Bhate C, Schwartz RA. Lyme disease: Part I. Advances and perspectives. *J Am Acad Dermatol.* 2011;64(4):619–636.

▶ **Objectives: Did you learn to …**

- Generate a differential diagnosis for a young patient presenting with polyarthritis?
- Diagnose Lyme disease?
- Describe the stages of Lyme disease?
- Implement appropriate therapy for Lyme disease?
- Discuss preventive strategies for Lyme disease and describe some of the complications of the disease?

▶ CASE 11.7

A 42-year-old female who was referred by an orthopedic surgeon presents to your office with multiple joint complaints. The orthopedist has seen her for left knee pain, intermittent swelling, occasional "clicking and locking," present for about 10 years. After knee radiograph and examination, the orthopedist diagnosed a chronically damaged meniscus, but he wants the patient evaluated by you for her other joint complaints.

Laboratory data ordered by her orthopedist (apparently, just to confuse you) show an ANA 1:320 (speckled pattern), an elevated rheumatoid factor, and an ESR 20 mm/hr. The patient moved to the United States from Guam 4 years ago. She reports poor sleep and feeling quite depressed. She feels that she has no friends, and she has had trouble adjusting to the colder weather. You notice she has a bottle of water with her and upon your specific questioning she states, "I have to sip some water throughout the day. I've done this for the last 15 years because my mouth gets so dry." Over the past 20 years, she has had numerous fillings for dental cavities. She denies problems with skin rash, swallowing, and eye pain. She does not use artificial tears.

Question 11.7.1 Which of the following findings in *this* patient is most likely to be a *sign of inflammatory* arthritis?
A) Spider angiomas (telangiectasia) on the back and abdomen
B) A small cool left knee effusion ("bulge sign") with crepitus
C) Presence of 16/18 fibromyalgia tender points, with non-tender control points
D) Incomplete left grip
E) Presence of a holosystolic murmur at the left sternal border, without radiation

Answer 11.7.1 The correct answer is "D." Although her symptoms are suggestive of fibromyalgia and depression, it is critical to differentiate between an inflammatory and a noninflammatory condition, especially since many inflammatory disorders (e.g., SLE, RA, Sjögren syndrome) may masquerade as fibromyalgia. An incomplete grip in an otherwise healthy woman is suggestive of synovitis, which can be further assessed by careful small joint examination. When synovitis is present, it is always abnormal and suggests an inflammatory arthritis, requiring further evaluation. "A" is incorrect because telangiectasias on the abdomen and trunk are typically related to liver disease,

while those found on hands and nail beds are associated with systemic sclerosis and other rheumatic diseases. "B," a positive knee "bulge sign" (swelling of the knee joint that bulges inferiorly when compressed superiorly) indicates fluid in the left knee joint. But from the patient's history and your orthopedic colleague's determination, this finding is chronic and mechanical in nature. "C," the presence of 16/18 tender points, would argue for fibromyalgia but is not a sign of inflammatory arthritis. Additionally, identifying greater than 11 out of 18 tender points is no longer part of the diagnostic criteria for fibromyalgia (keep reading for details). Finally, a holosystolic murmur ("E"), localized to the left sternal border and present in a healthy young woman, is nonspecific and most likely functional. If there were other signs and symptoms of cardiac disease, the murmur might indicate a more serious disorder.

On physical examination, you find a "bulge sign" on the left knee, but no other joint swelling. She has 16/18 tender points and normal range of motion and strength. The neurological examination is grossly normal, except for poorly defined numbness and pain to touch on the left side of her face. You also notice a mildly tender, hard, nodular swelling behind the angle of the mandible on the left in the area of the parotid gland. Her oral mucosa appears dry. Her conjunctiva is mildly, symmetrically injected.

Question 11.7.2 All of the following studies and interventions are appropriate EXCEPT:
A) CBC, transaminases, ESR, CRP
B) Anti-SS-A (Ro), anti-SS-B (La), anti-dsDNA, RF, serum protein electrophoresis
C) Prescribe trazodone 50 mg PO at bedtime and recommend aerobic exercises
D) Prescribe prednisone 20 mg PO daily, with calcium and vitamin D supplement
E) Maxillofacial MRI

Answer 11.7.2 The correct answer (and the thing to avoid right now) is "D." Although prednisone may be used to treat symptoms of autoimmune diseases, at this time the diagnosis is not secure, and initiating corticosteroid therapy exposes the patient to potentially unnecessary risk. She has findings of Sjögren syndrome—red (possibly dry) eyes, dry mouth, and enlarged parotid glands. However, the differential of mass in the parotid gland must include malignancy (e.g., lymphoma), sarcoidosis, and other autoimmune diseases. The laboratory tests offered in answers "A" and "B" may help assess other organ involvement of Sjögren syndrome and also aid in confirming the diagnosis. Other potential manifestations of Sjögren syndrome include generalized vasculitis, interstitial lung disease, cirrhosis, peripheral and cranial neuropathies, possibly thyroid disease, and renal disease leading to proteinuria and renal tubule dysfunction. Although not listed as an option, chest radiograph may also be helpful, assessing for findings associated with the diseases on your differential: Sjögren syndrome (interstitial lung disease), sarcoidosis (adenopathy and interstitial disease), and lymphoma (adenopathy). "E" is also important because although parotid enlargement may be seen in Sjögren syndrome, it is usually symmetrical and nontender. An imaging study is appropriate to rule out a neoplastic process. Finally, "C" is correct. Her symptoms of fibromyalgia, which it sounds like she also has, may respond to trazodone and exercise, and these low-risk interventions are appropriate at this juncture. Remember, the presence of one disease, in this patient likely Sjogren, does not protect against another disease (fibromyalgia).

She starts trazodone and exercise and feels better. The tests you order return as follows: negative SSA, SSB, and dsDNA; elevated RF; no monoclonal protein on SPEP but diffusely elevated globulins. A chest x-ray is normal. Her ESR is 35 mm/hr and CRP 0.5. A maxillofacial MRI shows an enlarged left parotid, with an ill-defined 2 × 3 × 1.5 cm dense signal in the center without neurovascular compromise.

Question 11.7.3 What is the most appropriate next step in the management of this patient?

A) Continue your current management and adopt a "watchful waiting" approach
B) Refer for biopsy of the left parotid
C) Initiate prednisone 20 mg PO daily, with calcium and vitamin D
D) Refer for minor salivary gland biopsy (lip biopsy)
E) MRI of the head and neck

Answer 11.7.3 **The correct answer is "B."** Wait… We're performing biopsies on masses in the rheumatology chapter? Yes. Even though her presentation is suggestive of Sjögren syndrome, the presence of a mass-like formation on MRI is concerning for lymphoma, and further evaluation (e.g., biopsy) is required. In addition, the negative SSA and SSB, while not excluding Sjögren syndrome, will make a biopsy necessary for diagnosis. Although a minor salivary gland biopsy ("D") is the most specific way to confirm a diagnosis of Sjögren syndrome, the first priority is to evaluate the parotid gland mass. The elevated RF and polyclonal gammopathy are consistent with Sjögren syndrome, and the ESR may be elevated due to increased globulins. MRI of the head and neck ("E") may provide some structural information, but it is not in the diagnostic criteria for Sjögren Syndrome.

Results of the parotid gland biopsy report read, "Lymphocytic infiltrate, no malignant cells noted." You then order flow cytometry, and it has no markers for lymphoma. Her biopsy scar has healed nicely, and she has no pain or numbness. You believe that she probably has Sjögren syndrome.

Question 11.7.4 What would you do next?

A) CT chest/abdomen/pelvis
B) Start prednisone 20 mg by mouth daily, with calcium and vitamin D
C) Recommend sugarless lemon drops and artificial tears as needed and continued trazodone and exercise
D) Wide excision of the parotid gland

Answer 11.7.4 **The correct answer is "C."** Lemon drops (or anything sour for that matter) will stimulate saliva production, helping with her dry mouth. Artificial tears may also be indicated for dry eyes. At this time your working diagnosis is Sjögren syndrome, and definitive diagnosis by minor salivary gland biopsy (from the buccal mucosa of the lower lip) is not likely to alter your therapy; and "D" is way too aggressive anyway. Since she has responded to trazodone and exercise and there is no evidence of systemic involvement, no further anti-inflammatory therapy ("B") is warranted. If she were to develop arthritis or other signs of systemic involvement (e.g., cognitive dysfunction or peripheral neuropathy), prednisone would be an option. Further workup for lymphoma, such as CT scanning ("A"), does not appear warranted. However, she will require active surveillance, since patients with Sjögren syndrome carry an increased risk of developing lymphoma.

HELPFUL TIP:
Sicca symptoms (dry eyes and mouth) are extremely common, especially in the elderly, and should be confirmed by objective physical findings. The diagnosis of Sjögren syndrome is suggested by presence of anti-SS-A, *or* positive ANA titer (1:320 or greater) with elevated RF (as in the patient above), but definitive diagnosis of Sjögren syndrome relies on histopathologic gland findings on minor salivary gland (lip) biopsy.

▸ **Objectives: Did you learn to …**
· Describe the appropriate evaluation of polyarthralgia and sicca symptoms?
· Evaluate a patient with probable Sjögren syndrome?
· Implement appropriate therapy for Sjögren syndrome?

▶ CASE 11.8

Once again, your fabled diagnostic and therapeutic abilities have earned you a well-deserved referral. Your previous patient is so pleased with the way things are going that she refers her sister-in-law to you. The sister-in-law is 46 years old and reports having been diagnosed with fibromyalgia several months ago. She reports having all-over pain, all the time, which has been worsening for the last 5 years. "Great," you think to yourself, "Thanks for the referral." She takes only acetaminophen and codeine as needed for pain (she typically needs it four times per day). She does not exercise because it hurts too much. She drinks 2 liters of Mountain Dew a day, from sun-up to sundown. Her sleep is reported as poor and nonrestorative.

Question 11.8.1 Which of the following statements is true regarding management of fibromyalgia?

A) Fibromyalgia pain is increased during exercise, so exercise should be avoided
B) Regular low-impact exercise, and nonpharmacologic measures to improve sleep are more effective than medications for improving fibromyalgia-type pain

C) SNRI agents such as duloxetine and milnacipran lead to rapid and long-term remission of fibromyalgia-type pain

D) Both NSAIDs and prednisone are helpful in reducing fibromyalgia pain

E) Opioids act on the central nervous system, which is why they are the most effective agents for treatment of fibromyalgia pain

Answer 11.8.1 The correct answer is "B." Improved sleep through good sleep hygiene and regular low-impact exercise are often more effective than medications for reducing fibromyalgia-type pain. Indeed, improving sleep and exercise (and identifying any underlying sleep disorder) are central to long-term management. "A" is incorrect: even when exercise is poorly tolerated due to pain, a program of stretching and gradually increasing exercise is very helpful in reducing pain over time. SNRI agents are helpful for reducing central pain sensitization, and are important adjunctive treatment to sleep and exercise, but they are not curative and do not provide rapid pain relief. "D" is incorrect: NSAIDs and prednisone are not effective for fibromyalgia-type pain. Opioids do act on the central nervous system and can lead to short-term reduction of fibromyalgia-type pain, but at the same time they increase central pain sensitization which can actually lead to worsening of pain (opioid-induced hyperalgesia).

Question 11.8.2 Which of the following is NOT an appropriate medication for treating fibromyalgia-type pain?

A) Hydrocodone/acetaminophen

B) Gabapentin or pregabalin

C) Amitriptyline

D) Duloxetine

E) Combination duloxetine and pregabalin

Answer 11.8.2 The correct answer is "A." Is there a theme emerging here? Opioids will provide a short-term reduction in pain, but tend to worsen central sensitization and actually increase fibromyalgia pain over time; they should be avoided in managing this type of pain. All of the other agents have shown modest efficacy in improving pain associated with fibromyalgia. Low dose tricyclic antidepressants have the best efficacy. SNRI agents such as duloxetine may be combined with a gabapentin or pregabalin, as can tricyclics.

HELPFUL TIP:
Fibromyalgia is a common syndrome characterized by diffuse chronic pain accompanied by other somatic symptoms such as poor sleep, fatigue, and stiffness, in the absence of another identifiable disease. In order to diagnose fibromyalgia, symptoms must be present for at least 3 months and other chronic pain conditions must be excluded. However, an exhaustive search for occult disease is not recommended. Most diagnoses can be made with history, physical examination, and minimal labs (e.g., CBC, CRP, ESR to rule out inflammatory disease).

The 1990 American College of Rheumatology criteria included identification of pain on palpation at 11 or more of 18 tender points (Fig. 11-2), but as of 2010, this minimum number is no longer required to establish a diagnosis. There is still value in examining these tender points, and a higher number of tender points are associated with higher likelihood of fibromyalgia. However, you need not have 11 of 18. Also, self-administered scales, such as the Widespread Pain Index, may be useful in diagnosing fibromyalgia. There is a female predominance in fibromyalgia, with up to 75% of patients being women.

Question 11.8.3 All of the following are associated with fibromyalgia EXCEPT:

A) Irritable bowel syndrome

B) Subjective fullness/swelling of hands and feet

C) Paresthesias

D) Fatigue

E) Night sweats

Answer 11.8.3 The correct answer is "E." All of the others are associated with fibromyalgia. Additional symptoms include headaches, depression, sleep disturbance (which may actually be the etiology), other GI symptoms, and urethral spasm with dysuria and urgency.

HELPFUL TIP:
Although some SNRIs (Duloxetine, Savella, Venlafaxine) are FDA approved for fibromyalgia, they are not as effective as the TCAs.

▶ **Objectives: Did you learn to …**
· Identify typical symptoms of fibromyalgia?
· Define diagnostic criteria for fibromyalgia?
· Implement appropriate therapy for fibromyalgia?

 QUICK QUIZ: SECONDARY OSTEOARTHRITIS

All of the following diseases and conditions are secondary causes of osteoarthritis EXCEPT:

A) Fibromyalgia

B) Hemochromatosis

C) Hyperparathyroidism

D) Amyloidosis

E) Previous joint trauma

The correct answer is "A." One of the most common secondary causes of osteoarthritis is previous joint trauma. Systemic diseases that can lead to osteoarthritis include hemochromatosis, hyperparathyroidism, and amyloidosis. Fibromyalgia does not cause osteoarthritis. Any disease that leads to a neuropathy, such as diabetes, can predispose to osteoarthritis (e.g., Charcot arthropathy).

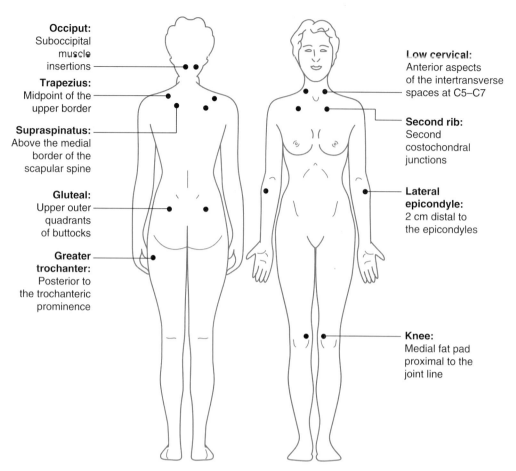

Occipit:
Suboccipital muscle insertions

Trapezius:
Midpoint of the upper border

Supraspinatus:
Above the medial border of the scapular spine

Gluteal:
Upper outer quadrants of buttocks

Greater trochanter:
Posterior to the trochanteric prominence

Low cervical:
Anterior aspects of the intertransverse spaces at C5–C7

Second rib:
Second costochondral junctions

Lateral epicondyle:
2 cm distal to the epicondyles

Knee:
Medial fat pad proximal to the joint line

FIGURE 11-2. Tender points in fibromyalgia.

▶ CASE 11.9

A 25-year-old female presents to your office complaining of bifrontal headaches, occurring intermittently over the last year. Also, she complains of fatigue that seems to be slowly worsening. Over the last 2 to 3 months, she has developed generalized joint pain and stiffness. The remainder of the history, including a detailed review of systems, is unremarkable.

On physical examination, you find a thin female in no acute distress. She is afebrile with a blood pressure of 110/62 mmHg and a pulse of 72 bpm. The joint examination shows full range of motion and no swelling. There is mild anterior cervical lymphadenopathy. Close inspection of her skin reveals erythema of the malar eminences and the nose laterally, *with involvement of the nasolabial folds.* You note flaking and scaling in the eyebrows.

Question 11.9.1 The RASH is most characteristic of which of the following diagnoses?
A) Dermatomyositis
B) Systemic lupus erythematosus (SLE)
C) Seborrheic dermatitis
D) Psoriasis

Answer 11.9.1 The correct answer is "C." The classic rash of SLE is the malar, or "butterfly," rash with erythema over the malar eminences, bridging over the base of the nose. **However,**

the nasolabial folds are spared with the lupus malar rash. Involvement of the nasolabial fold characteristically occurs in seborrheic dermatitis. Additionally, the flaking of the eyebrow skin would be consistent with seborrheic dermatitis. In dermatomyositis ("A"), facial lesions involve the upper lids and have a light reddish-purple hue (the so-called "heliotrope rash"). Flat-topped, violaceous papules over the knuckles (Gottron papules) are classic features of dermatomyositis. The typical lesions of psoriasis ("D") include erythematous papules and plaques with silvery scales, noted more commonly on extensor surfaces.

Question 11.9.2 Which of the following diagnoses or descriptions most accurately describes your patient's disease process at this point in time?
A) Fibromyalgia
B) Somatoform disorder
C) Polyarthritis
D) Polyarthralgia
E) Rheumatoid arthritis

Answer 11.9.2 The correct answer is "D." Your patient complains of pain in multiple joints but has no findings of inflammation of the joints; therefore, the designation of "polyarthralgia" fits best at this time. If multiple joints were inflamed, you would use the term polyarthritis. At this time, you do not have enough information to make any of the other diagnoses.

You screen for depression and anxiety and find neither. You recommend acetaminophen for joint pain and headaches and encourage her to exercise regularly. She returns 2 months later feeling worse. She has severe fatigue and joint pain, most commonly involving her hands and knees. She has taken a leave of absence from her job as a high school English teacher. New symptoms include sores in her mouth as well as chest pain, which is worse with inspiration. On examination, you note the presence of a cardiac friction rub. There is diffuse tenderness to palpation of both knees and a small effusion apparent in the left knee. Her left hand demonstrates slow, incomplete grip. The facial rash is barely noticeable. There are two nontender ulcerations of the oral mucosa. The remainder of the examination is unchanged from her previous visit.

Question 11.9.3 Her disease process and current findings are most suggestive of which of the following diagnoses?
A) Lymphoma
B) SLE
C) Fibromyalgia
D) Reactive arthritis
E) Limited scleroderma (CREST syndrome)

Answer 11.9.3 The correct answer is "B." While she does not meet all the criteria for a diagnosis of SLE, this presentation is more consistent with SLE than any of the other options. Several findings point toward SLE: arthritis, cardiac friction rub (presumably due to pericarditis), and painless oral ulcers. Keep reading for more on the diagnostic criteria for SLE.

Based on your history, you recognize that your patient may be at higher than normal risk for developing SLE.

Question 11.9.4 All of the following groups have a higher incidence of SLE than the general population EXCEPT:
A) Family members of patients with SLE
B) Females
C) Asian Americans
D) Age in the third to fifth decades
E) Caucasians

Answer 11.9.4 The correct answer is "E." Compared to Blacks, Asians, and Latinos, Caucasians have a lower risk of SLE. The peak incidence of SLE occurs in the third to fifth decades of life. Women are 5 to 10 times more likely than men to be diagnosed with SLE. First-degree relatives of patients with SLE are at higher risk as well. Twin studies have shown a 25% to 50% concordance rate among monozygotic twins.

You consider that this might represent drug-related lupus, but your patient denies using any medications except for acetaminophen.

Question 11.9.5 In drug-related lupus, you expect to see all of the following EXCEPT:
A) Negative ANA
B) Rapid resolution of symptoms after discontinuing the drug
C) Polyarthralgia
D) Negative anti-dsDNA
E) Low-grade fever

Answer 11.9.5 The correct answer is "A." Patients with drug-induced lupus will generally have a positive ANA. However, it can be differentiated from SLE by a negative anti-dsDNA. Drug-related lupus presents with a lupus-like syndrome, with the most common features being arthralgias, myalgias, fatigue, malaise, and low-grade fever. Pericarditis and pleuritis are occasionally present. Skin, renal, and neurologic involvement are rare. Some common drugs that cause drug-induced lupus include hydralazine, diltiazem, hydrochlorothiazide, phenytoin, glyburide, infliximab, and etanercept.

Your patient returns with a painful, swollen left knee, and she wants to do something about it. You also discuss the following laboratory test results: WBC 5,100 cells/mm^3, Hgb 11.0 g/dL, platelets 309,000 cells/mm^3; BUN 10 mg/dL, creatinine 1.0 mg/dL; ESR 77 mm/hr; ANA 1:1,280 with a nucleolar pattern; urinalysis +1 protein, otherwise negative; urine microscopic examination shows no RBCs or casts; chest x-ray shows no cardiomegaly and normal lung fields; ECG shows normal sinus rhythm. You believe that your patient has SLE.

Question 11.9.6 Which of the following management plans do you suggest to the patient?
A) Start ibuprofen 600 mg by mouth three times daily and refer to a rheumatologist (3–6 month wait—sheesh, they are busy)
B) Start prednisone 20 mg by mouth daily and hydroxychloroquine 400 mg by mouth daily, schedule for follow-up in 1 month, and refer to a rheumatologist (3–6 month wait)
C) Start methotrexate 10 mg by mouth weekly, prednisone 60 mg by mouth daily, and hydroxychloroquine 400 mg by mouth daily, and schedule follow-up in 1 month
D) Start prednisone 60 mg by mouth daily and refer to a rheumatologist (3–6 month wait)
E) Start ibuprofen 600 mg by mouth daily and adopt a "watchful waiting" approach with follow-up in 6 months

Answer 11.9.6 The correct answer is "B." Your patient now meets diagnostic criteria for SLE, according to the American College of Rheumatology. See Table 11-6 for the diagnostic criteria for SLE. *Note that a positive ANA is only one of the criteria and is not required for the diagnosis of lupus*; however, the vast majority of patients with SLE will have an elevated ANA and negative results should make you re-think the diagnosis. Prompt treatment of her symptoms is important. NSAIDs, such as ibuprofen, are useful in treating arthralgias, mild arthritis, and mild pleurisy and pericarditis. In this case, oral (or perhaps intra-articular) corticosteroids are indicated for immediate symptomatic relief

TABLE 11-6 CLASSIFICATION CRITERIA FOR SYSTEMIC LUPUS ERYTHEMATOSUS

SLE requires the presence of 4 of the 11 following findings, not necessarily occurring at the same time.

1. Malar rash
2. Discoid rash
3. Photosensitivity
4. Oral ulcers (usually painless)
5. Nonerosive arthritis (involving 2 or more peripheral joints with tenderness, swelling, or effusion)
6. Serositis (pericarditis or pleuritis)
7. Renal disorder (persistent proteinuria >0.5 g/day or cellular casts)
8. Neurologic disorder (seizures or psychosis)
9. Hematologic disorder (hemolytic anemia, leucopenia <4,000/mm^3 on 2 occasions, lymphopenia <1,500/mm^3 on 2 occasions, or thrombocytopenia <100,000/mm^3 in the absence of offending drugs)
10. Immunologic disorder (anti-DNA, anti-Smith, or antiphospholipid antibodies, or a false-positive serologic test for syphilis)
11. Positive ANA

Adapted from Tan EM, Cohen AS, Fries JF, et al. The 1982 revised criteria for the classification of systemic lupus erythematosus. *Arthritis Rheum.* 1982;25:1271–1277 and Hochberg MC. Updating the American College of Rheumatology revised criteria for the classification of systemic lupus erythematosus [letter]. *Arthritis Rheum.* 1997;40:1725.

of her arthritis, and a low-to-moderate oral dose should be used (10–20 mg rather than 60 mg). Vitamin D and calcium supplements should be prescribed with the corticosteroids. Methotrexate can be used in recurrent, persistent arthritis. In the event of more serious renal, hematologic, or neurologic disease, high-dose corticosteroids are employed. Hydroxychloroquine may provide relief of musculoskeletal and constitutional symptoms and may also have a corticosteroid-sparing effect, but most important is the observation that SLE patients who take hydroxychloroquine have fewer organ-threatening lupus manifestations and fewer disease flares over time. Lupus patients who take hydroxychloroquine live longer than those who do not. Ideally, this patient should also be referred to a rheumatologist, but appropriate treatment should be started in a timely fashion. Close follow-up is necessary due to the potential adverse effects of these medications (e.g., diabetes with prednisone).

Over the next year, your patient does very well. She establishes care with a rheumatologist and is in remission when she sees you next. She is interested in becoming pregnant and wishes to seek your advice prior to trying to conceive. ("Start a college fund early," you say. "Oh, that's not what you meant?") Fortunately, she has been able to discontinue prednisone and continues to tolerate hydroxychloroquine.

Question 11.9.7 With regard to pregnancy and SLE, your patient is at higher risk for all of the following EXCEPT:
A) Premature birth
B) Infertility
C) Intrauterine fetal demise
D) Spontaneous abortion

Answer 11.9.7 **The correct answer is "B."** Women with SLE have a greater risk of premature birth, spontaneous abortion, and intrauterine fetal demise compared with otherwise healthy women. However, these patients appear to have comparable rates of fertility. Pregnancy outcomes are best when the patient is in remission 6 to 12 months before conception. Pregnancy appears to have a variable effect on SLE, with some patients experiencing exacerbations of the disease.

Your patient does well with her pregnancy but develops recurrent DVTs in the subsequent few years. You wish to evaluate her for antiphospholipid antibody syndrome.

Question 11.9.8 Which of the following results would you expect to find in a patient with antiphospholipid antibody syndrome?
A) Elevated PT/INR
B) Low PT/INR
C) Prolonged dilute Russell viper venom time (DRVVT) that corrects with addition of platelets
D) Elevated aPTT that corrects with addition of normal serum
E) High-fibrin degradation products

Answer 11.9.8 **The correct answer is "C."** The DRVVT assay is highly sensitive to the presence of proteins that block phospholipids, because the viper venom depletes phospholipid action. The DRVVT may be prolonged when the less sensitive aPTT is normal. When the DRVVT is prolonged, addition of platelets (as source of phospholipid) will correct the DRVVT when prolongation is due to a lupus anticoagulant.

Even though they are prone to clotting, patients with antiphospholipid antibody syndrome often have a paradoxically elevated aPTT. If this abnormality does NOT correct in vitro with addition of normal serum, it is supportive of the presence of a "lupus anticoagulant," which is presumptive evidence of antiphospholipid antibody syndrome. If the aPTT DOES correct, think about the presence of heparin, an acquired factor deficiency secondary to an antibody (often factor VIII). These antibodies are presumptively present if mixing the patients serum with normal serum causes a prolongation of the aPTT (the opposite of anticardiolipin antibody syndrome where normal serum is mixed with the patient's serum). "D" is incorrect, as correction of a prolonged aPTT with normal serum implies factor deficiency, not a lupus-anticoagulant, as noted above. Besides venous thrombus formation, women with antiphospholipid antibody syndrome are more likely to have late fetal demise and multiple spontaneous abortions. "A" is incorrect, as a lupus anticoagulant will not affect the prothrombin time.

HELPFUL TIP:
Antiphospholipid antibody syndrome is a clinical syndrome caused by autoantibodies to phospholipids that modulate the coagulation cascade. The term "lupus anticoagulant" refers to a subset of these autoantibodies that interfere with clotting tests such as aPTT; these

can be detected by the DRVVT. Alternatively, the presence of antiphospholipid antibodies can be determined by ELISA for anticardiolipin or beta-2-glycoprotein antibodies. However, there is only an 85% concordance between the presence of antiphospholipid antibody syndrome and laboratory detection of the causative antibodies. Antibodies must be detected on two occasions at least 12 weeks apart, and there needs to be a clinical manifestation, such as pregnancy morbidity or vascular thrombosis (arterial, venous, or small vessel). Pregnancy morbidities include: (1) more than one fetal death of a morphologically normal fetus beyond 10 weeks of gestation, (2) more than one premature birth before the 34th week of pregnancy due to pre-eclampsia, eclampsia, or placental insufficiency, or (3) more than three consecutive (pre)embryonic losses prior to 10 weeks of gestation.

HELPFUL TIP:
Only about 10% of patients with lupus have antiphospholipid antibodies.

Question 11.9.9 Which of the following statements is (are) true?
A) Patients with anticardiolipin antibodies should be treated prophylactically even if they have never had an abnormal clotting event, in order to prevent venous thrombosis, stroke, or other abnormal clotting events
B) Percent factor II activity is an appropriate way to monitor the response to heparin in patients with antiphospholipid antibody syndrome
C) Antifactor Xa should be used to monitor the activity of enoxaparin if monitoring is required
D) A and C
E) B and C

Answer 11.9.9 The correct answer is "E." Both "B" and "C" are true statements. Since patients with antiphospholipid antibody syndrome have an elevated aPTT, this value cannot be used to monitor anticoagulation with standard heparin. Percent factor II activity is the most appropriate way to monitor these patients if they are on standard heparin. Antifactor Xa is used to monitor anticoagulation with enoxaparin. "A" is incorrect because there is no evidence that prophylactic treatment reduces complications (although there is significant controversy in this area). Clearly, after a patient has had a thrombotic event, or has another indication, she needs anticoagulation.

HELPFUL TIP:
Unfractionated heparin, low-molecular-weight heparin, and aspirin are all used in the treatment of antiphospholipid antibody syndrome in pregnancy. Warfarin is teratogenic and is contraindicated in pregnancy

(remember, it is rat poison!). The newer anticoagulants such as dabigatran, rivaroxaban, and apixaban should not be used in pregnancy: There is not enough experience with their effectiveness, and safety is uncertain.

Question 11.9.10 Which of the following drugs used to treat lupus is associated with macular damage, corneal opacities, and ciliary muscle dysfunction?
A) Azathioprine
B) Prednisone
C) Hydroxychloroquine
D) Cyclophosphamide
E) Methotrexate

Answer 11.9.10 The correct answer is "C." Hydroxychloroquine is associated with macular damage, corneal opacities, and ciliary muscle dysfunction, and its use requires a baseline eye examination, and then yearly exams *after 5 years of continuous use.* The risk for significant ocular toxicity is reduced if the daily hydroxychloroquine dose is kept below 5 mg/kg/day of actual body weight which is approximately 400 mg/day for most women, and 300 mg/day for smaller women. Daily use of an Amsler grid to detect ocular toxicity had been recommended in the past. It is ineffective. Other SLE drugs and side effects are noted in Table 11-7.

▶ **Objectives: Did you learn to …**
- Identify clinical manifestations of SLE?
- Define diagnostic criteria for SLE?
- Recognize the waxing and waning course of SLE?
- Implement appropriate treatment of the patient with SLE?
- Recognize adverse effects of medications used in the treatment of SLE?
- Describe some characteristics of antiphospholipid antibody syndrome?

TABLE 11-7 TOXICITIES ASSOCIATED WITH MEDICATIONS USED TO TREAT SLE

- NSAIDs: gastrointestinal bleeding, renal dysfunction, hypertension
- Steroids: diabetes, hypertension, hyperlipidemia, osteoporosis, cataract formation, weight gain, infections
- Hydroxychloroquine: macular damage, ciliary muscle dysfunction, corneal opacities, myopathy
- Azathioprine: infections, myelosuppression, hepatotoxicity
- Cyclophosphamide: infections, myelosuppression, hemorrhagic cystitis
- Methotrexate: infections, myelosuppression, hepatic fibrosis

▶ **CASE 11.10**

A 22-year-old white female presents to your office with the chief complaint of "blue fingers." She reports a history of intermittent bluish discoloration of the fingertips on both hands when they are exposed to cold temperatures. Although she believes the symptoms are worse now, she cannot recall

how long they have been present. She has never had ulcers on her fingers or toes.

Question 11.10.1 With no further information, what is the most likely explanation for these digital color changes?
A) Atherosclerotic disease of the extremities
B) Acrocyanosis
C) Scleroderma
D) Physiologic response to cold

Answer 11.10.1 **The correct answer is "D."** At this point all we know is that this patient's fingers turn blue upon exposure to cold. This is a normal physiologic response—vasoconstriction in response to cold. If you've never experienced this, you live very close to the equator and never venture far from home. "A" is incorrect. Peripheral vascular disease is the result of atherosclerotic disease of the extremities and typically occurs in older individuals; manifestations include claudication and skin ulceration. "B" is incorrect. Raynaud phenomenon must be distinguished from acrocyanosis (a rare vasospastic disorder of persistent coldness and bluish discoloration of the hands and feet, not just fingers and toes, sometimes following a viral infection). "C" is also incorrect. Scleroderma by itself does not cause blue fingers.

HELPFUL TIP:
Over 80% of cases of Raynaud phenomenon that present to a primary care physician's office are due to an exaggerated physiologic response to cold or emotional distress, which we call primary Raynaud phenomenon. In most primary cases, patients report the onset of symptoms in their teens or twenties. Although Raynaud phenomenon occurs in most patients with scleroderma (90–95%), scleroderma is a rare disease and is much less common than primary Raynaud phenomenon, so the converse is not true. Thus, the presence of Raynaud phenomenon is not synonymous with the presence of scleroderma. A very important clue to suggest that Raynaud is due to an underlying systemic rheumatic disease is onset after the age of 40—these patients should always have a thorough evaluation for underlying systemic causes. Other clues suggesting secondary Raynaud phenomenon include a history of severe disease (e.g., difficult to reverse attacks, digital ulcerations) or concurrent onset of new cutaneous, musculoskeletal, gastrointestinal, or cardiopulmonary problems. In these patients, an ANA titer may be helpful in further evaluation.

HELPFUL TIP:
Buerger disease (thromboangiitis obliterans) is strongly associated with tobacco abuse and presents with distal small vessel ischemia and symptoms that are similar to Raynaud phenomenon. It eventually progresses to infarction of tissue, frequently requiring digit amputation.

Further history reveals that the patient uses no medications. She has been healthy all of her life. Her mother and aunt have had blue fingers in cold temperature, too. She denies tobacco use. The review of systems is unremarkable.

Question 11.10.2 All of the following are expected findings in patients with primary Raynaud phenomenon EXCEPT:
A) Symmetric involvement of the hands
B) Well-demarcated cyanosis
C) Digital ulcerations
D) Normal ESR

Answer 11.10.2 **The correct answer is "C."** Primary Raynaud phenomenon is diagnosed when other causes of Raynaud phenomenon have been eliminated. Primary Raynaud phenomenon is not typically destructive, and digital ulcerations generally occur when the phenomenon is secondary to some other disease process (e.g., scleroderma and SLE). Primary Raynaud phenomenon is almost always symmetric. Raynaud phenomenon can be differentiated from a normal response to cold temperatures by the demarcation between pale or cyanotic fingertips and normal-appearing skin. A normal response to cold may include mottling, with indistinct borders between pale and purple-colored skin, and paresthesias of the involved area. In patients with Raynaud phenomenon, the distal most portion of the involved digit is pale or cyanotic, and the transition to normal skin color is abrupt. Since primary Raynaud phenomenon is not due to an inflammatory condition, markers of inflammation such as the ESR are usually normal.

HELPFUL TIP:
Nailfold capillary microscopy (NCM) can be used to examine the nailfold capillaries of patients with Raynaud phenomenon. NCM involves placing a drop of oil (a drop of surgical lubricant also works well) on the cuticle of one or more digits and visualization of the nail fold capillaries through an ophthalmoscope set at +40 diopters (40 green). Usually the ring and middle fingers (or symptomatic fingers) are examined. Normal capillaries are symmetric, nondilated loops. Distorted, dilated, or absent capillaries suggest secondary Raynaud phenomenon.

You perform a physical examination, including NCM which is essentially normal. There is currently no discoloration of the fingers.

Question 11.10.3 What is the next most appropriate step in the evaluation and management of this patient?
A) Cold provocation
B) Doppler ultrasound of the extremities
C) Blood viscosity testing
D) ANA
E) A trial of therapy, nonpharmacologic and/or pharmacologic

Answer 11.10.3 The correct answer is "E." Given that she is symptomatic, a trial of drug therapy is warranted. Cold provocation ("A") is not recommended, as results are inconsistent. Rather, the diagnosis is based on a convincing history of episodic cyanosis. Doppler ultrasound ("B") might be useful if you were considering large vessel disease from atherosclerosis, etc. However, it is not likely to be helpful in this patient. Blood viscosity testing ("C") is not something that is done routinely. Measurement of ANA ("D") can be helpful in ruling out underlying autoimmune disease since patients with Raynaud phenomenon and a positive ANA may have a higher risk of developing a systemic autoimmune disease. However, based on her age, symmetric involvement, lack of ulcerations, and lack of other symptoms, this patient most likely has primary Raynaud phenomenon unrelated to an underlying disease. A secondary cause (e.g., scleroderma) is more likely with any of the following: patients who are age 30 years old or older; attacks are asymmetric or associated with skin ulcers; there are symptoms suggestive of systemic involvement (e.g., arthralgias, dyspnea, reflux, or weight loss). In addition to abnormal nailfold capillaries, other subtle findings to suggest secondary Raynaud include puffy hand swelling and telangiectasias on the fingers or around the mouth. If you are concerned about secondary Raynaud phenomenon, an ANA would be indicated.

HELPFUL (FINGER) TIP:
Most patients with secondary Raynaud phenomenon will develop symptoms of their underlying autoimmune disease within a few years of onset of Raynaud phenomenon. But Raynaud phenomenon may occur years before other symptoms are prominent or bothersome enough for the patient to report them to a doctor.

After reviewing the diagnosis with your patient, you make several recommendations to help reduce the frequency of attacks: avoid cold temperatures, reduce emotional stress (like taking the boards?), and avoid tobacco and medications that cause vasoconstriction (e.g., sympathomimetic drugs).

Your patient returns 10 months later with new complaints. Both hands are swollen, stiff, and painful. She complains of multiple joint aches and fatigue despite sleeping well. Her appetite is normal, and she has no GI complaints. Although she has no rash, she complains of itchy hands (surely a sign of cancer, she thinks). On examination, you note that there is diffuse, nonpitting edema on her fingers and hands. She has difficulty making a fist. She has no skin findings. Her CBC is normal. Her ANA is strongly positive with a nucleolar pattern.

Question 11.10.4 Which of the following is the most likely explanation of these findings and the most appropriate provisional diagnosis?
A) Raynaud phenomenon
B) RA
C) Scleroderma
D) CREST syndrome
E) Osteoarthritis

Answer 11.10.4 The correct answer is "C." This patient is now presenting with symptoms of scleroderma, also called systemic sclerosis. Scleroderma encompasses a heterogeneous group of conditions, which are variable in severity, but share a common pathophysiologic mechanism—fibrosis of the skin and other organs. The pathology of scleroderma also involves small vessel vasculopathy, a process that leads to Raynaud phenomenon and ischemia of other tissues. Scleroderma may affect the joints, skin, lungs, kidneys, heart, and GI system. Fifty percent of patients with scleroderma have depression so don't overlook this comorbidity.

A positive ANA can be helpful when you suspect scleroderma based on clinical findings. ANA by indirect immunofluorescence will report the type of nuclear staining pattern. Centromere or nucleolar patterns are most highly associated with systemic sclerosis, but other patterns (such as speckled) are also seen. Patients with systemic sclerosis may have a negative ANA.

These findings are now much more than you would expect to see with Raynaud phenomenon; thus, "A" is incorrect. Diffuse swelling and stiffness are present rather than specific synovitis, so "B" (RA) is less likely. Also, osteoarthritis ("E") should have identifiable specific joint involvement rather than diffuse hand edema. CREST syndrome ("D") is an acronym standing for calcinosis cutis, Raynaud phenomenon, esophageal dysmotility, sclerodactyly, and telangiectasia, which are all manifestations that can occur in patients with systemic sclerosis. CREST should be used as a mnemonic to help remember the manifestation of systemic sclerosis, and not as diagnostic criteria. Of note, calcinosis is a relatively uncommon and late manifestation of systemic sclerosis.

HELPFUL TIP:
Further diagnosis and categorization of scleroderma can be accomplished with the aid of more specific serologic tests such as anti-RNA polymerase III antibodies (which predict high risk for renal crisis) and anti-topoisomerase antibodies (Scl-70) that predict higher risk for interstitial lung disease. Treatment for scleroderma is evolving, with some immunosuppressive therapies showing promise in the long-term management (methotrexate, mycophentolate, or cyclophospomide for skin involvement, prokinetics for pseudo-obstruction due to GI involvement, etc.). Finally, the greatest treatment breakthrough for scleroderma patients is the finding that ACE inhibitors can treat scleroderma renal crisis, leading to sharp reduction in mortality and preservation of renal function. Monitor renal function every 3 months for 4 to 5 years after diagnosis; this is when renal crisis is most likely to occur. Check for CrCl as well as urinary protein-to-creatinine ratio.

Because of digital ulcers you observe and the increasing pain of her Raynaud phenomenon attacks, you decide to prescribe medication for Raynaud phenomenon.

Question 11.10.5 Which of the following is the best therapy for reducing the frequency of attacks of Raynaud phenomenon?
A) Amlodipine 5 mg daily
B) Nifedipine 10 mg as needed
C) Nitroglycerin 2% ointment daily
D) Diltiazem 30 mg as needed
E) Prazosin 1 mg twice daily

Answer 11.10.5 The correct answer is "A." All of the medications listed are potentially helpful treatments when Raynaud phenomenon does not respond to conservative measures. However, the most appropriate choice is daily amlodipine. Dihydropyridine calcium-channel blockers, like amlodipine, have been shown to reduce the frequency of attacks by about 50% compared with placebo. They must be scheduled, rather than used as needed. In the case of nifedipine, it is best to use an extended-release version, as the short-acting preparation is more likely to cause hypotension; it also should not be used PRN (thus, "B" is incorrect). Diltiazem is not as effective as the dihydropyridine calcium-channel blockers. In systemic sclerosis, the benefit of calcium-channel blockers is often offset by their exacerbation of GERD. Alternatives include (in order of recommendation) sildenafil and other phosphodiesterase inhibitors, topical nitrates, ACE inhibitors, and ARBs. In addition, all patients should get aspirin in antiplatelet doses (81 mg daily). There is less evidence that prazosin is effective, but alpha-antagonists have a role if other therapies are unsuccessful. Sympathectomy is a last resort.

Question 11.10.6 Which of the following is NOT indicated for acute ischemic crisis related to Raynaud phenomenon?
A) Aspirin
B) Beta-blocker
C) Nifedipine
D) Digital or wrist nerve block
E) Topical nitroglycerin

Answer 11.10.6 The correct answer is "B." Beta-blockers are not indicated in the treatment of an ischemic crisis related to Raynaud phenomenon. Beta-blockers actually cause peripheral vasoconstriction and may worsen the problem. Peripherally, **beta-agonists** cause vasodilatation. When a beta-blocker is used, the patient ends up with an unopposed alpha-adrenergic response, which worsens vasoconstriction. All of the other therapies are useful in acute ischemic crisis. Of particular note is "D." A nerve or wrist block with lidocaine effectively causes a sympathectomy, leading to decreased vascular tone. As mentioned above, sildenafil appears to be beneficial in healing ischemic ulcers and for acute ischemic crisis.

▶ **Objectives:** Did you learn to ...
• Identify complications of Raynaud phenomenon and diseases associated with it?
• Develop a strategy for the prevention and treatment of symptoms of Raynaud phenomenon?
• Recognize clinical features of scleroderma?

▶ **CASE 11.11**

A 17-year-old male presents to your office with a history of low–back pain worsening over the past few months. He recalls having intermittent back pain for at least a year. The pain does not radiate. He runs cross-country and track without exacerbating his back pain. He denies fevers, weight loss, weakness, incontinence, and history of trauma. He is unaware of any family history of back pain. He is otherwise healthy.

Question 11.11.1 What further information will help you differentiate between potential causes of his back pain?
A) Relief with acetaminophen
B) Morning stiffness
C) Relief with rest
D) A and C
E) B or C

Answer 11.11.1 The correct answer is "E." Determining the pattern of the pain is critical. Inflammatory causes of back pain are characterized by morning stiffness and improvement with activity. In contrast, degenerative back disease causes pain that is exacerbated by activity and relieved with rest. Inflammatory back pain typically presents in younger patients; degenerative back pain typically does not present before age 30 or 40. Acetaminophen and other analgesics may relieve pain from either category of disease and so will not help you narrow the diagnosis.

 HELPFUL TIP:
In a young patient with back pain, also consider fractures (e.g., spondylolysis, a bilateral pars defect), infection (discitis, osteomyelitis), disc disease, and osseous malignancies.

On further questioning, your patient reports morning stiffness and pain that improves with stretching. Activity does not seem to aggravate his back but inactivity does. He has had no penile discharge, rash, or conjunctivitis, and denies diarrhea or other GI symptoms. On physical examination, your patient is surprised to find that he cannot reach his toes as he had been able to do just a few months ago in track practice. Range of motion in the neck, arms, and legs is normal. A focused neurologic examination is normal. There is mild, diffuse tenderness over the lumbosacral spine and with percussion over the sacroiliac joints. When supine on the examination table, a FABER maneuver (flexion, abduction, external rotation) reproduces sacral pain.

Question 11.11.2 The history and physical examination are most consistent with a diagnosis of:
A) Reactive arthritis (formerly termed Reiter syndrome)
B) Osteoarthritis of the lumbar spine
C) Degenerative disc disease
D) Ankylosing spondylitis
E) Vertebral body tumor

Answer 11.11.2 The correct answer is "D." The history and physical examination are most consistent with ankylosing spondylitis, a seronegative (RF negative) spondyloarthropathy. Ankylosing spondylitis is the most common form of spondyloarthropathy and is thought to have a prevalence of 1% in Caucasian populations. Historically, there is a 5:1 male-to-female ratio (but this may also be because ankylosing spondylitis is less recognized in women). Studies based on radiographic appearance and human leukocyte antigen (HLA) B27 typing show a much lower male:female ratio. In addition to the historical features mentioned in the answer to the previous question, there is often a family history of ankylosing spondylitis in patients ultimately diagnosed with the disease.

"A" is incorrect. Reactive arthritis occurs in reaction to an infection (*Chlamydia* urethritis, GI infection, etc.), and presents with mono- or oligoarthritis, usually of the joints in the leg. Note that chronic GI disease (e.g., Crohn, ulcerative colitis, celiac disease) may be associated with arthritis, but this is not considered "reactive arthritis." This patient's age makes osteoarthritis and degenerative disc disease less likely, so "B" and "C" are wrong. Also, he has no neurologic findings that you might expect with disc prolapse. Malignancy is associated with constitutional symptoms (fever and weight loss), neurologic involvement, and steadily worsening pain that is not relieved by activity—none of which are present in this case. Physical examination findings of spondyloarthropathies are listed in Table 11-8.

HELPFUL TIP:
The FABER (Flexion, Abduction, External Rotation) test, also known as the "figure 4" test, is performed by having the patient lie supine, passively flexing the knee to 90 degrees, resting the patient's foot on the contralateral thigh just above the knee, and applying pressure laterally and downward on the ipsilateral knee.

TABLE 11-8 PHYSICAL FINDINGS IN THE SPONDYLOARTHROPATHIES

- Limited range of motion in the axial spine
- Peripheral arthritis
- Tenderness at the sacroiliac joints
- Enthesopathy (pain at tendon site insertion, particularly the Achilles tendon and plantar fascia synovitis)
- Extra-articular symptoms (anterior uveitis in 30–40%, psoriasis, inflammatory bowel disease)

When viewed from above, the patient's legs take on the "figure 4" appearance. The pelvis should be stabilized by the examiner. A positive test occurs if ipsilateral hip or sacroiliac (SI) joint pain is reproduced. It is nonspecific and can be positive in many diseases of the SI joint and hip.

Question 11.11.3 Time for some tests! Which of the following is the best initial test to confirm the diagnosis of ankylosing spondylitis?
A) ANA
B) Lumbar spine radiographs
C) HLA-B27
D) ESR
E) Sacroiliac joint radiographs

Answer 11.11.3 The correct answer is "E." The hallmark of ankylosing spondylitis is sacroiliitis on pelvic radiographs. Although there are no universally accepted criteria for diagnosing spondyloarthropathies, x-ray evidence of sacroiliitis in the setting of a consistent clinical picture is sufficient to diagnose ankylosing spondylitis. Unfortunately, in early ankylosing spondylitis, x-rays are often inconclusive. MRI is more sensitive for detecting early sacroiliitis, but the cost is higher and may not be necessary when plain x-ray images are strongly supportive of sacroiliitis. The rest of the answers are incorrect. Ankylosing spondylitis is not associated with a positive ANA. Lumbar spine x-rays may be useful in ruling out other conditions and do show some changes in ankylosing spondylitis but may miss early disease. HLA-B27, a class I HLA gene, is present in about 90% of white patients and 50% to 80% of non-white patients with ankylosing spondylitis and is generally associated with spondyloarthropathies. However, HLA-B27 is not specific. It is present in many normal individuals as well and is of very little diagnostic value (although it does have a good negative predictive value). ESR is slightly elevated in most cases of spondyloarthropathy, but again it is not specific.

. . . .

Lumbar spine x-rays show squaring of the vertebral bodies. Pelvic x-rays identify mild symmetric sacroiliitis. You are now confident of the diagnosis of ankylosing spondylitis.

Question 11.11.4 Which of the following management plans is best for this patient?
A) Aspirin 650 mg by mouth four times daily (or Zorprin or other extended-release aspirin twice daily) and physical therapy referral
B) Naproxen 500 mg twice daily and physical therapy referral
C) Orthopedic referral for early surgical consideration
D) Prednisone 40 mg daily and fitting for a back brace
E) Naproxen 500 mg twice daily and fitting for a back brace

Answer 11.11.4 The correct answer is "B." NSAIDs are the mainstay of medical therapy for active phases of spondyloarthropathy. Patients generally experience significant relief from NSAIDs, and any additional benefit from systemic corticosteroids is questionable. Sulfasalazine is a second-line drug. Interestingly, aspirin tends to be less effective in these patients; thus, "A" is incorrect. The management of ankylosing spondylitis should also include an exercise regimen designed specifically for the patient, and physical therapy may play a key role. The use of braces is not helpful and may actually exacerbate the patient's symptoms. Orthopedic surgery only becomes necessary in cases of advanced ankylosing spondylitis when kyphosis or peripheral joint symptoms become severe.

....

After 3 months of physical therapy and NSAIDs, your patient returns. He has noticed minimal benefit, and now you find limitation of his neck range of motion.

Question 11.11.5 What is the most appropriate next step in the evaluation and management of this patient?
A) Discontinue naproxen and switch to indomethacin 50 mg three times daily
B) Begin methotrexate 15 mg per week and folic acid 1 mg daily
C) Begin prednisone 60 mg daily
D) Order MRI of the cervical spine
E) Continue naproxen and refer to rheumatology

Answer 11.11.5 The correct answer is "E." The patient is losing range of motion despite NSAID therapy. Referral to a rheumatologist to consider anti-TNF therapy (e.g., infliximab, adalimumab, or etanercept) is the best next step. Anti-TNF agents can halt disease progression and often improve range of motion in early disease *but are not considered first-line agents.* "A" is incorrect. Switching NSAIDs may provide some minor additional benefit but is unlikely to arrest disease progression. "B" is incorrect. Methotrexate may be beneficial for the peripheral arthritis of spondyloarthropathies but not for the axial skeleton disease. "C" is incorrect since systemic corticosteroids have no value in treating spondyloarthropathies. Local corticosteroid injections are often beneficial for enthesopathy and peripheral arthritis. "D" is incorrect. MRI of the cervical spine will show inflammatory changes of the spine but will not change your management.

....

The patient fails to keep his rheumatology appointment and returns to you 1 year later. He is taking over-the-counter naproxen. His neck is very stiff, with even less range of motion. He relates that he has been having crampy abdominal pain, and loose stools with bloody mucus. He is having dyspnea with mild exertion. On examination, his neck range of motion is worse, and back flexion is limited with straightening of his lumbar lordosis.

Question 11.11.6 What is the next most appropriate step in the evaluation and management of this patient?
A) Discontinue naproxen
B) Check CBC with differential and iron panel
C) Consult gastroenterology for EGD and colonoscopy
D) Consult rheumatology and tell patient he must keep his appointment
E) All of the above

Answer 11.11.6 The correct answer is "E." The patient could have enteropathic arthritis in association with inflammatory bowel disease. He could also have chronic GI blood loss from an NSAID-induced ulcer. For this reason and because NSAIDs can exacerbate inflammatory bowel disease, the naproxen must be discontinued ("A"). A CBC and iron panel may reveal iron deficiency anemia, which would explain the patient's dyspnea on exertion. Subspecialty evaluations by a gastroenterologist and rheumatologist are indicated both to confirm the diagnosis and to help with long-term disease management. Anti-TNF agents—like infliximab and adalimumab—but not etanercept—are beneficial **for both** the spondyloarthropathy (in this case, ankylosing spondylitis) and associated inflammatory bowel disease in enteropathic arthritis.

 HELPFUL TIP:
The most common spondyloarthropathies are ankylosing spondylitis, psoriatic arthritis, enteropathic arthritis, and reactive arthritis. These are pathogenically similar diseases that may be difficult to differentiate in early stages, but lack of differentiation does not generally affect therapy.

 HELPFUL TIP:
Enteropathic arthritis occurs frequently in patients with inflammatory bowel disease, and has features in common with ankylosing spondylitis, including inflammatory back pain and sacroiliitis. However, a reactive spondyloarthropathy may also occur after a GI infection such as *Salmonella*, *Yersinia*, *Shigella*, or *Campylobacter* and other infections such as chlamydia. Finally, other illnesses such as celiac disease may cause a reactive spondyloarthropathy.

▶ **Objectives: Did you learn to …**
- Recognize clinical manifestations of spondyloarthropathies, particularly ankylosing spondylitis?
- Name some of the different types of spondyloarthropathies?
- Develop an appropriate evaluation for the patient presenting with inflammatory back pain?
- Appropriately manage a patient with ankylosing spondylitis?

 QUICK QUIZ: SPONDYLOARTHROPATHIES

Which of the following is NOT a characteristic of reactive arthritis?
A) Conjunctivitis
B) Keratoderma blenorrhagicum
C) HLA-B8
D) Urethritis
E) Arthritis

The correct answer is "C." Reactive arthritis (formerly Reiter syndrome) is associated with HLA-B27 and not HLA-B8 (which is found in sclerosing cholangitis). All of the other choices are seen with reactive arthritis, including keratoderma blenorrhagicum, which is a rash found especially on the soles of patients with reactive arthritis. The urethritis is generally due to *Chlamydia trachomatis.*

HELPFUL TIP:
The onset of reactive arthritis is less insidious than that of ankylosing spondylitis, with some patients presenting with an acute illness that includes fever, acute joint swelling, and rash (keratoderma blenorrhagicum). Generally, reactive arthritis resolves within 12 months. Antibiotics are not effective as a treatment of reactive arthritis (although may be indicated for the underlying infection).

▶ CASE 11.12

A 52-year-old female presents to your office for an initial visit and complains of mild pain and weakness in her hips and thighs. The symptoms have been present for months. About 2 years ago another doctor diagnosed her with psoriasis because of a rash on her hands and elbows, which has since resolved. Otherwise, she reports being relatively healthy and taking no medications. She is a smoker. She has had no recent health screening. On physical examination, her vitals are normal. She has considerable difficulty getting out of her chair. Her strength is symmetrically diminished in the quadriceps and hip flexors. The rest of the examination is unremarkable.

Question 11.12.1 Which of the following diagnostic tests do you order first?
A) Muscle biopsy
B) Electromyography (EMG)
C) TSH
D) ANA
E) Troponin-T

Answer 11.12.1 The correct answer is "C." Hypothyroidism (along with many other diseases—see below) can cause a proximal muscle weakness and is very common in middle-aged females. A muscle biopsy or EMG study is premature without first evaluating for myopathy with serum enzyme levels (CK, aldolase). "D," an ANA, is not likely to be helpful. Autoimmune diseases such as polymyositis and dermatomyositis cause myopathy, but ANA is not specific for diagnosing these diseases. Finally, although CK-MB may be elevated in patients with myopathy, troponin-T ("E") is an enzyme relatively specific to cardiac muscle and should be normal.

You order TSH and CBC, which are both within normal limits. ESR, CK, and AST are elevated. You proceed to order that EMG which demonstrates abnormalities of the paraspinal

muscles. Your patient returns to discuss her test results and complains that her psoriasis is back. There are violaceous plaques on her knuckles and elbows and around her eyes.

Question 11.12.2 You recommend the following management plan for the disease:
A) Ultraviolet light therapy
B) Topical corticosteroids
C) Oral corticosteroids
D) Topical emollients
E) Acetaminophen

Answer 11.12.2 The correct answer is "C." This patient now has findings that support a diagnosis of dermatomyositis. To diagnose idiopathic inflammatory myopathy, such as dermatomyositis or polymyositis, certain criteria must be present (see Table 11-9). This patient has three of these criteria plus skin changes consistent with dermatomyositis. Violaceous plaques on the knuckles are commonly called Gottron papules. Similar lesions are often observed over pressure points (e.g., elbows). Because dermatomyositis is a systemic condition, treatment should likewise be systemic. Local topical therapies do not treat the disease, and oral corticosteroids are typically the first-line agents. Hydroxychloroquine is helpful when the rash does not respond to corticosteroids. Addition of immunosuppressive drugs, such as methotrexate or azathioprine, may be indicated.

Question 11.12.3 You diagnose dermatomyositis. Which of the following tests and exams should now be ordered?
A) Pap and pelvic examination, CA-125, and pelvic ultrasound
B) Screening mammogram
C) Chest radiograph
D) Fecal occult blood screening
E) All of the above

Answer 11.12.3 The correct answer is "E." Patients with adult-onset dermatomyositis have a sixfold increased risk of developing cancer. Therefore, upon diagnosing dermatomyositis, a thorough history and physical examination must be performed. All patients should undergo age-appropriate cancer screening tests (e.g., Pap smear, fecal occult blood testing, and mammography in this patient). Also, other tests generally recommended include CBC, metabolic profile, liver function tests, urinalysis, and chest x-ray—especially important in smokers. Since the patient is over age 50, colonoscopy is indicated. The cancers most commonly associated with dermatomyositis include

TABLE 11-9 DIAGNOSTIC FEATURES OF POLYMYOSITIS AND DERMATOMYOSITIS

- Elevated muscle enzymes (CPK and aldolase)
- Symmetrical proximal muscle weakness
- Abnormal EMG
- Consistent findings on muscle biopsy

Note: Skin findings must be present in order to diagnose dermatomyositis.

ovarian and gastric cancers and lymphoma. Therefore, it is reasonable to consider CA-125 and pelvic ultrasound.

HELPFUL TIP:
The association of dermatomyositis with GI malignancy is particularly strong. You may consider endoscopies and an alpha-fetoprotein (for gastric cancer). Some authorities also suggest CT of the abdomen and pelvis to rule out malignancy.

HELPFUL TIP:
Other causes of proximal muscle weakness include alcohol use, muscular dystrophy, medications (e.g., penicillamine and HMG-CoA reductase inhibitors), Cushing syndrome, viral infections, hypothyroidism, and diabetes mellitus. The list goes on, including myasthenia gravis and Eaton–Lambert syndrome.

▶ **Objectives: Did you learn to …**
- Recognize symptoms and signs of dermatomyositis and polymyositis?
- Describe how inflammatory myopathies are evaluated and diagnosed?
- Appreciate the relationship between malignancy and inflammatory myopathy?

QUICK QUIZ: ARTHRITIS AND JOINT INVOLVEMENT

Compared with RA, osteoarthritis has a greater predilection for which of the following joints?
A) MCPs
B) DIPs
C) Knees
D) Wrists

The correct answer is "B." Osteoarthritis tends to affect the DIP and PIP joints in the hand, sparing the MCP joints, whereas RA affects the MCPs and spares the DIPs. Both disease processes may involve the knees and wrists.

Clinical Pearls

○ Aspirate a monoarthritis and send synovial fluid for cell count with differential, Gram stain, culture and crystal analysis for evaluating and ruling out a septic joint. Remember that those with crystalline arthritis may also have a septic joint.

○ Begin supplementation with calcium and vitamin D for osteoporosis prevention with initiation of corticosteroids in the treatment of rheumatologic disease.

○ Do not delay initiation of high-dose corticosteroids for treatment of giant cell arteritis while awaiting a temporal artery biopsy.

○ Do not rely upon serum uric acid levels to diagnose or refute a gout attack.

○ Do not routinely order "rheumatology panels." Order appropriate rheumatologic tests based on clinical evaluation and specific disease under consideration.

○ Do not routinely screen for Lyme disease for chronic musculoskeletal pain. Repeat after us: "There is no such thing as chronic Lyme disease responsive to antibiotics. Once the patient is appropriately treated, additional courses of antibiotics are worthless."

○ Do not use opioid pain medications in treating chronic pain related to fibromyalgia as they tend to worsen central sensitization and increase fibromyalgia pain over time.

○ Ensure that women of child-bearing age on methotrexate have reliable contraception.

○ Prescribe a trial of DMARDs (disease modifying anti-rheumatic drugs) as first-line therapy in rheumatoid arthritis.

○ Use the lowest and minimum effective prednisone dose for acute symptomatic relief of inflammatory arthritis.

BIBLIOGRAPHY

Aletaha D, et al. Rheumatoid arthritis classification criteria: an American College of Rheumatology/European League Against Rheumatism collaborative initiative. *Arthritis Rheum.* 2010;62(9):2569–2581.

Álvarez-Lario B, MacArrón-Vicente J. Is there anything good in uric acid? *Q J Med.* 2011;104(12):1015–1024.

Bhate C, Schwartz RA. Lyme disease: Part I. Advances and perspectives. *J Am Acad Dermatol.* 2011;64(4):619–636.

Bhate C, Schwartz RA. Lyme disease: Part II. Management and prevention. *J Am Acad Dermatol.* 2011;64(4):639–653.

Black R, et al. The use of temporal artery ultrasound in the diagnosis of giant cell arteritis in routine practice. *Int J Rheum Dis.* 2013;16(3):352–357.

Botzoris V, Drosos AA. Management of Raynaud's phenomenon and digital ulcers in systemic sclerosis. *Joint Bone Spine.* 2011;78(4):341–346.

Clauw DJ. Fibromyalgia: a clinical review. *JAMA.* 2014;311(15):1547–55.

Dasgupta B, et al. Provisional classification criteria for polymyalgia rheumatica. *Arthritis Rheum.* 2012;64(4): 943–954.

Dejaca C, et al. EULAR recommendations for the use of imaging in large vessel vasculitis in clinical practice. *Ann Rheum Dis.* 2018;77(5):636-643.

Dougados M, Baeten D. Spondyloarthritis. *Lancet.* 2011;377:2127–2137.

Firestein GS, et al., eds. *Kelley's Textbook of Rheumatology.* 10th ed. Philadelphia: Elsevier Saunders; 2016.

Hu HJ, et al. Clinical utility of dual-energy CT for gout diagnosis. *Clin Imaging.* 2015;39:880–885.

Khanna D, et al. American College of Rheumatology guidelines for management of gout part II: therapy and anti-inflammatory prophylaxis of acute gouty arthritis. *Arthritis Care Res*. 2012;64(10):1447–1461.

Marmor MF, et al. Revised recommendations on screening for chloroquine and hydroxychloroquine retinopathy. *Ophthalmology*. 2011;118(2):415–422.

Nam JL, et al. Efficacy of biological disease-modifying antirheumatic drugs: a systematic literature review informing the 2013 update of the EULAR recommendations for the management of rheumatoid arthritis. *Ann Rheum Dis*. 2014;73:516–528.

Pincus T, Gibson KA, Shmerling RH. An evidence-based approach to laboratory tests in usual care of patients with rheumatoid arthritis. *Clin Exp Rheumatol*. 2014;32 (suppl 85):S23–S28.

Singh JA, et al. 2012 updated to the 2008 American College of Rheumatology recommendations for the use of disease-modifying antirheumatic drugs and biologic agents in the treatment of rheumatoid arthritis. *Arthritis Care Res*. 2012;64(5):625–639.

Stone JH, et al. Trial of tocilizumab in giant-cell arteritis. *N Engl J Med*. 2017; 377:317–328.

Van Hecke O. Polymyalgia rheumatic-diagnosis and management. *Aust Fam Physician*. 2011;40(5):303–306.

Villa-Forte A. Giant cell arteritis: suspect it, treat it promptly. *Cleve Clin J Med*. 2011;78(4):265–270.

Orthopedics and Sports Medicine

12

Britt L. Marcussen, Tameem A. Shoukih, and Mark A. Graber

General note: On the test if you have a choice between acetaminophen and an NSAID for an acute injury or noninflammatory arthritis, acetaminophen will always be the right choice. Most acute injuries are not inflammatory, and acetaminophen is a lot safer without gastropathy or platelet inhibition. If you do use an NSAID, naproxen is the safest from a cardiovascular standpoint but carries the same gastrointestinal risks as other NSAIDs. With that said, in 2012 the FDA recommended that the maximum daily dose of acetaminophen in otherwise healthy adults be reduced from 4,000 to 3,000 mg/day. In addition, the number needed to treat and get a 50% reduction in pain is 4.6 for 650 mg of acetaminophen compared to 1.7 for 600 mg of ibuprofen! So… well there is a quandary for you!

▶ CASE 12.1

A 5-year-old boy presents with acute onset of left anterior thigh and hip pain that began 2 days ago with no known prior trauma. He reports that it initially "loosened-up" after he had been out of bed for a few hours but has become worse again by afternoon. His pain is exacerbated by weight bearing and active or passive range of motion (ROM). His mother notes that he had a cold 7 to 10 days ago, but has been asymptomatic until he complained of thigh pain two nights ago. She also notes that he has had a low-grade fever. He has no other significant constitutional symptoms and appears to be in some pain, but otherwise he appears well.

Question 12.1.1 **Based on the information obtained thus far, which of the following is the most likely diagnosis?**
A) Osteomyelitis
B) Rheumatic fever
C) Slipped capital femoral epiphysis (SCFE)
D) Legg–Calve–Perthes disease (LCPD)
E) Transient (toxic) synovitis

Answer 12.1.1 **The correct answer is "E."** This presentation is classic for transient (toxic) synovitis. This is the most common cause of hip pain in children aged 3 to 10 years, with peak occurrence in ages 5 to 6 years. It is more commonly seen in boys (male:female ratio of 2–3:1) and is often preceded by a viral respiratory infection, although numerous studies have failed to demonstrate a specific viral or bacterial agent. Physical examination reveals a limp or refusal to walk and complaint of pain over the groin and/or proximal thigh. There is pain with ROM testing, especially during abduction. Most children will be afebrile with a temperature of ≤38°C.

Question 12.1.2 **Appropriate diagnostic workup might include which of the following?**
A) Joint aspiration
B) Plain film radiographs
C) Inflammatory markers including erythrocyte sedimentation rate (ESR) and C-reactive protein (CRP)
D) CBC with differential
E) All of the above

Answer 12.1.2 **The correct answer is "E."** All of the above may be appropriate as transient synovitis is a diagnosis of exclusion. Patients with mild symptoms may be observed without further investigation. However, if the pain is significant, ROM is significantly impaired, or if the temperature is >37.5°C, further diagnostic workup is indicated. Laboratory findings consistent with transient synovitis include: clear joint fluid aspirate, normal CBC, and a mildly increased ESR. Blood cultures, antistreptolysin O (ASO) titer, bone scan, and MRI may also be of benefit to rule out other possibilities (e.g., septic arthritis, rheumatic fever, and SCFE). *It is of extreme importance to differentiate transient synovitis from septic arthritis. Unfortunately, there is no combination of physical findings and laboratory tests short of joint fluid that will definitively rule out septic arthritis.* There are published clinical decision tools, but these are generally based on observational data and often have conflicting results. It requires clinical judgment; decide which patients you are worried enough about that you want to commit them to hip joint aspiration.

HELPFUL TIP:
Septic arthritis is an orthopedic emergency and commonly presents with an elevated temperature, general malaise, and inability to bear weight—often with pain, spasm, and guarding. Generally, you will also see an elevated white blood cell (WBC >12K), CRP (>20), and ESR, **although neither these or fever (>38.5) is a good enough indicator to rule out a septic joint by their normality or absence**. Joint fluid will have numerous WBCs (classic teaching is >50,000 WBC/mm³; however, counts lower than this do not rule out septic arthritis); 50,000 WBC/mm³ is only 62% sensitive with 25,000 WBC/mm³ still only 77% sensitive. Blood cultures are positive in 30% of patients. Remember Lyme arthropathy Chikungunya in your differential diagnosis in the proper geographic location!

Question 12.1.3 What is the most appropriate treatment for this patient with transient synovitis?
A) Open fixation
B) Immobilization
C) Antibiotics
D) Surgical decompression
E) Ibuprofen and rest

Answer 12.1.3 The correct answer is "E." Conservative treatment is warranted: the appropriate initial treatment is rest, weight bearing as tolerated, and observation. Transient synovitis generally responds well to oral NSAIDs. Home care is acceptable; however, admission is indicated if the diagnosis is equivocal or if significant pain management is required. For septic arthritis, prompt administration of an intravenous (IV) antibiotic—directed at the most likely infecting pathogen (*Staphylococcus aureus*, Group A and B *Strep* [more common in infants], *Hemophilus influenza*, and rarely *Salmonella* and *N. gonorrhea*) and altered as necessary based on culture results—is indicated. Surgical irrigation of the joint is often necessary and early orthopedic consultation is needed.

▶ **Objectives: Did you learn to …**
 · Recognize the clinical presentation of transient synovitis?
 · Differentiate transient synovitis from septic arthritis?
 · Treat a patient with transient synovitis?

▶ CASE 12.2

A 6-year-old white male is brought into clinic by his parents because he is complaining of pain in his hip and anterior thigh. He is walking much less than usual since the pain began about 4 weeks ago. You order a plain radiograph, which shows mild sclerosis with some increased density of the femoral head. An MRI is ordered (which is denied three times by the insurance company, but eventually obtained after 4 hours on hold), which shows osteonecrosis of the femoral head.

Question 12.2.1 What is the most likely diagnosis in this patient?
A) Osteomyelitis
B) Septic arthritis
C) SCFE (slipped capital femoral epiphysis)
D) LCPD (Legg–Calve–Perthes disease)
E) Sickle cell anemia

Answer 12.2.1 The correct answer is "D." LCPD is idiopathic osteonecrosis of the femoral head. It is unilateral in 90% of cases, and the typical age range is 4 to 8 years, but patients may be as young as 2 years and as old as 12 years. "A" is a possibility, although there should be evidence of osteomyelitis on MRI. "B" is discussed in the previous case. "C," SCFE, classically occurs in obese children (male predominance) who are 10 to 16 years old (see more below). "E," sickle cell anemia, can cause osteonecrosis of the femoral head also, but the disease is rare in white populations. LCPD is less common in black populations.

Question 12.2.2 Which of the following factors best predicts a poor outcome for patients with LCPD?
A) Later age at onset of illness
B) Findings of subchondral fractures or fragmentation
C) Early appropriate treatment
D) Severity of pain and in ability to bear weight
E) Bilateral involvement

Answer 12.2.2 The correct answer is "A." Compared to older children, younger children generally have a longer time for remodeling to occur via molding of the femoral head within the acetabulum; and therefore, younger children have less flattening of the femoral head.

Question 12.2.3 Which of the following is the best initial treatment for this patient with LCPD?
A) Joint replacement
B) Osteotomy
C) Rest and physical therapy
D) Opioids
E) Corticosteroid injection of the hip joint

Answer 12.2.3 The correct answer is "C." The initial treatment for a patient with LCPD typically includes rest, activity restriction, and physical therapy. The objectives are to increase ROM in the hip and to reduce the risk of significant deformity. In general, patients should be seen by an orthopedic specialist. The likelihood of a good outcome with nonoperative treatment is significantly higher in younger patients, less than 8 years of age. "A" is incorrect because joint replacement is not an option. "B" is incorrect. While osteotomy may be used, it is typically reserved for older children and patients who are not progressing well with conservative therapy. "D" and "E" are not appropriate interventions in this patient with mild pain and no joint inflammation.

LCPD is difficult to treat largely because of the long duration of treatment and activity restrictions required. Periods of rest with activity restriction, physical therapy, and surgical intervention may be indicated over **1 to 2 years of treatment** and observation. Even with the best of care, prognosis is fair with need for total hip replacement reaching approximately 50% by middle age due to severe degenerative arthritis.

▶ **Objectives: Did you learn to …**
- Recognize the clinical presentation of LCPD?
- Manage a patient with LCPD?

▶ CASE 12.3

A 15-year-old female cross-country runner presents to your clinic with the chief complaint of bilateral knee pain. She describes a gradual increase in her symptoms during the first 3 weeks of the season. She wants to run varsity this year and has done extra running and hill training after practice each day. She describes anterior knee pain in the patellar region with little or no swelling, but complains of crepitus and pain exacerbated by running, squatting, stair climbing, and prolonged sitting with the knee bent.

Question 12.3.1 The most likely diagnosis for the condition described is:
A) Osgood–Schlatter disease
B) Chondromalacia patellae
C) Patellofemoral pain syndrome (PFPS)
D) Femoral stress fracture
E) Jogger's joints

Answer 12.3.1 The correct answer is "C." PFPS is a common overuse syndrome seen more frequently in runners and female athletes (thus the moniker "runner's knee"). This condition is due to forces across the knee that lead to biomechanical overload of the patellofemoral joint and other anterior knee structures. Maltracking and malalignment of the patellofemoral joint can contribute to this overload, as can training errors, core weakness, and muscle imbalance. "A," Osgood–Schlatter disease, is also related to overuse but is two to three times more common in males, particularly in athletes engaging in repetitive jumping. The pain of Osgood–Schlatter is generally well localized to the tibial tubercle. Radiographic evidence of fragmentation of the epiphysis or heterotropic ossification anterior to the tubercle may be seen, but is not necessary for diagnosis. "B," chondromalacia patella, is softening of the articular cartilage of the patella as seen on arthroscopy and may be a result of long-term patellofemoral dysfunction. This is a surgical diagnosis and the term should be avoided clinically. Femoral stress fracture ("D") would be unlikely to present bilaterally. "E" is not a real thing but has nice alliteration.

Question 12.3.2 What is the preferred treatment for this female runner?
A) Arthroscopic debridement
B) Decreased activity level along with quadriceps and hip strengthening exercises

C) Evaluation for "Female Athlete Triad"
D) Casting or immobilization
E) Corticosteroid injection

Answer 12.3.2 The correct answer is "B." The most effective treatment modality is a combined physical therapy regimen consisting of strength training of the hip abductors and quadriceps, as well as quadriceps stretching. Quadriceps strengthening is usually initiated by resisted straight leg raises (SLRs) to minimize patellofemoral compressive forces. NSAIDs, cross-training, and core strengthening may also be of benefit. Adjunctive trials of therapeutic modalities such as orthotics and taping may be considered, but should not be used in isolation. Recalcitrant cases and patients with recurrent dislocation/subluxation should be referred to your friendly neighborhood orthopedic surgeon for consideration of surgical intervention. "A," "D," and "E" are all unnecessarily invasive for PFPS. As for "C," while it would be good to explore her general health in more detail, screening for the female athlete triad will not treat her current problem.

Three months later, the same patient presents complaining of unilateral right knee pain over the medial knee joint. Again, this pain is exacerbated by knee flexion and she notes popping and snapping when she stands from sitting. She notes that the pain is worse after prolonged sitting or going up or downstairs. Your examination shows a tender band of tissue about 1 cm medial to the patella.

Question 12.3.3 The most likely diagnosis is:
A) Osteosarcoma
B) Medial collateral ligament (MCL) strain
C) Plica syndrome
D) Recalcitrant PFPS
E) Meniscal tear

Answer 12.3.3 The correct answer is "C." This is the typical presentation of plica syndrome. Plicae are synovial remnants that did not resorb properly during development. They can be irritated, usually chronically or subacutely, especially in sports that require repeated flexion of the knee (e.g., rowing, cycling, running, etc.). Typical symptoms include popping or snapping sensation with knee flexion; there may also be knee locking and catching as well as having the knee "give." Treatment includes rest, ice, quadriceps strengthening, and NSAIDs. If conservative management fails, steroid injection or arthroscopy may alleviate the symptoms.

HELPFUL TIP:
The plica should be palpable. A medial/inferior plica is the most common (between the patella and the medial joint line). It can also occur laterally and either above or below the midpole of the patella. Adolescents and young adults are more frequently affected than patients of other ages.

▶ **Objectives: Did you learn to …**
- Identify and manage PFPS?
- Recognize plica syndrome?

▶ CASE 12.4

A mother brings her 18-month-old son in for a well-child check. Her only new concern today is that he seems to walk "bow-legged." He has been somewhat pigeon-toed since he could pull himself up and cruise along walls and furniture at home. On examination, you find the child's feet to be pointing inward. The foot is flexible and looks normal. The patellae are in a neutral position facing directly forward.

Question 12.4.1 What is the most likely diagnosis in this patient?
A) Cerebral palsy
B) Excessive femoral retroversion
C) Forefoot varus
D) Internal tibial torsion
E) Bilateral developmental dysplasia of the hip (DDH)

Answer 12.4.1 The correct answer is "D." This represents a case of intoeing (pigeon-toeing), which has several causes, and internal tibial torsion is frequently the culprit. Internal tibial torsion is characterized by a flexible, normal foot, with the patellae in a neutral position. The condition can be diagnosed by examining the child on his knees (feet dangling) or prone with knees flexed. Normally, there should be approximately 30 degrees of external rotation of the feet in this position. With internal tibial torsion, the toes will be pointing inward. In addition, when the child is sitting with legs dangling over a table, the lateral malleolus will be anterior to the medial malleolus, which is the opposite of what is normally observed. Finally, the hips must be normal in order to confirm this diagnosis. "A" is incorrect because you would expect other findings in a patient with cerebral palsy. "B" is incorrect. In fact, femoral retroversion is synonymous with "out-toeing," which is the opposite of intoeing (of course!). Excessive **femoral anteversion** can be a cause of intoeing. "C" is incorrect because the foot examination does not show varus deformity. Finally, "E" is incorrect, although bilateral DDH can be quite difficult to diagnose if not caught early in the newborn period. With DDH, one would expect external rotation of the leg rather than intoeing.

Question 12.4.2 What is the treatment of choice for this child?
A) Referral for bilateral osteotomy
B) Shoe modification and bracing (The Forest Gump Treatment Plan)
C) Physical therapy referral
D) Serial casting
E) Reassurance and watchful waiting

Answer 12.4.2 The correct answer is "E." Spontaneous resolution is the norm for most intoeing and out-toeing deformities. Most will spontaneously correct by age 6. Children continuing to have difficulty with persistent trips and falls or grossly unsightly gait beyond this time may benefit from a rotational osteotomy. Children with neuromotor disorders and cerebral palsy are more likely to require surgical intervention.

HELPFUL TIP:
Another cause of intoeing is femoral torsion. Femoral torsion is diagnosed by placing the patient prone with the hips in neutral and knees flexed to 90 degrees. Feet are rotated away from midline to measure internal rotation (anteversion). For external rotation (retroversion), place one hand on the buttocks and move one leg through midline until the pelvis begins to tilt. Typically, normal external rotation is 45 degrees, and normal internal rotation is 35 degrees. Rotation greater than this is considered excessive if it is accompanied by a limited ROM in the opposite direction. *In addition, when a patient with femoral torsion is seated with legs dangling, the patellae will not face forward (they face inward for intoeing from femoral torsion and outward for out-toeing from femoral torsion).*

▶ **Objective: Did you learn to …**
- Evaluate and manage intoeing and out-toeing in children?

▶ CASE 12.5

A 13-year-old male presents to the clinic with his mother for difficulty walking. He is unsure of when the problem first began, but has noticed it getting worse over the last week. It has forced him to stop playing sports. He reports a dull pain in the left hip but denies trauma. On examination, you find an obese male in no distress. There is loss of internal rotation, abduction, and flexion at the left hip joint. When his hip is flexed to 90 degrees, this loss of ROM is more pronounced.

Question 12.5.1 What is the most likely diagnosis in this case?
A) Osteoarthritis
B) Septic arthritis
C) SCFE
D) LCPD
E) Juvenile idiopathic arthritis

Answer 12.5.1 The correct answer is "C." SCFE occurs most commonly in active, overweight, adolescent males. Shear forces across the relatively weak physis cause displacement. **Slippage is generally gradual but may occur acutely.** Mean age at presentation is 12 for females (range 10–14) and 13 for males (range 11–16). Endocrinopathies, such as hypothyroidism and osteodystrophy, should be considered in those presenting atypically or outside the typical age range. Watch for development of a similar process in the contralateral hip over time, which has been reported anywhere from 20% to 80% of the time.

Question 12.5.2 Which of the following is the first study you order to confirm the diagnosis?
A) AP and frog-leg lateral radiographs of the hip
B) CT scan of the hip/pelvis
C) MRI of the hip/pelvis
D) ESR
E) None; physical examination is sufficient

Answer 12.5.2 The correct answer is "A." Radiographs of the hip should demonstrate displacement of the femoral head, which can then be classified as mild, moderate, or severe. "B" and "C" are incorrect because the radiograph is diagnostic in most cases. "D" is incorrect since SCFE is not an inflammatory condition. "E" is incorrect. Imaging should be obtained in order to confirm the diagnosis and rate the severity. MRI may be able to diagnose an early SCFE when radiographs are negative and you should have a low threshold for pulling the MRI trigger, given the consequences of missing this one!

Question 12.5.3 The treatment of choice for this patient is:
A) Antibiotics
B) Immobilization
C) Physical therapy
D) Surgical decompression
E) Surgical fixation

Answer 12.5.3 The correct answer is "E." The goals of treatment of SCFE are to prevent further slippage, promote closure of the physis, and to minimize the risk of osteonecrosis or chondrolysis. These aims are best accomplished through referral to an orthopedic surgeon and, ultimately, surgical fixation. "B" and "C" are incorrect because they delay definitive therapy and will not produce the desired result. "A" and "D" are incorrect because SCFE is not an infectious process.

▶ **Objectives: Did you learn to …**
- Recognize the clinical presentation of a child with SCFE?
- Treat a patient with SCFE?

▶ CASE 12.6

A worried mother presents with her 4-year-old son for evaluation of lower extremity pain. She reports the boy has complained of some vague bilateral leg pains over the past several weeks after vigorous physical activities. She became alarmed after he had awakened the past two nights crying in pain. The boy reports the pain is hardly noticeable during the day. Recently, the pain has been in the bilateral distal thighs; however, his mother notes times of unilateral pain. The boy and his mother both deny constitutional symptoms now or over the past several weeks. Examination reveals an afebrile, well-developed male in no distress. The musculoskeletal examination is normal.

Question 12.6.1 The most likely diagnosis for the condition described here is?
A) Ewing sarcoma
B) Growing pain
C) Kohler disease
D) Leukemia
E) Osteochondritis dissecans

Answer 12.6.1 The correct answer is "B." "Growing pain" is a diagnosis of exclusion, although history and physical examination usually suffice for excluding more serious diagnoses. It is a condition of unknown etiology, but is thought by some to be a result of overuse/overactivity on an immature musculoskeletal system. It is most frequently seen in otherwise healthy, active children aged 2 to 5, with some older children affected as well. Pain is commonly bilateral and localized to the calf, but may be felt at the ankle, knee, or thigh. Pain is more common in the evening and often causes awakening at night. Less commonly, patients have pain during the day after vigorous activities. Presentation with constitutional symptoms should lead to further evaluation with imaging and lab tests.

Question 12.6.2 Which of the following should you entertain when a patient presents with typical growing pain?
A) Osteomyelitis
B) Malignancy
C) Juvenile idiopathic arthritis
D) All of the above
E) None of the above

Answer 12.6.2 The correct answer is "D." It is important to consider other potential causes of what would otherwise appear to be growing pain. Although you may not find it necessary to perform any laboratory or radiologic studies, you should at least keep these and other diagnoses in mind when taking your history and performing your examination. Remember, growing pain is a diagnosis of exclusion.

 HELPFUL TIP:
Severe or persistent pain during the day **is not** "growing pain." By definition, "growing pain" occurs primarily at night and is better during the day.

Question 12.6.3 Treatment for growing pain includes:
A) Reassurance, rest, and short-term use of NSAIDs
B) Amputation
C) Chemotherapy and radiation
D) Casting and bracing followed by physical therapy
E) Staging of the disease is required prior to initiation of therapy

Answer 12.6.3 The correct answer is "A." OK, so this was just a fun one. Do not do anything drastic for a benign condition! Those of you who chose "B," amputation, will find themselves in one of Dante's circles (or in court—which is worse?) … and clearly need a coffee break.

The same boy returns with his mother years later. He is now 12 years old; the mother has noticed that one shoulder seems to be higher than the other (truncal asymmetry).

Question 12.6.4 Which of the following methods is the most sensitive for detecting scoliosis?
A) Observe the patient from the front with a loose-fitting shirt on; measure the difference in shoulder height
B) Observe the patient from behind, with shirt off, while he bends forward at the waist; look for elevation of the ribs or paravertebral muscle mass on one side
C) Observe the patient from the front, with shirt off, while he bends forward at the waist; look for elevation of the ribs or paravertebral muscle mass on one side
D) Observe the patient from the side, with shirt off, while he bends forward at the waist; look for elevation of the ribs or paravertebral muscle mass on one side

Answer 12.6.4 **The correct answer is "B," which is known as the "forward bending test."** This test is more sensitive than the other methods described. The forward bending test is accomplished by having the patient bend at the waist with feet together and hands hanging free. Observe the patient from behind and note any elevation of the ribs or paravertebral muscle mass on one side. The elevation should be measured in degrees (inclinometers are available), and an inclination of 5 degrees or more should be evaluated further. Options "A," "C," and "D" are **not** accepted methods of screening for scoliosis.

HELPFUL TIP:
Until 2018, routine screening for scoliosis was a recommendation "D" by the US Preventative Services Task Force (not recommended). In January 2018, USPSTF released an updated recommendation of "I" (insufficient evidence to assess balance of risks and benefits). For screening of otherwise healthy adolescents, it is reasonable to skip it, but scoliosis evaluation may be appropriate in patients who have noticed pain or some other abnormality.

HELPFUL TIP:
Scoliosis is a lateral curvature of the spine, usually accompanied by rotation and generally occurring in the thoracic or lumbar areas. It can occur with excessive kyphosis (posteriorly convex curvature) or lordosis (anteriorly convex curvature).

On forward bending test, you find slight elevation of the left paravertebral muscles mass, which you estimate to be 7 degrees. The remainder of the examination is normal.

You decide to obtain radiographs that show 12 degrees of angulation (Cobb angle).

Question 12.6.5 This patient's scoliosis is most likely:
A) Congenital
B) Idiopathic
C) Related to a tumor
D) Secondary to infection
E) Secondary to demonic possession

Answer 12.6.5 **The correct answer is "B."** Most scoliosis that develops during adolescence is idiopathic. When there is no pain, fever, weight loss, or other warning signs (e.g., neurologic symptoms), the curvature is unlikely to be due to tumor or infection. "A," congenital scoliosis, typically presents earlier in life. Infection, malignancy, and demons are not known to cause scoliosis.

Question 12.6.6 The most appropriate initial management plan for this patient includes:
A) Bracing
B) Observation
C) Physical therapy
D) Surgery
E) Any of the above are equally appropriate initial management plans

Answer 12.6.6 **The correct answer is "B."** In an otherwise healthy patient with a curvature measured at <25 degrees, observation is appropriate. "C" is incorrect because physical therapy and exercise regimens do not seem to limit the progression of scoliosis. "A" and "D" are incorrect because bracing and surgery are typically not warranted for this degree of scoliosis. Repeat examination and possibly repeat radiographs are warranted, but if the scoliosis remains stable and mild, the patient is not likely to experience any significant progression of disease with aging.

HELPFUL TIP:
Bracing for scoliosis should be limited to those with idiopathic scoliosis and greater than 30 degrees of angulation. Bracing is only effective if the child is still growing and <1 year past menarche if female. You should not go for this one alone…get help!

The mother returns now with her 2-year-old daughter who is refusing to move her right arm. Earlier today she threw a tantrum at the store when her father refused to buy her the new "princess toy" (advertising hits them young). Dad was holding on to her arm when she flopped to the floor. She immediately began crying and refusing to move her right arm. In the office, she is well but holds her right arm adducted, flexed, and pronated. (The princess toy is in the other hand. Guilt is a powerful weapon.) Despite every trick you know, you can't get her to move that arm. You inspect and palpate the

entire extremity and clavicle and find no crepitus, swelling, or tenderness.

Question 12.6.7 What is your next diagnostic step?
A) Obtain an x-ray of the elbow
B) Actively supinate the forearm and flex the elbow while applying pressure over the radial head
C) Actively twist the forearm at the elbow 360 degrees
D) Consult orthopedics
E) Perform a skeletal survey, mostly to bide time

Answer 12.6.7 **The correct answer is "B."** This child has a "nursemaid's elbow" that is due to subluxation of the annular ligament rather than subluxation or dislocation of the radial head. It occurs in toddlers due to traction via pulling on a pronated and extended arm. Symptoms are immediate and care is sought due to the child's refusal to move the arm. The diagnosis is clinical. Manual reduction may be done via supination/flexion or hyperpronation. Sedation is not needed. A palpable click may be felt. The child usually regains immediate movement of the arm and relief of discomfort. Immobilization is not needed, but parents should be told that recurrent subluxations may occur and therefore pulling on the arm should be avoided. "A" would be correct if there was concern for a fracture based on findings of swelling, history of trauma, or focal tenderness. "C" is impossible: Can you really rotate a joint 360 degrees? "D" is incorrect as any primary-care provider may manage this. "E" is unnecessary as a nursemaid elbow is not a marker of abuse, although traumatic injuries in children should always make one consider abuse.

HELPFUL TIP:
Reducing a nursemaid's elbow is gratifying. The patient with nursemaid's elbow should be using the arm normally within minutes. If the child still refuses to use the extremity after adequate observation, reconsider your diagnosis and whether the reduction was successful. Note that many will spontaneously reduce while radiographs are being done (therapeutic x-ray?). Both flexion and supination and extension and pronation have been used to reduce nursemaid's elbow.

HELPFUL TIP:
When dealing with pediatric orthopedics, always remember that child abuse is in the differential diagnosis. Be sure that the reported mechanism of the injury is consistent with the findings on examination and radiograph.

After successful reduction, you see the same 2-year-old child a month later presenting to your clinic with the parents who state that the child has been crying and has refused to walk since tripping over a toy a couple of hours ago. You look at the child and find no signs of abuse. The injured area is represented by the lower leg image in Figure 12-1.

Question 12.6.8 Your approach at this point is to:
A) Consult Child Welfare since this is almost always abuse
B) Consult orthopedics for casting and further treatment
C) No treatment necessary for this particular fracture in a 2-year-old
D) Obtain an MRI

Answer 12.6.8 **The correct answer is "B."** This is a typical "toddler's fracture" that consists of a spiral fracture of the tibia usually from insignificant rotational trauma (e.g., running and falling with a twisting motion). There should not be an associated fibular fracture. "A" is incorrect because this type of fracture is not usually from abuse. A midshaft fracture would more likely be from abuse. "C" is incorrect because this fracture needs to be treated. For a quick summary of fracture terminology, see Table 12-1, and keep these in mind—we'll use them later.

▶ **Objectives: Did you learn to …**
- Consider a broader differential diagnosis in a patient presenting with typical "growing pain?"
- Initiate conservative treatment for a patient with growing pain?
- Screen a patient for scoliosis?
- Develop an approach to the adolescent with scoliosis?
- Recognize the clinical presentation and treatment of a "nursemaid's elbow" (radial head subluxation)?
- Recognize a toddler's fracture (tibial spiral fracture)?

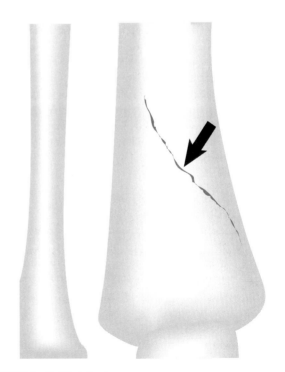

FIGURE 12-1. Toddler's Fracture.

TABLE 12-1 TERMINOLOGY FOR DESCRIBING A FRACTURE

Avulsion fracture: Fragment of bone pulled from its normal position by a muscular contraction or resistance of a ligament
Closed fracture: A fracture that does not communicate with the external environment (i.e., not through the skin)
Comminuted fracture: Consisting of three or more fragments
Greenstick fracture: Incomplete, angulated fracture of a long bone, particularly in children
Open fracture: Fracture that communicates with the external environment
Torus (Buckle) fracture: Described as a buckle fracture or compression of the bone without cortical disruption; seen especially in the distal forearms of children

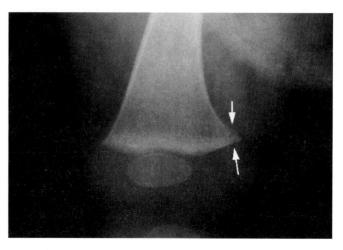

FIGURE 12-2. From Case 12.2.

▶ CASE 12.7

A mother presents to your clinic with her 10-month-old son. She is concerned that he has been very irritable since she arrived home from work, particularly when his legs are touched. She states that he has been crying "nonstop" since she arrived home. He was well when she left for work this morning, leaving the patient under the care of her boyfriend, Tony "the Hustler" O'Neil. The patient's mother denies any fevers, vomiting, diarrhea, or cough. On examination, he is generally fussy, worsening with palpation of his left leg, particularly around his knee. You also note five bruises on his chest and back. The remainder of the examination is unremarkable. You obtain the following radiograph of his left knee (Fig. 12-2).

Question 12.7.1 Which of the following mechanisms is most likely responsible for the fracture seen on x-ray (marked with the helpful arrow sign)?
A) A low-energy fall (fall off a low couch)
B) A high-energy fall (fall out of a second-story window)
C) A low-energy rotational force (tripping causing the foot to twist inward)
D) A high-energy tension or shearing force (a violent twisting of the leg)
E) Any of the above could result in the injury

Answer 12.7.1 **The correct answer is "D," a high-energy tension or shearing force.** The above radiograph depicts a metaphyseal corner fracture that is highly specific for nonaccidental trauma (that's the nice way to say "child abuse"). These fractures are typically caused by shaking of the child with flailing of the extremities or with forceful yanking or twisting of the arm or leg. The incidence of these fractures decreases substantially as children grow beyond 1 year of age.

Question 12.7.2 In which of the following patients is a skeletal survey indicated for concern of nonaccidental trauma?
A) A 2-month-old male with multiple bruises but no other localizing injuries
B) A 2-year-old female with an intracranial injury on brain CT
C) A 6-month-old male with a known metaphyseal corner fracture

D) An 18-month-old female with burns consistent with nonaccidental trauma
E) A skeletal survey is indicted for all the above patients

Answer 12.7.2 **The answer is "E," all of the above.** The American Academy of Pediatrics consensus guidelines on the radiographic evaluation of child abuse state that a skeletal survey should be obtained for all children younger than 2 years of age who may have experienced maltreatment. Skeletal surveys should also be considered for children between the ages of 2 and 5 depending on the clinical scenario. The following images are generally included in a skeletal survey: humeri, forearms, lower legs, hands, feet, skull, cervical spine, thorax (including oblique views), lumbar spine, and pelvis.

Question 12.7.3 Which of the following fractures is considered highly specific for nonaccidental trauma?
A) Posterior rib fractures
B) Clavicle fractures
C) Distal radius fractures
D) Spiral fractures of the tibia
E) Supracondylar fractures

Answer 12.7.3 **The correct answer is "A," posterior rib fractures.** In addition, the following fractures have moderate to high specificity for nonaccidental trauma: metaphyseal fractures, multiple fractures (especially if bilateral), fractures of different ages, epiphyseal separations, vertebral body fractures, digital fractures, scapular fractures, sternal fractures, and complex skull fractures.

▶ **Objectives: Did you learn to …**
• Recognize a metaphyseal corner fracture and what implications this fracture has?
• Know the indications to perform a skeletal survey when suspecting nonaccidental trauma and what images are included?
• Understand which fractures are specific for nonaccidental trauma?

QUICK QUIZ: THE BURNIN' HIP O' FIRE

A 35-year-old obese female with a large pannus presents with a burning pain in anterior–lateral thigh. It started when she bought a new wide belt (ornate with skulls and Harley–Davidson logos) and started wearing hip hugger pants in order to display her tasteful sacral tattoo (… and society thanks her). The pain seems worse on days when she wears the belt and seems better on days when she hangs out *au naturel* at home.

The most likely diagnosis is:
A) Meralgia paresthetica
B) Trochanteric bursitis
C) Tropical pyomyositis
D) Ruptured plantaris muscle
E) Polymyositis

The correct answer is "A." Meralgia paresthetica is described as a burning pain in the anterior–lateral thigh and is caused by compression of the lateral femoral cutaneous nerve. It is most common in those who wear tight jeans or wide belts and who are obese. Treatment is to relieve the inciting cause. Tricyclic antidepressants or other medication for neuropathy may also be helpful. "B," trochanteric bursitis, occurs when there is inflammation of the bursa over the greater trochanter of the femur. Patients complain of pain in the lateral hip and outer thigh. There is point tenderness over the greater trochanter. Treatment is physical therapy for core strengthening and a steroid injection of the bursa. "C," tropical pyomyositis, is a deep infection of a single muscle group that is often caused by *Staphylococcus aureus* and is generally in the muscles of the lower extremities. It is increasingly recognized in the United States. Predisposing factors in temperate climates include immunosuppression (especially HIV), malnutrition, IV drugs use, etc. In the tropics patients usually have a normal immune system. "D," a ruptured plantaris muscle, occurs in the calf and is not related to the thigh. It is often caused by planting of the foot forcefully (such as in tennis or basketball) and patients may report a "pop" followed by calf/gastrocnemius pain. "E," polymyositis, would cause bilateral pain and weakness in the proximal legs, but the pain would not be burning in nature.

▶ CASE 12.8

A concerned father presents to your clinic with a 1-month-old daughter. He is worried that his daughter appears to be pigeon-toed, and his mother-in-law is sure (as most mothers-in-law are) that the child will need immediate surgery for correction. Your examination reveals a pleasant, well-developed 1-month-old female with moderate medial deviation of the forefoot bilaterally. A line bisecting the heel passes through the fourth toe on each foot. The lateral borders of the feet are convex; the heels are in a normal neutral position. The feet are flexible and the deformity can be passively corrected to the midline.

Question 12.8.1 This description is best characterized as?
A) Clubfoot
B) Internal tibial torsion
C) Flexible flatfoot
D) Excessive femoral anteversion
E) Metatarsus adductus

Answer 12.8.1 **The correct answer is "E."** The above is a classic description of the foot shape of metatarsus adductus. In the normal foot, a line bisecting the heel would pass through the second and the third toe webspace. In those with metatarsus adductus, it passes more laterally depending on the severity. In those with the most severe deformity, a line bisecting the heel would pass through the fourth and the fifth toe webspace. In addition to the heels remaining in a neutral position—indicating that the problem is isolated to the shape of the foot and **not** to an internal rotation of the tibia—the forefoot is flexible and easily straightened into normal position.

Question 12.8.2 The most appropriate treatment for the above case would be?
A) Surgical reconstruction
B) Serial casting
C) Physical therapy referral for stretching and exercise
D) Watchful waiting and reassurance
E) Orthopedic outflare shoes

Answer 12.8.2 **The correct answer is "D."** Spontaneous correction occurs in most children. The mother-in-law can begin a regimen of gentle foot stretching. It will give her something to do but does not change the outcome. Care should be taken to avoid keeping the child in the prone position with the feet in an inward position—which the parents should be doing anyway ("back to sleep" for SIDS prevention). **If the deformity is severe and inflexible, serial casting and/or surgical intervention may be indicated.** A rigid metatarsus adductus in a child >3 months or a residual problem in a child with a flexible metatarsus adductus >6 months is an indication for pediatric orthopedic referral.

 HELPFUL TIP:
Clubfoot (talipes equinovarus) is observed at birth. Patients are more often males (2:1 male:female ratio) and present with the following findings: calcaneus seems to be drawn inward and upward, moderate forefoot adduction, and the foot can be placed in a neutral position by passive manipulation. These patients can be treated successfully with early referral for serial casting and manipulation, typically via the Ponseti method, which we are obligated to promote since Dr. Ignacio Ponseti developed it at the University of Iowa. Actually, it really is an extremely important advance in clubfoot treatment and is now the standard of care used around the world.

▶ **Objectives: Did you learn to …**
- Identify a patient with metatarsus adductus?
- Discuss treatment approaches to metatarsus adductus?

▶ CASE 12.9

A 5-year-old girl who has recently recovered from chicken pox ("Thank you, anti-vaccine parents!") presents with her mother for evaluation of left leg pain and refusal to walk. The mother reports that she has complained of worsening pain over the last 4 to 5 days. She started to limp noticeably yesterday and refused to walk this morning. Also, the mother reports general malaise and subjective fever. The patient complains of pain over the distal thigh and knee. The mother has not seen any swelling of the knee, and the patient denies trauma.

Examination reveals a pleasant 5-year-old female who appears uncomfortable, but nontoxic and in no acute distress. Her temperature is 38.5°C. The left distal thigh (not the joint) is painful to palpation, and slightly warm. The knee joint has no effusion and the ROM is full with only mild discomfort on knee motion. There is no hip joint involvement.

Question 12.9.1 What is the most common bacterial pathogen associated with this patient's condition?
A) Group A *Streptococcus*
B) Group B *Streptococcus*
C) *Haemophilus influenzae*
D) *S. aureus*
E) None of the above; this is not an infection

Answer 12.9.1 The correct answer is "D." The acute nature of the symptoms, presence of fever, and minimal involvement of the joint makes osteomyelitis the most likely diagnosis. In addition, osteomyelitis is associated with chicken pox in children. There is clearly an increase in the prevalence of MRSA as a pathogen in osteomyelitis (two-thirds of cases in a recent review). Thus, it is wise to choose an antibiotic with MRSA coverage.

 HELPFUL TIP:
Pseudomonas aeruginosa is commonly associated with osteomyelitis in the setting of a plantar puncture wound through a tennis shoe.

Allow us to digress.

Question 12.9.2 The most common organism causing osteomyelitis in patients with sickle cell disease is:
A) *Neisseria gonorrhoeae* (Gonococcus)
B) Polymicrobial
C) *Salmonella* species
D) *S. aureus*
E) *Streptococcus* species

Answer 12.9.2 The correct answer is "C." Staphylococcus is responsible for the majority of bone infections *in the general population*. *Salmonella* species are responsible for up to 85% of bone and joint infections in patients with a history of sickle cell disease, with *E. coli* being another important player.

 HELPFUL TIP:
Most cases of childhood osteomyelitis are the result of hematogenous spread rather than by direct contamination of the bone (as opposed to our middle-aged or elderly diabetic foot ulcer patients).

Question 12.9.3 Identification of the pathogen in a case of osteomyelitis is most commonly made by:
A) ASO titer
B) Blood culture
C) Joint aspiration, culture, and Gram stain
D) Pathology report following open biopsy
E) Witchcraft

Answer 12.9.3 The correct answer is "B." A blood culture will reveal the offending organism in 40% to 50% of cases. However, empiric treatment is often the rule, and antibiotics are selected based on most likely pathogens expected in a given clinical scenario. Joint aspiration is not typically indicated unless there is strong evidence of joint involvement. It can take weeks for changes to be seen on plain film radiographs. Therefore, MRI is the imaging modality of choice. CT or bone scan can also be used if MRI is not available or contraindicated. If changes are identified and a neoplastic process is ruled out, aspiration at the site of periosteal elevation and bony destruction should be considered if a pathogen has not yet been identified by blood culture. "A," an ASO titer, would not be helpful here since this test is for *Streptococcus pyogenes* infection. An ASO titer would be helpful if looking for rheumatic fever. "D," surgical biopsy, may be required if blood cultures do not reveal a pathogen and the patient is not responding appropriately to empiric antibiotics.

 HELPFUL TIP:
Treatment of osteomyelitis requires 4 to 6 weeks of antibiotics. Surgical debridement is usually (if not always) required as well. Several acute phase reactants can be useful in these cases including CRP and ESR. CRP rises rapidly and normalizes with successful treatment. ESR will decline steadily over 2 to 3 weeks with treatment.

▶ **Objectives: Did you learn to …**
- Diagnose osteomyelitis in a child?
- Identify common pathogens involved in osteomyelitis?

▶ CASE 12.10

A 45-year-old female with a history of rheumatoid arthritis, on chronic low-dose prednisone, presents to your clinic with 2 days of right knee pain. The patient reports that her knee has been swollen and painful to touch, and she now is having difficulty bearing weight due to the pain. She has had previous knee pain, but nothing this severe. She denies any trauma, fevers, chills, knee surgery, illegal drug use, or risky sexual behavior. On examination, she is well appearing, afebrile, and has a moderate right knee effusion with limited ROM. There is no overlying erythema, but the knee feels warm to touch.

Question 12.10.1 Which of the following diagnostics is the most valuable to rule in or rule out the diagnosis with the highest potential morbidity?
A) Plain films of the affected knee
B) WBC count
C) ESR
D) Arthrocentesis
E) MRI

Answer 12.10.1 The correct answer is "D." The most concerning diagnosis with the highest potential morbidity in this patient is septic arthritis. Her history of rheumatoid arthritis as well as long-term steroid use put her at high risk. In a patient in whom you are concerned about septic arthritis, the most important piece of diagnostic data that you can obtain comes from synovial fluid analysis. While plain radiographs, a WBC count, an ESR, and CRP may be obtained (your friendly neighborhood orthopedic surgeon will surely want to know them), they are neither sensitive nor specific enough to rule in or rule out septic arthritis in a high-risk patient.

Question 12.10.2 Which of the following signs or symptoms has sufficient sensitivity to rule out septic arthritis if *absent*?
A) Joint edema or effusion
B) Fever
C) Sweats
D) Significantly restricted ROM
E) None of the listed signs or symptoms has sufficient sensitivity to rule out septic arthritis, if absent

Answer 12.10.2 The correct answer is "E." Unfortunately, there are no clinical signs or symptoms that have sufficient sensitivity to rule out septic arthritis. Signs and symptoms should raise clinical suspicion; however, the only definitive diagnostic modality is arthrocentesis.

You effortlessly obtain 10 mL of cloudy synovial fluid that is sent to the lab for Gram stain, culture, cell count with differential, and crystal analysis. The Gram stain is

TABLE 12-2 SENSITIVITY AND SPECIFICITY OF SYNOVIAL FLUID ANALYSIS IN SEPTIC ARTHRITIS

Synovial Fluid WBC Count	Sensitivity (%)	Specificity (%)
>100,000/mm³	30	>99
>50,000/mm³	62	92
>25,000/mm³	77	73

negative with cultures pending. The synovial WBC count is 51,000/μL with >90% polymorphonuclear cells. The crystal analysis shows calcium pyrophosphate crystals. You obtain a peripheral WBC count that is 11,000/μL and an ESR is 55 mm/hr.

Question 12.10.3 What is the most appropriate next course of action based on these findings?
A) Prescribe high-dose prednisone for a flair of her rheumatoid arthritis
B) Start IV antibiotics and obtain emergent orthopedic consultation
C) Treat her for pseudogout
D) Recommend rest, ice, compression, and a prescription for oxycodone

Answer 12.10.3 The correct answer is "B." Various cutoffs for synovial WBC counts have been proposed, ranging from >25,000/μL to >100,000/μL in native joints, with sensitivities ranging from 30% to 77% (Table 12-2). Cutoffs are much lower in patients with prosthetic joints. A prosthetic joint with WBC count of >1,700/μL may be up to 94% sensitive for septic arthritis. When the percentage of polymorphonuclear cells is >90%, this significantly increases the likelihood of septic arthritis. Don't let the calcium pyrophosphate crystals dissuade you from suspecting septic arthritis as both gout and pseudogout can coexist with septic arthritis up to 25% of the time (*J Rheumatol.* 2012;39:157).

▶ **Objectives: Did you learn to …**
  · Recognize the clinical presentation of septic arthritis?
  · Understand the limitations of using signs and symptoms to rule out septic arthritis?
  · Describe the appropriate workup for a patient with suspected septic arthritis?

⌛ QUICK QUIZ: MY BIG FAT GREEK KNEE PAIN

A 55-year-old obese female comes to your office complaining of knee pain when she walks. She had an MRI at an urgent care center, which showed some meniscal damage. She is tender inferiorly and medial to the patella on the proximal tibia (but not on the joint line).

Which of the following is true?

A) Washing out her knee by arthroscopy will help to relieve her symptoms

B) The finding of a meniscal injury on MRI correlates well with symptoms of pain

C) Based on its location, pes anserie bursitis is the likely cause of her pain

D) Baklava is Dr. Wilbur's favorite food

The correct answer is "C." The pes anserine ("goose's foot") bursa is located on the medial, proximal aspect of the tibia and is where the tendons of the sartorius, gracilis, and semitendinosus attach. It often becomes inflamed causing significant and chronic knee pain. Conservative therapy with rest, ice, NSAIDs, and stretching may be tried initially. However, these often fail, and most patients experience significant improvement with corticosteroid injections. "A" is incorrect. Several studies have found that washing out the knee and trimming the cartilage is of no benefit in either meniscal injury or osteoarthritis. "B" is also incorrect. MRI of the knee is not particularly useful for determining whether a meniscal injury is the source of pain. Similar to herniated disks, many asymptomatic patients have meniscal injuries on MRI, limiting our ability to assign symptoms to an MRI finding. This is especially true in the elderly with arthritis where >90% will have meniscal damage. As to "D," it obviously does not relate to the case. We call that "test taking skill." If you chose "D," woe is with you.

 QUICK QUIZ: ORTHOPEDIC INFECTIONS

The most common organism causing septic arthritis in the teenage years is:

A) *N. gonorrhoeae*

B) Polymicrobial

C) *Salmonella* species

D) *S. aureus*

E) *Streptococcus* species

The correct answer is "A." Gonococcus is the most common organism isolated from the joints of sexually active, teenage individuals.

▶ CASE 12.11

A 28-year-old male presents to your clinic for evaluation of lower-back pain (LBP). Yesterday morning he first noticed the discomfort, manifesting as stiffness and soreness in the lower back. The day before had been spent running a floor polisher. He describes his pain as sharp in nature and 8/10 in intensity. He denies radiation of the pain, sensory changes, and constitutional symptoms. He is concerned after consulting Dr. Google that this may be an injury to a disk and that he may be permanently disabled due to his extreme pain. In fact, he helpfully printed the disability forms and hands them to you to complete.

Question 12.11.1 Which of the following signs or symptoms would be "red flags" indicating the need for early imaging and/or referral?

A) Pain radiating down one or both legs into the posterior thigh

B) Severe pain, prompting the patient to request narcotics

C) Pain greater with active lumbar extension than with forward flexion

D) New-onset erectile dysfunction with back pain

E) Pain worse with bending over

Answer 12.11.1 **The correct answer is "D."** The onset of erectile dysfunction is suggestive of neurologic involvement and warrants further investigation. None of the other options are suggestive of significant disease requiring immediate intervention ("A" certainly could represent disk disease; however, this does not require immediate intervention). Of note, spontaneous erections without sexual stimulation can also be a sign of neurologic involvement.

Question 12.11.2 Early imaging should be obtained in all of the following presentations of LBP EXCEPT:

A) Neurologic symptoms such as bowel or bladder dysfunction and impotence

B) History of fever, night sweats, and weight loss

C) History of cancer

D) Trauma

E) Age > 50 years

Answer 12.11.2 **The correct answer is "E."** Patients over the age of 50 should have early imaging. See Table 12-3 for other criteria that should prompt early imaging.

TABLE 12-3 CRITERIA SUGGESTING THE NEED FOR EARLY IMAGING FOR BACK PAIN

Bowel or bladder dysfunction
New onset of erectile dysfunction
Fevers or night sweats (suggestive of infection or malignancy)
Unplanned weight loss
Night pain
Personal history of cancer
Saddle anesthesia
History of recent trauma (e.g., fall or direct blow, NOT twisting or lifting)
Age >50 or <18 years
Patient with current or recent use of steroids
Any suspicion of an infectious or neoplastic cause for low-back pain
Pain for >6 weeks

HELPFUL TIP:

Several of the indicators listed in Table 12-3 are associated with cauda equina syndrome. Cauda equina syndrome is the product of an acute reduction in the volume of the spinal canal which can lead to compression and paralysis of multiple nerve roots in the S-1 to S-5 area resulting in urinary retention, saddle anesthesia, and lower extremity weakness. It is often caused by central disk herniations, epidural abscesses and hematomas, fractures, and other trauma. Incomplete syndromes are common; the patient may not have all of the clinical findings above. Cauda equina syndrome is an *orthopedic emergency*. An MRI and surgical consultation should be sought without delay.

HELPFUL TIP:

Patients who **do not** have films done initially for mild back pain from twisting, etc. actually have better outcomes than those who do. When we order imaging studies, we "medicalize" the illness, causing the patient to expect a longer recovery and the need for intervention in order to get better. Don't do films unless they have one of the red flag symptoms above.

Upon physical examination, you note the vital signs are normal. Straight leg raise (SLR) testing on the right leg at 55 degrees reproduces the patient's pain in the lower back and a painful "tightness" in the posterior thigh. He complains of the same discomfort on the left at 30 degrees.

Question 12.11.3 Based on these findings, which of the following statements is true?
A) This is a positive SLR test bilaterally and is specific for disk herniation
B) This is a positive SLR test on the left and is specific for disk herniation
C) This is a positive SLR test on the right and is specific for disk herniation
D) This is a negative SLR test bilaterally

Answer 12.11.3 **The correct answer is "D."** The SLR test can be performed in several ways, which are listed here.
- **Seated active:** with the patient seated on the examination table, the patient dorsiflexes the foot and extends the knee.
- **Seated passive:** with the patient seated on the examination table, the examiner passively extends the knee, and radicular symptoms will be exacerbated with passive ankle dorsiflexion.
- **Lying passive:** with the patient in a supine position, the examiner holds the knee in full extension and passively flexes the hip, and radicular symptoms will be exacerbated with passive ankle dorsiflexion.

In all cases, the test is positive when radicular symptoms occur (e.g., pain and paresthesias down the leg below the level of the knee—not back or thigh pain from muscle stretching) between 25 and 75 degrees of hip flexion while lying or with knee extension while seated. The symptoms will be exacerbated with active or passive ankle dorsiflexion. However, SLR is neither sensitive nor specific for disk disease. "Crossover" pain with radicular symptoms in the leg not lifted is very specific for disk disease but is not very sensitive.

Even though SLR is negative, you continue your neurologic examination. You note symmetric patellar reflexes, diminished Achilles reflex on the right, and symmetric strength in the legs except for decreased strength with right foot plantar flexion. You also note decrease in gross sensation to light touch over the right lateral foot.

Question 12.11.4 Which of the following nerve roots is most likely compromised?
A) L3
B) L4
C) L5
D) S1
E) S2–S4

Answer 12.11.4 **The correct answer is "D."** A summary of nerve root innervation is given in Table 12-4.

TABLE 12-4 EXAMINATION FINDINGS OF LUMBAR AND SACRAL SPINAL NERVE ROOTS

Nerve Root	Reflex	Motor	Sensory	Test
L2–L3	None	Quadriceps	Anterior thigh	Knee extension
L4	Patella	Tibialis anterior (foot dorsiflexion, inversion)	Medial lower leg and foot	Walk on heels
L5	Medial hamstring (difficult to assess)	Extensor hallucis longus (dorsiflexion of big toe)	Dorsal foot	Hold up great toe
S1	Achilles	Peroneus longus and brevis (ankle eversion) and plantar flexion of foot	Lateral foot	Walk on toes
S2–S4	Anal wink	Intrinsic foot muscles, anal sphincter tone	Perianal	

Question 12.11.5 Appropriate initial treatment for this patient's acute back pain should include which of the following?
A) Strict bed rest
B) Pain control
C) Corset or lumbar belt
D) Referral for epidural steroid injection or endoscopic disk resection
E) A and B

Answer 12.11.5 The correct answer is "B." In acute mechanical back pain (no longer than 6 weeks), regardless of the method of treatment, 40% are better within 1 week, 60% to 85% in 3 weeks, and 90% in 2 months. Negative prognostic factors include more than three episodes of back pain, gradual onset of symptoms, and prolonged absence from work. *Bed rest does not contribute to a return of function and may worsen outcomes.* Early mobilization of the patient is best for allowing him to continue activities as tolerated. Acetaminophen can be used for pain control and may have fewer side effects than do the NSAIDs. (However … see NNT in the first paragraph of this chapter!) Chiropractic care may be useful (but not for the neck where it may result in carotid or vertebrobasilar vessel dissection). Data on acupuncture are mixed.

HELPFUL TIP:
For LBP, early mobilization and walking is important. Epidural steroid injections, while intuitively appealing for disk disease, have been shown to be of no long-term (and little short-term) benefit (*J Bone Joint Surg.* 2012;94:1353–1358; *BMJ.* 2015;350:h1748).
    For **spinal stenosis**, surgery has not been shown to be particularly better than conservative, nonsurgical treatment (*Ann Intern Med.* 2015;162:465). Steroids have also not been shown to be of any benefit in spinal stenosis. Gabapentin and other anticonvulsants are not helpful for back pain (*CMAJ.* 2018; Jul 3).

You prescribe your pain medication of choice (as long as it's not an opioid) and recommend rehabilitation exercises.

Question 12.11.6 Which of the following has been shown to be effective at reducing the recurrence of back injury in the workplace?
A) Back support belts
B) "Back School" that teaches proper lifting techniques, stretches, etc.
C) Increasing physical fitness and muscle tone
D) A and C
E) B and C

Answer 12.11.6 The correct answer is "C." The only thing that has been unequivocally shown to reduce further back injuries is improving the overall fitness of the patient and their muscle tone. Of special note, back support belts, long worn in industry, have equivocal data with most studies being negative. "Back School" also does not seem to help.

HELPFUL TIP:
Physical therapy modalities such as application of heat, cold, ultrasound, and muscle stimulation may have short-term benefit. Rehabilitation exercises focusing on trunk extensors, abdominal muscles, and aerobic conditioning promote early mobilization, which is critical in treating acute back pain. **The specific exercise does not matter as much as the mobilization.** Sham therapy works as well as specific exercises as long as the patient is mobile.

▶ **Objectives: Did you learn to …**
· Generate a differential diagnosis and understand the etiology of lumbar spine pain?
· Evaluate and treat acute LBP?
· Recognize warning signs of LBP?

 QUICK QUIZ: BACK PAIN

Spondylolysis commonly occurs in which part of the spine?
A) Cervical spine lateral processes
B) Thoracic spine pars interarticularis
C) Thoracic spine lateral processes
D) Lumbar spine pars interarticularis

The correct answer is "D." Spondylolysis is characterized by pars interarticularis stress fractures and most commonly occurs in the lumbar region.

 QUICK QUIZ: MORE BACK PAIN

Anterior slippage of one vertebra on another is called:
A) Spondylolysis
B) Spondylolisthesis
C) Spondylitis
D) Spondyloarthropathy
E) Scheuermann disease

The correct answer is "B." Slippage of one vertebra on another is called spondylolisthesis. "A," spondylolysis, is discussed above. Spondylolysis can lead to spondylolisthesis. Spondyloarthropathy is a nonspecific term referring to inflammation of the spine and encompasses such diseases as ankylosing spondylitis, Reiter disease, enteropathic arthritis, etc. Spondylitis is a more specific term for the same thing (e.g., ankylosing spondylitis). "E," Scheuermann disease, is a benign process causing kyphosis by compression of the vertebrae (at least 5 degrees of wedging in three consecutive vertebrae). The cause is unknown but it tends to present in adolescence.

QUICK QUIZ: EVEN MORE BACK PAIN

Spondylolisthesis is graded based on the degree of slipping of one vertebra on the other. Which of the following patients would need surgical consultation?
A) Grade one (<25% slip) with no symptoms in an early teen (12–14)
B) Grade 2 (25–50% slip) with no symptoms in an early teen (12–14)
C) Grade 3 (50–100% slip) with mild pain in a 20-year-old college gymnast
D) When slippage is 10% to 15% with no symptoms in a patient >60 years old
E) When slippage is 25% with no symptoms in a patient >60 years old

The correct answer is "C." Sondylolisthesis can be a problem int th late teens and twenties, especially in athletes. Patients often become symptomatic when there is 25% slippage or greater. Mild degrees of slip can be treated conservatively, although surgical treatment threshold varies considerably among orthopedic surgeons. Predisposing factors for spondylolisthesis include recurrent lumbar hyperextension (gymnasts, football players, etc.), although many patients do not have an identifiable cause. Any adolescent athlete who presents with back pain that is made worse by hyperextension should raise your suspicion and spondylolisthesis. Older patients who are asymptomatic do not need to be considered for surgical treatment unless the slip is grade 4 (100% or greater).

QUICK QUIZ: BACK PAIN IN CHILDREN

A 4-year-old boy presents to your office accompanied by his mother who says he has a limp and LBP. This has been getting progressively worse over the past 2 weeks. When the patient sits, he sits in a "tripod" position supporting his weight on his hands. Vitals are normal without a fever and a CBC is normal.

This history is most consistent with:
A) Discitis
B) Occult fracture
C) Growing pains
D) Juvenile idiopathic arthritis
E) Mechanical low-back strain

The correct answer is "A." This history is most consistent with discitis. Discitis is an inflammatory process of the disk usually found in children age infancy to 3 years but may occur at any age. The etiology is usually *Staphylococcus* (low-grade infection, 60%) but there may be sterile inflammation. Fever is usually absent in discitis (seen in only 25%), and blood cultures are sterile.

The white count is usually normal, although ESR is elevated in 90%. Treatment is not standardized, but most experts would include anti-staphylococcal antibiotics. "B," occult fracture, is unlikely in a child this age. "C," growing pains, does not present with back pain (see the discussion of growing pains earlier in this chapter). Juvenile idiopathic (previously rheumatoid) arthritis presents with small joint involvement as opposed to back pain.

▶ CASE 12.12

A 24-year-old male presents to the clinic 2 days after a collision during a softball game in which he fell on his outstretched right hand ("But I made the play!" he exclaims). He reports he could not continue playing and that his pain has not improved. He has some general edema around the right wrist, poor grip strength secondary to pain, point tenderness over the radial aspect of the wrist ("snuff box tenderness"), and decreased ROM. There is no obvious deformity, and he is neurovascularly intact.

Question 12.12.1 **Of the following, what would be the most likely diagnosis for this patient?**
A) Colles fracture
B) Scaphoid fracture
C) Smith fracture
D) Extensor carpi radialis strain
E) Scapholunate sprain

Answer 12.12.1 **The correct answer is "B."** Although all of these could be in the differential diagnosis, "B" is the most likely based on mechanism of injury and clinical findings. The scaphoid spans both the proximal and distal carpal row. In this position, it is quite vulnerable to high-impact injuries, such as a fall on an out-stretched hand, and is the most commonly fractured carpal bone. The absence of deformity makes a Colles or Smith fracture ("A" and "C") less likely. Further, a sprain or a strain (options "D" and "E") are less likely, given the bony point tenderness, decreased range of motion, and overall nonimprovement with conservative measures.

HELPFUL TIP:
Palpating for snuffbox tenderness with the wrist in slight ulnar deviation increases the sensitivity of the physical examination. An additional physical examination finding consistent with a scaphoid injury is pain at the scaphoid with axial loading of the thumb.

Plain film radiographs, including AP and lateral of the hand and wrist as well as scaphoid views, are negative for fracture.

Question 12.12.2 **What is the most appropriate next step for this patient?**
A) Short-arm thumb spica cast with follow-up in 10 to 14 days
B) NSAIDs, ice, compression, and elevation followed by physical therapy

C) MRI or CT to rule out an occult fracture
D) Orthopedic referral
E) Return to play within the week

Answer 12.12.2 The correct answer is "A." Scaphoid fractures are often occult acutely and usually will be evident on plain films after 10 to 14 days due to bony resorption along the fracture line. If repeat films are negative but suspicion remains high, an MRI or CT should be considered.

> **HELPFUL TIP:**
> Although not the standard of care, early MRI or CT (neither is definitively superior to the other) to evaluate for occult scaphoid fractures may allow patients to return to full activity sooner than would be possible if they were splinted for 10 to 14 days. This may be cost-effective for certain patients (i.e., concert violinists or the Iowa Hawkeyes' starting quarterback). Both MRI and CT are better at excluding fractures than they are at confirming them (they can be ruled out, but not necessarily ruled in). It should be noted that **splinting** does not eliminate motion at the scaphoid; thus, there can be shear forces across the fracture line making avascular necrosis more likely…so, if you are worried they will be better off **casted** or in the MRI machine.

Repeat wrist radiographs including scaphoid views 2 weeks post injury indicate a nondisplaced fracture of the proximal pole of the scaphoid.

Question 12.12.3 You recommend which of the following treatment plans?
A) Wrist and thumb spica splint and physical therapy because good blood supply at the proximal pole allows fast healing
B) Thumb spica cast for 6 weeks then repeat x-rays
C) Short-arm cast excluding the thumb for 4 to 6 weeks
D) Orthopedics referral for open reduction/internal fixation
E) B or D

Answer 12.12.3 The correct answer is "E." It is clear that a spica cast with the thumb included is important; whether a short- or long-arm cast is optimal is still a matter of debate. Open fixation is another option. Generally, an orthopedic surgeon should oversee treatment of scaphoid fractures since the complication rate is high. A proximal pole fracture has high risk for nonunion and avascular necrosis (90%). **The blood supply to the scaphoid is through the distal pole, putting the proximal pole at high risk for complications.** Evidence of healing may not be well visualized on plain films, and a CT or MRI may be needed to confirm the degree of healing. The closer the fracture line is to the proximal pole, the lower the threshold for orthopedic referral.

> **HELPFUL TIP:**
> Healing time for a distal pole scaphoid fracture is 6 to 8 weeks, for middle third or waist fractures 8 to 12 weeks, and proximal pole fractures can take 12 to 24 weeks.

▶ **Objectives: Did you learn to …**
· Recognize a patient at risk for scaphoid fracture?
· Manage a patient with a scaphoid fracture?

 QUICK QUIZ: HAND INJURIES

A patient presents after "jamming" his index finger while playing basketball. He has mild swelling at the DIP joint. At rest, his DIP is flexed. He has full ROM of all joints except he cannot extend at the DIP.

What is the appropriate treatment and follow-up?
A) RICE therapy, PRN follow-up
B) A full extension splint of the DIP joint worn at all times with orthopedic follow-up in 1 to 2 weeks
C) A removable aluminum splint to be worn for comfort, follow-up in clinic in 1 month
D) Ibuprofen and return to full activities, PRN follow-up

The correct answer is "B." The patient has suffered an injury to his extensor tendon mechanism, known as a "mallet finger." X-rays are indicated to evaluate for a bony fracture/avulsion. The initial treatment is an extension splint at the DIP joint, and follow-up with an orthopedic surgeon as surgical correction is sometimes required. The splint must be worn at all times. See Figure 12-3 for the anatomy of a mallet finger.

> **HELPFUL TIP:**
> Surgical indication for a Mallot finger include: volar subluxation, >30% of the articular surface involved, >2 mm gap of the avulsed bone, chronic injury >12 weeks. An extensor lag of 10 degrees or less can be tolerated unless you are a professional pianist. If greater than 10 degrees, it increases the chance of a swan neck deformity down the road.

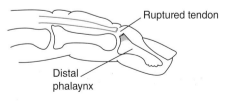

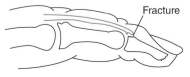

MALLET FINGER

FIGURE 12-3. Mallet Finger.

QUICK QUIZ: FRACTURES

A Colles fracture consists of:
A) Fractures of the midshaft of the radius and ulna
B) Fractures of the head of radius and ulna that is displaced dorsally and is angulated
C) Fractures of the head of the radius and ulna that are displaced ventrally and is angulated
D) Fracture of the distal radius at the metaphysis, dorsally displaced and often angulated

The correct answer is "D." OK, some of you may have chosen "B." However, the head of the radius is at the *elbow* and not at the wrist. A Colles fracture is a fracture of the distal radius at the metaphysis, which is displaced dorsally and often angulated. It is the most common wrist fracture in adults. The ulnar styloid is often involved, and there may be intra-articular involvement as well.

 HELPFUL TIP:
Finkelstein's test can be painful regardless of tendonitis so check both sides when doing your exam or you will get fooled.

 QUICK QUIZ: ANGER MANAGEMENT ISSUES

A 19-year-old male was mad at his computer and decided to punch the wall. "He fought the wall and the wall won." Radiographs demonstrate a fifth metacarpal fracture with some angulation.

What is the maximal acceptable angulation and rotation for a boxer fracture, fourth or fifth metacarpal, to maintain full hand function?
A) 10 degrees of dorsal angulation and 10 degrees of rotation
B) 30 degrees of dorsal angulation and 5 degrees of rotation
C) 40 degrees of dorsal angulation and 0 degrees of rotation
D) 90 degrees of dorsal angulation and 0 degrees of rotation

The correct answer is "C." Any degree of rotation, or **>40 degrees of dorsal angulation**, may result in significant functional deficits. Reduction should be attempted if angulation is >10 degrees. Patients should be advised that with angulations >10 to 15 degrees, there will likely be a loss of metacarpophalangeal (MCP) prominence, although there should be no loss of function. If this is unacceptable to the patient, referral is recommended.

 HELPFUL TIP:
Any "scissoring" or crossing of the patient's fingers while they clench their fist should raise your suspicion for a rotational deformity.

 HELPFUL TIP:
If you can't beat your computer at chess, don't get frustrated; try changing sports. We are sure you can beat your computer at mixed martial arts.

▶ **CASE 12.13**

The next patient in the ED is an 18-year-old high school football player. He was playing in a football game this evening when he was tackled from the side and landed directly on the lateral aspect of his right shoulder. He states that he can actively move his arm, but is limited by pain on the top of his shoulder. He has also noticed a small painful bump on top of the right shoulder and is concerned that he "broke his collarbone."

Question 12.13.1 Based on the mechanism of injury and patient history, the most likely injury would be?
A) Acromioclavicular (AC) sprain
B) Biceps tendon rupture
C) Glenohumeral dislocation
D) Rotator cuff tear
E) Scapula fracture

Answer 12.13.1 The correct answer is "A." Although any of these injuries may be present, an AC sprain is the most likely based on the history and the way the patient fell. A thorough examination should be able to further distinguish between these injuries. "B" is not likely, given the mechanism of injury. The deformity associated with biceps tendon rupture (a defect in tendon with pain and deformity in the muscle belly representing the contracted, detached muscle) would be on the upper arm or at the elbow, not on the "top" of the shoulder. "C" is incorrect. The deformity and loss of ROM of a glenohumeral dislocation (shoulder dislocation) is usually obvious. The mechanism of injury is typically a forced abduction and external rotation. "D" is less likely. A rotator cuff tear will present with pain more laterally over the subacromial space and should not have an associated deformity. The ROM is generally markedly limited by pain. "E" is unlikely. Scapula fractures are uncommon and are usually the result of high velocity blunt trauma such as a blow from a baseball bat or motorcycle accident. Plain film radiographs should be obtained to rule out a clavicle fracture, especially when any deformity is present.

Question 12.13.2 Your patient is worried that he broke his "collarbone." If he did sustain a nondisplaced clavicle fracture, which of the following would be appropriate treatment?
A) Rest, ice, and NSAIDs for pain control
B) A sling for comfort only
C) A figure-of-eight splint
D) A and B
E) Any of the above is an equally valid treatment

Answer 12.13.2 The correct answer is "D." While the traditional teaching has been that a figure-of-eight splint is required, it adds nothing to the treatment of a clavicle fracture. Pain control and using a sling works just as well. Additionally, figure-of-eight splints often increase a patient's pain and can cause a brachial plexus injury. Thus, a sling is preferable. Complete immobilization is not necessary for nondisplaced clavicle fractures—keep the patient moving.

Question 12.13.3 The proper treatment for a clavicle fracture that is minimally displaced is:
A) Closed reduction and then a sling
B) Open reduction and immobilization
C) Open reduction and **early** mobilization
D) A sling
E) Clavicular disarticulation

Answer 12.13.3 The correct answer is "D." The ends of a displaced clavicle fracture need not be 100% approximated for healing to occur and for function to return. Thus, reduction is generally not necessary.

HELPFUL TIP:
The paradigm of the treatment of clavicle fractures is shifting. More patients are getting surgical intervention (an internal fixation), especially athletes when a quick return to sport is desired. This decision depends on the degree of displacement and the occupation of the patient (Surgeons? Yes. Car Salesmen? Not so much). Greater degrees of fracture displacement and bayoneting have higher rates of fracture nonunion. Thus, discussion with an orthopedist is appropriate for patients with displaced clavicle fractures.

You send the patient for x-rays. AP radiographs show *slight widening of the AC joint on the injured side*. The examination and radiograph confirm your suspicion of an AC injury.

Question 12.13.4 For *this* patient with an AC sprain, you offer:
A) Sling for comfort, ice, and NSAIDs or analgesics for pain control
B) Referral for open fixation
C) Figure-of-eight strap for 4 to 6 weeks
D) Corticosteroid injection followed by physical therapy
E) Manual reduction, then sling-and-swath immobilization for 6 to 8 weeks

Answer 12.13.4 The correct answer is "A." Conservative management is appropriate for low-grade AC joint sprains. AC sprains are graded I to VI. Grades I to III are generally treated conservatively, while grades IV–VI may need to be treated surgically. Signs of high-grade (IV–VI) AC sprains include posterior or inferior displacement of the clavicle and widening of 100% or more of the coracoclavicular space. Just like with clavicle fractures, figure-of-eight straps have largely fallen out of favor for treatment of AC joint injuries. Corticosteroid injections are not the treatment of choice for acute AC joint injuries. An injection may be considered as an adjunct treatment for degenerative arthritis of the AC joint at some distant point in the future. Sling-and-swath immobilization is not indicated.

▶ **Objectives: Did you learn to …**
  · Differentiate between causes of shoulder injuries?
  · Treat a clavicular fracture?
  · Manage AC injuries?

▶ **CASE 12.14**

A 65-year-old male presents with left shoulder pain and weakness, which started 2 weeks ago after he put a new roof on his house. He does not recall a specific injury. The pain is worse with reaching for and lifting objects as well as with overhead activities. Nighttime pain is present. He describes himself active and healthy, and he only takes acetaminophen when needed for shoulder pain. You suspect that he may have rotator cuff tendinopathy.

Question 12.14.1 If this is the case, what do you expect to find on examination?
A) Tenderness to palpation of the greater tuberosity of the humerus
B) Limited active ROM
C) Normal passive ROM
D) Shoulder shrug with attempted abduction (such as with a frozen shoulder)
E) Any of the above

Answer 12.14.1 The correct answer is "E." Ok, so this might fit under the category of "trick question," but the shoulder examination can be normal in a patient with a rotator cuff tear or tendinopathy, or it can include any of the elements listed in "A" through "D." Notably, normal PASSIVE ROM ("C") does not rule out rotator cuff pathology.

Question 12.14.2 Which of the following muscles is NOT a part of the rotator cuff?
A) Supraspinatus
B) Infraspinatus
C) Subscapularis
D) Teres major
E) Teres minor

Answer 12.14.2 The correct answer is "D." The rotator cuff consists of the other four muscles listed and functions to rotate the arm and stabilize the humeral head.

Question 12.14.3 Which of the following muscles is the most commonly torn in the rotator cuff?
A) Supraspinatus
B) Infraspinatus
C) Subscapularis
D) Teres minor

Answer 12.14.3 The correct answer is "A." The supraspinatus is generally the point of origin for most tears.

HELPFUL TIP:
Full-thickness tears of the rotator cuff are uncommon in individuals below the age of 40, unless associated with trauma. Asymptomatic rotator cuff tears are very common in those over the age of 60 and are not always the pain generator—in other words—order MRIs judiciously in this population!

Based on your history and physical examination, you diagnose a rotator cuff tendinosis.

Question 12.14.4 Appropriate initial management of this 65-year-old male should be:
A) Acetaminophen and physical therapy
B) Oral corticosteroids and physical therapy
C) Subacromial injection with corticosteroid and physical therapy
D) Surgical repair and physical therapy
E) Figure-of-eight strap

Answer 12.14.4 The correct answer is "A." For initial management in an individual >60 years of age, acetaminophen and physical therapy for 6 weeks is the best answer. If the patient has no improvement or inadequate response, a corticosteroid injection may be used judiciously. Injection likely will result in at least short-term pain relief, but there is no good evidence that it helps long term. In addition, it is thought to weaken the tendon and may accelerate extension of a tear, if present. Patients with significant symptoms or failed therapy should be considered for MRI, orthopedic referral, and surgical management. Patients under the age of 60 with acute traumatic tears should be considered for surgery, with best results within 6 weeks of injury.

HELPFUL TIP:
The old adage about corticosteroids causing weakening of the tendon has recently been questioned. It is now thought that the steroid injection provides enough relief of the pain that the patient will start using the extremity in ways he or she had not done before. This leads to tendon rupture from the additional load. However, the point remains that steroid injections may be associated with, but not causative of, tendon rupture.

Your patient is successful in rehabilitating his left shoulder, but then he returns 2 years later with right shoulder problems. The right shoulder has become progressively stiff and painful, and his ROM is now significantly limited in all directions. **Your examination is consistent with "frozen shoulder" or adhesive capsulitis.**

Question 12.14.5 Adhesive capsulitis is most commonly associated with which of the following?
A) Diabetes
B) Hyperthyroidism
C) Spondyloarthritis
D) Nondominant arm
E) Male gender

Answer 12.14.5 The correct answer is "A." Adhesive capsulitis has no clear predilection as to gender, race, arm dominance, or occupation. It is characterized by loss of ROM of the shoulder in all directions, with loss of both passive and active motion. It has a high incidence in patients with diabetes and tends to be more recalcitrant in those patients, of whom up to 50% will have bilateral involvement—although not necessarily concomitantly. Adhesive capsulitis is not typically related to trauma, but it can be associated with disuse due to pain, osteoarthritis, sling use, etc. Other conditions that are associated with adhesive capsulitis include **hypo**thyroidism and Parkinson disease.

HELPFUL TIP:
Adhesive capsulitis is considered to be idiopathic and separate from posttraumatic or postoperative joint stiffness or adhesions.

Question 12.14.6 What initial treatment do you recommend for this patient with adhesive capsulitis?
A) Arthroscopic debridement
B) Oral corticosteroids
C) NSAIDs and a sling for comfort
D) Extended progressive physical therapy
E) Mobilization under anesthesia

Answer 12.14.6 The correct answer is "D." A progressive stretching program with heat and NSAIDs or acetaminophen to improve comfort is the most appropriate early treatment. A corticosteroid injection of the glenohumeral joint (under ultrasound guidance or fluoroscopy) may be beneficial but should be used cautiously in diabetic patients. Oral steroids have no greater benefit than NSAIDs. "C" is incorrect because a sling will contribute to further immobilization and worsening of the problem. Mobilization or capsular release under anesthesia may be a last resort in adhesive capsulitis.

HELPFUL TIP:
The typical clinical course for adhesive capsulitis evolves over 1 to 2 years with an initial "painful" phase followed by a "freezing" phase characterized by continued pain and worsening stiffness followed by a slow "thawing" phase with decreasing pain and increasing ROM.

▶ **Objectives: Did you learn to …**
  - Define the muscles of the rotator cuff?
  - Identify, evaluate, and treat a rotator cuff injury?
  - Recognize the presentation, associations, and treatment of adhesive capsulitis?

▶ **CASE 12.15**

A 58-year-old male presents after sudden onset of right upper arm pain. He was working in the yard, cutting and pulling out some bushes, when he heard a "snap" and felt the pain. He has a history of rotator cuff tendinosis and osteoarthritis.

Question 12.15.1 You should look for all of the following on physical examination EXCEPT:
A) A positive elevated arm stress test ("Roos" test)
B) A palpable biceps muscle defect
C) Normal grip strength
D) An asymmetric bulge in the affected arm

Answer 12.15.1 The correct answer is "A." The elevated arm stress test is used to evaluate a patient for thoracic outlet syndrome. Have the patient abduct and externally rotate both shoulders, flex the elbows, pull their scapulae together, and repeatedly grip and relax the hands—for 3 minutes. The test is positive if neurological or vascular symptoms are reproduced. If you think to yourself, "Well, that might irritate my shoulder or arm," you would be right to then suppose that this test has a high rate of false positives. In fact, the specificity for thoracic outlet syndrome is around 30%. And anyway, this patient's presentation is not consistent with thoracic outlet syndrome. However, the history is consistent with biceps tendon rupture. "B" through "D" would be expected in a patient with biceps tendon rupture. Yes, there is usually normal grip strength. The injury is, of course, in the upper arm.

Question 12.15.2 Which portion of the biceps is most commonly involved in ruptures?
A) Distal tendon
B) Proximal short head tendon
C) Proximal long head tendon
D) Midmuscle belly
E) Proximal short head belly

Answer 12.15.2 The correct answer is "C." The long head is most commonly affected due to its position and risk for weakening secondary to rotator cuff tendinosis and shoulder impingement.

You decide this patient has a rupture of the long head of the biceps tendon.

Question 12.15.3 How is this injury treated initially?
A) Immediate surgical repair
B) Delayed surgical repair

C) Immobilization for 4 to 6 weeks with sling
D) NSAIDs and physical therapy
E) Biceps muscle transplant, preferably from a retired NFL player

Answer 12.15.3 The correct answer is "D." For most isolated proximal long or short head tears (with the exception of some young athletes and heavy laborers who would not tolerate the slight decrease in strength), treatment is conservative. Analgesics and physical therapy typically suffice. Surgical repair may be indicated if conservative therapy fails. Of note, you should discuss with patients the cosmetic deformity that will be permanent when these injuries are unrepaired versus scarring associated with surgery. Generally, there is approximately a 20% loss of elbow flexion and supination strength with an isolated proximal tear.

HELPFUL TIP:
Although proximal biceps tendon ruptures are treated conservatively, distal ruptures should be referred for early surgical repair, as the continuity of the entire muscle is lost and function at the elbow joint is significantly impaired with a 30% to 40% loss of strength across the elbow joint.

▶ **Objectives: Did you learn to …**
  - Identify the clinical presentation of biceps tendon rupture?
  - Manage a patient with biceps tendon rupture?

▶ **CASE 12.16**

A 25-year-old male presents to you with a history of a soccer injury. Someone evidently fell on his right foot while trying to steal the ball. The patient rapidly and forcefully twisted around the fixed foot. Since then he has had significant pain and swelling of the foot. His x-ray is shown in Figure 12-4.

Question 12.16.1 Which of the following is true regarding this radiograph?
A) It shows a step-off between the base of the second metatarsal and the middle cuneiform
B) It shows midfoot boney instability
C) It may require weight-bearing films to identify this injury
D) The abnormality is named after a French gynecologist
E) All of the above are true

Answer 12.16.1 The correct answer is "E," all of the above. This is a Lisfranc injury, which occurs as a result of ligamentous rupture between the metatarsals and the tarsal bones (the space between the metatarsals and the tarsal bones is known as the Lisfranc joint). Look for a widened space between the first and second and/or second and third metatarsals. There may also

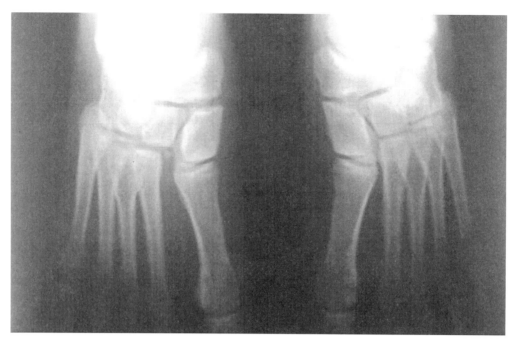

FIGURE 12-4. X-ray for Case 12.16.

be a step-off between the second metatarsal and middle cunei-form. These injuries may be difficult to identify, but obtaining weight-bearing films or stress views may help. Significant foot pain should be a tip off. See Figure 12-5 for further explanation. And, yes indeed, Dr. Lisfranc was a surgeon and gynecologist in Napoleon's army! Why did Napoleon need a gynecologist on campaign with him? That is a matter of debate.

Question 12.16.2 Appropriate treatment for this type of injury should include:
A) Weight bearing as tolerated in a post-op or hard-soled shoe
B) Rest, ice, compression, elevation, NSAIDs, and activity as tolerated. Will heal well and can be treated like a midfoot sprain
C) Orthopedic referral for open reduction/internal fixation (ORIF)
D) Walking boot that can be removed for several weight-bearing hours a day
E) Early 19th century French legionnaire's boot

Answer 12.16.2 The correct answer is "C." This injury/dislocation will lead to significant long-term pain and mid-foot instability if not recognized and treated appropriately. Any significant displacement (>2 mm) should be referred for surgical consideration. These are generally complex injuries prone to poor outcomes and should be managed by an ortho-pedic consultant.

▶ **Objectives: Did you learn to …**
  • Identify a Lisfranc injury?
  • Manage a patient with a Lisfranc injury?

▶ **CASE 12.17**

An 18-year-old female gymnast lands her dismount from the balance beam awkwardly. She reports the knee buckling, hearing a pop, and experiencing immediate right knee pain. She presents to your office 45 minutes after the injury. She is able to bear some weight on the leg but reports it is already swollen and feels "loose." On examination, there is a knee effusion present.

Question 12.17.1 Based on the information above, the most likely isolated injury experienced by this athlete is:
A) Medial meniscus tear
B) MCL sprain
C) Distal quadriceps/patellar tendon rupture
D) Anterior cruciate ligament (ACL) rupture
E) Distal femur fracture

Answer 12.17.1 The correct answer is "D." Did the patient or someone else hear a pop? If yes, suspect ACL tear (80%), meniscal injury (15%), and rarely a fracture. When did you notice swelling? If 0 to 12 hours after the injury, suspect ACL tear, fracture, or patellar dislocation/subluxation; if 12 to 24 hours, suspect meniscal injury. If there is hemarthrosis on aspiration, suspect ACL injury (>75%), patellar subluxation, or intra-articular fracture. A history of, "My knee gives way; buckles; feels loose; or comes apart," may be secondary to patel-lar subluxation/dislocation, ACL deficiency, or arthritis. Medial and lateral collateral ligament injuries do not typically present with significant effusion and typically feel stable with forward ambulation but are painful with side-to-side movements.

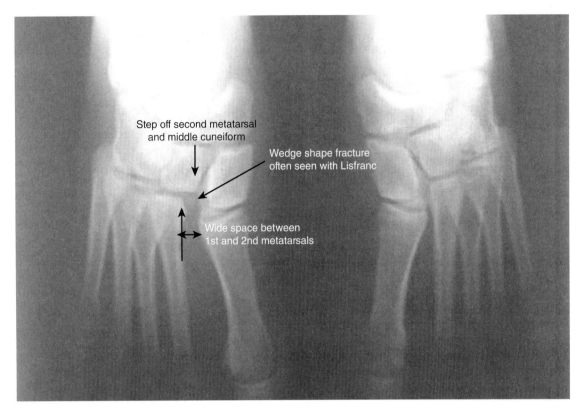

FIGURE 12-5. Case 12.16. Annotated Lisfranc Injury.

Muscle or tendon rupture may cause buckling, but will not typically cause effusion and will generally have an obvious deformity and inability to bear weight.

Question 12.17.2 Of the following, which is the best test to confirm the diagnosis of an ACL injury?
A) Plain film radiographs
B) McMurray test
C) Lachman test
D) Anterior drawer test

Answer 12.17.2 **The correct answer is "C."** In the hands of an experienced clinician, the Lachman test is the most sensitive test for ACL insufficiency (sensitivity 80–95%). The anterior drawer sign is negative in about 50% of acute ACL tears, and often is negative subacutely. McMurray test is used to evaluate for a meniscal tear. Plain films should be obtained for all patients with acute knee injury with effusion or suspected ACL tear. A Segond fracture (small avulsion of the lateral tibial plateau) is an x-ray finding associated with ACL tears. Although an MRI may be considered a gold standard test, its sensitivity has been reported as 97% when compared against arthroscopy findings and is positive in only 82% in cases of complete rupture. An orthopedic consult is generally indicated if ACL injury is suspected, and obtaining one is less expensive than MRI.

HELPFUL TIP:
The Lachman test is performed with the knee flexed at 20 to 30 degrees with the patient in a supine position. The examiner then attempts to anteriorly displace the tibia on the femur while stabilizing the femur. Always remember to check the contralateral side. Some patients have naturally lax ligaments.

You feel that this patient is very appropriate for radiographic evaluation, and you obtain x-rays of the knee.

Question 12.17.3 Which of the following is NOT one of the criteria of the Ottawa knee rules predicting the need for knee radiographs?
A) Age <18
B) Pain isolated to the patella
C) Tenderness at the head of the fibula
D) Inability to flex the knee 90 degrees
E) Inability to bear weight for four steps

Answer 12.17.3 **The correct answer is "A."** The age criterion for the Ottawa knee rules is age >55 years. All of the other options are correct. If **any** of these criteria are present (including a patient >55 years of age), a radiograph should be obtained. These rules have been validated and are 97% sensitive for fracture. The Pittsburgh rules, which are reportedly 99% sensitive, have only two criteria: (1) age <12 years or age >50 and (2) inability to bear weight in the clinic or ED. Of the two, the Ottawa rules are the more commonly accepted.

. . . .

The x-ray shows no fracture. You prescribe a knee immobilizer, rest, ice, NSAIDs, and refer the patient to an orthopedic surgeon. The patient returns 2 days later with marked effusion and pain. To help relieve the pain, you perform an arthrocentesis and 90 mL of bloody aspirate is obtained. As per your clinic's standard protocol, the joint fluid is sent for analysis. The analysis returns with the only abnormalities being blood and fat droplets.

Question 12.17.4 Based on the effusion, you suspect what diagnosis?
A) Complete ACL rupture
B) Meniscal tear
C) ACL and PCL tear
D) Intra-articular fracture
E) Patellar subluxation

Answer 12.17.4 **The correct answer is "D."** Fat from bone marrow may be seen even with a small intra-articular fracture. Consider CT or MRI if fracture is not noted on plain film. If a fracture is still not demonstrated, consider referral for orthopedic consultation.

HELPFUL TIP:
There is no need to refer for an ACL injury acutely (though they still should be referred). In fact, outcomes are the same regardless of whether the ACL is repaired or not (*BMJ.* 2013;346:f232). So, waiting a couple of days or a week for an orthopedic appointment is OK; give them crutches (partial weight bearing) and a hinged brace for comfort and stability. Of course you get an unhinged parent who demand a referral NOW.

▶ **Objectives: Did you learn to …**
- Generate a differential diagnosis for knee pain in an athlete?
- Diagnose ACL injury?
- Determine when knee radiographs are appropriate?

 QUICK QUIZ: KNEE PAIN

The best clinical test for determining the presence of a meniscal injury is:
A) Posterior sag test
B) Apley test
C) McMurray test
D) Pivot shift test
E) Thessaly test

The correct answer is "E." The best meniscus test is the Thessaly test with a diagnostic accuracy in the range of 61% to 96% compared to McMurry at 56% to 84%. It is performed standing with the knee bent 20 to 30 degrees. Then with the heal planted and fixed, the patient "does the twist." Pain (or a locking or clicking sensation) localizing to the joint line is considered a positive test. The McMurry test is done by flexing the knee and then extending the knee while performing internal and external rotation of the tibia/fibula. Keep one hand on the knee. The test is positive when the examiner feels a pop during the maneuver or when there is significant pain during internal or external rotation. The Apley test is done with the patient in a prone position. Move the knee to 90 degrees of flexion. Put downward pressure on the tibia/fibula while internally and externally rotating the lower leg. Pain suggests a meniscal tear. Pain should be relieved by distracting the joint. The posterior sag test is used to detect PCL injury, while the pivot shift test is used to detect ACL injury.

▶ **CASE 12.18**

A 24-year-old female presents to the clinic 24 hours after slipping on a patch of ice outside her home. She reports feeling a "pop" and immediate pain on the lateral aspect of the ankle. She reports significant swelling in the first few hours with pain and inability to bear weight initially, but now she is able to walk with a significant limp. She reports no significant past injuries to the foot or ankle. On examination, you note edema/effusion over the lateral ankle, some ecchymosis, tenderness, but no laxity on anterior drawer and inversion stress. There is no bony tenderness on palpation of the foot and ankle, but there is tenderness anterolaterally in the soft tissue.

Question 12.18.1 The most likely injury this patient has suffered is?
A) Fracture of the distal tibia
B) Fracture of the distal fibula
C) Sprain of the lateral ligament complex
D) Sprain of the medial ligament complex
E) Syndesmosis sprain

Answer 12.18.1 **The correct answer is "C."** A sprain is most likely because there is no bony tenderness. And, since she is tender laterally, the lateral ligament complex is most likely sprained.

Question 12.18.2 In this case, the most likely structure injured would be the:
A) Anterior talofibular ligament
B) Distal fibula
C) Distal tibia
D) Deltoid ligament
E) Achilles tendon

Answer 12.18.2 **The correct answer is "A."** This is a sprain of the anterior talofibular ligament. This is the first ligament injured with an inversion ankle sprain. It is followed by the calcaneofibular ligament if enough force is involved. "E," Achilles tendon injury (specifically rupture), is of special note. First, this injury presents as pain in the Achilles tendon area. With a complete Achilles tendon tear, the patient will have marked weakness of plantar flexion. A diagnostic test (Thompson test) is to squeeze the posterior calf, with the patient lying supine on the bed and the feet dangling off. In response, the foot should plantar flex. If this does not occur, consider Achilles rupture. Operative and nonoperative treatments can be used.

HELPFUL TIP:
The Ottawa criteria reliably predict who needs an ankle radiograph and who does not. This has been validated in ages 5 to 55. The Ottawa foot and ankle criteria are listed in Figure 12-6.

Question 12.18.3 **Which of the following is the most appropriate management of this patient's sprained ankle?**
A) Cast for 4 weeks followed by physical therapy
B) Crutches, non-weight-bearing for 2 weeks, and then progressive physical therapy
C) Rest, ice, elevation, and early mobilization using external support, crutches, or cane if needed; progress to activity as tolerated
D) Refer for orthopedic consultation

E) Immobilization with short-leg walking cast, heat for comfort, analgesics or NSAIDs, and progress to activities as tolerated

Answer 12.18.3 **The correct answer is "C."** Treatment for most sprains includes an external supportive brace, ice application, and elevation; early mobilization is critical and will hasten recovery. NSAIDs or acetaminophen should be used for pain control. The patient should be allowed partial weight bearing as tolerated with crutches or a cane. Patients with recurrent problems of instability should be referred to an orthopedist for evaluation.

HELPFUL TIP:
Early mobilization and weight bearing reduces the time of disability for ankle sprains. Rest and nonweight bearing should be minimized. Allow the patient to advance activities as tolerated.

▶ **Objectives: Did you learn to …**
- Identify a patient with an ankle sprain?
- Differentiate ankle sprain from fracture based on history and examination?
- Use the Ottawa ankle rules to determine when to obtain an ankle radiograph?
- Manage a patient with an ankle sprain?

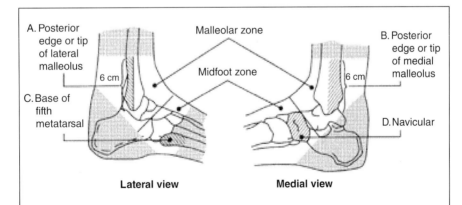

FIGURE 12-6. Ottawa Foot and Ankle Rules.

▶ CASE 12.19

A 27-year-old male presents to your clinic following an inversion-type injury to the foot and ankle. He cannot bear weight on the foot on presentation. He complains of pain and swelling laterally on the foot and ankle. There is some soft-tissue swelling but no obvious deformity. There is tenderness over the lateral ankle ligaments as well as over the base of the fifth metatarsal. AP and lateral films of the foot and ankle are obtained and reveal a nondisplaced fracture at the base of the fifth metatarsal. The radiograph is available for your review in Figure 12-7.

Question 12.19.1 **What is the name of this fracture?**
A) Jones fracture
B) Maisonneuve fracture
C) Colles fracture
D) Avulsion fracture of tuberosity, base fifth metatarsal

Answer 12.19.1 **The correct answer is "D."** This is an avulsion fracture of the base of the fifth metatarsal that may result from an inversion ankle injury. Classically, this has been thought to occur due to an attempt at dynamic stabilization by the peroneus brevis, causing an **avulsion of the proximal portion of the metatarsal base**, but may also be due to avulsion of the lateral band of the plantar fascia. A **Jones fracture** is a transverse fracture of the proximal fifth metatarsal at the metaphyseal–diaphyseal junction and typically extends into the inter-metatarsal facet (see Fig. 12-8). Jones fractures have a high incidence of nonunion because they occur in a watershed area of blood supply. A maisonneuve fracture is a fracture of the proximal one-third of the fibula associated with an external rotation injury of the ankle. A Colles fracture is a fracture of the distal radius (not involving the joint) with dorsal angulation of the distal fracture fragment.

HELPFUL TIP:
An unfused apophysis in children and adolescents may be confused with a fifth metatarsal avulsion injury. Tuberosity avulsion fractures are transverse, while the unfused apophysis is oriented vertically along the long axis of the metatarsal.

Question 12.19.2 **Appropriate treatment for the fracture described above would be:**
A) A hard-soled postoperative shoe bearing weight as tolerated
B) Nonweight-bearing short-leg cast for 6 to 8 weeks
C) Operative internal fixation
D) Walking boot with crutches for 6 to 8 weeks
E) None of the above

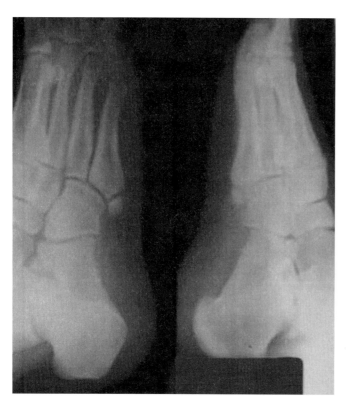

FIGURE 12-7. Fracture of the 5th Metatarsal.

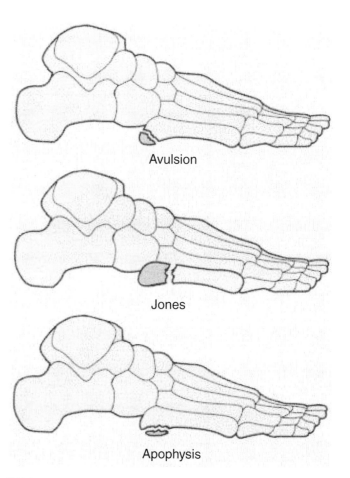

Avulsion

Jones

Apophysis

FIGURE 12-8. Fractures of the 5th Metatarsal.

Answer 12.19.2 The correct answer is "A." Nondisplaced tuberosity fractures generally heal well with conservative measures. These may be managed with a postoperative shoe with weight bearing as tolerated. A walking boot may be needed initially if there is significant pain present preventing ambulation in a hard-soled shoe; however, ankle immobilization is generally not needed for these avulsion fractures to heal. For a fracture with a displaced fragment >3 mm, orthopedic referral should be considered. Fractures to the metaphyseal–diaphyseal junction (**Jones fractures**) result from a vertical load placed on the lateral foot, such as an inversion injury or a stress injury. Jones fractures may potentially be managed with 6 to 8 weeks in a nonweight-bearing short-leg cast if nondisplaced; however, many require surgical intervention. **Jones fractures should be referred due to the high incidence of nonunion.**

HELPFUL TIP:
Stress fractures of the forefoot are common in competitive and recreational athletes, especially after a sudden increase in activity, intensity, duration, frequency, or a change in surface type. They may be occult on plain films acutely, but some subtle periosteal change may be evident on close examination in the area of maximal tenderness. If plain films are negative but suspicion remains high, treat as if a fracture is present. You may consider an MRI or repeat plain films and re-examination in 10 to 14 days. The same treatment considerations apply to metatarsal stress fractures as to any other nondisplaced forefoot fracture.

HELPFUL TIP:
Be alert for midfoot tenderness over the navicular. All navicular fractures, including stress fractures, should be referred to an orthopedist due to potential for avascular necrosis.

▶ **Objectives: Did you learn to …**
- Evaluate foot injuries?
- Describe fifth metatarsal fractures?
- Manage straightforward metatarsal fractures and identify which fractures should be referred?

▶ **CASE 12.20**

A 40-year-old female factory worker presents with progressively worsening heel pain. She has pain when she first gets out of bed in the morning. The pain tends to subside after 20 to 45 minutes, but is worsened by standing on the concrete floor of the factory where she works. She has a history of diabetes and hyperlipidemia. On examination, you find an obese female with a normal stance and gait. She has exquisite tenderness to palpation just distal to the heel on the underside of the foot. Pain is exacerbated by extension of the toes.

Question 12.20.1 Which of the following is the most likely diagnosis?
A) Tarsal tunnel syndrome
B) Achilles tendon rupture
C) Charcot foot
D) Plantar fasciitis
E) Plantar fascia rupture

Answer 12.20.1 The correct answer is "D." Plantar fasciitis, the most common cause of heel pain in adults, is a degenerative condition of the origin of the plantar fascia. "A" is incorrect. Tarsal tunnel syndrome is due to posterior tibial nerve entrapment and presents with diffuse pain at the medial ankle and arch of the foot. Paresthesias and dysesthesias often occur as well. "B," Achilles tendon rupture, is incorrect because the pain should be sudden, stabbing, and located in the calf (not the plantar aspect of the heel). "C" is also incorrect. Charcot foot does occur in diabetics, but it is actually the result of neuropathy and so generally does not present with pain. Instead, Charcot foot presents as an inflammatory condition (e.g., warmth, erythema, and edema) and progresses to joint instability and severe foot deformities. Finally, "E" is incorrect because plantar fascia rupture should have a sudden onset and is often related to trauma.

Question 12.20.2 Which of the following is true of plantar fasciitis?
A) It more commonly occurs in individuals with pes cavus
B) It is more common in women
C) It is commonly an acute injury
D) Radiographic identification of a "heel spur" or osteophyte is pathognomonic

Answer 12.20.2 The correct answer is "B." Plantar fasciitis is not associated with any particular foot type. It is nearly twice as common in women as men. It is also more common in overweight individuals. A rupture of the plantar fascia may occur acutely. Spurring may be seen in up to 50% of patients with plantar fasciitis but is present in 20% of age-matched asymptomatic adults. Thus, the finding of a spur is not diagnostic.

Question 12.20.3 Appropriate initial treatment for this patient's plantar fasciitis should include:
A) A heel cup or silicon pad
B) Achilles stretching
C) Ice or heat
D) NSAIDs
E) All of the above

Answer 12.20.3 The correct answer is "E," all of the above. Other initial treatments to consider include night splints to maintain ankle dorsiflexion and stretch the Achilles tendon and plantar fascia. Physical therapy modalities such as ultrasound may be helpful as well. Advanced treatments, such as corticosteroid injections, may be considered after failure of initial conservative therapy. However, injections are not without risk, including plantar fascia rupture, loss of the fat pads of the feet causing significant pain and disability, and infection.

HELPFUL TIP:
Not all heel pain is plantar fasciitis. Remember these others: tarsal tunnel syndrome (described above), painful heel pad syndrome (pain located over the heel secondary to breakdown of fibrous septae from overuse and which may take up to 6 months to heal), and piezogenic papules (pain over medial/inferior aspect of heel, tender papules noted when patient standing).

▶ **Objectives: Did you learn to …**
  • Diagnose plantar fasciitis and consider other causes of heel and foot pain?
  • Describe the natural history of and treatments for plantar fasciitis?

 QUICK QUIZ: HAND INJURIES

A "gamekeeper's thumb" would likely be seen as the result of which of the following injuries?
A) Fall on an outstretched hand
B) Crush injury, for example, between two pieces of machinery
C) Fall by a skier using a ski pole
D) Excessive electronic gaming (e.g., Nintendo and Xbox)
E) Fall from a mountain bike

The correct answer is "C." A gamekeeper's thumb is defined as an injury (partial or complete tear) of the ulnar collateral ligament of the first MCP joint. This injury can occur with a valgus force on the thumb, which may occur when falling with a ski pole. Plain films should be obtained to evaluate for fracture. Treatment is immobilization of the thumb, such as with a thumb spica splint. Displaced fractures and/or the presence of a Stener lesion (when a piece of the torn ulnar collateral ligament displaces superficially to the adductor pollicis aponeurosis, preventing healing of the ligament) will require surgical referral. "Gamer's thumb," "D," is a repetitive use syndrome caused by playing (appropriately enough) video games. It is an overuse syndrome often presenting with swelling at the base of the thumb.

 QUICK QUIZ: ELBOW FRACTURE

The most specific finding on radiograph for a radial head fracture is:
A) Anterior fat pad sign
B) Posterior fat pad sign
C) Trousseau sign
D) Medial fat pad sign

The correct answer is "B." The posterior fat pad sign, which indicates an effusion in the joint, is the most **specific** of the findings for a radial head fracture. An **anterior** fat pad sign is the most sensitive. Figure 12-9 demonstrates both the anterior and posterior fat pad signs. There is no medial fat pad sign, and Trousseau sign is related to hypocalcemia and is carpal spasm with arterial occlusion (as with a blood pressure cuff).

 QUICK QUIZ: RADIAL HEAD FRACTURE

The proper treatment of a nondisplaced, fractured radial head is:
A) Internal fixation
B) Sling with early mobilization
C) Short-arm cast
D) Long-arm cast

The correct answer is "B." For a nondisplaced radial head fracture, the treatment is simply a sling for comfort and early mobilization. Mobilization is especially important to avoid a stiff elbow. Orthopedic referral should be considered if there is any sense of a mechanical block to the elbow motion.

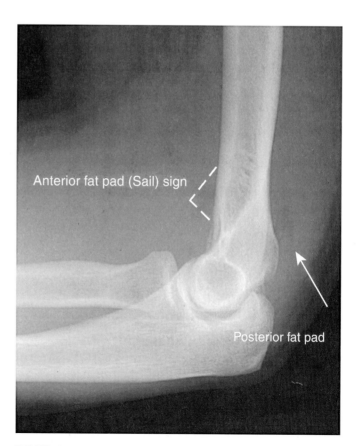

FIGURE 12-9. Fat Pad Signs in the Elbow.

QUICK QUIZ: PEDIATRIC FRACTURES

The most common elbow fracture in the pediatric population with a positive "fat pad sign" but no obvious fracture on x-ray is:
A) Radial head fracture
B) Supracondylar fracture
C) Medial condyle fracture
D) Lateral condyle fracture
E) Olecranon fracture

The correct answer is "B." Although in adults the most common occult elbow fracture is of the radial head, in the pediatric population it is a supracondylar fracture. These may be significantly displaced, but if nondisplaced they can be very subtle and the only sign of a fracture may be a displaced posterior (or anterior) fat pad.

 QUICK QUIZ: HIP PAIN

A 76-year-old female nursing home resident is brought to clinic after rolling out of bed last night. She is normally able to ambulate independently, but today cannot bear weight due to pain in her hip. She has significant hip tenderness and pain with any movement of her leg. She is unable to perform a SLR secondary to pain. Plain x-rays of her pelvis and hip are read as osteopenia with no obvious fracture.

What is the most appropriate next step?
A) Conservative treatment with acetaminophen and bed rest until able to ambulate
B) Admission for observation
C) Hip MRI
D) Physical therapy
E) Fentanyl patch

The correct answer is "C." The patient may have an occult hip fracture. Rates of occult hip fractures range from 2% to 10% of all hip fractures. To miss the diagnosis of a hip fracture may lead to displacement of the fracture and a worse outcome. Both CT and MRI can be used to evaluate for occult fracture, but most studies indicate that MRI has a greater sensitivity.

▶ CASE 12.21

A 45-year-old female hospital clerk presents with bilateral aching pain in the forearms and thenar eminences. The pain is made worse with driving and typing. She also has intermittent numbness over the same areas. She tried to ignore the symptoms, but today she dropped her coffee mug on her computer keyboard and became alarmed at her loss

of strength. She has hypothyroidism and is obese, but she reports that her health is otherwise good.

Question 12.21.1 Based on the history alone, which of the following is the most likely diagnosis?
A) Carpal tunnel syndrome
B) Osteoarthritis
C) Ulnar neuropathy
D) Diabetic neuropathy
E) Stroke

Answer 12.21.1 The correct answer is "A." Carpal tunnel syndrome is due to median nerve entrapment in the carpal tunnel of the wrist. Typical symptoms include numbness, paresthesias, and pain at the palmar/radial aspect of the hand, quintessentially the thenar eminence. In more severe or long-lasting cases, you may see atrophy of the thenar eminence. Patients may also develop weakness of thumb opposition. Osteoarthritis of the wrists does not usually cause nerve symptoms, but can cause spondylosis and nerve root impingement on occasion. Ulnar neuropathy involves the ulnar aspect of the hand, especially the fourth and fifth fingers, rather than the radial aspect, which is involved with carpal tunnel syndrome. Diabetic neuropathy typically presents in the feet since they are innervated by the longest nerves in the body. *Note:* This could represent cervical disk disease as well, especially given that it is bilateral.

Phalen sign is positive (placing the wrists in a flexed position causes aching and numbness in the median nerve distribution).

Question 12.21.2 What is the best next step in the continuing evaluation and management of this patient?
A) Nerve conduction studies
B) Radiograph of the wrist
C) MRI of the cervical spine
D) Orthopedic referral
E) Initiation of treatment

Answer 12.21.2 The correct answer is "E." In a clear-cut case of carpal tunnel syndrome, there is no need for further studies. If the diagnosis is in doubt, electromyogram and nerve conduction studies (EMG-NCS) may be of benefit. If the ROM in the wrist is limited, x-rays may be helpful. At this point in time, MRI and orthopedic referral are not likely to add much.

Question 12.21.3 Which of the following IS NOT associated with carpal tunnel syndrome?
A) Hypothyroidism
B) Diabetes mellitus
C) Amyloidosis
D) Polycythemia vera
E) Rheumatoid arthritis

Answer 12.21.3 The correct answer is "D." All of the above are associated with carpal tunnel syndrome except for polycythemia vera. Polycythemia vera can cause erythromelalgia which is a burning pain of the hands and feet associated with erythema, pallor, or cyanosis. It responds to aspirin. Other conditions associated with carpal tunnel syndrome include pregnancy, menopause, obesity, acromegaly, and end-stage renal disease. The point here is that patients with carpal tunnel syndrome should have a systemic cause ruled out, either clinically or with labs.

Question 12.21.4 What is the most appropriate initial treatment?
A) Thumb spica splint
B) Steroid injection
C) NSAIDs and neutral position wrist splints
D) Short-arm casts
E) Bilateral figure-of-eight splints

Answer 12.21.4 The correct answer is "C." Conservative therapy should be initiated first, unless there is some compelling reason for more aggressive therapy (e.g., severe weakness of the hands and loss of function). Most patients respond well to NSAIDs and the use of neutral position splints. The traditional cock-up splints are not as effective as neutral position splints. The splints should be worn at night. The patient may wear the splints during the day, too, but should take them off for several hours per day to avoid disuse muscle atrophy. "A" is incorrect since a thumb spica is not needed. "B," steroid injection, might be tried if initial conservative measures fail. However, the benefit is generally limited to 1 month. "D" is just wrong—don't cast patients with carpal tunnel syndrome! "E" is a terrible idea as well since a bilateral figure-of-eight splint is basically a straight jacket.

HELPFUL TIP:
Oral and injectable steroids have been used for carpal tunnel with limited success. Unfortunately, most modalities (NSAIDs, splints, steroids, etc.) are no better than placebo in randomized trials.

HELPFUL TIP:
Phalen and Tinel signs are crude tools at best. Tinel sign, which is a painful sensation of the fingers induced by percussion of the median nerve at the level of the carpal tunnel, may be positive, but is only 50% sensitive (flip a coin) and 54% specific. Phalen sign, keeping both wrists in a palmar-flexed position, may reproduce symptoms. Sensitivity varies from 10% to 88% depending on study; its specificity is 80%.

▶ **Objectives: Did you learn to …**
- Diagnose carpal tunnel syndrome and consider other causes of wrist pain?
- Manage a patient with carpal tunnel syndrome?

QUICK QUIZ: CASTING

A few days ago, your partner placed a cast on the arm of a 20-year-old male for a distal radial fracture. He calls your office today, when your partner has gone fishing (darn her, anyway). The patient is complaining of increasing pain and numbness of his fingers in the casted arm.

Which course of action is most appropriate?
A) Have the patient follow up tomorrow, when your partner is back in the office
B) Send the patient to the emergency room for compressive Doppler examination of the arm to rule out venous thrombosis
C) Ask the patient to come to clinic to have the cast replaced
D) Tell the patient that these are expected symptoms and advise him to take some aspirin
E) Recommend that he have his cast signed by as many friends as possible to take his mind of these clearly psychosomatic symptoms

The correct answer is "C." This patient has symptoms that are most likely due to an improperly fitted cast. The problem here could be vascular compromise, nerve compression, or a compartment syndrome. He should be seen without delay to evaluate for these, and the cast should be adjusted or replaced. The cast can be bivalved or have a window cut into it, then be observed for improvement in symptoms if the cast does not need to be completely removed to rule out the pathology noted above.

▶ **CASE 12.22**

A 30-year-old new mom presents to your office with back pain, pubic pain, fatigue, sore nipples, and fatigue, saying, "This mom stuff is rough!" However, what she really wants to address is her wrist pain. She has pain with lifting her daughter, doing the laundry (which never stops, by the way), carrying the car seat, and breastfeeding. Pain is at the base of the thumb and radiates up the arm. On exam, you can feel crepitus as she flexes and extends the thumb. Pain is exacerbated by ulnar deviation of the wrist when she is gripping her thumb (positive Finkelstein test).

Question 12.22.1 What is the most likely diagnosis?
A) Triangular fibrocartilage complex (TFCC) injury/tear
B) Extensor carpi ulnaris tendinitis
C) Intersection syndrome
D) De Quervain's tenosynovitis

Answer 12.22.1 The correct answer is "D." De Quervain's is a tendinosis of the abductor pollicis longus (APL) and/or extensor pollicis brevis (EPB) that often present in the setting of wrist overuse (although it can occur out of the blue). It is more common in women and during the postpartum period. Feeling crepitus over the tendons makes the diagnosis in this case but is not required finding. A positive Finkelstein's test is the classic physical exam finding (have the patient grip their own thumb and ulnar deviate, which will cause exquisite pain). "A," a triangular fibrocartilage complex (TFCC) tear usually occurs in the setting of a fall on an outstretched hand (FOOSH) injury and presents similar to a meniscus tear of the knee with painful clicking and catching *on the ulnar side of the wrist.* For TFCC tears, the tenderness is distal to the ulnar styloid. Extensor carpi ulnaris (ECU) tendinitis ("B") causes pain on the ulnar side of the wrist and the tendon can be palpated on the dorsal aspect of the ulnar wrist. ECU pain is often caused by repetitive motion (tennis, squash). The patient will have worsening of the pain with resisted supination and will be tender over the tendon. "C," intersection syndrome can present similarly to de Quervain, but the pain is several centimeters proximal to the wrist joint and not at the base of the thumb. The pain is on the dorsal side of the forearm.

Question 12.22.2 How would you initially treat this patient's de Quervain's tenosynovitis?

A) Steroid injection in the area of the tendon
B) Thumb spica splint
C) Give up the infant for adoption, thus removing stress on the tendons
D) NSAIDs as needed
E) A, B, and D

Answer 12.22.2 **The correct answer is "E."** Treatment is immobilization in a thumb spica, NSAIDs for pain, and injectable steroids. Be realistic—splinting and NSAIDs often have a low success rate in patients with moderate-to-severe pain. Some practitioners use injectable steroids as first-line. Surgery can be done in recalcitrant cases.

HELPFUL TIP:
For wrist pain, it helps to know where it hurts.
• Diffuse pain at the dorsal aspect: think of osteoarthritis (OA)
• Ulnar side pain: ECU tendinitis, chronic TFCC injury
• Radial side pain: OA of the wrist or base of the thumb, de Quervain's tenosynovitis, intersection syndrome

▶ **Objectives: Did you learn to …**
• Diagnose de Quervain's tenosynovitis and consider other causes of wrist pain?
• Manage a patient with de Quervain's tenosynovitis?

 QUICK QUIZ: AN ULTRA PAIN IN THE FOOT

A 30-year-old ultra-marathon runner presents to your office after an unusually long training block of 200 miles in the last week… that's a lot of books on tape! She complains of pain in the distal right foot. Pain is diffuse over the second and third metatarsal heads and does not radiate. On exam, she has a large, firm callus under the second metatarsal head. There is no swelling or redness over the joint. Pain is not reproduced with lateral compression over the distal metatarsal region. Her gait is normal and her arches are well supported. The second digit has a bit of a hammertoe deformity. Her x-rays are normal.

Based on the presentation, which of the following is true about her diagnosis?

A) This is most consistent with a Morton's neuroma and a corticosteroid injection might help
B) This is a stress fracture and she should cancel her registration for her upcoming event the "Death on Two Legs Ultramarathon"
C) She suffers from mania, and you should start lithium
D) This is metatarsalgia, and the treatment is conservative including RICE and a metatarsal pad/lift to take the pressure off the area

The correct answer is "D." In this case her callus (indicating increased load and friction) and her hammertoe (which further drives the metatarsal head down) are contributing to the biomechanical overload of the area and pain. Metatarsalgia is not just a running injury but can present in many patients and is considered an overuse injury. Patients with metatarsalgia are generally tender over the metatarsal head and may complain that they feel as though they are walking on a stone or rock. The treatment is, as noted in answer "D," a metatarsal lift or pad. Changing shoes may also help. Occasionally, in severe cases, boot immobilization and/or crutches will be needed to cool things off. "A," Morton's neuroma, typically presents with neuropathic pain that radiates into the toes. The squeeze test done by lateral compression across the metatarsals can reproduce the pain associated with Morton's neuroma. Stress fracture is also a possibility in this patient, given her mileage, and can be hard to differentiate from metatarsalgia. If you are concerned and need an answer right away, start with an x-ray, but you may need an MRI as x-rays miss a lot of these.

 QUICK QUIZ: EXERCISE PRESCRIPTION

Which of the following is true regarding current exercise recommendations for general health and disease prevention?

A) Patients should get at least 30 minutes of moderate intensity exercise five or more times per week
B) As an alternative to moderate intensity exercise, patients can get 20 minutes of high-intensity exercise three to four times per week
C) For older adults, 2 to 3 days per week of resistance training is recommended
D) For kids age 6 years and older, AAP recommends 60 minutes of moderate-to-vigorous activity daily
E) All of the above are true

The correct answer is "E." This is an important topic as obesity and inactivity rates have skyrocketed. Obesity is currently the fourth leading cause of death in the United States. More than 56%

of adults do not meet the recommended amount of exercise, and 36% of adults do no exercise at all. This costs our healthcare system over $300 per person per year and over $100 billion dollars annually. When suggesting exercise, recommend a warm-up period and a cool-down period. Remember the mnemonic "FITT":

Frequency: at least 3 days per week to start and build up from there

Intensity: moderate to intense effort (but remember to build up to this ... nobody will keep it up if you start them doing wind sprints on the first day)

Time: ideally 30 minutes or more five times per week, but this can be broken up in other ways, and the target of 150 minutes per week works better for some patients

Type: involve major muscle groups (walking, core training, weights, bicycling, etc.)

Moderate exercise is defined as 50% to 70% of your maximum heart rate, such as a brisk walk. Shorter bouts of more intense exercise have the same benefit as longer slower regiments. Patients can break exercise into shorter blocks throughout the day if that works better (e.g., walking rapidly for 10 minutes three times per day). Contrary to popular belief, resistance training also has cardiovascular benefit (*Mayo Clinic Proc.* 2017;92:1214–1222).

> **HELPFUL TIP:**
> So, what's your excuse? Take a study break and get out there. Exercise is good for your brain! Also, it has been shown that inactive and overweight doctors are less likely to prescribe exercise.

Clinical Pearls

- Do not let the presence of calcium pyrophosphate crystals or uric acid dissuade you from suspecting septic arthritis as both gout and pseudogout commonly coexist with septic arthritis.

- Do not routinely order plain films for low-back pain unless trauma, abnormal physical examination findings, or "red flag" symptoms are present.

- Do not routinely screen for scoliosis in asymptomatic adolescents.

- Maintain a high suspicion for a scaphoid fracture if there is trauma with snuffbox tenderness present.

- To achieve faster recovery, recommend early mobilization for low-back pain and ankle sprains.

- Maintain a high degree of suspicion for the orthopedic emergencies of septic arthritis and cauda equina syndrome.

- Avoid knee arthroscopy as initial therapy for meniscal tears.

- Do not prescribe opioids for chronic musculoskeletal pain as first-line therapy. Opioids should only be used as a last resort—if at all—and monitored closely.

- Use the Ottawa Ankle, Knee, or Foot Criteria to determine whether plain films are needed for evaluation of ankle, knee, or foot injuries.

BIBLIOGRAPHY

Alshryda S, et al. Acute fractures of the scaphoid bone: systematic review and meta-analysis. *The Surgeon.* 2012:10(4):218–229.

Aminoshariae A, Khan A. Acetaminophen: old drug, new issues. *J Endod.* 2015;41(5):588–593.

Dartness J, et al. Haematolgenous acute and subacute paediatric osteomyelitis. *J Bone Joint Surg Br.* 2012;94-B:584–595.

DeVries JG, et al. The fifth metatarsal base: anatomic evaluation regarding fracture mechanism and treatment algorithms. *J Foot Ankle Surg.* 2015;54:94–98.

Dixit S, et al. Management of patellofemoral pain syndrome. *Am Fam Physician.* 2007;75(2):194.

Griffin LY, et al. eds. *Essentials of Musculoskeletal Care.* 3rd ed. Rosemont, IL: American Academy of Orthopaedic Surgeons; 2005.

Margaretten ME, et al. Does this adult patient have septic arthritis? *JAMA.* 2007;297(13):1478–1488.

McCrory, et al. Consensus statement on concussion in sport: the 5th international conference on concussion in sport help in Berlin, October, 2016. *BJSM.* 2017;51:838–847.

McGillicuddy DC, et al. How sensitive is the synovial fluid white blood cell count in diagnosing septic arthritis? *Am J Emerg Med.* 2007;25(7):749–752.

Mirabelli, et al. The preparticipation sports evaluation. *Am Fam Physician.* 2015;92 (5):371–376.

Osmon DR, et al. Diagnosis and management of prosthetic joint infection: clinical practice guidelines by the Infectious Disease Society of America. *Clin Infect Dis.* 2013;56(1):e1–e25.

Reid D, et al. Acromioclavicular Joint Separations grades I-III: a review of the literature and development of best practice guidelines. *Sports Med.* 2012;42(8):681–696.

Rixe JA, et al. A review of the management of patellofemoral pain syndrome. *Phys Sportsmed.* 2013;41(3):19–28.

Rutz E, Spoerri M. Septic arthritis of the paediatric hip: a review of current diagnostic approaches and therapeutic concepts. *Acta Orthop Belg.* 2013;79(2):123–134.

Sawyer JR, Kapoor M. The limping child: a systematic approach to diagnosis. *Am Fam Physician.* 2009;79(3):215.

Simons R, Sherman S, eds. *Emergency Orthopedics.* 6th ed. New York, NY: McGraw-Hill Professional; 2010.

Simpson MR. Tendinopathies of the foot and ankle. *Am Fam Physician.* 2009;80(10):1107.

Steill IG, et al. Prospective validation of a decision rule for the use of radiography in acute knee injuries. *JAMA.* 1996;275:611.

Will JS, et al. Mechanical low back pain. *Am Fam Physician.* 2018;98(7):421–428.

Wilson JJ, Best TM. Common overuse tendon problems: a review and recommendations for treatment. *Am Fam Physician.* 2005;72(5):811–818.

Pediatrics

Guru V. Bhoojhawon and Patrick J. McCarthy

CASE 13.1

A 6-year-old male presents to your office with his mom. He has been soiling his underwear frequently and it is causing stress at home and school. His parents are frustrated and think he is old enough to know better. At school, he is being teased and being called "stinky pants." He reports feeling embarrassed. Mom asks you if there is something medically wrong with him.

Question 13.1.1 What percentage of chronic encopresis is functional (meaning no underlying medical or organic cause)?
A) 10%
B) 25%
C) 50%
D) 75%
E) 90%

Answer 13.1.1 The correct answer is "E." Ninety percent of chronic encopresis is functional. Functional encopresis is the repeated involuntary passage of stool into underwear in a child who is 4 years of age or older and at a developmental level appropriate for toilet training in the absence of an underlying medical cause. The most common reason is retentive constipation with overflow incontinence. Frequently, the child has an associated psychological problem. Boys are affected more often than girls. Children with this disorder withhold feces voluntarily thereby avoiding defecating. As stool stays in the colon, more water is absorbed, creating harder stool that is more difficult to pass. This leads to a self-perpetuating cycle. The excess stool stretches the rectum with eventual loss of sensation to defecate. Liquid stool may leak around the impacted mass, which parents often mistake as diarrhea. In some, a triggering event, such as passage of a painful stool leading to fear of stooling, forced toilet training before the child is ready, or sexual abuse, may have occurred. Often, children will dislike using public toilets, leading to voluntary holding, inciting the functional constipation cycle. A common theme is parental misunderstanding of the problem, thinking it is due to an undiagnosed medical condition, attention-seeking behavior, or child laziness.

HELPFUL TIP:
Some definitions ... **Non-retentive encopresis** is the *voluntary* stooling of one's pants. Once a medical cause has been ruled out, this is purely a behavioral or psychiatric problem. **Primary encopresis** is when stool continence has never been achieved. **Secondary encopresis** occurs when accidents began after a period of successful toilet training.

Question 13.1.2 Which of the following conditions is(are) associated with encopresis?
A) Urinary tract infections
B) Enuresis
C) Social isolation
D) Attention-deficit hyperactivity disorder (ADHD)
E) All of the above

Answer 13.1.2 The correct answer is "E." Encopresis is an independent risk factor for urinary tract infections. Feces in the underwear allows for close contact with the urethra and introduction of bacteria. Chronic contracting of pelvic floor muscles to withhold stool may lead to dysfunctional voiding and urinary stasis. Enuresis occurs in up to 40% of patients with chronic constipation. A mass of stool in the rectum can compress the bladder leading to uncontrolled voiding. The chronic odor of feces makes socialization rough and teasing frequent. ADHD frequently is associated with functional constipation and encopresis due to other stimuli diverting the child's attention from the urge to defecate.

HELPFUL TIP:
Encopresis or daytime enuresis should prompt you to rule out a spinal cord lesion with a detailed examination and further imaging, such as an MRI, if indicated by examination.

Question 13.1.3 Which of the following is(are) medical (organic) cause(s) of constipation?
A) Hypothyroidism
B) Hypercalcemia
C) Cystic fibrosis
D) Lead poisoning
E) All of the above

Answer 13.1.3 **The correct answer is "E."** All of the above can cause constipation and fecal incontinence. Organic causes account for only 5% to 10% of encopresis cases and can be anatomical (anteriorly displaced anus), neurological (Hirschsprung disease), immunologic (celiac disease), or iatrogenic (medications such as narcotics or anticholinergics). The first step in evaluating a child with encopresis is to rule out an underlying medical condition starting with a good history and physical examination. Do not forget to ask about timing of meconium passage in the past medical history, as delayed meconium passage may suggest cystic fibrosis or Hirschsprung disease. Rectal examination is useful to evaluate rectal sphincter tone and assess for fecal impaction. Look at the back for signs of an occult spina bifida such as sacral dimple or hair tuft. Lack of anal wink, cremasteric reflex, or deep tendon reflexes is suggestive of a neurologic cause. Often a painful fissure may initiate a vicious cycle of pain with stooling, leading to the withholding of stool, and leading to even more painful defecation, etc.

HELPFUL TIP:
Fecal impaction is a clinical diagnosis made by feeling a hard stool mass on rectal examination. It is not made by abdominal x-ray. Though guidelines do not recommend the *routine* use of digital rectal exams in diagnostic evaluation *of functional constipation,* if a fecal impaction is suspected, a rectal examination must be done. Yes … a rectal examination on a child. No one's happy about it, but it can be performed comfortably with lubrication and proper positioning (i.e. knee-chest positioning).

HELPFUL TIP:
Abuse may be a triggering event for constipation and encopresis. If abuse is suspected, contact child protective services.

Question 13.1.4 All of the following are useful in the treatment of functional encopresis EXCEPT:
A) Polyethylene glycol (PEG) 3350 (MiraLAX®)
B) Oral sodium phosphate solution (OsmoPrep)
C) Mineral oil
D) Lactulose
E) Milk of magnesia

Answer 13.1.4 **The correct answer is "B."** In 2008, the FDA placed a black box warning on oral sodium phosphate solutions due to risk of acute kidney injury from deposition of calcium phosphate crystals. As a result, oral non-phosphate-containing medications are frequently used. Treatment begins with disimpaction with enemas or with an oral medication such as PEG 3350 (MiraLAX®) or mineral oil. Many treatment guidelines prefer disimpaction using oral PEG 3350 (MiraLAX®) solutions over enemas or manual disimpaction. **Use of high-dose PEG 3350 (1.5 g/kg/day) or enemas for 6 consecutive days were equally effective in treating fecal impaction.** Manual disimpaction may be effective, but often requires general anesthesia in order to be tolerated. PEG 3350 (MiraLAX®) is generally preferred over enemas, given the widely accepted oral route of administration.

Treatment should be individualized. After disimpaction, patients require maintenance therapy (combination of medical, behavioral, dietary, and counseling). Evidence suggests that PEG 3350 (MiraLAX®) is most effective for maintenance therapy, though lactulose, milk of magnesia, or mineral oil may also be used. PEG 3350 (MiraLAX®) 0.2 to 0.8 g/kg/day should be initiated and incrementally increased until the patient is having regular, soft bowel movements. The normal recommended daily allowance of fiber and fluid intake should be encouraged. Behaviorally, the child should sit on the toilet with active pushing after each meal to make use of the gastrocolic reflex. Even if the child does not stool, they are learning to use the toilet and training their bowels. Use of a footstool may improve Valsalva maneuvers (kinda like the McRobert's maneuver!). A sticker chart can give visual reinforcement. Families need to understand that there is no quick fix and relapse is common (about 50%). It takes months for the rectum to return to normal size and sensation. But it may comfort readers to know that one of your editors witnessed a 19-cm colonic distention return to normal after aggressive use of PEG 3350; so, it happens. Patients who fail to improve after 6 months of compliant treatment should be referred to a pediatric gastroenterologist.

HELPFUL TIP:
Remember never to use mineral oil enterally in any child who is at risk of aspiration. It can cause a chemical pneumonitis.

▶ **Objectives: Did you learn to …**
  • Describe encopresis, including its presentation, diagnosis, and causes?
  • Differentiate between organic and nonorganic causes of encopresis?
  • Medically manage constipation and encopresis?

QUICK QUIZ: NEONATAL POLYCYTHEMIA

Causes of neonatal polycythemia (central venous hematocrit of 65% or greater) in the immediate postpartum period include all of the following EXCEPT:
A) Delayed umbilical cord clamping
B) Twin–twin transfusion

C) Congenital adrenal hyperplasia
D) Maternal diabetes
E) Sepsis

The correct answer is "E." Neonatal polycythemia can be caused by all of the above except for sepsis. Other causes include chronic intrauterine hypoxia (e.g., mother is a heavy smoker), intrauterine growth restriction, maternal hypertension, congenital hypothyroidism, and chromosomal abnormalities (e.g., trisomy 21, 18, and 13).

 QUICK QUIZ: MORE ON NEONATAL POLYCYTHEMIA

Patients with neonatal polycythemia are at risk for hyperviscosity syndrome including respiratory distress, hypoxia, cyanosis, hyperbilirubinemia, and hypoglycemia. Heart failure, stroke, renal vein thrombosis, and necrotizing enterocolitis may also occur.

The best treatment for these patients is:
A) Phlebotomy
B) Exchange transfusion with normal RBCs
C) Exchange transfusion using D5W
D) Exchange transfusion using normal saline
E) Aspirin

The correct answer is "D." Partial exchange transfusion using normal saline is the treatment of choice. "A" is incorrect since phlebotomy alone will reduce overall circulating volume and may exacerbate the problem. "B" is incorrect. If you chose this, back home for you! What is the point of taking out cells and then putting more in? "C" is incorrect because large amounts of D5W can cause fluid shifts, electrolyte abnormalities, cerebral edema, and hemolysis. Isotonic solution, such as normal saline, would be appropriate. Of note, patients with a hematocrit of 65% to 70% can be observed if they are asymptomatic. Samples obtained via heel-stick may have a falsely elevated hematocrit and should be confirmed with a venous draw. There is no one-to-one predictable relationship between hematocrit and blood viscosity. Also of note, there is no evidence that long-term outcomes are improved in *asymptomatic* patients with partial exchange transfusion versus observation.

▶ **CASE 13.2**

Amy, a 4-day-old infant, is brought to clinic because "she is yellow." She was born at term to a 25-year-old woman. Maternal lab results are as follows: blood type A+, syphilis negative, rubella immune, group B streptococcus (GBS) negative. Amy has been breastfeeding every 3 to 5 hours. She has had one stool and three wet diapers per day. Her weight is 15% less than her birth weight. On your examination, you notice jaundice from the head to the thighs. Her total bilirubin level is 21.6 mg/dL. The conjugated (direct) fraction is 0.4 mg/dL.

Question 13.2.1 **Of the following, the infant most likely is experiencing:**
A) Breastfeeding failure jaundice
B) Physiologic jaundice
C) Biliary atresia; you must consult pediatric gastroenterology
D) Alloimmune hemolysis due to ABO incompatibility

Answer 13.2.1 **The correct answer is "A."** Amy most likely has breastfeeding failure jaundice (often referred to as "breastfeeding jaundice"). *This occurs within the first several days of birth* before the mother's milk supply is adequate. This must be distinguished from **breast milk jaundice,** which **usually occurs later** without evidence of dehydration. One sign that Amy is not receiving adequate breast milk feedings—and that this is **breastfeeding failure** jaundice instead of breast milk jaundice—is the fact that she is 15% below birth weight, having fewer than six wet diapers per day and fewer than two to five stools a day. Remember that a well-hydrated infant of Amy's age should generally lose no more than 10% of birth weight. You should try to evaluate the mother's milk supply by asking about the mother's feeling of engorgement, feeling of breast emptying with feeding, seeing milk on the infant's lips and tongue immediately after feeding, and hearing the infants swallow with feedings. "B" is incorrect. Even though physiologic jaundice peaks at this age, the level of 21.6 mg/dL is higher than would be expected with physiologic jaundice (which should not be higher than 17 mg/dL in a term infant). "C" is incorrect because biliary atresia presents with **conjugated** hyperbilirubinemia (the liver can appropriately conjugate bilirubin, but there is obstruction to the outflow of the conjugated bilirubin—essentially an obstructive process). "D" is incorrect because ABO incompatibility is unlikely in a mother whose blood type is something other than O (who can make both anti-A and anti-B antibodies). In addition, Rh incompatibility is impossible due to the mother being Rh+. However, minor antigen incompatibility remains a possibility.

 HELPFUL TIP:
Causes of an elevated direct (conjugated) bilirubin: infection (including congenital), metabolic abnormalities (cystic fibrosis, galactosemia, Dubin–Johnson and Rotor syndromes, glycogen storage disease, etc.), anatomic abnormalities (biliary atresia, etc.), and cholestasis (especially from total parental nutrition). Note that *conjugated bilirubin does not cause kernicterus.* To remember this, think about conjugated molecules being bigger and thus not able to cross the blood-brain barrier.
Causes of an elevated indirect (unconjugated) bilirubin: increased breakdown of RBCs (ABO/Rh incompatibility, cephalohematoma, thalassemias, etc.), prematurity, hypothyroidism. Basically, overwhelming the liver from RBC breakdown.

Question 13.2.2 Which of the following is NOT a risk factor for severe neonatal hyperbilirubinemia?
A) Exclusive breastfeeding
B) Gestational age ≥41 weeks
C) Significant birth trauma
D) Visible jaundice in first 24 hours of life
E) East Asian race

Answer 13.2.2 **The correct answer is "B."** Post-dates gestational age is not associated with jaundice. Rather, premature infants are at a greater risk of jaundice. "A" is true, and exclusively formula-fed infants are less likely to have severe hyperbilirubinemia (but this is not a reason to recommend bottle feeding). Cephalohematoma and large bruises result in increased bilirubin production from heme breakdown, so "C" is true. The earlier jaundice occurs, the higher the peak is likely to be, so "D" is also true. Other major risk factors for severe hyperbilirubinemia include: a sibling who required phototherapy, East Asian race, and blood group incompatibility.

HELPFUL TIP:
Infants with total serum bilirubin levels >5 mg/dL typically have visible jaundice. The jaundice usually starts at the head and progresses distally to the feet. It resolves in the opposite pattern with the distal extremities resolving first.

HELPFUL TIP:
Jaundice present in the first 24 hours of life is pathologic and usually due to hemolytic disease such as ABO incompatibility.

Amy's CBC is unremarkable and blood type is A+.

Question 13.2.3 Which of the following is the most appropriate initial treatment for this patient (remember the *conjugated [direct]* fraction is 0.4 mg/dL)?
A) Admission for exchange transfusion
B) Admission for IV fluids alone to improve hydration
C) Admission for phototherapy
D) Discharge to home with recommendations for formula feeding, light exposure, and follow-up bilirubin tomorrow

Answer 13.2.3 **The correct answer is "C."** Amy should be treated with intensive phototherapy, given her level of hyperbilirubinemia that exceeds the recommended threshold. "A" is incorrect because the infant does not meet exchange transfusion threshold. Even if mildly above exchange threshold, some providers may attempt intensive phototherapy first if the infant does not have signs of bilirubin encephalopathy. An exchange transfusion would follow if phototherapy failed to lower the bilirubin level or signs of acute bilirubin encephalopathy developed. "B" is incorrect since phototherapy is the definitive

treatment. Adjunctive therapy with intravenous fluids is considered if weight loss exceeds 12% of birth weight. "D" is incorrect because the serum bilirubin level is above threshold for hospital admission and phototherapy. You should not recommend putting the baby in sunlight, as the ultraviolet radiation exposure is an unacceptable risk.

HELPFUL TIP:
The American Academy of Pediatrics (AAP) has established threshold values for hyperbilirubinemia treatment with phototherapy and exchange transfusion. Decisions regarding treatment vary depending on the infant's risk, age (in hours after delivery), gestational age, and total bilirubin level. There are graphs, tables, and nomograms (such as the Bhutani curve) to assist with decision-making. A free decision-making tool is available online (http://www.bilitool.org/).

You admit Amy for further management. You confirm Amy's current weight, which is indeed down 15% from birth weight. Children often lose weight after birth while effective feeding is being established.

Question 13.2.4 Beyond what point in time is it considered problematic if the patient has not returned to his or her birth weight?
A) 5 days
B) 7 days
C) 10 days
D) 14 days
E) None of the above. Don't worry, be happy.

Answer 13.2.4 **The correct answer is "D."** Children should regain their birth weight by age 2 weeks. If they don't, it isn't always abnormal, however. Fourteen percent of infants resulting from vaginal deliveries and 24% of Cesarean babies will not regain their birthweight by 14 days (*Pediatrics* 2016 Dec; 138:e2016–2625). Nonetheless, a detailed feeding history and evaluation of breastfeeding adequacy (if breastfed) and assessment of health and social situation should be performed.

Amy does well under your care (and the bili lights) and returns at 2 months of age for her well-baby visit. Mom questions the need for immunizations, reasoning, "We never see these archaic diseases anymore—I mean, come on, I can't even find a chicken pox party." Plus, she's read information on the Internet and has concerns about immunization safety. And wasn't there a study about kids who suffered autism because of thimerosal in a vaccine? And another study that vaccines transformed children into space aliens? Unfortunately, Amy's mother's concerns are not unusual. Parents—and ill-informed politicians—often harbor misconceptions about vaccinations.

Question 13.2.5 What is a common side effect that Amy might have after her immunizations at her 2-month visit?
A) Fever to 104°F
B) Autism
C) Diabetes
D) Erythema at the site of immunization
E) Symptomatic shedding of virus in her stool

Answer 13.2.5 The correct answer is "D." Vaccine side effects, such as **low-grade fevers** (not to 104°F as in "A"), induration and redness at the site, and fussiness are common. However, they are self-limited. "B" and "C" are incorrect. Autism and diabetes **have NOT** been linked to vaccines in **many large, well-designed studies**. "E" is incorrect because the DTaP, HIB, and IPV vaccines are inactivated. Thus, the virus or bacteria is killed and purified for a specific component. The hepatitis B vaccine is constructed with genetic engineering in a yeast cell. Thus, one would not shed virus in the stool. *The MMR, oral polio, oral rotavirus, and varicella vaccines are live attenuated vaccines.* With these immunizations, the virus has been weakened but can still replicate and be shed. In an immunocompetent host, this usually is not of clinical significance. Thus, "E" is incorrect. In patients who have an immunodeficient state (either innate or iatrogenic, such as immunosuppression or chemotherapy), care must be taken with provision of live vaccines, as they may cause illness in a susceptible host. When in doubt, consult the CDC website and ask a specialist before giving live vaccines! Also, oral polio vaccine is no longer used in the United States because the risk of disease from the vaccine is greater than the risk of disease from wild-type polio; IM polio vaccine only, please.

HELPFUL TIP:
The article "linking" MMR vaccine to autism was withdrawn by the authors (and *Lancet*) years ago, and the lead author (Andrew Wakefield) has lost his medical license because of fraudulent data. *He* turned out to be a space alien bent on world conquest by infecting the earth. Despite this there are continued misconstrued thoughts about vaccines.

Amy's mother accepts your advice but still has concerns.

Question 13.2.6 What other factually correct information can you share with her about vaccines at her 2-month visit?
A) Giving a child multiple vaccines at the same time weakens her immune system
B) The fever and rash side effects of the MMR are from the measles component and usually occur 1 week after the vaccine is given
C) If Amy receives her MMR at a 9-month visit (before she travels to visit Aunt Tilley who lives in an area where measles has re-surfaced due to lack of vaccination), her MMR immunization would be considered complete after this dose and another one at 5 years old

D) If Amy had an acute otitis media and fevers of 100.4°F, we should delay her immunizations until she is afebrile
E) Immunizations are not important, since these diseases are rare in the United States

Answer 13.2.6 The correct answer is "B." The measles component can cause a fever and rash 5 to 10 days after the immunization. This occurs in 5% to 15% of infants. Up to 25% of adults have arthralgias after receiving the vaccine and up to 10% develop arthritis. The MMR dosing schedule includes two doses of MMR. However, the first must be **after** 1 year of age. It may be given sooner if the child is at risk (such as with travel or with a measles outbreak) but must be **repeated after the first birthday**. Thus, "C" is incorrect. Minor illnesses should not prevent vaccination. True contraindications include anaphylactic reactions to a vaccine or vaccine constituent, moderate-to-severe febrile illness, and encephalopathy within 7 days of DTaP. Live virus vaccines are contraindicated in immunocompromised patients.

HELPFUL TIP:
As a general rule, if a patient misses a vaccine, just start up where you left off. There is no need to increase the number of vaccines given. If you have questions, you may consult the CDC website on catch-up immunization recommendations (and can even create a personalized catch-up schedule). There is a *free* app for that: Search the iPhone app store for "CDC immunizations." It is called "CDC Vaccine Schedule" (appropriately enough). There is also an Android version (same search words … though why you would want to immunize Androids is beyond us).

Amy continues her scheduled well-child examinations. At one of those visits, she was babbling and crawling around the office. She poked her fingers at the outlets (which thankfully were covered) and used a pincer grasp to pick up a raisin off the floor—at least, it looked like a raisin (ew, gross!).

Question 13.2.7 These behaviors are appropriate for the development of a child at approximately age:
A) 6 months
B) 9 months
C) 15 months
D) 24 months

Answer 13.2.7 The correct answer is "B." Take a moment to review the developmental milestones in Table 13-1. Children who are not meeting their milestones appropriately should be referred for developmental assessment and early intervention services. Note that premature infants' developmental stage may correspond with their corrected gestational age instead of their chronological age.

TABLE 13-1 DEVELOPMENTAL MILESTONES

Age	Gross Motor	Visual Motor	Language	Social
1 mo	Raises head slightly from prone, makes crawling movements, lifts chin up	Has tight grasp, follows to midline	Alert to sound (e.g., by blinking, moving, startling)	Regards face
2 mo	Holds head in midline, lifts chest off table	No longer clenches fist tightly, follows object past midline	Smiles after being stroked or talked to	Recognizes parent
3 mo	Supports on forearms in prone, holds head up steadily	Holds hands open at rest, follows in circular fashion	Coos (produces long vowel sounds in musical fashion)	Reaches for familiar people or objects, anticipates feeding
4–5 mo	Rolls front to back and back to front, sits well when propped, supports on wrists, and shifts weight	Moves arms in unison to grasp, touches cube placed on table	Orients to voice; 5 mo: orients to bell (localized laterally), says "ahgoo," razzes	Enjoys looking around environment
6 mo	Sits well unsupported, puts feet in mouth in supine position	Reaches with either hand, transfers, uses raking grasp	Babbles; 7 mo: orients to bell (localizes indirectly); 8 mo: "dada/mama" indiscriminately	Recognizes strangers
9 mo	Creeps, crawls, cruises, pulls to stand, pivots when sitting	Uses pincer grasp, probes with forefinger, holds bottle, finger-feeds	Understands "no," waves bye-bye; 10 mo: "dada/mama" discriminantly; 11 mo: one word other than "dada/mama"	Starts to explore environment, plays pat-a-cake
12 mo	Walks alone	Throws objects, let's go of toys, hand release, uses mature pincer grasp	Follows one-step command with gesture, uses 2 words other than "dada/mama"; 14 mo: uses 3 words	Imitates actions, comes when called, cooperates with dressing
15 mo	Creeps upstairs, walks backward	Builds tower of 2 blocks in imitation of examiner, scribbles in imitation	Follows one-step command without gesture, uses 4–6 words and immature jargon (runs several unintelligible words together)	Indicates some simple needs by pointing, hugs parents
18 mo	Runs, throws toy from standing without falling	Turns 2 or 3 pages at a time, fills spoon and feeds self	Knows 7–20 words, knows 1 body part, uses mature jargon (includes intelligible words in jargon)	Copies parent in tasks (e.g., sweeping, dusting), plays in company of other children
21 mo	Squats in play, goes up steps	Builds tower of 5 blocks, drinks well from cup	Points to 3 body parts, uses 2-word combinations, has 20 word vocabulary	Asks to have food and to go to toilet
24 mo	Walks up and down steps without help	Turns pages one at a time, removes shoes, pants, etc., imitates behavior of others	Uses 50 words, 2-word sentences, uses pronouns (I, you, me) inappropriately, points to 5 body parts, understands 2-step command	Parallel play
30 mo	Jumps with both feet off floor, throws ball overhand	Unbuttons, holds pencil in adult fashion, differentiates horizontal and vertical line	Uses pronouns (I, you, me) appropriately, understands concept of "one," repeats 2 digits forward	Tells first and last names when asked, gets drink without help
3 yr	Pedals tricycle, can alternate feet when going up steps	Dresses and undresses partially, dries hands if reminded, draws a circle	Uses 3-word sentences, plurals, and past tense. Knows all pronouns. Minimum of 250 words, understands concept of "two"	Group play, shares toys, takes turns, plays well with others, knows full name, age, sex
4 yr	Hops, skips, alternates feet going downstairs	Buttons clothing fully, catches ball	Knows colors, says song or poem from memory, asks questions	Tells "tall tales," plays cooperatively with a group of children
5yr	Skips, alternating feet, jumps over low obstacles	Ties shoes, spreads with knife	Prints first name, asks what a word means	Plays competitive games, abides by rules, likes to help in household tasks

Amy continues her scheduled well-child examinations. However, at 14 months old, mom brings Amy for a sick visit because she turned blue. After taking a complete history and doing a complete physical examination, you appropriately diagnose breath-holding spells.

Question 13.2.8 **Which of the following statements about breath-holding spells is true?**
A) The incidence of breath-holding spells for children between 6 months old and 6 years old is 50%
B) If a color change occurs, it occurs after loss of consciousness
C) Seizure-like activity may occur with breath-holding spells
D) A child typically takes 60 to 90 minutes to return to her baseline after a breath-holding spell
E) The evaluation should include an echocardiogram (ECG) and electroencephalogram (EEG)

Answer 13.2.8 **The correct answer is "C."** A typical breath-holding spell begins with an inciting event (like Santa did not bring the right toy or mom refused to buy a Happy Meal). Breath-holding spells occur in up to 4% of children and 80% start before 18 months. The child begins to cry, holds his or her breath, turns blue, and (may) lose consciousness. After loss of consciousness, some rhythmic jerking of the extremities may occur. The loss of consciousness is brief, and the child returns quickly to normal activity (no post-ictal state). The differential diagnosis includes cardiac arrhythmias, seizures, and apnea. If the history is classic for breath-holding spells, no further evaluation is necessary. The treatment is parental reassurance. Parents should be encouraged to ignore the episodes and not to give in to the child's requests in an attempt to avoid the spells. Iron supplementation may decrease the frequency of spells if anemia or iron deficiency is present.

HELPFUL TIP:
This type of spell **in a child under 1 year of age** may be referred to in the literature as a brief resolved unexplained event (BRUE). Until 2016, BRUEs were referred to as apparent life-threatening events (ALTEs). The term BRUE is nonspecific and is defined by what the parents observe: apnea, cyanosis, decreased responsiveness, etc. There is no relationship between a BRUE and sudden infant death syndrome (SIDS). The most common causes of a BRUE include lower respiratory tract infections, GERD, and seizure, though as many 50% occur without an identifiable cause. Additional causes include breath-holding spells, electrolyte abnormalities, cardiac dysrhythmias, metabolic diseases, and CNS problems. Always consider child abuse in your differential. A good history and physical examination are the most important evaluation tools. Diagnostic testing should be guided by history and physical examination findings. See Tieder JS, et al. *Pediatrics* 2016, for BRUE guidelines.

Question 13.2.9 **Between 12 and 15 months of age, Amy should receive all of the following vaccines, as per Centers for Disease Control and Prevention (CDC) recommendations, EXCEPT:**
A) MMR
B) Varicella
C) Hepatitis A
D) Rotavirus
E) Influenza

Answer 13.2.9 **The correct answer is "D."** Vaccination schedules and recommendations seem to represent quickly moving targets, so a regular review is required to keep up-to-date. At 12 to 15 months, the CDC recommends initial MMR, varicella, and hepatitis A vaccinations for all U.S. children. Influenza recommendations are updated annually and have become progressively more inclusive over time. The CDC recommends that all children ages 6 months through 18 years receive the influenza vaccine annually during the appropriate season. If the child is receiving her *first* year of influenza vaccination and is between 6 months and 8 years of age, she should receive two doses about 1 month apart to help boost immunity. Following this, the child may receive one dose of influenza vaccination annually. Of note, rotavirus vaccine should not be administered to children older than 32 weeks, and the first dose should not be given after 15 weeks.

Of course, the vaccine schedule is updated periodically but does not usually change drastically from year to year. For the most up-to-date version, go to the CDC website (http://www.cdc.gov/vaccines/schedules/hcp/child-adolescent.html) or use the app.

Amy's breath-holding spells resolve by the time she is 3 years old, and she continues to grow and develop normally. Amy's next issue comes when she is 5 years old and in your office for her pre-kindergarten physical.

Question 13.2.10 **You notice a new murmur. Of the following, which suggests that this is a benign murmur?**
A) Murmur is grade II/VI
B) Murmur has a thrill
C) Murmur radiates to the apex
D) Murmur is diastolic
E) Murmur is holosystolic

Answer 13.2.10 **The correct answer is "A."** Not all murmurs need to be referred to a cardiologist. There are features that can help differentiate pathologic from benign murmurs. A murmur that is diastolic, grades III to VI, pansystolic, or associated with cardiac symptoms is likely pathologic and requires further investigation. A benign murmur typically is systolic, soft (grades I–II, occasionally III), nonradiating, and short. A "benign" murmur is not a diagnosis of exclusion. You should try to decide about which innocent murmur it is. See Table 13-2.

On Amy's examination, you hear a grade III/VI systolic murmur in the pulmonic area with wide, fixed splitting of the

TABLE 13-2 BENIGN CARDIAC MURMURS OF CHILDHOOD

Still murmur: A grade I–III murmur heard best in left middle sternal border or between left lower sternal border and apex. It is a "musical," vibratory, or buzzing systolic ejection murmur, which is louder when the patient is supine, compared with when upright, and decreases in volume with a Valsalva maneuver. A Still murmur may get louder as blood flow increases with fever, exercise, or excitement.

Venous hum: A grade continuous I–III murmur heard best in the supraclavicular area. It should resolve when the patient is recumbent or with pressure over the jugular vein.

Pulmonic murmur: Heard as a grade I–III systolic ejection murmur in the first half of systole. It is generally best heard in the left upper sternal border.

Murmurs that change with respiration are generally, but not always, benign.

second heart sound. She is otherwise healthy without any cardiac symptoms.

Question 13.2.11 What is the appropriate next step in management of this issue?
A) Family reassurance
B) Endocarditis prophylaxis at the dental visit next week
C) ECG and chest radiograph
D) Limit physical activity
E) Refer for immediate operative repair

Answer 13.2.11 **The correct answer is "C."** Most likely, Amy has an ASD or atrial septal defect. The murmur is a systolic ejection murmur heard best at the upper left sternal border. The sound you hear is caused by increased flow across the pulmonic valve creating a relative stenosis (more volume needs to get through a relatively fixed outlet) and NOT from flow across the ASD. The increased flow across the pulmonic valve causes a wide, fixed split S2. There may be a mid-diastolic rumbling murmur at the lower left sternal border from increased flow across the tricuspid valve if the ASD is very large. The chest x-ray may demonstrate cardiomegaly with increased pulmonary vascular markings. The ECG can be normal or may show mild right ventricular hypertrophy, right axis deviation, and/or right bundle branch block with the characteristic rsR' pattern in the right precordial leads. Children with an ASD do NOT need endocarditis prophylaxis (except for the first 6 months after their surgical repair) and rarely need to limit their physical activity. Most small ASDs will close spontaneously by age 4 years. Closure by one of a variety of methods is recommended for symptomatic and significant left-to-right shunts with right ventricular enlargement.

▶ **Objectives: Did you learn to …**
· Describe the causes of neonatal hyperbilirubinemia?
· Manage an infant with breastfeeding failure jaundice?
· Identify risk factors for severe hyperbilirubinemia?
· Recommend vaccines for children in accordance with CDC guidelines?
· Identify vaccine misconceptions, list MMR side effects, and identify contraindications to immunization?

· Recognize stages of child development?
· Describe and manage breath-holding spells?
· Differentiate benign from pathologic cardiac murmurs in childhood?

 QUICK QUIZ: JAUNDICE

The current recommendation for the treatment of breast milk jaundice (NOT breastfeeding failure jaundice as per the previous case) is:
A) Continue to breastfeed
B) Stop breastfeeding and change to a cow's milk formula
C) Stop breastfeeding and change to soy milk formula
D) Stop breastfeeding and treat with rehydration solution (e.g., Pedialyte)

The correct answer is "A." Patients with hyperbilirubinemia due to breast milk jaundice should continue to breastfeed. Breast milk jaundice begins on days 5 to 7 of life, peaks by 2 weeks of age, and usually resolves by 10 weeks of age; monitor to make sure that the jaundice remains unconjugated and there is no need to look for a second source. Bilirubin levels will gradually decline while breastfeeding is continued. If breastfeeding is discontinued, serum bilirubin levels decline rapidly. Kernicterus is rare. The etiology is unclear, but it is hypothesized that glucuronidase in breast milk may lead to de-conjugation and increased enterohepatic recirculation of bilirubin.

▶ **CASE 13.3**

A family has moved into the area and brings their 12-month-old girl in for a well-child examination. They bring her medical records with them. Her parents have no concerns, and she has been healthy. Her growth chart (Fig. 13-1) concerns you, however. Her length tracks along the 25th percentile. But her weight has gone gradually from around the 25th to 50th percentile at 0 to 6 months old down to the 10th percentile at 9 months old, and now is at the 5th percentile at 12 months.

Question 13.3.1 **Which of the following most likely explains her pattern of growth?**
A) Normal variant
B) Familial short stature
C) Prenatal insult such as exposure to drugs or infection
D) Hypothyroidism
E) Inadequate nutrition

Answer 13.3.1 **The correct answer is "E."** This patient's pattern of growth is consistent with failure to thrive (FTT), now termed "weight faltering" or faltering growth (*Am Fam Physician.* 2016;94(4):299). The criteria for diagnosis of FTT include weight less than the third to fifth percentile (depending on the source) **or** a fall of weight of more than two major percentile lines in 6 months **or** weight less than 80% of ideal weight for age

Birth to 24 months: Girls
Length-for-age and Weight-for-age percentiles

NAME _____

RECORD # _____

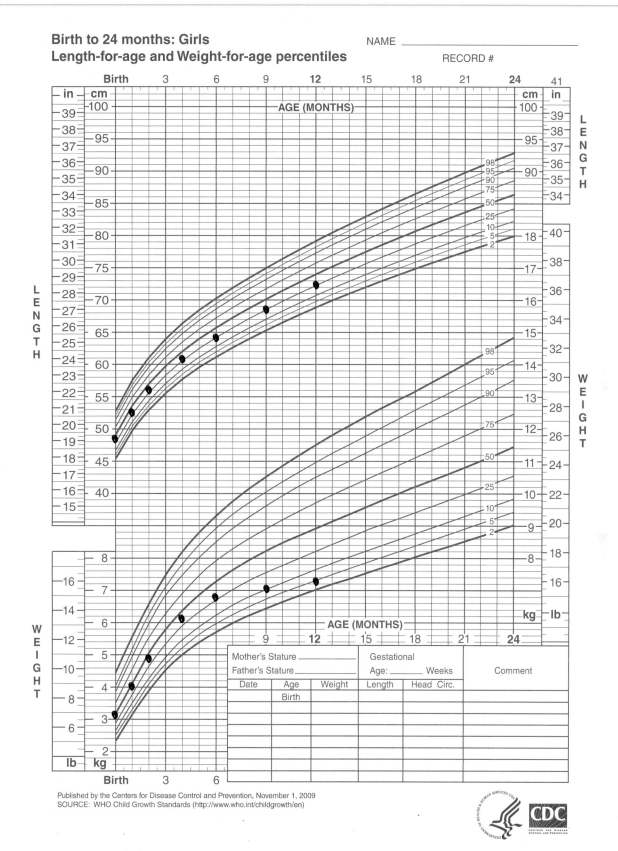

Published by the Centers for Disease Control and Prevention, November 1, 2009
SOURCE: WHO Child Growth Standards (http://www.who.int/childgrowth/en)

FIGURE 13-1. Your patient's growth chart

and/or weight for height less than fifth percentile. The patient meets more than one of the criteria for FTT, so "A" is incorrect. In "B," both height and weight would be affected. In this child, only the weight (and not the height) is affected. "C" is incorrect because a child with a prenatal insult tends to be smaller globally in both height and weight, and the weight percentile would not be expected to drop so dramatically from birth. "D" is unlikely because, in general, the endocrinological causes result in "stunting" where a child stops gaining height but continues to gain weight. Thus, "E" is the most likely cause of this patient's FTT.

Taking more history, you discover that the patient eats mostly rice and fruit. She does not like meat. She is picky. She drinks about 12 oz of whole milk and 12 oz of apple juice each day. She is active and developmentally appropriate. Her review of systems is negative as is her past medical history.

Question 13.3.2 **What is the LEAST appropriate way to proceed with evaluation and management of this patient?**
A) Allow the child to feed herself whenever she is hungry or thirsty. Parents should offer food and drink frequently throughout the day
B) Obtain CBC, iron studies, and urinalysis
C) Limit juice intake
D) Consult a registered dietitian
E) Prescribe a multivitamin

Answer 13.3.2 **The correct answer (and least appropriate approach) is "A."** The goal of management of failure to thrive is to ensure appropriate caloric intake, identify treatable causes of failure to thrive, and look for effects of her malnutrition. Thus, a CBC, iron studies, electrolytes, bicarbonate, glucose, and urinalysis may be helpful to investigate possible iron deficiency, anemia, lead poisoning or renal tubular acidosis. Generally, however, extensive diagnostic workup is not needed until after a period of confirmed appropriate caloric provision. If the patient's weight continued to falter, despite appropriate calories, more extensive workup is needed. Juice should be limited (due to its low nutritional value), meals scheduled, and caloric intake boosted. Although children should feed themselves, they take in more calories when given a set schedule for meals and snacks instead of being allowed to graze on food or drink throughout the day as in "A." A registered dietitian can help educate the family on appropriate food choices for a toddler and ways to boost calories. A child with a restrictive eating pattern, especially poor in iron-containing foods (such as meats), may benefit from a multivitamin with iron.

HELPFUL TIP:
For infants with failure to thrive, increased caloric provision is often needed to "catch-up" and sustain growth. Encourage the parents to increase the caloric density of foods and drinks. In children older than 1 year, you may ask them to use whole milk rather than reduced fat milk, add butter to food, etc. In children under 1 year of age who are exclusively breastfed, evaluation of maternal milk supply and breastfeeding adequacy is needed. In babies who are bottle-fed, fortification of breast milk or enrichment of formula (e.g., from standard 20 kcal/oz to 24 kcal/oz) may be needed. Most formulas can be used for this purpose, and recipes are readily available.

Your patient presents to the emergency department (ED) at 14 months old. Mom states that she has had several episodes of emesis over the last 48 hours and today began to have watery, foul-smelling diarrhea (as opposed to the yummy-smelling diarrhea to which we are so accustomed). Mom has lost track of number of episodes of emesis and diarrhea. She cannot tell if the child has had urine output because of the watery diarrhea. On your examination, the temperature is 102.5°F, heart rate 180 bpm, respiratory rate 50, blood pressure 80/50 mm Hg. Her weight is 8 kg. She has dry, cracked lips and dry skin. She lies in her mom's arms and is not very interested in your examination. Her capillary refill is about 4 seconds with some mottling of the extremities.

Question 13.3.3 **What is the most appropriate next step in the management of this patient's condition?**
A) Evaluate for underlying bacterial infection with blood, urine, and stool cultures
B) Admit to an inpatient unit and begin maintenance IV fluids
C) Infuse 20 mL/kg of normal saline IV rapidly
D) Begin oral rehydration with Pedialyte
E) Infuse 10 mL/kg of D5/half-normal saline over 2 hours

Answer 13.3.3 **The correct answer is "C."** This patient is severely dehydrated (estimated 15%) with signs of compromised tissue perfusion; therefore, she should have parenteral fluid resuscitation quickly with a 20 mL/kg isotonic fluid bolus. The bolus should be run over a few minutes and not administered with an infusion pump. Appropriate isotonic fluids include normal saline or lactated Ringer's. Although she will likely need admission as suggested by "B," she should be stabilized in the ED before transfer to the inpatient unit. Starting with maintenance fluids or a slow infusion, as suggested by "E," is incorrect, as repletion of intravascular volume is needed immediately. Oral rehydration, as in "D," is cost-effective in less severe dehydration, but is not recommended in the setting of compromised tissue perfusion. There are several tables published listing the clinical examination associated with various degrees of dehydration. See Table 13-3 for clues in determining the degree of dehydration.

HELPFUL TIP:
Dehydration is a clinical diagnosis, but laboratory findings can be helpful. The serum sodium classifies the dehydration as hypotonic, isotonic, or hypertonic. Metabolic acidosis is often present, and calculation of the anion gap may help determine the cause. Blood urea nitrogen and serum creatine concentrations can be helpful to assess for acute kidney injury but may be affected by other conditions.

TABLE 13-3 SIGNS AND SYMPTOMS OF DEHYDRATION[a]

Mild (5% in an infant, 3% in a child): Normal skin turgor, moist lips, tears present, normal vital signs, consolable

Moderate (10% in an infant, 6% in a child): Dry skin and lips, skin tenting, slightly increased pulse, decreased urine output, normal capillary refill

Severe (15% in an infant, 9% in a child): Parched lips, sunken eyes, decreased or no urine output, cool skin, elevated pulse, prolonged capillary refill, lethargic or obtunded

[a]Because of the poor association of physical findings with a particular percent dehydration use the terms "mild," "moderate" or "severe" is preferred over trying to assign a percent dehydration.

After completing the initial management, the patient is more interested in her surroundings. Her vital signs are pulse 160 bpm, respiratory rate 36, and blood pressure 80/50 mm Hg. Her lips are still dry, and she is irritable. The capillary refill is 2 to 3 seconds. She is more interactive with her mother.

Question 13.3.4 What further treatment is indicated for her dehydration?
A) 80 mL/hr × 2 hours of D5-1/4-NS
B) 33 mL/hr × 24 hours of D5-1/2-NS with 20-mEq KCl
C) 50 mL/hr × 24 hours of D5-1/4-NS
D) 20 mL/kg NS over 20 minutes
E) 10 mL/kg D5-1/2-NS over 2 hours

Answer 13.3.4 **The correct answer is "D."** After an initial bolus, the patient should be reassessed. This patient is still moderately dehydrated. Although she has responded to her initial bolus of normal saline, she still has abnormal vital signs as well as signs of dehydration on examination. Therefore, the normal saline bolus should be repeated. **Hypotonic solutions (e.g., 1/2 NS) or those containing glucose (D5) and/or potassium should *NEVER* be used as a bolus. Note the bold—we mean it!** Boluses of hypotonic solution can lead to hyponatremia, seizures, and cerebral edema. Boluses of potassium-containing solutions (especially in the setting of reduced urine output) can lead to life-threatening hyperkalemia. Potassium (if needed at all) should be withheld until the patient urinates and has better hydration status.

HELPFUL TIP:
Maintenance fluids can be used in patients with decreased oral intake to keep up with their daily water needs. Maintenance fluids can be calculated using the Holiday–Segar method: daily water needs for the first 10 kg of body weight is 100 mL/kg/day; water needs for the next 11 to 20 kg is 50 mL/kg/day; each additional kg over 20 kg is 20 mL/kg/day. You can also calculate the hourly fluid requirement by the "4, 2, 1" method. Children should get 4 mL/kg/hr for the first 10 kg body weight, 2 mL/kg/hr for the next 10 kg, and 1 mL/kg/hr for every kg over 20 kg. Assess for dehydration and/or a fluid deficit prior to starting maintenance fluids.

Fluid deficit (L) = usual weight (kg) − current weight (kg)

If a patient is dehydrated, utilize isotonic fluid boluses to correct this, then start your maintenance fluids! Remember, boluses "fill the tank" and maintenance fluids "keep it from running low." You've gotta' attain (euvolemia) before you can maintain! Also, replace ongoing losses from diarrhea, emesis, etc., if present.

HELPFUL (AND IMPORTANT) TIP:
Historically, hypotonic "peds" solutions (1/4 or 1/2 NS with 5% dextrose) had been used for maintenance fluids in children. In susceptible children, this can lead to hyponatremia, seizures, and cerebral edema. Fluids with a sodium content similar to that of plasma (135–145 mEq/L) should be used (*Lancet.* 2015;385(9974):1190–1197; 28). Recent literature suggests use of D5-NS (sodium content 154 mEq/L) or similar solutions are generally safer than hypotonic solutions when used as a maintenance fluid (*Cochrane Database Syst Rev.* 2014;12:CD009457; *Pediatrics.* 2014;133:105–113). Maintenance fluids in children should generally contain dextrose (5%) to maintain euglycemic and prevent catabolism. Care should be taken to prevent hyperglycemia in children with impaired glucose metabolism (e.g., metabolic syndrome, PCOS, diabetes mellitus).

The patient recovers well from her GI illness, but she returns a few months later to your clinic with a new illness. She has had temperatures of 103°F at home for 2 to 3 days. She has had no upper respiratory symptoms. Her oral intake has decreased, but she is maintaining good urine output. She has had no vomiting or diarrhea. Your examination reveals a febrile child who is slightly irritable. She is nontoxic and not dehydrated. Her oral cavity shows increased tonsil size with ulcers on her tongue and lips but not on the tonsillar pillars; *there are no other skin lesions.* Her anterior cervical lymph nodes are enlarged. The rest of her examination is noncontributory.

Question 13.3.5 What is the most likely diagnosis?
A) Streptococcal pharyngitis
B) Hand, foot, and mouth disease (HFMD)
C) Herpetic gingivostomatitis
D) Varicella
E) Infectious mononucleosis

Answer 13.3.5 **The correct answer is "C."** Primary oral herpes (herpetic gingivostomatitis) is associated with a relatively high fever and anteriorly placed ulcerations and vesicles (gums, tongue, and lips). Symptoms tend to start relatively abruptly with pain, salivation, refusal to eat, and fever. Herpes gingivostomatitis may recur during life in the form of "cold sores." "B" is incorrect because the patient does not have hand and foot lesions, which are required for a diagnosis HFMD. Oral lesions in HFMD often occur on the tongue and buccal mucosa. Like herpangina (see below), HFMD is caused by enteroviruses, most commonly coxsackieviruses. "D," varicella, can occur in the oral pharynx, but would have lesions elsewhere in various stages and respiratory symptoms as well. Infectious mononucleosis is not associated with vesicular lesions or mucosal ulcerations.

> **HELPFUL TIP:**
> The poorly named "herpangina," caused by enteroviruses (usually coxsackie A), is another consideration in the child with fever and mouth sores. Herpangina is associated with fewer vesicles and **ulcers located in the posterior oropharynx along the posterior soft palate and tonsillar pillars and fossa.** Headache, vomiting, and abdominal pain may be present as well. Note that this is a different clinical entity from hand, foot, and mouth disease despite the enteroviral cause.

Next, you see the patient's sister who is age 10 and presenting for a school physical. Her mother is concerned because this patient has pubic hair, which her mother thinks is premature (and scary … her baby can't be growing up yet!). On your examination, she has enlarged areola and a small amount of breast tissue. She also has sparse, dark, but mostly straight pubic hair.

Question 13.3.6 This patient's sexual maturity rating or Tanner stage is:
A) 1
B) 2
C) 3
D) 4
E) 5

Answer 13.3.6 **The correct answer is "B."** Breast buds and sparse, downy pubic hair put the patient in Tanner stage 2. Tanner stage 1 is prepubertal. Any sign of puberty moves a child from Tanner 1 to Tanner 2. Tanner stage 5 is adult or fully matured secondary sexual characteristics. See Table 13-4 for details.

TABLE 13-4 TANNER STAGES

Stage 1: Prepubertal
Stage 2: Sparse growth of downy hair at base of penis or along labia
- Girls: Breast bud development
- Boys: Enlargement of scrotum and testes with reddening and thickening of scrotal skin

Stage 3: Darkening, coarse hair sparsely in pubic area
- Girls: Enlargement of breasts (primary mound)
- Boys: Elongation of penis and increased size of testes

Stage 4: Adult pubic hair distribution (triangle) but smaller area covered with no extension to medial thighs
- Girls: Areola and papilla begin to mound above the level of the breast (secondary mound)
- Boys: Increase in breadth and development of penis, darkening of scrotal skin, enlargement of testes

Stage 5: Adult breasts, genitals, and hair distribution

The mom has a lot of questions about puberty. She is nervous about beginning to discuss sexual development with her daughter.

Question 13.3.7 What is a developmental fact that you can provide the mom for discussion with her daughter?
A) Typically, in females, the first sign of puberty is pubic hair
B) At 10 years old, the patient is experiencing premature puberty
C) The height spurt occurs early during puberty and is almost complete at menarche
D) Menarche occurs approximately 1 year after breast budding
E) Schools discuss puberty and relieve mom or dad of that duty (whew!)

Answer 13.3.7 **The correct answer is "C."** In girls, the growth spurt occurs early and is almost complete at menarche. Females begin puberty about 1 to 2 years before males. "A" is incorrect as thelarche, or breast budding, marks female onset of puberty. "B" is incorrect. The average age of breast budding is 10.9 years. Thus, the child is appropriate in her pubertal timing. "D" is incorrect. Menarche typically begins 2 years after breast budding. "E" is incorrect. Sex education in schools is highly variable, and these discussions are often limited in the time and content. It is important for the child to hear her mother's opinions on puberty and sex.

> **HELPFUL TIP:**
> Precocious or early puberty is defined as the onset of secondary sexual characteristics before age 8 for girls and age 9 for boys. Delayed puberty is the lack of such changes by age 14.

▶ **Objectives: Did you learn to …**
- Define failure to thrive in a child?
- Evaluate a child with failure to thrive?
- Evaluate a dehydrated child and determine severity of dehydration?
- Manage dehydration in the ED?
- Calculate rehydration fluids for a dehydrated child?
- Generate a differential diagnosis for pharyngitis with blisters?
- Describe changes of puberty and Tanner staging in a female?

 QUICK QUIZ: FEEDING INFANTS

Which is *not* an indication for use of soy formula in an infant?
A) Galactosemia
B) Congenital lactase deficiency
C) Cow milk protein intolerance
D) Parental desire for a vegan diet

The correct answer is "C." Few indications exist for use of soy-based formula over cow milk–based formula. Soy formula is lactose free and therefore should be used in conditions "A," "B," and "D." Galactosemia is a metabolic disorder characterized by the inability to break down galactose. Dietary galactose comes from lactose found in human and cow milk. Remember, lactose is a disaccharide composed of galactose and glucose. An extensively hydrolyzed or amino acid formula should be used for cow milk protein intolerance. Infants who are sensitive to cow milk protein have an approximately 10% to 15% chance of also being sensitive to soy proteins. Reflux deserves special note. There is no data supporting the use of soy formula for reflux.

▶ CASE 13.4

A 2-year-old male presents to your office with his father complaining that the patient has had intermittent crying followed by episodes of profound lethargy during which he is difficult to arouse. The father relates that the patient will sometimes clutch at his abdomen and roll into the fetal position during episodes. These episodes have been going on for about 4 hours. He has had no fever, no vomiting, and no diarrhea. Nobody else at home has been sick. He is developmentally normal and has no significant past medical history. His examination reveals that he is afebrile and sleepy but can be aroused. *His abdominal examination is benign.* The rest of the examination is unremarkable.

Question 13.4.1 Given his presentation, your clinical suspicion is for:
A) Meningitis
B) Renal colic
C) Intussusception
D) Gastric outlet obstruction
E) Appendicitis

Answer 13.4.1 The correct answer is "C." The patient may have intussusception. The combination of abdominal colic **plus** mental status changes should suggest intussusception. The etiology of the mental status changes is not clear, but mental status changes are one of the classical findings of intussusception. "A," meningitis, should still be a consideration in a patient with mental status changes, but he is afebrile and his symptoms are intermittent, making meningitis less likely. "B" is not associated with mental status changes. "D" and "E" usually present with some abnormal findings on abdominal examination.

HELPFUL TIP:
Fewer than 15% of patients with intussusception present with the classic triad of colicky abdominal pain, palpable sausage-shaped abdominal mass, and currant jelly stool.

Question 13.4.2 Which laboratory finding will help you to confirm the diagnosis of intussusception?
A) CBC
B) Urinalysis
C) Glucose
D) Serum lactate
E) None of the above

Answer 13.4.2 The correct answer is "E." None of the above will help to make the diagnosis of intussusception. Early in the course, the CBC may be normal and only 75% will have heme-positive stools.

HELPFUL TIP:
"Currant jelly stools" are a late finding in intussusception and are a reflection of mucosal ischemia. You really want to make the diagnosis before you see "currant jelly" per rectum. (Hey, have you ever actually seen currant jelly? It is bright red and gloopy, kind of like grandma's cranberry sauce.)

Question 13.4.3 You decide that this patient probably has intussusception based on your history and physical examination. The next step in diagnosing this patient is:
A) Upper GI with barium
B) A plain film of the abdomen
C) An air enema
D) An abdominal ultrasound
E) Administration of IV antibiotics

Answer 13.4.3 The correct answer is "D." In general, an ultrasound is the diagnostic modality of choice. An ultrasound may show a typical "bull's eye" lesion helping to make the diagnosis. "C," an air enema, is a diagnostic and therapeutic intervention. An air enema can be used to reduce the intussusception obviating the need for surgery. In general, however, a diagnosis is first made by ultrasound. An upper GI, "A," will be of no use since intussusception is a distal process. A plain film of the abdomen, "B," will most likely be nondiagnostic as is the case in most abdominal processes (except perhaps bowel obstruction or free air).

HELPFUL TIP:
For intussusception, an air or water-soluble contrast enema is preferred over traditional barium enema. Bowel perforation is the main risk of nonoperative reduction. Air and water-soluble contrast enemas are much less harmful than barium if leaked into the peritoneum. Air enemas have also been noted to have a higher success rate compared to hydrostatic enemas, with rates of successful reduction around 83% and 70%, respectively (*Am J Roentgenol.* 2015;205(5):W542–549).

Well, the ultrasound tech is in the Cayman Islands, so you opt for an air enema, which simultaneously diagnoses and reduces the intussusception. The patient appears well with no signs of perforation. He is eating goldfish crackers by the fistful in the ED and generally making a mess of the examination room. Recommendations vary as to the patient's disposition. Recurrence rate is less than 5% in the first 24 hours and about 10% in the first 48 hours after reduction. Some authors recommend admission for 24 hours post-reduction, but this does not change the recurrence risk. The child's clinical picture, access to care, and reliability of caregiver should be taken into account (*Pediatrics.* 2014;134(1):110). We suspect admission will be the right answer for the test.

HELPFUL TIP:
Most cases of intussusception are idiopathic. Less than 10% of patients have a pathologic lead point such as a Meckel diverticulum, intestinal polyp, or lymphoma. Increased age of child increases the risk of a lead point.

HELPFUL TIP:
Different types of intestinal obstructions occur at different ages. Obstruction at birth is typically an anatomic atresia, meconium ileus, or Hirschsprung disease. Volvulus due to malrotation can occur at any age, but most commonly appears in infancy (even within the first month of life … watch for bilious vomiting, a sign of volvulus). Between birth and 5 weeks of age, hypertrophic pyloric stenosis appears. Intussusception is the most common cause of GI obstruction between 3 months and 6 years of age.

▶ **Objectives: Did you learn to …**
 · Recognize the clinical presentation of intussusception?
 · Evaluate and treat a child with intussusception?

▶ CASE 13.5

Benjamin, a 4-month-old male, comes to your office for a well-baby examination. His parents have no concerns. Development and feeding are progressing as expected. Looking at him, you think to yourself, "My gosh. Infants have such big heads relative to their bodies." On your examination, his head is >95th percentile, but his weight and height are still at the 50th percentile. His previous head circumferences have all been at the 50th percentile. He is a social infant but is having difficulty supporting his large head.

Question 13.5.1 What is the imaging study LEAST likely to assist in the diagnosis of the macrocephaly?
A) X-ray
B) CT scan
C) MRI scan
D) Ultrasound

Answer 13.5.1 The correct answer is "A." Because the relative head size is so dramatic, an imaging study is needed, but skull radiographs are not likely to assist you in arriving at a diagnosis. The other modalities are used in this setting, and each has its benefits and detractions. Ultrasound is often used in infants when the anterior fontanelle is still patent and offers the advantage of no radiation exposure. Ultrasound is primarily used to assess fluid-filled spaces (ventricles in hydrocephalus, subdural hematoma, etc.). CT scan is a rapid and readily available test that can detect hemorrhages, intracranial calcifications, skull fractures, Chiari malformations, and more, but given the concern for radiation exposure and the risk of future malignancy, it is not the first-line imaging technique. CT is also limited in its ability to delineate soft-tissue problems, which is where MRI becomes important.

HELPFUL TIP:
The differential diagnosis of macrocephaly is long and includes hydrocephalus, brain tumor, benign familial macrocephaly, benign enlargement of the subarachnoid space (BESS), neurocutaneous disorder (e.g., neurofibromatosis, tuberous sclerosis), hemorrhage, and metabolic disorders (e.g., Tay–Sachs disease, mucopolysaccharidoses).

Question 13.5.2 The ultrasound tech is still on vacation (why can't we have his job?) and your MRI is undergoing scheduled maintenance, so you order a CT scan, which shows subdural hematomas. What is your next step in managing this patient?
A) Admit to the hospital
B) Examination of eyes in an ophthalmologist's office
C) "Babygram" to view entire skeleton of infant for fractures
D) Alert the department of human services within the next week
E) Send the patient to a neurosurgeon's office for the next available appointment

Answer 13.5.2 The correct answer is "A." Subdural hematomas in an infant are highly suspicious of abusive head trauma. **Your priority is to protect the child by admission to the hospital.** A retinal examination and skeletal survey are important in the evaluation but are secondary to protection of the child. A "babygram" should never be done to evaluate for skeletal trauma. There is a specific procedure for performing a formal skeletal survey for abuse, which should be completed in cases of suspected abusive head trauma. Your state agency responsible for investigating child abuse must be notified within **24 hours** (although clinicians are encouraged to know their legal responsibilities in the state in which they practice). Protection of the child is most important; if the family flees, calling the police or the appropriate state agency would be the first step. Suspicion of abuse, especially abusive head trauma, is an emergency, and it should not wait for a neurosurgeon's next available appointment.

HELPFUL TIP:
Retinal hemorrhages generally require a significant acceleration–deceleration mechanism to occur (e.g., shaking) and are *highly* suspicious for abuse. Nonabusive causes of retinal hemorrhages are very rare. Vaccinations, mild head trauma (such as falling off a sofa), CPR, seizures, and routine play do **not** cause retinal hemorrhages.

As you have done in this case, radiological studies should always be obtained in the evaluation of suspected child abuse. However, the cause of fractures has a broader differential than abuse.

Question 13.5.3 Which patient's injuries and/or radiological studies would be pathognomonic of abuse?

A) A 9-month-old male with widened distal radius and ulna with fraying and cupping evident on radiograph
B) A 21-month-old female with multiple fractures at different ages on radiograph. She has delayed tooth eruption and sparse hair
C) A colicky 1-month-old male infant with callus on the left clavicle radiograph
D) A 2-year-old female with a spiral fracture of the distal right tibia
E) None of the above

Answer 13.5.3 The correct answer is "E." None of these injuries is diagnostic of abuse. Although each of these children would make you think of possible abuse, none of them have been abused. "A" is a child with rickets. "B" is a child with osteogenesis imperfecta. "C" is a child who sustained a clavicle fracture at birth. "D" is a child with a "toddler's fracture." A toddler's fracture is a spiral tibial fracture found in children age 9 to 36 months (see Chapter 12). These fractures are found in the distal one-third of the tibia. Long bone fractures in nonambulatory children, distal metaphyseal "wedge" fractures (often called "bucket-handle fractures"), and posterior-rib fractures (from squeezing) are among injuries that are VERY concerning for abuse.

Benjamin's evaluation shows bilateral subdural hemorrhages and retinal hemorrhages. His skeletal survey is negative. The state agency removes him from the home and places him in foster care. Benjamin then returns for his 6-month well-child examination. He has been in foster care since you last saw him. His vision is being followed by an ophthalmologist. He smiles and squeals. His foster mother says, "Looks like he's right-handed. Does that mean that he's advanced for his age?" He rolls both ways. He has started on rice cereal and bananas. He sleeps well. On your examination, he continues to have macrocephaly but a soft fontanelle. His left hand is fisted. The rest of the examination is unremarkable.

Question 13.5.4 What is your assessment and plan for Benjamin?

A) Normal 6-month-old: Routine anticipatory guidance and immunizations
B) Infant with history of head trauma: Delay pertussis vaccination because of the autism risk
C) Infant with history of head trauma: Perform Denver Developmental Screening Test and document findings; repeat in 3 months
D) Hypertonic left upper extremity: Monitor progress at next well-child examination
E) Hypertonic left upper extremity: Refer for further evaluation and treatment of his delay

Answer 13.5.4 The correct answer is "E." Benjamin is at risk of developmental delays due to his abusive head injury. He should be monitored closely for delays. One way to monitor for delays is by performing a screening test, such as the Denver Developmental Screening Test. However, Benjamin has concerns that go beyond screening. His tightly fisted left hand with corresponding favoring of his right hand suggests spastic hemiplegia. Early hand preference is a worrisome sign. Typically hand preference is not definite before 18 to 24 months. Hand preference should prompt the physician to examine the other extremity. In this case, there is hypertonicity resulting from his trauma. Any child with concern of developmental delay should be referred for further evaluation. Some local and state agencies offer a free service to families to evaluate development and offer therapy. Do NOT watch and wait with a suspected delay. The earlier intervention begins, the better the outcome.

▶ **Objectives: Did you learn to ...**
- Recognize and evaluate macrocephaly in an infant?
- Generate a differential diagnosis of macrocephaly in an infant?
- Determine when child abuse should be included in the differential diagnosis?
- Describe some aspects of developmental delay and its management?

 QUICK QUIZ: DEVELOPMENTAL DELAY

A mother brings her 18-month-old son in for a routine visit, but is concerned that he is not as verbal as he was 3 months ago. She reports that he eats well. He just started walking. You wish to screen him for a pervasive developmental disorder (which includes autism spectrum disorder, Rett syndrome, childhood disintegrative disorder, and others).

What is the most appropriate office tool to use with this patient given his age and presenting symptoms?

A) Ages and Stages Questionnaire (ASQ)
B) Conner's Rating Scale—Revised Short Form
C) Denver Developmental Screening Test
D) Modified Checklist for Autism in Toddlers (M-CHAT)
E) Parents Evaluation of Developmental Status (PEDS)

The correct answer is "D." The Modified Checklist for Autism in Toddlers (M-CHAT for short) is a validated office screening tool for autism spectrum disorders. It would be the most appropriate tool of the options given. Of note, the AAP recommends screening all children for autism spectrum disorders using a standard screening tool such as the M-CHAT at ages 18 and 24 months. "A" is incorrect as the Ages and Stages Questionnaire is a broad-based developmental screening tool, as is "D," the Denver Developmental Screening Test. "B" is incorrect because this test is used to detect ADHD. Note that the USPSTF does not recommend for or against autism screening between 18 and 30 months noting that there is insufficient evidence to take a position on such screening. However, most practitioners follow the AAP recommendations.

▶ CASE 13.6

A 7-year-old male presents to your clinic with his mother with a complaint of enuresis. Evidently, this child has never been completely continent at night, wetting his bed several times per week. This has become somewhat of a problem for him now that his friends are having sleepover birthday parties. Plus, his mother confides that she's tired of paying for pull-ups and cleaning sheets. His incontinence is monosymptomatic (meaning no overactive bladder symptoms or daytime wetting).

Question 13.6.1 **What percentage of 7-year-olds continue to have enuresis?**
A) 1%
B) 10%
C) 20%
D) 40%
E) 75%

Answer 13.6.1 **The correct answer is "B."** About 10% continue to have enuresis at age 7 years which tapers to 1% to 2% at age 15 years or greater. Even though this would suggest that it is a variant of normal, there is extreme social pressure on children by age 7 to remain dry at night. Parental expectations may depend on their experience with other children. For example, if an older sibling was dry at night at age 3 or if a younger sibling is dry while an older child has enuresis, parents may not accept the bed wetting as normal. Age 7 is considered the cutoff for "normal" enuresis; therefore, beyond age 7 years, it is considered a problem.

HELPFUL TIP:
Note that the child in this case is male. Enuresis affects twice as many males as females.

Because he has had no period of nocturnal dryness, this patient has primary enuresis.

Question 13.6.2 **Which of the following is likely to be part of this child's history?**
A) A family history of enuresis
B) A stressful event in the family such as the birth of a new child or parental divorce
C) Increased fluid intake over the past 2 months
D) History of urinary tract infections

Answer 13.6.2 **The correct answer is "A."** Enuresis is divided into primary and secondary enuresis. Primary enuresis occurs in cases where there is **never** a consistent period of dryness at night. Secondary enuresis occurs when there is a period of dryness (by convention, 6 months) before the patient develops enuresis. "B," "C," and "D" would more likely be seen in children with **secondary** enuresis. Primary enuresis tends to be a familial trait. Secondary enuresis requires some investigation.

HELPFUL TIP:
About 15% of patients have primary enuresis at age 5. About 15% of patients with enuresis become dry each year thereafter. The longer enuresis persists, the less likely it is to resolve.

This patient's examination is essentially normal including neurologic evaluation.

Question 13.6.3 **Further evaluation of this patient should include all of the following EXCEPT:**
A) Asking about a history of bowel problems
B) Assessment of growth and development
C) Investigation into family history of nocturnal enuresis
D) Spine MRI to rule out pathologic lesion
E) Urinalysis

Answer 13.6.3 **The correct answer is "D."** Patients with enuresis who have an otherwise normal neurologic examination need not have an MRI done. If on examination this child had neurologic findings, an MRI would be indicated. All of the remaining options are part of a thorough evaluation of nocturnal enuresis. The assessment of growth and development is important to determine if the child is neurologically delayed, which could be contributing to enuresis. Attention to bowel problems is also important. Bowel and bladder dysfunction are common causes of enuresis. Fecal impaction can lead to incontinence. Asking about snoring can help to identify obstructive sleep apnea, which can be associated with enuresis.

You find no indication of a pathologic cause, and you decide that this is primary enuresis. The parents are desperate for some sort of intervention to fix the problem, since it is becoming a major source of anxiety in the home and of teasing at school (of course _anything_ can be a source of teasing at school).

Question 13.6.4 Which of the following should constitute the initial treatment of this patient's primary enuresis?
A) Patient education and motivational training (e.g., rewards for staying dry)
B) Over-learning
C) Enuresis alarm
D) Nasal desmopressin (DDAVP)
E) Oral desipramine

Answer 13.6.4 The correct answer is "A." All of the above have been found to be useful in the treatment of enuresis; however, the best initial approach includes education. Patients and parents should be informed of how common this condition is, how to reduce fluid intake in the evening without getting dehydrated, and how to schedule voiding. Motivational training plays a role as well. The other interventions are secondary. It is important to make sure the child knows that enuresis is not their fault! A child should never be punished for enuresis, as it is outside of their control. "B," over-learning, is thought to help prevent relapses in patients *who have been successful with an enuresis alarm*. Once continence is achieved with the alarm, the child drinks a set amount of fluid before bedtime. The amount is successively increased once dryness is achieved until a maximum is reached. The idea is that the patient is conditioned to respond to his increasing bladder capacity. "C," an enuresis alarm, is an effective treatment but relatively expensive and requires significant motivation on the part of the family. The enuresis alarm increases success of the other options, and when used in combination with other modalities, it has shown the best long-term results. "D" and "E" are incorrect in this scenario although they are used to treat enuresis. Relapse is more common when pharmacologic therapy is discontinued than with the other modalities. However, medications are effective as a short-term treatment option, but are felt to be second tier and used when the urine alarm fails or is impractical (think sleepover or summer camp). Of note, "D" is wrong for another reason: **nasal** DDAVP is no longer approved for nocturnal enuresis due to problems with hyponatremia. Oral DDAVP still carries the enuresis indication, but it can cause hyponatremia as well—it just occurs less often. Oral DDAVP may be used on an "as needed" basis for special events. Trying it at home on a "normal" night before the special event will help determine efficacy. Sometimes dose adjustment is required.

> **HELPFUL TIP:**
> Retention control training is no longer recommended as it was not found to significantly decrease wetting. Retention-control training was based on the (faulty) premise that enuretic children had smaller bladder capacities. The child would hold urine in an attempt to stretch the bladder and increase capacity. Retention control training can increase bladder capacity but does not improve enuresis. But maybe if you are a truck driver or a surgeon …

▶ **Objectives: Did you learn to …**
- Define primary and secondary enuresis?
- Describe some of the epidemiologic characteristics of enuresis?
- Evaluate a patient with enuresis?
- Develop a management strategy for enuresis?

 QUICK QUIZ: MECONIUM

Delayed meconium passage occurs in which of the following conditions?
A) Encopresis
B) Hirschsprung disease
C) Cystic fibrosis
D) Hyperthyroidism
E) B and C

The correct answer is "E." Seventy percent of newborns will pass meconium within the first 12 hours of life. More than 90% of newborns pass meconium within the first 24 hours. In those with delayed passage of meconium (generally defined as >24 hours of life), consider Hirschsprung disease, cystic fibrosis, hypothyroidism, sepsis, intrauterine narcotic exposure, or imperforate anus.

 QUICK QUIZ: RASH

Your next patient is a 3-year-old female with a rash. After playing outside (could playing outside be a red herring? The editors think so …), her father found spots on her legs, and she did not want to walk because her knees hurt. On examination, she is afebrile with normal vitals, slightly irritable, but otherwise interactive. She has slight nasal drainage, which her father says is residual from a cold last week. Her legs and buttocks have palpable purpura. Her knees are mildly swollen and are painful with range of motion. Her CBC (including platelets) and coagulation studies are normal, and her urinalysis is significant for 2+ hematuria.

The most likely diagnosis in this patient is:
A) Acute exposure to lawn chemicals
B) Henoch–Schönlein purpura (HSP)
C) Juvenile idiopathic arthritis (JIA)
D) Meningococcemia
E) Rocky Mountain spotted fever

The correct answer is "B." This is classic HSP (also known as "immunoglobulin A vasculitis"), an IgA-mediated, generally self-limited, leukocytoclastic vasculitis. The symptoms and signs of HSP are a rash (typically nonthrombocytopenic purpura), abdominal pain (from submucosal hemorrhage and edema), arthritis/arthralgia, and renal disease. Typically, the vasculitis follows an upper respiratory infection, as in this case, or streptococcal pharyngitis. Treatment for HSP is supportive, and

NSAIDs are first line. Monitoring for renal disease with serial UAs and blood pressure measurements after HSP is important.

"A," lawn chemical exposure, usually results in nothing acute but may cause acute cholinergic symptoms if organophosphates are used. "C," JIA, is not likely because the rash of systemic onset JIA is evanescent salmon-pink rash on the trunk and axilla that classically occurs when the patient spikes a fever. "D," meningococcemia, is incorrect because the patient is afebrile, alert, and nontoxic appearing without laboratory evidence of disseminated intravascular coagulopathy. "E" is unlikely because Rocky Mountain spotted fever presents with headache, high fever, petechial rash involving the palms and soles, and the patients will appear toxic. In addition, patients with Rocky Mountain spotted fever have thrombocytopenia when their petechiae appear.

HELPFUL TIP:
The rash of HSP is frequently initially urticaria with surrounding edema. The rash tends to be symmetric and occur in dependent areas developing first on the legs or on pressure points (buttocks). A discussion of treatment is beyond the scope of this book. However, common involvements include renal failure, GI bleeding, and more rarely CNS involvement such as seizures, CNS hemorrhage, etc.

▶ CASE 13.7

A 7-month-old fully immunized female presents to the office with fever. Mom reports she has "not been herself" and felt "a bit warm on the forehead." Vitals reveal a temperature of 39.2°C. Physical examination reveals an ill-appearing, nontoxic, and well-hydrated infant. You perform a complete history and physical but are unable to identify a source of the fever.

Question 13.7.1 After ensuring appropriate hemodynamics, what is the first step in your approach to this child?
A) Obtain a urinalysis and urine culture
B) Admit for observation and perform blood, urine, and CSF for culture
C) Give an intramuscular dose of ceftriaxone
D) Order acetaminophen 30 mg/kg and discharge the patient if the temperature comes down
E) Admit for IV fluids overnight

Answer 13.7.1 **The correct answer is "A."** At this age, occult serious bacterial infection is less likely than during the neonatal period especially when vaccinated against *Haemophilus influenzae* type b and *Streptococcus pneumoniae*. In a well-appearing child older than 90 days with a fever without a focal source, most experts recommend a screening urinalysis and urine culture as the initial diagnostic test. "B" is overly aggressive in a nontoxic patient, and "C" is not indicated and can make cultures more difficult to interpret should this child become

sicker. Use of antipyretics is reasonable, but in "D" the dose of acetaminophen is wrong (it should be 15 mg/kg/dose by mouth every 4–6 hours). Antipyretics may decrease fever of any cause, and "response" to acetaminophen would not negate the need for further evaluation. Since you are not seeing signs of dehydration, "E" is inappropriate.

HELPFUL TIP:
Studies have shown that the incidence of occult bacteremia is less than 1% in well-appearing **fully immunized** infants 3 to 36 months of age presenting with fever without localizing signs. Sometimes, a positive blood culture is due to contamination, which results in unnecessary additional testing, treatment, and cost. Some of you may be thinking, "What about a CBC?" In this patient, the WBC count can be equally misleading. The most important factors in decision-making are the patient's age, immunization status, and clinical appearance. Procalcitonin and/or CRP have not been found to be particularly predictive in outpatients and are *not* part of the routine evaluation of febrile pediatric outpatients.

Question 13.7.2 What is the most appropriate method of obtaining a urine specimen in this child?
A) Midstream "clean-catch"
B) Bag specimen from sterile plastic bag taped to the perineal region
C) Bladder catheterization
D) Suprapubic aspiration
E) C or D

Answer 13.7.2 **The correct answer is "C."** The gold standard test for the diagnosis of urinary tract infection is a quantitative urine culture. While the urinalysis and microscopy may suggest UTI, no component, or combination of components, is as sensitive or specific as an appropriately collected culture. Therefore, if a child is likely to require antimicrobial therapy, one should attempt to obtain urine for culture in a manner not likely to cause contamination. The midstream "clean-catch" may be obtained in older children who are toilet trained, making certain that the perineum is cleansed first. Bag specimens are prone to contamination and should NEVER be used for culture. If UTI is suspected or the source of fever is unknown, diapered children should ALWAYS have a catheterized urine sample obtained BEFORE starting antibiotics. Suprapubic aspiration is the gold standard, but it is typically more uncomfortable for the child and should only be performed by experienced providers.

HELPFUL TIP(S):
A negative bag-collected urinalysis and microscopy in a nontoxic infant may be helpful. If this is positive (not completely normal), it must be followed up with urine obtained by catheterization or suprapubic aspirate for urinalysis, microscopy, and culture. Any

nontoilet-trained child who will need antibiotics on a relatively emergent basis for a UTI should have urine obtained by catheterization or suprapubic aspiration sent for culture.

How many WBC/HPF are necessary to call it a UTI you might wonder? The answer is "zero." Thirteen percent of children with culture-proven UTI have no white cells in the urine (*Pediatrics*. 2016;138:e20160087). So, if you clinically think it is a complicated UTI, treat while awaiting the culture. Any delay in treating a *febrile* UTI in children leads to additional renal scaring (*JAMA Pediatr.* 2016 Jul 25).

Question 13.7.3 The patient has positive leukocyte esterase and nitrates on UA as well as 20 WBC/hpf on urine microscopy. Without knowing the culture and susceptibility results, which antibiotic would be the MOST appropriate choice for the treatment of a UTI in this child?
A) Trimethoprim/sulfamethoxazole (TMP/SMX)
B) Amoxicillin
C) Amoxicillin/clavulanate
D) Cefdinir
E) Ciprofloxicin

Answer 13.7.3 The correct answer is "D." The majority of urinary tract infections are due to Gram-negative organisms such as *Escherichia coli* in children and the resistance rate to amoxicillin is high (up to 40%). Thus, amoxicillin is not a good choice for empirically treating a UTI in children—or anybody, for that matter. The usual choice for empiric oral antibiotic treatment of UTI in children is a third-generation cephalosporin, such as cefdinir ("D"), cefixime, or cefpodoxime. Caution should be used with empiric use of first-generation cephalosporins, TMP/SMX ("A"), and amoxicillin/clavulanate ("C") due to increasing resistance of *E. coli* to these agents, though these agents may be appropriate if local resistance is low. Fluoroquinolones, such as "E," may be considered in adolescents or children with a *complicated* UTI. **No fluoroquinolones for cystitis**: The benefit is outweighed by the risk (persistent neurologic problems, hypoglycemia, etc.). Fluoroquinolones do seem to be as safe in children as in other patients but should be saved for situations where other drugs are suboptimal or ineffective, such as UTI caused by *Pseudomonas*. The duration of treatment should be 7 to 10 days for uncomplicated UTI. If the child appears clinically ill, has vomiting, or is less than 2 months old, initial parenteral treatment with ceftriaxone would be an appropriate first-line agent. After urine cultures return, coverage may be changed to a narrower-spectrum antibiotic, if possible. Note that nitrofurantoin is an acceptable alternative *for cystitis (but not pyelonephritis)* but is QID in children and expensive as a suspension.

Her urine culture reveals *Escherichia coli* susceptible to third-generation cephalosporins and resistant to narrower-spectrum drugs. You treat her appropriately.

Question 13.7.4 Following her initial treatment, what diagnostic study should be performed next?
A) Abdominal supine and upright radiographs
B) Renal ultrasound
C) Voiding cystourethrogram (VCUG)
D) Urology consultation for urodynamic studies
E) Both B and C

Answer 13.7.4 The correct answer is "B." In **febrile infants** with UTI, it is important to look for anatomic abnormalities of the urinary tract. Ultrasound imaging *(not VCUG)* is recommended following a first febrile UTI to identify those at risk for recurrence and subsequent damage to renal parenchyma (male or female). Urinary tract ultrasonography should be performed at the earliest convenient time. Ultrasound is useful in the evaluation for kidney size and hydronephrosis, but it is limited in the evaluation of vesicoureteral reflux (VUR), a common abnormality associated with recurrent UTI. VUR is evaluated with a VCUG or radionuclide cystogram (RNC). VCUG should be done after a first febrile UTI *only* when there is evidence of renal abnormality on the ultrasound, including scaring, hydronephrosis, abnormal anatomy, etc. Routine VCUG is NOT recommended. Thus, choices "B" and "E" are incorrect.

Right hydronephrosis was noted on ultrasound, and a VCUG is done. Your patient is found to have right-sided grade II reflux (see Table 13-5).

Question 13.7.5 Which of the following would be the most appropriate initial management of her grade II reflux?
A) Prescribe prophylactic antibiotics
B) Refer for surgical intervention
C) Perform renal scintigraphy to assess renal scarring
D) Observe for now with repeat ultrasound in 6 months
E) None of the above

Answer 13.7.5 The correct answer is "E." This remains a controversial topic. It seems (most) everyone agrees that children with grade I–II reflux with bladder and bowel dysfunction (BBD) benefit from prophylactic therapy in addition to treatment for the BBD. In those with grade I–II reflux and no bladder or bowel dysfunction, the benefit is less clear. Grade I and II reflux tends to resolve with maturity. It gets a bit trickier with grade III–IV. Overall, children with III–IV reflux seem to have

TABLE 13-5 INTERNATIONAL REFLUX STUDY COMMITTEE GRADING OF VESICOURETERAL REFLUX

Grade I: Involves the ureter only
Grade II: Involves the ureter, pelvis, and calyces without dilatation
Grade III: Involves the ureter, pelvis, and calyces with mild ureter and pelvis dilatation
Grade IV: Involves the ureter, pelvis, and calyces with significant dilatation and blunting of the calyceal fornices
Grade V: Demonstrates dilatation and tortuosity of the ureter as well as loss of the calyceal fornices

about half the number of infections with prophylactic therapy (typically with TMP/SMX); the benefit is most pronounced in those with a febrile first episode and bowel or bladder dysfunction. However, there is no difference in renal scarring and 63% develop resistant organisms vs. 19% in the placebo group (*N Engl J Med.* 2014;370;2367–2376; 2440–2441). The bottom line is to have a discussion with the parents and to promptly treat any UTIs to prevent renal scarring (particularly a risk in those with a temperature of >39°C or a non–*E. coli* organism). Renal scarring is best detected by radioisotope scanning with 99 m-technetium dimercaptosuccinate, but it is not indicated at this time. Therefore, "C" is incorrect. "D" is incorrect, as ultrasound would not be used to assess for resolution of VUR. Follow-up VCUGs are recommended only in presence of reflux, and generally are performed in 12- to 24-month intervals, though this is also (not surprisingly) variable.

HELPFUL (OR CONFUSING) TIP:
We don't know what the board examination will want as an answer. Historically, ultrasound *and* VCUG have been done after a first UTI in a male infant and a second UTI in a female infant. This gender differentiation no longer exists; do an US on every child with a first febrile UTI. Even though the AAP guidelines do not support doing a VCUG, the Section on Urology of the American Academy of Pediatrics published a statement in April 2012 disagreeing with the recommendation to not obtain a VCUG in children aged 2 months to 2 years after the first febrile UTI. Surgical intervention is generally reserved for those with severe reflux (grades IV and V) or recurrent UTI despite prophylactic antibiotics. See AAP guidelines in *Pediatrics.* 2011;128(3):595–610 (reaffirmed in 2016) for more information.

▶ **Objectives:** Did you learn to …
- Evaluate an older (>3 months old) infant with fever?
- Diagnose and treat a child with an initial urinary tract infection?
- Recognize that urinary tract infection is often a marker for urinary tract abnormalities in children?
- Manage a patient with VUR?

▶ **CASE 13.8**

Anthony is a 2,300-g male infant born at 35 weeks gestation to a 23-year-old G2P2 mother. The mother did not seek prenatal care and routine screening labs were not available. She presented to the ED in active labor shortly following spontaneous rupture of membranes at home. Upon transfer to the obstetric ward, she was noted to be febrile (38.8°C) and tachycardic. She was diagnosed with chorioamnionitis and received intravenous antibiotics. Five hours later, Anthony was delivered via spontaneous vaginal delivery.

Question 13.8.1 Management of this newborn infant whose mother was diagnosed with chorioamnionitis should include which of the following?
A) Empiric therapy with ampicillin and gentamicin
B) Empiric therapy with ampicillin
C) Empiric therapy with vancomycin
D) Empiric therapy with ceftriaxone
E) Empiric therapy with ampicillin and erythromycin

Answer 13.8.1 **The correct answer is "A."** Maternal chorioamnionitis is an important risk factor for early onset sepsis in the newborn. Based on the 2010 CDC guideline on the prevention of perinatal group B streptococcal disease (which remains current at the time of this edition), all infants born to mothers with chorioamnionitis should have screening labs and blood cultures at birth followed by minimum of 48 hours of antibiotic therapy. Antibiotic therapy may be extended and/or modified depending on the clinical course and culture results. Of note, there is significant institutional variation in this area, and some institutions utilize clinical prediction tools, such as the Kaiser Permanente Neonatal Sepsis Calculator, to guide decision-making and antibiotic treatment. Data suggests that a risk-based approach (compared to current CDC guidelines) may markedly reduce antibiotic use in infants without increasing the rate of early-onset sepsis (*JAMA Pediatr.* 2017;171(4):365–371). Updates to the CDC guidelines are in process, but for now we suspect that the test will follow current CDC guidelines. A lumbar puncture for CSF culture and analysis should be performed if the child is ill-appearing. Ampicillin and gentamicin ("A") as empiric therapy covers the most likely organisms including Group B streptococcus (GBS) and Gram-negative pathogens, respectively. Ceftriaxone ("D") should not be used in neonates, at it may displace bilirubin from albumin, leading to severe hyperbilirubinemia. Other third-generation cephalosporins, such as cefotaxime, can be used as an alternative to gentamicin in conjunction with ampicillin.

Anthony is started on appropriate antibiotics. Examination of this neonate reveals hepatosplenomegaly, lymphadenopathy, petechiae, and white mucocutaneous patches in the infant's mouth. His CBC reveals hemoglobin of 12 g/dL and a platelet count of 85,000/mm³ with evidence of hemolysis on the peripheral smear.

Question 13.8.2 The most likely pathogen infecting this infant is:
A) Rubella
B) Cytomegalovirus
C) *Toxoplasma gondii*
D) *Treponema pallidum*
E) *Candida albicans*

Answer 13.8.2 **The correct answer is "D."** Neonatal manifestations of congenital syphilis include hepatosplenomegaly, lymphadenopathy, jaundice, rash, hemolytic anemia, and thrombocytopenia. Unfortunately, these findings overlap considerably with many of the other congenital TORCH (toxoplasmosis, rubella, CMV, herpes) infections. *Abnormalities more specific to congenital syphilis* include white, patchy mucocutaneous lesions (think "condylomata lata"), edema, rhinitis (snuffles), osteochondritis, and pseudoparalysis. Congenital syphilis is caused by transplacental transmission of the spirochete *T. pallidum* ("D"). Intrauterine infection can result in stillbirth, hydrops fetalis, or prematurity.

HELPFUL TIP:
Late sequelae of congenital syphilis involve the bones and joints, teeth, eyes, and CNS and include bowed shins (Saber shins), frontal bossing, saddle nose, pegged central incisors, interstitial keratitis, and sensorineural deafness. The Hutchinson triad includes interstitial keratitis, deafness, and notched, peg-shaped teeth.

In addition to the laboratory data obtained above, you order an ultrasound of the patient's head, which appears normal.

Question 13.8.3 Intracerebral calcifications are CLASSICALLY associated with which congenital infection(s)?
A) Cytomegalovirus
B) Toxoplasmosis
C) *Treponema pallidum*
D) Rubella
E) A and B

Answer 13.8.3 The correct answer is "E." The clinical manifestations of congenital cytomegalovirus and toxoplasmosis are often similar. Infants are typically asymptomatic at birth, but a significant number ultimately develop visual impairment, learning disabilities, and developmental and intellectual delays months to years later. Those infants who are symptomatic at birth may demonstrate intrauterine growth retardation, hepatosplenomegaly, jaundice, hemolytic anemia, and thrombocytopenia. Intracerebral calcifications also occur in both CMV and toxoplasmosis. The calcifications tend to be periventricular in CMV (remember this by the fact that the calcifications look like a "C" in CMV) and more dispersed throughout the cortex in toxoplasmosis (remember by noting the "X" in both cortex and toxoplasmosis). Additional central nervous system abnormalities include microcephaly, chorioretinitis, and sensorineural hearing loss.

▶ **Objectives:** Did you learn to …
• Appropriately manage the neonate born to a mother who has evidence of chorioamnionitis?
• Recognize that many congenital TORCH infections may have overlapping signs and symptoms?
• Recognize that many infants with congenital TORCH infections are asymptomatic at birth?

 QUICK QUIZ: CONGENITAL INFECTIONS

A small-for-gestational age newborn infant is found to have hepatosplenomegaly, jaundice, and thrombocytopenia. Cardiac examination reveals a grade II/VI continuous murmur heard best at the left upper sternal border. An ophthalmologic examination demonstrates microphthalmia and cataracts.

The result of which maternal prenatal screening lab is likely to have been concerning in the above case?
A) VDRL
B) Rubella immunity status
C) HIV status
D) Varicella zoster immunity status
E) Group B streptococcal (GBS) cultures

The correct answer is "B." Cardiac, ophthalmologic, auditory, and neurologic findings predominate in the symptomatic infant with congenital rubella. Up to 85% of infants infected during the first 12 weeks of gestation will have some form of congenital defect. This decreases to 5% when the primary infection occurs after the third to fourth month of gestation. Ophthalmologic findings include microphthalmia, cataracts, glaucoma, and salt and pepper retinopathy. Infants are often microcephalic and develop sensorineural hearing deficits, meningoencephalitis, and developmental delay. **Deafness, cataracts, and cardiac anomalies are the classic findings with congenital rubella.** Additional findings of hepatosplenomegaly, thrombocytopenia, and osteitis may be present. A characteristic "blueberry muffin" appearance may be present due to the combination of jaundice and extramedullary (skin) hematopoiesis. Syphilis and GBS infections are described above and they do not typically cause the ophthalmologic findings described in this case. "C" is incorrect because congenital HIV infection is commonly asymptomatic. Evidence of immune deficiency may present later in the child's life with failure to thrive, generalized lymphadenopathy, hepatosplenomegaly, and recurrent infections. "D" is incorrect because congenital herpes infections do not cause cardiac abnormalities.

HELPFUL TIP:
USPSTF recommends (Grade A) universal newborn screening for hemoglobinopathies and congenital hypothyroidism as well prophylactic ocular topical medication for gonorrhea in all newborns. The USPSTF had previously recommended universal hearing screening for all newborns (Grade B) but are now silent on the issue. The AAP and AAFP still support universal hearing screening in all newborns. An eye exam is now recommended at age 3 to 5 years for all patients (https://www.uspreventiveservicestaskforce.org/).

 QUICK QUIZ: CONGENITAL RUBELLA

Which of the following cardiac lesions is most likely to be found in an infant with congenital rubella?
A) Patent ductus arteriosus (PDA)
B) Tetralogy of Fallot
C) Transposition of great vessels
D) Coarctation of aorta
E) Bicuspid aortic valve

The correct answer is "A." The most common cardiac lesions associated with congenital rubella are PDA and peripheral pulmonary artery stenosis. PDA is characterized by a continuous "machine-like" murmur heard best over the left upper sternal border. *Tetralogy of Fallot and transposition of great vessels are classically cyanotic heart defects that have no known association with congenital infections.* Coarctation of the aorta and bicuspid aortic valve both cause harsh systolic murmurs. The murmur of coarctation radiates to the back. Both coarctation and bicuspid aortic valve are commonly found in females with Turner syndrome.

▶ CASE 13.9

A term newborn infant is noted to have a solitary, tense bulla located on the dorsum of his wrist. The underlying skin is nonerythematous. Pregnancy was uncomplicated; however, the infant was delivered via cesarean section for failure to progress. The infant appears to be a vigorous feeder and is noted to frequently suck on his hands and wrists while in the nursery. He is otherwise asymptomatic.

Question 13.9.1 Which of the following is MOST appropriate at this time?
A) Start acyclovir
B) Perform lumbar puncture and send a sample of the CSF for HSV PCR
C) Perform a Tzanck smear of the bulla fluid
D) Obtain CBC and blood cultures
E) Observation with no intervention at this time

Answer 13.9.1 The correct answer is "E." Nothing needs to be done at this time. The appearance and location of the bulla is consistent with a sucking blister. A solitary bulla or blister on normal-appearing skin located on the upper limbs may be present at birth from in utero sucking. Often when presented with the affected extremity, the infant will demonstrate the sucking behavior in that location. Such blisters are often mistaken for herpes simplex, but the solitary nature and location help to establish the correct diagnosis—although there may be multiple blisters at times. Additional history of cesarean section makes HSV less likely in this scenario. Nonetheless, a sucking blister is a diagnosis of exclusion, and other more serious diagnoses should be ruled out by history and examination and further testing as indicated.

Question 13.9.2 The FALSE statement regarding neonatal herpes simplex virus infection is:
A) The majority of infants with neonatal HSV are born to mothers with symptomatic herpetic lesions
B) The incidence of neonatal transmission is higher when the pregnant woman experiences primary infection versus secondary reactivation
C) Most neonatal HSV infections are caused by HSV 2
D) Intrauterine exposure accounts for the minority of perinatal HSV infection
E) Herpetic skin lesions are often present in infants with CNS or disseminated HSV

Answer 13.9.2 The correct answer is "A." Less than one-third of infants with neonatal HSV are born to mothers with active genital lesions. In fact, most cases of neonatal HSV are found in infants of *asymptomatic mothers who are shedding the virus.* Neonatal herpes simplex virus often results in serious morbidity and mortality. Infants with HSV present with one of the following three disease patterns with overlapping features: localized disease involving the skin, eyes, and mouth; CNS disease; or disseminated infection. Encephalitis may occur with or without skin involvement; therefore, HSV infection should be suspected in any infant from birth to approximately 4 weeks of age that presents with fever, seizure, or mental status abnormalities such as lethargy, irritability, or poor feeding.

The other options are correct. A woman who contracts a primary infection during the pregnancy has a greater than 30% chance of transmitting the virus to her infant ("B"). There is less than 2% transmission if she experiences a secondary reactivation intrapartum. The majority of neonatal HSV is due to infection with HSV 2 ("C"). Only 5% of congenital infections occur in utero ("D"), as the majority occurs via exposure to infected cervical secretions during birth. Skin lesions ("E") are present in 60% of CNS cases and about 75% of disseminated cases.

HELPFUL TIP:
Most neonates with HSV infection do not present with skin findings at birth. It is more typical for neonates to develop HSV skin lesions 5 to 14 days after delivery.

HELPFUL TIP:
Infants born vaginally or via cesarean delivery to moms with active genital HSV lesions need HSV cultures or PCR of the mouth, nasopharynx, conjunctiva, and rectum obtained at 12 to 24 hours of age. In infants born to moms with a **primary** outbreak at time of delivery, guidelines recommend empiric acyclovir therapy after obtaining surface cultures/PCRs, blood PCR, and CSF PCR. Asymptomatic infants of mothers with a recurrent outbreak do not require empiric acyclovir treatment but still should receive surface swabs and blood PCR and be monitored closely for signs of infection. Symptomatic infants additionally require CSF for HSV PCR and acyclovir treatment.

▶ **Objectives: Did you learn to …**
- Differentiate between a herpes lesion and a sucking blister?
- Recognize rates and modes of transmission of herpes in neonates?
- Identify some of the clinical manifestations of neonatal herpes?

▶ CASE 13.10

A bunch of parents in your neighborhood decide to have a "chickenpox" party (prompting you to consider moving to a place where people believe in modern medicine). They want to synchronize their kids' chickenpox outbreaks with their busy schedules (heaven forbid we should get immunized—after all, it isn't natural!). One of the mothers, who has never had chickenpox herself, finds out that she is pregnant the day after being exposed to chickenpox. She is not yet symptomatic—from the pregnancy or the chickenpox

Question 13.10.1 The best advice for this potential mother about her pregnancy is:
A) Consider termination since it is likely that the child will have congenital varicella
B) Get treated within 96 hours of exposure with varicella immune globulin
C) Get treated within 96 hours of exposure with varicella immune globulin plus varicella vaccine
D) Get treated within 96 hours of exposure with IVIG plus varicella vaccine
E) No further action is needed

Answer 13.10.1 The correct answer is "B." Women who are varicella-susceptible (nonimmune), pregnant, and exposed to chickenpox should be treated with varicella immune globulin (VariZIG) within 96 hours of exposure, though some sources recommend administration up to 10 days post-exposure. If VariZIG is unavailable, IVIG may be given instead. The vaccine should be avoided during pregnancy (thus "C" and "D" are incorrect). It is a live, attenuated virus and still carries some risk to the fetus (although the degree of risk is unknown). It is safe to give the vaccine to mom in the *postpartum* period and is indicated if the mother is screened to be varicella nonimmune during her pregnancy. The risk of congenital varicella syndrome if the fetus is exposed in the first trimester is about 2%. The risk of neonatal infection is much higher if the mother is infected within 5 days of birth, and 30% of these cases result in severe neonatal varicella infection.

Question 13.10.2 You can let the mother know that:
A) Varicella immune globulin has been shown to reduce the risk of congenital varicella
B) Varicella immune globulin is aimed mostly at attenuating the case in the mother should she be infected
C) Varicella immune globulin has been shown to prevent congenital varicella
D) A and B
E) B and C

Answer 13.10.2 The correct answer is "B." Varicella immune globulin is aimed at reducing the symptoms in the mother and attenuating her case of varicella. Both "A" and "C" are false. There are no good data either way about how VariZIG will affect the child's outcome vis-à-vis congenital varicella. The theoretical benefit outweighs the risk of administration of VariZIG.

Question 13.10.3 Manifestations of intrauterine infection with varicella zoster include all of the following defects EXCEPT:
A) Optic atrophy
B) Congenital cataracts
C) Cardiac abnormalities
D) CNS abnormalities
E) Limb hypoplasia

Answer 13.10.3 The correct answer is "C." Cardiac abnormalities are not seen with varicella zoster exposure in utero. In addition to the findings above, patients with congenital varicella zoster will have cutaneous scarring called cicatrix. Intrauterine growth restriction is also a common finding.

Glory! The chickenpox party worked! Now that all of these children have been infected with varicella zoster, the question arises about how long they should be kept out of school.

Question 13.10.4 These children are considered infectious until:
A) 5 days after the first lesion appears
B) 10 to 14 days after the first lesion appears
C) New lesions are no longer forming
D) All lesions are crusted over
E) They are no longer febrile

Answer 13.10.4 The correct answer is "D." Patients are considered infectious until all lesions are crusted over. Lesions need not have healed entirely, only crusted over.

Question 13.10.5 The mother of your next patient has 4 children, and she is interested in having them vaccinated for varicella (At last, VICTORY!). In which of the following children is varicella vaccination contraindicated?
A) A 4-year-old with asthma on medium-dose inhaled corticosteroids
B) A healthy 3-year-old whose father is on immunosuppression for rheumatoid arthritis
C) A healthy 1-year old who has a newborn baby brother at home
D) A 8-year-old child with HIV and a normal CD4+ T-cell count
E) None of the above

Answer 13.10.5 The correct answer is "E." All of the above children may receive the varicella vaccine. Children with asthma and other conditions requiring *systemic* corticosteroids should not receive the varicella vaccine (remember, it is a live-attenuated vaccine) **if** they are on 2 mg/kg/day or more (up to 20 mg) of prednisone-equivalent for 14 days or more. Thus, "A" is incorrect. Children exposed to immunocompromised individuals, such as "B" should get the varicella vaccine to decrease risk of bringing wild-type varicella into the home. They do not need to be isolated from the immunosuppressed person, unless they develop skin lesions, at which time they should avoid direct contact until the lesions are resolved. Varicella-naïve siblings ("C") and mothers (even if breastfeeding) of infants should receive varicella vaccine. If a woman of child-bearing age obtains varicella vaccination, she should avoid pregnancy for 1 month after immunization, since the effect of the attenuated virus on a fetus is not known. Children with HIV, such as "D," may receive varicella vaccination if they have a normal CD4+ T-cell count (CD4+ T-cell percentage ≥15% for children 1 through 13 years of age and CD4+ T-cell count ≥200/mm³ for adolescents ≥14 years of age). Children with immunodeficiencies affecting T-cell mediated immunity should **not** receive the vaccine.

▶ Objectives: Did you learn to …
- Offer treatment for varicella exposure to a pregnant nonimmune female?
- Recognize the uses of varicella immune globulin?
- Identify symptoms of congenital varicella infection?
- Enumerate contraindications to varicella vaccination?

▶ CASE 13.11

A 3-year-old child presents to your office with a history of bright red cheeks. Over the past several days, she has had mild fever with mild muscle aches. Except for the rash, the child is now asymptomatic.

Question 13.11.1 **The most likely cause of this patient's illness is:**
A) Parvovirus B-19
B) Herpes virus 6
C) Rubeola
D) Rubella
E) Influenza virus

Answer 13.11.1 **The correct answer is "A."** A mild systemic illness followed by red, "slapped cheeks" is typical of erythema infectiosum or "fifth disease," caused by parvovirus B-19. The red, slapped cheeks are generally followed by a lacy, reticular rash on the extremities and trunk. This is usually a self-limited illness in children.

Question 13.11.2 **Which of the following is LEAST likely to be a complication of parvovirus B-19 infection—either congenital or acquired?**
A) Aplastic anemia
B) Birth defects, including CNS and limb disease
C) Hydrops fetalis
D) Inflammatory arthritis
E) Intrauterine fetal death

Answer 13.11.2 **The correct answer is "B."** Parvovirus B-19 causes all of the above except for birth defects. Fetal death, anemia, or nonimmune-mediated hydrops fetalis are potential outcomes of intrauterine exposure (one-third of infected women will pass the virus to their fetus). Most infants infected in utero are born normally at term, including those with evidence of hydrops earlier in the pregnancy. A small subset will acquire chronic or prolonged postnatal infection of unknown significance. "A," transient aplastic crisis, can occur in those with chronic hemolytic conditions such as sickle cell anemia. "D," inflammatory arthritis, is common in adults and adolescents with females more commonly affected. Although a few reports describe congenital abnormalities with parvovirus infection, most parvovirus infections do not cause congenital anomalies.

. . . .

The question of whether or not to exclude this child from preschool is raised. The patient still has the rash. There are a couple of pregnant teachers at the preschool.

Question 13.11.3 **You can tell the child's mother that:**
A) This child is infectious and should be excluded from preschool until the rash resolves
B) Since almost all adult women are already immune, there is no need to worry about transmission to the teachers
C) Since this virus is an enterovirus, careful hygiene in the school will prevent spread
D) This child can be allowed back into preschool and is no longer infectious

Answer 13.11.3 **The correct answer is "D."** Once the rash is present, this child is no longer infectious and can be allowed back into school. "B" is incorrect because only about 50% of adult women are immune. "C" is incorrect. First, this is not an enterovirus. Even though URI symptoms are often absent, transmission is mostly respiratory with vertical transmission of mother to fetus, and hematogenous spread (via transmissions) being much less common.

HELPFUL TIP:
Just try getting this child with a rash back in school and past the school nurse (we dare you); it can be difficult! On a related note, some schools are sure that there is a "magical effect" of topical antibiotics in preventing the spread of viral conjunctivitis. Don't drink the Kool-Aid.

▶ Objectives: Did you learn to …
- Recognize the clinical manifestations of parvovirus B-19 infection ("fifth disease")?
- Identify complications of parvovirus B-19 infection?

QUICK QUIZ: CHILDHOOD INFECTIONS

Which of the following is characterized by a high fever, possibly over 40°C, a bulging fontanelle, a maculopapular rash that begins *after* the fever abates, conjunctivitis, and upper respiratory symptoms?
A) Roseola infantum (erythema subitum)
B) Rubeola (measles)
C) Rubella (German measles)
D) Varicella (chicken pox)
E) Meningococcal meningitis

The correct answer is "A." Such a clinical presentation is typical of roseola infantum. Roseola infantum, which is caused by the human herpes 6 (and rarely herpes 7) virus, is characterized by a high fever for 3 to 5 days (often over 40°C), generalized malaise, a bulging fontanelle in up to 26% of infants, conjunctivitis, perhaps oral mucosal ulcers, and a rash that appears as the child begins to defervesce. Children usually look amazingly well given the degree of fever that they experience.

QUICK QUIZ: GASTROINTESTINAL SYMPTOMS

A young couple brings in their 18-month-old female for a 12-hour history of vomiting and diarrhea. The patient has felt warm, and her oral intake has been depressed. However, she continues to make tears with crying and has wet diapers. Her medical history is unremarkable. On examination, you find a tired-looking toddler who perks up slightly when you open a bag of toys (who *are* you anyway … Santa?). Her temperature is 38.5°C, and her capillary refill is less than 3 seconds. The remainder of the examination is unremarkable. You think that she has a viral gastroenteritis and give the parents some advice regarding rehydration.

Which of the following is the most appropriate advice for this patient?
A) Avoid all solid food for the next 24 to 48 hours
B) Use milk as the primary rehydration solution
C) Use only watered-down tea for rehydration
D) Use a commercially prepared oral rehydration solution and reintroduce foods as tolerated
E) Use cola beverages (e.g., Coca-Cola or Pepsi) because they contain more sodium than commercially available oral rehydration solutions

The correct answer is "D." Effective oral rehydration can be accomplished with any one of the rehydration solutions on the market (e.g., Pedialyte). "A" is incorrect. There is no need to limit the food intake of patients with vomiting or infectious diarrhea. They can have whatever they can tolerate *without vomiting*. The concept of "gut rest" is obsolete and leads to increased bowel permeability and prolonged diarrhea. So, early feeding is optimal and recommended. There is no need to avoid lactose-containing products. Transient lactase deficiency after gastroenteritis is usually self-limited (and generally limited to those <2 months of age) and does not require treatment unless symptoms are prolonged or severe after dietary re-introduction. "C" and "E" are incorrect. There is no role for weak tea, flat soda, "Jello water," sports drinks, juice, etc., in the management of gastroenteritis. The most common cause of hyponatremic seizures in the child is improper rehydration during gastroenteritis. Many commercial drinks, such as cola beverages and sports drinks, are not specifically designed for oral rehydration, and the sodium concentration is typically much lower than that in rehydration solutions, risking hyponatremia (in other words, the reverse of "E" is true). In addition, many of these have a high sugar content, which can worsen diarrhea due to osmotic effects.

HELPFUL TIP:
In the exclusively breastfed infant with vomiting and/or diarrhea, breastfeeding should be encouraged and not replaced with oral rehydration solutions. Similarly, use of formula or expressed breast milk in bottle-fed infants should be encouraged as long as it is tolerated.

HELPFUL TIP:
During a GI illness, advise parents to avoid nonabsorbable sugars, like those found in apple or grape juice. These can promote an osmotic diarrhea.

▶ CASE 13.12

A new mother and father bring their 2-month-old infant to your office with a complaint of inconsolable crying. This started at about 3 weeks of age and occurs about the same time every day. The crying will last for hours and is becoming quite disruptive. The child will draw up his knees and seem to be in quite a bit of pain. They have tried pretty much everything that they can think of, including car rides, swings, swaddling, various types of soothing music (such as death metal), etc., but to no avail. Shivers run up and down your spine as you recall your own early parenting experiences … or as you remember why you don't have kids (please apply the appropriate phrase for your personal experience).

Question 13.12.1 **The most likely diagnosis is:**
A) Colic
B) Intussusception
C) Hair around the penis or toes or corneal abrasion
D) Constipation
E) Cluster headache

Answer 13.12.1 **The correct answer is "A."** Colic generally begins at 3 weeks of age, peaks at about 6 weeks of age, and abates by 3 months of age. It is defined by a rule of 3s: intense crying for 3 hours per day, for 3 days per week, for 3 weeks. However, most parents, grandparents, nosy aunts, and pediatricians will describe any particularly fussy baby as "colicky." The cause is unknown. "B" is incorrect. While intussusception can certainly present with colicky abdominal pain, it is not likely to be recurrent for several days or weeks without a more significant problem (e.g., bloody stools) developing. "C," a hair or thread around a child's toes or penis or corneal abrasion, should be considered in any child with inconsolable crying. Again, this is not likely to result in crying that is daily and episodic. "D" is incorrect as this history is not consistent with constipation. And "E," a cluster headache, does not occur in this age group.

HELPFUL TIP:
While inconsolable crying has often been attributed to a corneal abrasion, recent data calls this into question. Just as many children who were NOT crying had corneal abrasions.

Question 13.12.2 You can advise the parents that:
A) Phenobarbital is safe and effective for controlling infant colic (when given to the parents to help them "chill out")
B) Elimination of cruciferous vegetables from the diet of breast-feeding mothers has been shown to reduce infant colic
C) Simethicone has been shown to be effective in infant colic
D) Anticholinergic drugs may be effective in treating infant colic, but the risks are unacceptable
E) Children who breastfeed are less likely to develop colic

Answer 13.12.2 **The correct answer is "D."** Anticholinergic drugs have been shown to be effective in the treatment of colic. However, the risks associated with the use of these drugs are generally considered unacceptable; thus, they should NOT be used for colic. The rest of the answers are incorrect. It does not seem as though breastfed infants are any less likely to develop colic than are bottle-fed infants ("E"). The evidence for elimination of cruciferous vegetables is inconclusive. Simethicone ("C") is NOT effective in treating infantile colic and can be expensive, but it is not harmful and gives the parents something to do.

HELPFUL TIP:
The cause of colic is unknown and likely multifactorial. Rarely is a medical explanation found. **It is important to identify alternative caregivers, since infant colic can be a major stress on parents and can possibly lead to abuse (particularly shaken baby syndrome).** Parent education is critical.

HELPFUL TIP:
There is evidence to support a trial of an extensively hydrolyzed infant formula (e.g., Nutramigen) for infant colic. Data isn't the strongest, though. Use of partially hydrolyzed or lactose-free formulas is of no benefit. Changing to a soy formula does not work.

HELPFUL TIP:
Data suggest that probiotics are *NOT* effective in infant colic (*BMJ.* 2014;348:g2107). However, they are safe and give the parents something to do. In breastfeeding women, elimination of common allergens (milk, eggs, nuts, wheat) can be tried. Again, the data isn't the greatest. Evidence for spinal manipulation in treating colic is inconclusive and may carry risk. As with most chiropractic studies, the data is poor. In a crossover study, 24% sucrose has been shown to be beneficial (Tootsweet and other brands ... or make it yourself), but is not routinely recommended. Finally, though the data is poor, acupuncture is standard in Sweden (of course they also eat lutefisk).

▶ Objective: Did you learn to ...
• Evaluate a patient with colic and offer management strategies to the parents?

 QUICK QUIZ: EPIGLOTTITIS 1

You have an anxious child in the ED who is toxic appearing with a history of sudden onset of high fever, drooling, and stridor. He is leaning forward, with his neck hyperextended, and chin thrust forward (tripod position). You suspect epiglottitis.

What is the FIRST step in the treatment of this patient?
A) Draw blood work including a CBC
B) Place an IV for access and fluids
C) Give a dose of IM steroids (e.g., dexamethasone 0.6 mg/kg) to help shrink the epiglottis
D) Put a face mask on the child and administer albuterol
E) Leave the child on the mother's lap and don't upset the child (you don't want a temper tantrum in the ED)

The correct answer is "E." Anything that upsets the child can lead to increased airway obstruction. Leave the child in the parent's lap and do not upset him. "A" and "B" are incorrect because they may upset the child, leading to increased work of breathing and increased obstruction. "C," dexamethasone, is indicated for croup and not for epiglottitis. "D" is also incorrect. However, it would **not** be wrong to give blow-by oxygen or blow-by nebulized epinephrine **if it did not agitate the child.**

 QUICK QUIZ: EPIGLOTTITIS 2

Which of the following is NOT needed in the optimal diagnosis and treatment of epiglottitis?
A) "Thumb sign" on radiograph
B) Antibiotics to cover *H. influenzae*
C) Antibiotics to cover *S. pneumoniae*
D) An operating room
E) Personnel able to emergently manage the airway

The correct answer is "A." The use of radiographs in suspected epiglottitis is fraught with problems and delays potentially life-saving therapy. DON'T DO IT. Epiglottitis is a clinical diagnosis that requires visualization of the epiglottis. This is preferably done in the operating room with a setup for both intubation and tracheostomy should that become necessary. If the child is mildly ill, looking at the epiglottis in the ED is permissible. However, be prepared to manage the airway. "B" and "C" are both correct. Since the advent of *H. influenzae B* vaccine, there is no longer a single organism causing most cases of epiglottitis. Bacteria that can cause epiglottitis include *H. influenzae*, *S. pneumoniae*, *S. aureus*, and groups A, B, and C beta-hemolytic streptococci. Epiglottitis may also be of viral origin.

 QUICK QUIZ: NEONATAL INFECTIONS

What is the most likely etiologic agent in this child: 2-week-old male with conjunctivitis, cough, rales, nasal congestion, infiltrate on radiograph, but no fever or wheezes?

A) Influenza
B) *Chlamydia*
C) Respiratory syncytial virus (RSV)
D) Parainfluenza
E) *Gonorrhea*

The correct answer is "B." This is a classic description of *Chlamydia trachomatis* infection in the newborn. Patients usually present between 5 and 14 days with exudative conjunctivitis and pneumonia. The gold standard for diagnosis of neonatal *Chlamydia* infection remains a culture obtained from conjunctival swabs of the everted eyelids; however, nucleic acid amplification tests of conjunctival scrapings have been found to have high sensitivity and specificity when compared with culture. Conjunctival cells must be present for an adequate specimen because *Chlamydia* is an intracellular pathogen. Exudates are not adequate for testing. Treatment is with systemic antibiotics **even if conjunctivitis is the only symptom present.** A macrolide is the appropriate treatment. Erythromycin (50 mg/kg/day divided four times daily for 14 days) or azithromycin (20 mg/kg/day for 3 days) may be used. Topical treatment may be used as an adjunct but alone is not sufficient for treatment of this patient. *Remember, the antibiotic eye ointment applied to the neonate at birth protects against ocular gonococcal infection but not Chlamydia.*

▶ CASE 13.13

A 12-month-old presents to your office in January with a 2-day history of runny nose and cough. The child now has wheezing with nasal flaring and retractions, and his oxygen saturation is 89%. There has been no fever, and several of the other children and adults in the family have had "a cold" over the past several weeks. On examination, you hear scattered wheezes and rales. You diagnose bronchiolitis.

Question 13.13.1 The MOST LIKELY virus involved in this child's illness is:
A) Rhinovirus
B) Adenovirus
C) Respiratory syncytial virus (RSV)
D) Parainfluenza
E) Human metapneumovirus

Answer 13.13.1 **The correct answer is "C."** The **most common** cause of bronchiolitis in children is RSV. All of the others can also cause bronchiolitis, as can influenza virus, but less commonly than RSV.

Question 13.13.2 Which of the following treatments has been unequivocally shown to be effective in bronchiolitis?
A) Nebulized albuterol
B) Nebulized epinephrine
C) Corticosteroids such as prednisone or dexamethasone
D) All of the above
E) None of the above

Answer 13.13.2 **The correct answer is "E."** None of the above has been shown to be effective in bronchiolitis. The mainstay of treatment is supportive care. Albuterol may transiently worsen hypoxia due to induction of V/Q mismatch and is not recommended.

 HELPFUL TIP:
Hypertonic saline was previously used in hospitalized infants and children as a treatment for bronchiolitis. It is no longer routinely recommended; it did not change duration of illness or hospitalization. Supportive care (maintenance of oxygenation and hydration) remains the mainstay of treatment.

Question 13.13.3 RSV is usually diagnosed by:
A) Nasal wash using immunofluorescence, antigen detection, or PCR
B) Baseline and convalescent antibody titers
C) Blood culture for RSV
D) Sputum Gram stain
E) Induced sputum culture

Answer 13.13.3 **The correct answer is "A."** A nasal wash for RSV immunofluorescence, antigen detection, or PCR is used to diagnose RSV. If a nasal wash cannot be obtained, a nasopharyngeal swab or throat swab offers the next best alternative. RT-PCR assays are becoming more cost-effective. Thus, they are being increasingly utilized as the first-line test at some institutions. Keep in mind that doing viral testing for children with bronchiolitis is **not** routinely recommended. In general, knowing which virus is causing the illness will not change management. Influenza testing may be useful at times of high prevalence in the community, as use of oseltamivir may be indicated. The other options are incorrect. Remember that "respiratory panels" can cost upwards of several hundred dollars.

HELPFUL TIP:
Bronchiolitis is a clinical diagnosis that does not require any diagnostic testing. Routine use of chest x-rays, CBCs, and viral testing is not recommended.

HELPFUL TIP:
Never give aerosolized ribavirin for the treatment of RSV. It doesn't work.

Question 13.13.4 Which of the following is indicated for the *prevention* of RSV in high-risk infants?
A) Vaccination against RSV
B) Oral ribavirin
C) Rimantadine or oseltamivir
D) Palivizumab (Synagis®)
E) RSV–IVIG (RespiGam)

Answer 13.13.4 **The correct answer is "D."** Palivizumab is a licensed prophylactic monoclonal antibody against RSV that is given via monthly intramuscular injection to high-risk patient populations during the RSV season. Administration of palivizumab is recommended before RSV season begins and then is given monthly for a maximum of five doses. RSV–IGIV, or RespiGam, is no longer used. There is no current RSV vaccine. None of the antiviral medications ("B" and "C") works for prevention or treatment of RSV.

HELPFUL TIP:
The following are the criteria for palivizumab:
• First year of life if born before 29 weeks, 0 day gestation.
• First year of life for infants born before 32 weeks, 0 day gestation with chronic lung disease of prematurity requiring oxygen for at least 28 days after birth.
• First year of life if cyanotic or hemodynamically significant heart disease.
• Second year of life if still requiring at least 28 days of oxygen and needing interventions such as steroids, diuretics, etc.
• Consider for immunosuppressed infants <24 months of age who will be immunosuppressed during RSV season.
• Keep abreast of RSV in your state; each state has specific rules for when Medicaid will cover palivizumab.

▶ **Objectives: Did you learn to …**
• Recognize the clinical presentation of a patient with RSV bronchiolitis?
• Diagnose and treat RSV bronchiolitis?
• Describe what patients may possibly benefit from RSV prophylaxis?

▶ **CASE 13.14**

A 4-week-old infant presents to your office with his parents. The parents note that he vomits every time he eats. His vomitus is mostly formula and is always nonbilious. He seems to be hungry and is demanding to be fed often. He does not have diarrhea. Examination reveals an afebrile and moderately dehydrated infant in no distress with tachycardia, a normal cardiopulmonary examination, and a relatively benign abdomen. His weight today is unchanged from a weight taken in your office 2 weeks ago. There is no "olive" palpable (really, have any of you actually felt the "olive")?

Question 13.14.1 Your working diagnosis is:
A) Midgut volvulus
B) Gastroenteritis
C) Pyloric stenosis
D) CNS injury with increased intracranial pressure

Answer 13.14.1 **The correct answer is "C."** This most likely represents idiopathic hypertrophic pyloric stenosis. The classic presentation of pyloric stenosis is nonbilious vomiting immediately after feeding, followed by a demand to feed again soon after (much the same as a teenager … the demand of feeding, not the vomiting). The symptoms are progressive. Initially, the vomiting may or may not be projectile and may occur after every feed or intermittently. Classically, pyloric stenosis occurs in infants 2 weeks to 2 months of age. Patients with prolonged symptoms are likely to have a hypokalemic hypochloremic metabolic alkalosis. "A," midgut volvulus, a surgical emergency, is unlikely because these patients have *bilious* vomiting. Our patient has nonbilious vomiting. "B," gastroenteritis, is not likely because there is no diarrhea, fever, or appetite loss. "D" is unlikely. While CNS injury with increased intracranial pressure and vomiting is a possibility, you would expect to see other evidence of CNS injury such as lethargy, possibly signs of head injury, etc. Note that this patient's weight is unchanged from 2 weeks ago, but it should be higher than 2 weeks ago.

Question 13.14.2 Which of the following patients is most likely to present with pyloric stenosis?
A) A first-born male
B) A first-born female
C) A second-born male
D) A second-born female
E) The rate of pyloric stenosis is equal in all of these groups

Answer 13.14.2 **The correct answer is "A."** There is a 4:1 male:female preponderance, and about 30% of all cases occur in a first-born child. Family history is important as infants born to a mother or father who had pyloric stenosis are at increased risk.

You give the patient a bolus of IV normal saline and decide to proceed with imaging to confirm the diagnosis.

Question 13.14.3 Of the following, which is the MOST appropriate initial study to assess for pyloric stenosis?
A) Plain abdominal x-ray
B) Upper endoscopy
C) Abdominal ultrasound
D) Upper gastrointestinal (UGI) contrast study
E) Abdominal CT

Answer 13.14.3 **The correct answer is "C."** In experienced hands, ultrasonography has greater than 95% sensitivity and specificity for pyloric stenosis. It has the additional advantage of avoiding radiation exposure. A pyloric muscle length, or thickness above the upper limits of normal, suggests the diagnosis. An UGI contrast study ("D") may be used as a secondary test if physical exam and ultrasonography are nondiagnostic (or ultrasonography is not available). The "string sign" on an UGI study suggests pyloric stenosis, and it is formed when contrast material trickles through the elongated pyloric channel (and thus looks like a thin string on x-ray). "A" and "E" are not indicated (or useful) for diagnosing pyloric stenosis. Endoscopy ("B") would only be indicated if other diagnostic studies were inconclusive and significant clinical suspicion remained. Palpation of the "olive" on physical exam is helpful if present; however, the diagnosis of infantile pyloric stenosis is increasingly being made by imaging studies before the olive becomes large enough to be palpable. Do an imaging study if you have any concern for pyloric stenosis.

HELPFUL TIP:
The definitive treatment for pyloric stenosis is surgical. However, it is an urgent, but not emergent, surgical indication. Make sure to take the time to correct fluid and electrolyte abnormalities prior to surgery.

You have a surgical consultant see the patient, pyloromyotomy is done, and everybody is happy.

▶ **Objectives: Did you learn to …**
 • Identify clinical manifestations of pyloric stenosis?
 • Diagnose and manage pyloric stenosis?

 QUICK QUIZ: PEDIATRIC BELLY PAIN

The treatment for midgut volvulus is:
A) Watchful waiting
B) Maneuver of Leopold
C) Emergent surgery
D) Air enema
E) Nasogastric suction and bowel rest

The correct answer is "C." Midgut volvulus is a surgical emergency. Midgut volvulus is an anatomical twisting of the bowel and needs to be surgically corrected. It presents with recurrent bilious vomiting; bilious vomiting in an infant should prompt you to rule out midgut volvulus. None of the others is correct. Watchful waiting is dangerous and risks ischemic bowel with perforation, so "A" and "E" are wrong. Leopold maneuvers are used to move a breech pregnancy to vertex and have nothing to do with the bowel. "D," air enema, can be used to reduce an intussusception but has no role in the treatment of midgut volvulus. "E" nasogastric suction and bowel rest are the treatment for a small bowel obstruction. Any bowel obstruction in a child demands investigation.

▶ **CASE 13.15**

A 5-year-old male who was recently diagnosed with influenza presents to your ED with complaints (via the parents) of intractable vomiting and mental status changes. On examination, the child is febrile and is vomiting but has neither meningeal signs nor focal neurologic findings. His liver is palpable. He takes no routine medications.

Question 13.15.1 Influenza is associated with which of the following complications?
A) Pneumonia
B) Rhabdomyolysis
C) Myocarditis
D) Encephalitis
E) All of the above

Answer 13.15.1 **The correct answer is "E."** All of the above can be a result of influenza. Pneumonia may be viral or due to a secondary bacterial superinfection. Patients may present with influenza-related severe leg pain secondary to rhabdomyolysis; the CK will be elevated. Myocarditis can present with CHF, arrhythmias, and sudden death; myocarditis can also be subclinical. Obviously, encephalitis will present with mental status changes.

You get labs on this patient. He is noted to be hypoglycemic and to have markedly elevated liver enzymes. His bilirubin is normal. The patient's white blood cell count is normal, and the differential indicates a lymphocytic predominance.

Question 13.15.2 The MOST LIKELY diagnosis based on this patient's history, physical, and laboratory findings is:
A) Reye syndrome
B) Bacterial meningitis
C) Transverse myelitis
D) Hepatic encephalopathy secondary to hepatitis
E) Diabetes mellitus in the "honeymoon" period

Answer 13.15.2 **The correct answer is "A."** This patient most likely has Reye syndrome (encephalopathy with fatty liver degeneration). Reye syndrome presents with intractable vomiting, elevated transaminases with a normal bilirubin level, hypoglycemia, and mental status changes (excitability, delirium, coma). Reye syndrome generally occurs in a genetically susceptible person who has been given aspirin in the setting of a viral illness such as influenza or chickenpox. This patient is not likely to have meningitis, given the absence of an elevated white count and lack of meningeal signs. Also, he clearly does not have transverse myelitis, an autoimmune condition producing rapidly progressive weakness and sensory disturbance. "E" is incorrect since he is not on insulin.

Question 13.15.3 **The medication MOST associated with Reye syndrome is:**
A) Ibuprofen
B) Celecoxib (Celebrex)
C) Aspirin
D) Acetaminophen
E) Naproxen

Answer 13.15.3 **The correct answer is "C."** The use of aspirin in a child with a viral illness, classically influenza or chickenpox, has been associated with the development of Reye syndrome. There is likely some inborn error of metabolism that predisposes to Reye syndrome. Of note, the incidence of Reye syndrome has been steadily declining (currently, less than 1/1,000,000 children) now that parents are aware that they should avoid aspirin use in children. Reye syndrome is most commonly seen on board exams and not in real life (but, still you should know it!).

HELPFUL TIP:
The treatment of Reye syndrome is supportive and includes controlling hypoglycemia and treating cerebral edema. There is no specific treatment of this illness. The mortality rate remains high. Surviving patients should be screened for an inborn error of metabolism.

For some reason, you found heme-positive stool in this patient. You must have been thinking that every patient deserves at least one rectal examination.

Question 13.15.4 **All of the following are relatively common causes of heme-positive stools in children 1 to 5 years of age EXCEPT:**
A) Colon polyps
B) Ulcers
C) Swallowed epistaxis
D) Gangrenous bowel
E) Intussusception

Answer 13.15.4 **The correct answer is "D."** Gangrenous bowel (e.g., necrotizing enterocolitis) tends to be found in neonates and infants <1 year old as a result of necrotizing enterocolitis, midgut volvulus, etc. All of the others are correct. See Table 13-6 for more causes of occult GI blood loss in children.

▶ **Objectives: Did you learn to …**
· Recognize sequelae of influenza infection?
· Describe Reye syndrome?
· Manage a patient with Reye syndrome (in the lottery-winning-chance that you'd ever really do that)?
· Identify some causes of heme-positive stools in children?

TABLE 13-6 CAUSES OF HEME-POSITIVE STOOLS IN CHILDREN

Less than 1 year: Swallowed maternal blood, anal fissure, intussusception, duodenal or gastric ulcers, gangrenous bowel (e.g., necrotizing enterocolitis), Meckel diverticulum, cow milk protein intolerance
More than 1 year: Juvenile colon polyps, ulcers, anal fissure, esophageal varices, intussusception, hemorrhoids, swallowed epistaxis, Mallory–Weiss tears, bacterial enteritis

▶ **CASE 13.16**

A mother comes to you with concerns about SIDS in her infant—not that her child has SIDS, which would be awful. Also, her sister had a child who died of SIDS, and she is concerned that her child is now at elevated risk.

Question 13.16.1 **You can tell her which of the following?**
A) Twin concordance studies suggest SIDS is passed as chromosomal recessive disorder.
B) Since her child is now 5 months old, there is no risk of SIDS as SIDS generally occurs before 3 months of age
C) Siblings of an infant with SIDS have a fivefold increase in the risk of SIDS
D) SIDS is more likely to occur in female infants
E) Young maternal age (<20 years old) is associated with **reduced** risk of SIDS

Answer 13.16.1 **The correct answer is "C."** A sibling of a child who died with SIDS has a fivefold increased risk of dying of SIDS (although the absolute risk is still less than 1%). "A" is incorrect. The cause of SIDS is unknown. Abnormal arousal from sleep may play a role with delayed brain maturation a factor. SIDS does not seem to be an isolated genetic disorder. "B" is incorrect. SIDS generally occurs between 2 and 4 months (median age 11 weeks). However, 90% of cases occur before 6 months of age, so a 5-month-old child is still at risk. "D" is incorrect as it is more common in males with a ratio of 3:2. Finally, the opposite of "E" is true: maternal age <20 years old is a risk factor as is maternal smoking and the infant's sleeping position.

Question 13.16.2 **All of the following have been associated with an increased incidence of SIDS EXCEPT:**
A) Side-sleep positioning
B) Prone-sleep positioning
C) Early introduction of solid foods
D) Premature birth
E) Intrauterine exposure to drugs

Answer 13.16.2 **The correct answer is "C."** The introduction of solid foods has nothing to do with the development of SIDS. All of the other factors increase the rate of SIDS including intrauterine environment. Of note, any nonsupine sleeping position is associated with an increased incidence of SIDS.

Question 13.16.3 The MOST important advice you can give to prevent SIDS is:

A) Allow the child to sleep in bed with the parent(s) so they can closely monitor the child during sleep
B) Bundle the child with blankets when sleeping
C) Use a child alarm in the room to alert the parent(s) if something is wrong
D) Place the child in the supine position (stomach and face up) when sleeping
E) Use sheepskin or polystyrene bedding to prevent suffocation

Answer 13.16.3 **The correct answer is "D."** Having the infant sleep in a supine position ("**back** to sleep") reduces the risk of SIDS by up to 50%. "B" (swaddling) and "E" (polystyrene or sheepskin bedding) **increase the risk** of SIDS. Smoking cessation is important as smoking during pregnancy or after increases the risk of SIDS. Co-sleeping ("A") should be discouraged as it increases the risk of SIDS. Home apnea monitors, oxygen monitors, etc. ("D") are not shown to prevent SIDS and do not perform as well as the types of monitors used in a hospital setting.

HELPFUL TIP:
The use of pacifiers in bed may actually decrease the risk of SIDS as well. Give it to the child when he or she is put down for sleep. Do not reinsert it once the child is asleep if he/she spits it out.

HELPFUL (AND SCARY) TIP:
Nothing is free (especially the board examination … how much are you paying for that?). Supine sleeping has increased the rate of positional plagiocephaly (flattening of the head, in this case in the occipital region). This risk can be minimized by placing the child in a **prone** position **while awake and supervised** (commonly referred to as "tummy time"). Helmets to reform the shape of the skull have been shown not to work (*BMJ.* 2014;348:g2741); and four out of five babies don't think they look very cool.

▶ Objectives: Did you learn to …
• Identify risks of SIDS?
• Give advice on how to reduce the risk of SIDS?

▶ **CASE 13.17**

The parents of a 1-month-old female bring the infant for her routine check-up. They are first-time parents and are concerned about feeding. Evidently, one of the grandmothers is "from the old country." Back in her day in the "old country," they would start children on solid foods at 2 months of age—usually starting with strained liver (lots of vitamins and stuff, plus it is disgusting and the adults wouldn't eat it). This grandmother also cannot figure out why the couple is wasting their money on formula when cow's milk (better yet, goat's milk when available) "worked just fine for me." They would like your advice about feeding.

Question 13.17.1 **You let them know that:**

A) Solid foods should be introduced at 3 months for all children. Two months of age is too soon. And grandma's right. Start with liver
B) Cow's milk is considered adequate only after 6 months of age
C) Early introduction of cow's milk has been irrefutably linked to type 1 diabetes mellitus
D) The first foods introduced should be strained meats
E) Children should have good head control before solid foods are introduced

Answer 13.17.1 **The correct answer is "E."** Doesn't "E" just sound best? Even if you hadn't a clue, you would still pick "E," right? Children should have good head control before starting solid foods. "A" is incorrect for a couple of reasons. First, solid foods are generally not recommended until 4 to 6 months of age. Second, note that the answer says "all children." "B" is incorrect. Cow's milk should be avoided for the first year of life. Breastfeeding is optimal and infant formula is another good option if mom decides not to breastfeed; formula contains additional nutrients not found in cow's milk. In addition, the early use of cow's milk has been linked to an increase in gastrointestinal blood loss and iron deficiency anemia. "C" is incorrect. There has been some observational evidence to suggest a connection between diabetes type 1 and cow's milk, but the data are quite suspect. "D" is incorrect. Foods should be introduced one at a time, but there is no requirement as to what the first food should be. Usually, iron fortified cereals are introduced first.

HELPFUL TIP:
A word on introducing foods and food allergy… Contrary to what many of us were taught, the early introduction of allergens, such as peanuts, seems to *reduce* the risk of subsequent allergy (*N Engl J Med.* 2015;372:803–813). Whether this extends to other foods is not known. But it is at least reasonable to introduce possibly allergenic foods (peanuts, wheat) early. Early introduction of solids at 3 months does help sleep (*JAMA Pediatr* 2018 Aug; 172:e180739.)

HELPFUL TIP:
AAP guidelines recommend 400 IU/day of vitamin D from birth through the teenage years, no exceptions. This can come either from supplements or foods. Breast milk does not contain enough vitamin D. Supplement vitamin D in exclusively and partially breastfed infants, formula-fed infants receiving less than 1 L of fortified formula per day, and children and adolescents obtaining <400 IU/day through fortified milk and foods.

The parents manage to fend off this grandmother (quite an accomplishment, eh?). The child continues with formula feedings. However, the child gets somewhat fussy on occasion and has bouts of diarrhea. The family wants to know what to do.

Question 13.17.2 **Your advice is to:**
A) Change formulas because this represents an allergy to the cow's milk formula
B) Do not change formulas
C) Change formulas because this likely represents lactase deficiency
D) Switch to a formula based on short chain fatty acids since this likely represents an inability to absorb and metabolize fats

Answer 13.17.2 **The correct answer is "B."** Children will occasionally be fussy and have occasional diarrhea. This does not indicate a formula allergy or intolerance. Reflux and spitting up are also common in infants. Again, this does not indicate a formula allergy. The parents should be reassured that as long as the child is growing and is not having significant difficulties, continuing the current formula is acceptable.

> **HELPFUL TIP:**
> Remember, as noted above, reflux or spitting up does not mean formula intolerance. **Do not make multiple formula changes!** This medicalizes a normal pattern in children. The majority of spitting up and reflux will resolve by 1 year of age. If the child looks well and is growing, there is no need to change the formula.

The parents decide that you are correct and continue to feed the child the cow's milk formula. Much as you predicted, the child does well on this formula. However, the child is now becoming "constipated" and the grandmother would like to give this child a laxative (preferably some concoction from the "old country" that no one else can pronounce or formulate). She (the infant, not the grandmother) is having only one bowel movement per day rather than the three to four per day that occurred during the first several months of life.

Question 13.17.3 **You let the parents know that:**
A) One stool a day is likely normal for this infant
B) An infant having less than two to three bowel movements per day is likely constipated since bowel transit time is only 8.5 hours or so
C) Infants fed soy-based formula tend to have softer stools than those fed cow's milk formula
D) Breastfed infants may normally have up to 10 stools per day
E) A and D

Answer 13.17.3 **The correct answer is "E."** The number of bowel movements in a normal infant can vary widely from 10 per day in a breastfed infant to 1 per day or every other day in a formula-fed infant. What is more important is whether the child has to strain to pass stool, how hard the stool is, etc. The number of stools per day is less important.

On further questioning, it becomes clear that the grandmother may be correct. This child is having a hard time passing stool and passes only small amounts of hard stool with great effort (red-purple face, lots of crying, etc.). The parents would like some advice.

Question 13.17.4 **Which of the following is a reasonable suggestion to treat this infant's constipation?**
A) Change to a formula with a preponderance of whey protein
B) Treat with corn syrup (whatever brand is cheapest)
C) Add fruit juices if the child is older than 2 months
D) Treat with lactulose

Answer 13.17.4 **The correct answer is "D."** Let's look at this in detail (since parents will tell you all of the details of their child's stools and often bring in a "selfie" of the stool...yes, it's happened!). "A," whey protein, was thought in the past to ease constipation. This has turned out not to be the case. "B" is problematic for a different reason. Many corn syrups in the past contained glycoproteins that were metabolized into nonabsorbable sugars. *This is no longer true for many corn syrups; the formulation has changed.* Fruit juices contain sorbitol and are effective. However, they should not be used under the age of 4 months. Beyond that age, sorbitol-containing juices such as pear, prune, or apple may be used to treat constipation. As an aside, glycerin suppositories can be used sparingly for very hard stool in the rectum. Routine use of glycerin suppositories may lead to tolerance (a dependence on manual stimulation to stool) as well as irritation of the rectal and anal mucosa. Finally, polyethylene glycol solution is reasonable in those greater than 4 months of age as are sorbitol-containing purees such as prunes (assuming the child is taking solids).

The child does well after the parents implement your lactulose plan, but she continues to have some reflux symptoms. This is getting worrisome to the parents although the child is growing well.

Question 13.17.5 **Which of the following is recommended as standard therapy in treating this child's reflux?**
A) Prone positioning of the child when sleeping
B) Use of a proton pump inhibitor
C) Elevating the head
D) Thickening the formula with rice cereal
E) None of the above

Answer 13.17.5 **The correct answer is "E."** This child has physiologic reflux. None of these interventions should be recommended as "standard therapy" for physiologic reflux. Treatment of uncomplicated reflux in infants without warning signs/symptoms is not routinely recommended and may medicalize a benign clinical variant. A watchful waiting approach is appropriate for these infants ("happy spitters"), though it may be messy!

Warning signs/symptoms include poor weight gain, excessive irritation with regurgitation, apnea, or wheezing. Children with concern for apnea or wheezing should have a thorough medical evaluation before attributing these symptoms to reflux. Of the interventions previously mentioned, thickening the formula ("D") may be helpful to prevent episodes of reflux and may be considered if reflux is concerning to the family. However, the benefit is often minimal. Addition of cereal increases the caloric density of feedings and should not be recommended for overweight infants. Thickening feeds with cereal may also be problematic for premature infants, as the increased viscosity may require increased energy expenditure and cause fatigue. Placing the child in prone position ("A") while sleeping increases the risk of SIDS. Neither an H_2 blocker, a proton pump inhibitor ("B"), nor elevating the head ("C") has been shown to reduce reflux. In fact, elevating the head (as in a car seat) may increase reflux.

HELPFUL TIP:
In infants with gastroesophageal reflux disease (defined as having symptoms such as weight loss and not just physiologic reflux), a trial of 2 to 4 weeks of extensively hydrolyzed ("hypoallergenic") formula or amino acid–based formula, increased caloric density of formula, or thickened formula is reasonable. H_2 blockers and PPIs have also been used but with very limited success. Prokinetic agents such as metoclopramide and erythromycin help improve gastric emptying, but studies have failed to show much efficacy for GERD. In 2009, the FDA issued a black box warning linking chronic metoclopramide use with tardive dyskinesia.

▶ **Objectives: Did you learn to …**
- Give appropriate advice for nutrition and feeding during infancy?
- Diagnose and manage constipation in infancy?
- Treat an infant with significant gastroesophageal reflux?

▶ CASE 13.18

A 23-year-old G2P1 female at 31 weeks of gestation presents to the ED and delivers precipitously. Her pregnancy was uncomplicated. The neonate is a 1.25-kg male. The helicopter is on its way to transport this premature infant to your regional pediatric hospital. However, it is going to be at least 3 hours because of weather concerns. The infant has moderate respiratory distress.

Question 13.18.1 **In the meantime, the BEST treatment for this newborn is:**
A) Antibiotics
B) Corticosteroids
C) High-flow 100% oxygen
D) Routine care (warmth, stimulation, etc.) and nothing else
E) Intubation and surfactant administration

Answer 13.18.1 **The correct answer is "E."** Without any further information, you must assume that this patient is at significant risk for neonatal respiratory distress syndrome (RDS). The appropriate treatment is surfactant. The dose of surfactant depends on the preparation, and the timing of administration varies by source (some authors favor immediate administration "prophylaxis," while others recommend "early rescue" treatment—usually within 2 hours of delivery). Surfactant therapy has good evidence for decreasing morbidity and mortality and should be used in all premature infants who are at risk for RDS (see next question) or acutely symptomatic. On the basis of synergistic interactions, experts recommend combination therapy with **antenatal** corticosteroids for the mother (if possible; see Chapter 15) and surfactant for the premature infant. "A" is incorrect as it is not the most important initial therapy although empiric antibiotic therapy is often indicated in premature infants due to difficulty in distinguishing between RDS and sepsis. "B" is incorrect because steroids for the **newborn infant** are associated with adverse neurodevelopmental outcomes. As for "C," excessive oxygen can be toxic to premature infants, and initial resuscitation should begin with blended oxygen or room air. "D" might be the second-best option if surfactant were unavailable but note that it says "and nothing else." It is highly unlikely this premature infant would need "nothing else" (college tuition may be nice). Surfactant is undoubtedly indicated here. Securing the airway for transport will likely also be needed anyway.

HELPFUL TIP:
Surfactant has been shown to decrease air leaks and mortality from RDS, but does not decrease the incidence of chronic lung disease or bronchopulmonary dysplasia.

Question 13.18.2 **All of the following are risk factors for neonatal RDS EXCEPT:**
A) Cesarean section
B) Gestational diabetes
C) Male sex of infant
D) Prolonged rupture of membranes

Answer 13.18.2 **The correct answer is "D."** Prolonged rupture of membranes is associated with a **decreased** risk of neonatal RDS. All of the others are associated with an increased risk. Of course, increasing prematurity is associated with increasing risk of RDS as is multifetal pregnancy, especially in the second fetus delivered in a twin pregnancy.

HELPFUL TIP:
The lecithin/sphingomyelin (L/S) ratio is the traditional method for assessing fetal lung maturity. If the L/S ratio is >2, the risk of RDS is low. Other options include phosphatidylglycerol level and direct surfactant measures. It is important to realize that these tests have fairly low-positive predictive values.

HELPFUL TIP:
As premature infants grow into adults, keep an eye on their blood pressures and glucose levels. Infants who were born prematurely and at very low birth weight (<1.5 kg) have more problems with hypertension and glucose intolerance as adults.

Because of your congenial bedside manner and amazing command of medical knowledge, this family returns to see you many times over the ensuing years. After looking at yourself in the mirror and reflecting on how awesome you are, you turn your attention to the newest addition to the family, a 4-day-old male infant you delivered—this time in the labor and delivery unit and at term. Gestation and delivery were uncomplicated. He is breastfed and was doing well until this morning. Unfortunately, his mother noticed today that he is breathing harder, eating poorly, and looking more yellow. You note a respiratory rate of 72 and crackles on lung examination, so you order a chest x-ray.

Question 13.18.3 Which of the following diagnoses is most likely?
A) Neonatal respiratory distress syndrome (RDS)
B) Persistent pulmonary hypertension (PPHN)
C) Pneumonia
D) Pneumothorax
E) Retained fetal liquid lung syndrome (RFLLS) (AKA transient tachypnea of the newborn).

Answer 13.18.3 **The correct answer is "C."** Pneumonia is more likely than the other options because of the timing of the symptoms. Neonatal pneumonia may be early (within the first week of life) or late onset. The pathogenic organisms involved are different for early and late disease. Patients presenting with early onset pneumonia are more likely to have acquired the infection in utero or during delivery; GBS is the most common pathogen in these cases. Patients presenting with late pneumonia may have acquired the disease during delivery, during hospitalization, or while in the community; GBS, *E. coli*, *S. aureus*, *Listeria*, HSV, and *Chlamydia* may all cause pneumonia in these patients. Temperature instability in the newborn is a good clue to an infectious etiology like pneumonia or sepsis. "A" is incorrect since RDS should not occur in a full-term infant nor present this late. "B" is incorrect because persistent pulmonary hypertension should present shortly after birth with hypoxemia and cyanosis. "D", pneumothorax, is a common result of birth trauma; up to 2% of infants may sustain a pneumothorax during delivery. However, very few infants with a pneumothorax are symptomatic, and you would expect the symptoms to occur shortly after delivery. In addition, breath sounds would be absent or diminished, and there would not be rales. RFLLS ("E"), previously known as transient tachypnea of the newborn, is incorrect because the "transient tachypnea" is a result of delayed reabsorption of alveolar fluid, occurs within 1 to 2 hours of birth and resolves on its own. RFLLS is more commonly seen in infants delivered by C-section and late-preterm infants.

You found your rectal thermometer (it was in your hand all along—just like your cell phone), and it turns out that your patient is febrile. The chest x-ray shows a left lower lobe infiltrate.

Question 13.18.4 After evaluation with a complete sepsis workup, which of the following is the MOST appropriate antibiotic selection in this setting?
A) Ampicillin
B) Ceftriaxone
C) Gentamicin
D) Vancomycin
E) A and C

Answer 13.18.4 **The correct answer is "E."** Pneumonia in the newborn period is most likely due to GBS or Gram-negative rods. Community-acquired bacteria are also possible, but less likely. The initial treatment regimen should cover the most common organisms. Ampicillin ("A") provides excellent coverage for GBS and *Listeria*, while gentamicin ("B") provides excellent Gram-negative coverage. In combination with ampicillin, a third-generation cephalosporin is a reasonable alternative to gentamicin. Ceftriaxone ("B"), however, is relatively contraindicated in neonates, as it displaces bilirubin from albumin-binding sites resulting in more severe hyperbilirubinemia and the risk of bilirubin encephalopathy (this infant is jaundiced). Ceftriaxone may also cause fatal precipitates in the lung and kidney when co-administered with calcium (perhaps not an immediate concern for this patient). And, *the risk of death may be higher with a cephalosporin when compared to gentamicin.* If absolutely necessary, cefotaxime or another third-generation cephalosporin may be used. It would be prudent to provide empiric antibiotic coverage for all likely bacterial pathogens. Staphylococcal pneumonia in the neonatal period is uncommon, but for severely ill infants, coverage for it should be considered. In this case, vancomycin ("D,") is reasonable which will cover MRSA, MSSA and streptococcus. It should not be used alone due to its lack of Gram-negative coverage. Given this infant's age, a complete sepsis evaluation (blood, urine, and CSF cultures) is indicated (and ideally before antibiotics, if the infant is stable).

HELPFUL TIP:
Remember the possibility of sustained paroxysmal supraventricular tachycardia with CHF in the infant who is tachypneic. These children often present with poor feeding, weakness, tachypnea, and rales. Treatment includes vagal maneuvers (such as placing a bag of ice over the face for 15 to 30 seconds…and watching the horror on the parents' faces as they think you are suffocating the kid). Other options include cardioversion and adenosine.

▶ **Objectives: Did you learn to …**
- Provide appropriate treatment to an infant at risk for neonatal RDS?
- Identify risk factors for neonatal RDS?
- Describe causes of respiratory distress in the neonatal period?
- Initiate treatment for neonatal pneumonia?

▶ CASE 13.19

A 20-day-old term male infant is brought to the clinic for evaluation of fever. He was born via uncomplicated vaginal delivery. Mom was GBS negative. In clinic, the infant has a temperature of 38.5°C but is otherwise vigorous with normal vital signs.

Question 13.19.1 What should be done next?
A) Discharge home with follow-up the next day
B) Treat with empiric antibiotics. Cultures are not necessary for this age group
C) Obtain a chest x-ray
D) Admit to the hospital
E) Treat with ibuprofen

Answer 13.19.1 The correct answer is "D." Fever in a neonate (younger than 28 days) or young infant (age 29–90 days) is defined as a temperature 38°C or 100.4°F (rectal) or higher. Up to 15% of febrile neonates and young infants will have a serious bacterial infection such as bacteremia, urinary tract infection, meningitis, pneumonia, osteomyelitis, septic arthritis, omphalitis, mastitis, or scalp abscess. UTI is the most common. The infant may appear well with fever being the only manifestation of a serious infection. Risk stratification is based on age, comorbidities, laboratory studies, and the presence of viral infection such as bronchiolitis. There is no clear consensus on the best approach to evaluating and managing febrile infants younger than 90 days. Currently, all febrile neonates, ill-appearing infants, or those not meeting low-risk criteria should be admitted for a full evaluation (including urinalysis with urine culture, lumbar puncture, CBC, blood cultures) and empiric antibiotic therapy. "B" is incorrect as cultures should preferably be obtained prior to initiation of antibiotic therapy. You may obtain a chest x-ray as part of your evaluation, but the best answer is admission. Ibuprofen is not approved for use in infants younger than 6 months. See Table 13-7 for evaluation of a fever in a child 7 to 90 days of age.

The patient is admitted. Blood work including a complete blood count and blood culture is obtained. Urinalysis and urine culture are obtained via sterile catheterization. A lumbar puncture (LP) is performed after obtaining consent (of course) and cerebrospinal fluid is sent for culture and analysis. (Use lidocaine for the LP, even in these young infants … it hurts!)

TABLE 13-7 EVALUATION OF THE FEBRILE NEONATE

Age < 7 days: ALL should receive full workup including urinalysis and urine culture, blood cultures, lumbar puncture with cultures, CBC, CXR, ampicillin + gentamicin. Admit.
Age 7–28 days: ALL should receive full workup including urinalysis and urine culture, blood cultures, lumbar puncture with cultures, CBC, CXR in those with respiratory symptoms. Ampicillin + cefotaxime or ampicillin + gentamicin. Admit.
Age 29–90 days:
Well-appearing: Urinalysis with culture and CBC (WBC of 5,000–15,000 *and* <500 bands suggests lower risk of infection); lumbar puncture not needed if child is well looking with reliable follow-up; CXR if respiratory rate >50 bpm, rales, rhonchi, other respiratory symptoms → If evaluation is low risk, consider ceftriaxone 50 mg/kg × 1 dose and return visit the next day for recheck. If high risk, based on CBC, clinical findings, then admit (see antibiotic choice below).
Ill-appearing: CBC, lumbar puncture with CSF culture, urinalysis with urine culture, and blood cultures; CXR if any respiratory symptoms (see above), Ceftriaxone + Ampicillin. Add vancomycin if CSF is abnormal. Admit to hospital.

Question 13.19.2 While waiting for your laboratory testing results what empiric antibiotics will you start?
A) Ampicillin and clindamycin
B) Gentamicin
C) Vancomycin and metronidazole
D) Ceftriaxone
E) Ampicillin and cefotaxime

Answer 13.19.2 The correct answer is "E." The choice of empiric antibiotics is based on most likely infecting bacterial organisms in a patient of this age. Bacterial infections in neonates likely were acquired during delivery. The most common organisms are GBS, *E. coli*, and *Listeria monocytogenes*. Empiric treatment should be with ampicillin and cefotaxime or ampicillin and gentamicin; not gentamicin alone as in "B" (you learned this from the case above!). Ampicillin provides coverage for *Listeria* and enterococci. Broadened coverage should be considered depending on focus of infection, and if Gram-positive cocci are seen on CSF Gram stain, vancomycin should be used instead of ampicillin. Empiric acyclovir treatment should be started if HSV risk factors are present.

While examining the patient, you notice he is not moving his right arm. When you ask the mom, she believes that it is new but is unsure when he stopped using it. Examination reveals tenderness over the right proximal humerus with overlying redness, swelling, and pain with moving the shoulder joint; a symmetric Moro reflex; and intact grasp reflex.

Question 13.19.3 Of the following, which is the MOST likely cause?
A) Erb palsy
B) Klumpke palsy
C) Humerus fracture
D) Osteomyelitis
E) Cerebral vascular incident

Answer 13.19.3 The correct answer is "D." Fever, pseudoparalysis (reluctance to move affected limb) and swelling with erythema of the affected area is concerning for osteomyelitis with associated septic arthritis. Osteomyelitis, an infection of the bone, usually results from hematogenous seeding. Infants have blood vessels that cross the growth plate allowing for bone infections to spread to the adjacent joint resulting in septic arthritis. *S. aureus* is the most common cause of osteomyelitis in all pediatric age groups. *H. influenzae* is less common since immunizations were begun; however, until culture results are available, it should be covered empirically in children aged 6 months to 4 years who have not yet completed their immunization series. GBS and Gram-negative rods such as *E. coli* are seen in neonates and should be covered empirically. "A" and "B" are types of brachial plexus injuries from birth trauma that result in paralysis and an *asymmetric* Moro reflex due to peripheral nerve injury. "C," a humerus fracture, though rare can occur as a result of birth trauma but is unlikely based on delayed presentation. "E" is incorrect as most neonatal strokes present with seizures and/or altered mental status. Of note, the normal Moro and grasp reflexes in this child point us away from true paralysis.

HELPFUL TIP:
Neonates with osteomyelitis are commonly afebrile and present with nonspecific symptoms such as irritability, decreased movement of a limb (pseudoparalysis), or pain with moving the affected extremity (think pain during a diaper change). Often the diagnosis is delayed and misdiagnosed at first as a traumatic injury.

HELPFUL TIP:
Neonatal osteomyelitis often involves multiple bones.

You discuss your concerns with the mother.

Question 13.19.4 She asks you how you will diagnose a bone infection. Your response is:
A) Clinically
B) With cultures
C) With x-ray
D) With MRI
E) All of the above

Answer 13.19.4 The correct answer is "E." Osteomyelitis is a clinical diagnosis requiring you to think about it in your differential. Cultures and imaging confirm the diagnosis. There is no *specific* laboratory test. Frequently, a leukocytosis with left shift and reactive thrombocytosis are present. Inflammatory markers, including C-reactive protein and erythrocyte sedimentation rate, are usually elevated; CRP can be followed to document response to therapy; ESR takes too long to change to be of much use in monitoring treatment. Cultures of the blood, joint fluid,

and/or bone are positive in 50% to 80%. Plain x-rays can rule out other causes such as a fracture but are often not useful in early osteomyelitis as it can take up to 10 days to see changes such as a lytic lesion. MRI is the best imaging study allowing for abscess detection and differentiation between bone and soft-tissue infection. MRI often requires sedation and is expensive. A radionuclide bone scan is helpful for poorly localized pain and/or concerns about multiple bone involvement. Ultrasound can be helpful in septic arthritis.

An x-ray shows a lytic lesion in the proximal humerus. An MRI is obtained, and it is consistent with osteomyelitis. You consult your pediatric orthopedic colleagues who take the infant to the operating room to wash out the joint and obtain cultures.

Question 13.19.5 Cultures of the joint and bone grow GBS. What is the length of antibiotic treatment?
A) 5–7 days
B) 10–14 days
C) 4–6 weeks
D) 6 months
E) 1 year

Answer 13.19.5 The correct answer is "C." Acute osteomyelitis is treated with antibiotics for a minimum of 3 weeks with most courses lasting 4 to 6 weeks. The majority of patients may be treated initially with intravenous antibiotics followed by transition to oral antibiotics after clinical improvement and lack of contraindication to oral therapy. In neonates, the entire course is frequently completed intravenously due to lack of clinical trials. Even with appropriate treatment, neonatal osteomyelitis may result in permanent deformities to the bone or joint with resulting decreased range of motion, asymmetric limb length, and abnormal gait; therefore, long-term follow-up is mandatory. *Note: Now that she has had one child with invasive GBS disease, mom will need GBS prophylaxis during* **all** *future labors if she were to get pregnant again.*

HELPFUL TIP:
Antibiotic prophylaxis during labor decreases the incidence of early onset GBS disease (within the first 7 days of life), but does not affect late onset GBS disease (7 days to 3 months of age). See Chapter 15 for indications for antibiotic prophylaxis for GBS during labor.

▶ **Objectives: Did you learn to …**
  · Initiate a diagnostic investigation and management strategy for a febrile infant younger than 90 days?
  · Diagnose and manage neonatal osteomyelitis?

 QUICK QUIZ: FEBRILE SEIZURE

You are evaluating a 10-month-old fully immunized child after a simple febrile seizure. The child has been previously healthy and has not taken antibiotics recently. Physical examination is unremarkable with no meningeal signs and a normal neurologic examination. The kid is cruising in the exam room trying to open drawers.

What diagnostic testing should be performed?
A) Lumbar puncture
B) EEG
C) Neuroimaging such as head CT or MRI
D) Serum electrolytes
E) None of the above

The correct answer is "E." The clue here is that the child looks normal and is cruising in the exam room. A child with a simple febrile seizure should rapidly return to normal mentation. Per the 2011 AAP guidelines, evaluation of a simple febrile seizure should focus on identifying the cause of the fever. Meningitis should always be considered, and a lumbar puncture should be performed if meningeal signs or symptoms are present. Previous recommendation was to perform a lumbar puncture on all infants younger than 12 months who presented with a simple febrile seizure. This recommendation was made before the widespread immunization against *H. influenzae* type b (Hib) and *S. pneumoniae*. Lumbar puncture (LP) is an **option** in infants 6 to 12 months of age who are not fully immunized or if the immunization status is unknown. Consider an LP in patients who have been on antibiotics because signs of meningitis may be masked. Routine evaluation with EEG, neuroimaging, serum electrolytes, or complete blood cell count should not be done if the only reason is to identify the cause of the febrile seizure.

▶ CASE 13.20

A previously healthy 3-year-old male presents to your clinic for evaluation of 6 days of fever. Mother has been checking axillary temperatures (and yes, not adding or subtracting a degree) which have reached at least 102°F each of the last 6 days. He is irritable. He was seen 2 days prior and given drops for "pink eye." He now has a new rash and his hands and feet are red and puffy. He has been drinking well and is well-hydrated. On exam, you find a large cervical lymph node on the right, peeling lips, and a red tongue and throat. He has not had cough or runny nose.

Question 13.20.1 **Which of the following represents the BEST treatment strategy for this child?**
A) Discharge home with watchful waiting
B) Discharge home with a prescription for amoxicillin-clavulanate
C) Referral to infectious disease for evaluation of prolonged fevers
D) Admission for further evaluation and treatment
E) Transfer to the emergency department for fluid resuscitation

Answer 13.20.1 **The correct answer is "D."** Based upon your evaluation, he meets criteria for classic Kawasaki disease (KD), which was formerly known as mucocutaneous lymph

TABLE 13-8 DIAGNOSTIC CRITERIA FOR CLASSIC KAWASAKI DISEASE

Diagnosis of Kawasaki disease can be made in the presence of at least 5 days of documented fever AND at least 4 of the following[a]:

1. Oral mucosal changes (lip erythema, lip cracking, "strawberry" tongue, oral mucosal erythema, pharyngeal mucosal erythema)
2. Nonexudative bilateral bulbar conjunctivitis (limbic sparing)
3. Rash (can be maculopapular, annular, or erythroderma)
4. Hand and foot changes (manifests ad edema and erythema in the acute phase and/or periungal peeling in the subacute phase)
5. Cervical lymphadenopathy of at least 1.5 cm (often unilateral)

[a]Careful history should be obtained, as some of the clinical features may have been present previously but resolved on presentation. Reported findings that have resolved should be counted.

node syndrome. The diagnosis of classic KD is based on the presence of documented fever for at least 5 days and the presence of at least four of five principal features (Table 13-8). KD is an acute vasculitis of childhood. The most feared complication of Kawasaki disease is coronary artery aneurysm. Prompt identification is needed so that further evaluation and treatment can occur to prevent this complication. Inpatient hospitalization is needed. Baseline echocardiography is needed to assess baseline cardiac structure, cardiac function, and coronary artery morphology, though should not delay initial treatment if not rapidly available. It would be inappropriate to send the child home ("A"), and antimicrobial therapy is not indicated ("B"). Infectious disease ("C"), rheumatology, and cardiology specialists may have additional expertise regarding KD; consultation is not necessary at this time. Since the child has adequate fluid status, fluid resuscitation ("E") is not indicated.

HELPFUL TIP:
Other illnesses may present with similar signs and symptoms as KD. Viral illnesses (adenovirus, measles, etc.), tick-borne illnesses, scarlet fever, toxic shock syndrome, drug reactions, and other rheumatologic conditions should be considered as differential diagnoses. Features not consistent with KD, such as oral ulcers, exudative conjunctivitis or pharyngitis, petechiae, or bullous rash, should prompt consideration of another diagnosis.

HELPFUL TIP:
Children who remain untreated for KD have an approximately 25% chance of coronary artery aneurysms. It is a major cause of acquired heart disease across the world.

Your patient is admitted to the hospital. A baseline echocardiogram is done, with no coronary artery dilation.

Question 13.20.2 Of the following, which is MOST appropriate initial treatment for KD?
A) Pulse-dose methylprednisolone
B) Intravenous immunoglobulin
C) Aspirin
D) A and B
E) B and C

Answer 13.20.2 The correct answer is "E." The 2017 American Heart Association guidelines for diagnosis and management of KD recommends treatment with IVIG (2 g/kg) "as soon as possible" after diagnosis. IVIG is disease-modifying, as it decreases the likelihood of coronary artery aneurysms. Use of moderate- (30–50 mg/kg/day) or high-dose (80–100 mg/kg/day) aspirin is recommended for its anti-inflammatory and antiplatelet effects, though it does not appear to decrease the occurrence of coronary artery aneurysms. Most clinicians will continue moderate- or high-dose aspirin until afebrile for 48 to 72 hours and then transition to low-dose aspirin (3–5 mg/kg/day). Low-dose aspirin is continued until echocardiograms at 1 to 2 weeks and 6 to 8 weeks post-treatment are negative for coronary artery abnormalities. Children with coronary artery abnormalities generally continue aspirin indefinitely. The use of steroids in KD is controversial and may be considered in high-risk children (which is beyond the scope of this review). However, steroids, if used, should be used at the time of initial treatment with IVIG and given daily with a long taper, not pulse dosed.

HELPFUL TIP:
Children treated with IVIG for KD may have fever related to the IVIG. If children have persistent fever beyond 36 hours after completion of IVIG, this represents IVIG-resistant KD. If this occurs, a second dose of IVIG is indicated. Consultation with a KD expert may be indicated. Steroids, infliximab, cyclosporine, and other biologics have been used for refractory cases. IVIG-resistance in KD does increase the risk of coronary artery aneurysms.

HELPFUL TIP:
Some children may not meet classic (or "typical") KD criteria, but they may have persistent fever and some signs and symptoms of KD without another clear cause. Such children should receive evaluation for incomplete (or "atypical") KD. If children have 5 days of fever and two to three of the KD criteria in Table 13-8, they should have further laboratory testing to determine if echocardiography and treatment for KD is needed. See the American Heart Association Guidelines for further information (*Circulation.* 2017 Apr 25;135(17):e927–e999).

You treated your patient with IVIG, and his fevers disappeared within 24 hours after completion of the infusion. He did not have recurrence of fevers. His echocardiograms at 2 weeks and 8 weeks post-treatment were normal, and aspirin was stopped. You are now seeing him 4 months post-treatment for his 4-year-old well-child visit. He is behind on some vaccines, including DTaP, hepatitis A, varicella, and influenza.

Question 13.20.3 Of the following, the most appropriate advice to give regarding administration of vaccinations is:
A) All needed vaccines can be given at this time
B) Inactivated influenza vaccine is contraindicated at this time
C) Live-virus vaccines should be delayed for at least 11 months after IVIG
D) Live-virus vaccines are contraindicated indefinitely
E) All vaccines are contraindicated indefinitely

Answer 13.20.3 The correct answer is "C." Vaccination remains important in children treated for KD. However, after IVIG, some circulating antibodies may persist for up to 11 months that may prevent the development of an adequate immune response to live-virus vaccines, such as measles and varicella. Thus, these should be delayed until 11 months after IVIG administration. One caveat: if a child remains on aspirin, varicella vaccination is NOT recommended due to the risk of Reye syndrome. The benefits of varicella vaccination while on low-dose aspirin may outweigh the risks if the likelihood of varicella exposure is high, and this should be discussed with the family. "B" is incorrect, as children should continue to receive the inactivated influenza vaccine. This is very important in children on aspirin, as influenza has been associated with Reye syndrome. "A," "D," and "E" are incorrect, as described above.

▶ **Objectives: Did you learn to …**
- Diagnose Kawasaki disease (KD)?
- Manage acute and IVIG-refractory KD?
- Describe the recommended timing of vaccines after IVIG administration?

 QUICK QUIZ: EYELID SWELLING

A 5-year old girl comes to your office with a 2-day history of right upper eyelid swelling, pain, and redness. She sustained an insect bite on her face when they moved into a new apartment last week. She has been afebrile. On examination, you can evert the eyelid and do not appreciate any conjunctival swelling, conjunctival injection, or proptosis. Her ocular movements are intact and painless.

Of the following, which is the MOST likely diagnosis?
A) Preseptal cellulitis
B) Orbital cellulitis
C) Acute viral conjunctivitis
D) Chalazion

The correct answer is "A." Preseptal (or periorbital) cellulitis refers to infection of the dermis anterior to the orbital septum, and needs to be differentiated from the more severe orbital cellulitis ("B") which refers to an infection of the contents of the orbit, posterior to the orbital septum (see "helpful tip," below). Well-appearing patients older than 1 year of age with preseptal cellulitis may be managed in the outpatient setting. Management is geared toward common infecting organisms (*Staphylococcus aureus*, *Streptococcus pneumoniae*, other streptococci and anaerobes). Oral clindamycin or amoxicillin-clavulanate are excellent choices for monotherapy. Alternatives include TMP-SMX with amoxicillin or a third-generation cephalosporin. Most patients improve within 24 to 48 hours. Treatment failure requires hospitalization for parental antibiotics. The infection can be caused by direct infection of the skin and soft tissues (i.e., insect bite) or from contiguous spread due to sinusitis or dental abscesses. Acute viral conjunctivitis ("C") not only may present with mild periorbital swelling, but also would present with conjunctival injection. Chalazion ("D") is a localized nonpainful swelling due to a blocked gland of the eyelid and would not affect the entire eyelid. This is noninfectious and is generally treated symptomatically with warm compresses. Curettage may be indicated for persistent lesions.

HELPFUL TIP:
Suspect orbital cellulitis in the presence of ophthalmoplegia, chemosis, proptosis, pain with eye movements, and decreased visual acuity! Orbital cellulitis requires urgent CT imaging, IV antibiotics, and consultation with an ophthalmologist.

▶ CASE 13.21

You receive telephone call from the mother of one of your patients, a 2-year-old previously healthy male. His mother is concerned that he had been walking around normally yesterday, but today will not stand or walk. This evening, he has become more irritable and cries if they try to put him in a standing position. He seems to be uncomfortable when they move his right leg while changing his diaper. There is no known trauma. He is eating and drinking less today. He feels warm, but they lost their thermometer and have not checked a temperature at home.

Question 13.21.1 **Of the following, what is the MOST appropriate advice to give to his mother?**
A) Give a dose of ibuprofen and call if symptoms worsen
B) Apply ice to his right leg and keep it elevated
C) "Double-diaper" him to prevent movement of the affected leg
D) Proceed to the ER for evaluation
E) Proceed with "watchful waiting" this evening and call in the morning if symptoms continue

Answer 13.21.1 **The correct answer is "D."** Failure to bear weight in an ambulatory child is NOT normal and requires further evaluation. The history is concerning for pathology of the

right hip and/or leg. The progressive nature of his symptoms and possible fevers raise concern for an infectious pathology, and requires urgent evaluation; thus, "E" would be incorrect. Symptomatic care, such as NSAIDs, rest, ice, and elevation ("A" and "B") may be appropriate for sprains and strains, but there is no known trauma history. Plus, can you imagine having a cranky toddler do those things? "Double-diapering" ("C") had historically been recommended for infants with concern for developmental dysplasia of the hip (DDH). This is not recommended treatment for DDH, as it does not provide enough limitation of hip movement. Infants with a positive screen for DDH (positive Ortolani or Barlow) should have appropriate imaging and be referred to an orthopedic surgeon and placed in a Pavlik harness.

. . . .

Your patient presents to the ER for further evaluation. There, he is ill-appearing, but not toxic. He is febrile to 103.1°F. He is tachycardic, but has a normal blood pressure for his age. He is well hydrated. On exam, he resists passive movement of his right hip and holds it slightly externally rotated and flexed. You can flex and extend the right knee without difficulty. There is no pain to palpation of the long bones of his legs. He will not stand, despite your best efforts. X-rays of the hip show possible joint widening. X-rays of the right femur and knee are without bone lesions or fracture. His dad asks you, "So, what do you think is going on, doc?"

Question 13.21.2 **Of the following, which is the MOST likely diagnosis?**
A) Transient synovitis of the hip
B) Septic arthritis of the hip
C) Femoral osteomyelitis
D) Spiral fracture of the femur
E) Slipped capital femoral epiphysis (SCFE)

Answer 13.21.2 **The correct answer is "B."** This child's presentation is most consistent with septic arthritis of the hip. Children with failure to bear weight, decreased range of motion, and new fever require thoughtful evaluation for possible osteoarticular infection. Children with septic arthritis of the hip often keep the hip flexed and mildly externally rotated, which widens the capsular volume, providing some comfort. Laboratory findings may be helpful in diagnosis and often include ESR > 40 mm/hr, CRP > 2.5 mg/dL, and WBC count > 12,000 cells/mm. Hematogenous seeding of the joint is the most common mechanism of infection. Transient synovitis ("A") of the hip is a benign self-limited condition characterized by hip pain with an antecedent viral illness. It is the most common cause of acute hip pain in children between ages 3 and 8. The symptoms typically last for 3 to 6 days. Patients are well-appearing and afebrile. NSAIDs are useful in transient synovitis. Osteomyelitis ("C") must be considered, but exam findings point more toward a septic hip. Osteomyelitis may present with fever without clear source and can be indolent. Osteomyelitis may have contiguous spread to adjacent joints. Femur fracture ("D") is less likely without trauma, and x-rays do not indicate fracture. SCFE

("E"), the displacement of the capital femoral epiphysis from the femur, is incorrect. This is most common in obese adolescents and requires surgical intervention.

You obtain an orthopedic surgery consult, and they agree that a septic hip is likely. They plan to obtain synovial fluid under ultrasound guidance to guide their therapy.

Question 13.21.3 Of the following, what synovial fluid findings would be MOST consistent with septic arthritis?
A) White blood cells (WBCs) <200/mm³ and <25% polymorphonuclear cells (PMNs)
B) WBCs 200 to 2,000/mm³ and <25% PMNs
C) WBCs 2,000 to 50,000/mm³ and >50% PMNs
D) WBCs >50,000/mm³ and >75% PMNs

Answer 13.21.3 **The correct answer is "D."** Immediate synovial fluid sampling should occur if septic arthritis is suspected. Septic arthritis presents with a high WBC count in the synovial fluid, usually >50,000 cells/mm³ with a predominance of PMNs. "A" represents normal synovial fluid. "B" represents a noninflammatory arthritis and may be seen in osteoarthritis in older folks. "C" represents a noninfectious inflammatory arthritis (i.e., juvenile inflammatory arthritis, reactive arthritis). In children, sampling of synovial fluid often requires sedation. If there is a high-suspicion for septic arthritis, sampling of synovial fluid is often done under anesthesia in the OR so operative intervention can occur if results are concerning.

HELPFUL (AND SOMEWHAT ANNOYING) TIP:
Lyme arthritis should be considered if travel to an endemic area has occurred. Travel to Wisconsin or Connecticut is a big clue! Lyme arthritis frequently presents with synovial fluid analysis showing 2,000 to 50,000 WBCs/mm³. Sometimes, however, Lyme may present with higher synovial fluid WBC counts (>50,000/mm³). Routine synovial fluid cultures are negative in Lyme arthritis. Additionally, while a WBC count of >50,000/mm³ is pretty specific for infection, it isn't terribly sensitive (61% sensitive); use clinical judgment (see Chapter 12). Finally, *Kingella kingae* (discovered and named by Elizabeth King… go figure), a Gram-negative organism, may be the most common cause of septic arthritis in children 2 to 3 years of age. PCR and meticulous cultures will reveal this organism. Yeah, we never heard of it either until researching for this book.

You obtain labs (which support septic arthritis) and blood cultures. The orthopedic surgeon takes the child to the OR and performs a joint aspiration. There are >100,000/mm³ WBCs with >75% PMNs, clinching the diagnosis. Your patient's dad has a lot of great questions. He next asks you, "Alright, so what are we going to do to fix this?"

Question 13.21.4 Of the following, which is the MOST appropriate therapeutic plan?
A) Joint aspiration alone
B) Urgent surgical irrigation and drainage of the hip
C) IV antibiotics
D) B and C
E) None of the above

Answer 13.21.4 **The correct answer is "D."** Prompt diagnosis and treatment is needed, as damage to the cartilaginous structures of the hip and blood supply to the femoral head can begin within 6 hours of infection and may be irreversible after 24 to 48 hours. Think of a hip infection like an abscess—source control is needed. Antibiotics are required to clear the infection from the joint and should be started immediately after obtaining blood and synovial fluid cultures. "A" is useful for diagnosis, but surgical drainage and irrigation of the hip is recommended, given possible morbidity of incomplete treatment.

Question 13.21.5 Of the following, which is the MOST appropriate empiric antibiotic regimen?
A) Cephalexin
B) Oxacillin
C) Ceftriaxone
D) Vancomycin
E) Linezolid

Answer 13.21.5 **The correct answer is "D."** Of the provided options, vancomycin is the most appropriate initial therapy for this toddler. The most common causal organisms are *Staphylococcus aureus*, *Streptococcus pyogenes*, and *Streptococcus pneumoniae*. In hemodynamically stable patients, vancomycin monotherapy is appropriate. This will cover resistant organisms, including MRSA and resistant *S. pneumoniae*. The high prevalence of community-acquired MRSA necessitates the inclusion of MRSA coverage, pending cultures. Clindamycin may be considered, often in conjunction with an anti-staphylococcal beta-lactam, such as nafcillin, but *S. aureus* resistance to clindamycin may limit its usefulness in some areas. "A" and "B" would provide excellent Gram-positive coverage, except for MRSA. "A" is additionally incorrect, as it is an oral medication, and parental therapy is indicated initially. "C" would be indicated in addition to vancomycin if there was concern for Gram-negative infection or Lyme. *Hemophillus influenzae* type B should be considered in nonvaccinated individuals. *Kingella kingae* is an indolent organism that is difficult to culture and may cause septic arthritis and osteomyelitis in young children. *K. kingae* often requires holding of cultures for up to a week to grow. Addition of a cephalosporin (e.g., cefazolin) may be needed to provide coverage for this organism if cultures are negative and the child doesn't improve as expected. "E" is an excellent Gram-positive drug and would be a great choice if there were a contraindication to vancomycin (e.g., renal failure). Linezolid is quite expensive, which limits its use. It can also be quite myelosuppressive. Antibiotic therapy should be tailored based on culture susceptibility data. In general, at least 3 weeks of total antibiotic therapy is indicated, with longer courses if complications or delayed improvement. Immunocompetent patients may be switched to enteral antibiotics once they show steady clinical improvement, decreased inflammatory markers, toleration of oral medication. In general, this is as effective as a prolonged parenteral course and avoids the complications of a central line. Special populations (i.e., neonates, immunocompromised patients) may require parenteral antibiotics for their full treatment course.

HELPFUL TIP:
In stable patients, blood and synovial fluid cultures should be obtained before starting antibiotics. Cultures and sensitivities will help guide antibiotic selection. Blood cultures are positive in ~40% of patients with septic arthritis. In rare cases, blood cultures may be positive when synovial fluid cultures are negative.

Your patient's synovial fluid cultures grew methicillin-sensitive *S. aureus*. After 4 days, he improved, was switched to oral antibiotics, and was discharged. On follow-up, his labs normalized, and he completed an appropriate 3-week course of antibiotics (sufficient if there is no associated osteomyelitis). You see the family again at his 3-year well-child visit in October and he is doing great! His dad asks you, "What shots does he need today?" You confirm that he has received vaccinations at prior well-visits according to the CDC recommended schedule.

Question 13.21.6 Of the following, which vaccines are indicated today?
A) MMR
B) DTaP
C) Influenza, if not obtained yet this season
D) All of the above
E) B and C

Answer 13.21.6 **The correct answer is "C."** We couldn't end without a final vaccination question. No vaccinations are routinely administered at the 3-year well-visit, except for the yearly influenza vaccine, if it had not already been administered. Review the CDC website again to refresh your memory!

▶ **Objectives: Did you learn to ...**
· Generate a differential for refusal to bear weight in a toddler?
· Differentiate between transient synovitis and septic arthritis?
· Manage a patient with septic arthritis of the hip?

Clinical Pearls

○ Do not agitate a child if you suspect epiglottitis as this may worsen airway obstruction.

○ Do not perform routine head imaging in a child with simple febrile seizure. Direct your investigation toward evaluation and treatment of the underlying fever.

○ Do not prescribe antibiotics for viral infections, including viral conjunctivitis and colds.

○ Do not routinely perform VCUG for the evaluation of first febrile UTI.

○ Do not use ceftriaxone in neonates as it displaces bilirubin from albumin-binding sites and can cause severe hyperbilirubinemia.

○ Obtain blood cultures at birth followed by a minimum of 48 hours of antibiotics in infants born to mothers with chorioamnionitis.

○ Perform universal hearing and metabolic screening in newborns.

○ Recommend placing babies "Back to Sleep" to reduce the risk of SIDS. The addition of infant home apnea monitors does not provide additional benefit.

BIBLIOGRAPHY

Advisory Council on Immunization Practices. Birth-18 years and "catch up" immunization schedules. Available at: http://www.cdc.gov/vaccines/schedules/hcp/child-adolescent.html. Accessed December 2, 2018.

Bekkali NL, et al. Rectal fecal impaction treatment in childhood constipation: enemas versus high doses of oral PEG. *Pediatrics.* 2009;124(6):e1108–e1115.

Brown ML, et al. Treatment of primary nocturnal enuresis in children: a review. *Child Care Health Dev.* 2011; 37(2):153–160.

Cohen-Silver J, Ratnapalan S. Management of infantile colic: a review. *Clin Pediatr (Phila).* 2009;48(1):14–17.

Committee on Infectious Diseases, American Academy of Pediatrics. Kimberlin DW, Brady MT, Jackson MA, Long SS, eds. *Red Book: 2018 Report of the Committee of Infectious Diseases.* 31st ed. Elk Grove, IL: American Academy of Pediatrics; 2018.

de Caen AR, et al. Part 12: Pediatric Advanced Life Support. 2015 American Heart Association guidelines update for cardiopulmonary resuscitation and emergency cardiovascular care. *Circulation.* 2015;132:S526–S542.

Du Toit G, et al. Randomized trial of peanut consumption in infants at risk for peanut allergy. *N Engl J Med.* 2015;372:803–813.

Gerber JS, Offit PA. Vaccines and autism: a tale of shifting hypotheses. *Clin Infect Dis.* 2009;48(4):456–461.

Gray MP, Li SH, Hoffmann RG, Gorelick MH. Recurrence rates after intussusception enema reduction: a meta-analysis. *Pediatrics.* 2014;134(1):110–119.

Herman MJ, Martinek M. The limping child. *Pediatr Rev.* 2015;36(5):184–195; quiz 196–187.

Hoberman A, et al. Antimicrobial prophylaxis for children with vesicoureteral reflux. *N Engl J Med.* 2014;370;2367–2376.

Ingelfinger JR, Stapleton FB. Antibiotic prophylaxis for vesicoureteral reflux-answers, yet questions. *N Engl J Med.* 2014;370:2440–2441.

Kuzniewicz MW, et al. A quantitative, risk-based approach to the management of neonatal early-onset sepsis. *JAMA Pediatr.* 2017;171(4):365–371.

Lauer BJ, Spector ND. Hyperbilirubinemia in the newborn. *Pediatr Rev.* 2011;32(8):341–349.

McCrindle BW, et al. Diagnosis, treatment, and long-term management of Kawasaki disease: a scientific statement for health professionals from the American Heart Association. *Circulation.* 2017;135(17): e927–e999.

McNab S, et al. Isotonic versus hypotonic solutions for maintenance intravenous fluid administration in children. *Cochrane Database Syst Rev.* 2014;(12):CD009457.

Mishori R, et al. *Chlamydia trachomatis* infections: screening, diagnosis, and management. *Am Fam Physician.* 2012;86(12):1127–1132.

Rappaport DI, et al. Should blood cultures be obtained in all infants 3 to 36 months presenting with significant fever? *Hosp Pediatr.* 2011;1(1):46–50.

Russell KF, et al. Glucocorticoids for croup. *Cochrane Database Syst Rev.* 2011;(1):CD001955.

Sadigh G, Zou KH, Razavi SA, Khan R, Applegate KE. Meta-analysis of air versus liquid enema for intussusception reduction in children. *Am J Roentgenol.* 2015;205(5):W542–549.

Subcommittee on Urinary Tract Infection, Steering Committee on Quality Improvement and Management, Roberts KB. Urinary tract infection: clinical practice guideline for the diagnosis and management of an initial UTI in febrile infants and children 2 to 24 months. *Pediatrics.* 2011;128(3):595–610.

Sung V, et al. Treating infant colic with the probiotic *Lactobacillus reuteri*: a double blind, placebo controlled randomized trial. *BMJ.* 2014;348:g2107.

Tabbers MM, et al. Evaluation and treatment of functional constipation in infants and children: evidence-based recommendations from ESPGHAN and NASPGHAN. *J Pediatr Gastroenterol Nutr.* 2014;58(2):258–272.

Tieder JS, et al. Brief resolved unexplained events (formerly apparent life-threatening events) and evaluation of lower-risk infants. *Pediatrics.* 2016;137:e20160590.

van Wijk RM, et al. Helmet therapy in infants with positional skull deformation: randomised controlled trial. *BMJ.* 2014;348:g2741.

Vandenplas Y, et al. Pediatric gastroesophageal reflux clinical practice guidelines: joint recommendations of the NASPGHAN and ESPGHAN. *J Pediatr Gastroenterol Nutr.* 2009;49:498–457.

Wan J, et al. Section on urology response to new guidelines for the diagnosis and management of UTI. *Pediatrics.* 2012;129(4):e1051–e1053.

Wang J, Xu E, Xiao Y. Isotonic versus hypotonic maintenance IV fluids in hospitalized children: a meta-analysis. *Pediatrics.* 2014;133(1):105–113.

Wyckoff MH, et al. Part 13: Neonatal resuscitation. 2015 American Heart Association guidelines update for cardiopulmonary resuscitation and emergency cardiovascular care. *Circulation.* 2015;132:S543–S560.

Adolescent Medicine 14

Stacey Appenheimer and Kelly Skelly

▶ **CASE 14.1**

A 14-year-old male presents to your clinic with his mother for a routine well-child examination. The patient's mother has some questions about puberty. Her son enjoys playing sports and she is concerned that he may be too small to play football. The past medical history is unremarkable.

Question 14.1.1 Which of the following can you tell the mother will likely be the first sign of puberty in this boy?
A) Increase in penile length
B) Enlargement of the testes
C) Deepening of the voice
D) Rapid increase in linear growth
E) Coarsening of pubic hair

Answer 14.1.1 **The correct answer is "B."** Increase in the volume of the testes is the first sign of pubertal development in boys. The age of onset of puberty in the past was 12 years (range 10–14), but recent studies have shown that the mean age of onset is now 1.5 to 2 years earlier than these historical norms. In a study including more than 4,000 healthy boys, the mean age for entering puberty was 10.14 years for Caucasian boys, 10.04 years for Hispanic boys, and 9.14 years for African-American boys. "E" is of special note. While pubic hair appears shortly after the onset of puberty, it is initially long and straight and not in a mature distribution. Coarsening of the pubic hair is a more advanced pubertal stage, occurring approximately 1.5 years after the onset of puberty, and an increase in penile length occurs simultaneously. The maximal growth spurt occurs approximately 2 years after the onset of puberty. Changing of the voice is a secondary hormonal effect that is quite variable in nature.

From the mother, you learn that the patient's father began going through puberty during high school, and he did not reach his adult height until he was in college at about age 20. The patient's father is 5′ 10″ tall (~178 cm). The mother is 5′ 3″ tall (~160 cm). Physical examination reveals that your patient is Tanner stage I for genitalia and pubic hair. His height and weight continue to track along their previously established curves on the growth chart, both at approximately the second percentile. The remainder of the examination is unremarkable.

Question 14.1.2 What is your next step in evaluation of this patient's short stature?
A) Obtain radiographs of the left hand and wrist to assess bone age
B) Draw blood to test for growth hormone and testosterone levels
C) Obtain an endocrinology consult
D) Order computed tomography (CT) imaging of the brain to rule out hypothalamic tumors
E) Order magnetic resonance imaging (MRI) of the brain to rule out hypothalamic tumors

Answer 14.1.2 **The correct answer is "A."** In the face of a normal physical examination and appropriate linear growth velocity, the likelihood of an intracranial process is very low. An assessment of bone age can be obtained easily with a radiograph—typically of the left hand and wrist. If there is discordance between bone age and physical exam findings, further testing may be indicated.

You decide to obtain a radiograph of the hand and the wrist to assess bone age, and the radiologist reports the patient's bone age as consistent with 12 years and 3 months (remember that our patient is 14 years old).

Question 14.1.3 What is the most likely diagnosis for your patient?
A) Growth hormone deficiency
B) Sella turcica tumor
C) Constitutional delay of growth and puberty
D) Idiopathic testicular atrophy
E) Testosterone receptor abnormality

Answer 14.1.3 The correct answer is "C." The bone age of 12 years and 3 months is reassuring. Since there is no fusion of the growth plates, his bones are immature and still have the ability to grow. Had the bone age been 14, it is likely that his adult height would be short; the bones would no longer have the inherent ability to grow. Bone age assessment is an accurate tool for determination of expected growth. Constitutional delay is the most common diagnosis for short stature, and it is often associated with a delayed onset of puberty. Constitutional delay is a diagnosis of exclusion; a complete history and physical often rules out other diagnoses. Family history often reveals a parent who was a "late bloomer" but eventually had normal pubertal development. This adolescent's history of normal linear growth velocity (albeit along the second percentile) is reassuring for the absence of growth hormone deficiency or intracranial abnormalities. This adolescent's combination of appropriate linear growth velocity, appropriate adjustment for bone age, and paternal history of late pubertal development is classic for a constitutional delay.

When your patient's height is plotted on a growth curve and adjusted for bone age rather than chronological age, the height now plots just below the 50th percentile. Your patient now has a question of his own. His biggest concern is that some of his classmates are starting to get taller, and he is afraid he will be too short to continue competing in sports. Once again, his mother is 5′ 3″ tall (~160 cm) and his father is 5′ 10″ tall (~178 cm).

Question 14.1.4 Based on what you know today, what is your best estimate of this patient's adult height?
A) 5′ 3″ ± 2 (160 ± 5 cm)
B) 5′ 5″ ± 2 (165 ± 5 cm)
C) 5′ 7″ ± 2 (170 ± 5 cm)
D) 5′ 9″ ± 2 (175 ± 5 cm)
E) 5′ 11″ ± 2 (180 ± 5 cm)

Answer 14.1.4 The correct answer is "D." You can provide a rough estimate of the patient's adult height using the calculation for mid-parental height (MPH). *Remember that the parent of the opposite gender—the mother in this case—must have the height adjusted for this calculation.* For boys, add 5 inches to the mother's height (12.5 cm) and then average this corrected maternal height with the paternal height to determine the MPH. For girls, subtract 5 inches from the paternal height and then average this corrected paternal height with the maternal height to calculate the MPH. In our patient's case, his mother's corrected height is 68 inches which averaged with his father's height of 70 inches, equates to an MPH of 69 inches. A margin of error of ±2 inches (5 cm) is often given with MPH estimates.

▶ **Objectives: Did you learn to …**
- Evaluate a patient with growth concerns?
- Identify the clinical presentation of constitutional delay?
- Calculate mid-parental height (MPH)?

▶ CASE 14.2

Your next patient is a 16-year-old female cross-country runner who you are seeing in follow-up for right shin pain. She was diagnosed in the local emergency department 1 week ago with "shin splints" and told to limit her activities. In your office, she tells you that the pain has been worsening over the last 3 months, and she has progressively decreased the distance and time of her runs (but, of course she's a runner, so she hasn't quit). She denies fever, swollen joints, or other systemic symptoms. She normally has regular menses, but notes that she has irregular menses during cross-country season. The patient's past medical history is significant for a stress fracture in her left foot 18 months ago. Your examination reveals tenderness at the middle one-third of the right tibia. In addition, she has pain on a single-leg hop. You are able to review her x-rays from the emergency department, which do not reveal any fractures or other abnormalities.

Question 14.2.1 What is the most appropriate next step to diagnose your patient's leg pain?
A) Ultrasound of the lower extremity
B) MRI of the lower extremity
C) Dual-energy x-ray absorptiometry (DEXA) scan
D) Thyroid-stimulating hormone (TSH) level
E) Urine pregnancy test

Answer 14.2.1 The correct answer is "B." MRI is sensitive and specific for stress fractures and has become the preferred study. The patient's history and examination are concerning for the presence of a tibial stress fracture. Stress fractures often present insidiously and cause gradual progression in symptoms over time until a critical point is reached in terms of sports participation. Half of stress fractures are not visible on plain radiographs.

Ultrasound is gaining popularity, but it is best used to rule out a stress fracture (given its high negative predictive value). DEXA scan can provide whole-body and site-specific measurement of bone mineral density, which may be related to the pathophysiology of stress fractures but does not help diagnose a site of injury. Radionuclide bone scans are often less expensive than CT or MRI, and they demonstrate sites of injury based on increased uptake of the radionuclide material. However, bone scans are not specific for stress fractures and are often falsely positive. Of note, plain radiographs may take months to become positive after a stress fracture and, while radiographs may be done, they will not be of use if the result is negative. Given the patient's other complaints, TSH and urine pregnancy test may be warranted but will not assist in the diagnosis of her leg pain.

An MRI is obtained and confirms the presence of a stress fracture in the middle one-third of the right tibia. Because of your patient's history, especially that of multiple stress fractures, you are concerned she may be suffering from the female athlete triad.

Question 14.2.2 What are the components of the female athlete triad?

A) Low-energy availability (with or without an eating disorder), menstrual dysfunction, altered bone mineral density
B) Depression, weight loss, sports-related injury
C) Poor sports performance, low self-esteem, injury
D) Weight gain, bony injury, mood changes
E) Fanatical attachment to sports, testosterone abuse, anger management issues

Answer 14.2.2 The correct answer is "A." The female athlete triad was first identified in the early 1990s and originally characterized as anorexia, amenorrhea, and osteoporosis. As more has been learned about the triad, the realization has been made that the triad likely represents a broader spectrum disorder within each category. Many young women with the triad will exhibit low-energy availability with or without disordered eating behaviors, such as caloric restriction or use of diuretics and diet pills, but would not meet the criteria for anorexia or bulimia nervosa. Menstrual dysfunction may include oligomenorrhea or irregular, intermittent menses, as well as amenorrhea. These young women may also have abnormal bone mineral density, with predisposition to bony injury, without having reached the strict criteria of osteoporosis.

The patient comes back to the office to receive her test results, and you take the opportunity to obtain more history. The patient admits that she is very concerned about her diet during her cross-country season, and she is very careful to choose foods that have very little fat but are often high in protein. She will occasionally "go overboard" and eat a lot, for which she compensates by taking part in extra workouts. She has also used laxatives in the past "to not gain weight when I eat too much."

Question 14.2.3 Which of the following findings is NOT classically found in bulimia nervosa?

A) Loss of dental enamel
B) Enlarged parotid glands
C) Metabolic acidosis
D) Skin changes over the dorsum of the hands
E) Maintenance of a significantly low body weight

Answer 14.2.3 The correct answer is "E." Loss of dental enamel, skin changes over the dorsum of the hands, and enlarged parotid glands may be seen as a result of repetitive self-induced vomiting. While self-induced vomiting would cause a metabolic alkalosis through loss of stomach acid, repetitive use of laxatives can cause gastrointestinal losses of bicarbonate, resulting in a metabolic acidosis. **Individuals with bulimia nervosa often maintain a normal weight,** while anorexia nervosa has strict diagnostic criteria requiring maintenance of significantly low body weight, often less than 85% of the ideal body weight.

Your patient also relates that she began having her periods around age 12. While they were initially irregular, they seemed to become more regular prior to starting high school. However, as she became more involved in high school sports, her periods became more irregular. During her off-season, her menses are "more regular," though she cannot predict when they will occur. She recalls that her last period was about 13 weeks ago.

Question 14.2.4 In evaluating your patient's menstrual dysfunction, what would be your next course of action?

A) Obtain serum LH, follicle-stimulating hormone (FSH), and estradiol levels
B) Order an abdominal and pelvic ultrasound
C) Perform a speculum-assisted pelvic examination with Pap smear
D) Obtain a urine beta-hCG
E) Prescribe an oral progestin-only pill (progestin challenge)

Answer 14.2.4 The correct answer is "D." The most common cause of secondary amenorrhea in women of childbearing age remains pregnancy. If pregnancy has been excluded, and the history and physical are reassuring, a progestin challenge can be helpful to determine if adequate estrogen is present; the progestin challenge should induce menses if adequate estrogen exists (see Chapter 15 for details on the evaluation of amenorrhea). Imaging studies and hormonal levels may help in excluding other diagnoses or may be warranted based on physical examination. A pelvic examination may be warranted based on history but is often not necessary in the *initial* evaluation of menstrual dysfunction. Pap smears are no longer recommended for women under the age of 21, regardless of sexual activity status.

Your patient's pregnancy test is negative and a progestin challenge induced menses, indicating adequate circulating estrogen. A comprehensive plan is developed that includes psychological counseling, dietary modification, physical therapy, consultation with a nutritionist, and frequent follow-up. Over the next several months, the patient recovers from her injury, and returns to running on a modified schedule. However, she now complains of heavy, painful menses and wants to go on the "shot" to stop them.

Question 14.2.5 In your counseling about birth control options, which of the statements below is FALSE?

A) The birth control pill can be used to treat irregular menses of the female athlete triad and will also increase bone deposition
B) The effect of Depo-Provera (medroxyprogesterone) is to suppress the hypothalamic–pituitary–ovarian axis, creating a low estrogen state akin to perimenopause
C) The FDA issued a "Black Box" warning on Depo-Provera that states "prolonged use … may result in loss of bone density that may not be completely reversible after discontinuation of the drug"
D) The risk of future fracture using Depo-Provera is unknown, as bone density is an incomplete measure of bone strength, and remodeling and recovery are significant
E) Use of a long-acting reversible contraception (LARC) should be offered as first-line contraceptive choice

Answer 14.2.5 The correct (and "false") answer is "A." The other statements are all true. Starting a combined estrogen/progesterone contraceptive pill will restart a menstrual cycle but may not increase bone density. As to "E," an American Academy of Pediatrics (AAP) policy statement from September 2014 recommends that a LARC be considered as a first-line contraceptive option in adolescents, including intrauterine device (IUD) or subdermal implant. These can provide 3 to 10 years of contraception and are effective and safe forms of birth control. Concerns about an increase in pelvic inflammatory disease (PID) with the IUD appear to be unwarranted.

In your routine anticipatory guidance, you discover that she avoids most dairy products due to a combination of prior concerns about fat content and lactose intolerance.

Question 14.2.6 What do you recommend for her daily intake of elementary calcium?
A) 900 mg
B) 1,100 mg
C) 1,300 mg
D) 1,700 mg
E) 2,100 mg

Answer 14.2.6 The correct answer is "C." While the absolute best intake of calcium for individuals is unknown, studies have shown positive calcium balance for adolescents with an intake of 1,200 to 1,500 mg daily. In its 2010 report, the Institute of Medicine (IOM) set 1,300 mg/day as the "adequate" dietary intake for boys and girls 9 to 18 years of age. This guideline was set to meet the needs of 95% of healthy children, with the upper limit of calcium intake set at 3,000 mg/day.

For most persons, 1,300 mg/day of calcium intake can be accomplished with four servings of dairy products (8 oz of milk = 8 oz of yogurt or cottage cheese = 1 inch cube of cheese) plus a varied diet that includes other calcium-rich foods (e.g., broccoli, collard greens, and turnip greens). It is generally preferable to achieve intake of calcium via diet, including fortified foods, because foods provide multiple nutrients that are important for bone health, such as phosphorus and magnesium. Unfortunately, adolescent girls' average calcium intake is only 700 to 800 mg/day, and adolescent boys' average intake is about 1,000 mg/day—and yet, we have an obesity epidemic. Ironic, but not funny.

Question 14.2.7 On average, what percentage of total body mineral content has a young woman deposited by the time she reaches 12 years of age?
A) 20% to 30%
B) 40% to 50%
C) 70% to 75%
D) 80% to 85%
E) 95% to 100%

Answer 14.2.7 The correct answer is "D." Research suggests that by age 12, a young woman has reached approximately 83%

of her peak bone mineral content, with 50% deposition happening from the time of "peak height velocity," which is premenarchal through 1-year postmenarche. The ability to absorb calcium from the diet is also enhanced during this period. Rates of deposition begin to decline approximately 2 years postmenarche and no significant gains are seen after the age of 17. These statistics emphasize that osteoporosis, while manifesting in older adults, is truly an issue of adolescent preventive medicine.

Your patient returns from a high-powered sports medicine clinic in Palm Springs (or Laguna Beach … or anywhere more likely to make TV than Iowa). She brings you her DEXA scan results that are consistent with osteopenia. She looks up from her Instagram feed and asks, "So, what are we gonna do about that, Doc?"

Question 14.2.8 You scour the literature and recommend:
A) Alendronate
B) Calcium and vitamin D
C) Vigorous weight-bearing exercise
D) Dehydroepiandrosterone (DHEA)
E) All of the above

Answer 14.2.8 The correct answer is "B." Alendronate has no proven benefit in adolescent osteopenic females. Recommending exercise is the usual course for older patients with osteopenia, but you need to be careful in the adolescent with weight concerns who may exercise excessively at baseline. DHEA is investigational and has not been shown to increase bone mineral density. Stick with the standard of care: calcium in the daily doses as recommended above and **vitamin D 600 IU daily** (note that this recommendation is a change in the 2010 IOM guideline—and, yes, that is the most recent guideline as of 2019).

▶ **Objectives: Did you learn to …**
- Evaluate a stress fracture in an adolescent runner?
- Identify the "female athlete triad?"
- Recognize the importance of calcium and vitamin D intake and osteoporosis prevention in adolescence?

 QUICK QUIZ: ADOLESCENT ATHLETES

According to most U.S. studies, what is the number one cause of sudden cardiac death (SCD) in adolescent athletes?
A) Marfan syndrome
B) Coronary artery disease
C) Congenital malformation of coronary arteries
D) Hypertrophic cardiomyopathy
E) Long QT syndrome

The correct answer is "D." Hypertrophic cardiomyopathy is an autosomal-dominant trait with highly variable penetrance that results in asymmetric septal wall hypertrophy. This may cause functional aortic outflow tract obstruction, as well as predispose the athlete to arrhythmias. Unfortunately, this condition is often asymptomatic prior to the terminal event, and screening tests such as electrocardiographs and echocardiograms have not been proven effective at early detection of this condition. Aberrant coronary arteries are thought to be the second leading cause of SCD in young athletes. Marfan syndrome and long QT syndrome are less common.

▶ CASE 14.3

As part of your group's community outreach, you are participating in a sports physical screening (somehow your partner got to throw out the first pitch at a baseball game, and you got this … we're guessing you must be new). One of the students is noted to be hypertensive with a blood pressure of 143/95 mm Hg. There is no family history of sudden death or early heart attack. He has never experienced any symptoms with exercise. His parents indicated on the form that they did not recall any history of previous heart murmur or high blood pressure. The remainder of the examination is unremarkable except for a I/VI systolic murmur. You ask the athlete to perform a Valsalva maneuver by holding his breath and bearing down while cardiac auscultation is repeated.

Question 14.3.1 Which of the following correctly describes the relationship between murmur intensity and the likely type of murmur?
A) Valsalva maneuver increases flow murmur, decreases outflow tract obstruction murmur
B) Valsalva maneuver increases both flow murmur and outflow tract obstruction murmur
C) Valsalva maneuver decreases both flow murmur and outflow tract obstruction murmur
D) Valsalva maneuver decreases flow murmur, increases outflow tract obstruction murmur

Answer 14.3.1 **The correct answer is "D."** The Valsalva maneuver decreases venous return to the heart, resulting in decreased diastolic filling. You would expect this to cause decreased flow through the outflow tract and thus a softer flow murmur. However, the decreased flow exacerbates the **functional** outflow tract obstruction of hypertrophic cardiomyopathy (there is less volume to push the septum out of the way resulting in a tighter functional stenosis), resulting in a louder murmur. In summary, benign flow murmurs will decrease in intensity with Valsalva maneuver, while the murmur of hypertrophic cardiomyopathy will increase with a Valsalva maneuver.

> **HELPFUL TIP:**
> The systolic crescendo–decrescendo murmur of hypertrophic cardiomyopathy increases in intensity when the patient moves from a supine to an upright position. S4 may be heard as well. Cardiac auscultation should be performed both supine and upright for a sports participation physical.

Reassured by a murmur that disappears with Valsalva maneuver and an otherwise unremarkable examination, you are now faced with an adolescent athlete with an elevated blood pressure confirmed by manual re-testing.

Question 14.3.2 What is the best recommendation for this athlete regarding sports participation and follow-up of his elevated blood pressure?
A) Qualified participation pending serial blood pressure checks over the next 3 weeks
B) Complete disqualification for 2 months, followed by return if ECG and echocardiogram are normal
C) Disqualification from competition only for 1 month, but allowed to practice once seen by a nephrologist
D) Full participation with no required follow-up based on reassuring history and examination
E) Full participation with blood pressure re-check prior to the next competitive sport season

Answer 14.3.2 **The correct answer is "A."** It is important to remember that the diagnosis of hypertension cannot be made at a single screening visit. The screening may be affected by patient anxiety ("white coat hypertension"), recent caffeine ingestion, drugs, or a number of other factors (including a common occurrence of scheduling examinations right after practice and standing half naked with your peers.). The National Heart, Lung and Blood Institute guideline recommends that hypertension be diagnosed if blood pressure is above the 95th percentile for children/adolescents on three separate recordings of blood pressure on different occasions after several minutes at rest, sitting comfortably.

Because exercise is beneficial for blood pressure control, continued aerobic activity should be encouraged while the serial blood pressure readings are obtained. Debate exists as to recommendations regarding static exercises, such as weightlifting. While lifting of heavy weights can exacerbate high blood pressure, there is some evidence to suggest that use of light-to-moderate weights with repetition is beneficial. Certainly, the presence of any additional symptoms with exercise, such as headache or lightheadedness, would require more significant limitations in activity.

▶ **Objectives: Did you learn to …**
· Identify important issues to address at the pre-participation physical examination?
· Evaluate an adolescent athlete with elevated blood pressure?
· Evaluate a cardiac murmur revealed on pre-participation physical examination?

▶ CASE 14.4

A 15-year-old female presents to your office for a well-adolescent examination. She is a healthy teenager with no complaints—well, she has the usual teenager complaints (her parents are "stupid," the teachers don't know anything, etc.).

You have incorporated into your routine a screening tool, the Guideline for Adolescent Preventive Services (GAPS) questionnaire, one of many such tools available. The questions cover all areas of adolescent development and are designed so that areas of concern are easily identified. See https://www.uvpediatrics.com/health-topics/stage/#GAPS for example.

Question 14.4.1 What are the three leading causes of mortality for adolescents?
A) Leukemia, suicide, accidental drowning
B) Childhood cancers, perinatally acquired HIV, suicide
C) Congenital malformations, childhood cancers, suicide
D) Accidental injury, homicide, suicide
E) Childhood cancers, SCD, suicide

Answer 14.4.1 The correct answer is "D." Accidental injury, homicide, and suicide are the three leading causes of death for adolescents and should be addressed during preventive health visits. As a category of accidents, motor vehicle fatality is the leading cause of death to teenagers, representing over one-third of all deaths. A high number of teens report unsafe driving behavior: 39.2% of teens have reported texting or emailing while driving. While most states have made texting and driving illegal, it is still important to discuss with your adolescent patients. Accidental injuries often involve the use of alcohol or other substances in combination with motor vehicle operation or other risk-taking behaviors. Ask about personal use of alcohol and if they are ever passengers of another teenager (or adult) who drives while impaired or intoxicated. The greater the number of teens in the car of a teen driver, the greater the likelihood of an accident. This argues for the law in some states that restrict the number of passengers in a teen driver's car.

You also noticed that your patient checked "yes" for a history of use of alcohol and marijuana.

Question 14.4.2 What is the approximate frequency of lifetime use of these substances among 9th to 12th grade students according to the Centers for Disease Control and Prevention (CDC's) 2017 Youth Risk Behavioral Survey (YBRS)?
A) Alcohol 10% to 20%; marijuana 5% to 10%
B) Alcohol 30% to 40%; marijuana 10% to 20%
C) Alcohol 50% to 60%; marijuana 20% to 30%
D) Alcohol 60% to 70%; marijuana 30% to 40%
E) Alcohol 70% to 80%; marijuana 40% to 50%

Answer 14.4.2 The correct answer is "D." The survey found 60.4% of adolescents reporting use of alcohol at some point in their lives, and 35.6% reporting use of marijuana. In addition, 28.9% have tried cigarettes (a decrease from 41.1% in 2013!).

HELPFUL TIP: A "NOT SO HEALTHY" ALTERNATIVE
Don't forget to ask about "vaping" when questioning an adolescent about substance use. While cigarette use is declining, vaping is quickly catching on with adolescents due to its marketing of flavorful nicotine that is supposed to be "healthier." These companies know their target audience and have made "cooler" delivery mechanisms (many actually look like flash drives, such as Juul®). In fact, many adolescents don't even equate vaping with use of tobacco products or health risks such as "popcorn lung" or potentially fatal lipoid pneumonia. The 2017 YBRS survey indicated 42.2% of adolescents surveyed have used vaping products. Eek!

HELPFUL TIP:
Screening tools for adolescent substance use include the "CRAFFT" questions, developed by the "Center for Adolescent Substance Abuse Research" (CeASAR), Children's Hospital Boston. Similar to the "CAGE" tool for adult alcohol assessment, the letters stand for:
- **C**—Have you ever ridden in a CAR driven by someone (including yourself) who was "high" or had been using alcohol or drugs?
- **R**—Do you ever use alcohol or drugs to RELAX, feel better about yourself, or fit in?
- **A**—Do you ever use alcohol/drugs while you are by yourself, ALONE?
- **F**—Do you ever FORGET things you did while using alcohol or drugs?
- **F**—Do your family or FRIENDS ever tell you that you should cut down on your drinking or drug use?
- **T**—Have you gotten in TROUBLE while you were using alcohol or drugs?

After eliciting a positive response to questions about drug use, you ask the patient about depression, and she states that she has been feeling "down" for several months now.

Question 14.4.3 What would your next step be?
A) Call the police and report the illegal use of substances by a minor
B) Reassure the patient about her confidentiality rights, counsel her to quit using drugs, and see her back annually
C) Negotiate next steps to guarantee the patient's safety and consider counseling referral and/or initiation of medication therapy
D) Obtain a nonconsented urine drug screen to document recent use of substances

Answer 14.4.3 The correct answer is "C." Most state laws, as well as HIPAA, guarantee teenagers confidentiality; it can only be broken when there is an issue of imminent danger to self or others or physical/sexual abuse. It is recommended that the patient be involved and consent to who and how the information is shared. Rarely is there a need to involve police, unless there is an issue of abuse requiring a report or concern over safety if the patient is returned to the home environment.

Psychotherapy, pharmacotherapy, or a combination of the two are all reasonable treatment options in adolescent depression. If a medication is started, SSRIs are considered first-line therapy by most published guidelines due to their proven efficacy. However, they ***should certainly be used with caution as studies suggest increased suicidality in teenagers treated with SSRIs. While there are increased attempts at suicide, there is NOT an increase in successful suicide.*** Fluoxetine has the most favorable benefit/risk profile in adolescents due to its long half-life. The American Academy of Child and Adolescent Psychiatry website has resources outlining patient and parent information about the risks and benefits of pharmacologic treatments. In any case, close follow-up of a depressed adolescent (weekly visits or phone calls) is recommended early in the treatment course.

HELPFUL TIP:
As of February 2016, the U.S. Preventative Services Task Force now recommends screening for mood disorders in teenagers aged 12 to 18 *as long as there are adequate resources available to aide in diagnosis, treatment, and follow-up.* They provide this a grade B practice recommendation. There is insufficient evidence at this point for screening children aged 11 years of age or younger.

HELPFUL TIP:
The American Academy of Pediatrics has a position statement against the use of nonconsented urine drug screens as a "screening" tool due to the lack of accuracy and the violation of patient trust.

(ONE MORE) HELPFUL TIP:
A study published in *Lancet* found that adolescent self-harm (cutting, burning, etc.) occurs in about 10% of adolescents. However, you can reassure parents that this declines to 3% as a young adult (Moran P, et al. *Lancet.* 2012).

▶ Objectives: Did you learn to ...
- Identify and employ useful screening tools for routine adolescent examinations?
- Recognize the importance of screening and treating depression in adolescents?
- Describe common causes of death in adolescents?
- Understand the common lifetime experience use of alcohol, tobacco, and marijuana?
- Describe screening and treatment options for mood disorders and substance abuse?

▶ **CASE 14.5**

Your afternoon has a number of patients with sports-related complaints. A 14-year-old wrestler has arrived in the office complaining of a rash on his left shoulder. The rash appears to consist of several small lesions with a vesicular appearance but no purulence and minimal erythema. There is neither tenderness to palpation nor tactile warmth in the affected area.

Question 14.5.1 **What would be your best test to confirm your diagnosis of these lesions?**
A) Microscopic evaluation with potassium hydroxide (KOH) preparation of the contents of one of the lesions
B) Gram stain of the contents of one of the lesions
C) Culture of the contents of one of the lesions
D) Tzanck smear of the contents of one of the lesions

Answer 14.5.1 **The correct answer is "D."** A Tzanck prep will give you immediate information about whether this represents herpes simplex. This is important information when deciding whether or not this patient can return to wrestling. HSV PCR assays are a more sensitive method to confirm HSV infection in clinical specimens obtained from genital ulcers and mucocutaneous sites and should also be obtained. These newer tests tend to be much quicker than older assays and typically return within 24 to 48 hours depending on your lab. The point here is that the lesions described have the appearance of HSV, and a confirmatory test for HSV should be obtained.

The lesions have appeared within the past day, and your laboratory testing confirms that the diagnosis is herpes simplex. Your patient does not recall any previous lesions like these. He denies any systemic symptoms.

Question 14.5.2 **What would be the best course of treatment for this patient?**
A) Cover the involved area to allow return to wrestling
B) Treat with topical acyclovir and return to wrestling when lesions have crusted over
C) Treat with oral acyclovir and return to wrestling when lesions have crusted over
D) Treat with oral steroids to suppress the response and promote quicker return to wrestling
E) Treat with topical antifungal medication and allow return to wrestling

Answer 14.5.2 **The correct answer is "C."** Cutaneous herpes, also referred to in wrestling as *herpes gladiatorum*, is a highly contagious illness. "B" is incorrect because topical acyclovir is **NOT** effective in treating herpes simplex. Most state high school athletic associations have specific rules regarding the treatment of cutaneous disorders in wrestling, including herpes, tinea corporis, and impetigo. With regard to herpes simplex, all lesions must be fully crusted over **and** the athlete must have had at least 3 days of oral antiviral therapy prior to returning to competition. One study has shown that use of prophylactic valacyclovir 1 gram daily may be efficacious in lowering the incidence of HSV outbreaks in wrestlers (*Clin J Sport Med.* 2016;26(4): 272–278). "D" is incorrect because oral steroids would suppress the athlete's immune response, which would allow for further spread of the lesions.

Your next patient is a 12-year-old male who is here for a sports physical. You review your patient's chart and scan his immunizations. The patient's mother remembers her son receiving his "kindergarten shots"; he has had no immunizations since. His records reveal the following vaccines: five doses of diphtheria–tetanus–acellular pertussis (DTaP), four doses of injectable polio vaccine (IPV), four doses of *Haemophilus Influenzae* Type B (Hib), three doses of hepatitis B; four doses of pneumococcal vaccine (PCV 13), two doses of measles–mumps–rubella (MMR), and two doses of varicella vaccine.

Question 14.5.3 **Which, if any, immunizations would you offer today?**
A) None. The patient is up-to-date for all immunizations
B) Conjugate pneumococcal vaccine
C) Hepatitis A/B vaccine, conjugate meningococcal vaccine, IPV
D) Hepatitis A vaccine; Tetanus, diphtheria, and pertussis (Tdap); conjugate meningococcal vaccine and start of the HPV series
E) Human papillomavirus (HPV) vaccine, Tdap, varicella vaccine

Answer 14.5.3 The correct answer is "D." Universal vaccination for hepatitis B is included in the primary immunization series for infants, so most adolescents have been vaccinated. However, it is still important to make sure this is up-to-date. Hepatitis A vaccine is now being required in many states before entry to school and is universally recommended for all children ages 12 months to 2 years. A catch-up vaccination schedule is now recommended for ages 2 to 18 years. For those not up-to-date with their hepatitis B vaccination, a combined hepatitis A/B vaccine exists.

Most children receive their last DTaP prior to entering preschool or kindergarten (age 4–5 years). Beginning in 2005, the CDC recommended giving the tetanus booster with pertussis (Tdap) at entry to middle school/junior high (ages 11–12) in place of the tetanus booster (Td).

For protection against some serotypes of *Neisseria meningitidis*, the CDC recommends universal vaccination with the conjugate meningococcal vaccine (e.g., Menactra) for teens, including a booster dose between ages 16 and 18 years.

The CDC recommends 9-valent HPV for routine vaccination of adolescents 11-12 years of age through age 26 (although you can start as early as 9 years of age). The upper age limit is now 45. For those 27–45 years of age, use shared decision making (MMWR 2019 Aug 16). "E" is incorrect because he has already had two doses of the varicella vaccine.

Question 14.5.4 **Which statement does NOT accurately describe how the conjugate meningitis vaccine (Menactra) differs from the older polysaccharide meningitis vaccine (Menomune)?**
A) **Menactra** elicits a T-cell immune response that gives long-term immunity and allows for herd immunity

B) **Menactra** protects against all the types of *N. meningitidis*: A, B, C, Y, W-135
C) **Menomune** does not elicit a booster effect, may only be given once, and is recommended only at the onset of high-risk activity, such as living in dorms or being a military recruit
D) **Menactra** should be offered at entry to middle school/junior high school (11–12 years) with a booster dose recommended between ages 16 and 23

Answer 14.5.4 The correct answer (and FALSE statement) is "B." Unfortunately neither Menomune nor Menactra protect against serogroup Type B. The other choices are correct. *N. meningitidis* Type B is endemic in North America and up until 2014, no vaccine was available. In 2014 and 2015, the FDA approved two meningococcal **Type B** vaccinations (three-dose MenB-FHbp (Trumenba®) and two-dose MenB-4c (Bexsero®)). The ACIP in October 2015 provided a grade B recommendation that MenB vaccination *may* be given *in addition* to Menactra and other indicated age-based vaccinations (preferably at a different anatomic site) between ages 16 and 23 with preferable dosing at 16 to 18 years to provide peak desired immunologic effect in the group that is at most risk. Additionally, high-risk populations including those with anatomic or functional asplenia, sickle cell disease, persistent complement component deficiency (including eculizumab use), or those in a serogroup B meningococcal disease outbreak should be vaccinated. Note that the two vaccines are not interchangeable.

HELPFUL TIP:
Review the vaccine recommendations since they are updated frequently by the CDC; vaccine recommendations can be found at http://www.cdc.gov/vaccines/schedules/.

▶ **Objectives: Did you learn to …**
· Identify herpes gladiatorum and describe its treatment?
· Recommend vaccines appropriate for adolescents?

▶ CASE 14.6

A 15-year-old pale Caucasian female returns for her annual well-child check and sports physical. She is well known to your clinic, and over the years she has steadily gained weight. Her parents and a younger sibling are overweight, and now she has become obese by measure of the pediatric BMI percentages. In recent years, you have become more diligent with watching the BMI on her growth curve. She is aware of her weight problem yet has not voiced any plan for attempting weight loss.

Question 14.6.1 **What defines "obesity" in adolescence?**
A) A BMI in the 85th to 94th percentile for age-sex-and-height-specific measures

B) A BMI ≥95th percentile for age-sex-and-height-specific measures
C) The child has the appearance of being heavy
D) The child complains of being fat or overweight
E) BMI >35 kg/m²

Answer 14.6.1 The correct answer is "B." A BMI at or above the 95th percentile is considered "obese." A BMI in the range of 85th to 94th percentiles is considered "overweight." The use of BMI allows for an objective measure, and although not perfect, can give a picture on the growth curve to patients and parents where they stand relative to age-sex-and-height-related norms. Strict BMI numbers (as in "E") are not applicable to children and adolescents. A subjective concern about weight ("D") is important but does not necessarily always warrant further evaluation.

Question 14.6.2 Her BMI is now at the 97th percentile, having jumped from the 86th percentile last year. What additional workup should be considered?
A) Fasting plasma glucose level or hemoglobin A1c
B) Fasting lipids
C) Renal function testing with BUN and creatinine
D) Liver function testing with ALT
E) All of the above

Answer 14.6.2 The correct answer is "E." Expert opinion suggests that once a child reaches a BMI at the 85th to 94th percentiles, a lipid panel and a fasting glucose or A1c should be obtained to evaluate for hyperlipidemia and early onset type 2 diabetes. When the BMI reaches the 95th percentile, renal function and blood pressure should be monitored, and liver function should be checked (for fatty liver). Fatty liver disease is possible at an early age and is reversible if weight loss can be achieved. Close attention to family history is essential. If family members are obese or have obesity-related comorbidities, early intervention and evaluation are even more crucial. For females who have started menses, it is important to assess for any changes in menstrual patterns.

Question 14.6.3 Which of the following is NOT a recommended early childhood intervention to prevent and/or treat obesity?
A) Encouraging breastfeeding
B) Decreasing screen time of electronic devices
C) Planning fewer family meals
D) Restricting calories from sweets and fast foods
E) Improving efforts for exercise and outdoor activity

Answer 14.6.3 The correct answer is "C." Helping with food preparation and sitting down as a family for meals can lead to consumption of more nutritious and lower caloric dense foods. Breastfeeding can lead to protection against obesity even into the teenage years. Formal recommendations suggest limiting TV, tablet, phone, computer use, and video games to less than 2 hours per day with minimal screen time for children under

age 2. Fast food, sweets, and desserts need to be limited to small servings or few servings per week. Finally, at least 60 minutes of exercise should be encouraged every day—doing a variety of activities will keep children more engaged and interested.

HELPFUL TIP:
If children do become overweight or obese, directed weight loss should be implemented. For kids with a BMI at the 85th to 94th percentiles, the goal is weight maintenance until they reach a BMI at the 84th percentile or less. For those with BMI at or above the 95th percentile, expert opinion recommends children age 2 to 11 years lose up to 1 pound per month and adolescents lose up to 2 pounds per week.

HELPFUL TIP: 5-2-1-0
The "5-2-1-0" mnemonic is a helpful way to counsel your patients and their parents on healthy lifestyle practices and has been a successful campaign supported by the American Academy of Pediatrics. The numbers stand for: **5** fruits and vegetables per day, **2** hours or less of screen time, **1** hour or more of physical activity, **0** consumption of sugary drinks.

During the examination of the patient, you notice acne, some coarse facial hair, and dark skin pigmentation around the base of her neck.

Question 14.6.4 What is another finding you may expect to see with further questions and tests?
A) Normal menses
B) Low free testosterone level
C) Low DHEA sulfate (DHEA-S)
D) Hypoglycemia
E) Abnormal hypothalamic–pituitary axis hormones

Answer 14.6.4 The correct answer is "E." While the earliest clinical manifestation is irregular menses, she is showing other signs of possible polycystic ovarian syndrome (PCOS). This can be associated with elevated prolactin, low TSH, and a marked elevation of FSH relative to luteinizing hormone (LH). PCOS can be associated with early menarche, dysmenorrhea, and amenorrhea. A pregnancy test should be done in any case of amenorrhea. PCOS is also associated with **elevations** of testosterone, DHEA-S, and androstenedione. If there are other significant physical examination findings such as elevated blood pressure, purple striae, and a "buffalo hump," consider testing for Cushing syndrome. See chapter 15 for more on PCOS.

Her obesity is discussed openly during the office visit. As expected, she is ashamed and embarrassed about her weight

gain. She admits to not knowing what to do and she asks if anything can be done to quickly lose weight.

Question 14.6.5 Which of these medications would you recommend now as a first-line therapy for weight loss?
A) Topiramate (Topamax)
B) Bupropion (Wellbutrin)
C) Orlistat (Xenical)
D) Metformin (Glucophage)
E) None of the above

Answer 14.6.5 The correct answer is "E." No medication is approved for children or adolescents as a first-line therapy. Antidepressants are not helpful if used primarily for weight loss. If there is comorbid depression, which is more common in obese children, a "weight loss" or "weight neutral" antidepressant may be appropriate. Antiepileptic medications have not proven helpful. Metformin has been used for weight loss in children but is not approved by FDA and has only small effect on weight with unclear clinical significance. Orlistat is approved for children age 12 and older; however, the benefits are limited to 2 to 3 kg of weight loss. Side effects are often intolerable and include loose, oily stools and stool urgency (just mention the phrase "fecal incontinence" to a teenager and see how far you get). Experts agree that orlistat is only appropriate for adolescents with comorbidities caused by obesity. Obesity ("bariatric") surgery (especially Roux-en-Y and gastric sleeve) is being performed more often on adolescents and is effective at reversing metabolic changes (insulin resistance, hypertryglyceridemia, etc.). It also improves sleep apnea and depression and improves quality of life.

 HELPFUL TIP:
The risk of becoming overweight can decrease by 4% for each month of breastfeeding up to age 9 months.

 HELPFUL TIP:
Weight loss in adolescence will likely lead to decreased cardiovascular disease as an adult (Juonala M, et al. *N Engl J Med.* 2011).

 HELPFUL TIP:
The USPFTF recommends counseling to minimize ultra-violent radiation exposure (e.g., sun tanning) in fair skinned adolescents in order to reduce the risk of skin cancer (Grade B recommendation).

▶ **Objectives: Did you learn to …**
· Define "overweight" and "obesity" in an adolescent?
· Identify risk factors associated with obesity in an adolescent?
· Manage an adolescent with a weight problem?

▶ **CASE 14.7**

You have watched your patient transform over the years from a rather normal-appearing boy into a very large, muscular, and intense young man. He is now 17 years old, and he has gained almost 45 lb in the last year alone as he prepares for his senior year of football and attempts to attract the attention of college recruiters (and potential mates). Without a doubt he has worked very hard on the field and in the weight room, but you also must raise the question of whether or not he has used some kind of supplement to help him change so drastically.

Question 14.7.1 Which of these substances is NOT prohibited by high school athletic associations or the NCAA?
A) Erythropoietin
B) Creatine
C) Androstenedione
D) Ephedrine
E) DHEA

Answer 14.7.1 The correct answer is "B." Creatine is allowed for use as a dietary supplement for athletes. However, the American College of Sports Medicine (ACSM) does NOT recommend the use of creatine in any athlete less than 18 years old. An estimated 8% of children 14 to 18 years old use creatine routinely. The NCAA does not allow colleges to provide athletes with creatine, but athletes can take it if they choose. All the other listed supplements are prohibited for use as performance-enhancing supplements. Other prohibited substances include anabolic steroids, pseudoephedrine, and blood transfusions.

Your patient does admit to using regular protein shakes and taking creatine. He denies the use of any illegal or prohibited substances and says he would never do anything dangerous. During his examination, his blood pressure is 146/92 mm Hg and his lab results show normal electrolytes, normal TSH, normal urinalysis, BUN 22 mg/dL, and creatinine 1.6 mg/dL (marked elevation for age 17).

Question 14.7.2 What is a possible side effect from the use of creatine?
A) Gastrointestinal discomfort
B) Edema
C) Muscle cramps
D) Acute kidney injury
E) All of the above

Answer 14.7.2 The correct answer is "E." All are potential adverse effects from creatine use. Most importantly, if used carelessly, creatine can lead to acute kidney injury. Creatine is excreted via the kidneys, and if overconsumed in the setting of dehydrating exercise, it can cause renal injury. Seventy-five percent of adolescent athletes who take creatine are either unaware of the proper dose or knowingly take too much. If used, plenty of water is required to help avoid troubling side effects.

Question 14.7.3 All of the following substances can provide potential athletic performance benefits EXCEPT:
A) Human growth hormone (HGH)
B) Caffeine
C) Creatine
D) Electrolyte replacements
E) Sodium bicarbonate

Answer 14.7.3 **The correct answer is "A."** HGH has no proven benefits for enhancing sports performance. Other substances with no proven benefits include amino acids, beta-hydroxy-beta-methylbutyrate, androstenedione, DHEA, chromium, and iron (when not iron deficient). The other substances listed above can provide short-term or long-term benefits. Caffeine has only a transient effect to help sharpen focus and intensity for brief periods of activity. Creatine can improve strength for adult male athletes in those sports that require very short bursts of intense effort. Electrolyte replacement drinks (or tablets) and sodium bicarbonate can help for more prolonged endurance activities where dehydration and resulting electrolyte imbalances are common.

Your patient denies using "steroids," but does know of older guys in the gym where he trains who have routinely used anabolic steroids.

Question 14.7.4 Besides the obvious added muscle girth, what are some other potential benefits of anabolic steroids for athletes?
A) Improved lipid profile
B) Taller stature
C) Anxiety relief
D) Lower blood pressure
E) None of the above

Answer 14.7.4 **The correct answer is "E."** There are no other clear benefits of anabolic steroids if used for athletics only. Potential negative effects include lower HDL, elevated blood pressure, left ventricular hypertrophy, gynecomastia, aggressive or even suicidal behavior, azoospermia, virilization of females, premature physeal closure in adolescents that could lead to shorter stature, and acute myocardial infarction. Approximately 33% of anabolic steroid users are not even athletes and use the substance to help improve physical appearance. Estimates in high school athletes show steroid use to be about 4% in males and about 2% in females. The temptation to use the illegal substance is driven by pressures to be better than peers, to fulfill one's "full potential," to live up to sports idols, and to help acquire college scholarships and/or sports contracts at a young age.

► Objective: Did you learn to …
  · Describe the effects of some common performance-enhancing drugs?

► **CASE 14.8**

A 14-year-old female comes into the office with a chief complaint of headache. She says the headache began after her soccer game yesterday. She recalls striking her head against an opponent when trying to head the soccer ball. During the remainder of the game, she began to feel a headache, and the harder she ran, the more "woozy" she felt. She denied any loss of consciousness, vomiting, visual symptoms, or neck pain. Today, she also has poor concentration and feels excessive fatigue.

Question 14.8.1 Which of the following is NOT a feature of a sports-related concussion (SRC)?
A) Caused by an impulsive force transmitted to the brain
B) Symptoms usually resolve spontaneously
C) There is a functional disturbance to the body
D) Neuroimaging always shows abnormalities
E) Clinical symptoms are highly variable and inconsistent

Answer 14.8.1 **The correct answer is "D."** There may be no evident structural brain injury with SRC. Evidence suggests that multiple concussions, or even lessor repetitive head injuries (such as with soccer "heading") can eventually lead to structural tissue damage. The symptoms of concussions have a rapid onset and while most athletes recover within the first month, some have a slower recovery from SRC. Some evidence suggests adolescents are at greater risk of persistent symptoms with pre-injury history of mental health issues or migraine headaches.

HELPFUL TIP:
Concussion is defined as a disturbance in brain function caused by trauma to the head. It does not require loss of consciousness or amnesia. Lightheadedness, disorientation, and nausea, etc. after head injury are all possible signs of concussion. Symptoms of post-concussion syndrome may include headaches, difficulty concentrating, "dizziness," lightheadedness, nausea, fatigue, irritability, anxiety, and depression. Symptoms generally resolve but may be long lived, especially in those over age 50, who may never return to baseline. In addition, the potential for developing chronic traumatic encephalopathy (CTE) is present and further study is ongoing.

HELPFUL TIP:
If an athlete sustains a head injury or a hard hit, the athlete should be removed from the game and a sideline assessment should be performed to assess for SRC. A simple standardized tool to use in the acute assessment of SRC and subsequent evaluations is the Sport Concussion Assessment Tool (SCAT-5) questionnaire (*Br J Sports Med*. 2018;51:838–847). The SCAT5 takes about 10 minutes to administer. **If a concussion is suspected, the athlete should NOT be allowed to return to the game.**

Question 14.8.2 Which of the following treatments is key for your patient with a concussion?
A) Early return to aerobic exercise—today if possible
B) Ibuprofen 800 mg every 8 hours as needed
C) Avoiding excessive sleep
D) Aspirin 325 mg daily as needed
E) Full cognitive rest (put down that smartphone, tablet, and social media!), even missing school if needed

Answer 14.8.2 The correct answer is "E." Caring for patients with an SRC requires graduated stepwise rehabilitation starting with full physical **and** cognitive rest. Once symptoms are clearly improving at rest, the student can get back to class and **slowly** be re-acclimated to physical activity. Sleep can provide a means of allowing the brain to rest and heal. No medications have proven helpful in alleviating the effects of a concussion. NSAIDs, aspirin, or acetaminophen may help with headache or pain.

HELPFUL TIP:
A recent randomized trial of early aerobic exercise in adolescents with concussion suggests that exercise is associated with more rapid recovery. In the study, randomized adolescents to exercise on a treadmill or stationary bicycle *at a speed that did not worsen or bring on their symptoms.* The group randomized to exercise returned to the classroom 4 days earlier (13 vs. 17 days) and had better long-term recovery (96% vs. 93%) (*JAMA Pediatr.* 2019 Feb 4 [e-pub]).

Question 14.8.3 In which case of head injury would neuroimaging be appropriate?
A) Ongoing mild headache for several days
B) Poor memory of the recent game and the events of the injury
C) Any new seizure activity
D) Loss of consciousness for less than 30 seconds
E) Mild irritability, depressed mood, and insomnia

Answer 14.8.3 The correct answer is "C." Seizure activity after head trauma or concussion requires imaging. Other symptoms that should prompt a head CT include severe headache, focal neurological symptoms, repeated emesis, difficulty arousing, slurred speech, prolonged poor orientation, concurrent neck pain, significant irritability, loss of consciousness for over 30 seconds, and any new neurologic or escalating symptoms. The initial study is normally a head CT, but if presenting after 48 hours from injury, a brain MRI is more suitable. Remember that the vast majority of concussion cases will **not** require imaging.

Question 14.8.4 Which of the following elements of past medical history may be relevant for this adolescent patient following her concussion?
A) Depression
B) Generalized anxiety disorder
C) Attention-deficit hyperactivity disorder (ADHD)
D) Migraine headaches
E) All of the above

Answer 14.8.4 The correct answer is "E." All of these conditions could be negatively affected by a concussion. Concussions can cause a temporary mood disorder and certainly aggravate depression and anxiety. Commonly, concussions will cause decreased concentration and inattentiveness. Teens who already have ADHD will likely have worsened symptoms and may need modification of their treatment. The headache of post-concussive syndrome may overlap or intensify an underlying headache diagnosis. Concussion may act as a trigger causing an increase in pre-existing migraines.

Your patient is an accomplished soccer player and feels a lot of pressure to return to action. She wants to play in the next game, and her coach and teammates are asking if she'll be back to practice this afternoon—which explains why your waiting room is so full of teenage girls wearing shin guards.

Question 14.8.5 What is your best advice about her return to practice and play?
A) "Go back to practice today, but take it slow and avoid full speed play"
B) "Try to participate in simple drills and just cheer on your teammates"
C) "Go home and engage in cognitive rest. You may return to activity with graded return to play regimen once symptoms resolve"
D) "Return to full, unrestricted team play as your soccer team needs you!"
E) "Do whatever you want"

Answer 14.8.5 The correct answer is "C." Her return to participation needs to be symptom guided. Each step of the recovery may be 24 hours. If she advances her activity with recurrence of symptoms, then she needs to go back to the prior step. The first step is no activity—complete physical and cognitive rest. The next step is return to full academic activities. Step three is light aerobic activity, followed by sport-specific drills. Next, the player can return to noncontact practice. If still symptom free, then she can return to full speed, contact practice. Finally, she can return to game action. If exertion causes any return of symptoms, then she is not ready and should return to the previous symptom-free stage. Even with normal neuropsychiatric tests, symptomatic athletes should not play. Additionally, academic accommodations may be necessary.

The above steps should be followed with the assistance of a healthcare provider or a qualified athletic trainer. The athlete cannot be put in the position of making the decision about how fast to return to regular play. SRC history should be obtained and considered for all athletes. Two or more concussions have been shown to lower grade point averages and three or more concussions may cause prolonged symptoms over 3 months in duration.

HELPFUL TIP:
If a concussion occurs, please do not allow return to play the same game or even the same day. The risk for second-impact syndrome is much greater if a player returns to play too early after a concussion. This is most likely to occur when a player does not report symptoms (more common in male athletes) after sustaining a concussion, and then has another head trauma. The rare second-impact syndrome can lead to cerebral vascular congestion, cerebral edema, and even death. The greatest risk athletes are those under age 20. See the Berlin (McCrory) guidelines for more detailed recommendations on returning to activity. The reference is in the bibliography.

Question 14.8.6 Which of the following risk factors is associated with a prolonged post concussive syndrome?
A) Younger athletes
B) Females
C) Poor social situation
D) Diet lacking in B vitamins
E) A and B

Answer 14.8.6 The correct answer is "E." Younger athletes and girls tend to have a longer recovery time. Kids with a history of concussion, mood issues, ADHD, and migraine headaches also take longer on average to recover. Luckily, most children get better spontaneously. If we are talking about adults, the older the adult the less likely they will fully resolve post-concussion syndrome and may have prolonged symptoms (e.g., dizziness, headaches, fatigue).

HELPFUL TIP:
"Cognitive rest" after a concussion may need to include avoidance of reading, computer games, TV, Internet, smartphone use, homework, school attendance, and driving. Here's the simple idea: pull back if the activity is exacerbating symptoms. Prevention of concussions is best accomplished by education of athletes, parents, and coaches, and by early recognition of more minor symptoms. Mouth guards do not have any proven benefit in preventing concussion, and helmets do not lessen the incidence of concussions; they just prevent more severe traumatic brain injuries.

▶ **Objectives: Did you learn to …**
  • Define concussion and recognize its importance in adolescent athletes?
  • Treat a patient with concussion?

Clinical Pearls

○ Consider long-acting reversible contraceptives (LARCs) as first-line therapy for contraception in adolescent females.

○ Do not allow an adolescent return to play after incurring a concussion. Keep the athlete out and prescribe cognitive rest. Once symptoms have improved, slowly allow the adolescent to return to play in a graduated and prescribed fashion.

○ Do not screen for substance abuse with nonconsented urine drug screens.

○ Routinely screen adolescents for substance abuse and mood disorders if adequate support resources are available. Use standardized screening tools.

○ Routinely vaccinate adolescents with Tdap, conjugate meningitis vaccine, and HPV series.

BIBLIOGRAPHY

American Academy of Pediatrics. Healthy active living for families. 2006. Available at: https://www.healthychildren.org/English/healthy-living/nutrition/Pages/Healthy-Active-Living-for-Families.aspx. Accessed February 2, 2019.

Colquitt JL, et al. Diet, physical activity, and behavioural interventions for the treatment of overweight or obesity in preschool children up to the age of 6 years. *Cochrane Database Syst Rev.* 2016;3:CD012105. Epub 2016 Mar 10.

Halsted ME, Walter KD, and The Council on Sports Medicine and Fitness. Clinical report: Sport-related concussion in children and adolescents. *Pediatrics.* 2010;126(3):597–615.

Ham P, Allen C. Adolescent health screening and counseling. *Am Family Physician.* 2012;86(12):1109–1116.

Harder T, Bergmann R, Kallischnigg G, Plagemann A. Duration of breastfeeding and risk of overweight: a meta-analysis. *Am J Epidemiol.* 2005;162(5):397–403.

Herman-Giddens ME, et al. Secondary sexual characteristics in boys: data from the Pediatric Research in Office Settings Network. *Pediatrics.* 2012;130(5):e1058–e1068.

Jenkinson DM, Harbert AJ. Supplements and sports. *Am Fam Physician.* 2008;78(9):1039–1046.

Kann L, et al. Youth risk behavior surveillance—United States 2017. *MMWR Surveill Summ.* 2017;67(SS-8).

Knight JR, Sherritt L, Shrier LA, Harris SK, Chang G. Validity of the CRAFFT substance abuse screening test among adolescent clinic patients. *Arch Pediatr Adolesc Med.* 2002;156(6):607–614.

McCrory P, et al. Consensus statement on concussion in sport: the 5th International Conference on Concussion in Sport held in Berlin, October 2016. *Br J Sports Med.* 2018;51:838–847.

Moran P, et al. The natural history of self-harm from adolescence to young adulthood: a population-based cohort study. *Lancet.* 2012;379:236–243.

Nwosu BU, Lee MM. Evaluation of short and tall stature in children. *Am Fam Physician.* 2008;78(5):597–604.

O'Connor EA, et al. Screening for obesity and intervention for weight management in children and adolescents: A Systematic Evidence Review for the U.S. Preventive Services Task Force. Evidence Synthesis No. 150. AHRQ Publication No. 15-05219-EF-1. Rockville, MD: Agency for Healthcare Research and Quality; 2017.

Office of Dietary Supplements. Calcium fact Sheet. National Institutes of Health. 26 Sept 2018. Available at: https://ods.od.nih.gov/factsheets/Calcium-HealthProfessional/. Accessed December 24, 2018.

Ott MA, et al. Policy statement: contraception for adolescents. *Pediatrics*. 2014;134(4):e1244–e1256.

Rao G. Childhood obesity: highlights from the AMA expert committee recommendations. *Am Fam Physician*. 2008;78(1):56–63.

Scorza KA, Raleigh MF, O'Connor FG. Current concepts in concussion: evaluation and management. *Am Fam Physician*. 2012;85(2):123–132.

Stephens MB. Preventive health counseling for adolescents. *Am Fam Physician*. 2006;74(7):1151–1156.

Thein-Nissenbaum JM, Carr KE. Female athlete triad syndrome in the high school athlete. *Phys Ther Sport*. 2011;12(3):108–116.

U.S. Department of Health and Human Services, Center for Disease Control and Prevention. Recommended immunization schedule for children and adolescents aged 18 years or younger, United States, 2018. Available at: www.cdc.gov/vaccines/schedules/hcp/child-adolescent.html. Accessed February 2, 2019.

U.S. Department of Health and Human Services, National Heart, Lung, and Blood Institute. Expert panel on integrated guidelines for cardiovascular health and risk reduction in children and adolescents: summary report. October 2012. NIH Publication No. 12-7486A. Available at: https://www.nhlbi.nih.gov/files/docs/peds_guidelines_sum.pdf. Accessed February 2, 2019.

U.S. Preventive Services Task Force, et al. Screening for obesity in children and adolescents: US Preventive Services Task Force Recommendation Statement. *JAMA*. 2017;317(23):2417–2426.

Wright H, Lenchik K, Santiago S. Diagnostic accuracy of various imaging modalities for suspected lower extremity stress fractures: a systematic review with evidence-based recommendations for clinical practice. *Am J Sports Med*. 2016;44(1):255.

Yan J, et al. The association between breastfeeding and childhood obesity: a meta-analysis. *BMC Public Health*. 2014;14:1267.

Yau PL, et al. Obesity and metabolic syndrome and functional and structural brain impairments in adolescence. *Pediatrics*. 2012;130(4):1–9.

Obstetrics and Women's Health

15

Meghan Connett and Brigit E. Ray

▶ CASE 15.1

A 24-year-old nulligravida female presents for her annual examination. Her gynecologic history is remarkable for irregular menses, menstruating every 4 to 8 weeks. She would like a more reliable form of contraception (currently using condoms) and would like to have predictable menses, but is very concerned regarding weight gain with various contraceptive methods.

Question 15.1.1 How would you counsel her regarding weight changes and contraception?
A) Studies show there is no significant difference in weight gain of women initiating oral contraceptive pills (OCPs) versus placebo
B) Weight gain of 10 lb is expected during the first year of use with any type of OCPs
C) Weight gain of 10 lb is expected during the first year of use with monophasic pills but not with triphasic formulations
D) Weight loss of 10 lb is expected during the first year of use with Depo-Provera (medroxyprogesterone acetate)

Answer 15.1.1 The correct answer is "A." Studies have shown no significant weight gain with OCP use when compared with placebo. Trials have been conducted evaluating estrogen components of 20 to 50 µg, both monophasic and triphasic. There is no evidence to support the premise that triphasic formulations offer improvement in weight changes. Depo-Provera has variable effects on weight gain. Several studies have shown a weight gain of 3 to 6 kg in the first year of Depo-Provera use; however, other studies have shown no difference in weight gain between Depo-Provera and placebo.

HELPFUL TIP:
Recall that in 2004 the FDA placed a "black box warning" on Depo-Provera for bone loss that "may not be reversible." However, subsequent studies showed bone gain after stopping Depo-Provera. ACOG notes in 2014 that Depo-provera can be used for more than 2 years if benefits outweigh the risks and bone mineral density will rebound when it is stopped. However, they also note that no high quality data exists about fracture risk later in life (Obstet Gynecol. 2014;123:1398-402)

Question 15.1.2 After reassuring her regarding the concerns of weight gain, you tell her about the additional potential benefit(s) of OCPs, which include:
A) Improvement in acne
B) Decreased dysmenorrhea
C) Decreased menstrual flow
D) Decreased risk of ovarian cancer
E) All of the above

Answer 15.1.2 The correct answer is "E." Besides these, additional potential benefits of OCP use include regulation and predictability of menses, decreased anemia, decreased hirsutism, and decreased risk of endometrial and colon cancers. *Note*: the cancer risk reduction is based on epidemiologic studies, not randomized controlled trials. A recently published Danish national registry study did find an increased risk of breast cancer with OCP use, even with lowest dose estrogen use. However, the magnitude of this risk remained small (*N Engl J Med*. 2017;377(23):2228–2239).

HELPFUL TIP:
After starting OCPs, patients should follow up within a few months for blood pressure checks, assuring compliance, etc. With pap smear guidelines having changed to every 3-to 5-year screening intervals for most women, the annual "pap" to get birth control no longer makes sense.

After further discussion, she reports that she has headaches every 1 to 2 months. She has never been evaluated for migraines, but reports that her headaches are bilateral, posterior, throbbing, and relieved with sleep and over-the-counter medication. She denies associated aura, nausea, or focal neurologic changes.

Question 15.1.3 How would you counsel her regarding OCPs and headaches?

A) Headaches are an uncommon reason for discontinuation of OCPs

B) She should not use OCPs because they are contraindicated in anyone with headaches

C) She should use progestin-only pills

D) She can use OCPs, as it is hard to predict whether her headaches will be affected

Answer 15.1.3 **The correct answer is "D."** Although headache is a frequently cited reason for women to discontinue OCPs, there is no strong correlation between headache frequency and intensity for most women. There is no evidence that the type of progestin or amount of estrogen will alter the headaches, except in women with menstrual migraines. Among women with migraines, headaches improve, worsen, or are unchanged after initiation of OCPs (helpful, right?). **There is an increased risk of stroke in women with a history of pseudotumor cerebri or migraines with aura or focal neurologic changes.** Therefore, OCPs are CONTRAINDICATED in these specific subgroups of women.

HELPFUL TIP:
Additional contraindications to combination OCP use include: any previous thromboembolic event or stroke, a history of estrogen-dependent tumor (e.g., some breast cancers), active liver disease, pregnancy (although accidental use of OCPs early in pregnancy has not been definitively linked to adverse outcomes), undiagnosed abnormal uterine bleeding, women older than 35 years who smoke (due to increased risk of cardiovascular disease), and **first 3 weeks postpartum** (2015 World Health Organization recommendation based on increased venous thromboembolism risk in the immediate postpartum period). See Figure 15-1 for quick reference guidance on contraceptive eligibility based on medical condition.

The patient wants to know how long she should use a backup method of contraception after starting the combination estrogen/progesterone OCP.

Question 15.1.4 You tell her the following regarding using a backup method:

A) If she starts taking the pill during the first 5 days of her menstrual period, no backup method is needed

B) If she starts taking the pill greater than 5 days after her the onset of her period, she needs a backup method for 30 days

C) She should use a backup method for 2 months after starting the pill regardless of when she started it

D) The OCP provides effective contraception immediately and no backup method is needed

Answer 15.1.4 **The correct answer is "A."** The old canard of requiring a month of backup contraception after starting OCPs or other hormonal birth control has fallen by the wayside. For combination estrogen/progesterone OCPs, for example, **no** secondary method of contraception is needed as long as the OCP is started within 7 days of the onset of the last menses. If the OCP is started greater than 5 days after the onset of the last menses, only 7 days of a secondary contraception method (e.g., condoms, diaphragm) is needed; combination OCPs work within 7 days of the start date. Please see Table 15-1 regarding CDC recommendations for backup contraception.

HELPFUL TIP:
Rifampin, rifaximin, and rifabutin are the only antibiotics that reduce the effectiveness of OCPs. Therefore, there is no need for a backup method when giving penicillin for strep throat, for example.

HELPFUL TIP:
The thinking about methods of contraception has changed in the last several years. The intrauterine device (IUD) is becoming increasingly popular for nulliparous teenagers. IUDs clearly decrease pregnancy in this group when compared to OCPs and do not seem to increase the risk of STDs (*N Engl J Med*. 2014;371:1316–1323). Nor do they result in increased risky sexual activity.

The American Academy of Pediatrics (2014) recommends that a long-acting reversible contraceptive (LARC) be considered as a first-line contraceptive in adolescents; options include implants and IUDs. LARCs can provide 3 to 10 years of contraception and are effective and safe forms of birth control. The use of condoms goes down with LARCs, however (*JAMA Pediatr*. 2016;170(5):428–434).

Eight months later, the patient calls to speak with your nurse regarding nausea and vomiting. Apparently, she decided to stop taking her OCP. Her last menstrual period was 10 weeks earlier, and she had a positive home pregnancy test 5 weeks ago. Over the last week, she has been vomiting once every day, at various times, but is nauseated throughout most of the day. She wants to know if there is anything else that is "safe" that she can do to decrease the nausea.

Question 15.1.5 What is your most appropriate response?

A) "This level of nausea and vomiting is abnormal and needs an immediate workup to rule out other pathology"

B) "This level of nausea and vomiting is very common, and there are several modifications and over-the-counter medications that are safe"

C) "This level of nausea and vomiting is very common; however, there are no medications that can be initiated in the first trimester"

D) "This level of nausea and vomiting is very common. Metoclopramide, promethazine, and ondansetron are our first-line therapies"

E) "Deal with it. You got yourself into this mess"

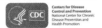

FIGURE 15-1 WHO medical eligibility criteria for contraceptive use. (Available from fhi360 at: https://www.fhi360.org/sites/default/files/media/documents/resource-chart-medical-eligibility-contraceptives-english.pdf.)

TABLE 15-1 BACKUP CONTRACEPTION WHEN INITIATING METHODS

Contraceptive Method	Backup Method: Initiation[a]
Copper-containing IUD (Paraguard)	None needed
Levonorgestrel-containing IUD	7 days; only needed if >7 days after starting menses
Implant	7 days; only needed if >5 days after starting menses
Injectable	7 days; only needed if >7 days after starting menses
Combined hormonal contraceptives	7 days; only needed if >5 days after starting menses
Progestin-only pill	2 days; only needed if >5 days after starting menses (per CDC reference below)

Note: Barrier methods or abstinence from intercourse may be used during the recommended backup interval.

[a]Any method may be initiated at any time if there is reasonable certainty the woman is not pregnant, based on the criteria of the Centers for Disease Control and Prevention.

Adapted from Klein DA, Arnold JJ, Reese ES. Provision of contraception: key recommendations from the CDC. *Am Fam Physician.* 2015;91(9):625–633 and Division of Reproductive Health, National Center for Chronic Disease Prevention and Health Promotion, Centers for Disease Control and Prevention (CDC). U.S. Selected Practice Recommendations for Contraceptive Use, 2013: adapted from the World Health Organization selected practice recommendations for contraceptive use, 2nd edition. *MMWR Recomm Rep.* 2013;62(RR-05):1–60.

Answer 15.1.5 The correct answer is "B." Mild-to-moderate nausea and vomiting are very common in the first trimester of pregnancy, often improving by 16 weeks of gestation. Several modifications can improve symptoms, including small, frequent meals, avoiding fatty foods, and avoiding environmental triggers (perfumes, smoking, position changes, or certain movements). Over-the-counter remedies include ginger root or ginger ale, vitamin B6 (10–25 mg three to four times daily) and doxylamine (10–12.5 mg three to four times daily). Vitamin B6 and doxylamine may be used separately or in combination. For those who do not respond, antiemetics including metoclopramide or promethazine should be considered (thus, "D" represents a next step, not a first step). Ondansetron would be third line due to slightly greater potential risk to the fetus. Up to 2% of the time, nausea and vomiting represent hyperemesis gravidarum, which involves weight loss of more than 5% of prepregnancy weight or dehydration and ketonuria.

HELPFUL TIP:
Diclegis (doxylamine succinate and pyridoxine hydrochloride) is now an FDA-approved medication for nausea and vomiting during pregnancy. Patients should take two tablets at bedtime as a starting dose and may increase to one in the morning, one in the mid-afternoon, and two

at nighttime, if needed. However, it is way expensive and has no advantage over the combination of OTC doxylamine and pyridoxine.

Question 15.1.6 If the patient had instead presented with six to eight episodes of emesis daily, an 8-lb weight loss since her last menses, and a urine specific gravity of >1.030 and ketonuria, your workup should have included:
A) Quantitative β-human chorionic gonadotropin (β-hCG)
B) Serum electrolytes, BUN, and creatinine
C) Thyroid-stimulating hormone (TSH)
D) Pelvic ultrasound
E) All of the above

Answer 15.1.6 The correct answer is "E." As with any other severely nauseated and vomiting patient, it is reasonable to check for electrolyte imbalances. Severity of nausea and vomiting correlates with higher levels of hCG, as would be seen with a molar or twin pregnancy. Gestational trophoblastic disease, although rare, should be evaluated for with an hCG level. The ultrasound would confirm a twin pregnancy and could provide evidence of a molar pregnancy. TSH can exclude hyperthyroidism.

Fortunately, your patient's symptoms improve with dietary changes, vitamin B6, and doxylamine. She presents for her initial prenatal visit at 12 weeks of gestation.

Question 15.1.7 You offer her the routine prenatal tests at this visit, which include all of the following EXCEPT:
A) Syphilis testing
B) HIV testing
C) 1-hour glucose tolerance test
D) Blood type and antibody screen
E) Fetal nuchal translucency with maternal hCG and plasma-associated pregnancy protein A (PAPP-A)

Answer 15.1.7 The correct answer is "C." Diabetes screening with a 1-hour glucose tolerance test (50-g carbohydrate load with blood glucose obtained at 1 hour) is typically performed between 24 and 28 weeks of gestation. Patients with risk factors for gestational diabetes, which our patient doesn't have, are candidates for earlier screening, even at the first prenatal visit. Risk factors include history of previous pregnancy with gestational diabetes, polycystic ovarian syndrome (PCOS), history of macrosomia, high pre-pregnancy BMI, first-degree relative with diabetes mellitus type 2, and certain ethnic groups such as East Asians, Hispanics, and Pacific Islanders. Syphilis and HIV testing ("A" and "B") are done to decrease the risk of perinatal transmission. The blood type and antibody screen ("D") are used to identify mothers with blood antibodies that could cause hemolytic disease of the fetus. Mothers who are Rh negative will subsequently receive RhoGAM at 28 weeks as well. Two maternal serum markers, hCG and pregnancy-associated plasma protein (PAPP-A, an early screen for Down syndrome), and one fetal marker (nuchal thickness) should be used between 11 and 14 weeks to evaluate for Down syndrome ("E"). This method offers a Down syndrome detection rate of approximately 85% with a 5% false-positive rate.

HELPFUL TIP:
Nuchal translucency looks at fluid collections in the posterior fetal neck. Increased translucency suggests increased fluid collection and is associated with abnormalities such as Down syndrome, Turner syndrome, and hemodynamic problems (cardiac abnormalities).

HELPFUL (AND IMPORTANT) TIP:
Since it does not screen for neural tube defects, first-trimester screening does not negate the need for a second-trimester maternal serum triple or quad screen. The triple screen, which screens for chromosomal abnormalities (e.g., Trisomy 21) and neural tube defects, includes levels for AFP (α-fetoprotein), HCG, and uE3 (unconjugated estriol). The quadruple screen adds an inhibin A. The triple or quadruple screen is done between 15 weeks 0 days and 19 weeks 6 days of gestation. The triple screen has a 70% sensitivity for neural tube defects and Down syndrome with a 5% false-positive rate. The quadruple screen has an 81% sensitivity and a 5% false-positive rate. See ACOG's patient chart for types of genetic testing and when to test (Fig. 15-2).

The patient has passed all of her screening tests with flying colors, and she returns at 36 weeks of gestation.

Question 15.1.8 What additional screening test(s) is/are obtained near 36 weeks of gestation?
A) Amniocentesis
B) 3-hour glucose tolerance test
C) Fetal fibronectin (FFN)
D) Group B streptococcus (GBS) culture or PCR
E) All of the above

Answer 15.1.8 The correct answer is "D." There have been several updates on how to reduce the transmission of GBS to newborns. Newer (2019) recommendations from ACOG and the AAP recommend to start screening for GBS now at 36 weeks and no longer at 35 weeks. The test results are valid for up to 5 weeks which would last through 41 weeks of gestation. Give prophylactic antibiotics of IV penicillin G every 4 hours from active labor until delivery in women who screen positive for GBS, have a prior history of a neonate with GBS infection (regardless of testing results....just treat them) or have GBS status unknown with risk factors (pre-term labor, premature rupture of membranes/ prolonged rupture of membranes> 18 hours, fever of >38C or GBS positive status in prior pregnancy).

Rapid GBS testing, should only be done on those who present in labor with an unknown GBS status and no risk factors; there are a lot of false negatives. As noted above, those with risk factors get treated anyway. For patients with a penicillin allergy, a beta-lactam such as cefazolin is preferred for those with low risk of anaphylaxis. Clindamycin and vancomycin are options in patients with a severe penicillin allergy. Vancomycin is now preferred as there has been growing resistance to clindamycin. Use clindamycin only if GBS cultures show susceptibility and no indication of inducible resistance on testing. We recommend to work closely with your pharmacist colleagues to order the proper vancomycin dosing. (Obstet Gynecol. 2019 Jul: 134(1):e19-e40 and Pediatrics. 2019 Aug; 144(2):e20191881)

▶ **Objectives: Did you learn to …**
- Describe contraception options?
- Provide appropriate routine prenatal care?
- Recognize nausea and vomiting of pregnancy and describe its appropriate management?

▶ **CASE 15.2**

You are taking obstetric calls for your group over Labor Day (Get it? Bad joke?) weekend. Labor and delivery calls you about a 27-year-old G1P0 at 38 weeks of gestation who awoke this morning complaining of wetness. However, when she went to the bathroom, she discovered significant vaginal bleeding that had soaked her bed. She denies any cramping or abdominal pain. She is on her way to the hospital—and so are you.

Question 15.2.1 You tell the nurses to call you with her vital signs and to initiate all of the following interventions immediately upon the patient's arrival EXCEPT:
A) Obtain IV access
B) Draw blood for type and screen
C) Perform a digital vaginal examination
D) Initiate fetal monitoring
E) Draw blood for complete blood count

Answer 15.2.1 The correct answer is "C." A small-to-moderate amount of bleeding is not unexpected during labor; however, the profuse bleeding described by the patient is an obstetrical emergency. The first priorities are to obtain IV access ("A") and ensure that the mother is hemodynamically stable. Baseline laboratory evaluation ("E") will give some indication of the amount of blood loss and establish that blood is available for transfusion if necessary ("B"). Monitoring of the fetal heart rate (FHR) will evaluate fetal status ("D"). Also, an ultrasound should be done to evaluate for placenta previa. *A digital vaginal examination should NOT be performed until the diagnosis of placenta previa has been excluded.* A consultation with someone skilled in cesarean section should be obtained if the initial evaluation suggests that immediate fetal delivery is necessary.

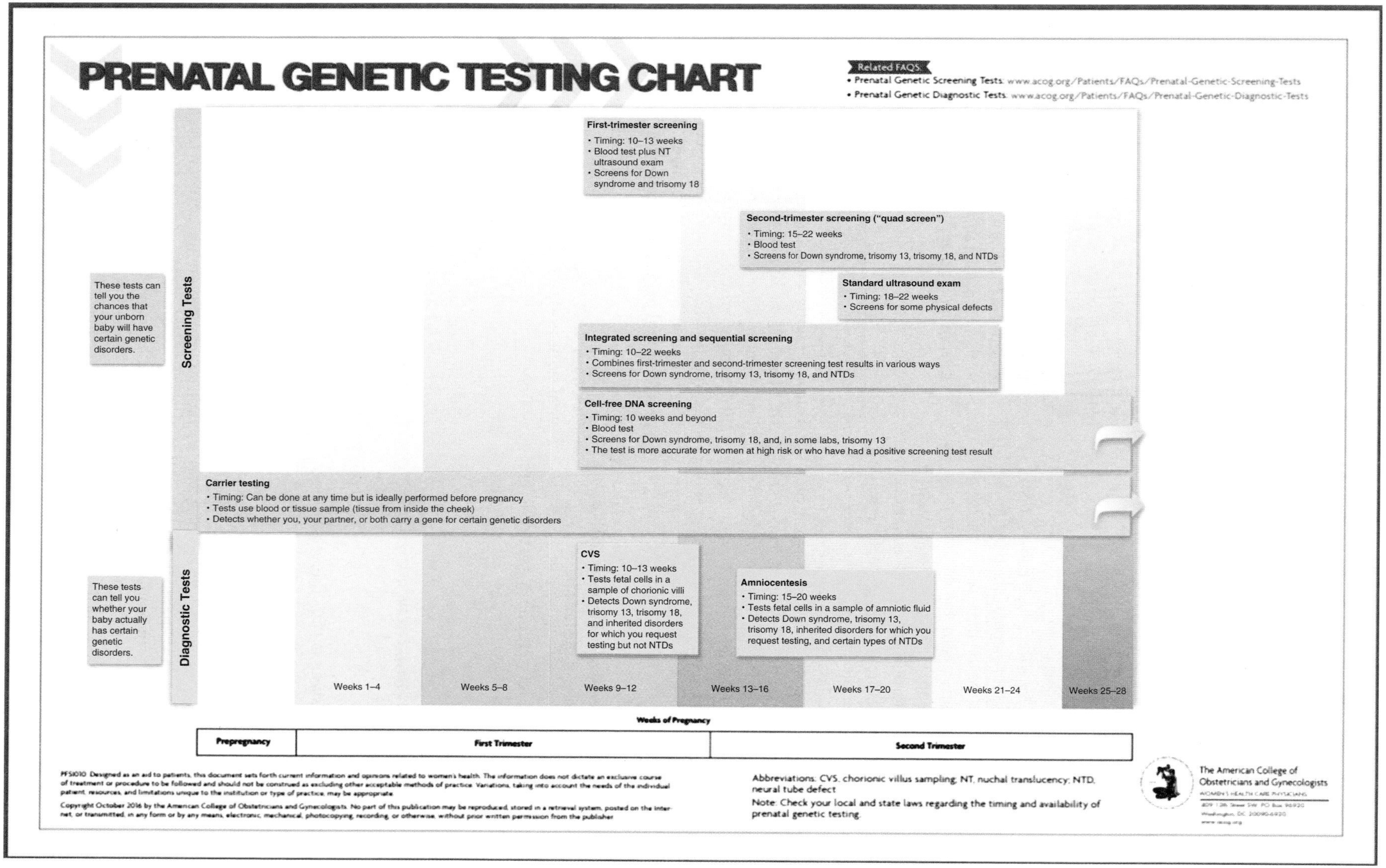

FIGURE 15-2 Prenatal genetic screening. Reprinted with permission from American College of Obstetricians and Gynecologists. Prenatal genetic testing chart (infographic). Washington, DC; American College of Obstetricians and Gynecologists; 2016. Available here: https://www.acog.org/Patients/FAQs/Prenatal-Genetic-Testing-Chart-Infographic. Retrieved September 11, 2019.

HELPFUL TIP:
Classically, placenta previa presents as *painless* third-trimester bleeding, whereas placental abruption classically presents as *painful* third-trimester bleeding. Note that these are the "classic" presentations, not pathognomonic.

When the patient arrives at the hospital, she alters her recollection of events (never happens in our practice) to say that the fluid soaking the bed sheets was blood-tinged and pink in color and first occurred 2 hours ago. She continues to have vaginal leakage but denies any bright red bleeding or contractions. Ultrasound reveals a fundal placenta (not a placenta previa) without any evidence of abruption. Fetal heart tones are in the 140s and reactive. Sterile speculum examination reveals fluid, which is nitrazine and ferning positive (both evidence of ruptured membranes). Her GBS culture performed 2 weeks ago is negative. She is still not feeling contractions, and there are no contractions on the monitor.

Question 15.2.2 What is the most appropriate next step in the management of this patient?
A) Begin an induction of labor
B) Send her home after 4 hours of reassuring fetal monitoring
C) Treat her with IV penicillin for GBS prophylaxis
D) Repeat her GBS test to confirm GBS status

Answer 15.2.2 The correct answer is "A." A patient should not be sent home after rupture of membranes. She is at risk for intrauterine infection, and induction is indicated to reduce the risk of infection at term. Induction of labor, even with an unfavorable cervix, is not associated with an increase in cesarean or operative vaginal delivery, but it is associated with fewer maternal infections (chorioamnionitis), shortened time from rupture of membranes to birth, and fewer neonatal intensive care unit admissions. "C" and "D" are incorrect. Her GBS status was negative 2 weeks ago. Although GBS colonization can be transient, since the test was collected after 35 weeks it should be reliable. Even if her membranes were ruptured for more than 18 hours, she would not require treatment with antibiotics unless she developed a fever (remember she is GBS negative … review the criteria in answer 15.1.8). *If a fever develops, think chorioamnionitis when choosing antibiotic therapy.*

Sterile vaginal examination reveals a cervix that is 3 cm dilated, 2 cm long (effacement), soft, anterior, and vertex at a −1 station. The patient agrees to an induction of labor.

Question 15.2.3 The best induction method for this patient is to:
A) Insert intracervical laminaria
B) Begin IV oxytocin at 2 milliunits per minute
C) Insert intravaginal dinoprostone (Prepidil, Cervidil)
D) Have her partner sit on her abdomen
E) Have her run a few laps around L&D (or walk around the hospital)

Answer 15.2.3 The correct answer is "B." The use of intravaginal and intracervical methods for cervical ripening could be cautiously considered in patients with premature rupture of membranes with an *unfavorable* cervix; but "C" is not the best choice—she is already 3 cm dilated with a Bishop score of 6! Drugs for cervical ripening may include prostaglandins which act in the cervix to facilitate smooth muscle relaxation resulting in softening and dilatation of the cervix. They also may induce myometrial contraction. Currently, the only prostaglandin labeled by the Food and Drug Administration (FDA) for such purpose is the prostaglandin E2 agents such as dinoprostone (Prepidil, Cervidil). Prostaglandin E1 agents such as misoprostol (Cytotec) inserted intravaginally are also commonly used for cervical ripening but *do not carry a label by the FDA for this indication.* Intracervical use of laminaria (an expanding pledget placed in the cervix, such as "A") is generally reserved for pregnancy termination. "D" would not be comfortable and may cause undue harm to mom and the fetus—and it's kind of weird. "E" is not the best choice. While walking may stimulate contractions (as can "stripping" the membranes if they are intact), she already has ruptured membranes and a more aggressive approach is warranted.

Oxytocin should be carefully titrated via IV route for labor induction or augmentation. The general starting doses are 0.5 to 2 milliunits per minute, increased by 1 to 2 milliunits every 20 to 40 minutes, to a maximum dose rarely exceeding 30 to 40 milliunits per minute.

The patient is currently in labor (success!), and now her cervical examination is 6 cm dilation, 1 cm effaced, and −1 station. The amniotic fluid is still clear, having ruptured approximately 22 hours ago. She has had an epidural placed for analgesia. The FHR baseline has increased to 165 beats per minute with minimal variability. Contractions occur every 3 minutes. Maternal temperature is now 38.6°C, and her pulse is 110 bpm. The patient denies any complaints.

Question 15.2.4 Given the history of prolonged rupture of membranes and fever, which of the following is the most likely diagnosis?
A) Normal labor
B) Epidural fever
C) Nosocomial infection
D) Chorioamnionitis

Answer 15.2.4 The correct answer is "D." Chorioamnionitis is the most likely diagnosis and the diagnosis of most concern given the prolonged rupture of membranes (we gave you this answer above—you got that, right?). Treatment should be initiated immediately. "A" is incorrect as fever is not a normal part of labor. "B" is possible, but not as likely and a dangerous assumption. There is an association between the use of epidural analgesia and a rise in maternal temperature. Etiologies proposed for this temperature increase include lack of pain-induced hyperventilation and decreased perspiration due to sympathetic blockade. "C" is extremely unlikely given her brief time in the hospital.

Question 15.2.5 What is the next step in the care of this patient?
A) Increase the oxytocin to hasten delivery
B) Remove the epidural
C) Initiate broad-spectrum antibiotics
D) Call your backup for cesarean section (or do it yourself)
E) Give acetaminophen 1,000 mg orally

Answer 15.2.5 The correct answer is "C." Initiation of antibiotics is associated with a decrease in both maternal and neonatal morbidity. Multiple organisms are isolated in more than 66% of cases; therefore, antibiotics should be broad. Approved regimens include ampicillin and gentamicin, ticarcillin/clavulanate, or piperacillin/tazobactam. If the patient is penicillin allergic, cefazolin and gentamicin may be used for mild penicillin allergy. For those with severe penicillin allergy, clindamycin OR vancomycin with gentamicin is recommended. There is no need to increase the oxytocin ("A"); she has already made good labor progress. There is also no need to proceed with a cesarean delivery ("D") unless there is another indication, such as non-reassuring FHR pattern. Although epidural anesthesia is associated with increased maternal temperature, it should only be removed if it is felt to be contributing to maternal pathology (e.g., meningitis, epidural abscess, or epidural bleed). Acetaminophen ("E") is fine, but it should not be used in lieu of antibiotics.

The patient's labor is progressing. Her cervix is 9 cm dilated, completely effaced, and station is +3. Her temperature is 39°C. The FHR pattern is shown in Figure 15-3.

Question 15.2.6 What is the FHR interpretation?
A) Baseline 165 beats per minute, reactive
B) Baseline 165 beats per minute, with periods of bradycardia
C) Baseline 165 beats per minute, with late decelerations
D) Baseline 165 beats per minute, with variable decelerations

Answer 15.2.6 The correct answer is "C." The FHR pictured is described as Category II (see Table 15-2) with a baseline of about 165 beats per minute. There is moderate variability present. Following each contraction, there are late decelerations to the 110s. "A" is incorrect since "reactive" refers to a nonstress test, not fetal monitoring during labor (see Helpful Tip below for more). "B" is incorrect as fetal bradycardia is defined as an FHR of less than 110 beats per minute for at least 10 minutes. "D" is incorrect. Variable decelerations vary with respect to timing, duration, and depth.

HELPFUL TIP:
Nonstress tests are performed outside of the intrapartum period. A reactive nonstress test is defined as two accelerations of at least 15 beats above baseline and lasting at least 15 seconds within a 20-minute interval in gestations **greater than 32 completed weeks**. In gestations less than 32 weeks, reactive is defined as two accelerations at least 10 beats above baseline and lasting at least 10 seconds.

Question 15.2.7 What is the likely etiology of the fetal heart rate (FHR) tracing in Figure 15-3?
A) Head compression
B) Placental insufficiency
C) Cord compression
D) Any of the above is equally likely to cause the tracing

Answer 15.2.7 The correct answer is "B." Late decelerations are believed to be secondary to transient fetal hypoxia in response to decreased placental perfusion. Prompt evaluation and intervention is warranted. Early decelerations are generally reassuring and attributed to fetal head compression. Variable decelerations are the most common decelerations seen in labor and indicate cord compression. Variable decelerations can sometimes be relieved by maternal repositioning or amnioinfusion (infusing saline or Ringers Lactate to "re-expand" the uterus and relieve the pressure on the cord).

Question 15.2.8 What is the LEAST appropriate course of action now?
A) Administer maternal oxygen
B) Stop oxytocin
C) Forceps or vacuum-assisted vaginal delivery
D) Consider cesarean delivery
E) Reposition mother (roll to one side or knee–chest)

Answer 15.2.8 The correct answer is "C." Increasing maternal oxygenation ("A") may improve fetal oxygenation. Oxytocin can decrease placental blood flow via uterine stimulation, and hence should be decreased or stopped if non-reassuring FHR changes are present ("B"). If there is evidence of maternal hypotension, maternal hydration may be indicated. Another option is position changes (left lateral) to improve placental perfusion ("E"). Maternal position can affect uterine blood flow and placental perfusion. The gravid uterus may compress the vena cava while supine. Because the patient is 9 cm dilated, forceps or vacuum-assisted vaginal delivery ("C," also known as operative vaginal delivery) is NOT indicated; dilation needs to be complete (10 cm) in order to use forceps or vacuum. Cesarean delivery ("D") should be anticipated if the above interventions do not improve the fetal heart tracing.

The FHR changes resolve with your appropriate interventions. The patient progresses to complete dilation and delivers vaginally 1 hour later. Maternal antibiotics are discontinued following delivery, and the maternal temperature 2 hours after delivery is 37°C. On postpartum day 1, your patient complains of sore breasts from breastfeeding but no particular swelling of the breast (beyond what is expected postpartum), and her abdomen is sore "all over." She is having a moderate amount of lochia, and her temperature is 38.4°C.

Question 15.2.9 The most likely cause of the fever at this time is:
A) Endometritis
B) Mastitis
C) Deep vein thrombosis
D) Septic pelvic thrombophlebitis

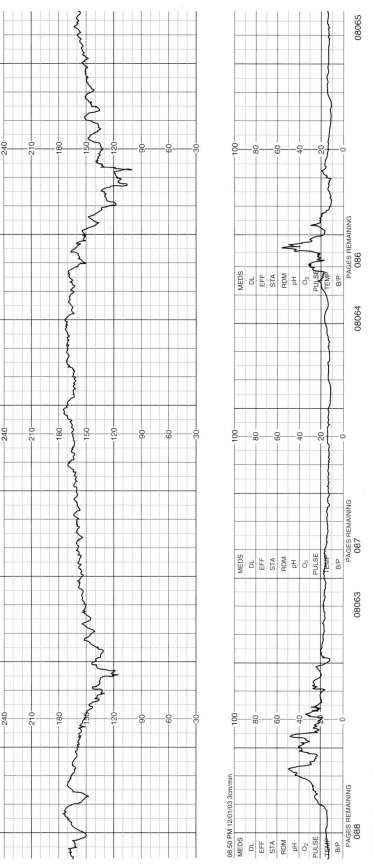

FIGURE 15-3 Fetal Monitoring Tracings.

TABLE 15-2 FETAL HEART TRACING CATEGORY DEFINITIONS

Category I Tracing (normal): FHR include ALL of the following:
- Baseline FHR within normal range at 110–160 bpm
- Moderate baseline FHR variability
- Absent late or variable decelerations
- Accelerations may be present or absent

CATEGORY II Tracing: Includes all FHR tracings that are not categorized as Category I or Category III. May represent an appreciable part of those encountered in clinical practice (atypical … may represent fetal hypoxia). Any of the following:
- Bradycardia with FHR <110 bpm **WITH** variability
- Fetal tachycardia with FHR >160 bpm
- Minimal baseline variability or absent baseline variability WITHOUT recurrent decelerations, or marked baseline variability
- Absence of induced accelerations after fetal stimulation
- Recurrent variable decelerations accompanied by minimal to moderate baseline variability
- Prolonged deceleration >2 minutes but <10 minutes
- Recurrent late decelerations with moderate baseline variability
- Variable decelerations with other characteristics such as slow return to baseline, "overshoots," or "shoulders"

CATEGORY III Tracing (abnormal):
EITHER
- Absent baseline FHR variability AND any of the following:
  - Recurrent late decelerations
  - Recurrent variable decelerations
  - Fetal bradycardia
OR
- A sinusoidal pattern

Adapted from American College of Obstetricians and Gynecologists. ACOG Practice Bulletin no. 106: Intrapartum fetal heart rate monitoring, nomenclature, interpretation and general management principles. *Obstet Gynecol.* 2009;114(1):192–202.

Answer 15.2.9 The correct answer is "A." Whenever fever occurs in the immediate postpartum period, endometritis should be suspected. The presence of intra-amniotic infection (chorioamnionitis) increases the risk of postpartum endometritis to 13% (or 1 in 8 women, if you prefer fractions). Antibiotics are not routinely continued for chorioamnionitis after a vaginal delivery because the "source" of the infection (the placenta) has been removed. Mastitis ("B") is characterized by a swollen, firm, tender breast with systemic symptoms including fevers, chills, and flu-like symptoms. However, it was stipulated that the breasts were normal for our postpartum patient, making mastitis unlikely (and bilateral mastitis is very unlikely, anyway). *Staphylococcus aureus* is the typical pathogen in mastitis. Pregnancy and the postpartum period increase a woman's risk of thrombogenesis. In fact, this persists up to 12 weeks postpartum. However, DVT ("C") is not a likely source of the fever. Septic pelvic thrombophlebitis ("D") is a diagnosis of exclusion and is usually entertained when fever spikes continue despite treatment for endometritis.

You start appropriate antibiotics and the patient does well. The family, in gratitude, names the child after you (adding the suffix "-tops" to the child's name, like "Triceratops") and makes you the godparent necessitating gifts for the next 18 years on the child's birthday.

HELPFUL TIP:
Infants born to women with chorioamnionitis have a fourfold increase in neonatal mortality and a threefold increase in the incidence of respiratory distress, neonatal sepsis, and intraventricular hemorrhage.

▶ **Objectives: Did you learn to …**
- Triage and manage third-trimester bleeding?
- Recognize and treat a patient with premature rupture of membranes?
- Evaluate and manage intrapartum fever?
- Interpret FHR patterns and begin initial management of abnormal patterns?
- Appreciate the risk factors, evaluation, and management of postpartum infection?

▶ CASE 15.3

You are seeing a 31-year-old G2P1 at 41 weeks of gestation by definite last menstrual period and 16-week ultrasound. She continues to note fetal movement and her examination is normal: BP 120/68 mm Hg, urine dipstick negative for protein and glucose, fundal height 42 cm, fetus is vertex, FHR 156 bpm. Her cervix is soft, anterior, 2 to 3 cm dilated, 50% effaced, and +1 station. She was induced with her first pregnancy, and this time she wants to have a "natural labor." You decide to calculate a Bishop score.

Question 15.3.1 The Bishop score helps to determine:
A) The health of the fetus
B) The need for cervical ripening agents for induction and helps to predict labor induction success
C) The maturity of the fetal lungs
D) The risk of fetal demise in the post-term fetus
E) The results of a Catholic intramural baseball game

Answer 15.3.1 The correct answer is "B." The Bishop score, which takes into account cervical dilation, effacement, consistency, and position, as well as fetal station, is a useful tool to determine if cervical ripening agents are needed for induction and to predict induction success. Calculators are readily available online.

....

The patient's Bishop score is favorable at 9–10.

Question 15.3.2 Which of the following is the most appropriate recommendations at this point?
A) She should be induced at once; there is a high chance of fetal mortality after 41 weeks of gestation
B) Since her antepartum course has been uncomplicated to date, it is safe for her to await spontaneous labor until 43 weeks of gestation
C) She should undergo a nonstress test and ultrasound for amniotic fluid index
D) She should plan for a cesarean section

TABLE 15-3 GUIDELINES FOR DATING BASED ON ULTRASONOGRAPHY

Gestational Age Range based on LMP	Method of Measurement	Discrepancy between Ultrasound Dating and LMP Dating that Supports Re-dating
≤13 6/7 weeks • ≤8 6/7 weeks • 9 0/7 weeks to 13 6/7 weeks	CRL	• More than 5 days • More than 7 days
14 0/7 weeks to 15 6/7 weeks	BPD, HC, AC, FL	More than 7 days
16 0/7 weeks to 21 6/7 weeks	BPD, HC, AC, FL	More than 10 days
22 0/7 weeks to 27 6/7 weeks	BPD, HC, AC, FL	More than 14 days
28 0/7 weeks and beyond[a]	BPD, HC, AC, FL	More than 21 days

AC, abdominal circumference; BPD, biparietal diameter; CRL, crown rump length; FL, femur length; HC, head circumference; LMP, last menstrual period.

[a]Because the risk of re-dating a small fetus that may be growth-restricted, third-trimester re-dating should be guided by careful consideration of the entire clinical picture and close surveillance.

Adapted from American College of Obstetricians and Gynecologists. Method for estimating due date. Committee Opinion No. 611. *Obstet Gynecol.* 2014;124:863–866.

Answer 15.3.2 **The correct answer is "C."** By definition, a term gestation is one completed in 38 to 42 weeks. There is no significant increase in fetal mortality in an uncomplicated pregnancy at term. Virtually all reports suggest an increase in perinatal morbidity and mortality when pregnancy goes beyond 42 weeks of gestation. Antenatal surveillance of post-term pregnancies should be initiated at 41 weeks of gestation.

HELPFUL TIP:
Accurate determination of date of conception is important in reducing the false diagnosis of post-term pregnancy. The estimated date of delivery is most reliably and accurately determined early in pregnancy. Ultrasound may assist in determining dates but has a standard of error that is dependent on the gestational age (see Table 15-3).

Question 15.3.3 **At 41 weeks she is really (really, really) tired of being pregnant and wants "a natural way" to induce contractions. Which of the following nonpharmacologic methods of inducing or augmenting labor is LEAST likely to be effective?**
A) Stripping the amniotic membranes
B) Prolonged walking
C) Amniotomy
D) Nipple stimulation

Answer 15.3.3 **The correct answer is "B."** Stripping membranes ("A") appears to be effective in initiating spontaneous labor within 72 hours. Amniotomy ("C") may be used for labor induction, especially if the Bishop score is favorable. However, a Cochrane review from 2013 did not find strong evidence supporting the use of amniotomy alone and it is not additive to oxytocin for induction. Nipple stimulation ("D") causes release

of oxytocin and may be utilized for labor induction, but its marginal benefit is only seen in patients with a favorable Bishop score. Walking ("B") does not result in labor induction or augmentation, but it's not harmful either.

HELPFUL TIP:
Sexual intercourse is sometimes recommended to induce labor. Studies are of low quality and use various endpoints ... also, it is difficult to standardize the intervention (a lesser editorial team might insert a joke here—but not us). One of the better quality studies (*Obstet Gynecol.* 2006;108(1):134–140) did find that coitus was associated with reduced need for labor induction at 41 weeks.

Question 15.3.4 **If induction becomes necessary, which of the following pharmacologic interventions would be the best approach to your patient who has a cervix that is soft, anterior, 2 to 3 cm dilated, 50% effaced, and +1 station?**
A) IV oxytocin
B) Intracervical PGE2 (dinoprostone, Prepidil)
C) Intravaginal PGE2 (dinoprostone, Cervidil)
D) Intravaginal PGE1 (misoprostol, Cytotec)
E) None of the above. All pharmacologic interventions are contraindicated

Answer 15.3.4 **The correct answer is "A."** This patient does not need further cervical ripening but is a candidate for induction of labor. If cervical ripening were needed, there are several available agents. Option "D," PGE1 (misoprostol, brand name Cytotec) can be administered intravaginally or orally (but note that the Food and Drug Administration [FDA] has not approved it for use in pregnancy). As to "B" and "C", PGE2 (dinoprostone, brand name Cervidil) is administered intravaginally. PGE2 gel (dinoprostone, brand name Prepidil) can be administered either intravaginally or intracervically. Because the cervix is favorable in this case, proceeding with oxytocin is the best option.

....

Your patient's husband is called up for active duty in Iraq (or Afghanistan … or Libya or … sadly, we are on the 5th edition of this book and have not needed to change this scenario) and is due to report in the next few days. She is now 41 2/7 weeks of gestation and desires induction so he can be with her for the delivery. You admit her to labor and delivery the following morning. The initial FHR monitoring before induction (also known as a nonstress test) is shown in Figure 15-4.

Question 15.3.5 What is the correct interpretation?
A) Baseline 150 beats per minute; not reactive
B) Baseline 150 beats per minute; reactive
C) Baseline 180 beats per minute; decelerations to 150s; not reactive
D) Baseline 180 beats per minute; moderate variability; reactive

Answer 15.3.5 The correct answer is "B." The baseline is about 150 beats per minute. There are two accelerations greater than 15 beats and lasting longer than 15 seconds, which meets the criteria for a reactive nonstress test. There is one contraction and evidence of uterine irritability noted as well.

HELPFUL TIP:
When interpreting FHR tracings, variability is an important element that demonstrates fetal cardiac response to parasympathetic input. The small waveform fluctuations within the baseline heart rate tracing represent the FHR variability. After 28 weeks of gestation, variability should be present. It is categorized as absent (no amplitude, flat tracing), minimal (0–5 beat amplitude), moderate (6–25 beat amplitude), or marked (>25 beat amplitude). The absence of variability is associated with fetal decompensation or distress.

....

You perform amniotomy with return of particulate meconium-stained fluid. Her cervix is now 5 cm dilated, 80% effaced, with vertex at +1 station. You elect to continue monitoring progress.

Question 15.3.6 Which of the following choices of labor analgesia is MOST appropriate at this point?
A) Epidural analgesia
B) Local perineal anesthetic infiltration
C) Bilateral pudendal nerve block
D) All of the above are equally appropriate

Answer 15.3.6 The correct answer is "A." Epidural analgesia offers the most effective form of pain relief and generally may be utilized once the patient is determined to be in active labor.

Various local anesthetic agents ("A") are available for local infiltration of the perineum and vagina to provide analgesia for **episiotomy or laceration repair following delivery but not for labor.** Bilateral pudendal nerve blocks ("C") are useful during the **second** stage of labor, as a supplement to epidural analgesia for anesthesia of the sacral nerves, or as an option for operative vaginal delivery anesthesia (e.g., forceps, vacuum). Opioid agonists and agonist–antagonists are also available and commonly employed. However, some reports suggest that the analgesic effect of opioids in labor is limited when using the lower doses that are generally regarded as safer for the fetus.

....

The nurse notices some changes on the fetal heart monitor. The current FHR is shown in Figure 15-5.

Question 15.3.7 What is the correct interpretation of this FHR tracing?
A) Baseline 160 beats per minute; reactive
B) Baseline 160 beats per minute; variable deceleration to the 90s
C) Baseline 160 beats per minute; late decelerations to the 90s
D) Baseline 160 beats per minute; early decelerations to the 90s

Answer 15.3.7 The correct answer is "B." A variable deceleration to the 90s occurs with the first contraction on this strip. Variable decelerations vary with respect to timing, duration, and depth—thus, the name "variable." They are not uniform. Variable decelerations represent changes in the FHR in response to cord compression. Please refer to Table 15-2 with definitions and FHR tracing categories.

HELPFUL TIP:
A systematic review in 2013 showed no benefit in outcomes for continuous FHR monitoring compared to intermittent FHR monitoring. Unfortunately, there are more cesarean sections and operative vaginal deliveries when continuous FHR monitoring is used. However, much of FHR monitoring use is dictated by local practice patterns, expert consensus, and medicolegal concerns.

Question 15.3.8 Given the findings in Figure 15-5, which of the following should be performed next?
A) Check the patient's cervix
B) Place a fetal scalp electrode
C) Begin IV oxytocin infusion
D) Place an intrauterine pressure catheter and begin an amnio-infusion
E) Take a coffee break; you've got a long night ahead

Answer 15.3.8 The correct answer is "A." Variable decelerations are common in labor, and brief variable decelerations are benign. When variable decelerations become recurrent, progressively deeper, and longer lasting with delayed return to baseline, they are non-reassuring and may reflect fetal hypoxia. A pelvic examination should be performed to determine if the

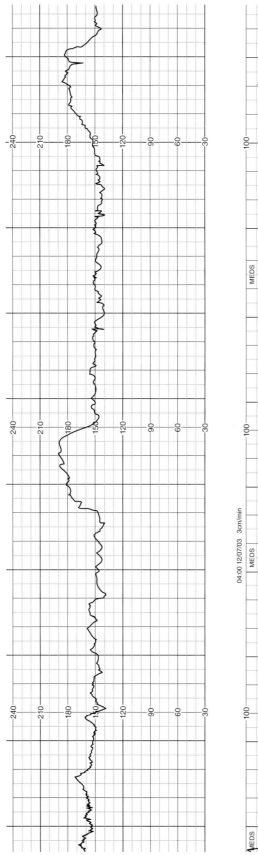
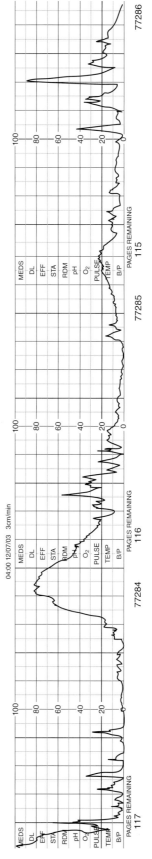

FIGURE 15-4 Fetal Monitoring Tracings.

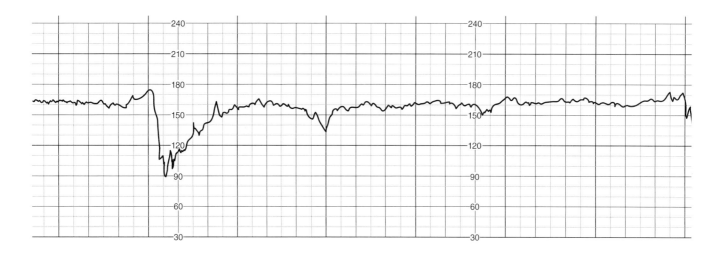

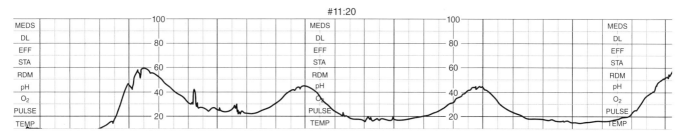

FIGURE 15-5   Fetal Monitoring Tracings.

umbilical cord is prolapsed or if there has been rapid descent of the fetal head or rapid progression of labor. Oxytocin, "C," should not be considered in this patient since she is having adequate contractions. Replacement of the amniotic fluid ("D," amnioinfusion) with normal saline infused through a transcervical catheter has been reported to decrease both the frequency and severity of repetitive variable decelerations and can decrease rate of cesarean section. However, it would first be helpful to assess the cervical status. *Of note, amnioinfusion is no longer recommended as a prophylactic intervention for moderate or severe meconium.*

Labor progresses without incident. Your patient is now completely dilated and effaced, with fetal head at +3 station. She is comfortable with her epidural and able to push with good effort. The FHR tracing is reassuring. Contractions are every 3 minutes.

Question 15.3.9 Appropriate management at this point is:
A) Continue pushing
B) Vacuum-assisted delivery
C) Forceps-assisted delivery
D) Midline episiotomy
E) Augment with oxytocin

Answer 15.3.9 **The correct answer is "A."** At this point, labor is progressing and maternal–fetal status is reassuring. You should continue expectant management. No intervention is indicated.

HELPFUL TIP:
Episiotomies should *not* be performed routinely. Indications for episiotomy are typically related to non-reassuring fetal status and shoulder dystocia. There is no evidence that episiotomies reduce perineal trauma, postpartum dyspareunia, etc. In fact, an episiotomy increases the risk of third- and fourth-degree tears and increase blood loss.

She pushes for 3 hours. She is now exhausted. The fetal head now separates the labia with contractions, and then recedes slightly. You consider offering assistance with delivery.

Question 15.3.10 In counseling your patient and her husband about the maternal risks of operative vaginal delivery, which of the following should you discuss?
A) Vaginal trauma
B) Shoulder dystocia
C) Fetal injury
D) Perineal and rectal trauma
E) All of the above

Answer 15.3.10 **The correct answer is "E."** Maternal risks of operative vaginal delivery include injury to the lower genital tract and rectal sphincter involvement in the case of a third- or fourth-degree laceration. In addition, fetal complications need to be discussed. Shoulder dystocia is more common with operative delivery than with a spontaneous vaginal delivery (see the following for more information).

Question 15.3.11 Each of the following is a fetal risk of operative vaginal delivery EXCEPT:
A) Cephalohematoma
B) Skull fracture
C) Brachial plexus injury
D) Respiratory distress syndrome
E) Facial nerve palsy

Answer 15.3.11 The correct answer is "D." Risk of respiratory distress syndrome is not increased by assisted delivery. Neonatal cephalohematoma, retinal hemorrhage, and jaundice (secondary to breakdown and reabsorption of the cephalohematoma) are more common with vacuum-assisted delivery than with forceps-assisted delivery. Skull fracture and facial nerve injury is more common with forceps-assisted delivery than with vacuum-assisted delivery. Shoulder dystocia with resultant brachial plexus injury is more common with vacuum-assisted delivery, prolonged time required for delivery, and increasing birth weight. Note that injury can occur before operative delivery as a result of abnormal labor forces (we don't think anyone has told the malpractice attorneys …).

Delivery of an 8-lb baby is accomplished without operative vaginal assistance. The mere presence of the vacuum on the table was enough to entice the uterus to perform one last massive contraction—assisted by the infant clawing its way out when it saw the vacuum coming. Following spontaneous delivery of the intact placenta 15 minutes later, you note a large gush of blood.

Question 15.3.12 Which of the following is the most likely source of the bleeding?
A) Uterine atony
B) Vaginal laceration
C) Cervical laceration
D) Retained placenta

Answer 15.3.12 The correct answer is "A." Postpartum hemorrhage is most commonly associated with uterine atony. Risk factors include prolonged labor, over-distended uterus (such as from two or eight gestations [remember Octomom?]), very rapid labor, high parity, chorioamnionitis, retained placental tissue, poorly perfused myometrium, halogenated hydrocarbon anesthesia, and previous uterine atony. Maternal trauma to the genital tract ("B" and "C") may result in postpartum hemorrhage and should be routinely investigated, particularly following operative delivery. A retained placenta cotyledon is another common source for postpartum hemorrhage. The placenta should be inspected, and if there is any question of retained products of conception, the uterus should be manually explored.

Question 15.3.13 Which of the following should be undertaken next?
A) Obtain IV access and initiate hydration
B) Begin bimanual uterine compression
C) Inspect vagina and cervix for lacerations
D) Obtain blood for type and screen for possible blood transfusion
E) All of the above

Answer 15.3.13 The correct answer is "E." Postpartum hemorrhage is an *obstetrical emergency* and must be addressed immediately. The gravid uterus receives 500 mL of blood per minute, which can lead to massive hemorrhage if not addressed quickly. Additional personnel should be notified to help with obtaining IV access and blood draws, while you quickly try to identify the source of bleeding.

After thorough exploration of the vagina and uterus, you suspect uterine atony is the cause of bleeding. While continuing uterine massage, you think about your options.

Question 15.3.14 Which of the following is/are options in treating this patient's bleeding?
A) Dilute oxytocin (Pitocin) IV
B) Methylergonovine (Methergine) IM
C) Carboprost tromethamine (Hemabate) IM
D) Misoprostol (Cytotec) PR
E) All of the above

Answer 15.3.14 The correct answer is "E." All of the drugs listed cause smooth muscle contraction of the uterus. Oxytocin can be given as a dilute IV solution or IM. It should never be administered as an undiluted IV bolus, due to the risk of **hypotension** and cardiac arrhythmia. Methergine (methylergonovine) is an ergot alkaloid and may be administered orally or intramuscularly (**not intravenously**). *Caution should be used in women with hypertension, as Methergine can cause hypertension.* Hemabate (carboprost tromethamine) is an F-2 prostaglandin analog that is administered IM or directly into the uterine myometrium. *Caution should be used in women with asthma, as Hemabate can cause bronchoconstriction.* Cytotec (misoprostol) is a prostaglandin E1 analog that works well and can safely be administered to women with asthma or hypertension. Rectal or oral administration can be used, but rectal administration is preferred in a patient with potential hemodynamic instability. This can be a lifesaver especially in third-world countries where other options may not exist. Please see Table 15-4 for further information on treatments on postpartum hemorrhage.

HELPFUL TIP:
A large, randomized international trial, the WOMAN trial, has shown the benefits of using tranexamic acid in setting of postpartum hemorrhage. There was significant reduction in mortality (1.5% vs. 1.9% [*P*=0.045] for tranexamic acid compared to placebo). The World Health Organization (WHO) recommends early use of intravenous tranexamic acid (TXA) *within 3 hours of birth* in addition to standard care for women with clinically diagnosed postpartum hemorrhage following vaginal birth or caesarean section (*Lancet.* 2017;389(10084):2105–2116). The sooner the better: TXA saves fewer lives as time goes on.

TABLE 15-4 MANAGEMENT OF POSTPARTUM HEMORRHAGE

Drug[a]	Dose and Route	Frequency	Contraindications	Adverse Effects
Oxytocin	IV: 10–40 units per 500–1,000 mL as continuous infusion or IM: 10 units	Continuous	Rare, hypersensitivity to medication	Usually none. Nausea, vomiting, hyponatremia with prolonged dosing Hypotension can result from IV push, which is not recommended
Methylergonovine	IM: 0.2 mg	Every 2–4 h	Hypertension, preeclampsia, cardiovascular disease, hypersensitivity to drug	Nausea, vomiting, severe hypertension particularly when given IV, which is not recommended
Carboprost (Hemabate)	IM: 0.25 mg Intramyometrial: 0.25 mg	Every 15–90 min, eight doses maximum	Asthma, relative contraindication for hypertension, active hepatic, pulmonary, or cardiac disease	Nausea, vomiting, diarrhea, fever (transient), headache, chills, shivering, hypertension, bronchospasm
Misoprostol	600–1,000 micrograms oral, sublingual, or rectal	One time	Rare, hypersensitivity to medication or to prostaglandins	Nausea, vomiting, diarrhea, shivering, fever (transient), headache

IV, intravenously; IM, intramuscularly; PG, prostaglandin.

[a]All agents can cause nausea and vomiting.

Modified from Lyndon A, Lagrew D, Shields L, Main E, Cape V, eds. Improving health care response to obstetric hemorrhage version 2.0. A California quality improvement toolkit. Stamford (CA): California Maternal Quality Care Collaborative; Sacramento (CA): California Department of Public Health; 2015.

She requires IV crystalloid and four units of packed red cells for symptomatic anemia following delivery. Both mother and infant eventually do well, and the patient and baby are discharged on postpartum day 2. You schedule a follow-up appointment in 2 days. You are concerned about Sheehan syndrome, given the severe postpartum hemorrhage.

Question 15.3.15 All of the following are characteristic of Sheehan syndrome EXCEPT:
A) Failure in lactation
B) Amenorrhea
C) Desire to be a punk rocker
D) Decreased LH/follicle-stimulating hormone (FSH)
E) Adrenal cortical insufficiency

Answer 15.3.15 The correct answer is "C." Severe intrapartum or postpartum hemorrhage may result in pituitary necrosis due to hypovolemia and hypoperfusion. This leads to a global hypopituitarism known as Sheehan syndrome. Sheehan syndrome is characterized clinically by endocrine deficiency syndromes as a result of loss of anterior pituitary function. Initial symptoms may be vague (lethargy, anorexia, weight loss, difficulty with lactation), and the syndrome can go unrecognized. Later manifestations include failure of lactation, amenorrhea, breast atrophy, loss of pubic and axillary hair, adrenal cortical insufficiency, and hypothyroidism. Desire to be a punk rocker is "Sheena syndrome." If you don't get it, you missed the Ramones.

▶ **Objectives: Did you learn to …**
• Recognize the risks of prolonged pregnancy and identify appropriate timing of intervention?
• Describe the indications and risks associated with induction of labor?

• Interpret intrapartum FHR patterns and choose appropriate management options?
• Evaluate analgesia options, contraindications, and risks during labor and delivery?
• Recognize the indications for and management of operative vaginal and abdominal delivery?
• Evaluate and manage postpartum hemorrhage?

 QUICK QUIZ: WHAT'S SCARIER THAN TWINS?

While on call for your small community hospital, a nurse on the labor and delivery ward calls you about a patient with preterm contractions. You come in to see the patient and find a 33-year-old G1P0 at 26 weeks of gestation by in vitro fertilization. She is usually followed at an academic hospital 400 miles away. She looks worried and says, "I'm going to have twins. But not now!" She recalls her prenatal lab results were unremarkable. She recalls her ultrasound showed "two heart beats."

All of the following risks are increased with a multifetal gestation EXCEPT:
A) Preterm labor
B) D-isoimmunization (Rh isoimmunization)
C) Preterm rupture of membranes
D) Intrauterine growth restriction
E) Twin–twin transfusion syndrome

The correct answer is "B." The most significant complication of multiple gestations is preterm labor resulting in preterm delivery. Preterm rupture of membranes and intrauterine growth restriction also occur more frequently in multiple gestations than singleton pregnancies. The risk of all these complications is directly proportional to the number of fetuses. Twin–twin transfusion syndrome rarely occurs and is associated with monochorionic gestations. Multifetal gestations do not increase the risk of D-isoimmunization.

▶ CASE 15.4

After a busy day in clinic, you get the traditional 5 PM call from labor and delivery. The nurse tells you that your partner's patient is presenting with concerns for preterm labor. She is a 24-year-old G1 at 26 weeks by LMP and first-trimester ultrasound. She is having contractions but no vaginal discharge. The contractions started about an hour ago and are 5 to 6 minutes apart. The nurse asks if you want to check fetal fibronectin (FFN).

Question 15.4.1 A NEGATIVE fetal fibronectin is associated with:
A) Fetal lung immaturity
B) Ruptured fetal membranes
C) A decreased risk of preterm birth
D) An increased risk of preterm birth

Answer 15.4.1 The correct answer is "C." FFN is a basement membrane protein produced by the fetal membranes. A negative test is useful in assessing the risk of preterm delivery during the following 2-week period. With a properly performed test in a symptomatic patient, up to 99.5% of patients with a negative FFN will not deliver in the subsequent 7 days. *A positive test is not useful as the test has low positive predictive value.* In performing FFN testing, the following criteria must be met: intact amniotic membranes, minimal cervical dilation (<3 cm), and sampling between 24 0/7 and 34 6/7 weeks. Recent sexual intercourse and the presence of vaginal discharge or bleeding may cause a false-positive test. Collect the swab in the posterior vaginal fornix before cervical checks and transvaginal ultrasound as these can also cause the test to be falsely positive. FFN does not assess fetal lung maturity ("A"). Ruptured membranes ("B") would cause a positive FFN.

You are wondering if this patient is a good candidate for corticosteroid therapy.

Question 15.4.2 Regarding the risks and benefits of corticosteroid therapy for fetal lung maturation, which of the following is FALSE?
A) Corticosteroid therapy is recommended for all pregnant women between 24 and 34 weeks of gestation who are at risk of preterm delivery within 7 days
B) Corticosteroid therapy has been associated with an increased risk of neonatal infection
C) Antenatal corticosteroid therapy reduces the incidence of respiratory distress syndrome, intraventricular hemorrhage, and necrotizing enterocolitis
D) Corticosteroids accelerate the production of pulmonary surfactant in the fetal lungs

Answer 15.4.2 The correct answer is "B." There is no evidence that antenatal corticosteroid therapy increases the risk of neonatal infection. However, maternal infection is a **relative** contraindication to corticosteroid therapy. Corticosteroids are recommended for all pregnant women between 24 and 34 weeks of gestation who are at risk of preterm delivery within 7 days. Corticosteroids may be given after 34 weeks if there is documented fetal lung immaturity and delivery will likely occur before lung maturation.

Question 15.4.3 Which of the following FDA-approved tocolytics is regarded as first-line therapy to abort preterm labor?
A) Nifedipine
B) Magnesium sulfate
C) Prostaglandin inhibitors
D) Ritodrine
E) None of the above

Answer 15.4.3 The correct answer is "E." Is this a trick question? Not really. The only FDA-approved agent for use as a tocolytic *was* ritodrine, a β-adrenergic receptor agonist, which was pulled from the market in the United States in 1993. There are no currently available FDA-approved tocolytics. Thus, other agents have been investigated. Terbutaline, magnesium sulfate, prostaglandin inhibitors, and calcium channel blockers have all been studied and may be utilized in select cases for tocolysis—but realize that these drugs are not approved by the FDA for this indication and that they carry substantial risks. Indomethacin has also been used successfully for tocolysis. Again, it is not approved for this indication.

HELPFUL TIP:
Tocolysis only staves off labor by 48 hours at best, so the real goal should be to prolong the pregnancy until steroids have time to be effective. Contraindications to tocolysis include: evidence of fetal distress, fetal anomalies, abruptio placentae, placenta previa with heavy bleeding, and severe maternal disease.

You examine the patient after ordering an FFN. Her cervix is 1 cm dilated at the external os and closed at the internal os, long, and posterior. Ultrasound shows that the infant is vertex. The monitor shows FHR baselines of 140 and 145 bpm. Contractions are irregular, occurring every 4 to 9 minutes. Urine dipstick shows a specific gravity of 1.030.

Question 15.4.4 The LEAST appropriate intervention in this 26 week gestation is:
A) Continuation of monitoring
B) Oral hydration
C) Obstetrical consult for cerclage placement
D) Test for group B streptococci, gonorrhea, and chlamydia
E) Administration of corticosteroids

Answer 15.4.4 **The correct answer is "C."** Cerclage (a stitch to hold the cervix closed) is indicated for incompetent cervix, not preterm labor. A cerclage is typically placed for incompetent cervix (two or more consecutive second-trimester losses with minimal or no symptoms) in the first part of the second trimester after fetal viability has been established. It would not be used at 26 weeks. The patient should be evaluated carefully, and the frequency of uterine contractions should be assessed during the initial management ("A"). Because dehydration may result in uterine irritability, rehydration ("B") may stabilize the uterus. There is no proven benefit of hydration in the patient who is euvolemic. Get cultures ("D") to prevent perinatal transmission, even though treatment of positive cultures has not been established to aid in the prevention of preterm birth. Corticosteroids ("E") are discussed earlier.

HELPFUL (AND USELESS IF NOT AT LEAST INTERESTING) TIP:
Delivery rates in Israel go up around Jewish holiday fast days likely because of the relative dehydration.

▶ Objectives: Did you learn to ...
 • Recognize preterm labor and manage it appropriately?
 • Understand the indications, contraindications, risks, and benefits of tocolytics and corticosteroids?

▶ **CASE 15.5**

A 33-year-old G1 at 35 2/7 weeks presents to labor and delivery. Her pregnancy has been complicated by preterm labor. Her GBS status is unknown. On admission, she is uncomfortable with regular contractions every 3 to 4 minutes. The FHR baseline is 135 bpm with moderate variability. Her cervix is 6 cm dilated, completely effaced, with a bulging amniotic sac and fetus in vertex presentation.

Question 15.5.1 **Which of the following is your best course of management?**
A) Administer corticosteroids
B) Administer tocolytics
C) Initiate GBS prophylaxis
D) Discharge her to home until she is in active labor
E) A, B, and C

Answer 15.5.1 **The correct answer is "C."** GBS prophylaxis is indicated for preterm delivery if GBS status is unknown. Appropriate antibiotics include penicillin or ampicillin or an alternative intravenous agent if the patient has a penicillin allergy as previously discussed in question 15.2.5. This patient is outside the window (24–34 weeks) for corticosteroid administration ("A"). Given the gestational age (>34 weeks), advanced cervical dilation, and high likelihood of imminent delivery, tocolysis should be avoided ("B").

HELPFUL TIP:
Indications for GBS prophylaxis: (1) GBS screen positive during current pregnancy; (2) GBS bacteriuria anytime during current pregnancy; (3) prior history of giving birth to a neonate with GBS disease; (4) unknown GBS status **plus** fever **or** preterm labor **or** prolonged rupture of membranes. No GBS prophylaxis is indicated in women who are **culture negative** with fever (but think about chorioamnionitis!), preterm labor, or prolonged rupture of membranes.

HELPFUL TIP:
The risk for recurrent premature delivery in subsequent pregnancies is about 15%. 17α-Hydroxyprogesterone caproate given IM (brand name Makena) *may* reduce the incidence of preterm birth when started at 16 to 20 weeks and can be offered to a woman with a singleton gestation and a history of a prior spontaneous preterm singleton birth. Recent data suggests that *vaginal* progesterone may be less effective than once thought (*Lancet.* 2016;387(10033):2106–2116). Remember that "may" is the logical equivalent of "may not". If prior preterm birth was secondary to an incompetent or shortened cervix, then a cerclage should also be considered (*Obstet Gynecol.* 2012;120(4):964–973).

▶ Objective: Did you learn to ...
 • Describe indications for GBS prophylaxis?

 QUICK QUIZ: PRETERM BIRTH

Risk factors for preterm birth include each of the following EXCEPT:
A) Multiple gestation pregnancy
B) Maternal bacteriuria
C) Maternal history of preterm contractions with term birth
D) Maternal smoking
E) Maternal hypertension

The correct answer is "C." While preterm contractions are concerning, a maternal history of preterm contractions with term birth does not increase the risk of preterm delivery in a subsequent pregnancy. Multiple gestations, history of preterm birth, smoking, cocaine use, asymptomatic bacteriuria, and hypertension are all risk factors for preterm birth.

▶ **CASE 15.6**

A 37-year-old G3 P0111 (all those numbers indicate the following: 0 full term, 1 preterm, 1 abortion/miscarriage for any reason, 1 living child) presents for routine obstetric care at 10 weeks of gestation. Her second pregnancy was complicated by preeclampsia with severe features at 35 weeks requiring induction of labor and magnesium sulfate therapy. Her past medical history is uncomplicated. Her blood pressure is 132/86 mm Hg, urine protein is negative, and physical examination is unremarkable. Uterine size is consistent with dates and fetal heart tones are auscultated. The patient wonders if she will need to deliver early and need magnesium again.

Question 15.6.1 You counsel her that her risk of recurrent preeclampsia with severe features is in the range of:
A) <5%
B) 10%–20%
C) 50% to 60%
D) >90%

Answer 15.6.1 The correct answer is "B." The risk of recurrence of preeclampsia is affected by both gestational age at diagnosis and the severity of preeclampsia. Preeclampsia at an early gestational age or preeclampsia with severe features increases the risk of recurrence. The overall recurrence risks are estimated at less than 10% for mild preeclampsia and greater than 20% (or more) for preeclampsia with severe features. Risk factors for preeclampsia include young maternal age, advanced maternal age, diabetes, and chronic hypertension, among many others.

The patient would like to do anything reasonable to prevent preeclampsia again.

Question 15.6.2 In addition to obtaining baseline laboratory evaluation (CBC, AST, ALT, creatinine, 24-hour urine for protein) to aid in early diagnosis, you recommend the following therapy:
A) Low-sodium diet
B) Diuretic for hypertension and edema
C) Aspirin 81 mg daily
D) Subcutaneous heparin therapy at prophylactic doses
E) None of the above

Answer 15.6.2 The correct answer is "C." ACOG's Task Force on Hypertension in Pregnancy from November 2013 recommends the use of 81 mg aspirin daily in patients who have a history of early-onset preeclampsia with preterm delivery **or** in patients with a history of preeclampsia in more than one prior pregnancy. USPSTF recommends the use of low-dose aspirin as a preventive medication after 12 weeks of gestation in women who are at high risk for preeclampsia. Calcium supplementation? Not so much.

Because of her age (37 years), the patient also inquires about her risk for delivering a baby with Down syndrome.

Question 15.6.3 What is her estimated risk of a Down syndrome baby with this pregnancy?
A) 1/9,000
B) 1/1,200
C) 1/150
D) 1/12

Answer 15.6.3 The correct answer is "C." The risk of Down syndrome begins to rise rapidly at age 35, with an estimated risk of 1/250 at age 35, 1/150 at age 37, and 1/70 at age 40.

After hearing her age-related risk for Down syndrome, the patient asks about what tests she should have to screen for Down syndrome.

Question 15.6.4 You counsel her regarding various tests and offer:
A) First-trimester triple screening (PAPP-A, hCG, and nuchal lucency)/integrated screening
B) Chorionic villus sampling (CVS)
C) Amniocentesis
D) Second-trimester quadruple screening (hCG, maternal serum alpha fetal protein [MSAFP], estriol, inhibin A)
E) Cell-free fetal DNA testing from maternal peripheral blood
F) All of the above

Answer 15.6.4 The correct answer is "F." All patients should be offered first-trimester screening, and if declined, they should be offered second-trimester quadruple screening. Because of her advanced age (>35 years at the time of delivery), the patient should be offered CVS and amniocentesis as well. Patients should understand that the first- and second-trimester screening tests are just that—**screening methods**. However, both CVS and amniocentesis can diagnose Down syndrome, in addition to other chromosomal abnormalities. CVS is typically completed between 10 and 13 weeks of gestation, whereas amniocentesis is performed after 15 weeks. Both are invasive procedures, which carry risks, including pregnancy loss, rupture of membranes, and fetal injury. Cell-free fetal DNA testing is a newer and noninvasive screening test that can be done after 10 weeks of gestation in patients at high risk for aneuploidy. If abnormal, it should be followed up with a diagnostic test, such as an amniocentesis. Please see Figure 15-3 for further information on prenatal screening options.

The patient has a negative first-trimester screening, which decreases her Down syndrome risk to 1/800. She declines an amniocentesis. You draw her MSAFP (maternal serum AFP) only at 17 weeks, because, as you learned above, the first-trimester screening does not evaluate for neural tube defects. The AFP is normal. She subsequently undergoes diabetes screening between 24 and 48 weeks with a 1-hour post-50-g glucose test, which shows a glucose level of 170 mg/dL.

Question 15.6.5 The next step is:
A) Order a 3-hour glucose tolerance test
B) Set up diabetes teaching and a consult with a nutritionist/dietician
C) Start glyburide
D) Start insulin
E) All of the above

Answer 15.6.5 The correct answer is "A." It is recommended to perform a 1-hour 50-g glucose load *screening* test for gestational diabetes between 24 and 28 weeks of gestation. Earlier testing *may* be suitable if risk factors are present (see Table 15-5) for gestational diabetes. However, the test should be repeated between 24 and 28 weeks as a proportion of women will have a negative screening test early on and then subsequently develop gestational diabetes. The cut-off for a "positive" test is somewhat controversial but is agreed to be between 130 and 140 mg/dL; typically cut-offs are based on individual institutional standards. Since hers is abnormal (≥140 mg/dL), the next step is to perform a second, *diagnostic* test which is the fasting 3-hour glucose tolerance test, utilizing a 100-g glucose load with measurement of blood sugars at 0 (fasting) and 1, 2, and 3 hours post glucose load. A woman with two out of three abnormal values on her 3-hour glucose tolerance test is diagnosed as having gestational diabetes. As with the 1-hour glucose tolerance test, there are variations in standards of "cut-offs" for a "positive test"; you should refer to your institution's standards.

HELPFUL TIP:
The International Association of Diabetes in Pregnancy Study Group has previously proposed a more aggressive universal screening approach using a *single* 2-hour OGTT after administration of a 75-g glucose load during the second trimester. A *single* glucose value meeting or exceeding the set thresholds (fasting <92 mg/dL, 1 hour <180 mg/dL, 2 hour <153 mg/dL) would equate to a "positive" screen for gestational diabetes. These proposed changes have been met with some resistance as there would potentially be a significant increase in the number of women diagnosed with gestational diabetes who would not be at risk of adverse outcomes (*Obstet Gynecol.* 2018;131(2):e49– e64).

TABLE 15-5 RISK FACTORS FOR GESTATIONAL DIABETES TO WARRANT PRE-/EARLY GESTATIONAL SCREENING

Body mass index > 25 (or > 23 in Asian Americans) with one of the following risk factors:
- First-degree relative with history of diabetes
- Previous history of gestational diabetes
- Prior birth of infant > 4,000 g (9 lbs)
- High-risk ethnicity (i.e., African Americans, Latinx, Native American, Asian American, Pacific Islander)
- Hypertension
- HDL < 35 mg/dL or triglycerides > 250 mg/dL
- PCOS
- Physical inactivity
- Impaired glucose tolerance or fasting glucose on prior testing (i.e., FPG or A1c)

Adapted from American College of Obstetricians and Gynecologists Committee on Practice Bulletins. ACOG Practice Bulletin No 180: Gestational Diabetes. *Obstet Gynecol.* 2018;131(2):e49–e64; and American Diabetes Association. Classification and Diagnosis of Diabetes. *Diabetes Care.* 2017;40(suppl. 1):S11–24.

The patient completes her glucose tolerance test with values of:
- **Fasting: 92 mg/dL**
- **1 hour: 194 mg/dL**
- **2 hours: 169 mg/dL**
- **3 hours: 148 mg/dL**

(Her institution's cut-offs are as follows: fasting 95 mg/dL; 1 hour 180 mg/dL; 2 hours 155 mg/dL; and 3 hours 140 mg/dL)

Question 15.6.6 The next step in management is:
A) Continue routine prenatal care
B) Set up diabetes teaching and a consult with a nutritionist/dietician
C) Start glyburide
D) Start insulin

Answer 15.6.6 The correct answer is "B." Your patient has three out of her four results above the accepted thresholds. If a patient has two or more glucose levels that are above the accepted cut-off ranges, she is diagnosed with gestational diabetes (GDM). The recommendation is to initiate dietary modifications including carbohydrate restriction with frequent blood sugar monitoring and exercise. If the target glucoses (<95 mg/dL fasting and <120 mg/dL 2-hours post-prandially) cannot be met with dietary changes alone, medical therapy should be started.

Although insulin has been the standard therapy and is still preferred as it does not cross the placenta, glyburide or metformin are also equally appropriate for first-line therapy and have been used with increasing popularity despite this being an "off-label" indication. Of note, metformin has been shown to cross the placenta with the long-term influence on neonates still unclear. Additionally, glyburide has been shown to have increased risk of hypoglycemia and has not been shown to be as effective as insulin or metformin. Therefore, remember: *Insulin is better than metformin, which is better than glyburide* (*BMJ.* 2015;350:h102 and *Obstet Gynecol.* 2018;131(2):e49– e64).

The patient is seen for her 32-week visit and her fundal height is only 28 cm (which surprises you, given her diagnosis of gestational diabetes … the babies of diabetic mothers tend to be large!). She has been compliant with the dietary changes and her blood sugars are usually 80s fasting and 120s 2-hour postprandial. She has gained 20 lb so far in the pregnancy. You send her for an ultrasound, which reveals an infant measuring only 28 3/7 weeks of gestation, weighing 1,168 g (<10th percentile). Amniotic fluid volume and umbilical artery Dopplers are normal.

Question 15.6.7 Appropriate follow-up includes:
A) Changing the estimated due date
B) Scheduling an induction
C) Repeating the ultrasound for growth in 1 week
D) Repeating the ultrasound for growth in 4 weeks

Answer 15.6.7 The correct answer is "D." Current ultrasound techniques are not sensitive enough to assess growth at weekly intervals ("C"), and therefore waiting 4 weeks would give a better assessment of growth rate. This infant demonstrates intrauterine growth restriction. The patient had a first-trimester ultrasound with her first-trimester screening, which establishes her due date. *It is inappropriate* to change her due date based on a 32-week ultrasound ("A"). Initiating an induction would be inappropriate without further investigation, given the early gestational age ("B"). You could do an ultrasound at 1 to 2 weeks to assess amniotic fluid and umbilical Doppler but not fetal size. Antenatal surveillance is indicated at this time with bi-weekly nonstress testing.

The patient continues with bi-weekly nonstress tests and her ultrasound at 35 weeks reveals appropriate interval growth but remains growth-restricted at a weight of 1,846 g (<10th percentile). Today her blood pressure is 146/88 mm Hg and urine protein on dipstick is +1. Ugh … she can't seem to catch a break.

Question 15.6.8 At this time, appropriate intervention includes:
A) Administering corticosteroids
B) Obtaining a 24-hour urine for protein
C) Following up with a routine appointment in 1 week
D) Starting labetalol
E) Starting lisinopril

Answer 15.6.8 The correct answer is "B." Given the patient's elevated blood pressure and 1+ protein on dipstick, you need to be concerned about recurrent preeclampsia. Urinary excretion of protein may be transient, and a 24-hour urine protein level is a more accurate reflection of proteinuria and the preferred method to diagnose preeclampsia (although, as noted below, urine protein is no longer required for a diagnosis of preeclampsia/eclampsia). Alternatively, a protein/creatinine ratio of at least 0.3 mg/dL can also be used for preeclampsia diagnosis. "A" is incorrect. The patient is at 35 weeks of gestation (although measuring smaller), which is beyond the recommended gestation at which corticosteroids are administered (24–34 weeks). This patient must be followed up in a couple of days so that you don't miss the diagnosis of preeclampsia. Although anti-hypertensives such as labetalol can be utilized in pregnancy, they are not routinely initiated for mild elevations in blood pressure at later gestations. We hope you avoided "E," as ACE inhibitors are contraindicated in pregnancy.

Serial blood pressure measurements in the clinic reveal no blood pressures greater than 146/88 mm Hg. Her nonstress test is reactive. The patient is sent home to collect her 24-hour urine and returns in 2 days. Her blood pressure is now 148/90 mm Hg and she has trace protein on urine dipstick. The 24-hour urine returns at 180 mg (her baseline 24-hour urine protein at the beginning of the pregnancy was 116 mg). She denies any headache, visual changes, nausea, or abdominal pain.

Question 15.6.9 Your diagnosis is:
A) Gestational hypertension
B) Preeclampsia
C) Preeclampsia with severe features
D) Acute renal failure

Answer 15.6.9 The correct answer is "A." She now has two blood pressure readings greater than 140/90 mm Hg and more than 6-hours apart, which satisfy the criteria for hypertension. Given that this elevation in blood pressure started after 20 weeks of gestation, it is likely pregnancy-related. She does not have protein >300 mg in a 24-hour urine collection, so she does not meet that diagnostic criterion for preeclampsia and does not have symptoms that would qualify her for a diagnosis of preeclampsia with severe features. *Note that proteinuria is no longer required to make the diagnosis of preeclampsia. Another abnormality such as elevated LFTs, thrombocytopenia, renal insufficiency, CHF, or CNS symptoms can make the diagnosis of preeclampsia even in the absence of proteinuria.* The diagnostic criteria for preeclampsia are outlined in Table 15-6.

TABLE 15-6 DIAGNOSTIC CRITERIA FOR PREECLAMPSIA

2013 Diagnostic Criteria for Preeclampsia
Blood pressure:
- ≥140 mm Hg systolic or >90 mm Hg diastolic on **TWO** occasions at least 4 hours apart **AFTER** 20 weeks of gestation in a woman with history of previously normal blood pressure
- ≥160 mm Hg systolic or ≥110 mm Hg diastolic; hypertension can be confirmed within a short interval (minutes) to facilitate timely antihypertensive therapy

AND
- Proteinuria:
  - ≥300 mg per 24-hour urine collection (or this amount extrapolated form a timed collection)

OR
- Urine protein:creatinine ratio greater than or equal to 0.3 with each measured in mg/dL

OR
- Dipstick reading of 1+ (used only if other quantitative methods aren't available)

OR

In the absence of proteinuria, new-onset hypertension with the onset of any of the following (laboratory values further defined under "Diagnosis of Preeclampsia with Severe Features" below):
- Thrombocytopenia
- Renal insufficiency
- Impaired liver function
- Pulmonary edema
- Cerebral or visual symptoms

Diagnose "Preeclampsia with Severe Features" when there is the presence of any of the following:
- Blood pressure >160 mm Hg systolic or ≥110 mm Hg diastolic on two occasions at least 4 hours apart while the patient is on bed rest (unless antihypertensive therapy is initiated before this time)
- Platelet count of less than 100,000/μL (thrombocytopenia)
- Serum creatinine concentrations greater than 1.1 mg/dL or a doubling of the serum creatinine concentration in the absence of other renal disease (renal insufficiency)
- Elevated blood concentrations of liver transaminases to 2× normal concentration, severe persistent right upper quadrant or epigastric pain unresponsive to medication and not accounted for by alternative diagnoses or both (impaired liver function)
- Pulmonary edema
- New-onset cerebral or visual symptoms

Adapted from American College of Obstetricians and Gynecologists. Executive summary: hypertension in pregnancy. *Obstet Gynecol.* 2013; 122(5):1122–1131.

She returns to the office for her appointment 5 days later at 36 weeks of gestation after having felt well over the weekend. However, today she developed a headache. Her blood pressure is 166/112 mm Hg and her urine dipstick reveals 3+ protein.

Question 15.6.10 **Your next step is to:**
A) Start oral labetalol and see the patient back in 2 days for a blood pressure check
B) Repeat the 24-hour urine for protein
C) Admit to labor and delivery for blood work and monitoring, with plans to move toward delivery
D) Immediate Cesarean section

Answer 15.6.10 **The correct answer is "C."** The clinical picture is now developing into preeclampsia with severe features (headache, systolic BP >160 mm Hg, diastolic BP >110 mm Hg, and 3+ proteinuria … see Table 15-6). The patient needs to be admitted for further monitoring of blood pressure and symptoms. In addition, blood work should be obtained including a CBC, and liver and renal studies. Starting oral labetalol would treat the patient's hypertension, but this step alone is not prudent for a patient who appears to have preeclampsia with severe features. The 24-hour urine protein collection may be helpful in meeting the technical criteria to diagnose preeclampsia and can be done during admission; however, the results would not change the immediate management of the patient. If a faster evaluation is needed, the protein/creatinine ratio could be done in this case. However, as noted above, preeclampsia with severe features can also be diagnosed without the presence of proteinuria in the presence of certain clinical and/or laboratory findings (see Table 15-6).

HELPFUL TIP:
In a preeclamptic patient, blood pressure can be controlled with labetalol, hydralazine, or **oral** nifedipine. Avoid nitroprusside. The downside of BP control is that it reduces placental flow. **Also, treating the BP has no effect on the course of preeclampsia.** *Therefore, treat BP only if >160/100 mm Hg* **or** *the patient is having end-organ symptoms.* Further information on acute and emergent management of severe hypertension can be found in *Obstet Gynecol.* 2019;133(2):e174–e180.

You admit her to the hospital. Repeat blood pressure is 164/98 mm Hg and urine dipstick shows 3+ protein. Her cervix is soft, 2 cm dilated, 50% effaced, with fetus vertex at −2 station.

Question 15.6.11 **What is the most appropriate intervention at this point?**
A) Begin induction of labor
B) Start magnesium sulfate
C) Prepare for a cesarean delivery in case it is needed
D) All of the above

Answer 15.6.11 **The correct answer is "D."** All of these options are important to consider at this time. Induction with oxytocin and treatment of preeclampsia with magnesium to prevent seizures are appropriate at this point. Obstetrical backup should be involved earlier rather than later unless you possess the skill to do the cesarean section yourself.

HELPFUL TIP:
Delivery of the baby (baby and placenta, really) is the ultimate treatment for preeclampsia and should be initiated as soon as feasible when the mother's condition demands it.

You begin magnesium sulfate for the preeclampsia and oxytocin for induction. The induction proceeds without incident, and she delivers a viable male infant.

Question 15.6.12 **How long will you continue the magnesium sulfate?**
A) Until delivery of the placenta
B) For 12 hours after delivery
C) For 24 hours after delivery
D) Until the urine protein dipstick is negative
E) Until discharge

Answer 15.6.12 **The correct answer is "C."** Treatment should be continued for 24 hours following delivery.

HELPFUL TIP:
Monitor deep tendon reflexes, level of consciousness, and urine output for all patients on magnesium. Turn off the magnesium infusion if signs of toxicity emerge (e.g., decreased mental status, hyporeflexia) or if the patient is at risk for impending toxicity (e.g., from renal failure).

ANOTHER HELPFUL TIP:
Remember all those "mag checks" you did every 2 hours as a medical student? Well, *for patients with preeclampsia without severe features, ACOG no longer recommends magnesium sulfate as a routine intervention* (again, look at Table 15-6). Not a total waste of time, right? "Mag checks" did improve your rapport with your patients … maybe… especially when you had to wake them up to check their reflexes. Remember that the purpose of magnesium sulfate infusion is to reduce the risk of seizures (i.e., the progression to eclampsia). The NNT for mild preeclampsia is 100.

YET ONE MORE HELPFUL TIP:
According to ACOG guidelines, bed rest should not be prescribed for patients with gestational hypertension or preeclampsia without severe features.

▶ **Objectives: Did you learn to …**
- Screen for, diagnose, and manage gestational diabetes?
- Evaluate, diagnose, and manage hypertension in pregnancy?
- Define and manage preeclampsia?
- Identify intrauterine growth restriction?

▶ CASE 15.7

Now, you have to rush from L&D back to clinic (this never happens, right?) where you meet a 31-year-old woman for preconception counseling. She has a history of hypertension and a heart murmur. She has dyspnea when climbing stairs, but performs normal activities of daily living with minimal difficulty. She takes lisinopril 10 mg daily for hypertension. On physical examination, heart rate is 82 bpm and blood pressure is 138/90 mm Hg. Her height is 5′ 6″ and weight 160 lb. She appears well.

Question 15.7.1 Regarding the management of her chronic hypertension during pregnancy, which is the most appropriate next step?
A) Discontinue lisinopril and begin methyldopa, labetalol, or nifedipine and recheck blood pressure in 2 weeks
B) Increase lisinopril to 20 mg daily and recheck blood pressure in 2 weeks
C) Make no changes at this time
D) Discontinue lisinopril; recheck blood pressure in 2 weeks
E) Either A or D is correct

Answer 15.7.1 The correct answer is "E." ACE inhibitors are contraindicated in pregnancy; therefore, a woman contemplating pregnancy should discontinue the medication or replace it with a safer alternative. In fact, for a woman capable of conceiving, ACE inhibitor use is discouraged unless no better alternative exists and the patient is using a reliable form of birth control. Women with mild chronic hypertension (systolic blood pressure 140–160 mm Hg) have a low risk for cardiovascular complications during pregnancy and can be managed with nonpharmacologic therapy as long as they are asymptomatic. In 2 weeks, when she has her return visit, if she is hypertensive (>140–160/>100 mm Hg), select a medication regarded as safe during pregnancy; methyldopa, nifedipine, or labetalol would be preferred. You could also start one of these at the current visit while discontinuing the ACE inhibitor ("A"). *Note that the ACOG recommendation is to treat chronic hypertension in pregnancy only if the BP is >160/105 mm Hg. If the patient has hypertension secondary to preeclampsia, ACOG would recommend treating the blood pressure only if the blood pressure is >160/110 mm Hg or if there are symptoms.* These recommendations are controversial, and many would initiate blood pressure control in both groups at a lower BP. Treating hypertension reduces the incidence of "severe" hypertension, but does not change outcomes (*N Engl J Med.* 2015;372:407–417). See also *Obstet Gynecol.* 2019;133(1): e26–e50 if you are interested in this topic.

Question 15.7.2 Which of the following statements about cardiovascular physiology in pregnancy is INCORRECT?
A) Blood volume and cardiac output increase by approximately 50% during pregnancy
B) Heart rate increases by 10 to 20 beats per minute, peaking in the third trimester
C) Systemic arterial pressure increases during the first trimester, reaches a peak in mid-pregnancy, and remains at that level until labor and delivery
D) Left ventricular ejection fraction remains constant or increases slightly throughout pregnancy
E) A temporary rise in venous return immediately following delivery may lead to a substantial rise in left ventricular filling pressure and cardiac decompensation in women with certain types of heart disease

Answer 15.7.2 The correct answer (and what does not happen in pregnancy) is "C." Systemic arterial pressure decreases during the first trimester, reaches a nadir during the second trimester, and returns to pre-pregnancy levels in the third trimester. The other statements are true. "E" deserves special mention. Immediately following delivery, relief of caval compression may cause a rise in venous return leading to clinical deterioration in some women with heart disease.

▶ **Objectives: Did you learn to …**
- Manage hypertension during preconception counseling?
- Recognize normal cardiac physiological changes associated with pregnancy?

▶ CASE 15.8

You are seeing a 28-year-old female whose LMP was approximately 7 days ago. She is complaining of vaginal bleeding and states that she is going through one pad every 20 minutes. Needless to say she is concerned. She is not using anything for contraception. Her vital signs and examination are unremarkable except for blood at the cervical os.

Question 15.8.1 After ruling out pregnancy and assuring that her hemoglobin is stable, what is your next step?
A) Fresh frozen plasma
B) Cyclic medroxyprogesterone 10 mg a day
C) DDAVP to maximize platelet function
D) Observation: nonintervention is the best policy if the hemoglobin is normal

Answer 15.8.1 The correct answer is "B." This patient has abnormal uterine bleeding, which is a broad term that includes different functional and structural causes of uterine bleeding. Dysfunctional uterine bleeding (DUB) secondary to anovulation is a very common cause of abnormal uterine bleeding. One popular regimen for DUB is medroxyprogesterone 10 mg/day for 10 days. This should be followed by a withdrawal bleed. This regimen can be repeated for the first 10 days of the next 3 months.

Other options include starting a monophasic OCP (three pills twice a day for 1 day, two pills twice a day for 1 day, one pill twice a day for 1 day, and then finish out the pack). Conjugated estrogens are a third option. Tranexamic acid (an antifibrinolytic) 1.3 g orally three times daily for 5 days is an additional alternative for patients with contraindications to hormonal therapy. Consider prescribing an antiemetic if using OCPs since they may cause nausea. **Always remember to rule out pregnancy (including ectopic) first**.

Question 15.8.2 The most common side effect of medroxyprogesterone at the above dose includes:
A) Bone marrow suppression
B) Thromboembolic disease
C) Depression
D) Sore breasts

Answer 15.8.2 **The correct answer is "C."** Many women will become depressed when taking this dose of medroxyprogesterone. They should be made aware of this ahead of time. The major side effect of the OCP regimen for abnormal uterine bleeding is nausea and vomiting. Consider giving the OCP regimen with an antiemetic. "B" is of note. Progesterones alone do not increase clot risk. They do inhibit thrombolysis, however.

HELPFUL TIP:
Another long-term option for patients with chronic abnormal uterine bleeding, after workup has been completed, is a levonorgestrel-containing IUD (e.g., Mirena, Skyla, Liletta).

Question 15.8.3 Causes of this patient's bleeding could include all of the following EXCEPT:
A) Hypothyroidism
B) Von Willebrand disease
C) Adenomyosis
D) Parathyroid disease
E) Uterine cancer

Answer 15.8.3 **The correct answer is "D."** All of the remaining can cause abnormal bleeding. Obviously, uterine cancer would be unlikely in a 28-year-old. Other causes of abnormal bleeding to consider are cervical polyps, endometrial polyps, adenomyosis, fibroids, PID and endocrine problems such as PCOS and thyroid abnormalities.

▶ **Objectives: Did you learn to …**
  · Evaluate a patient with abnormal uterine bleeding?
  · Treat a patient with abnormal uterine bleeding?

▶ CASE 15.9

A 37-year-old G3 P1112 (full term, preterm, abortions/miscarriage from any cause, living children) presents for an annual gynecologic examination and has questions regarding contraception. She is wondering if she is a candidate for an IUD.

Question 15.9.1 All of the following are contraindications to IUD placement EXCEPT:
A) Pregnancy
B) Acute pelvic infection
C) Undiagnosed vaginal bleeding
D) History of chlamydia infection

Answer 15.9.1 **The correct answer is "D."** Although active cervicitis and acute pelvic inflammatory disease (PID) are contraindications to placement of an IUD, a prior chlamydia infection does not exclude a patient from obtaining an IUD. Undiagnosed vaginal bleeding can be a sign of either endometritis or structural abnormalities of the uterine cavity, which must be addressed prior to considering an IUD. If you chose "A," some goons from the Board are coming to relieve you of your certification.

Your patient has none of these contraindications, and she would like to proceed with the IUD. Her friends have told her that IUDs work by causing abortions, and she is unsettled by this idea.

Question 15.9.2 The mechanism of action of IUDs (copper or progesterone) is:
A) Abortifacient
B) Causes a sterile inflammatory reaction to a foreign body
C) Impairs sperm transport from the cervix to the fallopian tube
D) B and C
E) All of the above

Answer 15.9.2 **The correct answer is "D."** Studies detecting levels of hCG reveal that this hormone is not present in IUD users during the luteal phase. Thus, the IUD is NOT an abortifacient. Studies suggest that the mechanism of action of IUDs includes interference with sperm transport from the cervix to the fallopian tube, inhibition of sperm survival, and endometrial inflammatory changes that inhibit implantation.

HELPFUL TIP:
The progesterone-releasing IUDs are approved for 3 to 5 years of contraception (depending on the brand) versus 10 years for the copper IUD.

After all of that counseling (that you can't bill for), her husband undergoes a vasectomy. During a routine appointment 2 years later, she complains of worsening menorrhagia. She denies intermenstrual spotting. She has not noticed any lightheadedness or dizziness but does complain of generalized fatigue. On physical examination, you find a normal sized thyroid and an enlarged, irregular uterus measuring 10 to 12 weeks in size. There are no distinct adnexal masses, but this is somewhat difficult to discern due to the irregular uterus.

Question 15.9.3 Your initial workup in this 39-year-old female should include all of the following EXCEPT:
A) CBC
B) TSH
C) CA-125
D) Pelvic ultrasound
E) Urine hCG (pregnancy test)

Answer 15.9.3 **The correct answer is "C."** A CBC ("A") will provide information regarding the hematocrit (and therefore the level of anemia) and platelet count—important information for someone with heavy menstrual bleeding. TSH ("B") will screen for hypothyroidism, which is a common cause of menorrhagia in a 39-year-old female. A pelvic ultrasound ("D") will aid in the evaluation of the mass palpated on examination and characterize the location and size of any uterine fibroids that may contribute to the bleeding; it will also evaluate for any adnexal masses. A pregnancy test ("E") is always a good idea to rule out possible pregnancy, ectopic pregnancy, and miscarriage as an underlying etiology. CA-125 ("C") is a nonspecific tumor marker that has a high false-positive rate in premenopausal women. Thus, CA-125 is **NOT** recommended as a screening test for ovarian (or endometrial) cancer. It can be used as an adjunct to pelvic ultrasound when a complex adnexal mass is identified.

The patient returns in 2 weeks following her ultrasound. Her hematocrit was 31% (indices are consistent with iron-deficiency anemia), platelets 195,000, and TSH 2.8 mU/L (normal). The ultrasound reveals a uterus measuring 12 × 8 × 6 cm, with multiple small intramural fibroids measuring less than 2 cm in diameter. There is one subserosal, pedunculated fibroid measuring 3.5 cm at the fundus.

Question 15.9.4 What is the most appropriate initial management?
A) Expectant management and reassurance
B) Nonsteroidal anti-inflammatory drugs (NSAIDs)
C) Gonadotropin-releasing hormone (GnRH) agonists
D) Blood transfusion
E) Hysterectomy

Answer 15.9.4 **The correct answer is "B."** Most fibroids are asymptomatic, although the most common symptom associated with leiomyomata (fibroids) is abnormal bleeding. This patient's fibroids are not impinging on the uterine cavity, but may be contributing to the patient's menorrhagia. Initial treatment of menorrhagia may include NSAIDs that inhibit prostaglandin synthesis. NSAIDs have been shown to reduce menstrual blood loss by 30% to 50% in women with menorrhagia. GnRH agonists ("C") may be utilized to produce a medical menopause. However, they are expensive, and long-term usage is associated with significant side effects (e.g., osteoporosis). Hysterectomy ("E") is the definitive treatment for leiomyomata in symptomatic women who have completed childbearing. However, the mortality associated with hysterectomy is approximately 0.5/1,000, at age 37. It is generally reserved for women who have failed medical management or have symptoms or signs related to fibroid size. This patient's lab values do not suggest a degree of anemia necessitating a blood transfusion ("D"). Of particular note, levonorgestrel-releasing IUD can be used as an alternative. Studies have shown a reduction in uterine volume and bleeding and an increase in hematocrit after placement of IUD. If the fibroids are intracavitary, an IUD should NOT be used.

You start an NSAID. She responds moderately well. You add an OCP, which adequately controls her symptoms. If the patient had not responded to medical therapy, you might have considered referral to a gynecologist for potential surgical therapy.

Question 15.9.5 What other characteristic(s) would have prompted evaluation for surgery?
A) Prolapsing fibroid through the cervix
B) 5-cm submucosal myoma protruding 50% into the uterine cavity
C) Rapidly enlarging uterus
D) 20-week sized uterus and pelvic pressure
E) All of the above

Answer 15.9.5 **The correct answer is "E."** A fibroid prolapsing through the cervix ("A") has a potential for necrosis and infection and may require surgical removal. A submucosal myoma, especially one that distorts the uterine cavity ("B"), can contribute to menorrhagia. A rapidly enlarging uterus ("C") would be concerning for a uterine malignancy and would require further investigation. Larger uterine fibroids are more likely to contribute to symptoms of pelvic pressure and pain ("D"), which may only respond to surgical correction.

The patient returns in 1 year for her annual examination, and her pelvic examination is unchanged. However, she expresses concern that these fibroids could become cancerous.

Question 15.9.6 What is the risk of uterine malignancy (leiomyosarcoma) in a patient with fibroids?
A) <1%
B) 5% to 10%
C) 40% to 50%
D) 90% to 95%

Answer 15.9.6 **The correct answer is "A."** The estimated incidence of leiomyosarcoma discovered at the time of surgery for fibroids is less than 1%. A leiomyosarcoma is a malignant tumor that does **not** arise from preexisting benign leiomyoma. Leiomyosarcomas typically arise in the fifth or sixth decade of life and are usually associated with abnormal bleeding or a rapidly enlarging uterus.

▶ **Objectives: Did you learn to …**
  · Recognize contraindications to IUD use?
  · Treat menorrhagia?
  · Describe management principles for uterine leiomyomas?

▶ CASE 15.10

A 20-year-old nulligravid female presents for evaluation of irregular menstrual cycles. Her past medical history is uncomplicated. Her gynecologic history is remarkable for menarche at age 12 years, irregular menses occurring every 21 to 40 days, and lasting 5 days, with last menstrual period 6 months ago. Her examination reveals no abnormal hair growth, no acne, normal Tanner stage V breast development, normal external genitalia and cervix, with a slightly enlarged uterus at 10 weeks size, and no adnexal masses.

Question 15.10.1 **What is the first test you should order?**
A) Pelvic ultrasound
B) Serum prolactin level
C) Urine hCG
D) Serum FSH
E) Serum TSH

Answer 15.10.1 **The correct answer is "C."** Primary amenorrhea is defined as either (1) the absence of menarche by 15 years with secondary sexual characteristics or (2) the absence of menarche by 13 years of age *with the complete absence* of secondary sexual characteristics. Secondary amenorrhea is defined as the absence of periods for three cycles in a woman who previously had menses. Pregnancy is the most common cause of secondary amenorrhea and thus must always be ruled out. After pregnancy has been excluded, the diagnostic focus is on differentiating between anatomic cause, ovarian failure, and endocrine abnormalities. The other tests may be done at some point, but a pregnancy test is first.

The urine pregnancy test is positive. Because of her irregular menses, you schedule her in 1 week for a vaginal ultrasound to confirm her gestational age. However, she calls your nurse in 3 days with vaginal spotting and lower pelvic cramping.

Question 15.10.2 **The most important diagnosis to confirm or exclude is:**
A) Spontaneous abortion
B) Incomplete abortion
C) Inevitable abortion
D) Ectopic pregnancy
E) Twin gestation

Answer 15.10.2 **The correct answer is "D."** Ectopic pregnancy is the leading cause of pregnancy-related death during the first trimester in the United States. Risk factors for ectopic pregnancy include prior PID, prior ectopic pregnancy, and prior tubal or other pelvic surgery. Spontaneous, incomplete, inevitable,

threatened, and missed abortions (or miscarriages) are terms to describe pregnancy loss occurring before 20 weeks of gestation. Each can result in significant maternal morbidity (including hemorrhage and infection) or death. However, these outcomes are less frequent than with an ectopic pregnancy.

Question 15.10.3 **Which of the following tests is/are important in the management of this patient?**
A) Progesterone level
B) Serum quantitative β-hCG
C) Hematocrit, blood type, and screen
D) Pelvic ultrasound
E) All of the above

Answer 15.10.3 **The correct answer is "E."** "A," progesterone level, helps to assess the viability of the pregnancy. A progesterone level <5 ng/mL is non-reassuring (85% spontaneous abortion, 14% ectopic pregnancy), and a level >25 ng/mL is reassuring (<2% ectopic pregnancies). Two serum quantitative β-hCGs obtained 48 hours apart help assess viability. A rise in level of >66% will occur in 85% of normal pregnancies, but only 17% of ectopic pregnancies. Transvaginal ultrasounds should be able to detect an intrauterine pregnancy at hCG levels of 1,500 to 2,000 IU. With hCG levels below 1,500 IU, an ultrasound is often still helpful for identifying an adnexal mass and potential ectopic pregnancy. A blood type and screen and hematocrit are important to evaluate for Rh status and anemia and prepare for transfusion should the hemorrhage be significant.

Upon presentation, the patient has normal vitals and appears clinically stable. The blood work returns with a hematocrit of 38% and blood type A negative, antibody screen positive for anti-D. The hCG level is 5,500 IU and progesterone is 18 ng/mL. She has not received any treatment for this bleeding prior to coming to your office.

Question 15.10.4 **While waiting for her ultrasound, you counsel her regarding her blood work, which indicates:**
A) She should receive RhoGAM immediately, given that she is Rh negative
B) She has previously been exposed to the D antigen and has developed antibodies
C) This fetus is D antigen positive and she has developed antibodies to *this* fetus
D) She should receive RhoGAM only after confirming that she has an intrauterine pregnancy

Answer 15.10.4 **The correct answer is "B."** Rh "negative" or "positive" refers to the D antigen, the antigen that is responsible for most cases of Rh sensitization. RhoGAM, or anti-D immune globulin, is used to prevent the development of Rh-D antibodies. If Rh-D antibodies are already present (i.e., the patient has already been sensitized), RhoGAM is not effective. This is why options "A" and "D" are incorrect. This patient has evidence of antibodies and has previously been exposed to the Rh-D

CHAPTER 15 · OBSTETRICS AND WOMEN'S HEALTH **477**

antigen. "C" is incorrect because not enough time has elapsed with her current bleeding to have induced antibody production to the D antigen. Without RhoGAM, 17% of mothers become sensitized. RhoGAM is recommended with ectopic pregnancies, spontaneous abortions, induced abortions, threatened abortions, amniocentesis, antepartum hemorrhage, and routinely at 28 weeks of gestation for Rh-D-negative women who are not already sensitized.

HELPFUL TIP:
If the Rh-D-negative woman is positive for D antibody, either she has previously been exposed to the D-antigen and mounted a response or she was given anti-D immune globulin during the previous 12 weeks (and it is still circulating).

The patient returns after her ultrasound, which reveals an intrauterine pregnancy measuring 6 weeks, 5 days gestation with cardiac activity at 110 beats per minute. The laboratory staff calls to report that the antibody screen was in fact an error, and the patient is A negative, antibody screen *negative* ("Oopsies!" says the lab tech). Therefore, you administer RhoGAM.

Question 15.10.5 You counsel the patient that her diagnosis at this time is:
A) Threatened abortion
B) Missed abortion
C) Complete abortion
D) Ectopic pregnancy
E) All remain in the differential

Answer 15.10.5 The correct answer is "A." Threatened abortion is defined as any vaginal bleeding in the first trimester but also incorporates those up to 20 weeks of gestation. 20 weeks of gestation, which accompanies a **currently viable** intrauterine pregnancy with a closed cervix. A missed abortion ("B") is retention of dead products of conception in utero. A complete abortion ("C") indicates the pregnancy and all products of conception have passed from the uterus. Ectopic pregnancy ("D") is incorrect as you have already confirmed by ultrasound (above) that this is an intrauterine pregnancy.

Over the next 2 days, her cramping and bleeding increase and she passes tissue (complete abortion). The patient is somewhat anxious regarding her fertility and is concerned that she may have something "wrong" with her that led to the miscarriage.

Question 15.10.6 What is the most likely etiology of this miscarriage?
A) Uterine anomalies
B) Maternal infection
C) Undiagnosed maternal diabetes
D) Embryonic chromosomal abnormality
E) Karmic retribution

Answer 15.10.6 The correct answer is "D." Approximately 50% of first trimester spontaneous miscarriages are due to chromosomal abnormalities. Some of these miscarriages will occur prior to clinical recognition of the pregnancy and will go unrecognized by the patient. "A"–"C" can be responsible for a first-trimester miscarriage as well but are less common. As to "E," ask your friendly neighborhood guru.

HELPFUL TIP:
The rate of spontaneous abortion increases with advancing maternal age. For women younger than 20 years with recognized pregnancies, the rate of spontaneous abortion is about 12%; the rate increases to 26% in women older than 40 years.

Question 15.10.7 The next step in the care of this patient is:
A) Hysterosalpingogram
B) Gonorrhea and chlamydia cultures
C) Glucose screening
D) Paternal chromosome testing
E) Counseling and reassurance

Answer 15.10.7 The correct answer is "E." Evaluation to determine the cause of this patient's pregnancy loss is not recommended. In general, evaluation is not recommended for a single first-trimester spontaneous loss if the woman is otherwise healthy. Patients with two to three *consecutive* spontaneous pregnancy losses are candidates for an evaluation to determine the etiology.

▶ **Objectives: Did you learn to …**
· Maintain a high degree of suspicion for pregnancy in a patient presenting with secondary amenorrhea?
· Identify causes of first-trimester bleeding?
· Define terminology used in spontaneous abortion (e.g., missed, completed, and threatened)?
· Manage early pregnancy loss?
· Describe Rh-D isoimmunization?

▶ **CASE 15.11**

You are now assuming care of a 28-year-old G3 P2002 at 38 3/7 weeks. Her pregnancy has been uncomplicated. On examination, you note her blood pressure is 102/66 mm Hg, urine dipstick is negative for protein and glucose, fetal heart tones are 154 beats per minute, and the fundal height is 44 cm. In reviewing her antepartum record, you note that her previous babies (Jimbo and Jumbo) weighed 8 lb 8 oz and 9 lb 6 oz at delivery. She has no history of shoulder dystocia. During this pregnancy, her lab results have been normal, and her 1-hour glucose after 75 g of glucose was 127 mg/dL at 28 weeks.

Question 15.11.1 Noting that she has a size–date discrepancy, what is your next step in the evaluation and management of this patient?
A) 3-hour glucose tolerance test
B) Nonstress test
C) Fetal ultrasound for growth and amniotic fluid index
D) Immediate induction of labor
E) Contraction stress test (CST)

Answer 15.11.1 The correct answer is "C." Size–date discrepancy can be caused by numerous maternal–fetal factors. Given the patient's history, the likely etiologies are either fetal macrosomia or polyhydramnios. Additionally, her body habitus could render the fundal height measurement inaccurate (her weight is not noted). To best determine the etiology, an ultrasound with amniotic fluid index is warranted. A 3-hour glucose tolerance test ("A") is not indicated since her screening glucose tolerance test was normal. A nonstress test ("B") may be warranted depending on the outcome of the fetal ultrasound and amniotic fluid index. However, if growth and fluid were normal, a nonstress test would not be indicated. The CST ("E") is utilized to assess fetal well-being in utero. A CST is done by administering oxytocin to induce contractions and observing the resulting FHR tracing. All else being equal, a CST is not warranted at this time.

HELPFUL TIP:
Controversy surrounds the issue of induction for fetal macrosomia. Induction for macrosomia has not been shown to improve maternal or fetal outcomes.

Question 15.11.2 Risk factors for fetal macrosomia include all of the following EXCEPT:
A) Gestational age
B) Maternal smoking
C) Excessive maternal weight gain
D) Multiparity (not a multiple gestation)
E) Macrosomia in a prior infant

Answer 15.11.2 The correct answer is "B." Maternal smoking is associated with restricted fetal growth. All of the others are associated with macrosomia. Additionally, male fetus and high maternal birth weight, and bad karma from a previous life are associated with macrosomia.

Ultrasound findings demonstrate a fetus in the vertex presentation with an estimated fetal weight of 4,200 g (9 lb 2 oz) and an amniotic fluid index of 12.6 cm (normal). You check her cervix and note that she is 1 cm dilated, 50% effaced, with vertex at 0 station.

Question 15.11.3 The optimal management at this time is:
A) Induction of labor
B) Cesarean section
C) Expectant management

D) Repeat the ultrasound weekly
E) Initiate a weight loss program

Answer 15.11.3 The correct answer is "C." Fetal macrosomia is generally defined as a birth weight greater than 4,500 g. Large for gestational age implies a birth weight greater than the 90th percentile for a given gestational age (or 4,000 g at delivery). Expectant management with spontaneous labor onset generally has been shown to have the best outcomes; all interventions entail an increase in fetal and maternal morbidity.

HELPFUL TIP:
According to ACOG (2009 and re-affirmed 2016), prophylactic cesarean section may be considered for estimated fetal weight >5,000 g in nondiabetic pregnancies and >4,500 g in diabetic pregnancies. While this practice does seem relatively common, it continues to remain controversial and has not been established in clinical trials nor appears to eliminate risk of birth-related trauma (*Obstet Gynecol.* 2016;128(5): e195–e209).

HELPFUL TIP:
Maternal risk from macrosomia is primarily related to labor abnormalities and includes postpartum hemorrhage, significant vaginal lacerations, cesarean delivery, and infection.

Contractions start spontaneously. Shortly after arrival to labor and delivery at 39 weeks, your patient has spontaneous rupture of membranes with clear fluid and requests an epidural for management of labor pain. Her cervix is 5 cm dilated, 90% effaced, and 0 station. FHR baseline is 145 bpm with moderate variability and no decelerations (a Category I tracing). Four hours later, she is comfortable after epidural is placed. *Her cervix is unchanged.*

Question 15.11.4 Appropriate intervention at this time is:
A) Induction of labor
B) Augmentation of labor
C) Cesarean section
D) Expectant management
E) Ultrasound to confirm vertex presentation

Answer 15.11.4 The correct answer is "B." Her labor has suffered from arrest of dilation and descent. At this time, the appropriate management is augmentation of labor. Induction of labor is the technical term for initiating uterine contractions before the onset of spontaneous labor, so "A" is incorrect. While expectant management ("D") may be acceptable at this point after counseling the patient, there is a risk of prolonged rupture of membranes and chorioamnionitis. Cesarean section ("C") at this point would be premature and unnecessary as dilation to 6 cm with failure of progression despite 4 hours of adequate contractions is considered the threshold for "active phase arrest" (*Obstet Gynecol.* 2016;123(3):693–711).

With IV oxytocin, she proceeds to complete and after 2 hours of pushing is ready to deliver. You anticipate a shoulder dystocia.

Question 15.11.5 Appropriate maneuvers to reduce a shoulder dystocia include all of the following EXCEPT:
A) McRoberts maneuver (flexing the patient's knees up against the abdomen)
B) Suprapubic pressure
C) Fundal pressure
D) Delivery of the posterior arm
E) Wood's corkscrew

Answer 15.11.5 The correct answer is "C." Fundal pressure may further worsen impaction of the shoulder and may result in uterine rupture—both are generally considered bad outcomes. All the others may be used to help relieve shoulder dystocia. To manage dystocia, the Advanced Life Support for Obstetrics (ALSO) course uses the "HELPERR" mnemonic: H—call for **h**elp (wait … aren't *you* the help? Call for more help!), E—**e**valuate for episiotomy, L—**l**egs flexed at the hip and knee (McRoberts maneuver), P—supra**p**ubic pressure, E—**e**nter to rotate fetus (Rubin II, Wood's corkscrew maneuver, reverse corkscrew maneuver), R—**r**emove posterior arm, and R—**r**oll the patient. There is no evidence that any one maneuver is superior to another in releasing an impacted shoulder or decreasing the chance of injury. Typically, McRoberts maneuver is used first. Last resort techniques include intentional fracture of the fetal clavicle, cephalic replacement (aka, the Zavanelli maneuver—pushing the head back up into the pelvis and performing a cesarean section), and transcutaneous symphysiotomy. Why obstetricians continue to use confusing eponyms is beyond us. But if you want to belong to the club, you need to know the secret passwords …

HELPFUL TIP:
Risk factors for shoulder dystocia include: previous shoulder dystocia, gestational diabetes, post-dates pregnancy, maternal short stature, abnormal pelvic anatomy, suspected fetal macrosomia, protracted active phase of first stage of labor, protracted second stage of labor, and assisted vaginal delivery.

In the same way that carrying an umbrella prevents a thunderstorm, merely being prepared for dystocia obviates the need for special maneuvers. The parents, happy with your care, name the baby after you but add "hotep" to the name, as in Graberhotep. Happy day! Time to talk to her about nursing.

Question 15.11.6 You tell her the benefits of breastfeeding, which include all the following EXCEPT:
A) Species-specific and age-specific nutrients for infants
B) Adequate iron for *premature* newborns
C) High level of immune protection from colostrum
D) Decreased risk of breast and ovarian cancer in mothers who breastfeed
E) Fewer illnesses while the infant is breastfed

Answer 15.11.6 The correct answer is "B." The benefits of breastfeeding for infants, women, families, and society are well documented. However, human milk may not provide adequate iron for **premature** newborns, term infants whose mothers have low iron stores, and infants older than 6 months. All the other choices are correct.

HELPFUL TIP:
Breast milk should only be kept at room temperature for 6 hours. However, it is safest to refrigerate it for 4 days maximum or freeze immediately. Do not heat refrigerated breast milk in the microwave, as it will destroy valuable micronutrients. Warming in hot water is a better way of reheating. And while we're at it, why do we assume babies want warm milk and then assume that toddlers want cold milk? Cold breast milk is OK for babies if parents want to try it—no need to warm the milk to body temperature.

Your patient and her infant do well and are discharged home on postpartum day 2.

Question 15.11.7 How do you counsel your patient regarding follow-up care after discharge?
A) She's good to go without follow-up. Baby is delivered and everybody is doing well! You can go for vacation on the beach in Costa Rica
B) Schedule follow-up in 3 weeks
C) Schedule follow-up in 6 weeks
D) Provide your "card" for any questions and see her in 1 year for her annual well-woman exam
E) B and C

Answer 15.11.7 The correct answer is "E." The immediate time period following birth is a critical period for both the woman and her infant, given the numerous new stressors and changes both are undergoing. Therefore, in 2018 ACOG recommended redefining postpartum care as a continuum instead of a single visit and thus affectionately labeling it the "fourth trimester" (and then the "fifth trimester" lasts until the kid graduates from college and starts paying for his or her own stuff, right?). It is recommended that women have contact with their maternal care provider within the first 3 weeks postpartum for an initial visit to address any acute issues following pregnancy and delivery and to further define and tailor ongoing care as needed ("B"). This initial visit should be followed by a more comprehensive well-woman visit to address ongoing care needs, psychological health, postpartum problems, and reproductive planning no later than 12 weeks following birth ("C"). "A" and "D" deserve particular mention as these would be poor delivery of care and you may as well say "Hasta la vista" to your practice.

She returns for her postpartum examination in 3 weeks and notes she is adjusting well. Her mood is doing great and she feels she has finally figured out "that whole breastfeeding thing." You schedule her for another visit in 6 weeks. At this visit, she notes incontinence of urine several times a day, especially with coughing, laughing, and sneezing. She has not experienced nocturia, dysuria, or hematuria.

Question 15.11.8 **These symptoms are indicative of which type of incontinence:**
A) Stress incontinence
B) Urge incontinence
C) Overflow incontinence
D) Functional incontinence
E) Psychogenic incontinence

Answer 15.11.8 **The correct answer is "A."** Stress incontinence is the involuntary loss of urine during physical activity such as coughing, laughing, jumping, running, and sneezing. Urge incontinence is the involuntary loss of urine associated with an abrupt and strong desire to void (detrusor overactivity). Overflow incontinence is the involuntary loss of urine due to under-activity of the detrusor muscle (e.g., neurogenic bladder) or obstruction (e.g., BPH in men) but this (urinary outlet obstruction, *not* BPH) is becoming more common in women. Functional incontinence is loss of urine associated with physical limitations (e.g., mobility restriction, arthritis, and dementia) in persons who have otherwise adequate bladder control. Psychogenic incontinence, incontinence secondary to severe depression or other psychological problem, is a rare disorder in this population and should be considered a diagnosis of exclusion. It is more frequent in patients with dementia.

Question 15.11.9 **Which of the following is most important prior to initiating incontinence therapy?**
A) Evaluate for a vaginal fistula using a dye instillation test
B) Obtain urinalysis followed by urine culture if abnormal
C) Refer for cystoscopy
D) Order urodynamic studies

Answer 15.11.9 **The correct answer is "B."** The first step in the diagnosis of incontinence is a detailed history and physical examination. A urinalysis and urine culture should be obtained to exclude urinary tract infection. Bacteriuria should be treated because the endotoxin produced by *Escherichia coli* may trigger abnormal detrusor activity or act as an α-adrenergic blocker causing urinary outlet obstruction as noted above (cool, huh?). Additional diagnostic tools may include a voiding diary, stress test (have the patient cough or bear down and see if there is leakage from the urethra), checking a postvoid residual, cystometry, and cystourethroscopy. If there is concern for a vaginal fistula elicited by the history and physical examination, dye instillation testing may be warranted (IV dye to evaluate for a ureteral fistula, bladder instillation to evaluate for a bladder fistula).

HELPFUL TIP:
Bariatric surgery (gastric banding, etc.) reduces the rate of urinary incontinence in women who qualify: body mass index (BMI) >40 or BMI >35 + comorbidities (DM, sleep apnea, severe joint disease, weight-related cardiomyopathy).

When you have completed your evaluation, you determine that she has stress urinary incontinence.

Question 15.11.10 **The best initial treatment option is:**
A) Pelvic muscle exercises
B) Trial of oxybutynin hydrochloride
C) Fitting of a pessary
D) Surgical consult
E) Incontinence pads

Answer 15.11.10 **The correct answer is "A."** Pelvic muscle exercises (e.g., Kegel exercises) facilitate improved urinary control in 40% to 75% of patients. The correct method can be taught during a routine pelvic examination. Pelvic physical therapy can be used to provide feedback on the patient's success with these exercises. "B" is incorrect. Oxybutynin hydrochloride is approved for detrusor instability (i.e., urge incontinence) and does not appear to be effective for stress incontinence. It also has significant anticholinergic side effects. "C" is incorrect. Several vaginal pessaries have been designed with the intent of providing differential support to the urethrovesical junction for treatment of stress urinary incontinence. This is an option for many women, especially those who want to avoid surgery, but a pessary would not be the initial treatment. "D" is incorrect. Surgical correction is typically reserved until 6 to 12 months postpartum, as the symptoms may continue to improve during that time. Note that surgical mesh has a very high rate of complications when used for the treatment of incontinence (mid-urethral sling) and, according to the FDA, has NO benefit over the traditional surgical treatment of stress incontinence. We would not subject our relatives (even our in-laws) to this treatment.

▶ **Objectives: Did you learn to …**
  · Evaluate and manage fetal macrosomia?
  · Manage a delivery complicated by shoulder dystocia?
  · Discuss the benefits of breastfeeding?
  · Classify urinary incontinence and treat stress-type incontinence?

▶ CASE 15.12

A 31-year-old nulligravid single female presents for a health maintenance examination. She has no gynecologic concerns, and her last menstrual period was 3 weeks ago. She uses oral contraception and has regular cycles. Her examination is unremarkable. The Pap smear returns with high-grade squamous intraepithelial neoplasia (HSIL).

Question 15.12.1 You notify her of the Pap smear findings and explain this indicates:
A) She has cervical cancer
B) She needs further diagnostic testing including colposcopy and possible biopsy
C) She needs treatment with cryotherapy or laser ablation
D) She should have the Pap smear repeated in 3 to 4 months
E) She should be enrolled in a hospice program

Answer 15.12.1 The correct answer is "B." Cervical cytology is the most effective cancer-screening program ever implemented. Both types of screening, liquid based and traditional Pap smears, have the same accuracy, and both types are endorsed for screening. Abnormal Pap smear findings require further investigation with colposcopy and directed biopsy, if indicated. Given the finding of high-grade intraepithelial neoplasia on the Pap smear, repeating the Pap smear in 3 months is inappropriate. An endocervical specimen (Pap smear or endocervical curettage) will need to be performed regardless of the appearance of the ectocervix to exclude endocervical pathology. Treatment with a non-excisional procedure ("C") is not acceptable and premature without a biopsy to confirm the diagnosis first.

You perform a colposcopy, and the cervix appears grossly normal. An endocervical Pap smear is obtained. There are acetowhite changes with areas of mosaicism at the squamocolumnar junction from the 4 o'clock to 11 o'clock position. The colposcopy is adequate.

Question 15.12.2 When you discuss the cervical findings you explain that:
A) She needs a biopsy of the abnormal area
B) Given the previous Pap smear, you recommend a "see and treat" loop electrosurgical excision procedure (LEEP)
C) The findings are consistent with dysplasia; no further therapy is warranted
D) She needs a repeat Pap smear in 3 to 4 months
E) Either A or B would be acceptable choices

Answer 15.12.2 The correct answer is "E." When acetic acid is applied to the cervix, abnormal cells tend to turn white ("acetowhite"), and as the acetowhite fades, the degree of vascularity can be appreciated. Mosaicism, or mosaic changes, refer to areas with increased vascularity and are indicative of abnormal changes, often dysplasia. However, "visual" findings at colposcopy are no more than suggestive, so "C" is incorrect. Biopsy of the area is warranted to obtain a tissue diagnosis. The

see-and-treat approach ("B") is an option for our patient since she is 31 years old; however, the see-and-treat approach should not be done in young women between the ages of 21 and 24 per the current ASCCP guidelines (yes, 21-24). In this age range, lesions often regress spontaneously. However, consider the "see-and-treat" approach in any patient who is unlikely to follow up.

The endocervical Pap smear is negative for dysplasia. You also performed a biopsy of the acetowhite change area, which revealed high-grade cervical intraepithelial neoplasia (CIN III).

Question 15.12.3 Which of the following do you recommend?
A) Hysterectomy
B) Trachelectomy
C) Cytological follow-up
D) LEEP or LASER ablation
E) 5-fluorouracil intravaginally

Answer 15.12.3 The correct answer is "D." While some patients with severe dysplasia (CIN III) may be candidates for a hysterectomy ("A"), it would be an overly aggressive approach in this 31-year-old female who has never been pregnant and may wish to conceive in the future. Additionally, women who had high-grade CIN before hysterectomy can develop recurrent vaginal dysplasia (VaIN) or cancer at the vaginal cuff. Likewise, trachelectomy (removal of the entire cervix) ("B") would be overly aggressive with no added benefit over a LEEP procedure. Cytological follow-up or "expectant management" ("C") is **NOT** recommended for high-grade dysplasia in this patient. The likelihood of regression is low in this patient's age demographic, while the likelihood of persistence or progression to cancer is unacceptably high. Young women between 21 and 24 do have the option proceeding with treatment (which is preferred with CIN III or inadequate colposcopy) OR observation with cytology and colposcopy at 6-month intervals for 12 months. A LEEP or ablation therapy would be the best recommendation in this patient. The use of 5-fluorouracil intravaginally ("E") is typically not recommended for initial treatment of **cervical dysplasi**a. It is used instead for **vaginal dysplasia**, when the extent of disease precludes complete excision or destruction.

Your patient wants to know the likelihood of regression to "normal" without treatment.

Question 15.12.4 What will you counsel?
A) About 90% of CIN III lesions will become invasive cancer without aggressive treatment
B) About one-third of CIN III lesions spontaneously regress
C) About two-thirds of CIN III lesions spontaneously regress
D) About 90% of CIN III lesions will remain CIN III on follow-up after 10 years

Answer 15.12.4 The correct answer is "B," although the data on prognosis varies due to variation in histologic diagnoses of CIN. In some studies, about one-third of untreated CIN III lesions will spontaneously regress, while about 50% will persist and the remaining will progress to invasive carcinoma. Other studies have shown progression to invasive carcinoma much higher.

She is concerned about future childbearing if she undergoes a LEEP.

Question 15.12.5 All of the following are possible complications of LEEP EXCEPT:
A) Cervical incompetence
B) Cervical stenosis
C) Cervical ectopic pregnancy
D) Decreased fertility
E) Premature rupture of membranes

Answer 15.12.5 The correct answer is "C." Cervical incompetence, stenosis, decreased fertility, and premature rupture of the membranes have been identified following all types of cone procedures, including LEEP, and are estimated to occur following less than 1% of procedures. Each of these complications seems to be related to the volume of tissue removed with the procedure rather than the procedure itself. Cervical ectopic pregnancy is quite rare and has **NOT** been associated with cone or LEEP procedures.

She undergoes LEEP treatment as recommended. The pathology reveals CIN III with margins uninvolved.

Question 15.12.6 What do you counsel her about follow-up?
A) She should return for a Pap smear and pelvic examination in 1 year
B) She should return for a Pap smear plus HPV co-testing in 12 and 24 months
C) She should return for a Pap smear in 2 to 3 months
D) She should return for a colposcopy and Pap smear in 2 to 3 months
E) She should just "chill out"; no follow-up is indicated

Answer 15.12.6 The correct answer is "B." The current recommendations for follow-up include a Pap smear plus HPV co-testing at 12 and 24 months. If both are negative, HPV co-testing should then be repeated 3 years later and if all remains negative, she then may return to routine age-based screening. If any of the Pap smears reveal atypical squamous cells (ASC) or higher grade dysplasia, or positive high-risk HPV, the patient should undergo repeat colposcopy.

At the follow-up evaluation at 12 months, her cervix appears normal, without lesions or discharge. The Pap smear returns as normal with negative high-risk HPV co-testing; however, testing is limited by absence of endocervical cells on the Pap smear.

Question 15.12.7 What is the best recommendation for management of this patient now?
A) Repeat Pap smear and co-testing in another 12 months
B) Cervical dilation and endocervical curettage
C) Cervical dilation and endocervical Pap smear
D) Repeat LEEP
E) Repeat the Pap smear as soon as possible

Answer 15.12.7 The answer is "A." Since the HPV test was negative, there is no need for further testing at this time and screening should proceed as previously outlined above for her CIN III. However, further evaluation now WOULD be necessary if the HPV were positive or unknown.

All your partners are on vacation and you are covering all their patients' test results. Suddenly you receive a STAT page from the pathology lab (a pathological emergency?). They wanted to notify you that they made a mistake when interpreting one of the Pap smear results on a 33-year-old patient and, in fact, the correct report should have been ASC-US (atypical squamous cells of undetermined significance) instead of ASC-H (atypical squamous cells, high grade). The lab technician is new here and is not quite sure if they can add on an "HPV test" to the Pap sample.

Question 15.12.8 As you prepare yourself to call the patient, what do you tell her is the next step?
A) Repeat Pap smear in 1 year
B) Ask the lab personnel to investigate if the HPV test can be done on that sample
C) Contact your malpractice attorney
D) Both A and B

Answer 15.12.8 The correct answer is "D," according to current ASCCP guidelines. If you are able to do HPV co-testing and it returns negative, she could have repeat co-testing in 3 years. If you choose to repeat cytology only in 1 year and it returns normal, she may return to age-appropriate screening. If the cytology returns with any other abnormalities greater than or equal to ASC then a colposcopy is indicated. Colposcopy would also be indicated if the HPV test returns positive. Make sure that the Pap report does not actually read ASC-H (atypical squamous cells: cannot exclude high-grade SIL). In this case, colposcopy would be indicated no matter the HPV status in this patient's age demographic. If the patient were pregnant, or between the ages of 21 and 24, management would be different. Making sure your malpractice insurance is current and up-to-date is always a good idea but probably is unnecessary in this case.

HELPFUL (MAYBE) TIP:
The guidelines for Pap smears are ridiculously complex and include differences based on patient age, pregnancy status, etc. We strongly recommend that you review the ASCCP guidelines and algorithms available at http://www.asccp.org/Default.aspx. There is also an app....but they charge you $10.00. It is cheaper to memorize it all. Some brief pearls:
• There is no need to start doing Pap smears until age 21 regardless of sexual activity; the great majority of patients with an abnormal Pap before age 21 will have regression of any lesion. HIV is an exception; see the following.

- Age 21 to 29: Screen every 3 years with cytology alone (not HPV).
- Age 30 to 65: Screen every 3 years with cytology and reflex HPV testing or every 5 years with HPV testing alone. Another option is every 5 years with cytology plus HPV ("co-testing").
- Age over 65: No screening necessary if past three consecutive Paps were normal and no risk factors.
- Hysterectomy: No need for screening unless was done for cancer or precancerous lesions. For a history of CIN 2/3 or higher, surveillance is recommended (see ASCCP guidelines).
- HIV positive: Pap smear twice in first year after diagnosis (regardless of age or mode of HIV transmission) and then yearly for 3 years. If negative, change to every 3-year testing.

▶ Objectives: Did you learn to …
- Manage an abnormal Pap test?
- Recognize the indications for colposcopy?
- Evaluate and manage cervical dysplasia?
- Recognize the risks and potential complications of LEEP?
- Manage the absence of endocervical cells on a Pap test?

▶ CASE 15.13

You are called to the emergency department to evaluate a patient with a 2-day history of abdominal pain. She is a 24-year-old G1 P1 female whose LMP was 1 week ago. On the "1–10" scale, her pain is a "12." She is on oral contraceptives for birth control. She has "never missed a pill" and "could not possibly be pregnant." Her pain is across her lower abdomen and a little more on the right side than the left. She has felt feverish. She has had some nausea but no vomiting. She denies bowel or bladder problems. Her pain improves with acetaminophen and worsens with activity.

On examination, she appears uncomfortable but not toxic. Her temperature is 38°C, but the rest of her vitals are normal. Her abdominal examination reveals decreased bowel sounds, with tenderness to palpation primarily across the lower quadrants. She has minimal guarding and no rebound tenderness. Her pelvic examination is remarkable for cervical motion tenderness. The uterus is of normal size and consistency with no masses.

Question 15.13.1 **Which of the following diagnoses can be absolutely excluded from your differential at this point?**
A) Ectopic pregnancy
B) Appendicitis
C) Pelvic inflammatory disease (PID)
D) Pyelonephritis
E) None of the above diagnoses should be excluded based on the information available

Answer 15.13.1 **The correct answer is "E."** The differential for lower abdominal pain in a young female includes all of the previously mentioned and more. Even though your patient seems unlikely to be pregnant due to her consistent use of contraceptives and recent menses, you should not exclude pregnancy without a negative urine hCG. Emergency department studies consistently show that women who claim to never have been sexually active can be pregnant. Either virgin births are a lot more common than we think or patient history cannot always be trusted.

You obtain cultures/PCR for chlamydia and gonorrhea. The urine pregnancy test is negative ("I told you not to waste healthcare dollars—especially in this economy," your patient complains). The urinalysis is negative for nitrites and leukocytes, and the WBC is 15,600/mm³ with an increase in bands. She reports that she's had an appendectomy.

Question 15.13.2 **What is the most appropriate next step?**
A) Consult surgery and gynecology to confirm your findings
B) Admit for IV antibiotics and IV hydration
C) Treat as an outpatient with antibiotics and schedule follow-up for 36 to 48 hours
D) Treat with IV antibiotics on an outpatient basis utilizing visiting nurse care
E) Obtain cultures, discharge the patient, and treat based on culture results

Answer 15.13.2 **The correct answer is "C."** The patient's history, examination, and diagnostic tests are most consistent with pelvic inflammatory disease (PID). PID is a clinical syndrome caused by the ascent of microorganisms from the lower genital tract (e.g., vagina) to the upper genital tract (e.g., endometrium). Most cases of PID can be managed in the outpatient setting. Indications for hospitalization are listed in Table 15-7.

 HELPFUL TIP:
The diagnosis of PID is a **clinical** one and not laboratory based! Untreated PID has significant morbidity and mortality; empiric treatment is recommended by the

TABLE 15-7 CRITERIA FOR ADMISSION FOR THE TREATMENT OF PID

- Uncertain diagnosis
- Surgical emergencies (e.g., appendicitis) cannot be excluded
- Suspected tubo-ovarian abscess
- Concurrent pregnancy (due to high risk of maternal mortality, fetal loss, and preterm delivery)
- Severe illness, intractable nausea and vomiting, or high fever
- Patient cannot tolerate or follow an outpatient regimen (e.g., severe vomiting)
- Lack of clinical response to oral outpatient antimicrobial therapy

Adapted with permission from Gradison M. Pelvic inflammatory disease. *Am Fam Physician.* 2012;85(8):791–796. Copyright © 2012 American Academy of Family Physicians. All rights reserved.

CDC if the patient meets the following minimal diagnostic criteria:

*   Uterine/adnexal tenderness **or**
*   Cervical motion tenderness **and**
*   No other cause for illness identified

Other helpful (but not necessary) criteria include:

*   Temperature ≥38.3°C
*   Abnormal cervical or vaginal mucopurulent discharge
*   Presence of an abundant number of white cells on saline microscopy of vaginal fluid
*   Adnexal mass
*   Laboratory evidence of gonorrhea or chlamydia infection
*   Elevated C-reactive protein and/or ESR

Question 15.13.3 For empiric antibiotic therapy for PID in this patient, you prescribe:
A) Amoxicillin 500 mg PO TID for 14 days
B) Ceftriaxone 250 mg IM once **PLUS** azithromycin 1 g
C) Ceftriaxone 250 mg IM once **PLUS** doxycycline 100 mg PO BID for 14 days
D) A and B
E) B and C

Answer 15.13.3 The correct answer is "C." Recommendations for treatment of PID include ceftriaxone (Rocephin) 250 mg IM once **PLUS** doxycycline 100 mg PO BID for 14 (yes, 14) days. Metronidazole may be added to this regimen to cover anaerobic bacteria. *Note that single-dose azithromycin is not indicated for the treatment of PID, only for cervicitis.* Thus, 14 days of doxycycline are indicated.

The current (2015) CDC treatment guidelines for rectal, oral, cervical, or penile gonorrhea include ceftriaxone 250 mg IM once **PLUS** azithromycin 1 g or 7 days of doxycycline. This is true even if the patient has **ONLY** gonorrhea. This is to prevent the development of resistant gonorrhea and also due to the high co-infection rate of gonorrhea with chlamydia. If ceftriaxone is not available, cefixime 400 mg orally in a single dose PLUS azithromycin 1 g orally in a single dose is an appropriate alternative. Of note, patients who have been treated for gonorrhea should be re-tested 3 months after treatment regardless of whether they believe their sex partners were treated as there is a high incidence of re-infection (CDC, 2015).

You administer ceftriaxone and instruct her to finish a 14-day course of doxycycline. She presents for follow-up a week later, at which time her symptoms have completely resolved.

Question 15.13.4 Which of the following is a potential consequence of PID?
A) Infertility
B) Chronic pelvic pain
C) Increased risk for ectopic pregnancy
D) Recurrent PID
E) All of the above

Answer 15.13.4 The correct answer is "E." All the choices previously listed are potential sequelae of PID. Additionally, a tubo-ovarian abscess may develop.

HELPFUL TIP:
The etiology of PID is polymicrobial, although sexually transmitted infections, predominantly gonorrhea and/or chlamydia, are implicated in up to two-thirds of cases. Antibiotic regimens are chosen for broad coverage. The CDC no longer recommends the use of fluoroquinolones for treatment of PID or gonorrhea due to increasing resistance. Of note, there is ceftriaxone-resistant gonorrhea in Japan and elsewhere with intermediate-resistant gonorrhea in the United States. There is also azithromycin-resistant gonorrhea in the United States.

Later she returns for a health maintenance examination. She quit taking her oral contraceptive 3 months ago after separating from her husband (the jerk gave her chlamydia, after all!). Subsequently, her periods have been irregular. She is not obese, has minimal acne, and no hirsutism or galactorrhea. Her physical examination is essentially normal. Urine hCG is negative (you *did* immediately think of an hCG, didn't you?) and a serum TSH is normal.

Question 15.13.5 What is the most likely etiology of the irregular cycles?
A) Anovulation
B) Pituitary tumor
C) Polycystic ovarian syndrome
D) Premature ovarian failure
E) Androgen-secreting tumor

Answer 15.13.5 The correct answer is "A." OCPs work by suppressing ovulation. Resumption of ovulation after pill cessation can take up to 6 months. In the absence of abnormal history, physical examination, or laboratory findings, the other choices are unlikely to be the etiology of the irregular cycles in this patient.

Question 15.13.6 Each of the following is appropriate initial management of this patient's irregular menses EXCEPT:
A) Expectant management
B) Reestablishment of cycle regulation with OCPs
C) Progestin-induced withdrawal cycles
D) Colposcopy with cervical and endometrial biopsies

Answer 15.13.6 The correct answer is "D." Anovulation is expected following OCP cessation; thus, expectant management is a reasonable option, as most people will resume regular cycling within 6 months. She could also opt to resume OCPs for cycle regulation if that is her goal. Withdrawal bleeds could be induced by cyclical progestin challenges. Colposcopy is not indicated in this patient as she has no cytologic abnormalities noted that would require follow-up with colposcopy and biopsy.

....

The patient is reluctant to resume "the pill" and elects expectant management. You next evaluate her 8 months later. Her last period was 7 weeks before. A urine pregnancy test is positive. Given her history of PID, you request a quantitative serum β-hCG and are considering a pelvic ultrasound to confirm intrauterine pregnancy.

Question 15.13.7 What is the minimum expected increase in quantitative hCG in early gestation in a normal pregnancy?
A) 20% increase in 24 hours
B) 66% increase in 48 hours
C) 100% increase in 24 hours
D) 10% increase in 48 hours
E) 75% increase in 72 hours

Answer 15.13.7 The correct answer is "B." hCG typically doubles (increases by 100%) every 48 hours in normal gestation. The minimum increase considered to be compatible with a viable pregnancy is 66% in 48 hours.

Question 15.13.8 If the quantitative serum β-hCG is 5,500 ng/mL and the pelvic ultrasound reveals no intrauterine pregnancy but a probable right tubal pregnancy, what would be the most appropriate management option?
A) Medical management with methotrexate
B) Laparoscopic surgery with evacuation of the products of conception
C) Consultation with someone able to do a salpingectomy if necessary
D) Dilation and curettage
E) Hysterectomy

Answer 15.13.8 The correct answer is "C." An ectopic pregnancy may rupture and become a life-threatening event at any point before complete resolution. If the patient becomes hemodynamically unstable, she will need emergent surgery. Thus, an early referral for management is warranted. Medical treatment with methotrexate may be indicated, but should be done under close supervision with surgical consultation available.

Question 15.13.9 If the quantitative serum β-hCG had come back at 1,000 ng/mL and no ultrasound were available, how would you have counseled the patient?
A) Given the history of PID, this is most likely an ectopic pregnancy. She should abort the pregnancy at once
B) Given the history of PID, she should remain on bed rest until a definitive diagnosis is made
C) She should be educated about ectopic pregnancy and miscarriage
D) She should have an urgent surgical consultation today for exploratory laparotomy

Answer 15.13.9 The correct answer is "C." This β-hCG level is consistent with an early gestation given her history of irregular cycles. However, with her history of PID, she is at risk for ectopic pregnancy. Thus, she should receive ectopic pregnancy and miscarriage precautions. While a history of PID increases the risk of ectopic pregnancy by 7- to 10-fold, only 8% of such patients will ever have an ectopic. So, it is still highly probable that the patient has a normal intrauterine pregnancy. If you chose "E," you may also want to hand her the pamphlet entitled "Choosing a Better Doctor."

....

Well, those were interesting thought experiments, but in reality, her quantitative serum β-hCG is 6,000 ng/mL. A pelvic ultrasound confirms a viable intrauterine pregnancy at 8 and 4/7 weeks of gestation and everyone is happy. She names the baby after you but with the suffix "lars," as in "Wilburlars."

 HELPFUL TIP:
Assisted reproductive technology substantially increases the risk of a heterotopic pregnancy (two pregnancies with only one inside the uterus) to about 1%, and in these patients, the rate of ectopic pregnancy is 4% to 8%, which is about fourfold higher than the general population. Having one ectopic pregnancy predisposes to having a subsequent one.

▶ **Objectives: Did you learn to …**
· Evaluate a patient with pelvic pain?
· Diagnose and treat PID?
· Evaluate and treat irregular menses?
· Diagnose and manage ectopic pregnancies?

▶ **CASE 15.14**

A 52-year-old female patient of yours presents for a health maintenance examination and Pap smear. Her last menstrual period was 3 months ago. She has intermittent hot flashes and night sweats. Her examination is remarkable for mild vaginal atrophy. She wonders about "estrogen testing" to see if she needs hormone replacement therapy.

Question 15.14.1 How will you counsel her about the role of estrogen testing?
A) Recommend against estrogen testing
B) Recommend buccal swab testing as it is the most accurate
C) Recommend fasting morning serum estradiol testing
D) Recommend estrogen testing with FSH to ensure menopause status
E) Recommend annual estrogen testing after the age of 55 years

Answer 15.14.1 The correct answer is "A." In a woman of the right age with symptoms consistent with menopause, no testing is recommended. Testing is only recommended if the diagnosis is unclear (e.g., a patient younger than 35). It can also be useful when a patient on OCPs presents with symptoms suggestive of menopause. In this case, an FSH could be done after the patient has discontinued hormonal contraception for 1 week (or on the last day of her placebo pills). If the FSH is high (>25 mIU/L), this indicates that the patient has likely entered the menopausal transition.

She jokes that you're probably getting kickbacks from the insurance company for ordering fewer tests, and then she asks, "How will you know if I'm going through menopause without an estrogen level?"

Question 15.14.2 How will you counsel her about menopause and its diagnosis?
A) FSH is the definitive test
B) There is no definitive test of menopause
C) 6 months amenorrhea, elevated FSH, and decreased estradiol confirm the diagnosis
D) 12 months amenorrhea, elevated FSH, and decreased estradiol are the definitive test
E) 2 years of mood swings and hot flashes will clinch the diagnosis

Answer 15.14.2 The correct answer is "B." Menopause is a clinical syndrome characterized by the cessation of spontaneous menstrual periods along with associated symptoms of estrogen deficiency such as hot flashes, vaginal atrophy, and psychological symptoms. As such, there is no definitive test.

She is concerned about menopause and wonders if she needs hormone replacement therapy.

Question 15.14.3 All the following are benefits of estrogen-containing hormone replacement therapy (HRT) EXCEPT:
A) Osteoporosis prevention
B) Decrease in colon cancer risk
C) Decrease in hot flashes and vasomotor symptoms
D) Decrease in stroke risk

Answer 15.14.3 The correct answer is "D." We have learned a lot about HRT in postmenopausal women with data from the Women's Health Initiative. Here's a quick summary. Proven benefits of HRT are limited to the following:

• Reduced risk of osteoporosis and related fractures
• Improvement of vasomotor symptoms such as hot flashes
• Decreased colon cancer risk (**not** seen in estrogen only arm). Data now suggest that even though the number of colon cancers is reduced, they are diagnosed at a more advanced stage. HRT is not recommended for chemoprevention of colon cancer in women

HRT may increase the risk of the following (variable findings):

• Breast cancer (estrogen-only arm showed a paradoxical **reduction** in risk of breast cancer)
• Myocardial infarction (estrogen-only arm showed no increase risk)
• Venous thromboembolic events
• Stroke

Only women with vasomotor symptoms appear to have improved overall quality-of-life scores with HRT. Given the

significant excess risks with HRT usage, many practitioners now recommend short-term HRT use only for vasomotor symptoms and not for osteoporosis prevention or other purported benefits.

Question 15.14.4 An absolute contraindication to use of HRT is:
A) Heart disease
B) Breast cancer
C) Endometrial cancer
D) Previous thromboembolic event
E) All of the above

Answer 15.14.4 The correct answer is "D." Previous thromboembolic disease is the only *absolute* contraindication to HRT. The others are *relative* contraindications. While HRT is not routinely recommended for women who have heart disease or a history of breast or endometrial cancer, it may be useful in women who have significant impairment in their quality of life from vasomotor symptoms refractory to other management methods. *Topical estrogens clearly have a lower risk of thromboembolic disease (vaginal rings or transcutaneous patches).*

You discuss menopause and the potential risks and benefits of HRT with your patient. She decides against HRT for now, but returns in 6 months with continued amenorrhea, hot flashes, and vaginal dryness—which seems to bother her the most.

Question 15.14.5 Options to treat the vaginal dryness include which of the following?
A) Systemic HRT
B) Vaginal estrogen
C) Lubrication
D) All of the above

Answer 15.14.5 The correct answer is "D." Systemic and local estrogen administration are both effective for treating vaginal dryness. Lubrication with vegetable/olive oil (preferably cold pressed, extra virgin, organic) and specifically manufactured lubricants can be effective.

HELPFUL TIP:
A new medication Osphena (ospemifene) is available for vaginal dryness and post menopausal dyspareunia. It claims to be "non-hormonal" but carries the same warnings about endometrial cancer and cardiovascular disorders as do the estrogens and is an estrogen receptor agonist/antagonist. It is about $9.00/pill. "We won't get fooled again!"

Question 15.14.6 How is vaginal atrophy most rapidly and *accurately* diagnosed?
A) Biopsy of vaginal mucosa
B) Culture of vaginal swab
C) Patient's history and physical examination
D) Serum hormone levels
E) KOH prep of vaginal swab

Answer 15.14.6 The correct answer is "C." The diagnosis of urogenital atrophy is clinical, based on history and physical examination findings. Tests such as microscopic examination of the vaginal smear will reveal an abundance of basal and para-basal cells and a paucity of mature squamous epithelium. A biopsy is a bit extreme. "B" and "E" are incorrect since atrophy is not an infectious issue.

....

Despite your tepid endorsement of HRT, she wants to try it to reduce hot flashes. You also counsel her on other options to treat hot flashes.

Question 15.14.7 Further options to treat symptomatic hot flashes include which of the following?
A) Progesterone alone
B) Clonidine
C) Exercise
D) Trial of an SSRI
E) All of the above

Answer 15.14.7 The correct answer is "E." HRT is the most efficacious treatment for vasomotor symptoms with almost 90% of women responding. Other options include progestins such as medroxyprogesterone (Provera) or megestrol (Megace), SSRIs, clonazepam, gabapentin (Neurontin), venlafaxine (Effexor), clonidine, exercise, and environmental modifications (e.g., thermostat settings, fans). *Note that we do not list estrogen alone. Unopposed estrogen can increase the risk of endometrial cancer and should be avoided unless the woman has had a hysterectomy.* There is no good evidence for the efficacy of vitamin E and black cohosh. Some phytoestrogens do reduce hot flashes (about one less per day) but not sweating, and the effect may not be clinically significant.

▶ **Objectives: Did you learn to ...**
  · Evaluate menopausal symptoms?
  · Describe hormone replacement therapy, including risks, benefits, and contraindications for its use?
  · Diagnose and manage atrophic vaginitis?
  · Treat menopausal symptoms?

▶ **CASE 15.15**

A 57-year-old postmenopausal patient presents for her annual examination. She is experiencing hot flashes and night sweats, as well as a recurrence of vaginal bleeding. Her medical history is otherwise unremarkable. She wants your opinion about resuming hormone replacement. Her pelvic examination is remarkable for atrophic vaginal mucosal changes, a stenotic cervix without lesions, normal size uterus, no adnexal masses, and no masses palpable on rectovaginal examination.

Question 15.15.1 All of the following are possible causes of her vaginal bleeding EXCEPT:
A) Cervical cancer
B) Uterine polyp
C) Polycystic ovary disease
D) Atrophic vaginitis
E) Endometrial cancer

Answer 15.15.1 The correct answer is "C." Polycystic ovarian disease does not cause vaginal bleeding in postmenopausal women. All the other choices are diagnostic considerations in a postmenopausal female with vaginal bleeding or spotting.

Question 15.15.2 Which of the following studies should you consider obtaining?
A) Urinalysis
B) Pap smear
C) Endometrial biopsy
D) Stool guaiac
E) All of the above

Answer 15.15.2 The correct answer is "E." The patient could mistake the source of the bleeding; thus, it is prudent to rule out a rectal or urinary source. Cervical and endometrial evaluations are necessary to rule out gynecological pathology, such as endometrial polyp, hyperplasia, or cancer.

Question 15.15.3 All of the following increase the risk of endometrial cancer EXCEPT:
A) Smoking
B) Obesity
C) Unopposed estrogen
D) Diabetes
E) Hypertension

Answer 15.15.3 The correct answer is "A." Endometrial cancer is believed to be caused by unopposed estrogen stimulation of the endometrium. Smoking decreases luteal phase estrogen and is epidemiologically linked to a **decrease** in the risk for endometrial carcinoma (of course, this risk is offset by the other adverse health effects of smoking—go figure!). Risk factors and protective factors for endometrial cancer are listed in Tables 15-8 and 15-9.

TABLE 15-8 RISK FACTORS FOR ENDOMETRIAL CANCER

Advancing age
Obesity[a]
Nulliparity
Early menarche
Late menopause
Chronic anovulation (e.g., PCOS)
Unopposed exogenous estrogen use
Tamoxifen
Hypertension
Diabetes
Estrogen producing tumor
Lynch Syndrome

[a]Obesity leads to increased estrogen levels from peripheral conversion of androstenedione. The presence of DM and HTN as risk factors may simply reflect the high incidence of obesity in patients with these disorders.

TABLE 15-9 PROTECTIVE FACTORS FOR ENDOMETRIAL CANCER[a]

Progesterone
Oral contraceptives
Cigarette smoking
Multiparity
Child bearing at an older age

[a]All reduce exposure to unopposed estrogens.

You review your patient's test results: normal Pap smear and urinalysis, stool guaiac negative for blood, and endometrial biopsy with fragments of benign polyp.

Over the next 3 years, she continues to have rare occurrences of vaginal spotting. She has declined further evaluation given the infrequency of the episodes. However, over the past several months, she has experienced an increase in the amount and frequency of the bleeding. Other than an interval weight gain of 27 lb, there has been no change in her examination. Repeat endometrial biopsy reveals complex hyperplasia with atypia, and the pathologist cannot rule out endometrial cancer.

Question 15.15.4 Of the following, the most appropriate intervention is:
A) Repeating the endometrial biopsy
B) Performing a transvaginal ultrasound to assess endometrial thickness
C) Starting high-dose progestin therapy
D) Starting high-dose selective estrogen receptor modulator therapy (e.g., tamoxifen)
E) Arranging for definitive management (e.g., hysterectomy)

Answer 15.15.4 The correct answer is "E." Her biopsy findings are highly abnormal and may indicate already existing carcinoma that was not contained in the sample examined. Referral to a gynecologist for definitive management is warranted at this time.

HELPFUL TIP:
In postmenopausal women, an endometrial stripe of greater than 5 mm on ultrasound is suggestive of endometrial cancer. With an endometrial stripe of 4 or 5 mm or less, malignancy is rare. In evaluation of postmenopausal women with vaginal bleeding, transvaginal ultrasound is an alternative to endometrial biopsy when an endometrial biopsy cannot be done. Further benefit of obtaining a transvaginal ultrasound, regardless of endometrial biopsy, is that it can detect structural lesions or masses. Often, both modalities are required to arrive at the right diagnosis for postmenopausal bleeding.

▶ **Objectives:** Did you learn to …
• Evaluate postmenopausal bleeding?
• Manage a patient with postmenopausal bleeding?
• Assess patient for risk of endometrial cancer?

▶ **CASE 15.16**

A 15-year-old nulligravid female presents with her mother for evaluation of painful periods. Menarche was at age 14. Her periods are typically every 4 to 8 weeks and are associated with severe cramping. She has missed 1 to 2 days of school with each menses because of pain. She denies intercourse. She has never had a pelvic examination. Her review of systems is otherwise negative.

Question 15.16.1 What is the MOST LIKELY etiology of the irregular cycles in *this* patient?
A) Pregnancy
B) Endometriosis
C) Anovulation
D) Hyperthyroidism
E) Imperforate hymen

Answer 15.16.1 The correct answer is "C." Abnormal uterine bleeding is common among adolescent girls who have reached menarche. The first few years of menstruation are often characterized by irregular cycles as a result of anovulation. Pregnancy and imperforate hymen ("A" and "E") lead to absence of menses, not irregular menses. While hyperthyroidism ("D") may lead to irregular cycles, it does not typically cause dysmenorrhea and is usually associated with other systemic complaints. Additionally, hyperthyroidism would be unusual, but not out of the question, in a patient of this age. Endometriosis ("B") may cause dysmenorrhea but is unlikely to occur in a patient this young; most cases of endometriosis present in patients aged 20s to 30s.

Question 15.16.2 What is the etiology of this patient's dysmenorrhea?
A) Prostaglandin release
B) Streptococcal endotoxin release
C) Estrogen release
D) Excessive testosterone production

Answer 15.16.2 The correct answer is "A." Dysmenorrhea is the term that describes excessive pain in association with menstruation. It is the most common gynecologic complaint, affects about half of all adolescent females, and is the leading cause of periodic school absenteeism. The pathogenesis of dysmenorrhea involves excess prostaglandin release, which causes prolonged, painful uterine contractions. It can be divided in two main subtypes: primary and secondary. Primary dysmenorrhea usually starts before the age of 20 and has a tendency to occur with menarche. It is caused by prostaglandin stimulation of the myometrium. Secondary dysmenorrhea typically arises after the age of 20 and is associated with pelvic pathology or other organic disease.

You perform a physical examination, revealing normal vital signs, normal weight, a benign abdomen, Tanner stage V, and no signs of androgen excess.

Question 15.16.3 Which of the following is the best next step in caring for this patient?
A) Offer reassurance and observation
B) Initiate combined hormonal contraception
C) Initiate a GnRH agonist
D) Prescribe a narcotic analgesic
E) Refer for diagnostic laparoscopy

Answer 15.16.3 **The correct answer is "B."** OCPs offer cycle regulation and a reduction in dysmenorrhea. "A," expectant management, is inappropriate, given the severity of symptoms and availability of safe and effective treatment. A further workup is not needed at this stage, as her history is straightforward, and her physical examination is reassuring. She certainly does not need surgery now ("E"). "C" is incorrect. GnRH agonists will induce amenorrhea, hot flashes, accelerated bone loss, are expensive, and require add-back estrogen when utilized longer than 6 months. Narcotic analgesics ("D") do not help reduce prostaglandin levels and are not appropriate for pain control in this case. *NOTE*: Although not listed in the answers, NSAIDs are quite effective at treating dysmenorrhea and should be considered as a first-line drug. Anecdotal evidence suggests that mefenamic acid (Ponstel) may be more effective for dysmenorrhea than other NSAIDs. Acetaminophen is not as effective as NSAIDs.

HELPFUL TIP:
The average age of menarche is 12.8 years in the United States, with the range from 10 to 15 years.

Your patient and her mother opt to try hormonal regulation with birth control pills. She returns for follow-up in 4 months and is doing well. She admits to being sexually active.

Question 15.16.4 In addition to reviewing the use of birth control pills, she should be questioned or counseled about which of the following?
A) Knowledge of sexually transmitted diseases and use of condoms
B) Age of her boyfriend
C) Consensual nature of her relationship
D) HPV vaccination
E) All of the above

Answer 15.16.4 **The correct answer is "E."** Visits for contraception are great opportunities for you to discuss safe sexual practices with the patient. Such an interview should include evaluation for sexual assault, coercion, or abuse. Although she is a little late for starting HPV vaccination, "D" is still correct

(better late than never—truly!). The ACIP recommends the routine use of 9-valent HPV vaccine (Gardasil 9) in all individuals age 11-26. Vaccination can start as young as age 9. 9-valent vaccines are given in three doses (0, 2, and 6 months from first dose). If patient gets their first two vaccines prior to age 15, they only need the first two doses at 0 and 6 months. HPV vaccine should also be considered for those 27-45 where the benefit may still outweigh the risk.

HELPFUL TIP:
HPV is the most common viral sexually transmitted infection in the United States with point prevalence in females ranging from 26% to 64%. Many patients have serial infections with different HPV types. Recent data suggests that there is herd immunity to HPV. Keep pushing those vaccines!

HELPFUL TIP:
The best time to check a pregnancy test is after the first missed menses. Otherwise, you risk having a false-negative test. Even on day 1 of a missed menses, the sensitivity is only 90% (thus, patients can present with an ectopic pregnancy with a negative urine pregnancy test).

You lose touch with the patient, and she discontinues her OCP. Years later when she returns for a health maintenance examination—and you're still paying off your student loans—she complains of increasing irritability along with intermittent bloating and swelling during the week before her period each month. Although she is annoyed by these symptoms, they are not so severe as to interfere with her usual activities. Her menses now occur monthly without intermenstrual spotting or missed periods.

Question 15.16.5 What is her most likely diagnosis?
A) Major depression
B) Premenstrual dysphoric disorder (PMDD)
C) Premenstrual syndrome (PMS)
D) Polycystic ovary syndrome (PCOS)
E) Hypothyroidism

Answer 15.16.5 **The correct answer is "C."** PMS is a constellation of physical, emotional, and behavioral symptoms. It is cyclical in nature, occurs during the second half of the menstrual cycle (luteal phase, 7–10 days before menses), and resolves soon after menses. A symptom-free interval occurs during the first half of the cycle (follicular phase). PMDD ("B") is more severe but occurs during the same time frame as PMS. Symptoms of PMDD include: labile mood, depressed mood, irritability, feelings of hopelessness, hypersomnia or insomnia, and decreased interest in usual activities. PMDD is diagnosed by DSM-V criteria and some functional impairment must be present.

HELPFUL TIP:
Premenstrual symptoms exist on a continuum with up to 90% of women affected by minimal PMS symptoms while 10% are severely affected. This group with more severe symptoms can be categorized as having PMDD.

Question 15.16.6 Each of the following is a key element of the diagnosis of PMS EXCEPT:
A) Physical symptoms of bloating, swelling, and/or fatigue
B) Elevated luteinizing hormone to follicle stimulation hormone (LH:FSH) ratio
C) Restriction of symptoms to the luteal phase of the menstrual cycle
D) Exclusion of other diagnoses that may better explain the symptoms

Answer 15.16.6 The correct answer is "B." PMS is a clinical entity and no laboratory data exist to aid in diagnosis. All other options described above are correct. An elevated LH:FSH ratio of 3:1 in the face of appropriate symptoms is suggestive of PCOS.

Question 15.16.7 Each of the following is a possible treatment option for PMS and PMDD EXCEPT:
A) Supportive therapy/counseling
B) Aerobic exercise
C) Selective serotonin reuptake inhibitors
D) Thiazide diuretics

Answer 15.16.7 The correct answer is "D." Thiazide diuretics are not helpful in PMS or PMDD, but all of the other options are potentially useful. Calcium has been used in the past, but the best data suggests that it is no more effective than placebo (30%). Treatment options that have been shown to help with PMS are listed in Table 15-10.

▶ **Objectives: Did you learn to …**
- Evaluate concerns about menarche and describe normal early menstrual patterns?
- Evaluate and manage dysmenorrhea?
- Diagnose and treat PMS?

▶ **CASE 15.17**

A frantic 25-year-old patient calls you. She and her boyfriend were having intercourse and the condom broke at the time of ejaculation about 16 hours ago. She does not use any other form of contraception. Her last menstrual period was about 2 weeks ago. You tell her that 8% of women become pregnant

TABLE 15-10 TREATMENT OPTIONS FOR PREMENSTRUAL SYNDROME

Nonpharmacologic
Aerobic exercise
Increased intake of complex carbohydrates and fiber
Reduction in sodium, caffeine, and alcohol intake
Supportive psychotherapy
Pharmacologic
Anxiolytics such as buspirone and benzodiazepines
Calcium and vitamin D supplementation
Danazol
Hormonal treatment (combination OCPs, GnRH agonists, progesterones)
NSAIDs
Serotonergic antidepressants such as SSRIs and venlafaxine
Spironolactone (NOT thiazide diuretics)
Vitamin B6 (pyridoxine)
Chasteberry

Adapted from Biggs W, Demuth RH. Premenstrual syndrome and premenstrual dysphoric disorder. *Am Fam Physician*. 2011;84(8):918–924.

after a single act of coitus. She is mortified, exclaiming, "I've always been in the top 8% of everything!"

Question 15.17.1 Appropriate methods of "emergency contraception" for this patient include:
A) Levonorgestrel (Plan B)
B) Ethinyl estradiol plus levonorgestrel (Yuzpe regimen)
C) High-dose ethinyl estradiol (Ivanapyuk method)
D) A and B only
E) A, B, and C

Answer 15.17.1 The correct answer is "D." Many OCPs are also effective if used at the right doses and within 72 hours (the Yuzpe method). Currently, only levonorgestrel (Plan B) and ulipristal (Ella) are FDA-approved for postcoital contraception. Plan B uses a high dose of levonorgestrel and is more effective than the combined OCPs for postcoital contraception. Plan B is available over the counter (in the United States). Ella (ulipristal) appears to be more effective than Plan B and may be taken up to 120 hours after unprotected intercourse but is only available by prescription. The Paraguard IUD (copper IUD) is another option and may be used up to 8 days after unprotected intercourse. "C" is incorrect as estrogen alone is not known to be effective as emergency contraception, and "Ivanapyuk" is a made-up name (but a good description of what happens to a patient who takes a massive dose of estrogen).

HELPFUL TIP:
Prescribe an antiemetic with postcoital OCPs as nausea and vomiting are common side effects. Plan B has fewer GI side effects. About the only contraindication to postcoital treatment is active pregnancy. Use a progestin-only regimen (Plan B) in women with a history of thromboembolism.

HELPFUL TIP:
Mifepristone (Mifeprex) is not approved in the United States **for postcoital pregnancy prophylaxis**, but is very effective (99–100%) and has a more favorable side-effect profile when compared with other regimens. Mifepristone *is* approved by the FDA to use in conjunction with misoprostol (Cytotec) for termination of early pregnancy (within 49 days of last menstrual period). Of note, there have been serious adverse events associated with this combination, including sepsis from *Clostridium* infections and even death. However, these events are very rare extremely rare and poses less of an overall risk than surgical abortion.

You recommend Plan B. Since she now trusts you, she schedules an appointment with you for evaluation of intermittent abdominal and pelvic pain. Her pain has gradually worsened over the last 2 years and is almost omnipresent. Now she complains of severe abdominal cramping and stabbing in the right lower quadrant. The pain radiates to the left lower quadrant at times and is worse during menstruation. Her periods have become heavier and occasionally irregular. She has no bowel or bladder symptoms. She has been missing work 1 or 2 days each month and is now concerned about her job.

Your examination reveals a well-developed woman who looks depressed and uncomfortable. Her abdomen is soft, nondistended, and diffusely tender to palpation in the lower quadrants. There is no evidence of guarding, rebound tenderness, or palpable masses. She has no back tenderness. The external genital and vaginal examinations show no lesions or erythema. There is a creamy discharge noted at the cervix. Bimanual reveals a retroverted uterus with uterosacral nodularity palpable. Both adnexal areas are tender to examination, but without masses.

You get a pregnancy test, cultures, and urinalysis, all of which are negative.

Question 15.17.2 Based on her symptoms and your physical examination, what is the most likely etiology of the patient's chronic pelvic pain?
A) Irritable bowel syndrome
B) Myofascial pain disorder
C) Endometriosis
D) Cervical dysplasia
E) Painful bladder syndrome (the disease formerly known as interstitial cystitis)

Answer 15.17.2 **The correct answer is "C."** There were no bowel symptoms elicited on the history to suggest irritable bowel syndrome ("A"). There were no signs elicited on the examination to suggest a myofascial pain disorder ("B"). The patient's history and physical examination, including uterosacral nodularity, is consistent with a diagnosis of endometriosis ("C"). Dysplasia ("D") is typically asymptomatic. There were

no bladder symptoms elicited on the history to suggest painful bladder syndrome ("E"). *Be truthful; have you ever actually felt ligament nodularity?*

HELPFUL TIP:
If after a careful assessment the diagnosis of endometriosis is highly likely, empiric therapy is considered a viable alternative to laparoscopy and preferred by many experts. However, definitive diagnosis relies upon direct visualization of endometrial implants confirmed by histologic examination.

She does not want laparoscopy. You offer alternatives, and she elects to undergo cycle suppression with a 3-month trial of leuprolide (Lupron) and to complete a pain calendar. You see her in follow-up in 3 months, and she is feeling much better. The pain has been almost completely suppressed, and she has missed only 1 day of work since you last saw her—but that was for a Star Trek convention. After all, the future birthplace of Captain Kirk is located in Iowa (Riverside, Iowa). She has hot flashes, but they are minor.

Question 15.17.3 What is the most appropriate management at this point?
A) Continue the Lupron for up to another 3 months (6 months total)
B) Stop the Lupron and monitor
C) Switch to a trial of cycle suppression using Depo-Provera (medroxyprogesterone acetate) or continuous low-dose OCPs
D) Switch to a trial of Premarin (conjugated estrogens)
E) A or C

Answer 15.17.3 **The correct answer is "E."** For pain relief, treatment with a GnRH agonist for 3 to 6 months is effective in most patients. Oral contraceptives, as well as oral or depo progestins (Depo-Provera), are more effective than placebo ("C"). Given the marked treatment success with the depo-Lupron, discontinuing treatment ("B") would likely result in recurrence of the patient's pain symptoms. Since endometriosis is estrogen dependent, use of estrogen (Premarin) ("D") theoretically could worsen symptoms. Another option is treatment with danazol. However, danazol is less well tolerated than GnRH agonists, Provera, or OCPs.

HELPFUL TIP:
NSAIDs are useful monotherapy in patients with mild endometriosis and are useful in combination with hormonal therapy (e.g., OCPs) for patients with more severe symptoms.

The patient is concerned about how endometriosis may affect her future fertility. You recall that she is 25 years old and has never attempted pregnancy (at least not intentionally). She has regular menstrual cycles.

Question 15.17.4 What will you tell her?
A) "You are surely infertile. Look into adoption"
B) "You just cannot know for sure until you have tried to conceive"
C) "What are you worried about? There is no association between endometriosis and infertility"
D) "Look at my face. See how tired I am? Do you really want kids?"

Answer 15.17.4 **The correct answer is "B."** It is impossible to predict fertility and infertility based on the available information. Early-stage endometriosis is not likely to be associated with alterations in fecundity. If the patient is willing, a diagnostic laparoscopy may aid in visualization of anatomic pathology and allow one to render a guess as to possible tubal disease.

HELPFUL TIP:
Chronic pelvic pain is a *symptom*, not a specific disease. By definition, chronic pelvic pain refers to pain that has been present for more than 6 months and for which a thorough investigation has been negative. Here is a helpful starting guide for eliciting the underlying causes of chronic pelvic pain:

- **Is the pain cyclic?** It may be related to endometriosis, dysmenorrhea, adenomyosis, or other diseases that respond to hormones, such as irritable bowel syndrome and interstitial cystitis.
- **Is the pain noncyclic?** It may be urinary, constipation, a myofascial trigger point in the abdominal wall, etc.
- **Always ask about sexual and physical abuse:** There is a high correlation between chronic pelvic pain and a history of sexual abuse.
- To go by the textbook, the "diagnosis" of chronic pelvic pain requires a negative diagnostic laparoscopy. However, laparoscopy may not be performed in all cases.

▶ **Objectives: Did you learn to …**
- Manage patients who desire emergency oral contraception?
- Define and evaluate chronic pelvic pain?
- Describe the ramifications, evaluation, diagnosis, and management of endometriosis?

 QUICK QUIZ: A "TRICHY" ONE

A 19-year-old sexually active female presents to your urgent care center with a foul-smelling vaginal discharge. She has noted the discharge for about 3 days. On examination, she is in no acute distress, and her vital signs are normal. Her pelvic examination is remarkable for mild vaginal erythema and a frothy gray discharge. You note a malodorous discharge and suspect *Trichomonas* (bacterial vaginosis can also be malodorous, of course, with a fishy smell). A wet prep confirms your diagnosis.

At this point in time, you recommend that she also be tested for:
A) Chlamydia and gonorrhea
B) Herpes simplex
C) Hepatitis A
D) All of the above

The correct answer is "A." Routine screening for chlamydia and gonorrhea infection is recommended for all sexually active adolescents. Given the presence of one STI, it is appropriate to offer testing for other STIs at this visit. Currently, herpes simplex virus (HSV) is not routinely tested for in asymptomatic persons, and the USPSTF recommends against serologic screening for HSV. Hepatitis A is not a sexually transmitted disease. Of note, *Trichomonas* has been found to be associated with a two- to threefold increase in acquisition of HIV (*Curr HIV Res.* 2012;10(3):202–210). Therefore, it would be appropriate to offer testing for hepatitis B, HIV, syphilis, etc., as individual cases dictate.

 QUICK QUIZ: PROLAPSE

An 80-year-old woman presents for evaluation of a "bulge" she noted after gardening over the weekend … or maybe it's been there for years—she's not sure. She has no discomfort and no difficulty with bowel or bladder elimination. On examination, you note her cervix extends 1 cm beyond the vaginal introitus with a Valsalva maneuver. There are no lesions or excoriations noted.

Of the following, what is the best initial treatment option?
A) Hysterectomy
B) Trachelectomy
C) Pessary trial
D) Bed rest
E) Hormone therapy

The correct answer is "C." Seventy percent of women who are fitted with a pessary are satisfied at 5-year follow-up. Hysterectomy and trachelectomy (removal of the cervix) are both unnecessarily invasive treatments without trying a conservative strategy.

 QUICK QUIZ: OVARIAN MASS 1

What is the best way to manage an *asymptomatic* 4-cm ovarian cystic mass found initially on pelvic examination and confirmed by pelvic ultrasound as a simple cyst in a 22-year-old female who is otherwise healthy?
A) Referral to a gynecologist
B) Start hormonal therapy to reduce ovulation
C) Expectant management with repeat ultrasound in 2 months
D) Serum CA-125 level

The correct answer is "C." A 4-cm ovarian mass likely represents a functional cyst in a woman who is cycling (reproductive age). In general, premenopausal women with simple cysts 10 cm or smaller may be managed conservatively with serial ultrasonography in 4 to 12 weeks. Since the mass is asymptomatic and without concerning ultrasound findings (complex mass, septations, solid components), expectant management is the best option. No further evaluation is warranted at this time. CA-125 is a tumor marker for epithelial ovarian cancer, but it is not useful as a screening test.

 QUICK QUIZ: OVARIAN MASS 2

What is the best first step in managing an asymptomatic palpable 4 cm adnexal mass in a 76-year-old postmenopausal woman (although why you are doing a pelvic exam on an asymptomatic 76 years old is a mystery)?
A) Referral to a gynecologist
B) Start hormonal therapy to suppress FSH and LH
C) Expectant management with repeat examination in 2 months
D) Serum CA-125 level
E) Pelvic ultrasound

The correct answer is "E." Unlike a relatively small palpable ovarian mass in a reproductive-age woman, a palpable ovarian mass in a postmenopausal woman represents ovarian malignancy until proven otherwise. The best initial imaging study for evaluation of a pelvic mass is ultrasound. Ultrasound will not only identify the location of the mass but will also identify its internal consistency. Characteristics suggestive of cancer include bilaterality, solid and cystic components, thick septations, and the presence of ascites. CA-125 is a marker for epithelial ovarian cancer and may assist in evaluation, but it cannot be relied upon to rule in or to rule out cancer as a diagnosis. (Best case scenario, in appropriately selected patients, CA-125 has a sensitivity around 95% and a specificity around 90% for the diagnosis of ovarian cancer.) CA-125 is useful in follow-up of patients with a history of ovarian cancer.

 QUICK QUIZ: GYNECOLOGIC CANCERS

What is the leading cause of death from a gynecologic malignancy in American women?
A) Ovarian cancer
B) Uterine cancer
C) Cervical cancer
D) Fallopian tube cancer
E) Vaginal cancer

The correct answer is "A." Ovarian cancer is the leading cause of death from gynecologic malignancy, is the second most common gynecologic malignancy, and is the fourth leading cause of cancer death in women. Endometrial cancer is the most common gynecologic malignancy but also one of the most treatable. Cervical cancer is the third most common gynecologic

malignancy. Both fallopian tube and vaginal malignancy are relatively rare.

 QUICK QUIZ: OVARIAN CANCER

How does ovarian cancer typically present?
A) Early satiety
B) Abdominal fullness and pain
C) Urinary obstruction
D) Asymptomatic mass noted on routine examination
E) A and B

The correct answer is "E." There are no specific early symptoms of ovarian cancer. Thus, most patients present with symptoms associated with increasing tumor mass: early satiety, abdominal fullness or bloating, and abdominal pain. Unfortunately, ovarian cancer is rarely identified at an early stage on routine annual examination.

 HELPFUL TIP:
An ovarian mass is more likely to be malignant if the patient is premenarcheal or postmenopausal. Other signs pointing to malignancy include mass greater than 10 cm in diameter and presence of solid or complex cystic features on ultrasound. Consider an ultrasound for otherwise unexplained bloating, abdominal distention, urinary frequency/urgency, abdominal or pelvic pain, early satiety, etc.

▶ **CASE 15.18**

While covering the emergency department on the graveyard shift, a 21-year-old college student presents sobbing with a friend. Her friend says, "She's been raped." Thankfully, your town has a rape crisis team who can come to the ED and provide emotional/psychological support, though they are not trained to do exams.

Question 15.18.1 Relevant history includes all of the following EXCEPT:
A) Whether force was used and what type
B) Physical characteristics of the assailant
C) Details regarding penetration (vaginal, anal, oral)
D) Number of sexual partners the victim has had in her lifetime
E) Condom use

Answer 15.18.1 **The correct answer is "D."** The patient's past sexual history is not relevant in the evaluation of sexual assault. The other issues are pertinent to the case. Although it may be difficult for the patient to relive the experience, you should try to obtain a detailed history of the assault. In order to assess her risk for pregnancy and infection, you need to ask about the area penetrated (e.g., vaginal, oral, or anal penetration) ("C"), whether the assailant ejaculated, and if a condom ("E") was used. In a sexual assault case, your job is also to collect evidence, including pertinent historical elements (e.g., number of assailants, names, physical appearance, whether force was used and what type—threat, restraints, weapons, etc.) ("A" and "B").

> **HELPFUL TIP:**
> Sexual assault includes genital, anal, or oral penetration by a part of the assailant's body or by an object. By definition, it occurs without the victim's consent (including inability to consent secondary to intoxication or drugs) and need not involve direct force or violence.

Question 15.18.2 Which of the following are important physical elements to collect for the forensic evaluation in this case?
A) Combed specimens from the scalp and pubic hair
B) Swabs of the oral, vaginal, and rectal mucosa
C) The patient's clothing
D) Fingernail scrapings
E) All of the above

Answer 15.18.2 The correct answer is "E." All of the items listed will be important to the investigation. Evidence collection kits for sexual assault cases ("rape kits") should be available in your emergency department.

Although apparently inebriated, the patient is able to give a coherent history. When you broach the subject of physical examination, her friend says, "Look, she was raped an hour ago. Can't you let her just recover a bit before you violate her all over again?"

Question 15.18.3 Which of the following is the most appropriate response?
A) "Of course. Come back tomorrow after you have sobered up and taken a shower"
B) "An examination is important for your health and in the event that this becomes a criminal case. The yield of the examination declines with time. Even if you don't feel like prosecuting now, you may decide to do so in the future, and the best evidence is gathered early"
C) "The examination has a fairly high yield even a week after the assault, so take your time on this"
D) "Under federal law I am required to perform this examination"

Answer 15.18.3 The correct answer is "B." The yield of a forensic examination declines with time. Even if a patient states that she does not want to prosecute the assailant, she should be encouraged to have the examination done in case she changes her mind. Also, you are concerned about her health, and she may be at risk for sexually transmitted diseases, pregnancy, and

traumatic injury. Despite the fact that yield does decline with time, reliable evidence may still be gathered up to 5 days after the assault. And remember that all patients with capacity have autonomy; you should not coerce or force someone to have an exam that they decline.

> **HELPFUL TIP:**
> "Rape trauma syndrome" generally occurs in three stages. The first includes anger, anxiety, guilt, shame, sleep disturbance, etc. The second stage includes somatic complaints (pelvic pain, other pain) and psychiatric complaints (depression, phobias, etc.). Some patients will resolve these issues while others will develop post-traumatic stress syndrome. The third stage is renormalization.

Question 15.18.4 Which of the following is the LEAST appropriate to offer this patient at this point in time?
A) HIV antigen/antibody testing
B) HSV antibody testing
C) Prophylactic treatment for gonorrhea and chlamydia
D) Mental health services referral
E) Emergency contraception

Answer 15.18.4 The correct answer is "B." Herpes virus antibody testing will only tell you if she has been exposed to HSV in the past. Further recommendations include syphilis testing, hepatitis B antibody testing, performing a wet prep of a vaginal sample, and checking a urine pregnancy test. Why HIV testing? You need to decide whether to provide prophylaxis. If the patient is HIV+, prophylaxis may just lead to resistance.

▶ **Objectives: Did you learn to …**
  · Evaluate a patient for sexual assault?
  · Manage a patient who has been the victim of sexual assault?

▶ CASE 15.19

A 21-year-old woman presents to your office complaining of pelvic pain with intercourse, worse over the last 2 weeks. She also complains of not getting pregnant, even though she's had several partners over her last 3 years of sexual activity and has been trying to get pregnant with the same partner for the past 6 months. She states she never has used birth control of any type—not even once. You commend her on commitment to her principles. She started her periods around age 14 but has only had a couple of periods since then. Apparently, this pattern of menstruation is normal for her family, as her mother was the same way.

On physical examination, you notice the patient is a centrally obese young woman, afebrile, with (culturally defined) excess hair noted down the side of her face and under her chin. She also has some erythematous pustules on her cheeks.

Question 15.19.1 Which of the following lab results would be most consistent with the history and examination findings?
A) Positive urine pregnancy test
B) Low TSH level
C) Elevated CA-125 level
D) Mildly elevated androgens
E) Prolactin level more than three times normal

Answer 15.19.1 The correct answer is "D." This patient gives a history and has an appearance consistent with polycystic ovarian syndrome (PCOS). The clinical features of PCOS include oligomenorrhea (90%), hirsutism (80%), obesity (50%), amenorrhea (40%), and infertility (40%). Early symptoms in an adolescent may consist only of irregular periods, acne, and central obesity. Clinical or laboratory evidence of androgen excess may be present, such as mildly elevated testosterone. Note that depending on the diagnostic criteria you are using for PCOS, an ultrasound may not be necessary. An LH:FSH ratio greater than 3:1 adds further support to the diagnosis. You should certainly do a pregnancy test, a TSH, and a prolactin level. However, this patient most likely has PCOS. There is no role for measuring CA-125 as this is a marker for ovarian cancer as per above.

> **HELPFUL TIP:**
> The most recent evidence points to insulin resistance as the underlying cause of PCOS, and these patients may have acanthosis nigricans. Insulin resistance can be quantified by calculating the ratio of fasting glucose to insulin. A ratio of less than 4.5 indicates insulin resistance. Insulin resistance stimulates ovarian androgen production, which leads to anovulation.

You proceed with the pelvic portion of the examination, noting the patient also has a diamond-shaped, rather than triangular-shaped, pubic hair pattern. You find no lesions on the vulva or in the vagina. However, the cervix appears reddened, with an almost strawberry texture. And, even though there is a generous amount of yellowish, malodorous leukorrhea in the vaginal vault, there is no notable pus at the cervical os. Bimanual examination is limited due to the patient's obesity.

Question 15.19.2 Of the following, which is the most likely cause of her cervicitis?
A) HSV infection
B) *Trichomonas vaginalis* infection
C) *Candida albicans* infection
D) PID
E) Bacterial vaginosis

Answer 15.19.2 The correct answer is "B." *Trichomonas* is a protozoan that is sexually transmitted and can cause urethritis in both sexes. However, in women, it most commonly causes ulceration of the cervical mucosa with punctate hemorrhages known as a "strawberry cervix." Signs and symptoms also include

a malodorous discharge and occasional vulvar and vaginal irritation. The cervix can be somewhat tender to touch, either during examination or intercourse, and patients often complain of a nonspecific pelvic pain. Males are often asymptomatic.

The wet mount demonstrates *Trichomonas*; there is no evidence of yeast or clue cells. You send samples for chlamydia and gonorrhea tests as well as a Pap smear. You recommend testing for HIV, syphilis, and hepatitis B, and she agrees.

Question 15.19.3 For her *Trichomonas* vaginal infection, you prescribe:
A) Flagyl (metronidazole) 2 g orally in a single dose
B) MetroGel-Vaginal (topical vaginal metronidazole) 5 g applied nightly for 5 days
C) Diflucan (fluconazole) 150 mg orally in a single dose
D) Zithromax (azithromycin) 1 g orally in a single dose
E) Levaquin (levofloxacin) 250 mg orally in a single dose

Answer 15.19.3 The correct answer is "A." The best choice is oral metronidazole. Topical antibiotic gels, creams, or ovules—either metronidazole or clindamycin (Cleocin)—only treat bacterial vaginosis, as the concentration is insufficient to reach the protozoa in the glands and urethral areas. The remaining options are all incorrect for treating *Trichomonas*. See Table 15-11 for more on diagnosis and treatment of infectious vaginitis.

> **HELPFUL TIP:**
> As with other STIs, a patient with *Trichomonas* should have her partner tested and treated (or just treated depending whether or not this is allowable under your state law). Males with *Trichomonas* infections will have symptoms in about 25% of cases. Symptoms consist of dysuria and clear or white urethral discharge, which can sometimes last for months if left untreated. If you see a male patient with dysuria, pyuria on urinalysis/micro, and negative cultures (including chlamydia and gonorrhea), consider *Trichomonas*.

> **HELPFUL TIP:**
> While it makes sense that single-dose azithromycin would work better in treating Chlamydial cervicitis because of compliance issues, the cure rate is the same whether azithromycin or the doxycycline is used. There is about a 3% failure rate with azithromycin which isn't seen with doxycycline. Both are first line per the CDC.

You now return your attention to her PCOS (remember, way back then, the reason she came in?). Her lab results demonstrated a LH:FSH ratio >3; normal TSH and prolactin; slightly elevated testosterone, but still well below the normal male range; fasting glucose:insulin ratio <4.5; and slightly elevated total cholesterol and triglycerides. Her LH:FSH

TABLE 15-11 VAGINITIS DIAGNOSIS AND TREATMENT

Organism	Discharge	Odor	Microscopy	pH	Treatment
Bacterial vaginosis	Thin, gray, homogeneous	Fishy with positive "whiff test"	Clue cells	>4.5	Metronidazole 500 mg BID × 7 days or clindamycin 300 mg BID × 7 days or topical metronidazole 1 applicatorful intravaginally daily × 5 days (lower success rate)
Candida	Adherent, white, "cottage cheese" like	Neutral	Pseudohyphae but only 65–85% sensitive	<4.5	Fluconazole oral, topical clotrimazole, miconazole, etc.
Trichomonas	Copious yellow, gray, green, foamy. Friable "strawberry" cervix	Malodorous	Trichomonads	>4.5	Metronidazole 2 g PO once (recommended), or 500 mg BID × 7 days (alternative)

Adapted with permission from Hainer BL, Gibson MV. Vaginitis: diagnosis and treatment. *Am Fam Physician*. 2011;83(7):807–815. Copyright © 2011 American Academy of Family Physicians. All rights reserved.

ratio was consistent with the diagnosis of PCOS. She has not menstruated for 4 months. A urine hCG is negative, and a repeat fasting glucose is 120 mg/dL.

Question 15.19.4 **Which of the following recommendations should you make now?**
A) Initiate metformin
B) Attempt weight loss through a nutritious diet and increased exercise
C) Initiate oral contraceptives to regulate menses
D) A and C
E) All of the above

Answer 15.19.4 **The correct answer is "E."** This patient has glucose intolerance (elevated fasting glucose and ratio of glucose:insulin <4.5), and it is reasonable to initiate dietary and medical therapy at this point in time. Another option is to start with lifestyle modifications and check fasting glucose again 3 to 6 months later. Due to increased risk of endometrial carcinoma in patients who have rare menses, it is important to regulate her cycles. OCPs ("C") can accomplish menstrual regulation.

HELPFUL TIP:
For hirsutism associated with PCOS, spironolactone is usually first-line therapy unless the patient has a contraindication; traditional hair removal techniques will still be required for the existing hair growth. Since spironolactone can result in feminization of a male fetus, patients taking spironolactone must be using reliable birth control.

HELPFUL TIP:
Not all women with PCOS are obese and hirsute. Many patients may be thin with sparse body hair and present with menstrual irregularities and fertility concerns.

▶ **Objectives: Did you learn to …**
· Identify the clinical presentation of PCOS?
· Diagnose and treat *Trichomonas* infection?
· Diagnose and manage PCOS?

 QUICK QUIZ: SCREENING IN TEENS

A 16-year-old female presents with her mother. They don't look happy. Her mother says, "She needs a Pap smear because she's been having sex with a couple of boys—in my house, I will have you know—for a year!" The patient rolls her eyes.

Consistent with published guidelines, you recommend:
A) Pap smear
B) Gonorrhea and chlamydia testing
C) Pap smear and gonorrhea and chlamydia testing
D) Return for a Pap after sexually active for 3 years (age 18 for this patient)
E) A chastity belt

The correct answer is "B." It is now recommended to delay cervical cancer screening until age 21, even if the woman has been sexually active. The reasoning: although adolescent females are frequently infected with HPV, they also easily clear these infections, with 95% of lesions spontaneously regressing. Exceptions to this rule include patients who are immunocompromised (e.g., organ transplant, HIV infection). For this patient, ensuring that she has completed her HPV vaccination series and counseling on safe sexual behavior is also warranted.

 QUICK QUIZ: AN ITCHY VULVA

A 65-year-old female presents for a health maintenance examination. She complains of a vulvar itching due to what she calls "recurrent yeast infections," and her symptoms have worsened over the last few months. She is sexually active with her husband

and has experienced dyspareunia with penetration lately. She always uses a water-based lubricant with intercourse. On examination, you find complete loss of the borders of the labia minora, constriction of the vaginal outlet, and several thin white plaques (like parchment paper) on the vulva. There is no other skin or mucosal involvement.

What is the most likely diagnosis?
A) Lichen planus
B) Lichen simplex
C) Lichen sclerosus
D) Vulvovaginal candidiasis
E) Squamous carcinoma

The correct answer is "C." The clinical description above is characteristic of lichen sclerosus, which occurs more commonly in older women but also has a peak in young girls. Almost all lichen sclerosus is intensely pruritic. As lichen sclerosus progresses, there may be loss of labial architecture, stenosis of the introitus, and obliteration of the clitoris. The lesions are usually multiple and appear as thin, shiny, white, wrinkled patches or plaques. The rest are incorrect. However, "E," squamous carcinoma, occasionally can be confused for lichen sclerosus but is more likely to present with ulceration and induration and is less common (though if you are suspicious of cancer, a biopsy is indicated). Patients with lichen sclerosus have a squamous cell cancer risk of 3% to 7% and should have an examination every 6 to 12 months with biopsies as indicated for persistent and non-healing lesions.

HELPFUL TIP:
Initial treatment for lichen sclerosus involves local steroid ointment application. High-potency steroids are initiated and then tapered to the lowest effective potency and frequency that maintain symptom control. Testosterone creams have fallen out of favor due to lesser efficacy and secondary virilization. Vaginal dilators can be used if there is constriction of the vaginal opening causing dyspareunia and it is of concern to the woman.

 QUICK QUIZ: VULVOVAGINAL CANDIDIASIS

A 48-year-old perimenopausal female presents with a 3-day history of vulvar pruritus. Her history is significant for mitral valve replacement and she is on warfarin with INR 2–3. A limited vulvar and vaginal examination reveals significant erythema with satellite lesions on the labia majora. Wet prep microscopy reveals abundant pseudohyphae and inflammatory cells. You somehow assemble all these clues into a diagnosis of candidal vulvovaginitis (and you can tell the patient is impressed when she says, "That's right, genius. I've got a yeast infection"). She enquires about use of oral therapy, as vaginal creams are "messy."

How will you counsel this patient regarding use of oral fluconazole (Diflucan)?
A) "You have no contraindications to oral fluconazole"
B) "Given your use of warfarin, you should not use oral fluconazole"
C) "You will need to stop warfarin while taking oral fluconazole"
D) "You should take extra warfarin if you take oral fluconazole"

The correct answer is "B." There are numerous drug interactions with oral fluconazole, including warfarin (both inhibit CYP3A4). The INR will increase after even one dose of fluconazole therapy. Similarly, the ubiquitous statins are affected by oral fluconazole with several case reports of rhabdomyolysis in the literature. In this case, stick with topical antifungals, although your patient satisfaction scores may plummet. (Incidentally, patient satisfaction has been inversely correlated with healthcare quality—although there appears to be a direct link between increased satisfaction and increased healthcare expenditure.) *Avoid fluconazole in pregnancy as well. A single dose can cause miscarriage or birth defects.*

 CASE 15.20

A 27-year-old female presents with her husband seeking advice regarding pregnancy loss. She recently had a miscarriage. Your patient states that this was her third miscarriage in the last 2 years. All three occurred at about 9 weeks of gestation.

Question 15.20.1 **Possible explanations for recurrent pregnancy loss in this patient include each of the following EXCEPT:**
A) Parental structural chromosome abnormalities
B) Uterine anatomic abnormalities
C) Anticardiolipin antibody syndrome
D) Idiopathic (unexplained etiology)
E) Conception while on oral contraceptives

Answer 15.20.1 **The correct answer is "E."** Conception while on oral contraceptives will not increase the risk of **recurrent** spontaneous miscarriages. Parental structural chromosome abnormalities (balanced structural chromosome rearrangement in one partner) are responsible for pregnancy loss in 2% to 4% of couples. Uterine anatomic abnormalities ("B") have been associated with 10% to 15% of pregnancy loss. "D" is true. The majority of couples with recurrent pregnancy loss will have an uncertain etiology despite extensive evaluation (>50%). See below for more on "C".

HELPFUL TIP:
Recurrent pregnancy loss is classically defined as loss of three or more **consecutive** pregnancies.

The couple desires testing for possible causes of the pregnancy losses.

Question 15.20.2 Of the following, which test(s) should be included in the evaluation?
A) Cultures for bacteria
B) Test for glucose intolerance
C) Maternal anti-paternal antibodies
D) Lupus anticoagulant and anticardiolipin antibody
E) All of the above

Answer 15.20.2 **The correct answer is "D."** Antiphospholipid syndrome is associated with pregnancy loss in 3% to 15% of women with recurrent pregnancy loss. The others are not useful. However, chromosomal testing of the parents (not given as an option in this question) may be useful. Other tests that can be considered include screening for thyroid abnormalities with anti-thyroid peroxidase (TPO) and TSH with free T4 as well as an ultrasound to look for uterine abnormalities

Evaluation of the recurrent pregnancy loss fails to identify a cause. Thus, like most couples with recurrent pregnancy loss, the etiology remains unexplained.

Question 15.20.3 What is the likelihood that this couple will have a successful pregnancy outcome in the next pregnancy?
A) Highly unlikely, they should consider adoption
B) Less than one in four chances of successful pregnancy
C) 60% to 70% chance of successful next pregnancy
D) You cannot hazard a guess. Amazingly, this has not been studied

Answer 15.20.3 **The correct answer is "C."** Studies suggest that 60% to 70% of couples with *unexplained* recurrent pregnancy loss will have a successful next pregnancy.

▶ **Objectives: Did you learn to …**
  · Define recurrent pregnancy loss and discuss some of its epidemiologic aspects?
  · Enumerate potential causes of recurrent pregnancy loss?
  · Identify etiologies and the workup of recurrent pregnancy loss?

 QUICK QUIZ: WEIGHT GAIN IN PREGNANCY

A 28-year-old primigravida female presents for an initial obstetric visit. Pelvic examination is consistent with a 6- to 8-week gestation uterus, and the remainder of the examination is unremarkable. As this is her first pregnancy, she has a number of questions. She wants to know how much weight gain is expected and whether she should "watch her weight."

You calculate her BMI as 24 kg/m² and recommend the following:
A) "Eat anything you want. You're eating for two!"
B) "Your BMI is normal. Your goal is to gain no more than 20 lb"
C) "Your BMI is low. Your goal is to gain 40 lb"
D) "Your BMI is high. Your goal is to gain no more than 15 lb"
E) "Your BMI is normal. Your goal is to gain 30 lb"

The correct answer is "E." The Institute of Medicine recommends weight gain in pregnancy based on pregravid BMI (see Table 15-12). In this patient, her BMI is in the normal range, so her goal for weight gain in pregnancy is 25 to 35 lb. Women with a normal pre-pregnancy BMI should gain about 1 lb per week during their second and third trimesters.

 QUICK QUIZ: AMENORRHEA

A 32-year-old female is coming to see you for amenorrhea. She had regular menses until the last year when they became irregular. She has not had any menses for the past 6 months. She is somewhat distraught because she wants to have a family. Being the smart doctor that you are, you know that a pregnancy test is the first thing to do: it is negative. Being the smart doctor that you are, you also think about the female athlete triad, but she does not meet this profile. You take more of a history and find out the following:

• There is no additional stress in her life (such as starting college or a new job), weight loss, or illness, etc., which might lead to hypothalamic amenorrhea.

• She has no galactorrhea (prolactinoma).

• She has no hot flashes, vaginal dryness, etc. (premature menopause).

• She denies headaches, visual changes, fatigue, polydipsia, or polyuria (pituitary problems).

• She has no acne, hirsutism, etc., suggestive of PCOS.

Hey, did you notice how we are cleverly giving you the workup of secondary amenorrhea in the question?

As recommended, you check a TSH and prolactin; they are normal.

TABLE 15-12 PREGNANCY WEIGHT GAIN GUIDELINES

BMI (kg/m²)	Goal Weight Gain (kg)	Goal Weight Gain (lb)
<18.5	12.5–18.0	28–40
18.5–24.9	11.5–16.0	25–35
25.0–29.9	7.0–11.5	15–25
>30	5–9	11–20

Adapted from Institute of Medicine, Resource Sheet, May 2009: Weight gain during pregnancy: reexamining the guidelines. Available at: http://www.iom.edu/Reports/2009/Weight-Gain-During-Pregnancy-Reexamining-the-Guidelines.aspx.

The next step in the evaluation of this patient's amenorrhea is:

A) A progestin challenge
B) Hysterosalpingogram to prove cervical patency
C) A trial of oral contraceptives to prove cervical patency
D) An LH to rule out menopause
E) All of the above

The correct answer is "A." A progestin challenge should cause a withdrawal bleed if there is still adequate estrogen (thus ruling out premature ovarian failure). If the progestin challenge does not result in menses, the step following this would be to start a combination oral contraceptive. Failure to induce menses with a combination OCP suggests a mechanical blockage such as Asherman syndrome (scarring of the endometrial lining with intrauterine adhesions). Failure to induce menses with a combination OCP can be followed by a hysterosalpingogram or hysteroscopy to identify any mechanical problems.

....

You did it! You successfully worked up secondary amenorrhea.

HELPFUL TIP:
But wait, there is more! If the progestin challenge is negative (no menses), check an FSH. If this is high, it might indicate ovarian failure. **If the FSH is normal or low in the absence of circulating estrogen** (a negative progestin challenge), consider a pituitary cause of amenorrhea including possible hypothalamic–pituitary axis dysfunction from weight loss, stress, pituitary tumor, empty sella syndrome, etc. No pituitary? No FSH.

Clinical Pearls

○ Do not perform elective deliveries (C-sections or inductions) that are not medically indicated prior to 39 weeks of gestation.

○ Do not perform routine screening for ovarian cancer in asymptomatic, low-to-average risk women.

○ Do not require a Pap and a pelvic examination to prescribe contraception. The only necessary requirement is to perform a detailed history to ascertain risk factors of using hormonal contraception, blood pressure check, and the performance of a urine pregnancy test to ensure the woman is not pregnant.

○ Do not routinely perform episiotomies; there is no evidence that episiotomies reduce perineal trauma, postpartum dyspareunia, etc.

○ In HIV-negative patients, do not begin cervical cancer screening before the age of 21 regardless of sexual activity status.

○ Due to the increased risk of endometrial cancer, do not use unopposed estrogen in a woman unless she has undergone a hysterectomy.

○ In a pregnant woman with third-trimester vaginal bleeding, do not perform a digital *or* speculum vaginal examination until you can rule out the diagnosis of placenta previa.

○ Perform routine GBS screening on pregnant women between 35 and 37 weeks of gestation UNLESS the woman has a documented history of GBS bacteriuria during current pregnancy or prior history of infant born with invasive GBS infection, in which cases they would be treated anyway.

○ Recommend folic acid in all women of childbearing age to prevent any risk of neural tube defects if she should become pregnant.

○ Use the ASCCP guidelines to determine frequency of Pap smears and management of abnormal smears.

BIBLIOGRAPHY

American College of Obstetricians and Gynecologists. ACOG practice bulletin no. 83: management of adnexal masses. *Obstet Gynecol.* 2007;110(1):201–214.

American College of Obstetricians and Gynecologists. ACOG practice bulletin no. 106: intrapartum fetal heart rate monitoring, nomenclature, interpretation and general management principles. *Obstet Gynecol.* 2009;114(1):192–202.

American College of Obstetricians and Gynecologists. ACOG practice bulletin no. 112: emergency contraception. *Obstet Gynecol.* 2010;115:1100–1109.

American College of Obstetricians and Gynecologists. ACOG practice bulletin no. 130: prediction and prevention of preterm birth. *Obstet Gynecol.* 2012;120(4):964–973.

American College of Obstetricians and Gynecologists. Obstetric care consensus no. 1: safe prevention of the primary caesarean delivery. *Obstet Gynecol.* 2014(reaffirmed 2016);123:693–711.

American College of Obstetricians and Gynecologists Committees on Adolescent Health Care and on Gynecologic Practice. ACOG committee opinion no. 602: depot medroxyprogesterone acetate and bone effects. *Obstet Gynecol.* 2014;123(6):1398–1402.

American College of Obstetricians and Gynecologists Committee on Practice Bulletins. ACOG practice bulletin no. 173: fetal macrosomia. *Obstet Gynecol.* 2016;128(5):e195–e209.

American College of Obstetricians and Gynecologists Committee on Practice Bulletins-Obstetrics. ACOG practice bulletin no. 180: gestational diabetes mellitus. *Obstet Gynecol.* 2018;131(2):e49–e64.

American College of Obstetricians and Gynecologists Committee on Practice Bulletins-Obstetrics. ACOG practice bulletin no. 188: prelabor rupture of membranes. *Obstet Gynecol.* 2018;131(1):e1–e14.

American College of Obstetricians and Gynecologists Committee on Practice Bulletins-Obstetrics. ACOG practice bulletin no. 203: chronic hypertension in pregnancy. *Obstet Gynecol.* 2019;133(1):e26–e50.

American College of Obstetricians and Gynecologists Committees on Adolescent Health Care and Gynecologic Practice. Committee opinion no. 602: depot medroxyprogesterone acetate and bone effects. *Obstet Gynecol.* 2014;123:1398–402.

American College of Obstetricians and Gynecologists Committee on Obstetrics. Committee opinion no. 611: method for estimating due date. *Obstet Gynecol.* 2014;124:863–866.

American College of Obstetricians and Gynecologists Committee on Obstetrics. Committee opinion no. 736: optimizing postpartum care. *Obstet Gynecol.* 2018;131(5):e140–e150.

American College of Obstetricians and Gynecologists Committee on Obstetrics. Committee opinion no. 767: emergent therapy for acute-onset, severe hypertension during pregnancy and the postpartum period. *Obstet Gynecol.* 2019;133(2):e174–e180.

Balsells M, et al. Gibenclamide, metformin, and insulin for the treatment of gestational diabetes: a systematic review and meta-analysis. *BMJ.* 2015;350:h102.

Biggs W, Demuth RH. Premenstrual syndrome and premenstrual dysphoric disorder. *Am Fam Physician.* 2011;84(8):918–924.

Centers for Disease Control (CDC). 2015 Sexually Transmitted Diseases Treatment Guidelines: Gonococcal infections. Available at: https://www.cdc.gov/std/tg2015/gonorrhea.htm. Accessed April 8, 2019.

Crossman SH. The challenge of pelvic inflammatory disease. *Am Fam Physician.* 2006;73:859–864.

Division of Reproductive Health, National Center for Chronic Disease Prevention and Health Promotion, Centers for Disease Control and Prevention (CDC). U.S. Selected Practice Recommendations for Contraceptive Use, 2013: adapted from the World Health Organization selected practice recommendations for contraceptive use, 2nd edition. *MMWR Recomm Rep.* 2013;62(RR-05):1–60.

Gradison M. Pelvic inflammatory disease. *Am Fam Physician.* 2012;85(8):791–796.

Hainer BL, Gibson MV. Vaginitis: diagnosis and treatment. *Am Fam Physician.* 2011;83(7):807–815.

Hatcher RA, et al. *A Pocket Guide to Managing Contraception.* 6th ed. New York: Ardent Media, Inc.; 2005.

Kirkham C, et al. Evidence-based prenatal care: Part I. general prenatal care and counseling issues. *Am Fam Physician.* 2005;71(5):1307–1316.

Kirkham C, et al. Evidence-based prenatal care: Part II. third-trimester care and prevention of infectious diseases. *Am Fam Physician.* 2005;71:1555–1562.

Klein DA, et al. Provision of contraception: key recommendations from the CDC. *Am Fam Physician.* 2015;91(9):625–633.

LeFevre ML. Low-dose aspirin use for the prevention of morbidity and mortality from preeclampsia: US Preventative Services Task Force recommendation statement. *Ann Intern Med.* 2014;161:819–826.

Magee LA, et al. Less-tight versus tight control of hypertension in pregnancy. *N Engl J Med.* 2015;372:407–417.

Magnotti M, Futterweit W. Obesity and the polycystic ovary syndrome. *Med Clin North Am.* 2007;91(6):1151–1168.

Massad LS, et al. American Society for Colposcopy and Cervical Pathology 2012 updated consensus guidelines for the management of abnormal cervical cancer screening tests and precursors. *J Low Genit Tract Dis.* 2013;17(5):S1–S27.

Mirmonsef P, et al. The role of bacterial vaginosis and trichomonas in HIV transmission across the female genital tract. *Curr HIV Res.* 2012;10(3):202–210.

Mørch LS, et al. Contemporary hormonal contraception and the risk of breast cancer. *N Engl J Med.* 2017;377(23):2228–2239.

Norman JE, et al. Vaginal progesterone prophylaxis for preterm birth (the OPPTIMUM study): a multicentre, randomised, double-blind trial. *Lancet.* 2016;387(10033):2106–2116.

Ott MA, et al. Policy statement: contraception for adolescents. *Pediatrics.* 2014;134(4):e1244–e1256.

Raina R, et al. Female sexual dysfunction: classification, pathophysiology, and management. *Fertil Steril.* 2007;88(5):1273–1284.

Rasmussen KM, et al. *Institutes of Medicine Report Brief. Weight gain during pregnancy: re-examining the guidelines.* Washington, DC: National Academies Press; 2009. Available at: http://www.iom.edu/Reports/2009/Weight-Gain-During-Pregnancy-Reexamining-the-Guidelines.aspx. Accessed April 8, 2019.

Secura GM, et al. Provision of no-cost, long-acting contraception and teenage pregnancy. *N Engl J Med.* 2014;371:1316–1323.

Steiner RJ, et al. Long-acting reversible contraception and condom use among female US high school students: implications for sexually transmitted infection prevention. *JAMA Pediatr.* 2016;170(5):428–434.

Tan PC, et al. Effect of coitus at term on length of gestation, induction of labor, and mode of delivery. *Obstet Gynecol.* 2006;108(1):134–140.

Tenore JL. Methods for cervical ripening and induction of labor. *Am Fam Physician.* 2003;67:2123–2128.

US Food and Drug Administration. Mifeprex (mifepristone) information. Available at: http://www.fda.gov/Drugs/DrugSafety/PostmarketDrugSafetyInformationforPatientsandProviders/ucm111323.htm. Accessed April 8, 2019.

WOMAN Trial Collaborators. Effect of early tranexamic acid administration on mortality, hysterectomy, and other morbidities in women with post-partum haemorrhage (WOMAN): an international, randomised, double-blind, placebo-controlled trial. *Lancet.* 2017;389(10084):2105–2116.

Workowski KA, Bolan GA. Sexually transmitted diseases treatment guidelines, 2015. *MMWR Recomm Rep.* 2015;64(RR-3):1–137.

World Health Organization. Medical eligibility criteria for contraceptive use, 5th ed. World Health Organization Updated 2015. Available at: https://www.who.int/reproductivehealth/publications/family_planning/Ex-Summ-MEC-5/en/. Accessed April 8, 2019.

Zolotor AJ. Update on prenatal care. *Am Fam Physician.* 2014;89(3):199–208.

Men's Health

16

Aaron R. Kunz and Jason K. Wilbur

▶ CASE 16.1

A 58-year-old black male presents to your clinic complaining of urinary hesitancy, frequency, and three to four episodes of nocturia per night, which have been worsening over the past few years. His urinary stream is weaker than it was a few years ago, and he feels he does not empty his bladder completely. He denies any history of urinary tract infections (UTIs) or painful urination. He is otherwise well with no significant past medical or surgical history. Currently, he takes no medications and has no allergies. On reviewing his family history, he notes his father and older brother died of prostate cancer in their fifties. His general physical examination is normal, and a genital examination is unremarkable. Digital rectal examination reveals a smooth prostate with no nodules or tenderness.

Question 16.1.1 Based on this patient's history and physical examination, all of the following would be appropriate at this stage EXCEPT:
A) Serum assay for prostate-specific antigen (PSA)
B) American Urological Association (AUA) symptom score
C) Post-void residual urine volume
D) Transrectal ultrasound with prostate biopsies
E) Urinalysis and microscopic examination of the urine

Answer 16.1.1 **The correct answer is "D."** Although your patient has an increased risk of prostate cancer, transrectal ultrasound with prostate biopsies is not indicated at this stage. This diagnostic test should be reserved for a higher suspicion of prostate cancer. Based on this patient's family history and the fact that he is black (black males have a 50% higher incidence of, and mortality from, prostate cancer compared with whites), PSA testing ("A") is appropriate in this setting, as opposed to general population screening, which is discussed later in the chapter. The AUA symptom score ("B") is a seven-item questionnaire about symptoms of urinary outlet obstruction, which can be used to assess severity and assist in management of prostate disease. It is not very useful for diagnosis, but, on the bright side, it is freely available online and can be used to follow the disease *symptomatically*. There is also the International Prostate Symptom Score, which is remarkably similar but has an additional question regarding how symptoms affect the patient's quality of life. Since your patient may not empty his bladder well, a post-void residual urine volume and urinalysis will help determine if he is experiencing urinary retention ("C") or an infection ("E").

Question 16.1.2 When considering benign prostatic hyperplasia (BPH), you reflect on the common symptoms of this syndrome, which include all of the following EXCEPT:
A) Urinary retention
B) Post-void dribbling
C) Frequency
D) Nocturia
E) Hematuria

Answer 16.1.2 **The correct answer is "E."** Hematuria is not usually associated with BPH. However, it can occur if a man's prostatic urethra is very enlarged and friable. Enlargement of the prostate often results in obstructive flow symptoms (e.g., hesitancy and slow, weak stream), which in turn can lead to irritative symptoms (e.g., frequency, urgency, and nocturia). Obstruction from an enlarged prostate alone can cause hypertrophy of the detrusor, or it can lead to an infection that results in detrusor instability—the cause of irritative symptoms. If irritative symptoms are present without obstructive symptoms, other diagnoses should be considered, including bladder cancer, urolithiasis, infection, and neurogenic bladder.

Your patient's urinalysis and PSA are normal. After emptying 250 mL of urine, the postvoid residual urine volume is 50 mL.

Question 16.1.3 With this information, you recommend which of the following strategies?
A) Urodynamic studies
B) Medical therapy
C) Surgical therapy
D) Scheduled bladder catheterization
E) Biofeedback

Answer 16.1.3 The correct answer is "B." You have enough information to diagnose symptomatic BPH and further studies ("A") are not necessary. Depending on the patient's preferences, the next step is to begin treatment, and, in most cases, medical therapy is initiated first. If medical therapy fails or if a patient has severe BPH with ongoing obstruction, retention of large volumes of urine, bladder stones, or recurrent UTIs, surgical therapy should be considered. The most commonly performed surgery is transurethral resection of the prostate (TURP), but other techniques can be employed as well, including transurethral incision of the prostate, minimally invasive procedures, and open surgery for very enlarged prostate glands. "D" is incorrect. Scheduled bladder catheterization is unlikely to benefit your patient since his post-void residual is not very large. A post-void residual greater than 200 mL is associated with an increased risk of UTIs, and such patients may benefit from scheduled catheterizations if medical or surgical interventions do not correct the problem or are contraindicated. Kegel exercises and biofeedback ("E") may be used to treat incontinence but are not used in BPH. Biofeedback is helpful for voiding dysfunction due to incomplete urinary sphincter relaxation.

Your powers of deduction lead you to the conclusion that the patient's urinary symptoms are due to BPH. He has always been proud of his bladder capacity (men can be proud of just about anything) and is embarrassed that he is taking frequent bathroom stops when driving with his wife on their road trips; your patient desires treatment.

Question 16.1.4 To give him the most immediate relief, you prescribe which of the following?
A) Finasteride
B) Oxybutynin
C) Tamsulosin
D) Imipramine
E) Furosemide

Answer 16.1.4 The correct answer is "C." Timing and type of intervention should depend on how much the patient is bothered by his symptoms and whether complications of BPH are present. If the symptoms do not significantly interfere with your patient's life, he may choose to wait and take no treatment once he is reassured that he does not have a life-threatening illness. In general, medical management begins with a selective alpha-1a receptor blocker, such as tamsulosin, which relaxes the prostate at the bladder neck. If the patient does not receive sufficient relief from maximum doses of an alpha-1a blocker, consider adding a 5-alpha-reductase inhibitor (e.g., finasteride, dutasteride). These drugs work by reducing the size of the prostate gland by interfering with the effects of androgens on prostate tissue. However, it may take up to 6 months for a 5-alpha-reductase inhibitor to result in a noticeable difference in symptoms (thus, "A" should not be the first treatment); the full benefit of an alpha-blocker will be apparent within 4 to 6 weeks. "B" and "D" are incorrect because these anticholinergic drugs are used for

incontinence due to detrusor instability and may make urinary retention worse in patients with outlet obstruction. Furosemide, "E," is a potent diuretic and would be a cruel joke to play on this patient.

HELPFUL TIP:
Since 5-alpha-reductase inhibitors shrink prostate tissue, they reduce the production of prostate-specific antigen (PSA). Be aware that PSA levels decrease by approximately 50% within 6 months of initiating one of these drugs. Therefore, if for some reason you check a PSA in a man on finasteride or dutasteride, the value should be doubled for the first two years when comparing to normal ranges. It should be multiplied by 2.5 thereafter.

Question 16.1.5 Before you tear up the prescription for terazosin you accidentally wrote, you review its side effects. Potential side effects of alpha-blockers include all the following EXCEPT:
A) Retrograde ejaculation
B) Hypertension
C) Intraoperative floppy iris syndrome
D) Priapism

Answer 16.1.5 The correct answer is "B." Hypotension (not hypertension) is the most commonly encountered problem with terazosin and other alpha-blockers, including the uroselective alpha-blockers, although to a lesser degree. In elderly males, the hypotension can be particularly problematic as the propensity for falling may increase. Additionally, alpha-blockers in combination with phosphodiesterase inhibitors (e.g., sildenafil) can cause dangerously low blood pressures. Retrograde ejaculation ("A") and priapism ("D") are not common but have been reported. And, as if we needed it, here is more evidence for a direct link between the male ocular and genital systems: intraoperative floppy iris syndrome ("C") describes a flaccid iris that protrudes out through the surgical incision in those undergoing cataracts surgery and has been reported with alpha-blocker therapy. Yes, you may have thought we made this up, but we didn't.

You start tamsulosin. Unfortunately, the patient is not able to tolerate it due to dizziness. His symptoms are bothersome enough that he wishes to try something else. You consider finasteride.

Question 16.1.6 Which of the following is true of finasteride?
A) It permanently reduces prostate volume, even after the drug is stopped
B) It is approved by the Food and Drug Administration (FDA) for abnormal hair growth in women
C) It may reduce the overall risk of developing prostate cancer, but increases the risk of developing high-grade prostate cancers
D) It improves symptoms within 1 week of starting the drug
E) None of the above

Answer 16.1.6 The correct answer is "C." *This is important:* 5-alpha-reductase inhibitors lower the overall risk of cancer, but increase the risk of those cancers diagnosed being high grade (Gleason score of ≥ 7). Finasteride (and dutasteride) works by inhibiting 5-alpha-reductase, which is the enzyme that converts testosterone to dihydrotestosterone. Dihydrotestosterone stimulates hyperplasia of the prostate gland, and removing this stimulus results in decreased prostate volume. However, removal of finasteride allows hyperplasia to continue, and thus answer "A" is incorrect. "B" is also incorrect because finasteride is not approved by the FDA for hirsutism in women. Additionally, finasteride is category X in pregnancy, with potential teratogenic effects on the fetus. "D" is incorrect because finasteride takes time to work—a lot of time. As previously mentioned, its peak effectiveness is not seen for 3 to 6 months after starting the medication.

> **HELPFUL TIP:**
> In comparison trials with alpha-blockers, 5-alpha-reductase inhibitors have shown variable results. The addition of a 5-alpha-reductase inhibitor to an alpha-blocker does not seem to have additional benefit over alpha-blocker therapy alone in the *near term*, but combination therapy has shown reduced incidence of clinical progression of BPH in *longer trials*.

You decide to add finasteride. You see him again 2 months later when he presents with a febrile illness. He thinks that he might have the flu, but his BPH symptoms worsened at the same time. For the last 2 days, he has felt feverish with back pain, perineal pain, and generalized malaise. He complains of dysuria and worsening urinary frequency and urgency.

Question 16.1.7 During your examination, you make sure NOT to:
A) Perform a rectal examination
B) Massage the prostate
C) Swab the urethra for chlamydia
D) Perform urinalysis and microscopic examination of the urinary sediment

Answer 16.1.7 The correct answer is "B." There is a risk of seeding bacteria into the bloodstream when an infected prostate is massaged. This patient has symptoms of prostatitis; thus, you should **avoid prostatic massage**. Nonetheless, you should perform a prostate examination. The following prostate examination findings are associated with prostatitis: tenderness, warmth, enlargement, and bogginess.

You suspect prostatitis and obtain urine for analysis.

Question 16.1.8 All of the following laboratory abnormalities are consistent with the diagnosis of acute prostatitis EXCEPT:
A) Leukocytosis
B) Hematuria
C) Bacteriuria
D) Elevated creatinine
E) Elevated PSA

Answer 16.1.8 The correct answer is "D." Tests of renal function should not be abnormal in simple, acute prostatitis. Chronic partial or complete urinary outlet obstruction may cause abnormal renal function but not acute prostatitis. Abnormal serum BUN and/or creatinine in the setting of prostatitis should prompt further investigation. The urine often shows bacteriuria ("C"), pyuria (and, therefore, leukocytosis ["A"]), and hematuria. However, the urine may also be negative. Urine should be sent for culture and sensitivity to definitively determine the pathogen and direct further treatment. "E" is true: the PSA is often elevated in prostatitis. However, it is not necessary nor is it recommended to obtain a PSA to diagnose prostatitis. When the PSA is elevated due to acute prostatitis, it may not return to normal levels for 1 month or more after the resolution of inflammation.

On examination, you find an uncomfortable appearing male in no distress. His temperature is 38.4°C, and the rest of his vital signs are normal. The prostate on digital rectal examination is tender, enlarged, warm, and boggy. The remainder of the examination is unremarkable. Urinalysis is consistent with an infection. He has a sulfa allergy.

Question 16.1.9 Which of the following is the most appropriate treatment plan for this patient?
A) Prescribe trimethoprim-sulfamethoxazole 160 mg–800 mg BID for 42 days
B) Prescribe ciprofloxacin 500 mg orally BID for 21 days
C) Admit for IV levofloxacin 500 mg daily for 14 days
D) Admit for IV levofloxacin 500 mg daily, followed by completion of therapy with oral levofloxacin 500 mg daily for 14 days when the patient is stable
E) Perform transrectal ultrasound to rule out prostatic abscess

Answer 16.1.9 The correct answer is "B." The most appropriate treatment for this patient is a fluoroquinolone, such as ciprofloxacin, for at least 21 days. Some authorities recommend longer treatment (up to 6 weeks) to reduce the risk of chronic prostatitis. In patients who are not allergic, a sulfa antibiotic ("A") could be considered as an alternative to a fluoroquinolone. In this case, "C" and "D" are overkill. Admission is appropriate for patients who appear septic, have not responded to oral antibiotics, or who have significant comorbidities. However, fluoroquinolones have 100% bioavailability PO. Thus, there is no indication for giving these drugs IV unless the oral route is unavailable (e.g., vomiting). Additionally, the treatment course for "C" and "D" is too short. "E" is incorrect because abscesses are rare and imaging for an abscess is only undertaken if the patient does not respond to appropriate antibiotics.

When you see this patient again, his symptoms of prostatitis have cleared, but he does not think that finasteride is really helping. His AUA symptoms score is 21 (severe). He is

wondering if a transurethral resection of the prostate (TURP) might help him, and he wants to discuss the downsides of the operation.

Question 16.1.10 Compared with watchful waiting, all of the following are observed at greater rates in men who undergo TURP EXCEPT:

A) Erectile dysfunction
B) Urinary incontinence
C) Urethral stenosis
D) Increased urine flow
E) Decreased post-void residual urine volume

Answer 16.1.10 The correct answer is "A." TURP is a commonly performed procedure for BPH. Indications for TURP include failure of medical therapy, recurrent infections, bladder calculi, renal insufficiency, and patient preference. Patients who undergo TURP typically experience decreased AUA symptom scores, increased urine flow rates ("D"), and decreased post-void residual volumes ("E"). There are downsides to TURP, including urinary incontinence ("B"), urethral stenosis ("C"), and the need to repeat the surgery. Strange as it may seem, several studies have shown that erectile dysfunction does NOT occur at increased rates in patients undergoing TURP compared with watchful waiting. However, men can have retrograde ejaculation status post-TURP.

HELPFUL TIP:
Daily low-dose Cialis (taladafil) has been approved by the FDA for treating BPH. But, the benefit over placebo is only 2.3 points on a 35-point scale ... don't expect miracles.

Your patient is so happy with his care that he shared his story over a few beers, and his friend comes to see you. This patient is a 50-year-old male, in no apparent distress, who presents with a 6-month history of recurrent irritative voiding symptoms (frequency, urgency, etc.), low back and distal penile pain, and recurrent UTIs with the same organism. Today he is afebrile with a mildly tender prostate on digital rectal examination.

Question 16.1.11 Based on this patient's history and physical examination, all would be appropriate at this stage EXCEPT:

A) Have the patient complete the NIH Chronic Prostatitis Symptom Index questionnaire
B) Perform a two-glass pre- and post-prostatic massage test
C) Obtain urine culture and if positive, treat based on sensitivities for at least 4 weeks
D) Obtain a pelvic MRI

Answer 16.1.11 The correct answer is "D." There is no indication for a pelvic MRI at this time. The two-glass pre- and post-prostatic massage test ("B") is a very useful method of

diagnosing chronic prostatitis. A mid-stream voided urine specimen is collected and sent for culture. If the urinalysis has greater than 10 WBCs per high-power field, next prostatic massage is performed, and then the first 10 mL of voided urine after the massage that should include expressed prostatic secretions should be sent for culture. Treatment is based on the culture and sensitivity results. A 4- to 6-week course of treatment is recommended with an appropriate antibiotic with good tissue penetration. The most common organisms isolated in chronic bacterial prostatitis are *E. coli, Klebsiella, Proteus, Pseudomonas,* and Gram-positive *Enterococcus.* The NIH Chronic Prostatitis Symptom Index questionnaire ("A") is a reliable, valid method to assess symptoms and quality of life impact in men with chronic prostatitis (http://www.prostatitis.org/symptomindex.html).

HELPFUL TIP:
To massage or not, that is the question. While there appears reasonable evidence not to massage the prostate in acute prostatitis (so as to avoid potentially seeding bacteria into the blood stream), prostate massage's role in chronic prostatitis remains evolving. Given the more multifactorial etiology of chronic prostatitis (which includes noninfectious etiologies), prostate massage's role in chronic prostatitis has been prevalent since the mid-1900s. Its benefits are thought to arise from draining theoretically occluded prostate ducts, improving circulation, and helping with antibiotic penetration. However, a 2018 Cochrane review noted uncertainty as to whether or not prostatic massage reduces or increases prostatitis symptoms compared with control (with a "very low quality of evidence" rating for the studies examined). Use your clinical judgment when recommending prostatic massage for your patients with chronic prostatitis.

▶ **Objectives: Did you learn to ...**
· Recognize the pattern of voiding dysfunction seen in BPH?
· Manage a patient with BPH and understand the potential adverse effects of medications used to treat BPH?
· Diagnose and treat acute prostatitis?
· Describe indications for and complications of TURP?
· Evaluate chronic prostatitis?

 QUICK QUIZ: SEXUALLY TRANSMITTED INFECTIONS

A 21-year-old college student and self-described as a "ladies' man" (interpret: jerk) presents because of a concerning spot that developed on his penis. He complains of pain at the spot but denies itching. He reports no fever. When asked further about his sexual practices, he reports no condom use because his partners are all "on the pill." He had chlamydia in high school but is otherwise healthy. His review of systems is negative. On examination of the penis, you find a 1-cm tender, erythematous papule with a deep central ulceration at the glans penis. There is

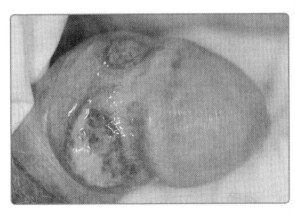

FIGURE 16-1. Chancroid lesions secondary to *H. ducreyi*. Notice the sharply demarcated borders and strongly erythematous appearance of the lesions. While it may look like syphilis, history is the key to distinguishing between the lesions, as chancroid lesions are painful while a chancre due to syphilis is nonpainful. (Used with permission from Kang S et al, eds. *Fitzpatrick's Dermatology*. 9th ed. New York: McGraw-Hill, 2019, Fig. 172-3.)

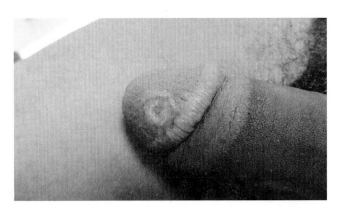

FIGURE 16-2. Chancre due to syphilis. Used with permission from Knoop KJ, Stack LB, Storrow AB, Thurman RJ (eds). *The Atlas of Emergency Medicine*. 4th ed. New York: McGraw-Hill, 2016, Fig 9.2. (Photo contributor: Larry B. Mellick, MD.)

some mild, tender lymphadenopathy in the inguinal area. The rest of the examination is unremarkable.

This lesion is most likely caused by:

A) *Haemophilus ducreyi*
B) *Neisseria gonorrhoeae*
C) *Staphylococcus aureus*
D) *Treponema pallidum*

The correct answer is "A." This is the lesion of *H. ducreyi*, otherwise known as chancroid. It can be confused with the chancre of primary syphilis, caused by *T. pallidum* ("D"), but the syphilis chancre is painless. Gram stain (Gram-negative rods in chains), culture, or biopsy may confirm the diagnosis. A few more notes: chancroid is rarely diagnosed in the United States and is probably under-diagnosed; it frequently co-infects with syphilis and tends to occur in clusters. A number of treatments are available including ceftriaxone (250 mg IM once), azithromycin (1 g PO once), ciprofloxacin (500 mg PO BID for 3 days), and erythromycin base (500 mg PO TID × 7 days). *Neisseria gonorrhoeae* ("B") and *Staphylococcus aureus* ("C") are incorrect because these pathogens do not form the type of lesion described in the questions stem. For more images of skin lesions associated with sexually transmitted infections, see Figures 16-1 through 16-7.

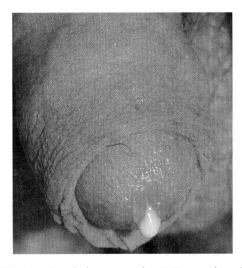

FIGURE 16-3. Purulent discharge secondary to *N. gonorrhoea*. Used with permission from Wolff K, Johnson RA, Saavedra AP, Roh EK. *Fitzpatrick's Color Atlas and Synopsis of Clinical Dermatology*. 8th ed. New York: McGraw-Hill Education, 2017, Fig. 30-22.

▶ **CASE 16.2**

A 22-year-old male presents complaining of a painless lump on his left testicle. He denies penile discharge, dysuria, or other urinary complaints. He underwent a left orchidopexy for an undescended testicle at age 6. Otherwise, his past medical history is unremarkable. On examination, the penis is circumcised with no lesion or discharge. There is adenopathy

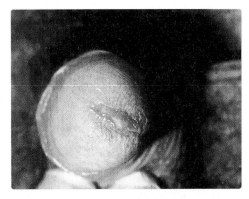

FIGURE 16-4. Clear discharge secondary to *C. trachomatis*. Source: https://commons.wikimedia.org/wiki/File:SOA-Chlamydia-trachomatis-male.jpg. Used with permission from SOA-AIDS Amsterdam.

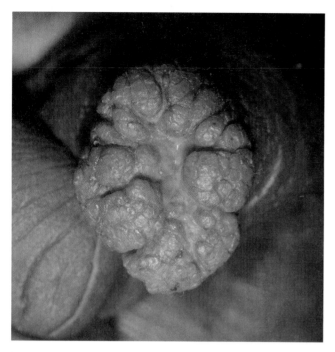

FIGURE 16-5. Cauliflower-like appearance of condyloma acuminata secondary to HPV infection. Used with permission from Knoop KJ, Stack LB, Storrow AB, Thurman RJ (eds). *The Atlas of Emergency Medicine*. 4th ed. New York: McGraw-Hill, 2016, Fig. 9.30. (Photo contributor: Lawrence B. Stack, MD.)

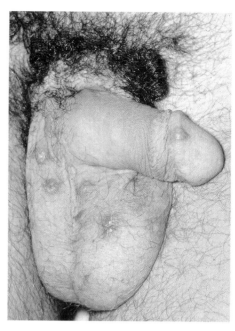

FIGURE 16-7. Reddish-brown papules and nodules characteristic of scabies. Used with permission from Wolff K, Johnson RA, Saavedra AP, Roh EK. *Fitzpatrick's Color Atlas and Synopsis of Clinical Dermatology*. 8th ed. New York: McGraw-Hill Education, 2017, Fig. 28-21.

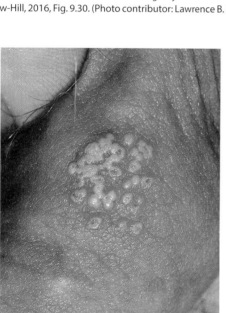

FIGURE 16-6. Grouped, vesicular lesions with overlying crust and erythematous base secondary to HSV. Used with permission from Wolff K, Johnson RA, Saavedra AP, Roh EK. *Fitzpatrick's Color Atlas and Synopsis of Clinical Dermatology*. 8th ed. New York: McGraw-Hill Education, 2017, Fig. 30-16.

in the left inguinal area. His testicles are descended bilaterally with a 1-cm palpable, irregular mass on the mid-lateral portion of the left testicle. His examination is otherwise unremarkable. Your patient is worried about testicular cancer and wants to know if he is at risk.

Question 16.2.1 **All of the following are associated with an increased risk of testicular cancer EXCEPT:**

A) Vasectomy
B) HIV infection
C) Cryptorchidism
D) Klinefelter syndrome
E) Family history

Answer 16.2.1 **The correct answer is "A."** Epidemiologic data do not support an association between testicular cancer and vasectomy. As is true of some other malignancies, males with HIV infection ("B") have an increased risk of testicular cancer. Also, males with cryptorchidism ("C"), defined as failure of one or both testicles to descend into the scrotum, and Klinefelter syndrome ("D") are at increased risk of testicular cancer. About 25% of testicular cancers occurring in patients with cryptorchidism arise in the contralateral (in the normally descended) testicle. While testicular cancer does not have as strong of a hereditary component, a positive family history ("E") is a risk factor for testicular cancer. Of note, black males have a much **lower** incidence of testicular cancer than do white males.

Question 16.2.2 **If your patient had not had an orchidopexy to repair the undescended testicle, he would be at risk for developing all of the following problems EXCEPT:**

A) Infertility
B) Inguinal hernia
C) Testicular torsion
D) Testicular malignancy
E) Impotence

Answer 16.2.2 **The correct answer is "E."** Organic impotence is not a consequence of cryptorchidism. All of the other problems listed occur at an increased frequency in males with an undescended testicle. The best time to begin treatment for an undescended testicle to minimize future sequelae is between 6 and 18 months of age and preferably by the end of the first year. The consequence of not treating an undescended testicle is a 20% to 40% increased risk of developing a testicular malignancy, which often presents as a painless mass (although it is not clear that fixing the undescended testicle lowers the cancer risk). Therefore, the reasons to treat cryptorchidism are (1) to better palpate the testicle to assess for potential malignant transformation; (2) to decrease the risk of malignant transformation (maybe); (3) to improve chances of fertility; (4) to decrease risk of testicular torsion; (5) to decrease psychological effects from having an empty scrotum; and (6) to repair an inguinal hernia at the same time, if it is present.

 HELPFUL TIP:
In patients with hypospadias and unilateral or bilateral empty scrotum, there is a higher rate of chromosomal anomalies.

Question 16.2.3 **After an appropriate history and physical examination, which of the following tests is the initial diagnostic study of choice in your patient with a scrotal mass?**
A) CT scan
B) Ultrasound
C) Complete blood count (CBC)
D) Alpha fetoprotein (AFP)
E) Pelvic x-ray

Answer 16.2.3 **The correct answer is "B."** The best initial diagnostic test would be a scrotal ultrasound to determine if this mass is cystic or solid. If it is determined to be a solid mass suspicious for malignancy, then other diagnostic studies would be warranted, such as β-hCG and AFP ("D"). In conjunction with a radical inguinal orchiectomy for testicular cancer, a CT scan would be indicated to evaluate for metastatic disease, but it is not the test of choice for initial diagnosis, so "A" is incorrect. CBC ("C") would have a role in suspected infection. X-ray ("E") has no role in the evaluation of this patient since this is a soft tissue mass.

 HELPFUL TIP:
If the ultrasound of a scrotal mass is equivocal, MRI or urological referral should be considered next.

Question 16.2.4 **In taking this patient's history, if he had described a *painful* lump in his scrotum, the LEAST likely cause would be:**
A) Chlamydia
B) Inguinal hernia
C) Hydrocele
D) Testicular torsion

Answer 16.2.4 **The correct answer is "C."** Spermatoceles and hydroceles are usually not painful. When a young, sexually active male presents with a painful scrotal mass or swelling, epididymitis from chlamydia ("A") or gonorrhea should be considered. Testicular torsion ("D") often has a very abrupt onset of pain and is a surgical emergency. Inguinal hernias ("B") can be intermittently painful if moving freely in the inguinal canal. However, if one becomes incarcerated, intense pain occurs. Of note, varicoceles are usually an incidental finding; however, large varicoceles may occasionally be painful. Likewise, testicular cancers are usually not painful but can become so if the tumor growth is rapid.

Your patient's ultrasound is concerning for testicular cancer, and you refer him to a urologist.

The next day the patient's 15-year-old brother presents with scrotal pain. You wonder if you are on the cusp of discovering an infectious cause of testicular cancer, but alas, it appears to be coincidence.

This patient's pain is on the right and he can localize it well to the front of the testicle. It has been present for 3 days and seemed to occur gradually over a few hours. There is no radiation of the pain. Running makes it worse, and cool packs seem to help. Yesterday he noticed a slight swelling of the scrotum on the same side. He denies trauma to the area, any history of sexual activity, other genitourinary complaints, fever, nausea, or vomiting. On examination you find normal vitals. He has a well-localized tender spot at the anterior superior right scrotum with a bluish discoloration under the skin ... as if it were some sort of sign ... a blue dot sign (Fig. 16-8).

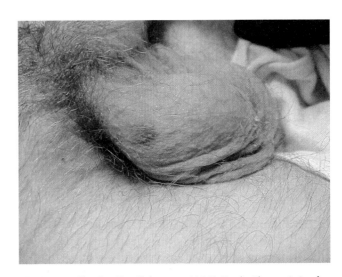

FIGURE 16-8. Blue Dot Sign (link to case 16.2.5). Used with permission from Knoop KJ, Stack LB, Storrow AB, Thurman RJ (eds). *The Atlas of Emergency Medicine.* 4th ed. New York: McGraw-Hill, 2016, Fig. 8.7. (Photo contributor: Alan B. Storrow, MD.)

Question 16.2.5 Which of the following is the most likely diagnosis?
A) Torsion of the appendix testis
B) Torsion of the testicle
C) Varicocele
D) Abscess
E) Spermatocele

Answer 16.2.5 The correct answer is "A." This is the classic presentation of a torsed appendix testis. The appendix testis is a pedunculated, vestigial structure at the anterior superior testicle. Torsion of the appendix testis is one of the most common causes of scrotal pain in children. The pain is usually well localized. There may be a reactive hydrocele. Diagnosis is confirmed by ultrasound. Unlike a torsed testicle ("B"), a torsed appendix testis is not an emergency. It may be treated by conservative therapy (rest, NSAIDs, ice) or surgical excision. The remainder of the options ("C," "D," "E") do not present with features of bluish discoloration under the skin.

▶ **Objectives: Did you learn to …**
· Recognize potential causes of a painless scrotal mass?
· Evaluate a testicular mass?
· Recognize the significance of cryptorchidism?
· Identify torsion of the appendix testis?

 QUICK QUIZ: HEMATOSPERMIA

A 28-year-old male presents to your office looking quite concerned. Several days ago after sexual intercourse with his girlfriend, he noticed bloody ejaculate in the condom. Since then he has masturbated twice ("just to check") and has not seen any more blood. He denies pain, hematuria, dysuria, fevers, night sweats, and weight loss. He reports that he is otherwise healthy. His examination, including genitourinary and rectal examination, is normal. A urinalysis is negative.

What is your next step in the evaluation and management of this patient?
A) Reassurance and follow-up
B) Scrotal ultrasound
C) Pelvic CT scan
D) Transrectal ultrasound
E) PSA

The correct answer is "A." Hematospermia, the name given to bloody penile ejaculate, is fairly uncommon. It can occur in men of any age and is perhaps most common after prostate biopsy or prostate surgery. In otherwise healthy young men, the cause is most often idiopathic and is almost always benign. History should focus on traumatic causes (e.g., a long bicycle ride), symptoms of prostate disease, and symptoms of infection. A genital and prostate examination should be performed. Urinalysis is helpful to exclude infection. Consider gonorrhea and chlamydia cultures in the appropriate patients, for example,

those with symptoms of urethritis. In this patient, reassurance is adequate. Persistent hematospermia, with symptoms present for over a month, may require further evaluation with PSA ("E"), imaging ("B," "C," "D"), and urologic consultation. Some experts recommend a more aggressive workup, especially in older males, but there is no evidence to support more extensive evaluations. Also, ask about recent travel, as schistosomiasis is a frequent cause of hematospermia and hematuria in other parts of the world. In most cases of hematospermia, semen analysis is not warranted, but it can be diagnostic in patients with schistosomiasis.

▶ **CASE 16.3**

A couple you have known for a few years comes to your office to announce that they are expecting and that they want you to be the baby's doctor (strange that they didn't ask you to be the mother's doctor, but you let it slide). According to an ultrasound, the fetus is male. The couple is ambivalent about neonatal circumcision and wants your advice.

Question 16.3.1 You start the conversation by saying:
A) "Circumcision is a relic of history and should be illegal"
B) "All major medical organizations (e.g., AAFP, AAP, AMA) recommend routine neonatal circumcision"
C) "The decision to perform circumcision is a personal one, influenced by a number of factors—but primarily by cultural, religious, and familial issues"
D) "Do whatever you want. I don't really care what you do with a tiny piece of skin"

Answer 16.3.1 The correct answer is "C." One of the strongest predictors of whether a newborn in the United States will be circumcised is the circumcision status of the father. There are other reasons cited by parents as well (discussed later in the case). "A" is incorrect simply because the statement is effused with emotion and lacks logic. "B" is incorrect. The AAFP has no policy statement on circumcision. In 2012 the American Academy of Pediatrics changed its statement on circumcision to the following: *the health benefits outweigh the risks, and circumcision should be made available to all families who choose it. However, 'routine' universal circumcision is still not recommended.* If you chose "D," you need to work on your bedside manner!

Question 16.3.2 Consequences of circumcision include which of the following?
A) Overall reduction in mortality of circumcised infants compared with uncircumcised infants
B) Reduction in UTIs in the first year of life
C) Reduction in the number of sexual partners
D) All of the above

Answer 16.3.2 The correct answer is "B." The rate of UTIs in uncircumcised males in the first year of life is about 10 times greater than the rate for circumcised males. In order to prevent one UTI in the first year of life, about 100 circumcisions need to be performed. The effect of circumcision on rates of UTI later in life is not well studied. The rate of UTI may be higher shortly after circumcision (within the first 2 weeks). "A" is incorrect because there is no data showing any difference in mortality between circumcised and uncircumcised infants. "C" is incorrect; some surveys have shown increased frequency and variety of sexual practices in circumcised males compared with uncircumcised (note that this is an association, not a causal relationship).

HELPFUL TIP:
Circumcision reduces the rate of cervical cancer in the female partners of males who were circumcised and previously had six or more sexual partners. This is thought to be due to decreased rate of HPV transmission. Of course, it is now recommended to provide vaccination to all young men and women with the HPV vaccination series. See the Chapters 13 and 14 for more information.

Question 16.3.3 Neonatal circumcision is associated with all of the following EXCEPT:
A) Risk of hemorrhage with the procedure
B) Psychological trauma and decreased sexual satisfaction later in life
C) Reduced risk of infection with STIs, such as HIV
D) Reduced risk of penile cancer

Answer 16.3.3 **The correct answer is "B."** Despite what some anti-circumcision websites maintain, circumcision does not appear to result in any significant psychological trauma or decreased sexual satisfaction for most men later in life. "A" is true. There is a small but real risk of hemorrhage with the procedure, and this occurs mostly in patients who have an unknown or unrealized coagulopathy. In fact, abnormal bleeding after circumcision is a common way in which sporadic cases of hemophilia are discovered (including one case discovered this way by one of the editors—and he still feels bad!). "C" is true. Several studies have demonstrated that circumcised men are less likely to have HPV infection. The data for the risk of other sexually transmitted infections (STIs) are somewhat contradictory, but generally favor a reduced risk of STIs in circumcised males. "D" is true. There is evidence that circumcision may decrease the transmission of HPV and penile cancer. Retrospective studies have shown that the rate of squamous cell carcinoma of the penis is about threefold higher in uncircumcised men, at least in the United States. However, penile cancer is exceedingly rare (about 0.6 cases/100,000) and the number of circumcisions needed to prevent one case of penile cancer is about 300,000. However, the American Cancer Society does **not** recommend routine neonatal circumcision for the prevention of penile cancer, but it does recommend that all risk factors be addressed.

HELPFUL TIP:
It is abundantly clear that circumcision reduces the transmission of HIV. This has led to a call for routine circumcision in high-risk populations (e.g., some parts of sub-Saharan Africa, etc.).

HELPFUL TIP:
In addition to uncircumcised status, risk factors associated with penile cancer include smoking, risky sexual behavior, poor hygiene, and genital warts.

You have a nice, long conversation with the couple, discussing the potential benefits and risks, and they decide to have their son circumcised. After the birth, you are performing a thorough examination when you find something slightly abnormal with the penis.

Question 16.3.4 Neonatal circumcision is indicated for:
A) Congenital phimosis
B) Micropenis
C) Hypospadias
D) Ambiguous genitalia

Answer 16.3.4 **The correct answer is "A."** Significant congenital phimosis rarely occurs and is an indication for circumcision. Phimosis is defined as the inability to retract the foreskin (prepuce) over the glans. This is a **normal** finding in uncircumcised infants. However, **significant** congenital phimosis may completely cover the urethra and not allow the normal passage of urine. "B," "C," and "D" are reasons to **avoid** routine circumcision and to call on the aid of a urologist.

HELPFUL TIP:
When performing circumcision, local anesthetic is recommended, and either dorsal penile nerve block or subcutaneous ring block is preferred. Other pain control modalities may be used as well, including pre-procedure acetaminophen, sucrose-coated pacifier, calming music, swaddling, etc.

▶ **Objectives: Did you learn to ...**
• Discuss the benefits and risks of circumcision with parents?
• Identify indications and contraindications for neonatal circumcision?
• Employ appropriate pain control measures for the procedure of circumcision?

▶ **CASE 16.4**

A 32-year-old male presents to discuss permanent sterilization. He clearly states that he wants a vasectomy, and sooner is better than later. He is married and has three children at home.

His wife just gave birth to twins. He is healthy and takes no medications. He looks tired and anxious. You examine him and find no abnormalities. The vas deferens is easily isolated bilaterally.

Question 16.4.1 What is your next step?
A) Refer him for psychological counseling as he is clearly under a great deal of stress
B) Provide him with detailed counseling on vasectomy, give him written material on the procedure, and ask him to discuss it with his wife
C) Do the vasectomy right now; the next patient can wait
D) Tell him that he is not an appropriate candidate for vasectomy because of his history of hypertension

Answer 16.4.1 **The correct answer is "B."** Patient education, counseling, and selection are very important aspects of vasectomy. When you counsel him on vasectomy, you should explore his reasons for wanting the procedure. You should not schedule a vasectomy without providing counseling and assuring that he understands the procedure in detail (thus, "C" is incorrect). This patient appears to be fatigued—an issue that should be explored further—and he has newborn twins at home (who the heck wouldn't be tired?). So, immediate referral for psychological counseling without investigating the underlying cause ("A") is not appropriate.

Question 16.4.2 While counseling this patient, you discuss which of the following issues?
A) Partner's desire for permanent sterility
B) Effect of the procedure on sexual function
C) Reversibility of the procedure
D) Complications
E) All of the above

Answer 16.4.2 **The correct answer is "E."** All these issues are important to discuss prior to scheduling the procedure. It is important that the couple agree on this procedure because it is *the couple*—not just your patient—who will be sterile. Aside from psychological effects of vasectomy, the procedure should not directly affect sexual function, orgasm, or ejaculation. Patients should be aware that vasectomy results in permanent sterility and that reversal procedures are only successful about half of the time. Potential complications include failure and unwanted pregnancy, infection, pain, bleeding, hematoma, etc.

Your patient decides to "get snipped" (as he puts it). You perform the vasectomy using a no-scalpel technique. The procedure was fairly easy, and the patient tolerated it well. One month after the procedure, the patient calls to complain about a painful swelling that has developed superior and slightly posterior to the left testis. He has no other symptoms.

Question 16.4.3 Which of the following is the most likely diagnosis?
A) Hematoma
B) Varicocele
C) Congestive epididymitis
D) Abscess

Answer 16.4.3 **The correct answer is "C."** Without any further information, congestive epididymitis is the most likely cause of this patient's current complaint. Congestive epididymitis occurs in about 3% of patients post-vasectomy, and the onset is usually within weeks to months after the procedure. "A," hematoma, can be avoided in most cases if hemostasis is achieved during the procedure and the patient does not overexert himself immediately post-operation. A hematoma is more likely to develop early rather than a month later. Likewise, an infection ("D") would be unlikely so far out from the procedure. "B" is incorrect because varicoceles do not develop after vasectomy (unless you are operating far away from where you are supposed to be). Overall, the most common scrotal pathology after vasectomy is sperm granuloma, which occurs in up to 40% of patients but is generally asymptomatic.

HELPFUL TIP:
The treatment of congestive epididymitis can be frustrating. Most men who have a vasectomy will have some element of congestive epididymitis, but most will have minor swelling without pain. For patients with painful congestive epididymitis, a trial of NSAIDs and sitz baths for several months is indicated. Failing conservative therapy, steroid injection or surgery may be indicated.

Two months after the vasectomy, your patient returns with a semen sample, showing no sperm. His surgery was successful, but failures do occasionally occur.

Question 16.4.4 Vasectomy failure is usually due to:
A) Failure to identify and transect the vas at the time of surgery
B) Recanalization
C) Infection
D) Immaculate conception

Answer 16.4.4 **The correct answer is "B."** Although "redundant systems" (removing a segment of the vas deferens, clipping or suturing the free ends, cauterizing the transected vas, suturing fascia around one free end while leaving the other outside the fascia) are employed to avoid this complication, recanalization can occur. A new pathway can form between the free ends of the transected vas deferens, allowing sperm into the ejaculated semen. Therefore, all patients should return post-vasectomy for semen analysis. "A" and "C" are potential, but infrequent, causes of failure. As to "D", only God knows.

Your patient is ultimately pleased with his vasectomy results. He returns to see you several years later because of concerns that he is balding. On examination, you find non-scarring hair loss at the vertex. The scalp appears normal otherwise.

Question 16.4.5 You should entertain all of the following diagnoses EXCEPT:
A) Androgenetic alopecia (yes, it is "androgenetic" and not "androgenic")
B) Telogen effluvium
C) Alopecia areata
D) Hypothyroidism
E) Tinea capitis

Answer 16.4.5 The correct answer is "E." Hair loss is common in males, affecting up to two-thirds of all men. Alopecia is often divided into scarring and non-scarring forms. Most infectious causes of hair loss (e.g., tinea capitis and folliculitis) are scarring if not treated, whereas the other causes listed ("A" through "D") are non-scarring. Without any signs of inflammation or hyperkeratosis, tinea capitis ("E") is unlikely. "A," androgenetic alopecia, is quite common in adult males (male balding). "B," telogen effluvium, presents with diffuse hair loss usually secondary to metabolic (including dieting) or emotional stress. This occurs as an abnormal percentage of hair enters the telogen phase during which they are shed. Grab some hair: if more than five hairs in telogen phase come out, you have your diagnosis. "C," alopecia areata, results in patchy hair loss in round or oval shapes. Metabolic conditions should also be in the differential diagnosis of hair loss, and these might include hypothyroidism ("D"), hyperthyroidism, and iron deficiency.

HELPFUL TIP:
Secondary syphilis causes a non-inflammatory, non-scarring hair loss that may be patchy or diffuse. Consider testing for syphilis in appropriate patients.

The patient reports a strong family history of baldness. On your examination, the patient has thin hair at the vertex and recession of the hairline in an "M" shape at the frontotemporal area. On the basis of the history and examination, you diagnose androgenetic alopecia. He would like to do something about his hair loss.

Question 16.4.6 Regarding androgenetic alopecia, which of the following statements is true?
A) Minoxidil must be used for at least 2 years to achieve permanent hair regrowth
B) Lower doses of 5-α-reductase inhibitors (e.g., finasteride) are used in treating androgenetic alopecia compared with BPH
C) Hair transplant should be avoided unless all other therapeutic attempts have failed
D) Topical steroids are an effective therapy for androgenetic alopecia
E) A toupee looks great on anyone

Answer 16.4.6 The correct answer is "B." Finasteride (Propecia) is FDA approved for androgenetic alopecia, and the dose is 1 mg/day rather than the 5 mg/day dose used to treat BPH symptoms. Minoxidil applied to the scalp is also an effective therapy for androgenetic alopecia. Both minoxidil and finasteride must be continued indefinitely to be effective (thus, "A" is incorrect). Hair transplant is a viable option for men and women with androgenetic alopecia, and it is sometimes used as a first-line therapy. Thus, "C" is incorrect. Topical steroids ("D") are not effective for this type of hair loss. "E" is clearly wrong; there are a lot of bad toupees out there.

▶ **Objectives: Did you learn to …**
· Provide pre-vasectomy counseling?
· Recognize complications of vasectomy?
· Identify causes of hair loss in men?
· Describe current treatment options for androgenetic alopecia?

 QUICK QUIZ: DEATH RATES IN MEN

For all the following causes of death, the age-adjusted death rate is higher for males than for females EXCEPT:
A) Liver disease
B) Alzheimer disease
C) Coronary artery disease
D) Suicide
E) Cancer

The correct answer is "B." When it comes to Alzheimer disease, men get a break; the death rate is higher for females. All of the other causes of death listed have greater death rates in males. For example, compared with women with liver disease, same age men with liver disease are twice as likely to die of their liver disease.

 QUICK QUIZ: MORE ABOUT DEATH IN MEN

The relative risk of death for males is greater throughout the life span. Compared with same age females, at what age range is the relative risk of death greatest for males?
A) <1 year
B) 5 to 14 years
C) 15 to 24 years
D) 25 to 34 years
E) >85 years

The correct answer is "C." Unfortunately, males aged 15 to 24 years have a relative risk of death of greater than 2.5 compared with same age females (usually preceded by a cry of, "Hey! Look what I can do!"). Mother Nature has a way of making up for boys and young men dying: more male fetuses are conceived than female. However, the miscarriage rate is also greater for male fetuses. Nonetheless, about 105 males are born in the United States for every 100 females. By age 35, enough males have died off that the number of males and females at that age is about equal, and thereafter the number of females exceeds the number of males (in other words, the singles scene improves markedly for the remaining males).

▶ CASE 16.5

A 14-year-old male presents with his mother, who is worried that he has growing breasts. Over the last 2 or 3 months, the patient has developed swellings beneath both nipples. He denies discharge or pain, but the nipples are tender at times.

Question 16.5.1 **You can tell this patient that physiologic gynecomastia (subareolar breast tissue) is a condition that affects:**
A) Newborns
B) Adolescents
C) Elderly males
D) All of the above

Answer 16.5.1 **The correct answer is "D."** The incidence of physiologic gynecomastia is trimodal, with peaks in the neonatal period, adolescence, and old age. Data can be contradictory at times, but clinically palpable breast tissue (either fat or true breast tissue) may be present in more than 50% of males in each of these three age groups.

Question 16.5.2 **Which of the following hormones is responsible for the proliferation of breast tissue?**
A) Testosterone
B) Estrogen
C) Androstenedione
D) Growth hormone
E) Progesterone

Answer 16.5.2 **The correct answer is "B."** Estrogens induce ductal hyperplasia and growth of glandular tissue. Testosterone ("A") and androstenedione ("C") inhibit the actions of estrogens on the breast tissue. Some men with gynecomastia have increased sensitivity of breast tissue to circulating estrogens. Others may have an increased proportion of estrogens compared with androgens. And others still may have a mixture of both processes or another process altogether.

Question 16.5.3 **Potential causes of gynecomastia include all of the following EXCEPT:**
A) Renal failure
B) Marijuana use
C) Testicular cancer
D) Hypothyroidism
E) Phenothiazines

Answer 16.5.3 **The correct answer is "D."** Hyperthyroidism, not hypothyroidism, can cause gynecomastia through increased aromatization of testosterone to estradiol and androstenedione to estrone. A number of drugs are associated with gynecomastia,

including marijuana ("B"), alcohol, 5-alpha-reductase inhibitors, phenothiazines ("E"), tricyclic antidepressants, androgens, estrogens, growth hormone, calcium channel blockers, and spironolactone. Other causes of gynecomastia include: hypogonadism, hyperprolactinemia, testicular tumors (some secrete estrogens), renal failure ("A"), and liver diseases (cirrhosis). Obesity is associated with gynecomastia, but obese patients may also appear to have gynecomastia while simply having excess fat deposition in the area of the breast (sometimes called "pseudogynecomastia").

A thorough drug history is negative. On physical examination, you find palpable, nontender tissue beneath the nipples, with slightly more prominent tissue mass on the right. The tissue is about 2 to 3 cm in diameter, and no discrete masses are palpable. There is no nipple discharge. An adult male's hair growth pattern is evident in the axillary and inguinal areas. The testicles are normal size without masses.

Question 16.5.4 **At this point in time, you recommend which of the following?**
A) Observation
B) Referral to a surgeon
C) Limited laboratory studies, including thyroid-stimulating hormone (TSH), testosterone, and liver enzymes
D) Biopsy of the tissue
E) Mammogram and/or ultrasound

Answer 16.5.4 **The correct answer is "A."** As previously mentioned, physiologic gynecomastia is quite common in adolescent males. The findings on examination are reassuring. This patient does not display any other signs of testosterone deficiency, and further workup ("C," "D," "E") is not indicated at this time. If there are no discrete masses on examination, a mammogram, ultrasound, or biopsy is not likely to be helpful. Referral to a surgeon is premature ("B"), as 90% of these patients experience spontaneous involution of the breast tissue over 3 years.

HELPFUL TIP:
In adolescent males with gynecomastia, further evaluation with laboratory studies and imaging is indicated if the breast tissue is rapidly enlarging or is greater than 5 cm in diameter, a mass (not normal breast tissue) is palpable, or other signs of under androgenization are present. Should the breast tissue be glandular, nonmalignant, and is causing significant embarrassment or pain, a trial of the selective estrogen-receptor modulator tamoxifen for gynecomastia may be reasonable, given its efficacy and safety profile. However, patients should be warned that use of this medication may not result in complete regression of the breast tissue despite potentially helping with pain.

You provide the patient and his mother with reassurance and have them return in a year. At follow-up, there is no palpable tissue. When you see the patient again, he is 17 years old.

He told his mother that he was having abdominal pain, but really he is worried that he may have contracted an STI. He has become fairly promiscuous and does not use condoms (after the gynecomastia disappeared, his mojo returned). In the last week he has developed dysuria and a yellowish urethral discharge. He has no other symptoms.

Question 16.5.5 Which of the following is the most likely diagnosis?
A) HPV
B) Syphilis
C) Gonorrhea
D) Trichomonas
E) Herpes simplex

Answer 16.5.5 The correct answer is "C." This patient's symptoms are typical of gonococcal urethritis. However, *N. gonorrhoeae* may be present in the urethra without any symptoms and *Chlamydia trachomatis* can present with a purulent discharge that is classically thought of as gonorrhea. Gonorrhea and chlamydia cannot be reliably distinguished on clinical grounds. "A" is incorrect as HPV causes genital warts, not urethritis. "B," syphilis, may present as a painless ulcer (primary syphilis). "D" is incorrect because most men infected with *Trichomonas vaginalis* are asymptomatic, although some will have mild urethritis. Finally, "E," herpes simplex, presents with painful vesicles at the area of inoculation.

You obtain urine for PCR for gonorrhea and chlamydia. You discuss other STIs and decide to perform some other tests (e.g., HIV, hepatitis B, syphilis antibody).

Question 16.5.6 At this point in time, you are compelled to do all of the following EXCEPT:
A) Recommend safer sexual practices
B) Inform the public health services if he tests positive
C) Treat him with antibiotics now
D) Encourage him to contact his partners and tell them to get tested
E) Inform his mother of your findings

Answer 16.5.6 The correct answer is "E." In general, adolescents can seek care for STIs and be treated without parental consent. However, clinicians should refer to the laws of the state in which they practice for ultimate legal authority in this matter. Of course, the time of diagnosis and treatment should be used as an opportunity to educate the patient regarding safer sexual practices ("A"). "B" is true. Gonorrhea and chlamydia are reportable diseases in every state. Again, clinicians should refer to the laws of their state and the reporting protocols of the clinic in which they practice. Empiric treatment is the rule here, so "C" is correct. "D" is also correct since all of this patient's partners should be contacted, tested, and treated. There are several ways to contact the partners and allowing the patient to do so is only one way. The clinician or the public health authorities could contact the partners as well.

HELPFUL TIP:
Expedited partner treatment, in which the patient being treated for an STI is also given medication for his/her partner(s), is recommended by the Centers for Disease Control and Prevention (CDC) and others. See http://www.cdc.gov/std/ept/ for more information and the legality of the practice in your state.

Question 16.5.7 Which of the following methods maintains a high degree of sensitivity and is also the quickest and least expensive way to diagnose gonococcal urethritis in a symptomatic male?
A) Culture
B) Gram stain
C) Serologic antibody assay
D) PCR
E) NAAT (nucleic acid amplification testing)

Answer 16.5.7 The correct answer is "B." In **symptomatic** males, Gram stain of a urethral sample can identify Gram-negative diplococci (*N. gonorrhoeae*) with a sensitivity of about 90% to 95%. The sensitivity drops to about 70% in asymptomatic males. If the materials and expertise are readily available, a Gram stain is quick and inexpensive. Culture ("A") of a urethral specimen on Thayer–Martin agar takes longer and false-negative tests can occur with high frequency (due to the need to have a CO_2-rich environment and to keep the culture in a narrow temperature range). PCR ("D") and other nucleic acid testing are more sensitive than cultures but still not 100%. PCR is particularly attractive as a screening test, as it can be performed on urine specimens instead of urethral swab specimens. Serologic assays ("C") for gonorrhea would not be helpful in diagnosing urethritis. "E," NAAT is actually the most sensitive technique for detecting gonorrhea. It can be used in asymptomatic individuals, is completed in hours, and works with patient-collected specimens (urine, self-collected vaginal swab). Overall it is the preferred test. But it is not as fast as a Gram stain and is more expensive.

HELPFUL TIP:
When obtaining urine for testing of gonorrhea and chlamydia, remind the patient to perform a first-catch urine and NOT a midstream clean-catch urine. A 20 to 30 mL sample should suffice. For men-who-have-sex-with-men, urethral, oral, and rectal samples should be sent.

Question 16.5.8 Your clinical suspicion of gonorrhea is high. What is your next step?
A) Single doses of ceftriaxone 125 mg IM
B) Single dose of penicillin G 1.2 million units IM and erythromycin 500 mg orally QID for 7 days
C) Tetracycline 500 mg orally QID for 10 days
D) Single doses of ciprofloxacin 500 mg orally and cefixime 400 mg orally
E) Single dose of ceftriaxone 250 mg IM and azithromycin 1 g orally

Answer 16.5.8 The correct answer is "E." If there is any concern for compliance, it is best to treat the patient in the office if you have access to the appropriate antibiotics. As of 2015, the CDC recommends ceftriaxone 250 mg IM as a single dose (rather than 125 mg, due to increasing resistance) PLUS azithromycin 1 g PO for uncomplicated gonococcal urethritis. The azithromycin is given for two reasons: increasing resistance among gonococcal isolates and to cover for possible chlamydia co-infection. If ceftriaxone is not available, cefixime 400 mg PO is an acceptable alternative. **Fluoroquinolones are not recommended for gonorrhea due to high rates of resistance in some communities.** "A" is incorrect because ceftriaxone alone will not provide empiric coverage for chlamydia, and the dose is too low anyway. "B" is incorrect because penicillin should never be used to treat gonorrhea (due to the prevalence of penicillinase-producing strains of the bacteria). "C" is incorrect. Tetracycline antibiotics provide adequate coverage for chlamydia and some strains of *N. gonorrhoeae*, but other strains of *N. gonorrhoeae* are resistant to tetracyclines, so these drugs are not used as first-line agents in treating gonorrhea. "D" is incorrect because fluoroquinolones are not recommended for gonorrhea and it contains nothing for the treatment of chlamydia.

HELPFUL TIP:
Another equally effective regimen for chlamydia is doxycycline 100 mg BID for 7 days. This is equal in efficacy to azithromycin despite the fact that some doses may be missed. Of note, doxycycline has been in short supply periodically.

You treat this patient with ceftriaxone and azithromycin and tell him to contact his partners so that they can get treated. When your patient returns to discuss his lab tests, he is feeling much better. You tell him that he was infected with both gonorrhea and chlamydia but that the rest of his tests were negative. He is relieved that he does not have HIV, but he wonders what problems chlamydia can cause.

Question 16.5.9 *C. trachomatis* **has been implicated in which of the following?**
A) Reiter syndrome
B) Lymphogranuloma venereum
C) Proctitis
D) Epididymitis
E) All of the above

Answer 16.5.9 The correct answer is "E." A small percentage of men with chlamydia urethritis develop reactive arthritis, and a subset of these will go on to have the triad of Reiter syndrome (urethritis, arthritis, and uveitis). Lymphogranuloma venereum is also due to a particularly virulent strain of *C. trachomatis*, but it produces genital ulcers and lymphadenitis and is generally seen in tropical areas. Lymphogranuloma venereum is treated with extended courses of doxycycline (100 mg PO BID for 21 days) or azithromycin (1 g PO weekly for 3 weeks). Chlamydia

proctitis occurs almost exclusively in homosexual men and presents with rectal pain, bleeding, and discharge. Diagnosis is confirmed by rectal swab, and the treatment is the same as for chlamydia urethritis. Epididymitis is most often the result of infection with *C. trachomatis* or *N. gonorrhoeae* in younger individuals (contrast to *E. coli* and *Pseudomonas* in those over the age of 35). Urethral strictures are also commonly related to prior STIs.

HELPFUL TIP:
The majority of males (and females) who are infected with chlamydia and/or gonorrhea **do not have symptoms.** Therefore, there is a good argument to be made for screening asymptomatic males (and females) in high-risk populations (e.g., adolescents, young adults, and those with multiple sexual partners). For females, see Chapter 15.

▶ **Objectives: Did you learn to …**
- Define gynecomastia and understand its causes?
- Identify when to initiate further evaluation in a patient with gynecomastia?
- Recognize symptoms of gonorrhea and chlamydia?
- Initiate treatment in a male with urethritis?
- Recognize manifestations of chlamydia infection in men?

 QUICK QUIZ: AN INFLAMED GLANS

A 36-year-old male diabetic patient presents with a 3-day history of irritation, itching, dysuria, and redness at the tip of his penis (Fig. 16-9). He is monogamous with his wife, and he denies any history of high-risk sexual behavior or STIs. On examination, you find an afebrile patient in no acute distress. The penis is circumcised, and the glans penis is red, tender, and edematous. There are numerous small, white papules on the glans.

Which of the following is the most appropriate treatment?
A) Sitz baths and improved hygiene
B) Oral doxycycline
C) Topical bacitracin
D) Topical miconazole
E) Topical steroids

The correct answer is "D." This patient has balanitis, which is defined as an inflammatory condition of the glans penis (balanoposthitis is the name applied to inflammation of the glans and foreskin). Some authors believe that balanitis is a noninfectious, inflammatory condition. Others implicate infectious causes. Of infectious causes, the most common is *Candida albicans*, especially in diabetic patients. This patient has classic findings of candidal balanitis and is diabetic. Therefore, the most appropriate therapy is a topical antifungal agent, such as miconazole ("D"). Fluconazole is an option. Topical and oral antibiotics ("B", "C") will not help, and topical steroids ("E") should be avoided. Sitz baths and improved hygiene ("A") should be encouraged, but they should not be employed without an antifungal agent.

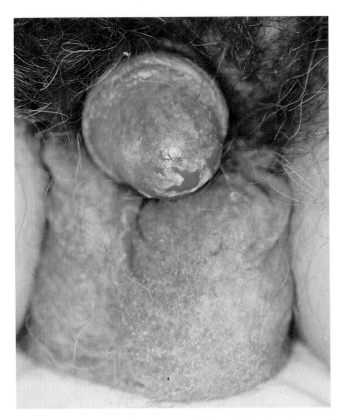

FIGURE 16-9. Candidal Balanitis. Used with permission from Knoop KJ, Stack LB, Storrow AB, Thurman RJ (eds). *The Atlas of Emergency Medicine.* 4th ed. New York: McGraw-Hill, 2016, Fig. 8.33. (Photo contributor: Kevin J. Knoop, MD, MS.)

► CASE 16.6

While covering the emergency department (ED), a 40-year-old male presents with a painful erection that began 4 hours ago "out of the blue" (perhaps after he took too many little "blue pills").

Question 16.6.1 Which of the following is true regarding priapism and normal erections?
A) Normal erections can last up to 12 hours, so this is not priapism
B) Abnormally prolonged sexual desire can "convert" a normal erection into priapism
C) The corpus spongiosum and glans penis are not involved in priapism
D) Acute urinary retention may lead to priapism and vice versa
E) All of the above are true statements

Answer 16.6.1 **The correct answer is "C."** Priapism is defined as the prolonged engorgement of the penis (or—rarely—the clitoris in females), unrelated to sexual desire or stimulation. The word priapism comes from the Greek god Priapus, apparently well known for his lasciviousness and generous genital endowment. In most cases of priapism, the corpus spongiosum and glans penis are not involved. Only the corpora cavernosa are engorged and rigid. Priapism typically lasts longer than 6 hours (thus making "A" incorrect), whereas normal erections

TABLE 16-1 DRUGS ASSOCIATED WITH PRIAPISM

Psychotropics
- Trazodone
- Chlorpromazine

Agents used to treat erectile dysfunction
- Intracavernosal injections (e.g., papaverine)
- Phosphodiesterase inhibitors (e.g., sildenafil)

Antihypertensives
- Hydralazine
- Prazosin

Anticoagulants
- Heparin

Drugs of abuse
- Alcohol
- Cocaine
- Marijuana

last minutes to hours. With normal erections, detumescence occurs after ejaculation or after the stimulus is removed. This is not the case with priapism, and sexual desire does not play a role in the development of priapism; thus, "B" is incorrect. "D" is also incorrect. Urinary retention is not thought to cause priapism, and priapism does not lead to urinary retention.

Question 16.6.2 Priapism may be secondary to all of the following EXCEPT:
A) Sickle cell disease
B) Penile trauma
C) Leukemia
D) Iron deficiency anemia
E) Trazodone use

Answer 16.6.2 **The correct answer is "D."** A number of different disease states and drugs have been implicated in the etiology of priapism. In one way or another, these diseases and drugs affect the balance of blood flow into the penis, leading to increased arterial blood flow and/or decreased venous outflow. Local malignancies, such as bladder and prostate cancers, can cause obstruction. Likewise, any condition that increases blood viscosity (e.g., sickle cell disease, polycythemia, leukemia) or results in thromboembolic phenomena (e.g., vasculitis) can cause priapism. Penile trauma that results in laceration of penile arteries can cause priapism. Numerous drugs have also been implicated (see Table 16-1), but, in most cases, the cause of priapism is not identified.

Question 16.6.3 What is your next step in management of this patient?
A) Reassurance
B) Call for emergent urologic consultation
C) Give oral alpha-blockers
D) Engage patient in guided imagery to lead his thoughts away from sex

Answer 16.6.3 **The correct answer is "B."** Priapism is a urologic emergency and needs to be treated ASAP. All the other answers ("A," "C," "D") could result in your undesired new title of "defendant." Until the urologist arrives, conservative measures are probably best, and you should try to make the patient comfortable using analgesics, oxygen, and hydration. Check a CBC since leukemia can rarely present with priapism. Some patients will respond to analgesics and ice packs. Oral or subcutaneous terbutaline may be helpful. Some authors recommend sedatives, such as benzodiazepines.

HELPFUL TIP:
If a urologist is not available and/or you are comfortable performing the procedure (and you have a good lawyer), you can attempt detumescence. A needle is inserted into the corpora cavernosa and blood is withdrawn. Then a vasoactive agent (e.g., phenylephrine) is injected. This procedure is repeated every 5 minutes until detumescence occurs. It should go without saying that the patient's vital signs must be closely monitored during this intervention because they will likely need sedation.

HELPFUL TIP:
After recovery, about 50% of men with priapism suffer erectile dysfunction. Penile implants are an option.

▶ **Objectives: Did you learn to …**
- Recognize priapism and its causes?
- Manage a patient with priapism?

 QUICK QUIZ: DEPRESSION AND SUICIDE

Which of the following groups has the highest rate of death by suicide?
A) Black males
B) White males
C) Black females
D) White females
E) Hispanic males

The correct answer is "B." In the United States, white males make up about 70% of all deaths due to suicide. Although females account for more suicide attempts, males are at greater risk of death from suicide. Men tend to use deadlier means, such as guns, hanging, and car collisions. In other words, men are very efficient at suicide. White men older than 85 years have one of the highest rates of death due to suicide: 59/100,000 (with the rate in the general public being 10.6/100,000). As a group, black males have the second highest rate of suicide. Of those groups listed above, black females have the lowest risk of death from suicide.

▶ **CASE 16.7**

A 78-year-old male presents for follow-up after an emergency department visit last week. He sustained a fall that resulted in a T11 compression fracture. You obtained a DEXA scan to confirm that he has osteoporosis and found that his T-score is indeed osteoporotic-range. Just to be on the safe side, you order a bunch of laboratory tests, all of which are normal except for serum testosterone. Lo and behold, his testosterone level is very low. He's also been tired, felt weak, and lost his libido. Because he knows we need to cover testosterone supplementation in this book, he asks you, "Should I be on one of those fancy testosterone supplements?"

Question 16.7.1 Which of the following testosterone supplementation products would you AVOID?
A) Transdermal testosterone patches
B) Buccal testosterone tablets
C) Oral testosterone tablets
D) Intramuscular testosterone injections
E) Transdermal testosterone gel

Answer 16.7.1 The correct answer is "C." Oral testosterone should be avoided due to significant first-pass metabolism and potential liver toxicity. The other choices listed are viable options for testosterone replacement (see Table 16-2). The IM option is not the best for a steady state, but patients often like it due to the peaks.

TABLE 16-2 TESTOSTERONE SUPPLEMENTATION PRODUCTS

Agents	Dosages	Comments
Buccal tablet (Striant)	Dosed 30 mg BID and must be kept beside buccal mucosa	The product does not dissolve completely
Transdermal gels (Androgel, Fortesta, Testim)	Dosed daily	Cover the application area to reduce risk of spreading by contact with others
Transdermal patch (Androderm)	Applied daily	Rotate sites to reduce skin irritation
Scrotal patches (Testoderm)		Now rarely used due to scrotal irritation and more acceptable alternatives
Intramuscular injections (Depo-testosterone, Delatestryl)	Dosed every 2–4 weeks	Serum testosterone levels fluctuate significantly between doses
Subcutaneous pellets (Testopel)		These are implanted (like Norplant) and are rarely used for supplementation
Oral agents (methyltestosterone)		Not available in the United States; significant first-pass metabolism, fluctuating serum levels, and risk of liver toxicity

HELPFUL TIP:
If a male patient with osteoporosis has testosterone deficiency, testosterone supplementation may be a reasonable treatment option, but the efficacy of testosterone in this scenario is **not** well established. Although testosterone contributes to peak bone mass in young men and low testosterone is associated with an increased fracture risk in older men, testosterone for the treatment of osteoporosis has been **disappointing**.

Question 16.7.2 Which of the following is true regarding testosterone supplementation in older men with testosterone deficiency?
A) Testosterone supplementation has markedly beneficial effects on depression
B) The effects of testosterone supplementation in young hypogonadal males and older testosterone-deficient males are the same
C) In testosterone-deficient older males with erectile dysfunction, testosterone supplementation dramatically improves erections
D) In testosterone-deficient older males with poor libido, testosterone supplementation improves libido
E) Testosterone supplementation has no effect on lean muscle mass or grip strength

Answer 16.7.2 The correct answer is "D." In testosterone-deficient older males, testosterone supplementation does improve libido. Unfortunately, "C" is incorrect: its effects on erectile dysfunction are not impressive. Even in testosterone-deficient men with erectile dysfunction, a phosphodiesterase inhibitor (e.g., sildenafil) is more likely to be successful. In terms of the neuropsychiatric effects of testosterone, many questions are as yet unanswered. However, testosterone supplementation does not appear to significantly affect depression, so "A" is incorrect. Furthermore, testosterone replacement does not replace the need for antidepressants if depression is the cause of symptoms. "B" is not true. Young hypogonadal males who are treated with testosterone have increased peak bone mass and virilization. But the effects on older males are different: older males have improved strength, libido, and sense of well-being without some of the effects seen in the young hypogonadal males. "E" is incorrect because testosterone has been shown to consistently improve lean muscle mass and grip strength.

HELPFUL TIP:
Hypogonadal males should **not** take testosterone replacement while trying to impregnate their partners because it will further decrease their sperm counts (due to the effect of exogenous testosterone feeding back on the hypothalamic–pituitary–gonadal axis). To improve fertility in these patients, unproven empiric therapy is often used, including clomiphene, human chorionic gonadotropin, and gonadotropin-releasing hormone.

HELPFUL TIP:
Topical testosterone can have an androgenizing effects on women and children if they come in contact with the gel on a male's skin. Patients should be warned of this.

You have a conversation with your patient about starting testosterone therapy. He would like to try it. Those direct-to-consumer marketing campaigns really work!

Question 16.7.3 You tell him about adverse effects and monitoring and tell him it is important to periodically check:
A) Hematocrit
B) Potassium
C) Alanine aminotransferase
D) A and B
E) A and C

Answer 16.7.3 The correct answer is "E." There are good reasons behind the recommendation for periodic monitoring with certain serum tests. Testosterone increases erythropoietin production and can cause erythrocytosis. In fact, testosterone should not be started in a patient with a hematocrit greater than 50% (or severe heart failure or untreated sleep apnea). Testosterone can cause elevated liver enzymes, increased cholesterol, and growth of prostate and breast tissue, including prostate and breast cancers. Prostate examination and PSA are recommended prior to starting therapy and periodically while on testosterone. Of course, it makes sense to periodically monitor serum testosterone levels to assure that the patient is in the normal range and not sub- or supratherapeutic. Potassium ("B") is not directly affected and no monitoring is recommended.

HELPFUL TIP:
In 2015, the FDA required updated labeling of testosterone products to add information about the possible increased risk of cardiovascular events. The risk–benefit ratio of testosterone products appears to NOT weigh in their favor.

▶ **Objectives: Did you learn to …**
• Identify testosterone replacement products and discuss how older males might benefit (or not) from them?
• Recognize some of the risks associated with testosterone supplementation?

▶ **CASE 16.8**

A 50-year-old male presents for a "get acquainted" visit. He has a history of hyperlipidemia treated with lovastatin. He takes no other medications and states that he is otherwise healthy. After watching a television feature called "What's

Killing Us Now: Prostate Cancer," he thought he should be screened.

Question 16.8.1 In order to assess his risk for prostate cancer, you should take into account all of the following factors EXCEPT:
A) Age
B) Race
C) Family history
D) Cigarette smoking
E) Ultraviolet light exposure

Answer 16.8.1 The correct answer is "E." Ultraviolet light exposure increases the risk of skin cancer but not prostate cancer (after all, it is located where "the sun don't shine"). Advancing age ("A") is strongly and directly associated with the development of prostate cancer. Between ages 50 and 70 years, the incidence of prostate cancer more than quadruples, and it continues to increase thereafter. Black ancestry ("B") and positive family history ("C") carry the strongest associations with prostate cancer. Cigarette smoking ("D") has been linked to an increased risk of prostate cancer, but not with the strength of association of age or family history. Interestingly, dietary factors may have a role in the development of prostate cancer, although the associations are not strong and studies conflict. A diet rich in fish and vegetables and low in red meat may reduce the risk of prostate cancer.

Your patient is Caucasian and denies any family history of prostate cancer. He has no urinary symptoms and denies sexual dysfunction.

Question 16.8.2 If he did have urinary symptoms, which of the following could be used to reliably distinguish BPH from prostate cancer?
A) Urgency
B) Nocturia
C) Frequency
D) Hesitancy
E) None of the above

Answer 16.8.2 The correct answer is "E." A male who presents with urinary symptoms of urgency, nocturia, frequency, and/or hesitancy is more likely to have BPH and not prostate cancer. These urinary symptoms are incredibly common in older persons in general and most often are benign in nature. In fact, "BPH symptoms" (better termed lower urinary tract symptoms or "LUTS"– really) are common in older women as well. However, urinary tract cancers (including prostate and bladder cancers) can present with these symptoms and must be considered. The point is that we cannot always attribute urinary symptoms in an older male to BPH.

You discuss prostate cancer screening with him, presenting the controversial and conflicting guidelines, discussing positive and negative values of lab tests (and what they

signify) using a dry erase board and giving a mini-lecture. Twenty minutes later he says, "It's just a blood test right? I think I want one ounce of prevention, you understand, Doc." He gets "the works": digital rectal examination and PSA. The examination is remarkable for a slightly enlarged, smooth, nontender prostate without nodules. The PSA level is 16 ng/mL (reference range for your lab 0–4 ng/mL).

Question 16.8.3 The most appropriate next step is to:
A) Repeat the PSA in 3 to 6 months
B) Order a transrectal ultrasound of the prostate
C) Refer to urology for further evaluation and prostate biopsy
D) Repeat the rectal examination and try to find the nodule that you missed
E) Order a free PSA

Answer 16.8.3 The correct answer is "C." To use the Monopoly® line: go directly to the urologist; do not pass GO. If he had symptoms of prostatitis, you might try treating with an appropriate antibiotic for 4 weeks and repeating the PSA to confirm elevation before referral. But this patient is completely asymptomatic. He is at relatively high risk of having prostate cancer based on his PSA level (16—that's high, in case you were uncertain) and age at presentation. Sending him to a urologist for prostate biopsy is the most prudent step. Follow-up PSA alone ("A") would be more defensible if the PSA level were <10 ng/mL and/or the patient were much older. "B," a transrectal ultrasound, is likely to miss more than it would find in this case. With this patient's PSA and current life expectancy, ultrasound should only be used as part of a larger urologic evaluation, including biopsy. "D," repeating the rectal exam, is just nuts. There is no need for this. Did you miss a nodule? Maybe. Would it hurt your ego? Who cares! You will eventually get over it. More likely, there was no palpable nodule. This patient could have stage T1 prostate cancer in which, by definition, no nodules are palpable. He could have a nodule located anteriorly in the prostate—a location you cannot palpate. He also may have a PSA elevation for reasons other than prostate cancer. Finally, "E" is incorrect. The free PSA is most helpful when the total PSA is in the intermediate risk zone (4.01–10 ng/mL). When the PSA is higher (>10 ng/mL), the risk of cancer is too great to make the free PSA useful. The fraction of PSA that is "free" (not bound to plasma proteins) is inversely proportional to risk of prostate cancer: the lower the free PSA compared with total PSA, the greater the risk of prostate cancer (cutoff percentages vary from 10% to 25%).

 HELPFUL (OR NOT SO HELPFUL) TIP:
The determination of when to send a patient for prostate biopsy is made on clinical grounds and must take into account the patient's risk, comorbidities, examination findings, PSA level, possibility of false-positive or -negative tests, patient's preference, etc. This decision cannot be made based on an arbitrary PSA value.

Question 16.8.4 Which of the following is true of the PSA test when used for screening purposes?

A) The positive predictive value approaches 100%
B) Since PSA testing has become widespread, prostate cancer incidence and mortality have increased
C) The false-negative rate is 20% to 25%
D) Age-specific cutoff values for PSA have proven to increase positive predictive value and specificity
E) Race-specific cutoff values for PSA have proven to increase positive predictive value and specificity

Answer 16.8.4 **The correct answer is "C."** There is a substantial false-negative rate—from 20% to 25%—limiting the use of PSA for screening purposes. "A" is incorrect by a long shot. The positive predictive value (likelihood of a positive test indicating true prostate cancer) ranges from about 20% to 60%, depending on the PSA level. The positive predictive value increases with increasing PSA level. "B" is incorrect. Since the PSA test has come into widespread use, the incidence of prostate cancer has increased, but mortality due to the disease has decreased. The reason for these trends has not been completely explained, and the role of the PSA test in these trends is not known. "D" and "E" are incorrect. Since older males seem to have higher PSA values in the absence of prostate cancer and black males tend to have prostate cancer found at lower PSA levels, age-specific and race-specific cutoff values have been proposed and investigated. However, the use of age-specific and race-specific PSA cutoff values is of questionable value.

HELPFUL TIP:
The 5-year survival rate of prostate cancer is about 99%. While the lifetime prevalence of prostate cancer is about 14%, the lifetime risk of dying of prostate cancer is less than 3%. For older men, we often hear, "You are more likely to die **with** prostate cancer than **of** prostate cancer." This saying appears rooted in reality.

Once again, your winning personality and reputation for thorough care has won you a referral! Your patient refers a friend to you. Your new patient is a 60-year-old male who presents to your clinic for advice regarding treatment after recently being diagnosed with prostate cancer. A urologist recommended surgery but he wants to know what you think. (Don't let it go to your head.)

Question 16.8.5 Possible treatment options for prostate cancer include all the following EXCEPT:

A) External beam radiation
B) Saw palmetto
C) Active surveillance
D) Robotic prostatectomy

Answer 16.8.5 **The correct answer is "B."** While over-the-counter saw palmetto is sometimes taken by patients for BPH even though it has not been proven to be effective, it is not used for prostate cancer treatment. External beam radiation ("A"), brachytherapy, surgery (open, laparoscopic, or robotic prostatectomy ["D"]), and androgen deprivation therapy are options considered for higher-risk prostate cancers. Watchful waiting and active surveillance ("C") are options considered for lower-risk prostate cancers. Active surveillance consists of scheduled PSA testing and digital rectal examinations every 3 to 6 months and repeat prostate biopsies at 1- to 3-year intervals.

HELPFUL TIP:
It is important to realize that there is great controversy over the role of digital rectal examination and PSA in screening for prostate cancer. They are not considered "good" screening tests (high rate of false positives and false negatives), but there is nothing else to offer at this time. In 2013, the American Urological Association (AUA) changed their guidelines to screening ages 55 to 69 every other year, and continue to recommend this over yearly screening in this population as of their 2018 review (though they note re-screening can be individualized based on a baseline PSA level). In 2012, the US Preventive Services Task Force recommended against prostate cancer screening. However, as of a 2018 update, USPSTF adopted a tiered screening approach like the AUA, with both organizations recommending: (1) a weighing of risks and benefits of prostate cancer screening between patient and healthcare provider to arrive at a shared decision on the matter for men ages 55 to 69 and (2) not routinely screening men > 70 years old. The AUA also notes screening should not be done for a man with a less than 10- to 15-year life expectancy as well as men ages 40 to 54 at average risk and any man <40 years old. The two largest studies of prostate cancer screening with PSA (the Prostate, Lung, Colon, and Ovarian Cancer Screening Trial [PLCO] and the European Randomized Study of Screening for Prostate Cancer [ERSPC]), done to answer the question of how PSA screening affects mortality, arrived at opposite conclusions (PLCO showed no mortality effect with screening, while the ERSPC showed a prostate cancer-specific mortality reduction with PSA screening). However you approach this issue, you're not alone, and the company you keep is just as confused.

▶ **Objectives: Did you learn to …**
· Identify risk factors for prostate cancer?
· Discuss prostate cancer screening with a patient?
· Interpret an elevated PSA?
· Recognize the limitations of prostate cancer screening?
· Recognize various treatment options for prostate cancer?

▶ CASE 16.9

A 32-year-old male accompanied by his wife presents for evaluation of infertility. They have been married for 5 years and have been attempting conception for 3 years without success. The patient's wife has a 7-year-old daughter from a previous marriage. The patient has no significant past medical or surgical history. He does not smoke, but he drinks a six-pack of beer and one cup of coffee daily—not necessarily in that order. He relaxes after work and on weekends by sitting in their hot tub for hours at a time. His BMI is 32 kg/m². He has normal facial and body hair and his testicles are descended bilaterally and of normal size. You note a moderate-sized varicocele on the left.

Question 16.9.1 Which of the following is *not* a modifiable risk factor for male subfertility?
A) Alcohol intake
B) Hot tub usage
C) Varicocele
D) Tobacco use
E) Obesity

Answer 16.9.1 The correct answer is "D." We should note that the study of infertility risk factors and treatments is complicated by inconsistent outcome measures (e.g., sperm count, sperm motility, conception, pregnancy resulting in live birth). However, there are no conclusive studies correlating tobacco use with male subfertility. The other answers are modifiable risk factors and have been directly linked to subfertility, either in decreased sperm count or in decreased sperm motility. It is important to ask about alcohol use ("A"). Other drug use, such as marijuana, should be investigated as well since it can affect sperm quality and motility (poor little guys can't swim straight when stoned). "B" is true. Hot tub usage, febrile illnesses, and the presence of a varicocele raise the temperature of the testicles, thereby decreasing the optimal environment for the maturation of sperm. But how about the boxers versus briefs controversy? Type of underwear does not seem to affect scrotal temperature significantly, and more to the point, tight underwear is not associated with decreased fertility. The presence of a varicocele ("C") is an interesting issue. It is certainly modifiable in that the patient could undergo a varicocelectomy, which might help if the varicocele is moderate to large in size. However, the degree to which a varicocele contributes to infertility is not well-known. Varicoceles are noted to occur more commonly in infertile men, but they also occur in 10% to 15% of the normal, fertile male population. Obesity ("E") contributes to the increased peripheral aromatization of testosterone into estradiol in fatty tissue. Other factors that contribute to subfertility/infertility include a history of cryptorchidism, hypospadias, viral orchitis after puberty, prior chemotherapy or radiation, intake of calcium channel blockers, and retrograde ejaculation associated with diabetes and multiple sclerosis.

HELPFUL TIP:
Infertility in a couple is defined as inability to conceive despite 1 year of frequent (how frequent is not defined), unprotected sexual intercourse. In the United States, the prevalence of infertility is 7% to 15% depending on how the statistic is measured.

Question 16.9.2 You order a seminal fluid analysis (SFA), and the sperm density is 12 million/mL with a motility of 35%. This finding is:
A) Normal for both sperm count and motility
B) Normal for sperm count but abnormal for motility
C) Abnormal for sperm count but normal for motility
D) Abnormal for both sperm count and motility
E) Scary; that seems like a lot of sperm

Answer 16.9.2 The correct answer is "D." As a general rule, normal sperm concentration for fertility is considered to be 15 million/mL or greater. However, as they say, it only takes one sperm to make a baby, so men with lower sperm counts can be fertile. At least 40% or more should be motile. Another finding of importance on SFA is the sperm morphology. Using strict criteria, normal morphology should be 4% or more (yes, unfortunately for men, only 4%).

You repeat the SFA 2 weeks later, and again it is abnormal. His testosterone level is low for his age, and his FSH and LH are high.

Question 16.9.3 Which of the following is most likely to be the cause of his decreased fertility?
A) Congenital absence of the prostate gland
B) Primary hypogonadism
C) Bilateral complete vas deferens obstruction
D) Androgen resistance

Answer 16.9.3 The correct answer is "B." A low testosterone level accompanied by elevated LH and FSH could indicate testicular failure (primary hypogonadism). "A" is not a known cause of infertility, and in fact it is not a known disorder as far as the editors can determine. The prostate gland's only important function is to provide a subject for an endless debate over screening so that epidemiologists have something to do. Just kidding… The prostate gland actually has a role in producing important substances that are part of the seminal fluid and assist sperm in their migration through the female genital tract. However, prostate problems do not seem to cause infertility. "C," an obstruction of the vas deferens, would most likely result in azoospermia with normal or high testosterone levels. "D" is incorrect. You would expect to see elevated testosterone levels in patients with androgen resistance. See Table 16-3 for a list of causes of infertility in males.

TABLE 16-3 A PARTIAL LIST OF CAUSES OF MALE INFERTILITY

Mechanism	Specific Examples
Hypothalamic–pituitary disorders	Congenital disorders (Kallmann syndrome), pituitary tumors, pituitary infarction, hormonal or psychotropic drug use
Primary hypogonadism	Klinefelter syndrome, cryptorchidism, alcohol use, chemotherapeutic agents, testicular torsion, hyperthermia
Disorders of sperm transport	Congenital absence of the vas deferens, epididymal dysfunction, spinal cord injury
Idiopathic infertility	Unexplained satisfactorily by history, examination, and laboratory evaluation

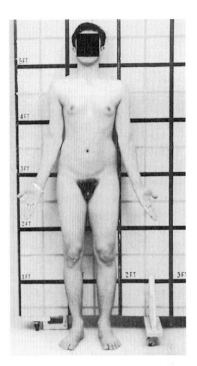

FIGURE 16-10. Klinefelter syndrome in a 20-year-old male. This photo demonstrates classic features of the syndrome, including gynecomastia, small penis, sparse body hair, and female pubic hair distribution. Used with permission from Gardner DG, Shoback D. *Greenspan's Basic & Clinical Endocrinology*, 10th ed. New York: McGraw-Hill Education, 2018, Fig. 12-7.

Question 16.9.4 How can you now best help this patient achieve fertility, assuming that there are no problems with his partner?
A) Empiric treatment for gonorrhea and chlamydia
B) Empiric treatment with testosterone injections
C) Empiric treatment with gonadotropin-releasing hormone
D) Referral to an infertility treatment center

Answer 16.9.4 **The correct answer is "D."** At this point of time, you have performed a reasonably complete evaluation and even arrived at a potential cause of infertility. However, treatments for male infertility are the subject of much debate, and the patient is probably best served by referral to an infertility treatment specialist. "A" is incorrect. Genital infections are not thought to play a major role in male subfertility/infertility, so, without clear evidence of gonorrhea and/or chlamydia, treating for these diseases is not recommended. "C" is incorrect because this patient does not appear to have a hypothalamic source for his infertility. "B," testosterone injection, can actually make the problem worse. The most effective therapy for patients with infertility and primary hypogonadism (i.e., this patient) may be sperm retrieval for intracytoplasmic sperm injection (not typically thought of as an office procedure for the family physician).

You refer this gentleman to an infertility treatment center in your neck of the woods. He is so pleased with your attention to detail and well-reasoned approach that he refers his best friend to you for the same problem—infertility. This new patient reports never conceiving, although his wife has had one child from a previous marriage. On physical examination, you note a thin frame, mild symmetric gynecomastia, and small, firm testicles. He has complete azoospermia on two semen analyses (Fig. 16-10).

Question 16.9.5 His most likely diagnosis is:
A) Cystic fibrosis
B) Psychosomatic azoospermia
C) Klinefelter syndrome
D) Testicular cancer
E) Turner syndrome

Answer 16.9.5 **The correct answer is "C."** The triad of small firm testicles, gynecomastia, and azoospermia are classic findings in patients with Klinefelter syndrome. Klinefelter syndrome occurs in 1 in 1,000 live male births and is responsible for 14% of cases of azoospermia. The most common (90%) chromosomal abnormality in Klinefelter syndrome is 47,XXY. "A" is incorrect. Although males with cystic fibrosis can have congenital absence of the vas deferens, these patients usually have normal-sized testicles and no gynecomastia. "B" is, of course, not a real thing. "D" is incorrect. Patients with testicular cancer usually have an enlarged testicle with a mass on the surface or inside the testicle. Although the treatments for testicular cancer may result in infertility, patients with testicular cancer do not typically present with infertility. "E" is incorrect. Turner syndrome (45,X) is associated with unambiguously female genitalia with no breast development.

▶ **Objectives: Did you learn to ...**
- Define modifiable risk factors for male subfertility/infertility?
- Recognize the significance (or lack of significance) of a varicocele?

• Identify the appropriate indications for obtaining laboratory studies in male patients with infertility concerns?
• Recognize some important causes of infertility?

▶ CASE 16.10

A 63-year-old male with a history of insulin-dependent diabetes complains of decreased libido and difficulty maintaining an erection, worsening over the past few years. He does have occasional erections sufficient for penetration and awakens with an erection at times. His medical history is also significant for hypertension and an appendectomy. His medications include insulin, lisinopril, and hydrochlorothiazide. He has been married for 30 years and has two grown children, ages 24 and 26.

Question 16.10.1 Which of the following historical elements is NOT likely to contribute to this patient's erectile dysfunction?
A) Diabetes
B) Depression
C) Hypertension
D) History of appendectomy
E) Antihypertensive medications

Answer 16.10.1 The correct answer is "D." We're checking to see if you're still awake. All the other options could cause some degree of erectile dysfunction. Any disease process that affects the nervous, vascular, endocrine, or smooth-muscle systems can result in erectile dysfunction. A partial list of other risk factors for erectile dysfunction includes advancing age, prostate disease or prostate surgery (if the nerves are cut … not an issue with TURP), pelvic fracture, alcohol or other substance abuse, medications (addressed later), spinal radiculopathy or spinal cord injury, multiple sclerosis, endocrine disorders (e.g., hypothyroidism, hyperthyroidism), smoking, cardiovascular disease, chronic renal failure, and Peyronie disease (a localized plaque-like fibrosis leading to possible erectile dysfunction, penis curvature, shortening of the penis).

 HELPFUL TIP:
There are two categories of erectile dysfunction—psychogenic and organic. In men younger than 35 years, psychogenic erectile dysfunction is much more common. In contrast, men older than 50 years are more likely to have an organic cause for their erectile dysfunction.

Question 16.10.2 What further historical element(s) is/are useful in the evaluation of erectile dysfunction?
A) Rapidity of onset of sexual dysfunction
B) Presence of nocturnal erections
C) Status of relationship with the sexual partner
D) Partner's interest in sex
E) All of the above

Answer 16.10.2 The correct answer is "E." Further history should involve all the elements listed. Patients with a sudden onset of erectile dysfunction often have a primary psychogenic erectile dysfunction. The presence of nocturnal erections establishes that the patient's neurologic and vascular mechanisms work to produce an erection. An organic disorder may still be playing a role, but the circuit is working. The status of the relationship with the patient's partner, his attraction to that partner, and the partner's interest in sex are important. If the patient and his partner are having relationship problems outside of the sexual arena, counseling may be the best first step in trying to address the erectile dysfunction.

Question 16.10.3 All of the following drugs or classes of drugs can adversely affect male sexual function EXCEPT:
A) Cimetidine
B) Chlorthalidone
C) Prednisone
D) Clonidine

Answer 16.10.3 The correct answer is "C." There are many drugs, prescription and recreational, which affect sexual function, and some of these include antihypertensives, antidepressants, antipsychotics, anxiolytics, hormonal agents (e.g., antiandrogens, estrogens, progestational agents, and anabolic steroids), and the H_2 blocker cimetidine (but apparently not ranitidine or famotidine). The effects range from decreased libido to impotence and/or ejaculatory dysfunction. Various recreational drugs such as alcohol, marijuana, heroin, and cocaine may initially cause a state of disinhibition and enhanced libido. However, excessive or chronic use leads to erectile dysfunction. Prednisone is not known to cause significant erectile dysfunction.

On physical examination, you find normal genitalia, normal femoral and dorsalis pedis pulses, appropriate virilization, and slightly diminished sensation at the plantar aspects of the feet with an otherwise intact neurological examination.

Question 16.10.4 Which of the following will be most useful in evaluating a cause for his erectile dysfunction and directing further therapy?
A) BUN and creatinine
B) TSH
C) PSA
D) Nocturnal penile tumescence study
E) Arterial and venous Doppler studies

Answer 16.10.4 The correct answer is "B." With the advent of safe and efficacious therapy for erectile dysfunction, many clinicians proceed directly to a medication trial without laboratory studies. In many patients, this approach is acceptable. Other patients may benefit from a limited laboratory evaluation—especially those men with other symptoms and/or comorbidities. Initial labs might include TSH, testosterone, and prolactin. If not done already, screening for diabetes and vascular risk (e.g., lipids) is appropriate. The role of nocturnal penile tumescence is debated, but it is not necessary prior to a therapeutic trial (additionally, this patient reported having nocturnal erections anyway). BUN and creatinine ("A"), and PSA ("C") are not likely to be helpful. Doppler flow studies ("E") of femoral vessels are unlikely to change therapy as long as the physical examination demonstrates normal distal blood flow. You know this patient has vascular disease (remember his diabetes, hypertension, and now erectile dysfunction), so his treatment should already involve lowering his vascular risk factors.

Question 16.10.5 Concurrent use of which of the following drugs is an absolute contraindication to taking a phosphodiesterase type 5 inhibitor (e.g., tadalafil, vardenafil, sildenafil)?
A) Hydrochlorothiazide
B) Isosorbide dinitrate
C) Testosterone
D) Finasteride
E) Saw palmetto

Answer 16.10.5 **The correct answer is "B."** In patients who take nitrates for coronary heart disease, phosphodiesterase inhibitors are contraindicated. The combination has been shown to cause hypotension, in rare cases severe enough to result in stroke. While concurrent use of finasteride ("D") is safe, the alpha-blockers used to treat BPH are another story (see below). Drugs that inhibit cytochrome P450 isoenzyme (such as cimetidine, erythromycin, clarithromycin, itraconazole, ketoconazole, and HIV protease inhibitors) may warrant phosphodiesterase inhibitor dosage reductions. Caution with phosphodiesterase inhibitors is advised in patients with uncontrolled hypertension, recent stroke or myocardial infarction, life-threatening arrhythmias, unstable angina, or heart failure. Other potential medical therapies for erectile dysfunction include testosterone supplementation ("C") and yohimbine. There are even more treatment modalities: sex therapy, vacuum erection devices, intracavernosal injection therapy, intraurethral pharmacotherapy, arterial revascularization (not routinely performed strictly for ED), penile prosthesis implantation, and combined therapy.

HELPFUL TIP:
There is not much difference between the various phosphodiesterase inhibitors on the market. The efficacy is about the same. Side-effect profiles are similar. Onset of action is about the same. Tadalafil has the longest half-life. In December 2017, sildenafil became generic, and in October 2018, tadalafil became generic. However, pills remain expensive even for generic medications—up to $25 to $50 per tablet, though coupons can reduce the price of the medication down to as little as $5 to $6 per tablet (prices per time of writing of this book). Want to be tricky? Prescribe the 20-mg tablets of sildenafil that are used for pulmonary hypertension. They are only about $1 each. Have your patient take three to five tablets. They will need to pay out-of-pocket, but they will very likely save money.

You start the patient on sildenafil. He discovers love again, but his wife finds out. Now you're in trouble!

▶ **Objectives: Did you learn to …**
· Evaluate a patient with erectile dysfunction?
· Describe various etiologies of erectile dysfunction?
· Identify medications that affect erectile function?
· Recognize indications, contraindications, and side effects of therapeutic modalities for erectile dysfunction?

Clinical Pearls

○ Do not delay an urgent urological consult for the treatment of priapism as this is a urological emergency.

○ Do not perform prostatic massage if there is a suspicion for prostatitis due to the risk of seeding bacteria into the bloodstream.

○ Do not use oral testosterone replacement therapy as there is a significant first-pass metabolism and potential for liver toxicity.

○ Engage in a shared discussion about the use of PSA in screening for prostate cancer, potential benefits, and potential negative consequences prior to deciding to perform screening. Do not offer screening PSA to patients with life expectancy less than 10 years.

○ Routinely screen young male patients for high-risk behaviors as trauma is the leading cause of death in young men.

○ Screen for potential secondary causes of erectile dysfunction prior to prescribing medication.

○ Screen young boys for cryptorchidism by doing a genital and testicular examination at well-child visits.

BIBLIOGRAPHY

American Urological Association Education and Research, Inc. (AUA). *Early Detection of Prostate Cancer: AUA Guideline.* Linthicum (MD): American Urological Association Education and Research, Inc.; 2013.

Bremner WJ. Testosterone deficiency in older men. *N Engl J Med.* 2010;363:189.

Centers for Disease Control and Prevention. Sexually transmitted diseases treatment guidelines, 2015. *MMWR.* 2015;64(3)59(RR-12):1–137.10.

Crawford P. Evaluation of scrotal masses. *Am Fam Physician.* 2014;89(9):723–727.

Dickson G. Gynecomastia. *Am Fam Physician.* 2012;85(7);716–722.

Edwards JL. Diagnosis and management of benign prostatic hyperplasia. *Am Fam Physician.* 2008;77(10):1403.

Heidelbaugh JJ. Management of erectile dysfunction. *Am Fam Physician.* 2010;81(3):305.

Lindsay TJ. Evaluation and treatment of infertility. *Am Fam Physician.* 2015;91(5):308–314.

Mohan R. Treatment options for localized prostate cancer. *Am Fam Physician*. 2011;84(4s):413–420.

Pearson R. Common questions about the diagnosis and management of benign prostatic hyperplasia. *Am Fam Physician*. 2014;90(11):769–774.

Sharp V. Prostatitis: diagnosis and treatment. *Am Fam Physician*. 2010;82(4);397–406.

Task Force on Circumcision. Male circumcision. *Pediatrics*. 2012;130(3):e758–e785.

Teichman JMH. *Urology: 20 common problems*. New York, NY: McGraw-Hill; 2001.

U.S.Preventive Services Task Force. Screening for prostate cancer: recommendation Statement, and rationale. *Ann Intern Med*. 2002;137(11):915.

U.S. Preventative Services Task Force. Screening for prostate cancer: recommendation statement. *Am Fam Physician*. 2013;87(4):1–7.

Wieder JA. *Pocket Guide to Urology*. 5th ed. Oakland, CA: J. Wieder Medical; 2014.

Dermatology

17

Megan H. Noe and Karolyn A. Wanat

Since dermatology is a visual science, take a look at pictures at www.dermnet.org.nz/sitemap.html or www.dermnet.com. We are not able to include pictures of every disease mentioned. See Table 17-1 for commonly used dermatology terms.

▶ CASE 17.1

A 37-year-old white female presents to clinic for her annual well-adult physical examination. After a complete skin examination, you find a suspicious lesion on her back (Fig. 17-1). It measures 16 mm × 8 mm. She has approximately 20 nevi that appear normal. The patient reports never performing self-skin examinations and does not know if the lesion is new. She denies any symptomatic lesions. Her family history is remarkable for "skin cancer" on her father's side. Many family members have "tons of moles." She frequented a tanning parlor in college (too much free time … probably majored in communications) and occasionally still does so before social events (didn't learn much about skin health in college).

Question 17.1.1 How do you evaluate the lesion?
A) Take a photograph and see her back in 2 months
B) Take a shallow shave biopsy of the lesion
C) Excise the entire lesion with 1- to 2-mm margins
D) Excise the entire lesion with 3-cm margins
E) All of the above are equally valid approaches

Answer 17.1.1 The correct answer is "C." This lesion is worrisome for malignant melanoma because of the different pigmentation colors and irregular borders. Any time you suspect melanoma, you are obligated to completely remove the entire lesion and send it for pathology either with a punch biopsy or excisional biopsy. "A" is not an option; if you suspect melanoma, the earlier you make the diagnosis the better. A shallow shave biopsy ("B") is also not recommended because in a shallow biopsy the deep margins are not visible, which is the most important factor in staging melanoma. Partial removal of a lesion may lead to a sampling error, which is why excisional biopsy with narrow (e.g., 1–2 mm) margins is preferred. "D" is preferable to "A" and "B";

TABLE 17-1 DERMATOLOGY TERMS

Abrasion: Partial-thickness loss of the epidermis
Abscess: Localized collection of purulent exudate
Annular: Grouped in a circular arrangement
Bulla: Fluid-filled cavity greater than 1 cm
Crust: Dried exudate on the skin surface; can be serous (yellow or honey-colored) or hemorrhagic (red-brown); when related to an infection the term impetiginization can be used
Desquamation: Skin cells coming off in scales or flakes
Erythema: A red color change that is blanchable with pressure
Herpetiform: Grouped in a dermatomal distribution
Macule/Patch: Circumscribed area of color-change without elevation or depression; a "macule" is <1 cm in diameter and a "patch" is >1 cm in diameter
Nodule: A solid subcutaneous mass
Nummular: Coin-shaped or circular
Papule/Plaque: A palpable, (elevated) **skin** lesion; a "papule" is <1 cm in diameter and "plaque" is >1 cm in diameter
Purpura: Bleeding into the skin; does not blanch with pressure
Pustule: A papule with purulent exudate
Ulcer: Full-thickness loss of the epidermis
Vesicle: A fluid-filled cavity in the skin less than 1 cm
Wheal: A round or irregular-shaped edematous plaque that tends to be transient (hive)

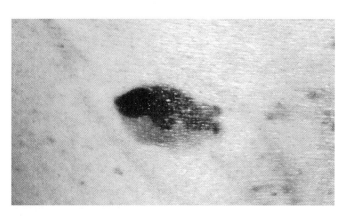

FIGURE 17-1. Malignant Melanoma.

however, it would be unnecessary to remove the lesion with such large margins when the histopathology is not yet known.

You excise the entire lesion with a small border. The pathology report reveals a malignant melanoma.

Question 17.1.2 Which of the following lesion characteristics will determine your patient's prognosis?
A) The depth and ulceration
B) The diameter of the lesion
C) The number of colors in the lesion
D) Whether or not it arose in a pre-existing mole
E) The number of lymphocytes in the biopsy

Answer 17.1.2 **The correct answer is "A."** As alluded to previously, the depth of the melanoma is the most important prognostic indicator. Breslow tumor thickness is most commonly used to arrive at a prognosis. Breslow tumor thickness measures the depth of the melanoma from the granular layer in the epidermis to the base of the melanoma in millimeters. A thinner melanoma correlates with a better prognosis, and melanomas with a Breslow depth <0.75 mm generally have the best prognosis. Ulceration is associated with more aggressive cancers and a poorer prognosis. Clark level (invasion based upon the anatomic structure of the skin) is still reported but is not as important in regards to prognosis as the Breslow depth. The diameter of the lesion ("B," or the size observed on the skin) has not been associated with prognosis (e.g., superficial spreading melanoma may be large but generally carries a good prognosis). A very large, clinically atypical pigmented lesion can often be benign. Melanomas can also be of one color, many colors, or nonpigmented; color does not correlate with prognosis. Up to two-thirds of melanomas arise in normal skin. They can be just as aggressive as those arising from moles. The number of mitoses in a lesion can help predict the outcome; the more the mitoses, the worse the prognosis. The number of lymphocytes observed within a lesion can provide some information regarding the inflammatory response, but does not possess the same prognostic value as the Breslow depth.

> **HELPFUL TIP:**
> If there is regional or distant spread of disease, the overall survival drops to less than 50% for regional metastases and less than 10% for distant metastases.

Question 17.1.3 In the United States, the lifetime risk of developing melanoma in a Caucasian is approximately:
A) 1/10
B) 1/38
C) 1/105
D) 1/1500

Answer 17.1.3 **The correct answer is "B."** The lifetime probability of developing melanoma for Caucasians is approximately 1 in 38. The lifetime risk is 1 in 172 for Hispanic Americans and 1 in 1,000 for African Americans.

Your biopsy reveals a melanoma in situ. You excise the entire lesion with 0.5-cm margins. There is no penetration of the epidermis.

Question 17.1.4 What additional evaluation is necessary?
A) Chest x-ray
B) CT scan of the chest
C) Serum lactic acid dehydrogenase (LDH)
D) All of the above
E) None of the above

Answer 17.1.4 **The correct answer is "E."** If the melanoma has not extended beyond the epidermis, it is referred to as a melanoma in situ. If excised with 0.5- to 1-cm margins, the long-term survival at 5 and 10 years approaches 100%. Therefore, any additional workup is not necessary according to the 2010 and 2017 reports from the American Joint Commission on Cancer. When the melanoma depth is greater than 1 mm, further workup may be performed depending on symptoms and stage of disease. A sentinel lymph node biopsy, although there is no proven therapeutic benefit, can provide additional prognostic information for melanomas with a depth >1 mm and is a diagnostic consideration. A CT scan of the chest and pelvis and MRI of the brain can be ordered if clinical symptoms exist or metastatic disease is suspected, but these studies are not routinely recommended. Metastatic disease has not been reported with melanoma in situ.

Question 17.1.5 Which of the following has NOT been associated with an increased risk of the development of melanoma?
A) Blistering sunburns in childhood
B) Sister with melanoma
C) Red or blonde hair color
D) More than 50 moles on a person's body
E) Smoking

Answer 17.1.5 **The correct answer is "E."** A history of blistering sunburns, melanoma in first-degree relatives, light hair, and more than 50 moles are all associated with an increased risk of developing melanoma. Also, high socioeconomic class (too much time to lay in the sun or tanning booth) and immunosuppression appear to be risk factors. Smoking has not *yet* been linked to malignant melanoma—unlike many other malignancies.

Question 17.1.6 The most common subtype of melanoma in people of African descent is:
A) Superficial spreading melanoma
B) Lentigo maligna melanoma
C) Nodular melanoma
D) Acral lentiginous melanoma
E) Amelanotic melanoma

Answer 17.1.6 **The correct answer is "D."** There are four classical subtypes of malignant melanoma. The subtype does not predict prognosis. **Superficial spreading melanoma ("A")** is the most common type in fair skin populations. It can occur at any site and clinically presents as a brown macule with irregular, notched borders. It grows radially (outward) initially. **Nodular melanoma ("C")** is the second most common type in fair skin individuals and, as the name suggests, is an exophytic nodule and often associated with deeper level of invasion and a vertical (downward) growth phase. **Amelanotic melanoma ("E")** is a subtype of nodular melanoma that presents with little to no pigment and may be red or pink in color. **Lentigo maligna melanoma ("B")** most often occurs in the elderly on sun-exposed areas, such as the face and hands and presents as a brown macule or patch with hue variations that spreads outward slowly. When there is dermal invasion, lentigo maligna is referred to as lentigo maligna melanoma. **Acral lentiginous melanoma ("D")** is the least common type in Caucasian populations but is the most common type in races with pigmented skin, such as people of African descent. Acral lentiginous melanoma occurs on the palms, soles, or near the nails. This is what killed Bob Marley.

▶ **Objectives: Did you learn to …**
- Evaluate a patient with suspected melanoma?
- Describe how the prognosis of melanoma is determined?
- Recognize the lifetime risk of malignant melanoma in the United States?
- Identify risk factors for the development of melanoma?
- Recognize the four classic subtypes of melanoma and which are the most common in African and Caucasian populations?

 QUICK QUIZ: ITCHY ELBOWS

A 22-year-old female presents with a pruritic rash on her elbows and extensor forearms. She's studying for finals, so she's been indoors for days eating Wheat Thins and drinking Mountain Dew. She has a history of celiac disease, but is otherwise healthy and takes no medications. On examination, she is afebrile and has 2- to 4-mm diameter vesicular lesions with numerous excoriations in a bilaterally symmetrical pattern on her extensor forearms, knees, and buttocks.

The most likely diagnosis is:
A) Dermatitis herpetiformis
B) Poison ivy (contact dermatitis)
C) Herpes simplex
D) Neurotic excoriations

The correct answer is "A." Dermatitis herpetiformis is the most common skin condition to occur in association with celiac disease (gluten enteropathy). This patient seems to have lapsed in her gluten-free diet, and her skin eruption has worsened as a result. Dermatitis herpetiformis presents with excoriated vesicles that are extremely pruritic. It can be confused with scabies. Often, only excoriations (and no blisters) are seen on examination. Dermatitis herpetiformis is also commonly symmetrical (as opposed to HSV) and may involve several body areas, most commonly extensor surfaces of the extremities. The cornerstone of treatment is a gluten-free diet. Dapsone can also help speed up

resolution of the rash, but a strict gluten-free diet will also lead to disease resolution. In this case, "B" is unlikely due to symmetric and diffuse eruption without linear lesions and no reported exposure to poison ivy (we didn't tell you this, but her college is located in Antarctica, making poison ivy very unlikely). "C" is incorrect since the eruption is diffuse and there is no pain. Neurotic excoriations ("D") do not present with vesicles.

▶ **CASE 17.2**

A 7-month-old male is brought to clinic for a "rash all over." Six weeks ago, his parents noticed him rubbing his legs against his crib and scratching his head frequently. They are concerned because they find blood on his sheets in the morning, and he has become increasingly irritable. He is eating and drinking normally. His past medical history is unremarkable. His father has sensitive skin and hay fever, but no one else in the family currently has a rash. He does not attend a daycare. On skin examination, you find lichenified and erythematous patches of skin with fissures and bleeding on the ventral heels, dorsal feet, hands, and a few areas on the scalp. His cheeks are bright red with scale. His diaper area is uninvolved and there are no lesions in the web spaces of the hands and feet.

Question 17.2.1 Based on the description, which of the following is the most likely diagnosis?
A) Seborrheic dermatitis
B) Atopic dermatitis
C) Scabies
D) Tinea corporis
E) Tinea versicolor

Answer 17.2.1 The correct answer is "B." The most likely diagnosis is atopic dermatitis, also known by the moniker "eczema." Atopic dermatitis is characterized by intense pruritus and an associated rash. Atopic dermatitis is often referred to as the "itch that rashes." It occurs in characteristic locations. In younger infants, the cheeks and neck are involved. As they begin to crawl, their extensor surfaces are involved. The diaper area, because it is moist, is not usually involved. In older children, the flexural areas, such as the antecubital and popliteal fossae, are involved. Seborrheic dermatitis ("A") is common in infants (cradle cap) and is usually seen on the scalp and face, although it can involve the whole body. Seborrheic dermatitis is usually associated with a yellow, greasy scale and is less erythematous than atopic dermatitis. Scabies ("C") typically affects certain locations (web spaces, wrists, waist, etc.) and uncommonly involves the scalp, except in infants or immunocompromised patients. Also, in this question, he does not appear to have any exposure to scabies. Tinea corporis ("D") presents with a ring of advancing erythema and a central clearing ("ringworm"). Finally, tinea versicolor ("E") typically involves the trunk and extremities with hypo- or hyperpigmented patches with superficial scale. It does not involve the scalp and is not very pruritic.

You diagnose the patient with atopic dermatitis.

Question 17.2.2 Which of the following is true about atopic dermatitis?

A) The prevalence of atopic dermatitis appears to be decreasing worldwide
B) Atopic dermatitis tends to worsen with use of emollients
C) In some patients, skin infections can exacerbate atopic dermatitis
D) Positive skin prick tests and RAST testing correlate highly with food challenges (e.g., those with positive tests will have worsening of their rash when given a food challenge)
E) In most infants, atopic dermatitis will not significantly improve or resolve by school age

Answer 17.2.2 The correct answer is "C." Skin infections (Staph or Strep infections) can be associated with worsening atopic dermatitis, and when children flare, impetiginization (superinfection) should be considered. In these situations, a course of antibiotics may improve the overall clinical course (cephalexin is often a good choice). Sixty percent of atopic dermatitis appears in the first year of life, usually after 2 months of age; and it will usually get somewhat better by school age. The cause of atopic dermatitis is not yet known. The role of specific allergens is controversial. In some patients, a food allergy can worsen the disease but is not thought to be the cause. However, in severe, unresponsive atopic dermatitis, food allergens should be evaluated. Most patients who have positive allergy testing to foods do not have improvement in their skin with removal of the allergen ("D"). Atopic dermatitis does tend to improve as the affected child ages ("E"), and the use of emollients ("B") is a cornerstone of therapy.

> **HELPFUL TIP (OR NOT):**
> The link between allergies of any kind, including food and environmental, and atopic dermatitis has been called into question. It does seem that a subset of patients have atopic dermatitis that flares in response to exposure to certain food and environmental triggers, but these patients are the minority. Random elimination diets are to be discouraged. Only patients with proven food allergy **and** an immediate worsening of symptoms when exposed to that food should eliminate that particular food from their diet.

Question 17.2.3 The clinical features of impetiginized atopic dermatitis include:

A) Lichenification of the skin
B) Pruritus and relapsing nature
C) Associated asthma or allergic rhinitis
D) Elevated IgE serum levels
E) Redness of the skin with honey crusting

Answer 17.2.3 The correct answer is "E." Although all of the above can be associated with atopic dermatitis, honey crusting implies a secondary bacterial infection (impetigo), which is common in atopic dermatitis and needs to be recognized and treated to get atopic dermatitis under control. Oral antibiotics and bleach baths can be used to help control the superinfection. However, bleach baths and emollients **in the bath** are not particularly effective. (Ann Allergy Asthma Immunol. 2017;119(5):435., BMJ 2018;361:k1332). Waxing and waning pruritus is what defines this common skin condition. Chronic scratching often leads to thickened skin with accentuation of skin lines (lichenification). Early lesions will not have lichenification, however. Asthma and allergic rhinitis can be associated with atopic dermatitis. This common hypersensitivity triad is referred to as atopy (although in most patients atopic dermatitis is not actually allergic in nature). "D," elevated IgE, does occur in patients with atopic dermatitis, and higher levels of serum IgE are associated with more extensive disease of greater chronicity. However, an elevated IgE level is merely an association and is not pathognomonic of atopic dermatitis. Erythema of the skin is a nonspecific sign of inflammation and is seen in many skin disorders.

Question 17.2.4 Your initial recommendation should include which of the following in the management of atopic dermatitis:

A) Daily use of thick emollients such as white petrolatum
B) Bathing with lukewarm water and mild cleansers
C) Topical corticosteroids or topical immunomodulators
D) Oral antibiotics if there is evidence of superinfection
E) All of the above

Answer 17.2.4 The correct answer is "E." The protective barrier of the skin is broken down in patients with atopic dermatitis. By frequently applying a protective barrier, such as petrolatum, the skin becomes less pruritic resulting in less itching-induced skin trauma and rash, thus decreasing the "itch-scratch cycle." This is the most important aspect of long-term management. Topical steroids and immunomodulators work well to decrease the inflammation in the skin and are first-line anti-inflammatory treatment; however, the goal is to protect the skin with thick emollients to re-moisturize and restore the barrier function of the skin. Daily bathing with mild cleansers and cool water followed by the application of emollients is recommended. Patients with atopic dermatitis have a higher bacterial count of *Staphylococcus aureus* on their skin. By bathing for short periods daily, the bacterial count is decreased, thus decreasing the risk of secondary infection. Oral antihistamines cause some level of sedation, which is often helpful at night when the child is awake and itching. Interestingly, there is almost no evidence to support the use of antihistamines in the treatment of atopic dermatitis, except small studies that have shown nonsedating antihistamines to be no better than placebo. If you choose to recommend an antihistamine, use an older drug (e.g., diphenhydramine) **but use extreme caution in children under 2 years of age**—there is no proven benefit for any indication in this age range and infants are more sensitive than adults and older children to the CNS depressant effects of diphenhydramine.

HELPFUL TIP:
Mid-potency steroid (e.g., triamcinolone) ointments are the mainstay of pharmacotherapy for atopic dermatitis flares. For the face, low-potency steroid (e.g., hydrocortisone) ointments can be used for a maximum of 2 to 3 weeks at a time. For severe, acute flares, systemic steroids can be employed for 10 to 14 days.

HELPFUL TIP:
Topical calcineurin inhibitors (e.g., tacrolimus, pimecrolimus) are recommended for use as a steroid-sparing agent in treatment of atopic dermatitis. They are generally safe and well tolerated; however, they carry a "black box warning" related to a theoretical risk of lymphoma. Studies since the black box warning was issued have failed to demonstrate a causal relationship between topical calcineurin inhibitors and lymphoma. They are not approved for children under the age of 2. However, the American Academy of Dermatology recommends **off-label use** of 0.03% tacrolimus or 1% pimecrolimus for patients with atopic dermatitis under 2 years of age if needed. Crisaborole (Eucrisa), a topical phosphodiesterase-4 inhibitor that is FDA-approved for mild-to-moderate eczema, can also be used as a steroid sparing agent. It is also only approved for children over 2 years of age. The NNT=8–14 is versus placebo vehicle and it is rather expensive.

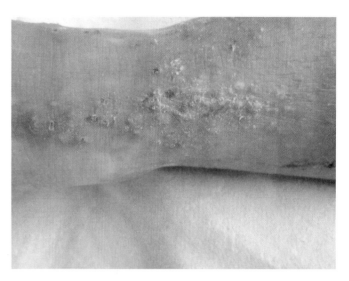

FIGURE 17-2. Lichenified, impetiginized, atopic dermatitis (Courtesy of Drs. Karolyn Wanat and Megan Noe.)

avoided in young children, as should fluoroquinolones (except in rare cases such as cystic fibrosis). Systemic therapy is necessary at this time due to clinical worsening and presence of lymphadenopathy.

HELPFUL TIP:
A subset of patients with severe, treatment refractory atopic dermatitis may require treatment with immunomodulatory agents including cyclosporine, azathioprine, methotrexate or mycopenolate mofetil, under the care of a specialist. Additionally, dupilumab (Dupixent), a monoclonal antibody that targets the IL-4 receptor, is a biologic medication FDA-approved for moderate-to-severe atopic dermatitis. Tofacitinib (Xeljanz), an oral janus kinase inhibitor, is another emerging therapy for severe atopic dermatitis.

A recent ear infection has caused your patient's skin to worsen. He returns to clinic and your physical examination reveals the skin lesion seen in Figure 17-2. He has appreciably enlarged cervical lymph nodes. The patient has no known drug allergies.

Question 17.2.5 Which of the following oral antimicrobials would be the best initial choice for this patient?
A) Cephalexin
B) Ciprofloxacin
C) Metronidazole
D) Tetracycline
E) No systemic treatment is necessary at this time

Answer 17.2.5 **The correct answer is "A."** Patients with atopic dermatitis are prone to certain skin infections that may exacerbate their disease. Ninety percent of patients with atopic dermatitis will grow *S. aureus* on swab cultures of their crusted lesions. By decreasing the bacterial count, inflamed lesions often heal faster. Depending on your community susceptibilities, community-acquired methicillin-resistant *S. aureus* (CA-MRSA) may be of concern. However, first-generation cephalosporins are a reasonable initial antibiotic choice for impetiginized atopic dermatitis because of excellent skin penetration and activity against Gram-positive cocci (both *Staph* and *Strep*). Tetracycline is another option for impetiginization; however, this should be

Your patient's culture results are consistent with methicillin-sensitive *S. aureus* (MSSA). With the appropriate antibiotics, the patient improves markedly. Time to rest on your laurels … Wait … there's this little thing called continuity of care, and 3 months later, your patient returns with a new eruption. Clinical appearance is shown in Figure 17-3.

Question 17.2.6 Which of the following is the most appropriate treatment at this time?
A) Acyclovir
B) Cephalexin
C) Ciprofloxacin
D) Metronidazole
E) A and B

Answer 17.2.6 **The correct answer is "E."** Patients with eczema may also develop **eczema herpeticum**, a particularly severe form of disseminated herpes simplex with punched

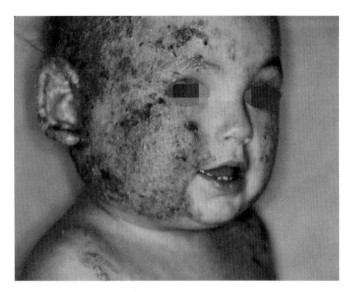

FIGURE 17-3. Eczema herpeticum.

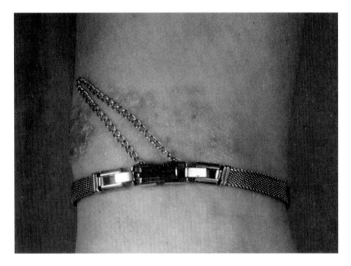

FIGURE 17-4. Allergic contact dermatitis.

out erosions and rapid spread of HSV within the areas of eczema. Patients can develop both eczema herpeticum and impetiginization, so treatment of both is important. The characteristic look of punched-out erosions requires immediate therapy with acyclovir, and often requires intravenous medications as the disease may be fatal. Treatment with cephalexin should be given, especially because the patient improved previously.

As the patient grows, he improves significantly. However, his skin continues to be sensitive to many products. As a teenager, he presents with a recurring rash near his wrist that is intensely pruritic. He has recently started wearing a bracelet … and he won't take it off despite the rash because he's too cool … (see Fig. 17-4).

Question 17.2.7 The test most likely to confirm your presumptive diagnosis is:
A) Potassium hydroxide (KOH) of a skin scraping
B) Tzanck preparation
C) Patch testing
D) Serum thyroid-stimulating hormone level
E) Serum IgE levels

Answer 17.2.7 **The correct answer is "C."** The patient most likely has an allergic contact dermatitis to the nickel in the metal bracelet on his wrist. Patients with a history of atopic dermatitis are more likely to have contact hypersensitivities. Nickel is a common contact allergen and can also be seen with contact to earrings, optical glasses, and buttons on jeans. Patch testing ("C") is a test for delayed-type hypersensitivity reactions that can identify many of the common contact allergens. KOH application to a skin scraping ("A") is used to identify fungal elements. KOH dissolves keratin, the protein in skin, to better identify the fungal elements. Tzanck preparations ("B") stain keratinocytes from the base of bullae to evaluate lesions suspicious for mucocutaneous herpes, primary varicella, or herpes zoster. Thyroid disease can cause many skin conditions but is not a known cause of allergic contact dermatitis. An abnormality in the TSH level ("D") is least likely to yield a diagnosis in this case. As to "E," serum IgE levels may be elevated in atopic patients, but this is not diagnostic as IgE can be elevated in many states (Iowa, Wyoming, New York.)

▶ **Objectives: Did you learn to …**
- Recognize atopic dermatitis by its classic presentations?
- Identify the hallmarks of atopic dermatitis?
- Manage a patient with atopic dermatitis and its complications?
- Recognize that eczema herpeticum in those with atopic dermatitis?

▶ CASE 17.3

A 49-year-old obese white male with poorly controlled diabetes mellitus, hypertension, and hyperlipidemia presents to clinic for a regularly scheduled visit. He complains that his left and right legs are extremely red and painful. He denies constitutional symptoms. His vital signs are within normal limits. He has warm legs with circumferential erythema extending from the ankle to the mid-calves with 2+ pitting edema bilaterally with hemosiderin staining (brownish macular lesions) of the ankles. There is no lymphadenopathy. There are no open sores or minor trauma noted (see Fig. 17-5). His complete blood count with differential is within normal limits. You send him for Doppler studies that fail to reveal venous thrombosis. You prescribe 7 days of oral antibiotics and send him home, confident that your therapy will not fail.

He returns 3 days later with modest improvement in the redness. After completing the antibiotic course, he presents to clinic 3 weeks later complaining of return of the redness. (Why don't patients just get better with a pill like they are supposed to?)

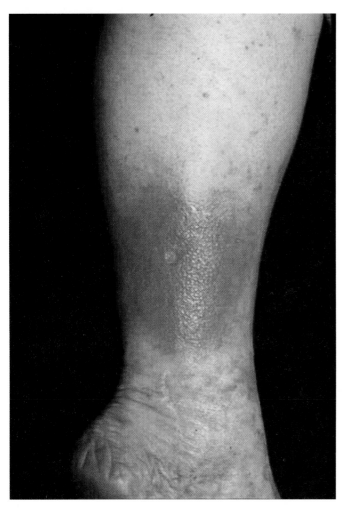

FIGURE 17-5. Chronic venous stasis (lipodermosclerosis).

Question 17.3.1 The most appropriate next step in the care of this patient is to:
A) Prescribe another course of oral antibiotics for 14 days
B) Admit the patient to the hospital for intravenous antibiotics
C) Send a punch biopsy of skin for bacterial culture
D) Recommend daily leg elevation and use of compression hose
E) Prescribe a diuretic (e.g., furosemide)

Answer 17.3.1 The correct answer is "D." This patient has a characteristic history of stasis dermatitis, a condition that is often misdiagnosed as recurrent or chronic cellulitis. **Remember cellulitis is almost always a unilateral disease.** Stasis dermatitis is a dermatitis of the lower extremities that results from chronic edema. It can start relatively abruptly and be unilateral or bilateral. The pitting edema with hemosiderin staining is a clue that there is chronic fluid extravasation from the vessels of the lower extremities. Ectatic veins may also be present. The goal of therapy is directed at resolution of the edema. Patients must lose weight and employ a strict routine of compression hose and leg elevation. In the short term, topical corticosteroids can improve the inflammation. In general, diuretics should

not be used simply to treat edema, as these drugs have numerous systemic effects. Paradoxically, diuretics can actually make edema worse in the long term by causing low circulating volume and renal retention of sodium and water to make up for the diuretic-induced hypovolemia. Chronic lower extremity edema can lead to local tissue necrosis, resulting in ulceration. With long-standing venous insufficiency, more chronic changes can also occur including lipodermatosclerosis (which is "woody" fibrosis-bound down skin) as well as overlying retention of the king and verrucous features (elephantiasis nostra verrucosum).

From years of diabetic nephropathy, the patient's kidneys eventually fail leading to transplantation (and use of immunosuppressants). After 5 years of stable renal function and improved control of his diabetes, he develops a new nonhealing lesion on the left forearm.

Question 17.3.2 What cutaneous malignancy is he at the highest risk of developing?
A) Basal cell carcinoma
B) Malignant melanoma
C) Squamous cell carcinoma
D) Metastases from an undiagnosed internal malignancy
E) Kaposi sarcoma

Answer 17.3.2 The correct answer is "C." All primary cutaneous malignancies are increased in immunosuppressed patients. However, squamous cell carcinoma is the most common in transplanted, immunosuppressed patients, surpassing basal cell carcinoma, which is most common in the general population. Depending on sun exposure and length of immunosuppression, the incidence of squamous cell carcinoma in transplant populations is as high as 45%. Any nonhealing lesion should be further investigated with a biopsy. There are also significantly increased rates of Kaposi sarcoma in immunocompromised patients.

You removed the lesion, which was indeed squamous cell carcinoma. Good job! The patient develops a shallow ulcer superior to the medial malleolus. "Is that another one of them cancers, Doc?" your patient asks.

Question 17.3.3 The most common cause of an ulceration at this location is
A) Arterial insufficiency
B) Diabetic neuropathy
C) Chronic venous stasis
D) Pyoderma gangrenosum
E) Prolonged pressure (e.g., "decubitus" ulcer)

Answer 17.3.3 The correct answer is "C." Your patient is at risk for many of the above diagnoses; however, venous ulcerations classically occur over the medial lower leg. In contrast to this patient's venous ulceration, arterial insufficiency ulcers ("A") classically have a punched-out appearance and occur over bony prominences (e.g., malleoli) or distal aspects (e.g., tips of toes) and are extremely painful (in the absence of neuropathy) and usually dry. Poor peripheral pulses, cool extremities, and hairlessness are clues to arterial insufficiency. Abnormal ankle–brachial indices help to confirm peripheral artery disease. Neuropathic ulcers ("B"), such as those associated with diabetic neuropathy, also occur over pressure points including the plantar surface of the foot. The patient may complain of burning or tingling of the foot, but the ulcer is asymptomatic (because of lack of pain sensation from diabetic neuropathy). Pyoderma gangrenosum ("D") is a rare cause of ulceration associated with systemic diseases including inflammatory bowel disease, connective tissue diseases, and hematologic malignancies. Pressure ulceration ("E") is common and results from tissue ischemia from prolonged pressure, usually over bony prominences, such as the sacrum, coccyx, and heels.

As you start to exit the examination room, the patient states "Oh by the way, Doc, can you do anything for my toenails?" Your examination reveals three, yellow heaped-up nails on the left foot. You suspect a dermatophyte infection.

Question 17.3.4 **What do you do next?**
A) Perform a KOH examination of toenail scrapings
B) Empirically treat with an oral antifungal
C) Empirically treat with a topical antifungal
D) Tell the patient that his nails are the least of his worries

Answer 17.3.4 **The correct answer is "A."** The cost of antifungal therapy has declined substantially over the past few years with generic options becoming available. Some experts now argue that "B," empiric therapy, is reasonable in otherwise healthy patients without contraindications. However, a board examination is not real life, and "A" would be the best choice. Here's the argument for testing prior to treating: all that looks fungal is not necessarily fungal. Dystrophic nails can mimic onychomycosis and may be the result of psoriasis, eczema, trauma, or other inflammatory conditions. KOH is an inexpensive and easy test to perform in the clinic setting. If it is negative, then a toenail clipping can be sent for fungal culture or pathologic study with periodic acid–Schiff staining if desired.

The KOH is negative, so you send a toenail clipping for culture. It grows a *Candida* species.

Question 17.3.5 **Which of the following would be the LEAST efficacious medication?**
A) Amphotericin
B) Fluconazole
C) Nystatin
D) Terbinafine
E) Voriconazole

Answer 17.3.5 **The correct answer is "D."** All the above medications have some *Candida* species coverage, but terbinafine (Lamisil) has the least yeast coverage. Of note, amphotericin would be the most toxic (but still would work well) and should

be avoided. *A plea from your editors*: the topical "paint-on" nail antifungals are relatively expensive, have a marginal benefit, and the recurrence rate tends to be high. Besides, who is really going to paint their nails everyday for a year?

HELPFUL TIP:
Terbinafine (Lamisil) is effective against most dermatophyte infections of the nails (except Candida). Most cases of onychomycosis are sensitive to terbinafine. Complete cure rates for systemic antifungals range from 50% to 75% (terbinafine has the highest rate), while cure rates for topical antifungals are less than 10% even under ideal conditions. For all-comers, recurrence after clearance is as high as 50%.

Another patient comes in with toenail fungus, but this time he has white changes, most prominent on his proximal nailfolds.

Question 17.3.6 **You would like to test him for:**
A) Diabetes mellitus
B) Kidney disease
C) Lupus erythematosus
D) HIV
E) Yum, let's go eat mushrooms

Answer 17.3.6 **The correct answer is "D."** This pattern of dermatophyte infection, proximal white subungual onychomycosis, is characteristic of immunosuppression and particularly HIV disease. Testing for underlying HIV is important with this clinical presentation. Other nailbed changes can be seen with diabetes, kidney disease, and lupus. As to "E," mushrooms might have this appearance but don't grow on toes—we hope. As an aside, there is a great restaurant in Jogjakarta, Indonesia, where everything is made out of various types of mushrooms (shelf fungus, etc.). It is pretty yummy. If you are in the area check out "Je Jamuran."

▶ **Objectives: Did you learn to …**
· Recognize the presentation of stasis dermatitis and describe its etiology?
· Treat stasis dermatitis?
· Recognize the cutaneous malignancies seen in transplanted, immunosuppressed patients?
· Differentiate between common causes and sites of lower extremity ulcerations?
· Diagnose and treat onychomycosis?

▶ **CASE 17.4**

You are working in the student health clinic at the local university when a previously healthy 19-year-old female presents with malaise for 3 weeks and a severe sore throat for 3 days. Yesterday, she took some old amoxicillin that her roommate

gave her. Today, she developed a diffuse macular, red skin eruption, starting on her chest and spreading to involve her extremities. Her mucous membranes, palms, and soles are free of lesions, but she has enlarged tonsils with exudates and large cervical lymph nodes, including prominent posterior nodes. A rapid *Strep* test is negative.

Question 17.4.1 You suspect:

A) An allergic reaction to the amoxicillin
B) An Epstein–Barr virus infection (mononucleosis)
C) An enterovirus infection
D) A gonococcal infection
E) Scarlet fever

Answer 17.4.1 **The correct answer is "B."** All of the above infections except for enterovirus can present with an exudative pharyngitis; enterovirus presents with gastrointestinal or meningeal symptoms. The clinical scenario describes the usual course of infectious mononucleosis: a college-age student, a few week prodrome of malaise, and posterior cervical lymphadenopathy. Amoxicillin or ampicillin given to patients with infectious mononucleosis can result in a macular, diffuse rash. This is not an allergy but can be mistaken for one. Scarlet fever, which this patient does not have, is a complication of group A streptococcal infection, which presents with an erythematous, coarse ("sandpaper") rash, strawberry tongue, and skin desquamation.

Later that same day, a (precocious) 16-year-old male presents with a mildly pruritic rash on his trunk. He had a cold a few weeks earlier but is otherwise healthy. He denies high-risk sexual activity or IV drug abuse (of course, your definition of "high-risk" and his may not be the same!). Your examination reveals the findings in Figure 17-6.

Question 17.4.2 You tell the patient:

A) This skin condition is usually chronic and relapsing
B) That topical corticosteroids are needed to speed up the healing
C) That the rash usually resolves within 6 to 8 weeks without treatment
D) That the rash is likely to be fatal
E) That he is living a Kafkaesque nightmare and slowly metamorphosing into an insect

Answer 17.4.2 **The correct answer is "C."** The rash is consistent with pityriasis rosea (PR), which is an acute, often asymptomatic, eruption on the trunk and proximal extremities. The etiology is (still) unknown. Secondary syphilis, which is on the rise in some areas of the United States, can mimic PR. A sexual history is necessary, and appropriate laboratory studies should be undertaken if a patient is sexually active, especially if high-risk behaviors have occurred or if local syphilis rates are high. PR, unlike syphilis, often resolves within 8 weeks without treatment and does not usually recur. Topical steroids are not necessary for healing but may be helpful in the minority of patients

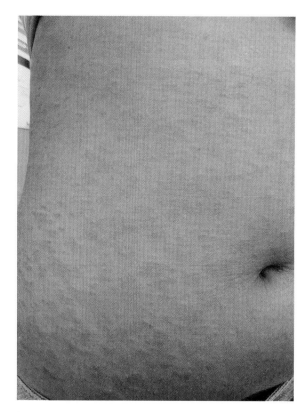

FIGURE 17-6. Pityriasis Rosea (Courtesy of Drs. Karolyn Wanat and Megan Noe.)

who experience itching. "E" is incorrect. This rash just isn't that serious.

HELPFUL TIP:
Pityriasis rosea starts with a "herald patch," a salmon-colored, 2- to 5-cm oval-shaped lesion on the back, neck, or chest. The herald patch may clear a bit and scale and is then followed by numerous smaller lesions that crop up mostly on the trunk. These lesions tend to be oval in shape and are oriented along skin lines, giving a "Christmas tree" appearance.

Your next patient is a 20-year-old female complaining of "a rash down there." You confirm that she is talking about a vulvar rash and ask about her sexual history. She says that she had not been sexually active with anyone for about 1 year until a recent spring break fling in Florida. On examination, you find a rash over the pubic region and extending into the inguinal areas and medial thighs. There is no pain or pruritus (see Fig. 17-7).

Question 17.4.3 Which of the following is FALSE?

A) These lesions are transmitted in adults only by sexual contact
B) If not treated, the lesions may resolve on their own
C) Topical corticosteroids do not improve this skin condition
D) The lesions are contagious and can spread readily and rapidly
E) The skin lesions are a result of a viral infection

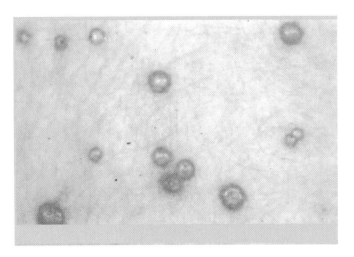

FIGURE 17-7. Molluscum contagiosum.

Answer 17.4.3 The correct (and false) answer is "A." These lesions, referred to as molluscum contagiosum, result from a pox virus. Molluscum is commonly spread via sexual contact in adults; however, **any** physical human contact can also spread it. Molluscum is extremely common in children in daycare settings. The lesions generally resolve in time without treatment. Because they can be auto-inoculated, the molluscum lesions can rapidly increase in number, and it is for this reason that treatment is recommended. Treatment consists of destructive methods, such as cryotherapy or curetting. The immune modulator imiquimod has been used, but is not approved by the Food and Drug Administration (FDA) for molluscum, and only small trials have been undertaken. Topical steroids are not indicated. In immunocompromised patients, molluscum lesions can be widespread and persist much longer.

HELPFUL TIP:
Other molluscum therapies appear effective in small trials but are not FDA approved, including podofilox 0.5%, KOH 5% to 10%, and cantharidin.

Your next patient is a healthy 18-year-old male who presents for treatment of plantar warts. He has tried topical salicylic acid 17% at home. He used it for a few weeks without significant improvement.

Question 17.4.4 Which of the following can be used for therapy for plantar warts (verruca plantaris)?
A) Cryotherapy (liquid nitrogen)
B) Duct tape occlusion
C) Imiquimod
D) Candida antigen injection
E) All of the above

Answer 17.4.4 The correct answer is "E." No therapy for cutaneous warts (plantar or otherwise) has been proven superior, and all of the options can be used with different pros and cons.

"A," cryotherapy, is easily performed in the office and is quick but may be too painful for children to tolerate. Also, cryotherapy may result in hypopigmented scarring in dark-skinned patients. As we all know, duct tape can be used for anything (e.g., holding your muffler together, preventing poison gas exposure) and has been used to treat warts, but the evidence is conflicting. "C," imiquimod, is initially painless, can lead to a brisk inflammatory response, and unlikely to cause scarring, so it is a good choice for facial warts or dark-skinned patients. However, it is the most expensive option. "D," candida antigen injection, is a therapy that aims at stimulating an immune response to the warts. Mumps antigen has been used as well. In the antigen injection studies, only one wart was injected to achieve treatment for all of a patient's warts. This can be effective but is a painful injection. Destructive methods are all approximately 70% effective at eradicating warts. It is important to remind patients that no single method is more likely to work than another, and warts can resolve on their own. In immunocompetent patients, most warts resolve in time without treatment. For young children, this is an important issue, since they cannot understand the pain associated with most treatment modalities.

HELPFUL TIP:
To use duct tape for warts, the patient should put a piece of duct tape on the wart and leave it on for 6 days. On day 7, remove the duct tape, soak, and abrade the wart with a pumice stone. Reapply the duct tape the next day.

▶ **Objectives: Did you learn to …**
• Recognize that ampicillin/amoxicillin given to patients with mononucleosis will often result in a macular rash?
• Diagnose pityriasis rosea (PR) and recognize secondary syphilis as a mimic?
• Recognize and treat molluscum contagiosum?
• Describe the treatment modalities for verruca plantaris?

 QUICK QUIZ: HYPERSENSITIVITY REACTION

Which of the following represents a type IV hypersensitivity reaction?
A) Serum sickness reaction
B) Contact dermatitis to poison ivy
C) Urticaria
D) Vasculitis

The correct answer is "B." Contact dermatitis has a geometric appearance and a characteristic immune-mediated reaction; someone may not react when they first encounter the agent and then develop stronger inflammatory responses with subsequent exposures. Contact dermatitis is an example of a delayed-type hypersensitivity reaction. The pruritus from contact dermatitis usually *does not* respond well to diphenhydramine or hydroxyzine. It is not histamine mediated. Serum sickness ("A") is a

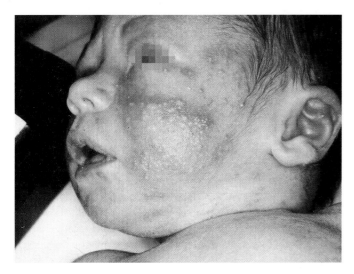

FIGURE 17-8. Erythema toxicum neonatorum.

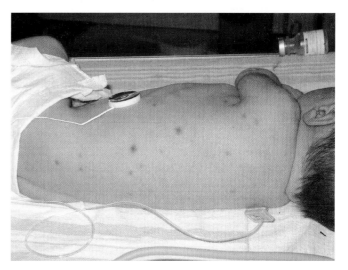

FIGURE 17-9. "Blueberry muffin" appearance from CMV (but also caused by Rubella, Parvovirus B-19, etc.)

type III immune complex reaction. Urticaria ("C") is a type I hypersensitivity response, mediated by mast cell degranulation. Vasculitis ("D") can be either immune complex, antibody, or complement mediated.

HELPFUL TIP:
Auto-eczematization or "id" reactions represent a hypersensitivity response of the body to a significant infection or dermatitis in another part of the body. For example, patients with severe tinea pedis can develop eczematous lesions on other parts of the body and treatment of the tinea pedis will resolve the eczematous eruption (or "id" reaction).

▶ **CASE 17.5**

You are rounding in the newborn nursery. A healthy 2-day-old term infant has a new rash characterized by yellow pustules on an erythematous base (Fig. 17-8) involving the trunk and extremities but sparing the palms and soles.

Question 17.5.1 **What is the diagnosis?**
A) Transient neonatal pustular melanosis
B) Herpes simplex
C) Miliaria
D) Erythema toxicum neonatorum
E) Epidermolysis bullosa

Answer 17.5.1 **The correct answer is "D."** Erythema toxicum neonatorum is a common, benign, self-limited rash seen in term infants. Lesions usually appear after 24 to 48 hours of age. Lesions may begin as erythematous macules that progress to yellow pustules on an erythematous base, may be sparse or numerous, and involve the trunk and extremities, sparing the

palms and soles. The etiology is unknown and the diagnosis is clinical. Transient neonatal pustular melanosis ("A") usually affects term African-American infants presenting at birth with pustules on a hyperpigmented macule that may involve the palms and soles. Neonatal herpes ("B") presents with blisters or erosions and an ill-appearing child. Diagnosis is made via a Tzanck preparation demonstrating multinucleated giant cells, viral culture, or direct fluorescent antibody for HSV 1 or 2. Commonly seen in warm climates, miliaria ("C") or "prickly heat" is due to blocked sweat ducts presenting as non-inflamed pinpoint clear diffuse vesicles. Epidermolysis bullosa ("E") is a chronic blistering disease presenting as blisters at sites of mild trauma.

HELPFUL TIP:
Neonatal acne presents as a pustular, facial eruption with a mean onset at 2 to 3 weeks of life. It is asymptomatic and diagnosed clinically. Fungal organisms have been found in some pustules. Treatment for acne is not necessary as most lesions resolve in several weeks; if severe, topical "azole" antifungals can be used. Besides, we doubt neonatal acne will affect the child's chance of landing a daycare prom date.

While taking care of the neonate in the newborn nursery, you notice a child in isolation. His skin catches your eye (see Fig. 17-9).

Question 17.5.2 **The most common cause of this rash in newborns in the United States is:**
A) Cytomegalovirus (CMV)
B) Rubella
C) Langerhans cell histiocytosis
D) Rh incompatibility
E) Parvovirus B19

Answer 17.5.2 The correct answer is "A." All of the listed can present as a "blueberry muffin baby"; however, CMV is the most common cause in the United States. CMV is the most common congenital viral infection, affecting about 1% to 2% of all births. Rubella was the most common cause in the pre-vaccination era (which, unhappily, seems to be returning). In most cases, the purple plaques represent extramedullary hematopoiesis.

....

Later that same morning, a previously healthy 2-month-old neonate presents to your clinic with peeling of the skin and a fever (Fig. 17-10). She had appeared well until 2 days ago when she became more irritable. Her mother noted a decrease in her urine output. The child was born vaginally without complications and has no known medical conditions. On physical examination, you notice a well-nourished, crying infant with large sheets of desquamating skin on her extremities. Her mucus membranes appear normal. You order complete blood count and urine analysis.

Question 17.5.3 **The most likely diagnosis is:**
A) Toxic epidermal necrolysis (TEN)
B) Burns
C) Staphylococcal scalded skin syndrome (SSSS)
D) Diffuse cutaneous mastocytosis

Answer 17.5.3 The correct answer is "C." This is Staphylococcal scaled skin syndrome (SSSS), which results from a distant Staphylococcal infection (often involving urinary tract, nasopharynx, eyes, perianal areas). The key features of SSSS in Figure 17-10

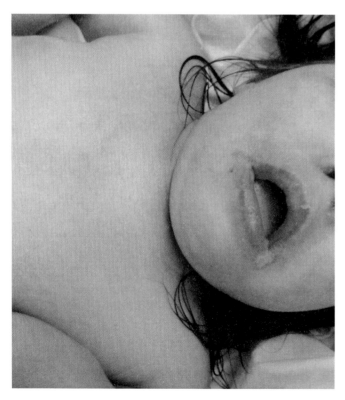

FIGURE 17-10. Staphylococcal scalded skin syndrome (Courtesy of Drs. Karolyn Wanat and Megan Noe.)

are bright red erythema with impending desquamation in the neck folds and periorificial areas with sparing of the oral mucosa. So what differentiates "C" from "A"? TEN presents with shedding of sheets of skin **and often has mucosal involvement that separates it clinically from SSSS**. Both can present with significant skin pain. However, TEN is a result of drug hypersensitivity or bacterial sepsis (in the case of the neonate children); and neonates with TEN are quite ill compared with children with SSSS. In TEN, a biopsy would show full-thickness necrosis of the epidermis versus an intraepidermal split in SSSS. Burns ("B") can mimic SSSS, but burns would not be likely to cause a diffuse red eruption and will often have a specific shape depending on what burned the skin. "D," diffuse cutaneous mastocytosis, can present with hemorrhagic blisters and erosions, but these are usually focal areas, not sheets of skin loss. Keep reading for more information on SSSS.

Question 17.5.4 **In this case of SSSS, peeling of the skin is a result of:**
A) Necrosis of the entire epidermis from lymphocyte attack
B) A widespread bacterial skin infection
C) Histamine released in the skin with edema and blistering
D) Toxin-mediated skin blistering from nonskin source of infection

Answer 17.5.4 The correct answer is "D." This clinical scenario describes SSSS, which is an epidermolytic toxin-driven disease. Extreme tenderness of the skin precedes superficial, widespread desquamation. The skin is usually bright red with areas of flakiness. Radial wrinkling of the mouth, giving an "old, sad man" appearance, is common. The source of infection is not the skin but rather an occult site such as nasopharynx, eye, perianal area, or urinary tract; therefore, investigation for a causative infection should be undertaken (e.g., blood, nares, ocular, perianal, and urine cultures).

▶ **Objectives: Did you learn to …**
  • Recognize neonatal benign cutaneous eruptions?
  • Identify a "blueberry muffin" neonate and know the common causes?
  • Recognize SSSS and consider its differential diagnosis?

 QUICK QUIZ: NAILS

Which of the following nail findings–systemic disease pairing is INCORRECT?
A) Muehrcke nails–nephrotic syndrome
B) Nail pitting–psoriasis
C) Periungual fibroma–tuberous sclerosis
D) Splinter hemorrhages–infective endocarditis
E) Koilonychia–systemic lupus erythematosus

The correct answer is "E." Koilonychia, otherwise known as "spoon nail," is a result of softening and thinning of the nail plate and is found in patients with long-standing iron deficiency anemia, Plumer–Vinson syndrome, Raynaud disease, hemochromatosis, and trauma. It can also be inherited as an autosomal-dominant trait. Connective tissue diseases, such as lupus, are more commonly characterized by nail fold abnormalities, such as nail fold telangiectasias, rather than koilonychia. Muehrcke nails ("A") have paired narrow horizontal (meaning perpendicular to the long axis of the finger) white bands, separated by normal nail, which remain static as the nail grows. They are most often seen in patients with nephrotic syndrome, and their presence reflects the degree of hypoalbuminemia. When you see onycholysis (separation of the nail plate from the nail bed that appears opaque), consider trauma, onychomycosis, psoriasis, and other systemic disease. Nail pitting can be associated with several conditions including psoriasis, atopic dermatitis, and alopecia areata. A periungual fibroma ("C") should prompt evaluation for tuberous sclerosis with brain imaging for tuberous lesions. Splinter hemorrhages ("D") are usually a result of trauma but can be a sign of infectious endocarditis.

HELPFUL TIP:
Paronychia, inflammation around the nail, may be acute or chronic. Acute paronychia is often due to bacterial infection and is treated with oral antibiotics, drainage, warm compresses, and soaks. Chronic paronychia is related to eczema and may have secondary *Candida* infection. Treatment is with topical steroids, topical antifungals, and oral antifungals.

 QUICK QUIZ: DERM PHOTO

A 52-year-old white male presents to clinic with a nonhealing, asymptomatic "pimple" on the cheek. It has been present for 6 months and has recently started to bleed when he shaves. On examination, you note his fair skin, blue eyes, and ruddy complexion. You find the lesion in Figure 17-11.

Your preliminary diagnosis is:
A) Sebaceous hyperplasia
B) Squamous cell carcinoma
C) Basal cell carcinoma
D) Metastases from internal malignancy
E) Merkel cell carcinoma

The correct answer is "C." The photograph is a classic picture of a basal cell carcinoma with its rolled, pearly pink borders and telangiectasias. It is found commonly on sites that get a lot of sun exposure, especially the head and neck. People with fair skin and light hair and eyes are at particular risk. Sebaceous hyperplasia ("A") can look similar but is ivory or yellow in appearance and has lobulated appearance with a central pore. Squamous cell carcinoma ("B") is usually a hyperkeratotic or ulcerated papule or plaque. Metastases from solid organ malignancies ("D") are subcutaneous, firm nodules, although they may ulcerate. Merkel cell carcinoma ("E") is a rare tumor on the head and neck that usually appears as an ill-defined, violaceous nodule.

▶ CASE 17.6

While working in the emergency department, a 6-month-old healthy female infant is brought in by her grandmother. She is bleeding from her birthmark on her buttocks (see Fig. 17-12). Her grandmother watches her during the day while her mother is at work and has noticed the lesion getting larger recently. After holding pressure on the lesion for about 20 minutes, the bleeding stops. You educate the grandmother about the natural history of the "birthmark."

Question 17.6.1 **Which of the following is NOT a true statement about this type of birthmark?**
A) This is the most common type of soft-tissue tumor of infancy
B) Most of these birthmarks undergo spontaneous involution
C) Treatment is indicated in all lesions lest they become malignant
D) β-Blockers are the most appropriate therapy for ulcerated lesions
E) Many are not present at birth but develop shortly thereafter

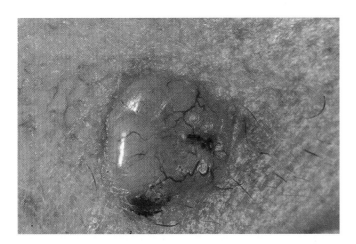

FIGURE 17-11. Basal Cell Carcinoma.

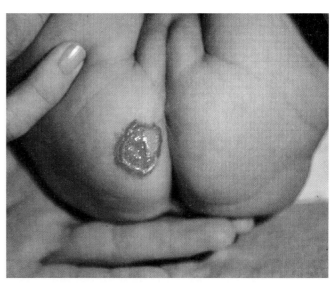

FIGURE 17-12. Ulcerated Hemangioma of Infancy.

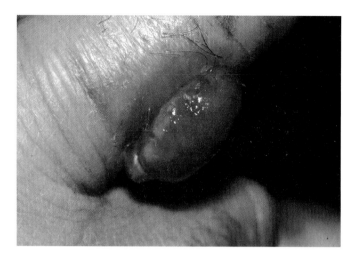

FIGURE 17-13. Pyogenic granuloma.

Answer 17.6.1 The correct (untrue) answer is "C." The child has an ulcerated hemangioma of infancy. Infantile hemangiomas are benign proliferations of endothelial cell lineage that are usually present at birth or soon thereafter. They are characterized by rapid growth in the first several months of life with a plateau occurring around 1 year of age. They spontaneously involute over years. Treatment options should be individually tailored, depending on the size and location of the lesion. Lesions located on the central face or in the diaper area should be treated, as should ulcerated hemangiomas at any body site. Topical timolol or oral propranolol is the standard of care for infantile hemangiomas that require treatment. Larger, segmental hemangiomas should be further evaluated with imaging studies to rule out syndromes with other associated anomalies such as PHACES syndrome (posterior fossa malformation, hemangioma, arterial anomalies, cardiac defects, coarctation of the aorta, eye abnormalities, sternal defects/supraumbilical raphe) and LUMBAR syndrome (lower body hemangioma, urogenital anomalies, myelopathy, bony deformities, anorectal malformation/arterial anomalies, and renal anomalies).

The same patient returns, this time with mom, at age 5. The hemangioma has involuted. About 2 months ago, the mother noticed a spot on the patient's left index finger, and now she is concerned that it is not resolving. The patient is not bothered by the lesion, except that it occasionally bleeds when she bumps it on something. On examination, you find a 3-mm dome-shaped, bright red nodule on the palmar aspect of the left index finger. It is nontender and smooth (see Fig. 17-13).

Question 17.6.2 The most likely diagnosis is:
A) Basal cell carcinoma
B) Squamous cell carcinoma
C) Acne
D) Pyogenic granuloma
E) Nodular melanoma

Answer 17.6.2 The correct answer is "D." This patient most likely has a pyogenic granuloma, which is essentially a nodular hemangioma arising at sites of trauma, especially the fingers

and toes. Although pyogenic granuloma is not cancerous, it can be confused with basal and squamous cell carcinomas as well as melanoma. For this reason, it is prudent to perform excision and histologic examination. After excision, the base of the lesion should be ablated (electrocautery or laser), or the pyogenic granuloma may return. Pyogenic granulomas are more common during pregnancy and have been associated with drugs such as oral retinoids, indinavir, methotrexate, sirolimus, and capecitabine. Acne ("C") should not be a consideration, as sebaceous glands are not found on the palms. By the way, did you notice that this poor child has developed coarse, dark hair growth on her knuckles? As it turns out, she's been playing with dad's Rogaine.

▸ **Objectives: Did you learn to …**
- Describe the natural history of infantile hemangiomas?
- Identify options for treating ulcerated hemangiomas?
- Describe the features and management of pyogenic granuloma?

▶ CASE 17.7

A 78-year-old female presents with a hive-like rash on her legs. It started 1 week ago and was preceded by itching of the legs without any visible changes. Red blotches rapidly developed that quickly became blisters. She denies pain or drainage. She also has some sores in her mouth. She reports overall good health and takes no medications. On examination, you find an afebrile, comfortable looking female. She has 1+ pitting edema at her ankles. You notice round, tense bullae erupting on erythematous patches on the abdomen and extremities. There are also scattered erosions present at the sites of previous bullae. The bullae contain clear fluid. There is no purulent material or blood (see Fig. 17-14).

Question 17.7.1 Which of the following is the most likely diagnosis?
A) Pemphigus vulgaris
B) Bullous pemphigoid
C) Varicella zoster
D) Dermatitis herpetiformis
E) Stevens–Johnson syndrome (SJS)

Answer 17.7.1 The correct answer is "B." Bullous pemphigoid is an autoimmune disorder and is primarily a disease of the elderly. Often patients will report pruritus or urticaria-like lesions, prior to the eruption of typical bullous lesions. When the bullae form, they are frequently asymptomatic but can be intensely pruritic and/or mildly tender. In contrast to pemphigus vulgaris ("A") and SJS ("E"), systemic symptoms are not part of bullous pemphigoid. Additionally, pemphigus vulgaris lesions are painful, and classically the bullae are flaccid rather than tense. SJS generally occurs in response to medications, and this patient is taking none. Varicella zoster ("C") should follow a unilateral dermatomal pattern rather than appear bilaterally; zoster is usually associated with pain and paresthesia.

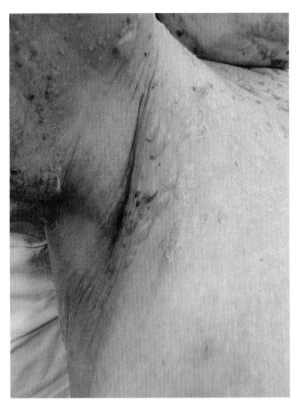

FIGURE 17-14. Bullous Pemphigoid (Courtesy of Drs. Karolyn Wanat and Megan Noe.)

Dermatitis herpetiformis ("D") presents with crops of vesicles and excoriations rather than bullae.

Although she feels well, the lesions are dramatic, and the patient is very concerned that she might have cancer. To confirm your diagnosis, you decide to biopsy the skin.

Question 17.7.2 The most appropriate way to perform a biopsy in this situation is:
A) 4-mm punch biopsy of the margin of an intact bulla for light microscopy
B) 4-mm punch biopsy of perilesional normal skin for light microscopy
C) 4-mm punch biopsy of perilesional normal skin for direct immunofluorescence
D) A and B
E) A and C

Answer 17.7.2 **The correct answer is "E."** Bullous pemphigoid is diagnosed definitively by demonstration of autoantibodies deposited along the basement membrane of **normal** skin. Direct immunofluorescence examination of normal-appearing skin ("C") can demonstrate linear depositions of IgG and C3 along the dermal-epidermal junction. A biopsy of the edge of an intact bulla ("A") will show the characteristic pathology of a subepidermal blister with eosinophils. For a definitive diagnosis, both "A" and "C" should be done.

You assure her that the lesions are not cancerous.

Question 17.7.3 What else can you tell her about the prognosis of bullous pemphigoid?
A) The average course resolves spontaneously in 5 to 6 years
B) It is associated with an increased risk of systemic malignancy
C) It is associated with a high mortality rate
D) It will likely spread to cover her entire body until she's one big blister, and her hair will fall out, and her friends will shun her, a la Job in the Old Testament

Answer 17.7.3 **The correct answer is "A."** Bullous pemphigoid may undergo complete resolution and never recur. Alternatively, the disease may have resolutions and exacerbations over time. It is not associated with an increased risk of cancer or a high mortality rate. Very extensive involvement may lead to skin infections and bacteremia, but diffuse disease is not common.

She seems miserable. You want to offer her the medication with the fastest onset of action.

Question 17.7.4 What is the most appropriate treatment option with a fast onset of action?
A) Oral azathioprine
B) Oral cephalexin
C) Oral prednisone
D) Topical antimicrobials

Answer 17.7.4 **The correct answer is "C."** Bullous pemphigoid is an autoimmune disease, so anti-inflammatory medications and immunosuppressive agents are used to treat it. Oral steroids are the first-line treatment because of the quick onset of action; however because of concerns for long-term side effects, patients should be transitioned to "steroid-sparing" agents as necessary. Once the disease is under control, oral steroids should be tapered to the lowest effect dose in combination with a tetracycline antibiotic or other immunosuppressive agent such as azathioprine, methotrexate, or mycophenolate. For patients with limited disease, high-potency topical steroids can also be used. Topical antimicrobials are used when treating infected, open bullae but are not effective for the treatment of the disease itself.

▶ **Objectives: Did you learn to ...**
  · Distinguish bullous diseases from one another?
  · Diagnose and treat bullous pemphigoid?

⧗ **QUICK QUIZ: PAPULAR ERUPTION**

A 30-year-old female presents with a several month history of bumps on her chin and around her mouth. Although she has never had problems with acne, she thought that she was developing acne and tried benzoyl peroxide. A month ago, she stopped the benzoyl peroxide because it did not seem to

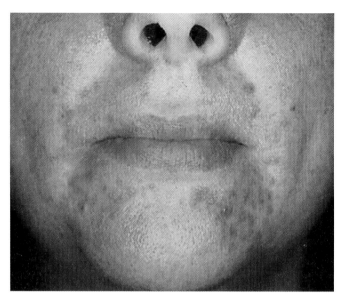

FIGURE 17-15. Perioral dermatitis.

work, and she switched to hydrocortisone cream, which has worsened the outbreak. The rash is neither itchy nor painful. She works in an office and cannot recall any contact irritants. On examination, you find erythematous papules with small pustules on the chin and laterally around her mouth (see Fig. 17-15). The neck and the remainder of the face are not involved.

Which of the following treatments do you recommend?
A) Oral tetracycline
B) Oral isotretinoin
C) Topical high-potency steroids
D) Topical triple antibiotic ointment
E) Topical retinoic acid

The correct answer is "A." This patient appears to have perioral dermatitis. Appropriate treatments for perioral dermatitis include topical metronidazole or topical erythromycin or oral tetracycline antibiotics (tetracycline, minocycline, or doxycycline). The etiology of perioral dermatitis is unknown. "B" and "E" are incorrect, since these are treatments of acne vulgaris. "C" is incorrect, since high-potency topical steroids can make the condition worse, with rebound erythema upon discontinuation. Topical triple antibiotic ointment ("D") is not likely to be effective.

▶ CASE 17.8

A 15-year-old male presents to your office complaining of "zits" on his face and back. He has several scattered comedones on his face and several deep nodules on his back. He also has some papulopustular lesions on his chin. You diagnose him with acne vulgaris.

Question 17.8.1 Which of the following is NOT TRUE about acne?
A) Non-comedonal acne is an inflammatory process
B) It commonly presents first in adolescence
C) It may first appear in adulthood
D) It is more severe in females than in males
E) The incidence is lower in Asians and Africans than in Caucasians

Answer 17.8.1 The correct (and untrue) answer is "D." Acne is an inflammatory process that involves the pilosebaceous units of the face and trunk. It can be comedonal, papulopustular, or nodulocystic in presentation. It typically presents first in adolescence with girls developing it from age 10 to 17 years and boys from 14 to 19 years. However, it may not appear until early adulthood. It is more severe in males than in females (thus "D" is not true), and it is less prevalent among Asians and Africans.

> **HELPFUL TIP:**
> Open comedones (blackheads) and closed comedones (whiteheads) are considered non-inflammatory lesions, whereas papular and cystic lesions are considered inflammatory. And no matter how tempting, patients should not pick at them! Picking may exacerbate scarring.

Your patient has heard many things about acne and wonders if they are true.

Question 17.8.2 Regarding acne, all of the following are true EXCEPT:
A) Acne is not caused by medications
B) Acne can be caused by industrial exposures such as cutting oils, aromatic hydrocarbons, and petroleum-based products
C) Infrequent facial cleansing does not cause acne
D) Emotional stress affects the course of acne
E) Acne can present at any age

Answer 17.8.2 The correct (and untrue) answer is "A." Acne can be caused by many medications including oral steroids, EGFR inhibitors (chemotherapeutic agents), lithium, isoniazid (INH), and phenytoin. Medication-induced acne presents as monomorphic papules on the face, chest, and back. Exposure to industrial chemicals that occlude the follicle can also lead to an acneiform eruption. Neither infrequent washing nor chocolate (or any other foods) cause acne—no matter what your mother told you. However, stress (like that homecoming dance in high-school) can often flare acne.

There are different types of acne that can affect individuals at various stages of life. Neonatal acne presents shortly after birth and is transient. Infantile acne presents at 6 to 12 months of age and resolves within 1 to 2 years. The most common time to develop acne is around puberty; however, women in their thirties and forties can also experience acne flares with hormonal fluctuations. As an aside, oral contraceptives (OCPs) go both ways with regard to acne: several OCPs are marketed to treat acne, but they have been reported to worsen acne in some patients. The result of OCPs may depend on the hormonal milieu of the specific patient (women with hyperandrogenism may benefit) and the type of progestin in the OCP. Acne is often improved in the summer months and worsen in the fall and winter. Many women also tend to flare up right before menses.

Question 17.8.3 For acne, which of the following treatment principles is correct?

A) Treatment can often lead to initial worsening of lesions
B) Therapeutic response often takes several months
C) Mild acne can be treated with topical medications
D) Often times, two or more therapeutic agents must be combined for effective treatment
E) All of the above are correct

Answer 17.8.3 **The correct answer is "E."** Topical retinoids, topical antibiotics, and benzoyl peroxide are the first-line agents and can be titrated as needed. Retinoids should be applied at bedtime. The main oral antibiotic agents are tetracyclines and should be used as **add-on therapy** to topical agents for moderate-to-severe inflammatory acne. OCPs with low androgenic progesterones can also be helpful. Since acne lesions may take up to 2 months to resolve, one may not notice a therapeutic response for several months (once the current crop of lesions resolve).

HELPFUL TIP:
Topical retinoids such as tretinoin are most effective for comedonal acne. Other topical retinoids include adapalene and tazarotene.

After a few months of topical therapy with benzoyl peroxide wash, topical clindamycin cream, and topical tretinoin, your patient returns with persistent lesions, including mild scarring and cystic lesions. You are considering isotretinoin, which is indicated for severe, recalcitrant, nodular acne.

Question 17.8.4 Which of the following is FALSE regarding the use of isotretinoin?

A) Two methods of contraception are required in all reproductive age women along with frequent pregnancy tests
B) It should not be used with tetracycline
C) Hypertriglyceridemia is a possible side effect
D) Patient should be monitored closely for changes in mood
E) A patient can only receive one course of isotretinoin

Answer 17.8.4 **The correct (or rather False) answer is "E."** Isotretinoin is an oral retinoid and is pregnancy category X. Because of this, the FDA has developed a mandatory patient registry called "iPLEDGE." All patients must enroll in his registry before receiving the medication and prescribers also need to be registered. Female patients of reproductive age are required to use two contraceptive methods *and have monthly pregnancy tests*. As both tetracycline and isotretinoin can lead to pseudotumor cerebri, they should not be used together. Hypertriglyceridemia, dry eyes, dry lips, and dry skin are common side effects. Less common side effects include decreased night vision, joint pain, and headaches. Isotretinoin has been reported to cause premature closure of growth plates rarely. There have been reports in the popular press and the scientific literature of suicide in patients on isotretinoin, though population-based studies have failed to demonstrate a causal relationship. Patients with a history of mental health issues should be followed carefully for any changes in their mood or behavior. Approximately one-third of patients who receive isotretinoin will require additional courses during their lifetime.

HELPFUL TIP:
Oral retinoids (isotretinoin) are vitamin A derivatives, so vitamin A supplements should be avoided as the combination may lead to vitamin A toxicity.

HELPFUL TIP:
Women should continue contraception for 1 month after discontinuing treatment.

▶ **Objectives: Did you learn to …**
- Diagnose and treat acne?
- Identify side effects of isotretinoin?

▶ CASE 17.9

A 26-year-old female patient presents to your office with painful, nonpruritic pink bumps that started last week on her shins. You find the firm lesions easier to palpate than to visualize (see Fig. 17-16).

Question 17.9.1 What is the most likely diagnosis in this patient?

A) Erythema multiforme
B) Urticaria
C) Erythema nodosum
D) Erythema migrans
E) Lumpy shin disease (aka, "footballer's disease" in England)

Answer 17.9.1 **The correct answer is "C."** This is erythema nodosum. Typically, these firm nodules occur first on shins and are often more easily palpated than seen. They may then spread to the thighs, trunk, and extensor surfaces of the arms. Erythema multiforme ("A") presents as erythematous, targetoid lesions usually affecting the distal extremities including palms

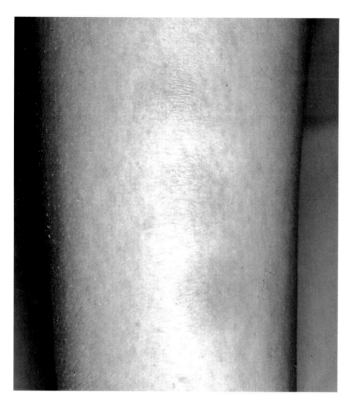

FIGURE 17-16. Erythema nodosum.

and soles. Urticaria ("B") is not tender but would be intensely pruritic. Erythema migrans ("D") is the quintessential lesion of Lyme disease: a nontender, nonpruritic red plaque with a central clearing. While "E" is technically correct in its description, we know of no such disease entity.

 HELPFUL TIP:
Erythema migrans is often thought of as a single "bull's eye" lesion in the area of the tick attachment. However, the "bull's eye" is present in a minority of cases, and erythema migrans can have multiple widespread lesions in some patients with Lyme.

Question 17.9.2 Which of the following can cause erythema nodosum?
A) OCPs
B) Streptococcal pharyngitis
C) Sarcoid
D) Viral upper respiratory infection
E) All of the above

Answer 17.9.2 The correct answer is "E." All of these entities may cause erythema nodosum, but viral URI and streptococcal pharyngitis are most common. Multiple medications can also be responsible.

This patient does relate a history of URI symptoms about 1 week prior to the onset of her symptoms.

Question 17.9.3 What advice are you going to give this patient?
A) The rash tends to be self-limiting and will resolve in 4 to 6 weeks
B) The rash will heal with scarring
C) The rash will likely spread to the face and upper extremities before it resolves
D) This is a chronic disease and no treatment is available

Answer 17.9.3 The correct answer is "A." In general, erythema nodosum heals spontaneously in 3 to 6 weeks without scarring. There are treatment options available if the patient is symptomatic. If erythema nodosum is caused by an infection, that infection should be treated appropriately. If it was caused by a medication, such as an oral contraceptive pill, it should be discontinued. Nonsteroidal anti-inflammatory agents can be used to help with the pain. For patients with severe painful disease, systemic steroids can be considered.

▸ **Objectives: Did you learn to ...**
• Recognize erythema nodosum?
• Describe some of the causes and natural history of erythema nodosum?

 QUICK QUIZ: ERYTHEMA MULTIFORME

Which of the following cause erythema multiforme?
A) Viral upper respiratory infection
B) Cimetidine
C) Herpes simplex outbreak
D) Nifedipine
E) All of the above

The correct answer is "E." All of the above are causes of erythema multiforme as are many, many other medications. **The most common precipitator of erythema multiforme is herpes simplex.** Look for this association in your patients.

 HELPFUL TIP:
Sunlight is a frequent precipitator of an outbreak of herpes labialis.

▶ **CASE 17.10**

A patient presents to your office with a 1-week history of a pruritic rash that comes and goes. No lesion is present for more than 24 hours. It involves his entire body except for his face. He cannot remember any new products with which he has been in contact (soaps, detergents, etc.). He is quite concerned. You correctly diagnose urticaria (Fig. 17-17).

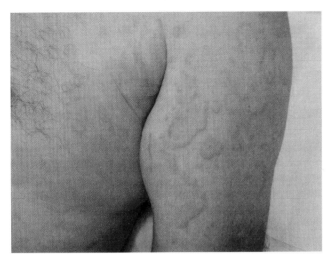

FIGURE 17-17.   Urticaria (Courtesy of Drs. Karolyn Wanat and Megan Noe.)

Question 17.10.1 **Your next step is:**
A) Skin testing for various commercial products
B) Viral titers for CMV, EBV, etc.
C) RAST test for common allergens
D) Recommend no further evaluation
E) Prescribe an epinephrine injection for emergency use at home

Answer 17.10.1 **The correct answer is "D."** No workup is needed at this time. Urticaria should be classified as "acute" (<6 weeks) or "chronic" (>6 weeks). Acute urticaria requires no further workup and should be treated symptomatically with antihistamines. Note that steroids do not add to antihistamines and should only be used in the case of angioedema (*Ann Emerg Med*. 2018;71(1):125–131.e1). In patients with chronic urticaria, a more detailed history should be taken looking for other symptoms or signs of infection, with laboratory testing as appropriate. In fact, beyond a good history, an extensive workup is pretty much futile. It is almost impossible to identify a cause of urticaria by laboratory testing. "E," an epinephrine injector, is not indicated for the treatment of urticaria but would be appropriate if this patient has experienced an anaphylactic reaction.

Question 17.10.2 **Urticaria is categorized as which of the following?**
A) Type I hypersensitivity reaction
B) Type II hypersensitivity reaction
C) Type III hypersensitivity reaction
D) Type IV hypersensitivity reaction
E) None of the above

Answer 17.10.2 **The correct answer is "A."** Urticaria is a clinical feature of a type I reaction. Other clinical presentations of type I reactions include anaphylaxis and angioedema. See Chapter 4 for a detailed answer on hypersensitivity reactions.

Question 17.10.3 **You decide to provide symptomatic care for this patient. Appropriate medications include which of the following?**
A) Ranitidine
B) Doxepin
C) Diphenhydramine
D) Cetirizine
E) All of the above

Answer 17.10.3 **The correct answer is "E."** All of the above can be useful in the symptomatic treatment of urticaria. Patients should be started on sedating and nonsedating antihistamines to control their symptoms. Doses greater than the recommended daily dose are frequently required. H_2-blockers are effective in the 10% to 15% of patients who do not respond to H_1-blockers. Of note, H_2-blockers also are used in anaphylaxis treatment, but the evidence is weak. Finally, doxepin is a particularly effective H_1- and H_2-blocker that can be used as a sedating antihistamine.

The patient returns to see you 6 weeks later and is still having symptoms. You are wondering a bit more about potential causes of this unfortunate individual's urticaria.

Question 17.10.4 **Which of the following are causes of urticaria?**
A) Sweating
B) Cold (OK, get over it. Move to Hawaii and quit whining!)
C) Water (So that is why you never shower and only drink beer?)
D) Pressure (OK, get over it. Use an antigravity unit and quit whining!)
E) All of the above

Answer 17.10.4 **The correct answer is "E."** All of the above can cause urticaria. In fact, these are not uncommon causes and can be identified by history. Patients may develop urticaria with exercise and sweating (cholinergic urticaria), cold (during the winter), and pressure (e.g., walking). Of particular note is water urticaria that occurs with water contact, including bathing and showering. See Table 17-2 for a more complete listing.

HELPFUL TIP:
Cold urticaria often starts with lesions appearing on exposed skin but may be worsened with rewarming.

You decide that this patient probably has cold urticaria (the fact that it is summer does not dissuade you as it may be related to all of that air conditioning!).

Question 17.10.5 **The next drug you might want to try on this patient is:**
A) Cyproheptadine (Periactin)
B) Prednisone
C) Montelukast
D) Nifedipine
E) Aspirin

TABLE 17-2 CAUSES OF URTICARIA: A PARTIAL LIST

Physical Urticaria	Allergic	Systemic	Medications (Direct Mast Cell Degranulators)
• Pressure	• Foods (nuts, fish)	• Malignancy	• NSAIDs
• Water	• Insect stings	• SLE	• Aspirin
• Vibration	• Drugs (IgE mediated)	• RA	• Opiates
• Cold		• Chronic Hep B and C	• ACE Inhibitors
• Sunlight		• EBV	• Contrast dye

Answer 17.10.5 The correct answer is "A." The physical urticarias (cold and pressure especially) *may* respond better to cyproheptadine than other modalities. If this patient had a "typical" urticaria, you might want to try prednisone, one of the leukotriene inhibitors or nifedipine (which interferes with mast cell degranulation). **Remember that leukotriene inhibitors, steroids, etc., are second line and should be used only when first-line drugs have failed or are not tolerated** (cyproheptadine for physical urticaria; doxepin, antihistamines, etc., for "typical" urticaria). There are no good studies on the effectiveness of leukotriene inhibitors (anecdotal evidence only), but they might be worth trying when all else fails.

HELPFUL TIP:
Any number of drugs can cause urticaria. Look at the medication list! Medications that act as mast cell degranulators should be avoided in patients with chronic urticaria, including aspirin, opiates, polymyxin B, NSAIDs, and systemic lidocaine.

▶ **Objectives: Did you learn to ...**
· Recognize urticaria?
· Identify potential causes of urticaria?
· Develop a treatment strategy for patients with urticaria?

 QUICK QUIZ: PRECANCEROUS LESIONS

Actinic keratoses (AKs) are precursors to what?
A) Nothing
B) Melanoma
C) Basal cell carcinoma
D) Squamous cell carcinoma
E) Granuloma annulare

The correct answer is "D." AKs are precursors to squamous cell carcinomas. As such, they should be treated. Options include cryotherapy, laser therapy, or 5-fluorouracil topically.

HELPFUL TIP:
Less than 1% of AKs progress to squamous cell carcinoma per year. Some spontaneously involute and some remain as AKs. However, in an individual, the risk of an AK developing into a squamous cell carcinoma increases with the number of AKs present.

 QUICK QUIZ: SKIN BARNACLES

What is the appropriate treatment for an asymptomatic seborrheic keratosis?
A) No treatment necessary
B) Cryotherapy
C) Surgical excision
D) Topical steroids
E) Topical antibiotic ointment

The correct answer is "A." Seborrheic keratoses are benign lesions that do not develop into malignancies. They are the greasy-looking, stuck-on growths that occur with age. They can be treated, if symptomatic, with cryotherapy. They look ugly, patients hate them, but they are harmless.

▶ **CASE 17.11**

A 50-year-old female with type 2 diabetes controlled with insulin complains of a rash that has developed on her legs over the past year. It started as a small patch on her left leg and then "spread" to her right leg. It is neither painful nor pruritic. You are impressed by the rash she shows you (Fig. 17-18).

Question 17.11.1 The most appropriate next step in the management of these lesions is which of the following?
A) A topical mid-potency steroid under occlusion or intralesional steroids
B) Discontinue insulin
C) Increase her insulin dose
D) Liberal use of emollients (e.g., petrolatum)
E) Leg elevation and application of compressive stockings

Answer 17.11.1 The correct answer is "A." This patient has developed necrobiosis lipoidica, a benign condition of the skin affecting a small percentage of patients with diabetes. Look for brownish red patches or plaques with yellowish areas through the center. The center is often shiny with telangiectasias. The legs are most often involved and the lesions may be painful. The name describes the pathology: necrobiosis refers to the inflammation around destroyed collagen, and lipoidica refers to the yellowish color associated with lipid deposits. It *does*

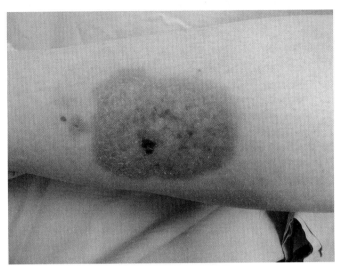

FIGURE 17-18. Necrobiosis Lipodica (Wolff K, Johnson RA, Suurmond D. *Fitzpatrick's Color Atlas & Synopsis of Clinical Dermatology.* 5th ed. New York: McGraw-Hill; 2005, Fig. 5-1. Copyright © The McGraw-Hill Companies, Inc. All rights reserved.)

not seem to be caused by insulin or affected by glucose control, so "B" and "C" are not appropriate choices. These lesions can be confused with eczema, and in fact may respond to topical steroids ("A"); however, emollients are not useful. Finally, necrobiosis lipoidica might be confused with the skin changes associated with venous stasis and chronic edema, which would be treated as in "E." Patients should know that necrobiosis lipoidica is often chronic and difficult to treat but benign. The diagnosis is clinical but can be confirmed by biopsy, and treatment is not always necessary.

Your patient also complains of thick, dark, velvety patches under her arms (Fig. 17-19). She's unsure of the duration, but states, "They've been with me a while. I just wondered if my medication might cause these." She gives you an accusing look, and you have to admit that she takes more than a few medicines related to her diabetes.

Question 17.11.2 Which medication provides a clue to the diagnosis?
A) Aspirin
B) Lisinopril
C) Insulin
D) Simvastatin

Answer 17.11.2 **The correct answer is "C."** The lesions are typical of acanthosis nigricans, a hyperkeratotic, hyperpigmented condition affecting skin folds (neck, inguinal area, axilla, etc.). The common causes of acanthosis nigricans are obesity, insulin resistance, and diabetes. From medical school, we all remember acanthosis nigricans as a cutaneous manifestation of internal malignancy. But such a presentation is rare. Cancer is more likely in patients with extensive and quickly progressing lesions, and as you might expect, it's not a good sign.

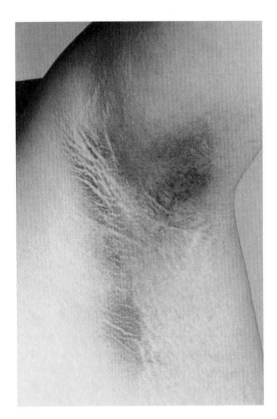

FIGURE 17-19. Acanthosis nigricans.

 HELPFUL (ISH) TIP:
Another cutaneous manifestation of internal malignancy is the sign of Leser–Trelat: a large crop of seborrheic keratoses that erupt quickly. Note that seborrheic keratoses themselves are benign and that knowing about Leser–Trelat is mostly good for looking smart.

Your patient returns a year later and the lesions on her legs have essentially disappeared. Now she has a new concern. She reports a sore on the bottom of her great toe. She's uncertain how it occurred and thinks it has only been present for a few days. You find a 1-cm circular ulcer at the plantar aspect of her great toe. Pulses are diminished.

Question 17.11.3 Which of the following should be the *next* step in treatment?
A) Culture the wound
B) Perform an MRI of the foot
C) Perform monofilament testing to check sensation in the foot
D) Debride the wound
E) Obtain ankle–brachial indices

Answer 17.11.3 **The correct answer is "E."** The described wound is most likely a diabetic foot ulcer, but the location and the patient's history of diabetes do elicit concern for an ulcer related to vascular disease. In addition, good vascular supply to the foot is necessary for wound healing. Therefore, you need to know the status of blood flow to the foot. This may be accomplished by physical examination. For patients at high risk for peripheral vascular disease or without strong pulses, ankle–brachial indices would be the next step. Culture of an open foot ulcer ("A") is pretty much worthless as it will likely return as polymicrobial. X-ray may be warranted as well as probing the lesion to see if it reaches the bone in order to evaluate for osteomyelitis, but starting with MRI ("B") is jumping the gun in this particular case. Knowledge of a patient's baseline monofilament sensation ("C") is important and good general foot care (shoes that fit, meticulous skin and nail care) can help in the prevention of future ulcers. Wound debridement ("D") will help to remove necrotic tissue and improve the speed of wound healing. The biofilm must be removed down to healthy tissue in order to maximize healing.

Ankle–brachial indices in both legs are normal. The rest of her skin is in good condition. Through her diligent care and control of her diabetes, the ulcer heals. She returns 3 months later with a new skin concern. On her anterior shin, she has developed a clear fluid-filled blister about 1 cm in diameter and irregular in shape. There is no erythema, no pruritus, and no pain. She denies trauma and new environmental contacts.

Question 17.11.4 Which of the following is the most likely diagnosis?
A) Dyshidrotic eczema
B) Contact dermatitis
C) Staphylococcal scalded skin syndrome (SSSS)
D) Bullosis diabeticorum
E) Drug eruption

Answer 17.11.4 **The correct answer is "D."** Bullosis diabeticorum, or bullous disease of diabetes, occurs in less than 1% of diabetic patients. However, patients may be alarmed by it and seek treatment. The cause is unknown, but it typically follows a benign course and resolves spontaneously over a few weeks or months. Because it requires no intervention, it is useful to distinguish bullosis diabeticorum from dyshidrotic eczema and contact dermatitis, both of which may mimic the disease except for pruritus and inflammation.

▶ **Objectives: Did you learn to …**
- Identify necrobiosis lipoidica, acanthosis nigricans, and bullosis diabeticorum?
- Treat these conditions (if necessary)?
- Evaluate a diabetic foot ulcer?

 QUICK QUIZ: SKIN SO ITCHY

A 60-year-old male who underwent pacemaker placement 3 days ago comes in with the pruritic rash seen in Figure 17-20.

This rash is most likely:
A) Grover disease
B) Lichen planus
C) Contact dermatitis

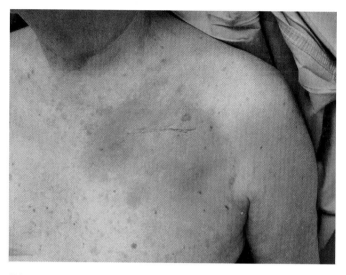

FIGURE 17-20. Contact dermatitis.

D) Atopic dermatitis
E) Pyoderma gangrenosum

The correct answer is "C." This is contact dermatitis, which may be acute, subacute, or chronic. It is an erythematous, pruritic eruption that usually blisters and leaves a crust. More chronic forms of contact dermatitis present with lichenification and scaling. The rash in Figure 17-20 does not look like any of the other choices. Grover disease (not related to the Sesame Street muppet but it would be cool if it were) ("A"), also known as transient acantholytic dermatosis, presents with small, sometimes pruritic, erythematous papules on the back and chest, which may blister. Lichen planus ("B") presents with pruritic, red-to-purple, flat-topped papules. Atopic dermatitis ("D") is discussed earlier in the chapter. Pyoderma gangrenosum ("E") presents with painful, red nodules and pustules that ulcerate. Again, since we cannot display pictures of all diseases mentioned, please look at one of the websites included at the beginning of this chapter.

 HELPFUL TIP:
Pyoderma gangrenosum is a diagnosis of exclusion but may be differentiated from other ulcer types by the exquisite pain it causes and the pathergic phenomenon it displays, where the wound will worsen in response to surgical manipulation (e.g., biopsy, debridement). It can be associated with inflammatory bowel disease, inflammatory arthritis, solid organ neoplasm (23%!), hematologic neoplasm or other hematologic disorders. Look at some pictures online. This is not one to miss.

 QUICK QUIZ: MR. SCRATCHER

A 76-year-old male comes to your clinic with a 1-year history of pruritic, eczematous rash on his chest and back. He has no atopic history or eczema as a child. He has no other active medical issues. He has tried moisturizers and over-the-counter hydrocortisone cream, which have provided minimal relief.

Which of the following is the most appropriate next step in his management?
A) Tacrolimus ointment
B) Skin scraping for KOH preparation
C) High-dose topical steroids
D) Punch biopsy
E) Oral antihistamines

The correct answer is "D." The development of a new, eczematous rash in an adult patient can be associated with more serious condition. This may be indicative of an underlying lymphoproliferative malignancy such as cutaneous T-cell lymphoma. In addition, a drug hypersensitivity reaction can also be a consideration. The most appropriate next step in this patient's management would be punch biopsy.

 QUICK QUIZ: DARIER SIGN

A 4-year-old girl comes to clinic accompanied by her mother for her yearly checkup. Her mother requests that you examine her daughter's skin because of a rash. Upon examination, you identify scattered reddish-brown macules on the back and chest. When stroked, the lesions urticate. There are no other complaints or abnormalities on physical examination.

What is the most likely diagnosis?
A) Atopic dermatitis
B) Contact dermatitis
C) Congenital nevi
D) Cutaneous lupus
E) Urticaria pigmentosa

The correct answer is "E." This child's rash is most likely secondary to urticaria pigmentosa, which is a cutaneous form of mastocytosis. Clinical findings include reddish-brown macules or slightly raised papules, which represent cutaneous accumulations of mast cells. These occur most commonly on extensor surfaces, thorax, and abdomen. When stroked, these lesions can urticate (Darier sign). Urticaria pigmentosa is the most common skin manifestation of mastocytosis in children and adults. Eighty percent of cases appear during the first year of life. Lesions resolve in >50% of patients by adolescence. The diagnosis is confirmed by skin biopsy. In children, urticaria pigmentosa is rarely associated with systemic disease.

▶ CASE 17.12

A 44-year-old female presents for a scaly rash for the past 6 months. It started on her knees and elbows and has spread to involve her scalp, abdomen, and gluteal cleft (Fig. 17-21). She has also noticed the appearance of "little holes" in her finger nails. She has tried moisturizers without improvement. She

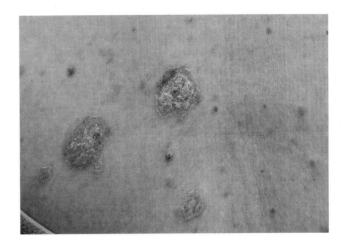

FIGURE 17-21. Herpes zoster.

also reports stiffness in her wrists and ankles that is worse in the morning. She denies smoking, but drinks three to four glasses of wine every night.

Question 17.12.1 What is the most likely diagnosis?
A) Cutaneous T-Cell Lymphoma
B) Psoriasis
C) Tinea Corporis
D) Contact Dermatitis
E) Eczema

Answer 17.12.1 The correct answer is "B." This clinical scenario is most suggestive of psoriasis. Psoriasis is a chronic inflammatory disease of the skin that affects about 3% of the population. Psoriasis is characterized by well-circumscribed plaques with silver scale. Common areas of involvement are the scalp, extensor surfaces, and gluteal cleft. Patients with psoriasis can also have nail involvement including pitting, oil spots and onycholysis (lifting of the nail plate from the nail bed), and subungual parakeratosis that can resemble onychomycosis. About 30% of patients with psoriasis also have psoriatic arthritis and any patient with joint symptoms should be referred to rheumatology for evaluation. Patients with psoriasis also are at higher risk of developing cardiovascular disease, diabetes, hypertension, and metabolic syndrome. Cutaneous T-cell lymphoma ("A") more commonly occurs in areas covered by a "bathing suit" on the trunk and on the scalp and extensor surfaces as above. Tinea Corporis ("C") can mimic psoriasis but is typically not as widespread. Adults with tinea corporis may also have concomitant tinea pedis. The rash associated with contact dermatitis ("D") should be more geometric—from contact with the allergen—and is typically not symmetric, as above. Finally, in adults, eczema more commonly occurs on the hands, feet, and flexor, not extensor, surfaces. Also, eczema is not associated with nail pitting.

Based on the clinical appearance, you diagnose the patient with psoriasis and estimate the plaques to cover about 5% of her body surface area. You prescribe a medium-to-high potency topical steroid. **She returns in 3 months and notes her psoriasis has not improved with regular use of the topical steroid.**

Question 17.12.2 Given the patient has not improved with topical steroids, what is an appropriate treatment option?
A) More topical steroids
B) Oral Steroids
C) Oral Antifungal agent
D) Phototherapy
E) Methotrexate

Answer 17.12.2 **The correct answer is "D."** Phototherapy is a well-established treatment option for patients with moderate-to-severe psoriasis. Most commonly, narrow band ultraviolet B (nbUVB) light (311 nm) is used. Other treatment options for severe psoriasis include: biologics—monoclonal antibodies that bind to inflammatory cytokines like tumor necrosis factor (adalimumab [Humira], certolizumab [Cimzia], etanercept [Enbrel], infliximab [Remicade]); IL-12/23 (ustekinumab [Stelara]); IL-17 (brodalumab [Siliq], ixekizumab [Taltz]; secukinumab [Cosentyx]) and IL-23 inhibitors (guselkuma [Tremfya], tildrakizumab [Ilumya]); and apremilast (Otezla), an oral phosphodiesterase-4 inhibitor. Methotrexate ("E") is also a treatment for psoriasis and psoriatic arthritis, but this women reports drinking three to four glasses of alcohol nightly, so she is not an appropriate candidate for methotrexate. While changing topical steroids can sometimes help to improve psoriasis ("A"), in patients with 5% BSA, who report good compliance, alternative therapies should be considered. While oral steroids ("B") may improve the redness of psoriatic plaques, *they should not be used for the chronic management of psoriasis* because of concern for rebound or pustular psoriasis flare upon completion of therapy. While tinea corporis can mimic psoriasis, in patients without evidence of superficial dermatophyte infection, like a positive KOH scraping, oral antifungal agents ("C") are unlikely to improve psoriasis.

▸ **Objectives: Did you learn to …**
- Diagnose psoriasis?
- Identify the various treatment modalities utilized, often with assistance from a dermatologist, to treat psoriasis?

 QUICK QUIZ: PATCHY HAIR LOSS

A 14-year-old female presents to your office with a circular, shiny bald patch on the parietal scalp. She did not know that it was there until her hairdresser first noticed it about a month ago. She is very anxious that she is going to lose all her hair. On exam, there are two circular alopetic patches on the left parietal and left occipital scalp with exclamation point hairs present around the border. Pitting is also present on several finger nails.

The most likely diagnosis is:
A) Tinea capitis
B) Alopecia areata
C) Androgenic alopecia

D) Trichotillomania
E) Telogen effluvium

The correct answer is "B." Alopecia areata is an immune-mediated disorder that causes non-scarring hair loss, typically presenting with circular, discrete patches on the scalp, but other hair-baring sites can also be affected. The clinical course of alopecia areata is unpredictable. About 50% of patients achieve hair-regrowth within a year, but recurrence is common. Uncommonly the hair loss can progress to involve the entire scalp (alopecia totalis) and/or all body sites (alopecia universalis). Intralesinsal or topical steroids are first-line therapy for localized alopecia areata.

The other diagnoses listed above are all in the differential diagnosis of patchy or diffuse hair loss. Tinea capitis ("A") is a superficial dermatophyte infection of the scalp, more common in children. While patients may present with circular patches or hair loss, there is typically an overlying crust or scale, which was not present in this case. Inflammation and cervical lymphadenopathy can also be present. Trichotillomania ("D") is an impulse control disorder where patients repeatedly pull out their own hair. While trichotillomania may present with discrete patches of hair loss, short or broken-off hairs are typically seen throughout the patch or at the periphery.

Androgenetic alopecia ("C") (male/female pattern hair loss) is a gradual loss of hair in adult men and women. Men typically develop gradual thinning of hair on the temporal and vertex scalp, often affecting the frontal hairline. Women most commonly report thinning of the hair on the frontal and vertex scalp, creating noticeable thinning around the part. Treatment in men includes finasteride (first line) and topical minoxidil. For women, treatment includes minoxidil with spironolactone (an antiandrogen) as second line. Telogen effluvium ("E") is diffuse hair thinning caused by a rapid shift in the follicular hair cycling leading to premature shedding of hair. Common triggers for telogen effluvium include childbirth, major illness/surgery, drugs, malnutrition, and severe emotional stress (death of a friend/family member, moving, starting a new job). Discrete patches of hair loss are typically not seen in androgenic alopecia or telogen effluvium. Evaluation of telogen effluvium includes "the hair pull test." Grasp 50 to 60 hairs and pull. The extraction of more than 6 to 10 hairs is abnormal. Treatment is to address the underlying cause.

▸ **CASE 17.13**

A 30-year-old stressed out medical student presents to your clinic with a worsening, painful rash on one side of her chest. She denies any prior spots like this and has no other medical problems. She is up-to-date on her vaccinations because of medical school and complains that this rash is interfering with studying for the upcoming final block of examinations (she wants to be a dermatologist, so she really has to "ace" her examinations). Physical examination demonstrates a linear group of vesicles with

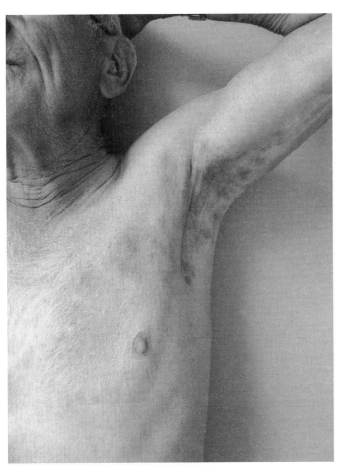

FIGURE 17-22. (Courtesy of Drs. Karolyn Wanat and Megan Noe.)

erythema on her left chest following a dermatomal pattern. See Figure 17-22 (in which the young medical student has turned into an older man).

Question 17.13.1 Treatment should be initiated with which of the following therapies:

A) Cephalexin
B) Mupirocin
C) Paroxetine
D) Valacyclovir
E) No treatment is necessary as this is self-limited

Answer 17.13.1 **The correct answer is "D."** This is most likely herpes zoster, which is reactivation of the varicella zoster virus. Valacyclovir is an effective treatment. Even in immunocompetent patients, herpes zoster can be reactivated from the dorsal root ganglion during periods of stress. Although it can be self-limited, treatment with antiviral (valacyclovir or acyclovir) is recommended during the first 72 hours to decrease outbreak and risk of postherpetic neuralgia. With the presentation of pain, agents such as gabapentin, amitriptyline, or pregabalin are also often prescribed. Post-herpetic neuralgia can also be treated with topical lidocaine patches; however, these should not be applied to open blisters/wounds on the skin. A live,

attenuated, vaccine to prevent zoster (Zostavax) is available. In 2017, a two-dose recombinant zoster vaccine (Shringrix) was FDA approved for healthy adults 50 years of age and older. It is more effective than Zostavax and is now considered preferable.

▶ **Objective: Did you learn to …**
  · Recognize and treat herpes zoster (Shingles)?

Clinical Pearls

○ Be sure to look for abnormal looking skin lesions on the palms, soles of the feet, and near the nails, as these lesions may progress to more aggressive forms of melanoma before they are discovered.

○ Confirm a toenail fungal infection prior to initiating systemic antifungal therapy.

○ Do not perform a shave biopsy on a skin lesion if you are suspecting melanoma as depth of the lesion is used to stage melanoma and determine prognosis.

○ Do not routinely recommend diuretics as general therapy to lessen the edema of venous stasis as they may make symptoms worse by decreasing circulating volume and increase renal retention of sodium. Instead, recommend weight loss, compression stockings, and leg elevation.

○ Do not use systemic antibiotics for first-line treatment of acne. Instead, employ topical agents as first-line therapy.

○ Do not use topical antifungal agents to treat fungal nail infections. They are relatively expensive, have marginal benefit, and a high recurrence rate.

○ Recommend regular sun protection using sunscreen, light protective long-sleeved clothing, hat, and sunglasses.

○ Recommend timely removal/biopsy of any suspicious looking nevi.

○ Refer infants with larger, segmental hemangiomas to dermatology and obtain imaging studies to rule out syndromes with other associated anomalies.

BIBLIOGRAPHY

Barniol C, et al. Levocetirizine and prednisone are not superior to levocetirizine alone for the treatment of acute urticarial: a randomized double-blind clinical trial. *Ann Emerg Med.* 2018;71(1):125.e1–131.e1.

Bruckner AL, Frieden IJ. Hemangiomas of infancy. *J Am Acad Derm.* 2003;48:477–493.

Di Lorenzo G, et al. Leukotriene receptor antagonists in monotherapy or in combination with antihistamines in the treatment of chronic urticaria: a systematic review. *J Asthma Allergy.* 2008;2:9–16.

Eichenfield LF, Tom WL, Berger TG, et al. Guidelines of care for the management of atopic dermatitis: section 2. Management and treatment of atopic dermatitis with topical therapies. *J Am Acad Dermatol.* 2014;71(1):116-132.

Gershenwald JE, et al. 2010 TNM staging system for cutaneous melanoma ... and beyond. *Ann Surg Oncol.* 2010;17:1475–1477.

Gershenwald JE, et al. Melanoma staging: evidence-based changes in the American Joint Committee on Cancer Eighth Edition Cancer Staging Manual. *CA Cancer J Clin.* 2017;67:472–492.

Hurwitz S, eds. Eczemetous eruptions in childhood. In: *Clinical Pediatric Dermatology.* 3rd ed. Philadelphia, PA: W.B. Saunders Co.; 2005.

Khumalo N, et al. Interventions for bullous pemphigoid. *Cochrane Database Syst Rev.* 2003;(3):CD002292.

O'Connor NR, McLaughlin MR. Neonatal skin: Parts I and II. *Am Fam Physician.* 2008;77:47–60.

Rager EL. Cutaneous melanoma. *Am Fam Physician.* 2005;72:269–276.

Ramsey HM, et al. Factors associated with nonmelanoma skin cancer following renal transplantation. *J Am Acad Dermatol.* 2003;49(3):397–406.

Usatine RP, et al. *The Color Atlas of Family Medicine. Part 13: Dermatology.* New York: McGraw-Hill; 2009.

Wolff K, Johnson RA. *Fitzpatrick's Color Atlas and Synopsis of Clinical Dermatology.* 6th ed. New York: McGraw-Hill; 2009.

Neurology

18

Daniel M. Anderson, Qiang Zhang, and Teri Thomsen

▶ CASE 18.1

A 75-year-old right-handed man presents to the emergency department (ED) with dizziness that started 5 hours ago. His dizziness consists of a spinning sensation and he feels off balance as he walks. He reports coughing when trying to drink water earlier, but otherwise notes no other symptoms. He has an unremarkable past medical history and is taking no medications. On examination, he is found to have left-sided ptosis and left facial numbness to pinprick. Gag reflex is absent. Motor examination is otherwise unremarkable. Sensory examination revealed decreased pinprick sensation of the right arm and leg. He is unsteady while walking, tending to lean leftward.

Question 18.1.1 What is the most likely diagnosis in this patient?
A) Acute vestibulitis/labyrinthitis
B) Benign paroxysmal positional vertigo (BPPV)
C) Cerebellar stroke
D) Brain stem stroke
E) Ménière attack

Answer 18.1.1 The correct answer is "D." Although dizziness can be associated with all of the above disorders, a brain stem stroke is the most likely answer. The associated symptoms of ptosis (suggestive of Horner syndrome: miosis, ptosis, hypohydrosis—generally from disruption of the sympathetic innervation), absent gag reflex with patient report of possible dysphagia, and crossed sensory findings (decreased sensation of the left side face and the right arm and leg) are most consistent with brain stem localization. In peripheral etiologies of vertigo ("A," "B," and "E"), one would not expect these findings (sensory phenomena, ptosis, or swallowing difficulties). In BPPV ("B"), one would expect brief attacks, lasting seconds to minutes, and not a prolonged attack. In Ménière's ("E"), there is often some history of tinnitus, ear fullness, and/or hearing loss (low frequency initially). Acute vestibulitis/labyrinthitis ("A") are resultant of

inflammation of the inner ear and most commonly present following a viral respiratory tract infection. Onset is typically sudden, about 1 to 2 weeks after resolution of infection, and consist of vertigo and loss of hearing vs. tinnitus without sensory findings. A pure cerebellar stroke ("C") would not be expected to have sensory findings.

HELPFUL TIP:
When a patient complains of dizziness, ask what the patient means by "dizziness." The term "dizziness" means different things to different patients. "Dizziness" may represent vertigo, lightheadedness, pre-syncope, disequilibrium when walking (e.g., falling to one side), anxiety, etc. Also, know that there is controversy among experts as to whether this delineation of dizziness is more misleading than it is helpful.

....

In conferring with your colleague, she asks if you are going to give tissue plasminogen activator (tPA).

Question 18.1.2 Which one of the following is NOT a contraindication to intravenous (IV) tPA?
A) Age >75
B) INR >1.7
C) Platelets <100,000
D) Stroke within last 3 months
E) Glucose <50
F) Hemorrhage seen on head CT

Answer 18.1.2 The correct answer is "A." Acute stroke treatment with thrombolytics **may be** of benefit if administered to carefully selected patients within **3 hours** of symptom onset, or **4.5 hours** of symptom onset if certain criteria are met (see Table 18-1). When administered properly, the number needed to treat for improvement at 3 months is **6**. However, there is no survival benefit. The risk of hemorrhage is 6%

TABLE 18-1 ELIGIBILITY AND CONTRAINDICATIONS FOR TPA FOR ACUTE ISCHEMIC STROKE, SYMPTOM ONSET 0–4.5 HOURS

Eligibility
- Age ≥ 18 years
- Clinical diagnosis of ischemic stroke causing measurable neurological deficit

Contraindications
- Intracranial hemorrhage on CT
- History of intracranial hemorrhage
- Clinical presentation suggesting subarachnoid hemorrhage
- Intracranial/intraspinal surgery within the past 3 months
- Stroke or serious head trauma within the past 3 months, or posttraumatic infarction
- Sustained blood pressure of SBP >185 or DBP >110 mm Hg
- Symptoms consistent with infective endocarditis
- Known or suspected aortic dissection
- Intra-axial intracranial neoplasm
- Active internal bleeding or known bleeding diathesis
- Recent GI bleeding within 21 days
- Platelet count < 100,000
- PTT > 40 or on anticoagulation with an INR of >1.7 or PT ≥ 15
- Current use of low–molecular-weight heparin (LMWH), direct thrombin inhibitors, or direct factor Xa inhibitors

Relative contraindications
- Symptoms minor or rapidly improving
- CT showing multilobar infarction (>1/3 middle cerebral artery distribution)
- Seizure at onset of acute stroke
- Glucose < 50 mg/dL or > 400 mg/dL
- Known arteriovenous malformation or aneurysm
- Major surgery or serious trauma, excluding head trauma, in the past 14 days
- History of GI (over 21 days ago) or genitourinary tract hemorrhage
- Recent arterial puncture at a non-compressible site in the preceding 7 days
- Recent lumbar puncture in the preceding 7 days
- Myocardial infarction in the past 3 months, pericarditis
- Preexisting disability or dementia
- Pregnancy or within 14 days after delivery
- Ophthalmic hemorrhagic conditions including diabetic hemorrhagic retinopathy

Additional relative contraindications for patients presenting in the window of 3–4.5 hours from symptom onset
- Age >80 years
- History of prior stroke and diabetes
- Any active anticoagulant use, even with INR ≤ 1.7
- NIH stroke score >25

AHA/ASA 2018 guideline.

HELPFUL TIP:
Make sure you are compulsive about inclusion and exclusion criteria! Thrombolytics **do not** seem to confer an advantage in those with a "mild, non-disabling stroke" (NIH stroke scale 0-5 *and* a deficit that *would not* preclude the patient from employment) (*JAMA*. 2018 Jul 10; 320(2):156–166). When in doubt, call the nearest stroke-accredited hospital to speak to the on-call neurologist.

The patient is outside of the 4.5-hour window for thrombolysis and has a blood pressure of 200/100 mm Hg.

Question 18.1.3 The best next step in treatment at this point is to:
A) Administer IV labetalol with a blood pressure goal of 140/90 mm Hg
B) Administer IV labetalol with a blood pressure goal of 130/85 mm Hg
C) Administer IV nitroglycerin with a blood pressure goal of 150/90 mm Hg
D) Administer sublingual nifedipine with a blood pressure goal of 160/95 mm Hg
E) Monitor the patient's blood pressure and avoid antihypertensives

Answer 18.1.3 The correct answer is "E." Do not treat this patient's blood pressure unless the blood pressure is >220 mm Hg systolic or >120 mm Hg diastolic; and even then the goal would be to reduce blood pressure by 15% over 24 hours. Treating blood pressure during the acute phase of ischemic stroke reduces central nervous system (CNS) perfusion and puts ischemic brain at risk. Obviously, this does not apply if the patient has a hypertensive urgency or hypertensive crisis (e.g., heart failure or other end-organ dysfunction). **Note that this is for *ischemic stroke* and not hemorrhagic stroke. Lowering the blood pressure to a systolic of around or below 160 mm Hg is indicated in hemorrhagic stroke.** In this scenario, if you use an antihypertensive, labetalol or nicardipine is preferred. You can also use hydralazine if the heart rate is low. Why not nitrates? Nitrates cause intracranial vasodilatation increasing intracranial pressure.

Question 18.1.4 After admission to a monitored bed, which of the following diagnostic evaluations is LEAST likely to be of further benefit in this patient?
A) Fasting lipid profile
B) Magnetic resonance angiography (MRA) of the head and neck
C) Fasting glucose
D) Hypercoagulable testing
E) Transesophageal echocardiogram

Answer 18.1.4 The correct answer is "D." Hypercoagulable states are an uncommon cause of stroke. If you are unable to determine the origin of a clot in a thromboembolic stroke and

(1 in 16). Of those with symptomatic hemorrhagic transformation, 60% are fatal. There is no upper age cutoff for administration of tPA. Strong contraindications include intracranial hemorrhage, minor or improving symptoms, as well as those listed in Table 18-1. The field of acute stroke care is highly dynamic and lots of progress has been made recently. In addition to tPA, thrombectomy has become standard of care for acute ischemic strokes with large vessel occlusion. When in doubt, please do not hesitate to contact your neurology colleagues.

the patient is otherwise low-risk (let's say a healthy 25-year-old male who runs marathons), then you can consider a workup for a hypercoagulable state. Such an evaluation is not useful in most stroke patients—like your typical 80-year-old hypertensive female, even if her carotid Doppler's and echocardiogram are negative. In addition to monitoring the patient for signs of neurologic decline or complications, evaluation of potential risk factors for recurrent stroke is an integral part of stroke care. Hypertension, hyperlipidemia, cardiac arrhythmia or structural defects, illicit drug use (IV drugs and stimulants), smoking, and diabetes mellitus are risk factors for recurrent stroke and should be evaluated. MRA allows noninvasive evaluation of intracranial and cervical blood vessels in both the anterior and posterior circulation. Echocardiography is also an important part in the evaluation of stroke, and **transesophageal** echocardiography is more sensitive for identifying thrombotic sources for stroke when compared with transthoracic echocardiogram.

The patient is found to have a lateral medullary stroke on MRI and has heavy atherosclerotic burden in his vertebral arteries. Echocardiogram and telemetry are normal.

Question 18.1.5 What would be the optimal antithrombotic medication in this patient for prevention of recurrent stroke?
A) Coumadin (warfarin)
B) Aspirin
C) Plavix (clopidogrel)
D) Aggrenox (aspirin/dipyridamole)
E) Pletal (cilostazol)

Answer 18.1.5 The correct answer is "B." In patients with a noncardiogenic source for their stroke, there is no data to support the use of anticoagulation (warfarin) for stroke prevention. Similarly, there is no prospective data to support a role for cilostazol or pentoxifylline in the prevention of stroke.

With regard to antiplatelet agents, low-dose aspirin is the first-line choice. **There has been little benefit shown in increasing the dose of aspirin to more than 81 mg every day, although this may change.** Newer data suggests higher doses of aspirin are needed (325 mg) for those over 70 kg (*Lancet.* 2018 Jul 12;392(10145):361–362). If a patient fails aspirin (recurrent stroke of same mechanism), either **change** to clopidogrel or Aggrenox (combination aspirin/dipyridamole); both are equally effective in stroke prevention.

Dual antiplatelet therapy is gaining favor in TIAs and minor ischemic strokes (NIH stroke scale <= 3 or ABCD2 score of 4 or more if patient had a TIA) (NOT major ischemic strokes). You may see aspirin and clopidogrel used together **for the first 21 days** after a minor ischemic stroke or TIA (*BMJ.* 2018;363:k5130). CHANCE study showed the use of aspirin and clopidogrel *within the first 24 hours after symptom onset* was effective and superior to aspirin alone for decreasing risk of stroke within the first 90 days without increase in hemorrhage

(*N Engl J Med.* 2013;369:11–19). A more recent study showed that dual antiplatelet for 90 days conferred an overall lower risk of major ischemic events (5% vs. 6.5%) but a higher risk of major hemorrhage (0.9% vs. 0.4%) (*N Engl J Med.* 2018;379:215–225). Stay tuned to see how this all plays out for the standard of stroke care moving forward.

HELPFUL TIP:
Patients with a cryptogenic stroke may have a patent foramen ovale. Current data suggests that repairing this can reduce stroke recurrence especially in those <60 years of age (*BMJ.* 2018;362:k2515); you still need to continue aspirin or another antiplatelet agent.

Your next patient is a 59-year-old male who appears to have had a simple TIA with left-sided focal weakness. The TIA lasted <10 minutes and the patient has a normal blood pressure and is nondiabetic.

Question 18.1.6 His risk of having a stroke in the 48 hours after a simple TIA is:
A) 1%
B) 5%
C) 10%
D) 20%
E) 30%

Answer 18.1.6 The correct answer is "A." The overall risk of stroke ranges from 4% to 20% in the 90 days after a TIA. This is a pretty wide range. To narrow down the range a bit, the ABCD^2 (Table 18-2) has been developed and takes into account age, duration of symptoms, blood pressure, and diabetes. This can be used to predict the 48-hour risk of stroke.

Rapid evaluation of the at-risk patient is warranted, as some of these patients may need anticoagulation or carotid endarterectomy for stroke prevention.

TABLE 18-2 ABCD^2 CRITERIA

Age: 1 point for age ≥60 years
Blood pressure: 1 point for systolic >140 or diastolic >90 mm Hg
Clinical features: Focal weakness (2 points) or only speech difficulty (1 point)
Duration of symptoms: >60 minutes (2 points), ≤59 minutes (1 point)
Diabetes: 1 point

ABCD^2 Score	Risk of Stroke in Next 48 Hours (%)
0–3 points	1
4–5 points	4.1
6–7 points	8.1

HELPFUL (AND UNFORTUNATE) TIP:
The initial MRI is falsely negative 13% of the time at 4.5 hours in nonposterior circulation regions (*Stroke.* 2013;44(6):1647–1651). It is even worse in the posterior circulation. The initial MRI picked up only 50% of strokes in the posterior circulation that were <1 cm in size and 92% of those >1 cm in size (*Neurology.* 2014;83(2): 169–173). What does this mean for you? If you think a patient has had a stroke but the MRI is negative, the patient may still have had a stroke.

▶ **Objectives: Did you learn to …**
- Identify signs/symptoms suggestive of acute ischemic stroke (cerebral infarction)?
- Initiate a diagnostic evaluation for a patient with a possible stroke?
- Describe the role of intravenous tPA in the treatment of acute ischemic stroke?
- Evaluate options for secondary prevention of stroke?
- Assess stroke risk after TIA?

 QUICK QUIZ: CAROTID ARTERY DISEASE: WHEN TO CUT?

Which of the following referrals for carotid endarterectomy is most likely to result in a benefit to the patient?
A) A symptomatic woman with 70% or greater stenosis to a surgeon who has a 5% complication rate
B) An asymptomatic man with 60% stenosis to a surgeon who has a 7% complication rate
C) A symptomatic woman with a 50% to 69% stenosis and a life expectancy of >5 years to a surgeon who has a 5% complication rate
D) None of the above
E) All of the above

The correct answer is "A." All sources agree that a symptomatic patient who has 70% stenosis of the carotid will benefit from surgery, provided that the surgeon's complication rate is sufficiently low. Men, but not women, seem to have a benefit with **symptomatic** stenosis of 50% to 69% if the life expectancy is >5 years **and** the surgeon's complication rate is <6% (NNT 22). In **asymptomatic** patients, those with >60% stenosis will benefit from carotid endarterectomy, but NNT is 33 and the benefit is less than those with symptomatic disease. Stenting is another option. It seems as though long-term outcomes with stenting and endarterectomy are about the same although more data is needed (*N Engl J Med.* 2016;374(11): 1021–1031). Stenting seems to be worse than endarterectomy in patients over 70, however (*Lancet.* 2016;387(10025):1305–1311), and there are more periprocedural complications in all ages.

 QUICK QUIZ: A PAIN IN THE NECK

A 35-year-old female presents for worsening right-sided posterior neck pain that radiates to her right occiput. The pain has been dull and intermittent for about a week and associated with some right posterior scalp tenderness. She became alarmed today because she felt dizzy after her workout. She describes several minutes of vertigo that resolved a few hours ago. Now, sitting in your examination room, she denies vision changes, muscle weakness, numbness, paresthesia, swallowing problems, and speech deficits. Since she's training for a "Viking's Valor Race," she has intensified her workouts in the past few weeks, lifting heavier weights. She is relatively healthy but does take lisinopril for hypertension due to fibromuscular dysplasia. Her vitals are normal. Her neurological examination is normal.

The most appropriate next step in the care of this patient is:
A) Reassurance, rest from exercise, ibuprofen
B) Referral to a neurologist
C) Initiation of aspirin 81 mg daily
D) Urgent head CT
E) Urgent MRI/MRA of the head and neck

The correct answer is "E." This patient is presenting with symptoms concerning for vertebral artery dissection. Extracranial arterial dissections of the head and neck are a relatively more common cause of stroke in young adults compared with older adults. Fortunately, many patients experience symptoms of dissection (typically head and/or neck pain, although a Horner syndrome can develop in patients with carotid artery dissection) prior to having a stroke and can be identified early if the physician is attentive and orders the appropriate test. In this case, "D" is not the right test. Head CT would be unlikely to show anything since she does not currently have neurologic signs or symptoms. Even with a CT angiogram of the brain, the extracranial neck arteries (where the problem exists) would not be visualized. Thus, the imaging must include the head and neck and must provide views of the arteries. If "E" is not available, CTA of the **head and neck** is a reasonable alternative. Classically, an angiogram was used to make the diagnosis, but it is more common now to use MRA or CTA. Of note, patients with fibromuscular dysplasia are more likely to have vertebral and carotid artery dissections, but the vast majority of patients with vertebral or carotid dissection do **not** have any known connective tissue disorder. Case series of dissections often describe a minor trauma (e.g., weight lifting, amusement park rides, various sports, "fender bender" accidents, chiropractic neck manipulation, etc.) prior to the onset of symptoms. Stroke often occurs 7 to 9 days after the dissection. Traditionally, anticoagulation has been used for carotid or vertebrobasial dissection. However, this practice has been called into question (*Lancet Neurol.* 2015;14(4):361–367).

QUICK QUIZ: DRIP AND SHIP

A 65-year-old female presents to the emergency room with sudden onset left-sided weakness that started 3 hours ago. She has a past medical history of atrial fibrillation, but her warfarin was held for the past 6 days due to a planned colonoscopy. On exam, she has moderate-to-severe dysarthria but is oriented to person, time, and place with intact language. She has a forced right gaze deviation and a left homonomous hemianopsia. She has profound weakness on the left arm and leg, and a left facial droop. She has decreased sensation on the left face, arm, and leg. Head CT shows no acute pathology, and INR is 1.1. You started IV tPA, and you do have the option to fly your patient to the university hospital with a 30-minute trip. When deciding on the need to contact the neurology/neurointervention team at the university hospital, which of the following neurological deficit is most specific for a large vessel occlusion that would potentially require emergent thrombectomy?

A) Left-sided limb weakness
B) Left facial weakness
C) Left-sided sensation loss
D) Right gaze deviation
E) Dysarthria

The correct answer is "D." While all of the findings are consistent with MCA stroke, right gaze deviation is consistent with a cortical lesion in the right frontal lobe. One of the major functions of the frontal eye field is to drive contralateral gaze; therefore, a lesion will cause gaze deviation to the ipsilateral side. When a patient presents with right MCA syndrome with gaze deviation, the patient needs to be evaluated for large vessel occlusion. Major clinical trials have shown that endovascular thrombectomy resulted in significantly better functional outcomes for patients with large vessel occlusion (proximal MCA or internal carotid artery). Initial trials indicated that thrombectomy is effective in patient within 6 hours of symptom onset. Recent trials have extended that time window to 24 hours in selected group of patients. The bottom line is that you should contact your neurology colleagues when you are concerned that your patient has a large vessel occlusion, as these patients usually do not respond well to IV tPA alone. "B," left limb and facial weakness may happen with right proximal middle cerebral artery (MCA) occlusion, but it can also happen with internal capsule stroke which is actually very common with small vessel disease. "C," left-sided sensation loss is part of the right MCA syndrome, but it can also happen with thalamic stroke which is also very common in small vessel disease. Dysarthria ("E") can occur with right proximal MCA occlusion but is not very helpful with localizing the lesion.

HELPFUL TIP (A BRIDGE TO NOWHERE):
According to the 2017 American College of Cardiology Expert Consensus, for a patient with nonvalvular atrial fibrillation and a low thrombotic risk, it is reasonable to hold anticoagulation without bridging before a procedure. For patients with moderate thrombotic risk (prior history of ischemic stroke, TIA, or systemic embolism more than 3 months ago), you should determine the bleeding risk (HAS-BLED score). If there is increased risk of bleeding, holding anticoagulation without bridging is recommended. If there is no significant bleeding risk, consider bridging. For patients with high thrombotic risk (CHA2-DS2-VADSc score 7 to 9, or if the patient had a stroke, TIA, or systemic embolism within the past 3 months), bridging should always be considered.

▶ CASE 18.2

A 24-year-old right-handed woman presents to you in the ED after her second episode of loss of consciousness. The first spell occurred 6 months ago and was associated with a 60-second loss of consciousness and jerking movements of her arms and legs. Following the spell, she was confused for about 15 minutes. At that time, her initial ED evaluation was unremarkable. She presents today following a spell that occurred about 45 minutes ago. Her friends observed her to have language difficulties with inability to communicate before falling to the ground with shaking of her arms and legs for about 2 minutes. They could not get her to respond during this time. Afterward, she was confused, and they brought her to the ED. Upon arrival in the ED, she is mildly drowsy but otherwise oriented. She has no memory of the earlier events. Her general medical and neurological examinations are unremarkable.

Question 18.2.1 Which of these tests would be LEAST helpful in determining the etiology of this spell?
A) Urine toxicology screen
B) Electrolytes
C) Neuroimaging (head CT or MRI)
D) Electrocardiogram (ECG)
E) Electroencephalogram (EEG)

Answer 18.2.1 The correct answer is "D." In this case, ECG would be the lowest yield, as this spell is most suggestive of a seizure. The major clue is the focal neurological deficit consisting of language difficulties preceding the bilateral tonic–clonic phase. This suggests a focal onset epilepsy. Syncopal episodes, which are often of primary cardiac etiology or other cause that reduces global circulation (orthostasis, for example), are generally of shorter duration without postictal confusion. It is common for syncope to be accompanied by movements that can look like seizure-like activity. This can include anything from myoclonus (brief single muscular contractions), tonic activity or tonic–clonic activity even with head turning (*Cardiol Clin.* 2015;33(3):377–385). However, this does not make it a primary seizure disorder.

All of the other tests would be useful. Evaluation of a first-time seizure should include assessment for alcohol or other drug withdrawal (especially benzodiazepines) as well as drug intoxication (cocaine, synthetic marijuana AKA "Spice" and

"K2," and methamphetamine) ("A"). Infection, including meningitis and encephalitis, can provoke a seizure. Hyponatremia, hypernatremia, hypocalcemia, hypoglycemia, hyperglycemia, hypomagnesemia, hypophosphatemia, and uremia are all associated with seizures ("B"). To rule out structural lesions (e.g., tumor and vascular malformation) and stroke, neuroimaging ("C") should be performed. Although MRI has greater sensitivity, it is often not available in a timely manner, and thus, CT is the modality of choice emergently, but this will not exclude acute ischemic stroke. EEG ("E") would be able to assess for any ongoing seizure activity or help classify the type of epilepsy to guide antiepileptic medication selection.

HELPFUL TIP:
All patients with **syncope**, including children, deserve at least one ECG in order to rule out prolonged QT interval, Brugada syndrome, etc. If the spell is not clearly a seizure and could be syncope, get an ECG. *Patients with simple syncope, no head trauma, and a normal neurologic examination do not need a CT scan (see www. choosingwisely.org).*

HELPFUL TIP:
The most common cause of status epilepticus in a patient with a known seizure disorder is noncompliance! One of the most common causes of breakthrough seizures in those with a known seizure disorder is sleep deprivation.

Evaluation in the ED, including electrolytes, CBC, brain CT scan, and urine toxicology, is unremarkable. An electroencephalogram (EEG) is obtained in the ED and read as normal. The patient is feeling well and does not wish to remain in the hospital. Her friends assure you that they will be with her over the next 24 hours.

Question 18.2.2 After reviewing her test results with her, what do you recommend for further management?
A) Continued follow-up with no further workup or treatment
B) Video/EEG monitoring
C) Initiate treatment with antiepileptic drug(s)
D) Tilt table testing
E) PET CT of the brain

Answer 18.2.2 **The correct answer is "C."** This is this patient's second presumed seizure. In adults with a first seizure, only 30% to 60% will go on to have a second seizure. In patients who have a second seizure, the likelihood of going on to have a third is 80% to 90%; therefore, after a second unprovoked seizure, treatment is recommended. Video/EEG monitoring ("B") is appropriate for classifying spells of unclear etiology. In order for video/EEG to be an effective tool, the patient should have spells frequently enough to capture them during a reasonable inpatient stay

(3 days average). Tilt table testing ("D") would not be of value, as syncope is unlikely to be the cause of these spells, and PET CT ("E") is reserved for patients undergoing workup for epilepsy surgery. This patient is a female of childbearing age; therefore, choosing a medication that is relatively safe during pregnancy and discussion of teratogenic side effects should occur prior to starting the medication.

You discuss her case with the neurologist, Dr. Lotta Branes, who agrees that she should start an antiepileptic drug (AED) since this is her second unprovoked seizure.

What is the sensitivity of a single interictal EEG for a seizure focus?
A) 20%
B) 30%
C) 50%
D) 60%
E) 90%.

The correct answer is "D." A single interictal (between seizures) EEG has only a 60% sensitivity for picking up a seizure focus. The sensitivity goes up to 90% after three interictal EEGs. However, this still means that an EEG will be negative in 10% of those with epilepsy even after three EEGs.

Question 18.2.3 Which of the following does not increase the sensitivity of EEG for epilepsy?
A) Multiple interictal EEGs on different days
B) 24-hour EEG monitoring
C) A period of sleep during the EEG
D) A large area of cerebral abnormality
E) A lesion deep in the temporal lobe

Answer 18.2.3 **The correct answer is "E."** Both prolonged EEG monitoring and a patient that falls asleep during the EEG increase the chances of finding an epileptic discharge. The size of the epileptic focus needs to be large enough and close enough to the scalp for extracranial electrodes to pick up the abnormality. Therefore, deep lesions such as mesial temporal lesions may have normal EEGs and may even have a normal EEG during a seizure if there is minimal seizure spread to adjacent regions.

She has multiple questions about AEDs … and so do you!

Question 18.2.4 Which of the following AEDs is *NOT* typically associated with weight gain?
A) Valproic acid (Depakote)
B) Lamotrigine (Lamictal)
C) Carbamazepine (Tegretol)
D) Gabapentin (Neurontin)

Answer 18.2.4 **The correct answer is "B."** Valproic acid ("A"), carbamazepine ("C"), and gabapentin ("D") are all associated with weight gain. Lamictal ("B") is typically weight neutral; Zonisamide and topiramate are associated with weight loss.

Question 18.2.5 Which of the following adverse effects is NOT typically associated with phenytoin (Dilantin)?
A) Cerebellar atrophy
B) Gingival hyperplasia
C) Stevens–Johnson syndrome
D) Hypertension
E) Bone demineralization

Answer 18.2.5 The correct answer (one that is not typically seen) is "D." Phenytoin (Dilantin) is associated with a number of idiosyncratic effects including cerebellar atrophy ("A"), hirsutism, Stevens–Johnson syndrome ("C"), and gingival hyperplasia ("B"). Diplopia and nystagmus can be prominent side effects, particularly with supratherapeutic doses. Dizziness, drowsiness, fatigue, headache, nausea, vomiting, weight loss, and urine discoloration (pink, red, or reddish-brown) are among some of the side effects seen with phenytoin. Many AEDs cause increased metabolism of vitamin D via the liver. Long-term use of AEDs may lead to osteoporosis ("E"), so vitamin D supplementation with calcium is routine. Phenytoin is associated with hypotension (NOT hypertension) and cardiac dysrhythmia (particularly with IV administration) and can cause "purple glove syndrome" if the peripheral IV infiltrates. This is due to the solution/carrier for the drug. Fosphenytoin (Cerebyx) does not have risk of "purple glove syndrome" and has much lower incidences of hypotension and arrhythmias, so is the formulation of choice when giving phenytoin IV.

Question 18.2.6 When starting antiepileptic drugs, which of the following needs to be titrated slowly to avoid a life-threatening dermatologic reaction?
A) Levetiracetam (Keppra)
B) Topiramate (Topamax)
C) Carbamazepine (Tegretol)
D) Lamotrigine (Lamictal)
E) Lacosamide (Vimpat)

Answer 18.2.6 The correct answer is "D." Although phenytoin, carbamazepine, and lamotrigine are all associated with Stevens–Johnson syndrome, lamotrigine should be titrated up slowly over several months. One of the most universally reported side effects with any antiepileptic medication is fatigue or drowsiness. Levetiracetam has been associated with mood irritability. Topiramate should be avoided in any patient with prior nephrolithiasis and has been associated with tingling of fingers/toes, weight loss, and changes the taste of carbonated beverages. Fast up-titration of topiramate can also cause confusion and speech issues. Carbamazepine at high levels will cause diplopia, nystagmus, and ataxia, which is also common with other drugs at supratherapeutic doses and is reversible when medication is adjusted. Carbamazepine can also cause hyponatremia. *Again, many AEDs cause increased metabolism of vitamin D via the liver. Long-term use of AEDs may lead to osteoporosis, so vitamin D supplementation with calcium is routine.*

Question 18.2.7 Which of the following AEDs is NOT Class D for pregnancy?
A) Valproic acid (Depakote)
B) Phenytoin (Dilantin)
C) Lamotrigine (Lamictal)
D) Phenobarbital
E) Primidone

Answer 18.2.7 The correct answer is "C." The newer AEDs including: gabapentin, lamotrigine, levetiracetam, oxcarbazepine, tiagabine, and zonisamide are currently Class C in pregnancy. Valproic acid, phenytoin, phenobarbital, primidone, and carbamazepine are all Class D drugs in pregnancy. Topiramate has been associated with birth defects and should be avoided. In particular, valproic acid has a known association with neural tube defects. As a result, it is recommended that **ALL women of childbearing age be on folate and a prenatal vitamin while on AEDs.** It is **NOT** recommended that women discontinue AEDs when pregnant, rather simplifying to monotherapy is recommended if possible. Antiepileptic drug levels need to be monitored during pregnancy as the blood level of medications like lamotrigine and levetiracetam can fall to subtherapeutic levels as pregnancy progresses. Adjusting dosing may be necessary to keep the patient close to their pre-pregnancy drug levels.

HELPFUL TIP:
In the third trimester, vitamin K 10 mg PO daily is recommended by some experts due to depression of clotting factor levels with many antiepileptics. This lowering of clotting factors has been associated with neonatal bleeding.

Question 18.2.8 Which of the following drugs does *NOT* have potential interactions with oral contraceptives?
A) Valproic acid (Depakote)
B) Carbamazepine (Tegretol)
C) Oxcarbazepine (Trileptal)
D) Phenytoin (Dilantin)
E) Topiramate (Topamax)

Answer 18.2.8 The correct answer is "A." Interactions with oral contraceptives, decreasing the efficacy of the OCP **not** the anticonvulsant, have been reported with oxcarbazepine (Trileptal), phenobarbital, phenytoin (Dilantin), lamotrigine (Lamictal), and topiramate (Topamax).

Zonisamide (zonegran), valproic acid (Depakote), tiagabine (Gabitril), levetiracetam (Keppra), gabapentin (Neurontin), and felbamate (Felbatol) do not interfere with oral contraceptives. A barrier method of contraception, in addition to oral contraceptives, is recommended in women on AEDs, particularly those with known interactions with oral contraceptives.

Question 18.2.9 **Which of the following is NOT part of routine counseling with epilepsy and the *initiation of therapy with an antiepileptic drug*?**
A) Work safety
B) Calcium and vitamin D supplementation
C) Driving
D) Alcohol consumption
E) Epilepsy surgery

Answer 18.2.9 **The correct answer is "E."** Epilepsy surgery is reserved for patients who are intractable to medical management and have failed at least two AEDs at doses used in clinical trials. Exceptions would include patients with focal pathology (e.g., malignancy or vascular malformation). "B," calcium and vitamin D supplementation, should be initiated in patients on AEDs due to increased risk of osteoporosis (*get the hint that this is important yet?*). "A" and "C," work and driving safety issues, should be discussed. Most states have specific laws regarding driving and seizures and the time before resumption of driving privileges varies greatly; check the laws in your state(s) of practice. Epileptic patients should be warned of potentially dangerous activities at work and home (e.g., working on ladders, with heavy equipment, bathing, and swimming). Patients should also be warned of potential factors that could lower their seizure threshold, including alcohol consumption ("D"), herbal ephedra supplements, sleep deprivation, infection, and medication noncompliance.

▶ **Objectives: Did you learn to …**
- Evaluate a patient with a potential new diagnosis of epilepsy?
- Identify some areas of specific concern regarding women's issues in epilepsy?
- Recognize commonly encountered or serious side effects with antiepileptic drugs?
- Counsel patients with epilepsy for daily activities and regarding medication management?

 QUICK QUIZ: SEIZURE DISORDERS

All of the following are indicated in the treatment of absence seizures (aka generalized nonconvulsive epilepsy) EXCEPT:
A) Ethosuximide (Zarontin)
B) Acetazolamide (Diamox)
C) Valproic acid (Depakene)
D) Clonazepam (Klonopin)
E) Phenytoin (Dilantin)

The correct answer is "E." Phenytoin is not indicated in the treatment of absence seizures. The other options are indicated. Other drugs known to be useful in absence seizures include lamotrigine (Lamictal), phenobarbital, and topiramate (Topamax).

 HELPFUL TIP:
Primary generalized epilepsy (epilepsy that tends to start in childhood/juveniles and is likely of genetic origin) typically responds to different medications than focal onset epilepsy (temporal lobe epilepsy, for example). Broad spectrum antiepileptics that are used for *generalized epilepsy* include: valproic acid (Depakene), topiramate (Topamax), levetiracetam (Keppra), and lamotrigine (Lamictal). Medications that are typically used for *focal onset epilepsy* include levetiracetam (Keppra), carbamazepine (Tegretol), oxcarbazepine (Trileptal), lacosamide (Vimpat), and lamotrigine (Lamictal).

▶ **CASE 18.3**

A 60-year-old left-handed man comes in with a complaint of numbness and tingling in his lower extremities for about 10 months. He notes no weakness. He has had type 2 diabetes mellitus for 6 years and has a 30 pack-year smoking history. Examination reveals decreased sensation to light touch, pin-prick, and vibratory sensation in the feet extending to 7 cm below the knees symmetrically. You also notice lack of hair on his leg to the same level. Chest, abdomen, and upper extremities have normal sensation. His reflexes are 1+ in the upper extremities and quadriceps with absent Achilles bilaterally. The remainder of his neurological and general medical examination is unremarkable. He says his diet is good but he always brings you a dozen doughnuts when he visits … with one or two missing.

Question 18.3.1 **This history is most consistent with:**
A) Stroke
B) Early mononeuritis multiplex
C) Guillain–Barré syndrome (GBS)
D) Brown–Sequard syndrome
E) Peripheral neuropathy

Answer 18.3.1 **The correct answer is "E."** This is the quintessential presentation of a patient with diabetic peripheral neuropathy. "A" is incorrect because of the distribution. Bilateral distal lower extremity sensory changes are not likely from a stroke. "B," mononeuritis multiplex, is—at least initially—not in a stocking-glove distribution. Patients with mononeuritis multiplex will notice a stepwise loss of sensation and motor ability in discrete peripheral nerve distributions. Eventually, these may become confluent and resemble a stocking-glove neuropathy. However, this is found late in the disease. Additionally, there is usually motor involvement. "C" is unlikely because GBS has a relatively rapid onset and is associated with motor findings. "D," Brown–Sequard syndrome, is the result of a lesion in one side of the spinal cord. Patients have diminished proprioception, vibration sense, and strength on the side of the lesion, and decreased sharp sensation and loss of temperature sense on the other side. Since our patient's findings are symmetrical in both distribution and manifestation, it is not Brown–Sequard syndrome. The finding of decreased reflexes also localizes to the peripheral nerve, which supports peripheral neuropathy.

Question 18.3.2 Which of the following laboratory tests would NOT be useful in helping to determine a particular cause of this patient's neuropathy?
A) Serum immunofluorescence electrophoresis
B) TSH/free T4
C) Hemoglobin A_{1C}
D) Electrolytes (Na, K, Cl, CO_2)
E) Vitamin B12

Answer 18.3.2 **The correct answer is "D."** Electrolytes are not likely to give us a diagnosis in this patient. The initial evaluation of a patient with "stocking-glove" sensory loss should focus on finding potentially modifiable causes of neuropathy. These would include hypothyroidism ("B"), diabetes ("C"), and vitamin B12 deficiency ("E"). In addition, serum immunofluorescence electrophoresis ("A") can help to identify monoclonal gammopathy, which is associated with neuropathy. Heavy metal testing may also be of use, although it is in the second round of testing.

HELPFUL TIP:
A history of alcohol use is important, as chronic alcohol abuse is commonly associated with polyneuropathy, even in the absence of vitamin B12 or other nutritional deficiencies.

Your patient is on a number of medications.

Question 18.3.3 Which of the following medications is known to cause a peripheral neuropathy?
A) Metronidazole
B) HMG-CoA reductase inhibitors
C) Amiodarone
D) Disulfiram
E) All of the above

Answer 18.3.3 **The correct answer is "E."** All of the above can cause a peripheral neuropathy. Some of the other drugs that can cause neuropathy include **fluoroquinolones**, phenytoin, isoniazid, several chemotherapeutic agents, nitrofurantoin, ddC, and D4T. See Table 18-3 for more causes of peripheral neuropathy.

Question 18.3.4 Electrophysiological testing (electromyography and nerve conduction studies or EMG/NCV) can be helpful for all of the following EXCEPT:
A) Localizing a compressive neuropathy
B) Identifying subclinical motor deficits
C) Identifying a specific etiology of the neuropathy (e.g., diabetic vs. B12 deficiency vs. syphilis)

TABLE 18-3 CAUSES OF PERIPHERAL SENSORY NEUROPATHY
Infectious
Syphilis
Lyme disease
Mycoplasma
West Nile virus
Leprosy
Nutritional
Vitamin B12 deficiency
Thiamine (vitamin B1) deficiency
Folic acid deficiency
Vitamin B6 toxicity
Celiac disease
Drugs
Metronidazole
Fluoroquinolones
Nitrofurantoin
Dapsone
Isoniazid
Phenytoin
Thalidomide
Disulfuram
Amiodarone
Vincristine/Vinblastine
Cisplatin
Hydroxychloroquine/Chloroquine
Statins
Entanercept
Infliximab
HIV therapies (didanosine, stavudine, zalcitabine)
Metabolic
Diabetes
Hypothyroidism
Toxic
Alcohol
Mercury
Thallium
Other heavy metals
Miscellaneous
Amyloid
Paraneoplastic syndromes
Mitochondrial disease
Chronic inflammatory demyelinating polyneuropathy (CIDP)
Monoclonal gammopathy

D) Determining axonal damage versus demyelination as the primary pathologic process
E) Differentiating between primarily myopathic and neuropathic processes

Answer 18.3.4 **The correct answer is "C."** EMG and NCS are *not* capable of yielding results specific to the etiology of neuropathy (e.g., identifying diabetic neuropathy vs. B_{12} vs. syphilis); however, they can yield a pattern suggestive of a particular etiology. For example, increasing motor reaction to repeated stimulation is classic Eaton–Lambert syndrome (a paraneoplastic syndrome), while a decreasing motor response with repeated stimulation is suggestive of myasthenia gravis. EMG can be helpful in confirming the presence of a radiculopathy in the proper clinical setting. They can also determine whether the process is primarily axonal (damage directly to the axons/reduction in the number of axons) versus demyelinating (damage to the myelin sheath). NCS can help localize a compressive lesion such as carpal tunnel syndrome or ulnar neuropathy at the elbow versus a brachial plexus injury or radiculopathy. EMG and NCS can be used to differentiate between myopathic and neuropathic processes.

HELPFUL TIP:
If electrophysiological testing shows an acquired primary demyelinating neuropathy, a neurologic consult is recommended. The differential diagnosis of demyelinating neuropathies is small and they may respond to immunotherapy in the right clinical setting.

After being followed in clinic for several years, the patient begins to complain of a painful, burning sensation developing in his feet and ankles. This pain developed gradually over the past few years in the areas that previously were numb. He has a friend who was started on gabapentin (Neurontin) for a similar problem and is wondering if this would be a good drug for him.

Question 18.3.5 Which of the following is NOT an adverse reaction or contraindication to gabapentin?
A) Dizziness
B) Peripheral edema
C) Fatigue and drowsiness
D) Hepatic disease
E) Paresthesias

Answer 18.3.5 The correct answer is "D." Gabapentin (Neurontin) is renally—rather than hepatically—cleared. In the setting of renal dysfunction, reduced dosing is necessary. Although gabapentin is generally well-tolerated, numerous side effects have been reported. Among the most prominent complaints are those of dizziness, vertigo, and ataxia. Fatigue and drowsiness are also relatively common adverse effects; paresthesias, myalgias, and weakness have also been reported. Peripheral edema (particularly lower extremities) and facial edema are also seen as a result of therapy with gabapentin. Titrating slowly to the target dose over several weeks can improve tolerance.

Your patient is concerned about swelling in his legs, as he has had problems with this in the past and does not want to try gabapentin at this time.

Question 18.3.6 All of the following medications would be a reasonable FIRST choice for treatment of painful neuropathy EXCEPT:
A) Amitriptyline
B) Topical lidocaine ointment
C) Oxycodone
D) Topical capsaicin cream
E) Pregabalin (Lyrica)

Answer 18.3.6 The correct answer is "C." Opiates are not the treatment of choice for peripheral neuropathy and tend not to be effective in this setting. Tricyclic antidepressants (TCAs) are commonly used in the setting of neuropathic pain, and along with gabapentin and pregabalin, they are recommended by the American Academy of Neurology. The evidence for TCAs suggests they are superior to other classes of drugs. If pain is confined to a small area, a topical treatment such as capsaicin cream or topical lidocaine may be effective. Lidoderm patches prescribed outside the setting of postherpetic neuralgia represent an off-label use.

HELPFUL TIP:
Other treatments for neuropathic pain include anticonvulsant drugs such as gabapentin, pregabalin, valproic acid, and carbamazepine. SNRIs such as duloxetine have also found to be reasonable treatments. **You want a number needed to treat? For a 50% pain reduction, the NNTs are as follows: TCAs: 3.6, strong opiates: 4.3, Duloxetine/SNRIs: 6.4, Gabapentin: 7.2–8.3, Pregabalin: 7.7** (*Lancet Neurol.* 2015;14(2):162–173). These drugs have different mechanisms of action and one type may work better for some patients than others. What does this mean for your patient? Basically, most of these drugs will not work for most patients. Don't expect success … as you well know from experience. Or maybe all your chronic neuropathy pain patients are all happy, smiley, and sunny!! Finally, gabapentin has become a drug of abuse which enhances the high of opiates and has been found as a co-intoxicant in cases of opiate overdose death. Several states list it as a controlled substance.

Question 18.3.7 What is the most common infectious cause of peripheral neuropathy in the *world* (not just in the United States)?
A) HIV
B) Lyme
C) Leprosy
D) Hepatitis C
E) Tuberculosis

Answer 18.3.7 The correct answer is "C." The most common infectious cause of peripheral neuropathy in the world is leprosy. Leprosy (Hansen disease) is caused by *Mycobacterium leprae*, an acid-fast bacillus. It usually presents with a hypopigmented anesthetic patch. The sensory deficits start with loss of temperature sensation followed by loss of pain and then tactile sensations. Modalities carried by the posterior columns (proprioception and vibration) are spared. Sensation in the palms, soles, mid-chest, and mid-back is preserved until late in the disease. "A,"

HIV, can cause peripheral neuropathy, most commonly being a symmetric, distal polyneuropathy. Autonomic dysfunction and mild weakness accompany distal paresthesias and burning sensations with sensory loss. Keep in mind that many of the medications used in HIV therapy are also associated with peripheral neuropathies. Early neurologic manifestations of Lyme disease ("B") include lymphocytic meningitis, cranial neuropathy (a Bell palsy–like picture), or painful radiculoneuritis. Guillain–Barré syndrome (GBS), and mononeuritis multiplex can be seen early in the course of Lyme disease. Advanced (late) neurologic complications of Lyme disease include peripheral neuropathy and encephalomyelitis. "D," hepatitis C (and hepatitis B) can cause peripheral nerve manifestations. Hepatitis B has been associated with GBS (demyelinating) and mononeuritis multiplex. Hepatitis C is also associated with multiple mononeuropathies. Tuberculosis has rarely been associated with neuropathy, but isoniazid is well-known to cause peripheral neuropathy (that's why we prescribe pyridoxine (B6) with it).

HELPFUL TIP:
In the United States, diabetes and alcohol use disorders are the most common causes of peripheral neuropathy.

▶ **Objectives: Did you learn to …**
- Recognize common etiologies of peripheral neuropathy?
- Identify appropriate uses of electrophysiological testing?
- Identify types of neuropathy that are potentially treatable?
- Prescribe medical therapy for painful peripheral neuropathy?

 QUICK QUIZ: WRIST DROP

Which of the following is most likely to cause an isolated wrist drop?
A) C3 disk lesion
B) Ulnar nerve compression
C) Radial nerve compression
D) C4 disk lesion
E) Median nerve compression

The correct answer is "C." Compression of the radial nerve (such as sleeping with someone's head on your arm) can cause an isolated wrist drop, the so-called "Saturday Night Palsy." Suspect alcohol or other drug abuse in patients with this lesion. It is pretty hard to get this type of compressive lesion if you are not passed out or very sedated. "B," ulnar nerve compression (cubital tunnel syndrome), presents with pain and numbness in the elbow and fourth and fifth fingers and weakness of the intraosseous muscles (weakness with spreading fingers). "E," median nerve compression (including carpal tunnel syndrome), leads to numbness on the palmar surface of the thumb and fingers two, three, and the radial half of four. There is weakness and perhaps atrophy of the thenar muscles (unable to maintain opposition of thumb to fifth finger against resistance).

▶ **CASE 18.4**

A 25-year-old woman presents to your clinic complaining of a bifrontal headache that started this morning. She describes the pain as throbbing and 8/10 in severity. She is complaining of photophobia and nausea. She has had similar headaches in the past, lasting a few hours to all day. She is unable to work during these headaches and prefers a dark, quiet room (as do we all). The physical examination, including neurological examination, is unremarkable.

Question 18.4.1 **Which of the following statements is most accurate?**
A) She likely does not have migraine headaches because her headache is bilateral
B) She likely does not have migraine headaches because they most commonly present in the fourth to fifth decade of life
C) She likely does not have migraine headaches because they rarely occur in the morning
D) She likely has migraine headaches

Answer 18.4.1 **The correct answer is "D."** She likely has migraine headaches. Migraine headaches may vary considerably in severity, time of day, and characteristics. The International Headache Society (IHS) has a useful classification system with criteria for the diagnosis of migraine headaches (Table 18-4). "B" is incorrect because migraine headaches typically present in the first three decades of life. Attacks typically last less than 1 day, although they may occasionally last longer. Migraine headaches are typically moderate to severe in intensity, may occur at any time during the day, and occur with or without aura. Most, but not all, migraine headaches are unilateral, and accompanied by nausea and vomiting. They are more prevalent among women, with a 1-year prevalence rate of approximately 18% in women, 6% in men, and 4% in children. Family history is important, as 80% of patients with migraine headache have a first-degree relative with migraines.

Migraine headaches are classified as migraine with aura and migraine without aura. Typical auras develop over several minutes and last for less than 60 minutes. Auras may involve visual, language, sensory, or motor deficits. The visual auras are by far the most common and may appear as photopsias (flashes of

TABLE 18-4 IHS CRITERIA FOR THE DIAGNOSIS OF MIGRAINE WITHOUT AURA

At least five attacks fulfilling the following criteria:

- Headache lasting 4–72 hours (untreated or unsuccessfully treated)
- Headache has at least two of the following characteristics:

  1. Unilateral location
  2. Pulsating quality
  3. Moderate or severe pain intensity
  4. Aggravation by or causing avoidance of routine physical activity
- During headache at least one of the following:

  1. Nausea and/or vomiting
  2. Photophobia and phonophobia
- No evidence of organic disease

light), scotomas (blind spots), or complex shapes that build or move across the visual field. The IHS criteria for migraine with aura are listed in Table 18-5.

> **HELPFUL TIP:**
> *Remember that the IHS criteria are research tools. Patients may have a migraine and not meet all of the criteria noted by the IHS.* While patients with a certain type of migraine headache will ideally meet all criteria, it is not necessary to meet all criteria to make a clinical diagnosis of migraine headache.

You have decided to treat this woman's migraine headache.

Question 18.4.2 Which medication would be LEAST appropriate for acute management of her headache?
A) Oral ibuprofen
B) Intranasal sumatriptan
C) IV meperidine (Demerol)
D) Intranasal DHE

Answer 18.4.2 The correct answer is "C." The least appropriate treatment from the above list would be Demerol (meperidine). The long-term use of opiates for rescue therapy has not been found to improve the quality of life in patients with migraines. Oral NSAIDs ("A"), including aspirin and combination analgesics containing caffeine, are a first-line choice for mild-to-moderate migraine attacks or severe attacks that have been NSAID responsive in the past. "B," the "migraine-specific" treatments, commonly called the "triptans" (e.g., sumatriptan, zolmitriptan, naratriptan, rizatriptan, almotriptan, eletriptan, and

---

TABLE 18-5 IHS CRITERIA FOR THE DIAGNOSIS OF MIGRAINE WITH AURA

At least two attacks fulfilling criteria A and B:

A. One or more of the following *fully reversible* aura symptoms:
   1. Visual
   2. Sensory
   3. Speech and/or language
   4. Motor
   5. Brainstem
   6. Retinal

B. At least three of the following six characteristics:
   1. At least one aura symptom spreads gradually over ≥ 5 minutes
   2. Two or more aura symptoms occur in succession
   3. Each individual aura symptom lasts 5–60 minutes
   4. At least one aura symptom is unilateral
   5. At least one aura symptom is positive
   6. The aura is accompanied, or followed within 60 minutes, by headache

History, physical, and appropriate diagnostic tests exclude a secondary cause

---

frovatriptan—wow, talk about "me too" drugs …), are effective and relatively safe for the acute treatment of migraine headaches. Triptans are an appropriate initial treatment choice in patients with moderate-to-severe migraines who have no contraindications to their use (see below). Alternative vasoconstrictive agents, including DHE nasal spray (dihydroergotamine, "D"), can provide a safe and effective treatment of acute migraine attacks. DHE can be administered IV as well. Vasoconstrictive side effects, including the risk of coronary artery spasm, should specifically be discussed with patients prior to initiation of therapy.

> **HELPFUL TIP:**
> Adding oral metoclopramide to aspirin or NSAIDs will improve their rate of success. Part of the nausea and vomiting from migraines (and the reason that oral medications often do not work) is from gastroparesis. Metoclopramide overcomes this problem and treats nausea as well. Our favorite drug to treat headaches is prochlorperazine, 10 mg IV or 25 mg PR. This works for both migraine and tension-type headaches. See Table 18-6 for a list of abortive treatments for migraine headaches.

Question 18.4.3 Which of the following statements is correct?
A) If a patient does not respond to sumatriptan, there is no point in trying another triptan because the patient will not respond
B) DHE and sumatriptan may be safely used within the same 24-hour time period
C) Sumatriptan use is contraindicated in patients with known coronary artery disease, regardless of age
D) Flushing, sweating, and paresthesias after a dose of sumatriptan is an indication of a severe reaction and continued use of this medication is contraindicated

Answer 18.4.3 The correct answer is "C." The triptans should not be used in patients with known coronary disease. Patients who do not respond to one triptan may respond to other triptans, and a trial of other triptans is appropriate. Also, a patient may respond initially to a triptan but not respond on other occasions. Each triptan has a maximum recommended dose, and a good rule of thumb is that the initial dose may be repeated once in a 24-hour period of time. However, avoid the use of DHE within 24 hours after a triptan has been given due to increased vasoconstriction and the possibility of vasospasm.

Question 18.4.4 Contraindications to the use of "triptans" include all of the following EXCEPT:
A) Lung cancer
B) Uncontrolled hypertension
C) Use of an MAO inhibitor within the last 2 weeks
D) Use of an ergot preparation within the last 24 hours

Answer 18.4.4 The correct answer is "A." Lung cancer is not a contraindication to the use of triptans. In addition to "B" to "D," caution should be used in patients with history of stroke, known cardiac risk factors, and impaired liver function.

HELPFUL TIP:
Common reactions to triptans include jaw tightness, flushing, anxiety, dizziness, and sweating. These are uncomfortable but not dangerous. Serious reactions to triptans include coronary vasospasm, anaphylaxis, or hypertensive crisis in patients with known CAD, hypersensitivity to triptans, or uncontrolled hypertension.

HELPFUL TIP:
Consider dexamethasone as an adjunct therapy in severe headache. A single dose of dexamethasone 10 mg PO, IV, or IM after abortive therapy in the ED may prevent headache recurrence in patients who have had a headache for more than 24 hours (NNT 9).

TABLE 18-6 AMERICAN HEADACHE SOCIETY GUIDELINES FOR ACUTE TREATMENT OF MIGRAINE

Level A: Established as effective (supported by at least two Class I studies)	• Acetaminophen (non-incapacitating) • Aspirin • Diclofenac • Ibuprofen • Naproxen • Sumatriptan PO/SC/IN • Almotriptan • Eletriptan • Frovatriptan • Naratriptan • Rizatriptan • Zolmitriptan • DHE (IN/Pulmonary inhaler) • Butorphanol IN
Level B: Probably effective (supported by one Class I study or two Class II studies)	• Prochlorperazine IV/IM/PR • Metoclopramide IV • Chlorpromazine IV • DHE (IV/IM/SC) • Ketorolac IV/IM • Magnesium Sulfate IV
Level C: Possibly effective (supported by one Class II study or two Class III studies)	• Valproate IV • Ergotamine • Codeine PO • Butorphanol IM • Tramadol IV • Dexamethasone IV

Headache 2015; 55:3–20 (Update since the American Academy of Neurology 2000 guideline).

Your patient has decided to take ibuprofen for her headaches. This medication seemed to be effective at first, but she notes that for the past several weeks she has been taking two to three doses of ibuprofen per day without significant headache relief. She has had a dull bilateral headache that is moderate in severity for the last 2 weeks. The medication dulls the headache but it comes right back. She has no personal or family history of coronary artery disease.

Question 18.4.5 Which of the following statements is correct?
A) She likely has a tension headache and should increase her frequency of ibuprofen and continue to take it on a daily basis
B) She likely has a medication-overuse headache in addition to chronic migraine headache (status migrainous) and should taper and then discontinue ibuprofen
C) A medication such as sumatriptan used on a daily basis does not increase the risk of rebound headache
D) She likely does not have medication-overuse headache because opiates are the only medications that increase the risk of these headaches

Answer 18.4.5 The correct answer is "B." See below for a detailed explanation.

Question 18.4.6 Which of the following medications taken on a frequent basis is LEAST likely to cause medication-overuse or rebound headache?
A) Sumatriptan
B) Morphine
C) Ibuprofen
D) Amitriptyline
E) All of the above are equally likely to cause rebound headache

Answer 18.4.6 The correct answer is "D." Frequent use of opiates, acetaminophen, NSAIDs, ergotamine, triptans, and any other analgesics may put a patient at risk for medication-overuse or rebound headache. Although analgesic rebound headache characteristics can vary significantly, the patient typically reports a pattern of headache that decreases modestly in severity with the use of their analgesic of choice, and then in 2 to 4 hours (depending on the medication), the headache returns to its previous severity or worsens further. Failure to repeat analgesic use results in a withdrawal headache (similar to the caffeine withdrawal headaches physicians often experience when they miss their morning coffee). In the case of triptans, the headache may not worsen for many hours or even until the next day, but a cycle of regular use of the medication is still established. At this time, no clear consensus on the duration of therapy necessary to produce analgesic rebound is reported. As a general rule, it is best to limit the use of analgesic medications to no more than two- to three-headache days per week. In addition, limit the patient's analgesic use to no more than 2 to 3 weeks per month. Patient education is the most important part of therapy in treating analgesic rebound or medication-overuse headaches.

HELPFUL TIP:
Treatment of rebound headaches consists of discontinuing the medication. Several approaches have been tried to reduce headaches after the analgesic has been withdrawn. These include IV or oral steroids, long-acting NSAIDs (naproxen), and elective admission, and therapy with IV DHE (dihydroergotamine) or Thorazine (chlorpromazine). These should be combined with a prophylactic medication such as amitriptyline (or other tricyclic) used on a daily basis. Patients can also take hydroxyzine and prochlorperazine when they have a breakthrough headache at home; these medications do not cause rebound headaches.

Question 18.4.7 Which of the following medications would be the LEAST appropriate for the preventative treatment of your patient's migraine headaches?
A) Verapamil
B) Propranolol
C) Amitriptyline
D) Clonazepam

Answer 18.4.7 The correct answer is "D." Clonazepam is not used as a preventive treatment for migraine headaches. Keep in mind the common side effects of these medications and the appropriateness in your specific patient. For example, valproate would be a bad choice for many patients secondary to weight gain or teratogenicity. Propranolol ("B") and verapamil ("A") may cause hypotension. Amitriptyline ("C") may cause cardiac arrhythmia in certain patients, while constipation and urinary retention are relatively common in elderly patients. Topiramate (Topamax) may actually cause weight loss, as well as kidney stones and impaired cognition.

HELPFUL TIP:
A number of medications are useful in the **prevention** of migraine headaches. The American Academy of Neurology evidence-based guideline classified these medications into different groups:
- Medications with established efficacy (with two or more class I trials) include: divalproex sodium (Depakote), propranolol/timolol/metoprolol, and topiramate (Topamax).
- Medications that are probably effective (with one class I or two class II studies) include: amitriptyline, venlafaxine (Effexor), and atenolol/nadolol.
- Medications that are possibly effective (with one class II study) include: cyproheptadine (Periactin), lisinopril, candesartan, clonidine, guanfacine, carbamazepine (Tegretol), and nebivolol/pindolol.
- Other medications such as nortriptyline, verapamil, fluoxetine (Prozac), gabapentin (Neurontin), magnesium, and vitamin B_2 have also been used in migraine prevention, but clinical studies were inadequate to establish efficacy or with conflicting data. Of note,

for some older medications, class I clinical studies are lacking mostly because they are not patentable or do not promise a financial return.
- More expensive approaches (not included in the AAN guideline) such as botulinum toxin injection and the newly approved Erenumab (Aimovig, an anti-CGRP receptor monoclonal antibody (*anti-calcitonin gene-related peptide*)) should be considered for patients with refractory migraine headaches. Erenumab (Aimovig) provides 2.5 additional headache free days/month at a cost of >$5,000/year. There are more drugs in this class on the near horizon.

HELPFUL TIP:
Combination products such as butalbital/caffeine/acetaminophen/codeine (e.g., Fiorinal with codeine) have no role in the treatment of migraine or other headaches. Addiction, abuse, and diversion and withdrawal are potential issues with these drugs.

Question 18.4.8 Which one of the following medications is rated Class B or better in pregnancy?
A) Phenergan (promethazine)
B) Imitrex (sumatriptan)
C) Codeine
D) Amitriptyline
E) None of the above

Answer 18.4.8 The correct answer is "E." Headache treatment in pregnancy remains a difficult problem. Although numerous medications are available for headache treatment, their safety in pregnancy has not been established. Amitriptyline, nortriptyline, venlafaxine, promethazine, prochlorperazine, codeine, hydrocodone, and meperidine are all Class C. The triptan class of medications, including sumatriptan, remains Class C, though pregnancy registries, retrospective, and observational studies suggest that sumatriptan is safe. Valproic acid is a class D in pregnancy. Ergotamine (DHE 45) is Class X.

Question 18.4.9 In which of the following patients is neuroimaging LEAST likely to be useful?
A) A 30-year-old woman with a headache typical of a migraine
B) A 23-year-old woman with a history of migraine headaches that is very concerned because her current headache of 1-week duration is more severe than her typical migraine headaches. She has been unable to sleep or concentrate at work because of her "headache anxiety"
C) A 60-year-old man with new headache, worse in the morning and of 6 weeks duration
D) A 40-year-old man with a headache and right-arm weakness

Answer 18.4.9 The correct answer is "A." According to the American Academy of Neurology, neuroimaging is not typically recommended in **migraine** patients with a normal neurologic examination. Imaging may be considered in patients who are disabled by their fear of serious pathology or if the provider is suspicious about underlying pathology. Factors that may lead one to consider neuroimaging include a new onset, atypical headache, or unexplained abnormal neurologic examination.

HELPFUL TIP:
Not all unilateral headaches are migraines. Think of occipital neuralgia, temporal arteritis, jolts and jabs (ice-pick) headache, temporalis muscle overuse/TMJ syndrome, chronic paroxysmal hemicrania, short-lasting unilateral neuralgiform headache attacks with conjunctival injection and tearing (SUNCT) syndrome, and cluster headaches, among others. We can't cover all of these in our limited space. We are trying our hardest, captain.

▶ **Objectives: Did you learn to ...**
- Recognize and diagnose migraine headaches?
- Initiate appropriate acute therapy for migraine headaches?
- Identify contraindications and adverse reactions of the triptan medications?
- Recognize and treat analgesic-related headaches?
- Identify appropriate preventive therapy for chronic headaches?

▶ CASE 18.5

A 30-year-old woman presents to your office with a 2-day history of progressive, unilateral arm (proximal and distal) numbness without weakness. She has been diagnosed with fibromyalgia in the past. She is taking fluoxetine for depression and has a history of previous hospitalizations for depression.

Question 18.5.1 Which of the following is the most appropriate next step?
A) Monitor her symptoms and reassure that her numbness is likely related to her fibromyalgia
B) Order nerve conduction velocity (NCV) studies
C) Order a head CT
D) Get additional history; ask about previous similar episodes or other neurological concerns
E) Order a chest radiograph (CXR) and complete blood cell count (CBC)

Answer 18.5.1 **The correct answer is "D."** Of course, the answer is "more history." With a progressive neurological deficit, the first step in the workup is to further explore the history. Frequently, patients will not mention previous neurological symptoms because they—the symptoms, not the patients—are vague (although, to be fair, some patients are vague).

....

When you ask about previous spells, she notes that she had an episode of left leg numbness that lasted about 1-week several years ago, but she thought nothing of it, as it was mild. Six

months ago, she had a 3-day visual disturbance in her right eye, during which she found it difficult to read and focus on objects; no blind spot was noticed. However, she had pain in the eye, especially when moving it.

Question 18.5.2 What is the most likely diagnosis based on the history given?
A) Multiple sclerosis (MS)
B) Fibromyalgia
C) Conversion disorder
D) Atypical migraine
E) Ischemic strokes

Answer 18.5.2 **The correct answer is "A."** MS would be the most likely diagnosis based on the history related above. MS most commonly presents in women 20 to 35 years old and in men 35 to 45 years old. It is almost five times more prevalent among women than men and is more common in the Caucasian population. MS is a CNS demyelinating disease that is thought to occur by an immune-mediated process. The demyelinating lesions of MS can occur anywhere in the CNS including the brain, brain stem, spinal cord, and optic nerves. The presenting symptoms of MS vary, but common symptoms are visual complaints, weakness, urinary retention, and sensory deficits. Although migraine ("D") can be associated with neurologic symptoms, one would expect more stereotypic events and a history of previous headaches. Fibromyalgia ("B") is associated with numerous somatic complaints, but is not typically associated with sensory deficits or visual problems. Conversion disorder ("C") can produce all of the symptoms described earlier but is a diagnosis of exclusion in the setting of a physical exam that doesn't follow anatomic localization. Ischemic strokes ("E") would present with sudden onset of symptoms that improve slowly over weeks to months. In contrast, MS lesions have a slower onset with symptoms building over a day or two and then improve over weeks to months.

HELPFUL TIP:
MS has a geographic predilection. The incidence of MS increases with increasing distance from the equator. (Alaskans are screwed.) Various theories have suggested an association with sunlight exposure, vitamin D, virus exposure, or ethnicity.

Question 18.5.3 If your patient indeed does have MS, which type is most likely?
A) Neuromyelitis Optica
B) Relapsing–remitting
C) Primary progressive
D) All of the above are equally likely

Answer 18.5.3 **The correct answer is "B."** The two common forms of MS are primary progressive and relapsing–remitting. The diagnosis of relapsing–remitting MS is based on clinical grounds and laboratory data. Clinically, symptoms of CNS dysfunction develop over hours to days, stabilize, and then improve. It is important to identify clinical events disseminated in space and time. In this case, your patient had a prior history of optic neuritis and lower extremity numbness and now has arm numbness. "A," neuromyelitis optica, is a CNS demyelinating disease that can have a similar presentation to MS but typically has long spinal cord lesions (greater than three vertebral segments) and tends to spare the subcortical white matter, which is a classic lesion location in MS. Neuromyelitis optica is treated slightly differently than MS and tends to be more aggressive, so a correct diagnosis is important.

Question 18.5.4 Which of the following tests would NOT be helpful in further diagnosing MS?
A) MRI brain with contrast
B) Lumbar puncture
C) Nerve conduction studies
D) Visual-evoked potentials
E) MRI cervical and thoracic spine with contrast

Answer 18.5.4 **The correct answer is "C."** MS is a central demyelinating process and does not produce abnormalities that would be seen on nerve conduction studies. "A" and "E," MRI of the brain, cervical and thoracic spine, would be helpful. Brain MRI is 85% to 97% sensitive in detecting MS plaques. Multiple areas of increased signal in the periventricular area are suggestive of, but not specific for, MS. Gadolinium-enhancing lesions suggest active disease. "B," lumbar puncture, can also be useful. Cerebrospinal fluid (CSF) abnormalities suggestive of MS include oligoclonal bands and increased synthesis of IgG and mild lymphocytic pleocytosis. A spinal fluid examination may be considered if the clinical diagnosis of MS is suspected but is not definite. However, the positive and negative predictive value of CSF oligoclonal bands is inadequate to do more than support the clinical diagnosis. Finally, "D," visual-evoked potentials, may be helpful if the etiology of prior vision loss is unclear. Evoked potentials may be used to aid in the diagnosis of MS by indicating prior demyelination of the optic tract (optic neuritis) if the clinical history is vague (e.g., eye pain without vision loss or no recollection of symptoms). This will aid in proving the occurrence of different events separated by space and time.

Question 18.5.5 Which of the following is not a recognized therapy for MS?
A) Corticosteroids
B) Interferon-β
C) Glatiramer acetate (Copaxone)
D) Sulfasalazine
E) Dimethyl fumarate (Tecfidera)

Answer 18.5.5 **The correct answer is "D."** Sulfasalazine is not useful in the treatment of MS. Immune-modulating therapy reduces the number of exacerbations and active lesions on MRI. These include interferon-β-1a (Avonex and Rebif) and interferon-β-1b (Betaseron), as well as glatiramer acetate (Copaxone). These medications are more efficacious if started early in the course of the disease. Common adverse effects of interferon include fatigue, depression, and myalgias.

Corticosteroids ("A") have a role in treating severe acute exacerbations (e.g., optic neuritis, severe neurological impairments limiting activities of daily living) in the form of a short burst and taper (typically methylprednisolone, 1 g/day often followed by an oral prednisone taper). Steroid use does not appear to offer long-term functional benefit, excluding the possible exception of IV pulsed steroid dosing. There have been oral and infusion immunosuppressant medications FDA approved for relapsing–remitting MS. The first FDA-approved treatment for primary progressive MS occurred in 2017, ocrelizumab (Ocrevus), an anti-CD20 monoclonal antibody.

Question 18.5.6 Which of the following treatments have NOT been associated with progressive multifocal leukoencephalopathy?
A) Natalizumab (Tysabri)
B) Ocrelizumab (Ocrevus)
C) Glatiramer acetate (Copaxone)
D) Dimethyl fumarate (Tecfidera)

Answer 18.5.6 **The correct answer is "C."** Progressive multifocal leukoencephalopathy is a serious brain infection by the JC virus that has a high mortality rate. The JC virus attacks immunocompromised hosts. (Yes, it is a polyomavirus virus and not the prion disease Creutzfeldt-Jakob. JC is not an abbreviation, it is the name of the virus). Dimethyl fumarate, ocrelizumab, and natalizumab are all immune-suppressing medications that carry a risk of PML. Ocrelizumab is new to the market but a few cases have emerged. In general, any medication that is immunosuppressive carries some risk of PML. Interferon and glatiramer are not associated with PML.

The patient is wondering what she can do to prevent exacerbations.

Question 18.5.7 Which of the following is associated with exacerbation of MS symptoms?
A) Cold temperatures (you could recommend she move to Florida)
B) Urinary tract infection
C) Influenza vaccination
D) Trauma

Answer 18.5.7 **The correct answer is "B."** Urinary tract infections can exacerbate MS. Unfortunately, urinary tract infections are particularly common in those with MS because of the frequent occurrence of neurogenic bladder and possible need for frequent intermittent self-catheterization. Systemic infection has also been reported to provoke MS exacerbations. "A" is of special note. Cold is not associated with exacerbations, **but heat is notorious**, and this phenomenon actually has a name—Uhthoff phenomenon. Patients with MS should be instructed to avoid hot tubs, saunas, steam rooms, etc. "C," vaccinations, including influenza vaccine, had been posited as a cause of exacerbations. However, a review of multiple clinical trials showed no increased risk of exacerbations in patients with MS receiving the influenza, hepatitis B, or tetanus vaccinations. **Note that we do not have experience with nasal influenza vaccine and MS. Since the nasal vaccine contains live virus, it should probably be avoided in patients with MS.** "D," trauma, has been suggested as a possible exacerbation trigger, but the American Academy of Neurology clinical practice guidelines state that the majority of class II evidence available on this issue supports no connection.

HELPFUL TIP (A WORD ON OTHER DRUGS FOR MS): Ampyra (dalfampridine) is supposed to increase walking distance. Nuedexta (dextromethorphan + quinidine) is designed to reduce pseudobulbar symptoms (emotional lability with spontaneous laughing, crying). Both are of marginal benefit.

There are many more "newer" therapies for relapsing–remitting MS (e.g., dimethyl fumarate [Tecfidera], mitoxantrone [Novantrone], natalizumab [Tysabri], teriflunomide [Aubagio], ocrelizumab [Ocrevus], and others), most of which require neurologic specialty care and carry high risk of adverse events.

▶ **Objectives: Did you learn to …**
- Identify epidemiologic characteristics of MS?
- Identify appropriate workup for patients with possible MS?
- Diagnose MS?
- Discuss potential treatment options available for long-term disease modification as well as acute exacerbations?
- Recognize factors that might result in exacerbations of MS?

▶ CASE 18.6

A 43-year-old woman with a history of myasthenia gravis presents to the ED while on vacation. She reports she is feeling tired and rundown and endorses flu-like symptoms in addition to some worsening of her proximal lower extremity weakness. On examination, she is afebrile with a respiratory rate of 18. She has mild diplopia with lateral gaze. Her strength is 4/5 proximally and 4+/5 distally bilaterally. Her sensory examination is normal. Plantar responses are down-going bilaterally.

Question 18.6.1 In determining this patient's further disposition, what is the most important test?
A) Arterial blood gas
B) CXR
C) Head CT
D) Spirometry (forced vital capacity [FVC] and negative inspiratory force [NIF])
E) CBC

Answer 18.6.1 The correct answer is "D." This patient is experiencing an exacerbation of myasthenia gravis. This could be occurring for any number of reasons including concurrent illness or possibly noncompliance with her regimen. The greatest morbidity and mortality for this patient lies in the potential for respiratory failure and arrest. In primary neuromuscular respiratory

failure (e.g., myasthenia gravis, acute inflammatory demyelinating polyradiculoneuropathy, Guillain–Barré syndrome), the arterial blood gas ("A") may remain normal despite impending respiratory collapse. The best way to evaluate respiratory status is with the FVC and NIF. If the FVC is less than 15 mL/kg or NIF less than −20 cm H_2O, elective intubation should be considered, although some centers will choose to monitor these patients closely in an intensive care setting. Once a patient with myasthenia gravis has been intubated, you should stop their pyridostigmine as it will increase respiratory secretions and GI motility leading to diarrhea. Neither of these is desirable in an intubated ICU patient (the nurses will love you for this one) and the pyridostigmine will not liberate them from the ventilator. Monitoring the FVC/NIF should be done regularly throughout the hospital course until the patient is clinically improved and stable.

You decide to give this patient a dose of edrophonium trying to reverse her symptoms. When you do this, she becomes increasingly weak, requiring intubation.

Question 18.6.2 The BEST explanation of this is:
A) Since she has missed multiple doses of her pyridostigmine, she has become desensitized and will have an overwhelming response to small doses of IV edrophonium
B) Influenza has made her particularly susceptible to edrophonium
C) The patient has taken too much pyridostigmine by accident
D) The alcohol that she has had on vacation has changed her pyridostigmine requirement

Answer 18.6.2 The correct answer is "C." Myasthenic crisis can be due to two causes. First, the patient may have not taken enough medication or may have missed doses. In this case, edrophonium will improve symptoms. The second cause is **too much** pyridostigmine. This will also cause weakness. In this case, the edrophonium will worsen the patient's symptoms. Here's how it works. Pyridostigmine and edrophonium are both cholinesterase inhibitors similar to organophosphates. They act by binding to acetylcholinesterase and preventing the breakdown of acetylcholine in the neuromuscular junction. Too much of either drug (or a combination of the drugs) will cause weakness and an organophosphate toxicity-like syndrome (salivation, lacrimation, defecation, urination, weakness, etc.).

Question 18.6.3 Which of the following IS NOT likely to contribute to the diagnosis of myasthenia gravis?
A) Tensilon (edrophonium) test
B) Nerve conduction studies
C) Anti-thymocyte antibodies
D) Anti-acetylcholine receptor antibodies

Answer 18.6.3 The correct answer is "C." Anti-thymocyte antibodies are used to treat renal rejection and have also been used in aplastic anemia, red cell aplasia, and other disorders. They have no relationship at all to myasthenia gravis … sorry. All of the others can be used in the diagnosis of myasthenia gravis. The edrophonium test ("A") is a functional test. One must be ready to intubate the patient when performing an edrophonium test, as weakness may get worse. Nerve conduction studies ("B") show a reduction in the amplitude of the response to repeated stimulation (thus, patients get weaker with repeated muscle use). Antiacetylcholine receptor antibodies ("D") are found in the majority (80–90%) of patients with myasthenia gravis. Children or adolescents presenting with myasthenia-like symptoms may be antibody negative, in that case congenital myasthenic syndromes should be considered as these are genetic diseases affecting the neuromuscular junction and will not get better with immune suppression. However, congenital myasthenic syndrome may either improve or worsen with pyridostigmine based on the genetic defect and may have other treatment options.

HELPFUL TIP:
Myasthenia gravis can be systemic or limited to the ocular muscles. It is often associated with a thymoma (or thymus hyperplasia), and patients with myasthenia gravis should have a chest CT scan to rule out thymoma or thymus hyperplasia. If present, removal of the thymoma will often "cure" the patient's disease.

Question 18.6.4 Which of the following is LEAST likely to be confused with myasthenia gravis on the basis of its neurologic symptoms?
A) Eaton–Lambert syndrome
B) Guillain–Barré syndrome (GBS)
C) Amyotrophic lateral sclerosis (ALS)
D) Botulism toxicity
E) Penicillamine-induced myasthenia gravis

Answer 18.6.4 The correct answer is "B." Remember that myasthenia gravis has no sensory findings. GBS includes sensory findings of pain, paresthesias, numbness, etc. that are generally absent in the other syndromes. "A," Eaton–Lambert syndrome, is a paraneoplastic process, which consists of weakness **that gets better with repetitive movement.** This is the exact opposite of what is seen with myasthenia gravis where repetitive tasks lead to increased weakness. Thus, Eaton–Lambert syndrome is often worse in the morning and better toward the afternoon—the reverse of what is seen with myasthenia gravis. Patients with amyotrophic lateral sclerosis ("C"), botulism ("D"), and penicillamine-induced myasthenia gravis ("E") do not have sensory symptoms. Thus, these can be confused with myasthenia gravis.

HELPFUL TIP:
ALS results in upper and lower motor neuron death. With upper motor neuron disease, reflexes remain intact and often times are brisk. Reflexes are generally lost in Guillain–Barré and other causes of lower motor neuron disease such as diabetes, Charcot–Marie–Tooth disease, polio and other causes of acute, flaccid paralysis (i.e., West Nile Virus, others).

The patient and her husband have some questions about myasthenia gravis and are wondering if there are any medications that might exacerbate this patient's weakness.

Question 18.6.5 Which of the following can worsen myasthenia gravis?
A) Fluoroquinolones
B) Verapamil
C) β-Blockers
D) Oral contraceptives
E) All of the above

Answer 18.6.5 The correct answer is "E." All of the above can worsen myasthenia gravis. Other drugs of note include: aminoglycosides, anesthetic and paralytic agents, diuretics, tetracyclines, and magnesium, among many others.

You decide to add to the treatment of this patient.

Question 18.6.6 Which of the following is considered a standard therapy for myasthenia gravis?
A) Plasmaphoresis for an acute myasthenic crisis
B) IVIG
C) Prednisone
D) Azathioprine
E) All of the above are used for myasthenia gravis

Answer 18.6.6 The correct answer is "E." Do you see a pattern here? All of the treatments are immunomodulators. The combination of high-dose prednisone with either IVIG or plasma exchange is used to treat acute myasthenia crises. The choice of IVIG or plasma exchange is based on the patient's comorbidities, tolerability, prior success, and hospital resources. Caution is advised when initiating prednisone acutely as some patients will have temporary worsening of symptoms before improving. Other options are cyclosporine and mycophenolate. The idea here is to reduce anti-endplate antibodies (although nobody is quite sure how IVIG works). Pyridostigmine is used only for mild symptomatic relief. Remember thymectomy as this may be a cure if a thymoma is present.

▸ **Objectives: Did you learn to …**
· Manage a patient with an exacerbation of myasthenia gravis?
· Understand the use of diagnostic tests in myasthenia gravis?
· Recognize diagnoses that can be confused with myasthenia gravis?

▶ **CASE 18.7**

A 29-year-old woman presents to the ED with sudden onset of a severe headache involving bilateral occipital pain associated with nausea. She has a history of migraine headaches consisting of right-sided throbbing pain that typically respond to sumatriptan but occasionally require IV ketorolac and metoclopramide. The headache has not responded to her sumatriptan (Imitrex) injection. She appears to be in moderate pain but otherwise has a normal general and neurological examination. This is the "worst headache of her life."

Question 18.7.1 What is the next step in the management of this patient?
A) Ketorolac (Toradol) and metoclopramide IV
B) Hot tea and soft pillow
C) Dihydroergotamine (DHE) IV
D) Head CT
E) Lumbar puncture

Answer 18.7.1 **The correct answer is "D."** Although this patient has a history of migraines, she is reporting a sudden onset headache that is markedly changed from her typical pattern of headache. In this setting—especially with the "worst headache of her life"—the diagnosis of subarachnoid hemorrhage (SAH) must be ruled out. None of the other answers are correct. While pain management can be given before CT (e.g., IV morphine or fentanyl), ketorolac ("A"), aspirin, and DHE ("C") are inappropriate if there is a question of SAH. Ketorolac and aspirin have antiplatelet effects, which can increase bleeding. DHE can cause vasospasm and worsen brain ischemia. Finally, if you recall, this patient tried her sumatriptan. One should not use DHE within 24 hours of a triptan. The need for a lumbar puncture is discussed below.

The patient's head CT is negative.

Question 18.7.2 What next?
A) Lumbar puncture
B) IV hydroxyzine and meperidine and discharge when she is comfortable
C) IV hydroxyzine and promethazine (Phenergan) and discharge when she is comfortable
D) Discharge home with prescription for acetaminophen and oxycodone (Percocet)
E) Discharge home with prescription for rizatriptan (Maxalt)

Answer 18.7.2 **The correct answer is "A."** In the setting of a "worst headache of life," a CT scan to rule out SAH is required. The sensitivity of CT scan of the brain for hemorrhage in the setting of SAH is 90% to 95% within 24 hours of the event (decreases to 80% at 72 hours). CT only picks up 50% of warning leaks. As a result, **a negative head CT does not adequately rule out SAH** and should be followed with a lumbar puncture. The CSF from the lumbar puncture must be spun down immediately to examine for xanthochromia. Xanthochromia is a yellow discoloration of the normally clear CSF resulting from degradation of hemoglobin. In addition to xanthochromia, markedly elevated RBC counts are indicative of SAH. If either the CT or LP is positive for SAH, MR angiogram or CT angiogram should be performed, and you should also contact your neurosurgery colleagues as some patients may need surgical intervention such as ventriculostomy.

HELPFUL TIP:
Thirty-nine percent of patients with an SAH have no neurologic signs or symptoms. Only 10% of patients with SAH have an initially focal examination. Patients with SAH may have a fever and leukocytosis. While looking at the patient's fundi is important, the *absence of papilledema does not rule out SAH.* SAH can present as back pain. Since each bleed carries a 50% mortality, this is one diagnosis you do not want to miss. Use LP liberally in appropriate patients.

HELPFUL TIP:
You may hear about a couple of studies that have shown that a CT scan done within 6 hours of headache onset is sensitive enough to rule out SAH without the need for an LP. This has definitely not yet become the standard of care.

You complete the LP, and it is normal. Apparently, this was just the worst migraine of her life. After loading her up on some good drugs, her pain subsides. Problem solved!

▶ **Objective: Did you learn to …**
· Identify a patient presenting with SAH symptoms and perform an appropriate workup?

▶ **CASE 18.8**

A 40-year-old man presents with a complaint of low-back pain that is dull in nature, which started 2 days ago. This morning he woke up with a feeling of numbness and tingling in his feet, which gradually seemed to worsen. By noon, he noted difficulty walking and decided to come to the ED. He denies bowel or bladder incontinence. On examination, he is in no acute distress and has a respiratory rate of 12. He has strength of 5/5 in his upper extremities, and in his lower extremities, strength is 4/5 proximally and 3/5 distally. Sensory examination reveals a mild decrease in pinprick and light touch in a stocking distribution to the mid-calf. Reflexes in the upper extremities are 2+ and in the lower extremities are trace at the knees and absent at the Achilles. Plantar response is down-going bilaterally.

Question 18.8.1 What is the most likely diagnosis?
A) Diabetic polyneuropathy
B) Guillain–Barré syndrome (GBS)
C) Diabetic amyotrophy
D) Stroke
E) Conversion reaction

Answer 18.8.1 **The correct answer is "B."** Of the choices given above, the most likely diagnosis is Guillain–Barré syndrome (GBS), an acute immune-mediated polyneuropathy. With an acute onset of bilateral lower extremity weakness and sensory deficits, the diagnosis of an acute cord-compressing lesion (e.g., tumor and epidural abscess) should also be considered and ruled out, especially when back pain is also present. The time course described previously is not consistent with diabetic polyneuropathy ("A") nor would one expect to see weakness as a prominent symptom. Diabetic amyotrophy ("C") is characterized by painful **proximal** muscle weakness with minor sensory loss. The onset of diabetic amyotrophy can be subacute or acute. The time course described above of gradually progressing deficits is not consistent with stroke ("D"). Additionally, the findings of a stroke should not be bilateral. Conversion reaction ("E") is a diagnosis only of exclusion.

Question 18.8.2 Which of the following is/are associated with GBS?
A) *Campylobacter jejuni* infection
B) Lyme disease
C) Epstein–Barr virus
D) CMV virus
E) All of the above

Answer 18.8.2 The correct answer is "E." All of these infectious agents are associated with GBS, especially *Campylobacter*. Other associations include viral URIs, HIV, immunizations (rare), mycoplasma, epidural anesthesia, sarcoid, lupus, etc. Add to this the Zika virus and the West Nile virus. The point here is that one should look for an underlying illness in patients with GBS.

HELPFUL (AND INTERESTING) TIP:
Antibodies to *Campylobacter* have been shown to cross-react with nerve tissue, thus the association of *Campylobacter* with GBS.

Question 18.8.3 Which of the following actions would NOT be appropriate for additional diagnosis and/or management of this patient with progressive weakness?
A) Cardiac monitoring
B) Forced vital capacity (FVC)
C) Discharge to home on steroids with a follow-up in the morning
D) EMG/NCV

Answer 18.8.3 The correct answer is "C." *This patient should not be sent home.* Did you even consider it? Discharge is a particularly bad idea because his disease has worsened rapidly over the last 12 hours. As with other potential causes of neuromuscular respiratory failure, an FVC and NIF are necessary to determine adequate respiratory reserve. The FVC and NIF should be monitored closely during the acute illness. GBS can have a rapid and catastrophic worsening that necessitates monitoring during the acute phase of illness. Typically, patients reach the peak of severity about 2 weeks into the illness. Autonomic dysfunction is associated with GBS, and close cardiovascular monitoring is important. EMG/NCV can be of value in diagnosing GBS—although early on in the course of the disease, these tests may be normal.

A diagnosis of GBS is made.

Question 18.8.4 Which of the following is NOT an appropriate treatment modality?
A) IVIG
B) Plasma exchange
C) Elective intubation if FVC is <15 mL/kg
D) Corticosteroids

Answer 18.8.4 The correct answer is "D." Corticosteroids are not used in the treatment of GBS. Multiple studies have shown no benefit to corticosteroids in this disease. Treatment options for GBS include careful monitoring of disease and supportive therapy with no intervention for mild cases but when patients develop motor deficits or respiratory failure, IVIG or plasma exchange are the two treatments that improve outcomes. If a patient requires ventilatory support or has weakness that precludes ambulation, treatment should be started immediately. Elective intubation is appropriate if the FVC is less than 15 mL/kg or the NIF is –20 cm H_2O. As discussed in regard to neuromuscular respiratory failure with myasthenia gravis, arterial blood gases are not reliable markers of impending failure, and the FVC must be closely monitored.

The family would like to know what the outcome in this patient with GBS will be, so you pull out your crystal ball.

Question 18.8.5 Well, instead of sarcasm, you actually opt for compassion and tell them that FULL RECOVERY can be expected in _____ percent of patients.
A) 15%
B) 50%
C) 80%
D) Greater than 95%

Answer 18.8.5 The correct answer is "A." Fifteen percent of all patients with GBS will have **complete** resolution of their symptoms. Sixty-five percent will be left with minor deficits, and about 10% will become disabled. Patients with GBS should survive the illness unless there are comorbidities present that make weaning ventilator support difficult, such as severe COPD or autonomic crisis leading to cardiovascular collapse.

HELPFUL TIP:
West Nile virus infection can present as either a GBS (symmetrical neurological symptoms with loss of reflexes) or a poliomyelitis-like syndrome (generally asymmetrical weakness with worse weakness proximally, loss of reflexes, fasciculations).

▶ **Objectives: Did you learn to …**
  • Recognize the clinical presentation of GBS?
  • Identify underlying illnesses that are associated with GBS?
  • Manage a patient with GBS?

▶ CASE 18.9

A 38-year-old woman is brought to the ED by her husband who expresses concerns over changes in her mental status over the past 2 days. She has become confused, forgetting the names of persons well-known to her, and forgetting what she is doing. Her conversations have become increasingly more difficult to follow, and over the past 12 hours, she has gradually become sleepier. On examination, she has a temperature of 38.5°C. She is drowsy but can be aroused. She has no meningismus. She is oriented only to person. She responds to questions slowly and incorrectly and follows only simple commands ("stick out your tongue"). The remainder of her neurological examination is essentially normal, given her limited ability to cooperate. CBC, coagulation studies, and electrolytes (including calcium, magnesium, and phosphorous) are normal.

Question 18.9.1 **What is the best next step in evaluating this patient?**
A) Lumbar puncture
B) Head CT
C) Electroencephalogram (EEG)
D) Chest x-ray (CXR)

Answer 18.9.1 **The correct answer is "B."** Although performing all of the above tests will be helpful in evaluating this patient, the most important test to do at this time is a head CT to rule out any mass lesion or hemorrhage. You could argue that "A," an LP, could be done first, and some experts would agree with that decision. However, the standard in the United States is to do the CT scan first if there is any possibility of a mass lesion. Once a mass lesion or hemorrhage has been ruled out, an infectious encephalitis or meningitis needs to be empirically treated with a goal of treatment within 30 minutes from the time of arrival in the ED. There is a possibility that nonconvulsive status epilepticus is causing these mental status changes. However, even if the EEG ("C") showed nonconvulsive status epilepticus, a head CT and lumbar puncture would remain necessary. Although pneumonia could cause confusion, a CXR ("D") is unlikely to be of high yield in this setting.

Her head CT is normal. You perform a lumbar puncture, which reveals 18 WBCs (all lymphocytes), 12 RBCs, CSF protein 67 mg/dL (elevated), and CSF glucose 70 mg/dL (normal). An EEG is normal.

Question 18.9.2 **What is the next step in managing this patient?**
A) Admit for viral encephalitis with close monitoring
B) Admit for viral encephalitis and start acyclovir *and* antibiotics
C) Admit for bacterial meningitis and start antibiotics
D) Discharge to home with close follow-up tomorrow at 8 am

Answer 18.9.2 **The correct answer is "B."** The probable diagnosis in this setting is herpes simplex encephalitis. Her CSF results are consistent with a viral process and are not consistent with bacterial meningitis (due to the normal glucose and only lymphocytes in the differential). Given the mortality of herpes simplex encephalitis (30–70%), all patients in whom the diagnosis is suspected should be started on acyclovir 10 mg/kg every 8 hours IV empirically (with appropriate dosage adjustments for renal failure), while further confirmatory testing is pending (CSF PCR for the herpes simplex virus). There can be false-negative tests so if there is high clinical suspicion for HSV encephalitis then treatment should continue. Treatment should be for a minimum of 10 days. It is important to recognize that the EEG and CT may be normal in herpes simplex encephalitis, particularly early in the disease. However, on CT, one may see evidence of temporal lobe hemorrhage and/or hypodensity in the temporal lobes. EEG can show either periodic lateralized epileptiform discharges or focal slowing in the temporal lobes. Temporal lobe changes may be even more prominently visualized on MRI, and this may be of benefit in cases in which the diagnosis remains unclear. Even with prompt, appropriate treatment, only 38% of patients returned to normal or near-normal neurologic functioning at 2 years. "B" includes antibiotics because most clinicians would cover for bacterial meningitis until the CSF cultures come back negative.

▶ **Objectives: Did you learn to …**
- Recognize the clinical presentation of and the laboratory findings in viral encephalitis?
- Initiate appropriate treatment in a patient with a presumptive diagnosis of herpes encephalitis?

▶ CASE 18.10

A 70-year-old male presents to your office as a new patient. He is with his wife, who assists in providing the history. His appetite is reduced, and he has lost 10 lb in the past 6 months. His only medication is aspirin, and he has no significant past medical history. On examination, his vital signs are normal, and he is in no acute distress. His gait is slow, and he takes eight steps to turn. He has retropulsion (takes two steps backward when you pull him from behind). There is a resting tremor in both hands but more prominently in the right. You find cogwheel rigidity in both arms as well, but again more prominently displayed on the right. His cognitive screening tests are normal.

Question 18.10.1 **The most likely diagnosis is:**
A) Essential tremor
B) Parkinson disease
C) Normal pressure hydrocephalus (NPH)
D) Progressive supranuclear palsy
E) Stroke

Answer 18.10.1 **The correct answer is "B."** This patient most likely has Parkinson disease. "A" is incorrect because essential tremor is typically worsened by activity and is not associated with the other neurologic findings seen in this patient. "C" is incorrect. The classic triad of NPH includes urinary incontinence, gait ataxia, and dementia. "D" might be a consideration, but there is no specific finding of progressive supranuclear palsy here (e.g., aggressive course, more severe axial rigidity, dysarthria, dysphagia, and downward gaze paresis). Stroke is quite unlikely to present in this insidious fashion with generalized findings.

Question 18.10.2 Which of the following is NOT a common feature of idiopathic Parkinson disease?
A) Rigidity
B) Extraocular movement paresis
C) Bradykinesia
D) Postural instability
E) Asymmetric resting tremor

Answer 18.10.2 The correct answer is "B." There are four cardinal features of Parkinson disease: tremor, bradykinesia, rigidity, and postural instability. Two or more of these features should be present to make the diagnosis. The tremor of Parkinsonism is classically a resting tremor (as opposed to the postural, intention, or action tremor) and is most common in the hands, typically with one side affected more than another. Rigidity ("A") is described as increased resistance to passive movement. Cogwheel rigidity is a ratchet-like sensation noted when testing a limb with concurrent tremor. Extraocular movement paresis ("B") is more commonly seen in progressive supranuclear palsy (PSP). Bradykinesia ("C") may be observed by monitoring the speed and amplitude of movements. Gait disturbance ("D") with reduced stride length and stooped posture is a common finding, but generally occurs later in the course of the disease. Postural stability and ability to rise from a chair are also impaired. Postural stability may be tested by retropulsion.

You are fairly certain that your patient has Parkinson disease.

Question 18.10.3 Which of the following is not common in idiopathic Parkinson disease?
A) Micrographia
B) Hypomimia
C) Hypophonia
D) REM sleep behavioral disorder
E) Alien limb phenomenon

Answer 18.10.3 The correct answer is "E." Alien limb phenomenon can be present in addition to parkinson*ism* in cortical basal syndrome, but it is not common in idiopathic Parkinson disease. Micrographia ("A"), writing in small letters, is associated with Parkinson disease. Decreased facial expression (hypomimia ("B")) with decreased rate of eye blink and diminished vocal volume (hypophonia ("C")) are also common with Parkinson disease. Other conditions that occur in patients with Parkinson disease include depression, cognitive impairment, and REM sleep behavioral disorder ("D") (e.g., kicking and screaming during REM sleep in response to vivid, disturbing dreams).

HELPFUL TIP:
There are "Parkinson plus" syndromes, so-called because they present with parkinsonian features with additional characteristics. Look for these syndromes in those that you believe may have Parkinson disease:
(1) **Progressive supranuclear palsy:** associated with supranuclear gaze palsy, dysarthria, dysphagia, postural instability, and axial rigidity.
(2) *Multiple system atrophy (formerly known as Shy–Drager syndrome):* notable for early autonomic dysfunction, including marked orthostatic hypotension.
(3) *Corticobasal syndrome:* associated with apraxia, cortical sensory dysfunction, and the **"alien limb phenomenon"** (ICD-10 code R41.4 if you are interested). Alien limb phenomenon occurs when the patient's arm moves by itself (e.g., will reach up to touch the patient's face). Sometimes the patient is not aware of what the alien limb is doing until the movement draws his or her attention. The patient may not believe that the limb belongs to them. Spontaneous limb movements also occur when the patient is startled or the limb is touched (anyone see Dr. Strangelove?).

Question 18.10.4 The diagnosis of Parkinson disease is most appropriately made:
A) With a brain MRI
B) By CSF analysis
C) Clinically
D) By a neurologist
E) At autopsy

Answer 18.10.4 The correct answer is "C." The diagnosis is based on a history and physical examination that are consistent with Parkinson disease. Additionally, a response to dopaminergic agents is *virtually diagnostic* of Parkinson disease. If the patient does not have some response to a dopaminergic agent, reconsider your diagnosis. "A" is incorrect because there are no findings on brain MRI that are specific for the diagnosis of Parkinson disease. Likewise, "B" is wrong because CSF analysis cannot provide the diagnosis. "D" is clearly wrong—do you really need a neurologist for this? The "gold standard" for diagnosis is neuropathologic examination, but you would rather not wait for the autopsy to diagnose Parkinson disease.

HELPFUL TIP:
Up to 10% of patients with Parkinson disease will have some degree of intention tremor in addition to their resting tremor. A DAT (123I-FP-CIT single-photon emission tomography) scan may be helpful in differentiating Parkinson spectrum disorders from essential tremor and drug-induced parkinsonism. It is positive for nigrostriatal dopaminergic denervation in Parkinson spectrum disorders and negative in essential tremor and drug-induced parkinsonism.

Your patient takes only aspirin, which you know does not cause parkinsonism.

Question 18.10.5 **Which of the following medications is frequently associated with a Parkinson-like syndrome in the elderly?**
A) ACE inhibitors
B) HMG-CoA reductase inhibitors
C) Calcium channel blockers
D) Metoclopramide
E) All of the above

Answer 18.10.5 **The correct answer is "D."** Metoclopramide is a frequent cause of the misdiagnosis of Parkinson disease in the elderly. Additional medications, such as SSRIs, antipsychotics, and others, can mimic Parkinson disease. Importantly, *drug-induced parkinsonism may last for up to 6 months after discontinuation of the offending agent*.

You think it is best to initiate treatment in this patient.

Question 18.10.6 **Possible treatments of Parkinson disease include all of the following EXCEPT:**
A) Levodopa
B) Deep brain stimulation
C) Pramipexole
D) Donepezil
E) Selegiline

Answer 18.10.6 **The correct answer is "D."** Donepezil is used to treat Alzheimer disease. The initial symptoms of Parkinson disease typically respond well to levodopa and the dopamine agonists. Selegiline is a monoamine oxidase B inhibitor and yields modest symptomatic benefits. Dopamine receptor agonists, such as pramipexole (Mirapex) and ropinirole (Requip), may be used in the initial treatment of Parkinson disease.

HELPFUL TIP:
Surgical options for advanced Parkinson disease include deep brain stimulation and pallidotomy. Subthalamic nucleus and globus pallidus internus are commonly used targets of deep brain stimulation in Parkinson disease treatment. Both reduce tremor and bradykinesia. Pallidotomy is rarely used these days, given the effective and reversible nature of deep brain stimulation.

Question 18.10.7 **Which of the following is *NOT* a common side effect of levodopa?**
A) Nausea
B) Paresthesias
C) Dyskinesia/dystonia
D) Hallucinations

Answer 18.10.7 **The correct answer is "B."** Paresthesias are not associated with the use of carbidopa/levodopa. Carbidopa inhibits peripheral metabolism of levodopa and therefore allows a higher proportion of levodopa to cross the blood–brain barrier for CNS

effect. Carbidopa helps to prevent levodopa-induced nausea ("A"). Dystonia and dyskinesia ("C") are common with therapy lasting more than 2 years or at peak dose responses and may necessitate lowering the doses. Psychiatric problems ("D"), including hallucinations and psychosis, can be seen with dopaminergic agonists and levodopa. Other common side effects of levodopa include hypotension, confusion, and other psychiatric disturbances.

HELPFUL TIP:
Levodopa is a dopamine precursor, and carbidopa is a peripheral dopadecarboxylase inhibitor that does not cross the blood–brain barrier. The symptoms of tremor, rigidity, and bradykinesia are initially relieved by levodopa. However, with time, larger doses and more frequent doses are required to maintain control of symptoms. Deep brain stimulation may be helpful in patients with advanced Parkinson disease to reduce doses of dopaminergic medications.

You decide to start levodopa/carbidopa (Sinemet) three times daily. At the follow-up visit, the patient is doing relatively well on this combination. However, he notices that in the mornings and prior to the next dose of medication, he tends to be stiff and has difficulty ambulating.

Question 18.10.8 **The most appropriate next step is to:**
A) Initiate a "drug holiday" to restore the patient's sensitivity to the drug
B) Add another dopaminergic agent such as ropinirole (Requip)
C) Add a catechol-O-methyl-transferase (COMT) inhibitor such as entacapone (Comtan)
D) Add an anticholinergic agent such as benztropine (Cogentin)

Answer 18.10.8 **The correct answer is "C."** The patient is experiencing the "wearing-off" phenomenon. There are several ways to address this. One option is to add a COMT inhibitor (like entacapone [Comtan]) in order to slow down the metabolism of levodopa. COMT inhibitors have no effect on their own and should only be used with levodopa. Another option is to switch the patient from immediate-release carbidopa/levodopa to a sustained-release product (e.g., Sinemet CR). Another common approach to the "wearing-off" phenomenon is altering the dosing of carbidopa/levodopa—either increasing the dose or shortening the interval between doses. Istradefylline (Nourianz), an adenosine receptor agonist, has recently been approved for wearing off phenomenon. There is also now inhaled levodopa (Inbriza) that can be used 5 times per day, though you have to question your management if your patient needs Inbriza 5 times per day.

HELPFUL TIP:
Tolcapone (Tasmar) is associated with fatal hepatic necrosis and requires monitoring of liver function tests (LFTs). Thus, entacapone (Comtan) is the preferred drug (though a benign side effect is urine discoloration). Alcapone is associated with tax evasion and "hits." This Capone should be avoided as well (get it? Al Capone??).

When you counsel your patient regarding medication use, you urge him not to stop taking his medication all at once.

Question 18.10.9 Which of the following is NOT a potential adverse effect of abrupt discontinuation of dopaminergic agonists and/or levodopa?
A) Neuroleptic malignant syndrome (NMS)
B) Severe rigidity
C) Confusional state
D) Severe dyskinesias

Answer 18.10.9 The correct answer (not a potential adverse effect) is "D." Levodopa and dopamine agonists should be tapered. Abrupt discontinuation of these medications may precipitate NMS ("A"). In addition, abrupt withdrawal is also associated with an acute confusional state ("C") separate from the mental status changes seen in NMS. Severe worsening of the patient's parkinsonism is expected, which can result in prominent rigidity ("B"). Dyskinesias are frequently seen with dopaminergic agonist/levodopa **therapy**, but are not exacerbated or triggered by **withdrawal** of these agents.

HELPFUL TIP:
Diagnostic criteria for definite NMS include hyperthermia, muscle rigidity, and five of the following: mental status changes, tremor, tachycardia, incontinence, labile blood pressure, metabolic acidosis, tachypnea/hypoxia, elevation of creatine kinase, diaphoresis/sialorrhea, and leukocytosis. Treatment includes supportive care as well as the use of benzodiazepines (lorazepam or diazepam… first line), dantrolene, bromocriptine, and amantadine, although there is limited data to support the use of any of these medications.

A year later your patient returns and seems to be doing well. You ask him about symptoms of Parkinson disease, if he is having any adverse effects of medications, and if he is experiencing any of the Parkinson-associated diseases.

Question 18.10.10 Which of the following is NOT associated with Parkinson disease?
A) Depression
B) Dementia
C) REM sleep disorder
D) Narcolepsy
E) Hallucinations

Answer 18.10.10 The correct answer is "D." Narcolepsy has not been associated with Parkinson disease. However, excess daytime sleepiness has been associated. This is likely due to a combination of factors, such as sleep disturbance, depression, dopaminergic drugs, and Parkinson disease itself. Depression is commonly seen in Parkinson disease and is reported to occur in up to 41% of patients. Dementia, typically with Lewy bodies

present on pathological analysis, is seen and can affect the decision to proceed with surgical treatment of Parkinson disease, as patients with advanced dementia get less benefit from surgery. Also, REM sleep behavior disorders are seen in Parkinson disease and can be a source of stress for families and caretakers. REM sleep behavior disorder is characterized by acting out of dreams that can consist of vocalizations as well as active and even violent movements. Typically, REM sleep behavior disorder responds to melatonin and clonazepam. Finally, hallucinations can be caused by Parkinson disease as well as by levodopa and dopamine agonists. Decreased visual contrast sensitivity and other visual changes as well can occur with Parkinson disease.

HELPFUL TIP:
The dopamine agonists (pramipexole, ropinirole, etc.) have been associated with compulsive behavior (sexual compulsion, compulsive gambling, etc.). This may explain why our elderly patients like to go to Las Vegas and Atlantic City … .

▸ **Objectives: Did you learn to …**
· Identify common features of Parkinson disease?
· Diagnose Parkinson disease?
· Manage a patient with Parkinson disease?
· Understand pharmacotherapy available for Parkinson disease and some of the potential adverse effects of drug therapy?

▶ **CASE 18.11**

A 45-year-old left-handed woman who is a busy executive for a Fortune 500 company presents with excessive daytime sleepiness. She is otherwise healthy and takes no medications.

Question 18.11.1 How do you approach this problem?
A) Reassure her that it is normal for people to be drowsy under stressful work conditions
B) Begin zolpidem at night for sleep
C) Schedule the patient for polysomnography
D) Discuss the patient's sleep hygiene
E) Administer modafinil (Provigil) prior to important board meetings

Answer 18.11.1 The correct answer is "D." It is essential that all patients with complaints of either insomnia or excessive daytime sleepiness have a thorough sleep history taken. Polysomnography may be necessary, but this test—like all diagnostic tests—should be driven by a hypothesis. A history is necessary to develop a hypothesis and determine a test's utility. Starting hypnotic agents ("B") or stimulants ("E")—or both—without thoroughly investigating the underlying problem may cover up a significant, treatable problem and is considered bad form.

Question 18.11.2 Which of the following is NOT an important aspect of a sleep history?
A) Sleeping and waking times
B) Use of stimulants and alcohol
C) Sleep interruptions (children, cell phones, pagers, etc.)
D) Snoring
E) Listening to "soft rock" ("easy listening" or "adult contemporary") and traumatic brain injury.

Answer 18.11.2 The correct answer is "E." Okay, maybe this one was too easy, but we hate "easy listening" music. The Geneva Convention prohibits its use on prisoners of war … we've been told. All ranting aside, this tidbit of her history has no bearing on her sleep. Important parts of the sleep history include the sleeping environment (alone, with spouse or other individual, in the daylight hours, etc.), nap history, family history of sleep problems, and symptoms of specific sleep disorders (snoring, hypnagogic hallucinations, etc.). A medication history is important as well as a history of watching TV in bed, eating in bed, playing with a cell phone in bed, working on a computer prior to bed (such as many of us commonly do) etc., which indicate poor sleep hygiene. Traumatic brain injury is not associated with sleep disorders.

Question 18.11.3 Which of the following is NOT part of a typical sleep study?
A) Monitoring of EEG
B) Monitoring respirations and oxygen desaturations
C) Evaluating the sleep latency in response to sleep aids, such as zolpidem and trazodone, to maximize effective pharmacologic therapy
D) Monitoring EMG
E) Video monitoring of sleep

Answer 18.11.3 The correct answer is "C." Sleep studies are generally done in the naive state without the use of medications. All of the rest are true. "D" and "E" deserve more attention. "D," monitoring EMG, allows informing the physician about muscle activity during sleep (e.g., restless limbs). "E," video monitoring and taping, allows the physician to look for problems, such as awakening, evidence of restless leg syndrome, and sleep apnea. Of note, in home sleep studies are becoming more commonly employed for evaluation of sleep disorders.

Question 18.11.4 In considering a diagnosis of narcolepsy, which of the following is NOT part of the diagnosis?
A) Cataplexy
B) Sleep paralysis
C) Hypnagogic hallucinations
D) Sleep myoclonus
E) Excessive daytime sleepiness

Answer 18.11.4 The correct answer is "D." Sleep myoclonus (hypnagogic jerks) is commonly seen in normal people as they begin to fall asleep (witness colleagues at grand rounds with sudden tossing of the head) and is not a part of narcolepsy. Narcolepsy is a disorder characterized by four cardinal traits, although not all need be present to make the diagnosis: cataplexy, excessive daytime sleepiness, sleep paralysis, and hypnagogic hallucinations. "A," cataplexy, is a sudden loss of voluntary muscle control during which the patient may appear to be asleep; however, cataplexy does not have to be accompanied by sleep attacks, and the patient may be aware throughout the attack. "B," sleep paralysis, can occur either at the onset of sleep or upon awakening and can be quite frightening to the patient. "C," hypnagogic hallucinations, are vivid and typically fearful dreams that occur at the onset of sleep but can also occur upon awakening (hypnopompic hallucinations). "E," excessive daytime sleepiness, is a hallmark of narcolepsy and can include sleep attacks as well as persistent drowsiness and "micro sleep" (brief intrusions of sleep during a waking state). The complete tetrad of symptoms is seen in only 10% of patients with narcolepsy.

Question 18.11.5 Which of the following is NOT a treatment for narcolepsy?
A) Amitriptyline (Elavil)
B) Clonazepam (Klonopin)
C) Fluoxetine (Prozac)
D) Modafinil (Provigil)
E) Atomoxetine (Strattera)

Answer 18.11.5 The correct answer is "B." Clonazepam is not a treatment for narcolepsy. The treatment of narcolepsy has two primary goals. The first goal is to address daytime sleepiness, which is primarily done with stimulants such as modafinil or methylphenidate. The second goal is to reduce the symptoms of cataplexy. This can be accomplished with agents such as tricyclic antidepressants, and to a lesser extent, SSRIs. Sodium oxybate (Xyrem) (sodium salt of gamma hydroxybutyrate acid, the "date rape drug") can be used for treatment of cataplexy as well as excessive daytime sleepiness, although a risk evaluation and mitigation strategy should be exercised due to its abuse potential (including date rape); it should not be prescribed to those with a history of drug abuse, etc. Atomoxetine (Strattera) is a norepinephrine reuptake inhibitor, and has no addiction liability or recreational effects.

After a thorough history, you find nothing to suggest narcolepsy besides daytime sleepiness. Of course, you are considering other diagnoses simultaneously—unless you are experiencing a sleep attack yourself (easy to do when studying for the boards).

Question 18.11.6 Which of the following would NOT suggest a possible diagnosis of obstructive sleep apnea?
A) Difficulty falling asleep
B) Frequent nighttime arousals
C) Obesity
D) Paroxysmal nocturnal dyspnea
E) Snoring

Answer 18.11.6 The correct answer is "A." Difficulty falling asleep is not one of the components of obstructive sleep apnea. Snoring, obesity, excessive daytime sleepiness, and paroxysmal nocturnal dyspnea are all associated with obstructive sleep apnea. Some patients will note frequent arousals from sleep with or without accompanied shortness of breath.

HELPFUL TIP:
It is important to note that not all patients with sleep apnea are overweight, and this diagnosis must be considered in all patients with excessive daytime sleepiness or other suggestive symptoms. Small oropharyngeal airway (especially in **thin** women) and gastroesophageal reflux are associated with sleep apnea.

Question 18.11.7 What treatment options would NOT be appropriate to consider in your patient if she has obstructive sleep apnea?
A) Bilevel positive airway pressure (BiPAP)
B) Continuous positive airway pressure (CPAP)
C) Positional therapy
D) Uvulopalatopharyngoplasty (UPPP)
E) Zolpidem

Answer 18.11.7 The correct answer is "E." Sleep aids, including benzodiazepines, do not have a role in the treatment of obstructive sleep apnea and *may actually worsen symptoms*. CPAP and BiPAP are both potential treatments. Polysomnography (sleep testing) with titration of CPAP or BiPAP should determine which modality to use and the pressure settings. These should not be arbitrarily set to the "normal settings" for a patient. Of note, auto-pap (APAP) therapies are becoming more popular and have been shown to have similar treatment effects and to improve patient adherence (*Syst Rev.* 2012;1:20). Positional therapy ("C"), avoiding sleeping on one's back, may be effective in some patients. Some techniques for achieving this goal include sewing an object on the back of the pajama shirt that will irritate the patient when they roll onto it (i.e., tennis balls in a sock). Weight loss, although not mentioned above, can provide improvement in symptoms as well. Surgical therapies including UPPP ("D") can also be considered based on the patient's symptoms and preferences. Guidelines suggest that not everyone needs a polysomnogram. Measuring the number of oxygen desaturations (home sleep apnea testing… HSAT) can be appropriate in patients without coexisting illness (COPD, CHF, cor pulmonale, etc.). HSAT is less sensitive than a formal polysomnogram. See *J Clin Sleep Med.* 2017;13(10):1205–1207 for more details.

HELPFUL TIP:
Just as Cookie Monster has learned that cookies are a "sometimes food," hypnotic medications should generally be considered a "sometimes medicine." Patients develop tolerance to all commonly used hypnotics with the possible exception of melatonin. Additionally, some hypnotics cause amnesia and others (like the orexin inhibitor class [e.g., suvorexant (Belsomra)]) cause prolonged daytime somnolence the next day. Suvorexant can also cause extremity weakness and some people carry out complex behaviors (such as driving) while unaware. Hypnotics only add about 15 to 30 minutes to a patient's total sleep time. For many patients, the risk–benefit ratio does not favor hypnotics. Start with sleep hygiene and CBT-I (Cognitive behavioral therapy for insomnia).

Further history leads you to suspect that she has restless legs syndrome, and you confirm the diagnosis with a sleep study.

Question 18.11.8 Which would be a *first-line* agent for treatment of restless legs syndrome?
A) Clonazepam
B) Codeine
C) Methadone
D) Pramipexole
E) Tramadol

Answer 18.11.8 The correct answer is "D." Restless legs syndrome is characterized by an urge to move the lower extremities due most often to an uncomfortable sensation. This sensation usually occurs during rest and is typically relieved by moving the legs. Dopamine agonists, such as ropinirole (Requip) and pramipexole (Mirapex), are the first-line treatments for restless legs syndrome. Gabapentin, gabapentin enacarbil (Horizant, a prodrug to gabapentin), and pregabalin can also be considered for RLS treatment. Levodopa (e.g., Sinemet) may be effective but the evidence is weak. A variety of other medications are used for restless leg syndrome but do not carry an FDA indication for it. Benzodiazepines ("A") and narcotic medications ("B" and "C") as well as tramadol have all been used as alternative therapies, though their effectiveness is unknown.

Question 18.11.9 What other workup would you suggest for this patient once the diagnosis of restless legs syndrome is made?
A) No further workup is indicated, initiate treatment as above
B) Serum calcium
C) Serum iron studies, including ferritin
D) Serum vitamin B12
E) Serum vitamin B6

Answer 18.11.9 The correct answer is "C." Studies have shown a link between low iron stores and restless legs syndrome. All patients with restless legs syndrome should have an iron profile performed, and low iron or ferritin levels merit iron supplementation (and workup for underlying cause, of course). Other associations are diabetes, pregnancy, end-stage renal disease, Parkinson disease, venous insufficiency, folate deficiency, and caffeine intake (dump that fourth cup of coffee …)

▶ **Objectives: Did you learn to …**
- Take an appropriate sleep history?
- Generate a differential diagnosis for daytime sleepiness?
- Gain familiarity with the diagnostic testing used in a sleep laboratory?
- Identify the presentations of and treatments for common sleep disorders, including narcolepsy, obstructive sleep apnea, and restless legs syndrome?

HELPFUL TIP:
One of the favorite parasomnias of the editors is "exploding head syndrome" (this is actually real, not a joke). Patients have the feeling of popping or explosions occurring in their head as they fall asleep.

▶ CASE 18.12

A 60-year-old right-handed gentleman presents with the complaint of head pain.

Question 18.12.1 Which of the following historical descriptions is of the LEAST VALUE in identifying a specific diagnostic classification for head/face pain?
A) Right-sided, electric, stabbing pain involving primarily the cheek, occurring for seconds to minutes repeatedly throughout the day
B) Right-sided, electric, stabbing pain involving primarily the throat, tongue, and right ear
C) Right-sided severe headache involving the orbit and associated with lacrimation and rhinorrhea typically occurring at the same time each day for a given period of time
D) "Sinus pressure" with a history of sinus headaches responsive to antibiotics in the past
E) Pattern of severe right-sided "stabbing and boring" headaches around the age of 30 that went away with scheduled indomethacin

Answer 18.12.1 The correct answer is "D." Sinus headaches are typically a diagnosis of exclusion. Acute sinusitis can cause severe head-and-face discomfort, but **sinusitis remains a relatively uncommon (and way overdiagnosed) etiology for recurrent head-and-face pain.** The specific headache syndromes described in "A," "B," "C," and "E" are described in more detail in the following questions.

Question 18.12.2 Let's say this patient gives you the history of right-sided severe headache involving the orbit associated with lacrimation and rhinorrhea typically occurring at the same time each day for a couple of weeks. Which of the following would you use for initial acute treatment of this headache syndrome?
A) Naproxen
B) Oxygen
C) Tylenol
D) Verapamil

Answer 18.12.2 The correct answer is "B." The type of headache syndrome described is most consistent with cluster headaches. These are most commonly seen in men and are characterized by exquisite pain, typically centered at the orbit. Conjunctival injection, rhinorrhea, and lacrimation frequently accompany the headache. Pain is often disabling. As the name suggests, the patient tends to have headaches in groups (or clusters). These headaches are more common at night, and REM sleep is thought to be a triggering factor. For acute treatment, conventional headache medications such as DHE and the triptans can be effective. Treatment with high-flow oxygen has also shown significant efficacy as an abortive treatment: typical protocol would be 8 L oxygen on nonrebreather for 15 minutes, with reports of 70% of patients achieving headache relief. Verapamil can be effective for prophylaxis but is not effective as an abortive. Other, more typical migraine prophylactic agents (propranolol, topiramate, indomethacin, valproic acid) have been tried, but no systematic studies have been done to evaluate their efficacy in cluster headaches.

Question 18.12.3 Let's say your patient describes a history of severe right-sided "stabbing and boring" headaches around the age of 30 that went away with scheduled indomethacin. This description would be most consistent with which of the following headache syndromes?
A) Tension headache
B) Paroxysmal hemicrania
C) Migraine without aura
D) Chronic daily headache
E) Analgesic rebound headache

Answer 18.12.3 The correct answer is "B." Paroxysmal hemicrania is classically described as a unilateral headache with a stabbing/boring character. Although age of onset can vary greatly, it classically occurs in women in their thirties (although it can be seen in men as well). Patients will have between 2 and 40 episodes during a given day, although they do not occur at the same time as is typical with cluster headaches. Although autonomic symptoms (rhinorrhea, lacrimation, conjunctival injection, and ptosis) can be seen in a majority of patients, these headaches can be differentiated from clusters by the pattern of recurrence (sporadic throughout the day versus a predictable time of day for a certain period of time); significant overlap between the two headache syndromes does exist and differentiation can be difficult. Paroxysmal hemicrania is typically exquisitely sensitive to indomethacin, and response to indomethacin is highly correlated with this diagnosis. Migraine headaches ("C") typically do not occur multiple times in one day and are usually described as a throbbing pain. Chronic daily headaches ("D") as well as analgesic rebound headaches ("E") are generally continuous in nature with limited, if any, periods of time without some degree of headache. Chronic daily headache in the setting of prolonged analgesic use is highly suggestive of analgesic rebound headache. The duration of analgesic therapy necessary to trigger and propagate these headaches remains uncertain. However, it can be as little as three times per week.

With further history, your patient describes right-sided, electric, stabbing pain involving primarily the cheek and occurring for seconds to minutes repeatedly throughout the day.

Question 18.12.4 What would be the first-line choice for therapy of this entity?
A) Carbamazepine
B) Amitriptyline
C) Ibuprofen
D) Morphine
E) Microvascular decompression (Jannetta procedure)

Answer 18.12.4 The correct answer is "A." This description is typical of trigeminal neuralgia. Carbamazepine has been shown to be effective in treating trigeminal neuralgia and was used for treatment of this disorder prior to being used for seizures. Tricyclic antidepressants, opioids, and nonsteroidal anti-inflammatory agents are not first-line agents for treatment. Typically, NSAIDs are of limited, if any, benefit in this setting. Other agents that have been used for treatment include gabapentin, pregabalin, oxcarbazepine, clonazepam, baclofen, phenytoin, lamotrigine, and topiramate. Microvascular decompression (the Jannetta procedure) can be effective in alleviating pain from trigeminal neuralgia. However, medical therapy remains the first-line treatment.

HELPFUL TIP:
A unilateral electric, stabbing pain occurring in the tongue, oropharynx, and occasionally extending to the ipsilateral ear has been described; this is known as **glossopharyngeal neuralgia**. Treatment of glossopharyngeal neuralgia is similar to the pharmacologic treatment of trigeminal neuralgia described above. If the patient complains of stabbing eye or temporal headaches lasting seconds, consider the diagnosis of primary stabbing "jolts and jabs" headaches (aka "ice pick" headache). They can occur 40 to 50 times a day or more and are likely a migraine variant.

▶ **Objectives: Did you learn to ...**
- Describe the features of various headache syndromes?
- Initiate treatment for cluster headaches, paroxysmal hemicrania, and trigeminal neuralgia?

▶ **CASE 18.13**

A 55-year-old male with a history of diabetes and *prostate carcinoma* presents to your office complaining of back pain, groin numbness, and an inability to initiate voiding. This has been worsening over the past 1 week.

Question 18.13.1 The most likely explanation for these symptoms is:
A) Cauda equina syndrome
B) Urinary outlet obstruction secondary to prostate carcinoma
C) Hydroureter and hydronephrosis secondary to urolithiasis
D) Neurogenic bladder from long-standing diabetes
E) All of the above are equally likely

Answer 18.13.1 The correct answer is "A." This is a presentation of cauda equina syndrome. Cauda equina syndrome is caused by compression of the cauda equina at the level of L4 or L5 by a protruding disk, tumor, etc. Symptoms include progressive fecal or urinary incontinence (secondary to inability to initiate voiding and loss of anal sphincter tone), impotence, distal motor weakness, and sensory loss in a saddle distribution. This patient's symptoms are not likely to be due to urinary outlet obstruction ("B"). Urinary outlet obstruction should not

be associated with sensory changes in a saddle distribution. The same is true of "C." "D," neurogenic bladder from diabetes, could be a possibility. However, this should not include back pain or perineal numbness.

Question 18.13.2 On examination of this patient, you would expect to find:
A) Increased rectal tone
B) Decreased rectal tone
C) Normal rectal tone
D) No rectum

Answer 18.13.2 The correct answer is "B." Patients with cauda equina syndrome should have decreased rectal tone. If you chose "D" ... well, there are a lot of things we could say but won't.

Question 18.13.3 The initial treatment of this patient with cauda equina syndrome should include which of the following?
A) Pain management with narcotics
B) Dexamethasone administered IV
C) Placement of a Foley catheter
D) Urgent neurosurgical consultation
E) All of the above

Answer 18.13.3 The correct answer is "E." Pain management ("A") is critical in any patient. Dexamethasone ("B") may reduce tumor-related edema leading to a reduction in cord compression—although high-dose steroids are no more effective than usual doses. A Foley catheter ("C") is indicated to treat the patient's urinary retention. Since this is a neurosurgical emergency, urgent neurosurgical ("D") or orthopedic consultation should be obtained. Local radiation may also be used acutely depending on your surgeon, oncologist, etc.

HELPFUL TIP:
The diagnosis of cauda equina syndrome is often delayed for months since many patients initially have incomplete syndromes, including only pain and mild neurologic symptoms. This is unfortunate since outcome depends on the degree of neurologic dysfunction at the time of diagnosis.

▶ **Objectives: Did you learn to ...**
- Recognize the clinical presentation of cauda equina syndrome?
- Identify causes of cauda equina syndrome?
- Initiate treatment of a patient with cauda equina syndrome?

 QUICK QUIZ: SEIZURE DISORDERS

Absence seizures are characterized by all of the following EXCEPT:
A) Loss of consciousness
B) Feeling of déjà vu

C) Rhythmic lip smacking or eye blinking
D) Staring spells
E) Occurrence up to hundreds of times per day

The correct answer is "B." Feelings of déjà vu and other "psychic" phenomenon such as hallucinations are associated with temporal lobe (aka simple partial) seizures.

▶ CASE 18.14

A 2-year-old female presents to the ED after having a seizure. The parents note that the patient was fine this morning, spiked a temperature to 39.9°C, and then had a 5-minute bilateral tonic–clonic seizure that resolved spontaneously. This is her second such episode in 18 months. On arrival, the patient is febrile, lethargic, and looks postictal.

Question 18.14.1 **Your next step is to:**
A) Reassure the parents that this is a simple febrile seizure
B) Obtain blood cultures and start ceftriaxone
C) Perform an LP if the CBC shows leukocytosis and elevated bands
D) Administer acetaminophen and wait for 2 hours to see if the patient returns to baseline before deciding on further treatment
E) Arrange for an outpatient EEG

Answer 18.14.1 **The correct answer is "B."** This patient **must** be assumed to have meningitis until proven otherwise. Treatment should be started immediately. "A" is incorrect. This is not a simple febrile seizure by history. The child is postictal and looks ill. While it may end up being a simple febrile seizure, you cannot make that conclusion at this point. If the child did not look lethargic and was up and running around, no further evaluation or treatment would be needed at this time. "C" is incorrect. First, the CBC may be relatively normal even with meningitis. Second, you do not want to delay antibiotics until the CBC and LP are done. "D" is incorrect for the same reason. **The standard of care in meningitis is antibiotics within 30 minutes of hitting the door.** Waiting to see the patient's response to acetaminophen for 2 hours will clearly put you out of this time window.

You do the right thing and treat the patient with ceftriaxone. The patient does look better in an hour or so, has returned to baseline and lumbar puncture was negative for infection. She is alert, attentive, and playing with toys. The parents are concerned about whether or not this patient has a seizure disorder. They would like a further evaluation.

Question 18.14.2 **Which of the following is indicated at this point for *a general patient* with a first-time seizure (*and not for this patient since she had a febrile seizure*)?**
A) EEG done on the same day
B) Admission to the hospital and EEG the next day

C) Serum electrolytes and glucose
D) Trial of antiepileptic drug
E) None of the above

Answer 18.14.2 **The correct answer is "C."** The workup of a seizure includes serum electrolytes, calcium, magnesium phosphate, glucose, etc. Note that these need not be done for someone with a known seizure disorder who has his or her typical seizure and returns to baseline. In these cases, only a drug level of their antiepileptic drug need be done unless there is some change in the seizure type, mental status, etc. "A" and "B" are incorrect. The EEG will be positive because of the recent seizure and may not reflect the underlying condition. Thus, waiting a couple of weeks after the seizure will give a better picture of what the brain's innate electrical activity looks like. Of course, an EEG or other workup is not necessary for a febrile seizure. "D" is incorrect because we have not yet proven this child has a seizure disorder. Prescribing antiepileptic drugs would be premature.

HELPFUL TIP:
A "stat" EEG can be helpful if you are not sure if a patient is having an active seizure versus a nonepileptic spell (formerly called a "pseudoseizure" now called a "psychogenic nonepileptic seizure," PNES). However, even a "stat" EEG will take several hours to be hooked up and read by a neurologist. A delay in therapy for hours would be unacceptable for a patient in status epilepticus and would lead to permanent brain damage or death. A "stat" EEG may also be helpful in a patient with mental status changes who you believe may be having nonconvulsive status epilepticus. Again, if there is clinical suspicion then waiting for the EEG should not delay therapy.

The parents are wondering what to do about treating this patient to prevent further febrile seizures.

Question 18.14.3 **Your recommendation to prevent further seizures is:**
A) Acetaminophen at the onset of fever
B) Ibuprofen at the onset of fever
C) Phenytoin until the child reaches the age of 5
D) Buccal midazolam at the onset of any fever
E) None of the above

Answer 18.14.3 **The correct answer is "E."** None of these choices are optimal in the management of this patient. "A" and "B" seem like a good idea but do nothing to reduce the occurrence of febrile seizures. Neither "C" nor "D" is effective. One study suggests that rectal diazepam at the onset of a fever will reduce the occurrence of febrile seizures. However, it is associated with some morbidity (e.g., sleepiness) and should be reserved for those with frequent febrile seizures.

HELPFUL TIP:
Daily phenobarbital **can** prevent febrile seizures but is associated with behavior and learning problems and is generally not recommended. Daily valproate may be effective as well. Neither of these is recommended because of side effects.

The parents have another child at home who has had one febrile seizure. He is now 12 months old. The parents want to know what his likelihood of having a seizure disorder is.

Question 18.14.4 You can let them know that he has *approximately*:
A) 1% to 5% chance of developing a seizure disorder
B) 10% to 15% chance of developing a seizure disorder
C) 40% to 50% chance of developing a seizure disorder
D) 80% to 90% chance of developing a seizure disorder

Answer 18.14.4 The correct answer is "A." Patients who have a single febrile seizure have approximately 1% to 5% chance of developing a seizure disorder. This is essentially the same risk as the general population.

HELPFUL TIP:
About 50% of patients who have their first febrile seizure under age 15 months will have a recurrent febrile seizure. This drops to 30% if the first seizure is after 15 months of age. Family history is also involved; 45% of those who have a first-degree relative with febrile seizures will have a second seizure.

▶ Objective: Did you learn to …
- Diagnose and manage febrile seizures in children?

▶ CASE 18.15

A 64-year-old man presents to the emergency department (ED) with confusion and hallucinations for the past 2 weeks. He has a history of end-stage liver disease due to NASH (non-alcoholic steatohepatitis) cirrhosis. He often sees rats running around and sometimes even feels the rats crawling on his body. He tries to get them off. General exam is significant for diffuse jaundice, asterixis, and prominent ascites. He is afebrile and does not have nuchal rigidity. O2 saturation, heart rate, and blood pressure are normal. He is oriented to time, place, and person, although he is easily distractible and he is unable to spell "world" backward. Neurological exam is unremarkable otherwise. You start initial workup, and he has elevated plasma ammonia at 82 (elevated). He also has elevated bilirubin, AST, ALT, INR (1.8), and decreased albumin, all stable compared to 2 months ago. CBC and BMP are within normal limits. Urine analysis and paracentesis are not suggestive of infection. Cultures of urine, ascites, and blood pending.

Question 18.15.1 In addition to treating hyperammonemia, the *best* next step is?
A) Lumbar puncture
B) Electroencephalography (EEG)
C) Check thiamine level
D) Brain CT
E) Brain MRI

Answer 18.15.1 The correct answer is "D." Hyperammonemia may cause brain edema which can be life threatening and require neurosurgery consultation and intracranial pressure monitoring. Brain CT is also very sensitive for acute intracranial hemorrhage which may also cause mental status changes. Patients with chronic liver disease can develop subdural hematomas with minor trauma due to decreased level of coagulation factors. Brain MRI is a better test when there is clinical suspicion of acute ischemic stroke or intracranial malignancy. However, patients with delirium frequently have trouble tolerating the MRI procedure while sedation can potentially worsen delirium. Lumbar puncture is indicated if there is concern of CNS infection. For patients with elevated INR, empiric antibiotic coverage can be started for suspected CNS infection if LP cannot be completed safely. In this case, patient's delirium is most consistent with hepatic encephalopathy. However, if a clear etiology of delirium is not identified, brain MRI, EEG, and lumbar puncture should be considered. The patient does not have a history of alcoholism, but poor nutrition status can also cause thiamine deficiency. It usually takes days for the thiamine level to come back; therefore, if there is any suspicion of thiamine deficiency, go ahead and give the thiamine.

HELPFUL TIP: HOURS TO DAYS
Delirium has five key features as defined in the American Psychiatric Association's *Diagnostic and Statistical Manual*, 5th edition (DSM-V):
1. Disturbance in attention
2. The disturbance develops over a short period of time (usually hours to days), represents a change from baseline, and tends to fluctuate during the course of the day
3. An additional disturbance in cognition
4. The disturbances are not better explained by another preexisting, evolving, or established neurocognitive disorder
5. There is evidence that the disturbance is caused by a medical condition, substance intoxication or withdrawal, or medication side effect

The bottom line is, if patient develops an acute or subacute change in cognition, you need to identity the underlying etiology, as the disease process is frequently reversible.

Brain CT is normal. The patient is admitted and his plasma ammonia level improves but remains elevated the next day. However, he continues to experience hallucinations. He is on the waiting list for a liver transplant. He is evaluated by the liver transplant team. During the interview, the liver team learns that patient might have been having occasional hallucinations for the prior 6 months, although he never had any psychiatric issues before. It is also noted that patient has a long history of "acting out" dreams. He fell off the bed during sleep a couple times in the past 6 months. Patient scores 12/30 on a MOCA test (a test for cognitive impairment; it takes 10-15 minutes to administer, has a better sensitivity than does the Mini Mental Status and it is available for free at www.mocatest.org).

Liver team raises the concern of dementia with Lewy bodies.

Question 18.15.2 All of the following are core clinical features of *early* dementia with Lewy bodies EXCEPT:
A) Fluctuating cognition with pronounced variations in attention and alertness
B) Recurrent visual hallucinations that are typically well formed and detailed
C) Cardinal features of parkinsonism: bradykinesia, resting tremor or rigidity
D) REM sleep behavior disorder
E) Profound memory loss

Answer 18.15.2 The correct answer is "E." Profound memory loss is a hallmark feature of Alzheimer's dementia. Patients with dementia with Lewy bodies usually have preserved memory *early on*. Dementia with Lewy bodies is the second leading cause of dementia but largely underdiagnosed clinically. The new diagnostic criteria from American Academy of Neurology in 2017 added REM sleep behavior disorder (RBD) as a core clinical feature, because studies have shown that up to 90% of patients with RBD will eventually develop synucleinopathies (including Parkinson disease, dementia with Lewy bodies, and multiple system atrophy [previously Shy–Drager]). RBD is a parasomnia and occurs when there is loss of atonia and patients "act out" their dreams including thrashing, kicking, and punching. Multiple system atrophy includes loss/attenuation of autonomic function, parkinsonism, cerebellar ataxia, pyramidal signs (increased lower extremity muscle tone, hyper-reflexia, positive Babinski, loss of fine motor skills), and urogenital dysfunctioning (though not all need be present... autonomic dysfunction is generally present, though). Fluctuating cognition, visual hallucination, and parkinsonism are all core clinical features of dementia with Lewy bodies. Neuroleptic sensitivity is no longer considered a core clinical feature of dementia with Lewy bodies.

HELPFUL TIP: SLEEP AND PSYCH
Dementia is a disorder that is characterized by a decline in cognition involving one or more cognitive domains (learning and memory, language, executive function, complex attention, perceptual-motor, social cognition). The deficits must represent a decline from previous

level of function and be severe enough to interfere with daily function and independence (DSM-5). Dementia patients are more vulnerable to delirium. Therefore, it is not uncommon to see patients with delirium superimposed on underlying dementia. Cognitive evaluations from a quick MOCA to a full neuropsychological test battery are important, but the results are unreliable during acute delirium. Another major part of dementia evaluation is to rule out reversible conditions like B12 deficiency, liver disease, syphilis (in high-risk patients only ... syphilis is making a comeback), or hypothyroidism. Don't forget obstructive sleep apnea and depression as both can mimic dementia and worsen cognitive symptoms in dementia.

Given that dementia with Lewy bodies is a neurodegenerative disorder with no effective disease-modifying therapy, the liver transplant team is wondering whether they should keep your patient on the liver transplant list. You contact the neurology team for further evaluation.

Question 18.15.3 All of the following tests are helpful with further evaluation for Lewy body dementia EXCEPT:
A) Brain MRI
B) DaTscan
C) Polysomnography
D) Electromyography (EMG)

Answer 18.15.3 The correct answer is "D." An EMG is not particularly helpful in the evaluation of dementia. Brain MRI ("A") is important in the evaluation of dementia as it can show a pattern of atrophy that could guide your diagnosis. DaTscanning ("B") is useful when evaluating nigrostriatal dopaminergic denervation such as is seen in Parkinson's disease (see earlier section on Parkinson's disease). A sleep study ("C") should be done (evaluating RBD). The diagnostic criteria for dementia with Lewy Bodies were updated in 2017. Please see Table 18-7 for current diagnostic criteria.

A behavioral neurology specialist evaluates your patient. More history from family members indicates a steady decline of his performance in activities of daily living over the past year. Neurology suggests that the patient's presentation is most consistent with hepatic encephalopathy. Neurology also indicates that underlying dementia with Lewy bodies is a possibility, but the diagnosis cannot be made given patient's ongoing delirium.

▶ **Objectives:** Did you learn to …
- Identify signs/symptoms suggestive of delirium?
- Initiate a diagnostic evaluation for etiology of delirium?
- Tell the difference between delirium and dementia?
- Initiate a dementia evaluation?
- Diagnose dementia with Lewy bodies?

TABLE 18-7 2017 DIAGNOSTIC CRITERIA FOR DEMENTIA WITH LEWY BODIES

Essential for a diagnosis of DLB is dementia, defined as a progressive cognitive decline of sufficient magnitude to interfere with normal social or occupational functions, or with usual daily activities. Prominent or persistent memory impairment may not necessarily occur in the early stages but is usually evident with progression. Deficits on tests of attention, executive function, and visuoperceptual ability may be especially prominent and occur early.

Core clinical features *(The first three typically occur early and may persist throughout the course)*

Fluctuating cognition with pronounced variations in attention and alertness.
Recurrent visual hallucinations that are typically well formed and detailed.
REM sleep behavior disorder, *which may precede cognitive decline.*
One or more spontaneous cardinal features of parkinsonism: these are bradykinesia (defined as slowness or movement and decrement in amplitude or speed), rest tremor, or rigidity.

Supportive clinical features

Severe sensitivity to antipsychotic agents; postural instability; repeated falls; syncope or other transient episodes of unresponsiveness; severe autonomic dysfunction, e.g., constipation, orthostatic hypotension, urinary incontinence; hypersomnia; hyposmia; hallucinations in other modalities; systematized delusions; apathy, anxiety, and depression.

Indicative biomarkers

Reduced dopamine transporter uptake in basal ganglia demonstrated by SPECT or PET.
Abnormal (low uptake) [123]iodine-MIBG myocardial scintigraphy.
Polysomnographic confirmation of REM sleep without atonia.

Supportive biomarkers

Relative preservation of medical temporal lobe structures on CT/MRI scan.
Generalized low uptake on SPECT/PET perfusion/metabolism scan with reduced occipital activity ± the cingulate island sign on FDG-PET imaging.
Prominent posterior slow-wave activity on EEG with periodic fluctuations in the pre-alpha/theta range.

Probable DLB can be diagnosed if:

a. Two or more core clinical features of DLB are present, with or without the presence of indicative biomarkers or
b. Only one core clinical feature is present, but with one or more indicative biomarkers.

Probable DLB should not be diagnosed on the basis of biomarkers alone.

Possible DLB can be diagnosed if:

a. Only one core clinical feature of DLB is present, with no indicative biomarker evidence, or
b. One or more indicative biomarkers is present but there are no core clinical features.

(continued)

TABLE 18-7 2017 DIAGNOSTIC CRITERIA FOR DEMENTIA WITH LEWY BODIES (Continued)

DLB is less likely:

a. In the presence of any other physical illness or brain disorder including cerebrovascular disease, sufficient to account in part or in total for the clinical picture, although these do not exclude a DLB diagnosis and may serve to indicate mixed or multiple pathologies contributing to the clinical presentation, or
b. If parkinsonian features are the only core clinical feature and appear for the first time at a stage of severe dementia.

DLB should be diagnosed when dementia occurs before or concurrently with parkinsonism. The term Parkinson disease dementia (PDD) should be used to describe dementia that occurs in the context of well-established Parkinson disease. In a practice setting the term that is most appropriate to the clinical situation should be used and generic terms such as Lewy body disease are often helpful. In research studies in which distinction needs to be made between DLB and PDD, the existing 1-year rule between the onset of dementia and parkinsonism continues to be recommended.

Source: Used with permission from McKeith IG, et al. *Neurology.* 2017;89(1):88–100.

Clinical Pearls

○ Be sure to follow the inclusion and exclusion criteria for administering tPA for acute stroke. If in doubt, call your nearest stroke-accredited hospital for recommendations.

○ For acute ischemic stroke, if you have any concern of a large vessel occlusion (such as, right gaze deviation with right MCA syndrome), call the closest neurological intervention team for recommendations on potential endovascular thrombectomy. Thrombectomy can be done after tPA is given. Drip and Ship!

○ Do not aggressively treat elevated blood pressures in an acute ischemic stroke as it decreases cerebral perfusion and puts ischemic brain at risk for further injury.

○ Do not perform neuroimaging in an individual with a history consistent with typical migraine headaches or simple syncope with a normal neurological examination and no evidence of head trauma.

○ Do not screen asymptomatic patients for carotid artery disease.

○ Enquire about sleep apnea signs and symptoms in all adults presenting with daytime somnolence and order a polysomnogram or nighttime oxygen desaturation test for evaluation if there is suspicion for sleep apnea.

○ Perform a lumbar puncture to rule out subarachnoid hemorrhage even in the context of a negative head CT as a head CT only detects about 50% of warning leaks.

○ Routine narcotics are not recommended for treatment of neuropathic pain or migraine headaches.

○ Routinely recommend good sleep hygiene as first-line therapy for insomnia and fatigue.

○ Start antibiotics early if you have a high suspicion for bacterial meningitis. This includes before the lumbar puncture if suspicion is high enough.

○ Use of triptans in patients with coronary artery disease is contraindicated due to increased risk of coronary vasospasm.

BIBLIOGRAPHY

American Academy of Neurology. The role of laboratory and genetic testing in diagnosing distal symmetric polyneuropathy. 2018. Available at: https://www.aan.com/Guidelines/home/GetGuidelineContent/322. Accessed July 23, 2018.

American Academy of Neurology. The treatment of painful diabetic neuropathy. 2018. Available at: https://www.aan.com/Guidelines/home/GetGuidelineContent/480. Accessed July 23, 2018.

Brott TG, et al. Long-term results of stenting versus endarterectomy for carotid-artery stenosis. *N Engl J Med.* 2016;374(11):1021–1031.

CADISS Trial Investigators, et al. Antiplatelet treatment compared with anticoagulation treatment for cervical artery dissection (CADISS): a randomised trial. *Lancet Neurol.* 2015;14(4):361–367.

Chronicle E, Mulleners W. Anticonvulsant drugs for migraine prophylaxis. *Cochrane Database Syst Rev.* 2004;3:CD003226.

Confavreux C, et al. Vaccinations and the risk of relapse in multiple sclerosis. *N Engl J Med.* 2001;344:319–326.

Doherty JU et al. 2017 ACC Expert Consensus Decision Pathway for periprocedural management of anticoagulation in patients with nonvalvular atrial fibrillation: a report of the American College of Cardiology Clinical Expert Consensus Document Task Force. *J Am Coll Cardiol.* 2017;69:871–898.

Emeriau S, et al. Can diffusion-weighted imaging-fluid-attenuated inversion recovery mismatch (positive diffusion-weighted imaging/negative fluid-attenuated inversion recovery) at 3 tesla identify patients with stroke at <4.5 hours? Stroke. 2013;44(6):1647–1651.

Fenstermacher N, et al. Pharmacological prevention of migraine. *BMJ.* 2011;342:d583.

Finnerup NB, et al. Pharmacotherapy for neuropathic pain in adults: a systematic review and meta-analysis. *Lancet Neurol.* 2015;14(2):162–173.

Goodin DS, et al. Disease modifying therapies in multiple sclerosis: report of the Therapeutics and Technology Assessment Subcommittee of the American Academy of Neurology and the MS Council for Clinical Practice Guidelines. *Neurology.* 2002;58:169–178.

Gronseth GS, Ashman EJ. Practice parameter: the usefulness of evoked potentials in identifying clinically silent lesions in patient with suspected multiple sclerosis (an evidence-based review). Report of the quality standards subcommittee of the American Academy of Neurology. *Neurology.* 2000;54:1720–1725.

Hassan-Smith G, Douglas MR. Management and prognosis of multiple sclerosis. *Br J Hosp Med (Lond).* 2011;72(11):M174–M176.

Howard G, et al. Association between age and risk of stroke or death from carotid endarterectomy and carotid stenting: a meta-analysis of pooled patient data from four randomised trials. *Lancet.* 2016;387(10025):1305–1311.

Hughes RA, et al. Pharmacological treatment other than corticosteroids, intravenous immunoglobulin and plasma exchange for Guillain–Barré syndrome. *Cochrane Database Syst Rev.* 2011;16(3):CD008630.

Ip S, et al. Auto-titrating versus fixed continuous positive airway pressure for the treatment of obstructive sleep apnea: a systematic review with meta-analyses. *Syst Rev.* 2012;1:20.

Jankovic J, Stacy M. Medical management of levodopa-associated motor complications in patients with Parkinson's disease. *CNS Drugs.* 2007;21(8):677–692.

Jausch EC, et al. Guidelines for the early management of patients with acute ischemic stroke: a guideline for healthcare professionals from the American Heart Association and American Stroke Association. *Stroke.* 2013;44:870.

Johnston SC, et al. National Stroke Association guidelines for the management of transient ischemic attacks. *Ann Neurol.* 2006;60(3):301–313.

Johnston SC, et al. Clopidogrel and aspirin in acute ischemic stroke and high-risk TIA. *N Engl J Med.* 2018;379:215–225.

Khatri P, et al. Effect of alteplase vs aspirin on functional outcome for patients with acute ischemic stroke and minor nondisabling neurologic deficits: the PRISMS randomized clinical trial. *JAMA.* 2018;320(2):156–166.

Kuijpers T, et al. Patent foramen ovale closure, antiplatelet therapy or anticoagulation therapy alone for management of cryptogenic stroke? A clinical practice guideline. *BMJ.* 2018;362:k2515.

Marmura MJ, et al. The acute treatment of migraine in adults: the American Headache Society evidence assessment of migraine pharmacotherapies. *Headache.* 2015; 55(1):3–20.

Martelletti P, Steiner TJ. *Handbook of Headache: Practical Management.* London, UK: Springer; 2011.

McKeith IG, et al. Diagnosis and management of dementia with Lewy bodies. *Neurology.* 2017;89(1):88–100.

Pahwa R. Understanding Parkinson's disease: an update on current diagnostic and treatment strategies. *J Am Med Dir Assoc.* 2006;7(Suppl 2):4–10.

Powers WJ, et al. 2018 guidelines for the early management of patients with acute ischemic stroke: a guideline for healthcare professionals from the American Heart Association/ American Stroke Association. *Stroke.* 2018;49(3):e46–e110.

Prasad K, et al. Dual antiplatelet therapy with aspirin and clopidogrel for acute high risk transient ischaemic attack and minor ischaemic stroke: a clinical practice guideline. *BMJ.* 2018;363:k5130.

Pringsheim T, et al. Prophylaxis of migraine headache. *CMAJ.* 2010;182:E269–E276.

Rosen IM, et al. Clinical use of a home sleep apnea test: an American Academy of Sleep Medicine position statement. *J Clin Sleep Med.* 2017;13(10):1205–1207.

Saber Tehrani AS, et al. Small strokes causing severe vertigo: frequency of false-negative MRIs and nonlacunar mechanisms. *Neurology.* 2014;83(2):169–173.

Sheldon R. How to differentiate syncope from seizure. *Cardiol Clin.* 2015;33(3):377–385.

Silberstein SD, et al. Evidence-based guideline update: pharmacologic treatment for episodic migraine prevention in adults: report of the Quality Standards Subcommittee of the American Academy of Neurology and the American Headache Society. *Neurology.* 2012; 78(17):1337–45.

Theken KN, Grosser T. Weight-adjusted aspirin for cardiovascular prevention. *Lancet.* 2018 Jul 12;392(10145):361–362.

Wang Y, et al. Clopidogrel with aspirin in acute minor stroke or transient ischemic attack. *N Engl J Med.* 2013;369:11–19.

Ophthalmology

19

Austin R. Fox

▶ **GLOSSARY OF TERMS**

Accommodation: Change in the shape of the lens to compensate for changes in focal length. The term may also be used to refer to the compensation of the eye to adjust to focusing on objects at different distances.

Amblyopia: Decreased monocular (or more rarely binocular) vision cortical in nature and not attributable to a structural abnormality of the eye or visual pathway. This may be a result of strabismus, high uncorrected refractive error, or visual deprivation during the critical period of cortical visual development during childhood.

Esotropia: Deviation of an eye/the eyes inward when compared with normal alignment.

Exotropia: Deviation of an eye/the eyes outward when compared with normal alignment.

Relative afferent pupillary defect (RAPD): A RAPD is detected when there is a relative difference in the initial pupillary response to a light stimulus between the two eyes. The "swinging flashlight test" done in a darkened room may be used to test for a RAPD; the initial pupillary response should be equal in both eyes. An eye with a RAPD will (abnormally) dilate with direct light to the eye but constrict normally in response to light shined in the fellow eye. **A patient may have poor vision but not a RAPD.** One will NOT get a RAPD from a refractive error, corneal disease, cataract, hyphema, or *isolated* vitreous hemorrhage. However, there will often be optic nerve or retinal pathology coexisting with a vitreous hemorrhage. So if there is an RAPD + vitreous hemorrhage, the nerve and retina need to be evaluated (generally by ophthalmology… though they should be seeing most all patients with a vitreous hemorrhage anyway). Go to http://www.webcitation.org/74lKatwTk for a really cool interactive animation.

Strabismus: A general term that refers to a misalignment of the eyes. Esotropia, exotropia, and hypertropia (one eye deviated upward) are all examples of strabismus. The term strabismus says nothing about etiology, which can be congenital, neurologic, or muscular.

Want more? See https://webeye.ophth.uiowa.edu/eyeforum/index.htm. It has great pictures, tutorials and quizzes.

▶ **CASE 19.1**

A mother presents with her healthy, 2-month-old male infant. She reports that for the past week his eyes have been noticeably crossed. He appears to fixate with either the right or left eye. She feels that aside from being cross-eyed, he seems to see well. On examination, his eyes are very crossed, but he has full motility. When either eye is covered, he fixes and follows with the fellow eye and appears to have normal motility.

Question 19.1.1 **The most likely diagnosis in this patient is:**
A) Pseudoesotropia
B) Congenital esotropia
C) Accommodative esotropia
D) Sixth nerve palsy

Answer 19.1.1 **The correct answer is "B."** Esotropia is more common than exotropia. Congenital esotropia is generally found in children younger than 6 months. "C," accommodative esotropia, which occurs when the patient tries to "accommodate" (both eyes move inward for convergence to look at something close at hand) is the most common cause of esotropia in childhood and develops between age 6 months and 7 years. In accommodative esotropia the eyes do not converge equally when accommodating, giving an esotropia. It is rare for accommodative esotropia to develop before 4 months or after 8 years of age. Pseudoesotropia is common in infants due to their flat nasal bridges and medial epicanthal folds, giving an appearance of esotropia. A simple way to assess children for a true strabismus is to shine a penlight in their eyes and evaluate the corneal reflection of your light (Hirschberg test). The light reflex will be in the same location on the eye bilaterally for pseudoesotropia,

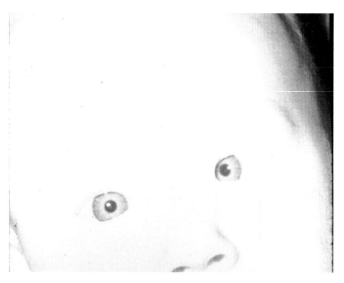

FIGURE 19-1 Congenital esotropia. Note the large deviation with abnormal corneal light reflexes. The corneal light reflex of the left eye appears more temporal than that of the right eye. Therefore, the left eye is deviated inward.

but reflect on different parts of the cornea or sclera with true esotropia or other forms of strabismus (see Fig. 19-1).

 HELPFUL TIP:
It is important to differentiate an esotropia due to sixth nerve palsy. A sixth nerve palsy affects the lateral rectus muscle, and the patient will have limited abduction (moving away from nose) on the affected side. This is usually the first cranial nerve affected in patients with increased intracranial pressure. In adults, the most common etiology is vasculopathic, and in children, the most common etiology is trauma. Other causes may include increased intracranial pressure, viral illness, brain tumor, inflammation, or infection.

Question 19.1.2 Which of the following statements is FALSE?
A) Congenital esotropia is nearly always present at birth
B) Alternating fixation (e.g., the ability to fix on an object with either eye) is characteristic of congenital esotropia
C) Patients with congenital esotropia generally have normal amounts of hyperopia (farsightedness) for their age
D) Patients with a high degree of uncorrected hyperopia (farsightedness) can develop an accommodative esotropia

Answer 19.1.2 **The correct answer (and the false statement) is "A."** Congenital esotropia presents by the age of 6 months but is rarely present at birth. If true esotropia is observed at birth, it may be due to another neurologic disorder, and further evaluation is indicated. Any form of strabismus may result in vision loss, and for this reason, it is important to treat strabismus early in life. The rest of the answers are true. As for option "B," since patients have two eyes with equal vision, neither is preferred, so they will use both eyes to focus on objects (although not at the same time, of course!). Option "C" is true; patients with congenital esotropia do

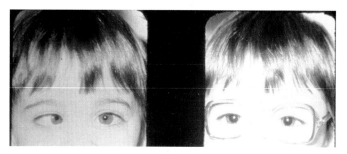

FIGURE 19-2 Accommodative esotropia improves when vision is corrected. Adaptation for near vision consists of accommodation (change in lens shape), miosis (constriction of the pupil), and convergence. This can eventually lead to an accommodative esotropia, which can easily be corrected with glasses. With glasses, the patient no longer uses the near response of accommodation and convergence so that the eyes resume normal alignment.

have a normal degree of hyperopia for their age. "D" is also a true statement regarding accommodative esotropia (see Fig. 19-2).

Question 19.1.3 Which of the following is NOT an appropriate treatment for strabismus?
A) Surgical correction if correction of refractive errors with full hyperopic spectacle does not resolve the strabismus
B) Patching the strabismic (misaligned) eye
C) Atropine drops or patching the non-strabismic eye *without* surgery
D) Atropine drops or patching the non-strabismic eye *plus* surgery

Answer 19.1.3 **The correct answer is "B."** The goal of the treatment of strabismus is to prevent amblyopia. Amblyopia is commonly caused by strabismus (ocular misalignment), significant uncorrected refractive error, or disorders that distort images from the eye to the brain (i.e., congenital cataracts). In amblyopia, the brain "turns off" or suppresses the vision in the affected eye. In addition to surgical treatment (realignment, removal of cataract, etc.), *amblyopia therapy and prevention is accomplished by blurring or impeding the vision in the unaffected (good) eye to strengthen the affected (bad) eye.* This can be done by physically patching the good eye (not the strabismic eye as noted in "B") or by pharmacologic "patching" of the good eye using atropine drops if compliance with a patch is an issue (although eye patches remind kids of pirates, and pirates are cool— aargh, mate!). NOTE: Terms such as "bad eye" and "good eye" are frequently confusing, so strabismic or deviated eye often replaces "bad eye" as no eye is truly bad, but rather a product of its environment, and "good eye" is usually reserved as a popular greeting in Australia (just say it like Russell Crowe would!).

Question 19.1.4 In which of the following situations would neuroimaging be necessary?
A) A 6-month-old with longstanding esotropia and equal visual acuity bilaterally
B) A 5-year-old with recent onset esotropia *correctable by glasses*
C) A 12-year-old with normal refraction and acute onset esotropia with diplopia
D) A newborn with a unilateral congenital cataract and an esotropia

Answer 19.1.4 The correct answer is "C." ANY unexplained new onset strabismus mandates an evaluation. A 12-year-old with acute esotropia, diplopia, and no evidence of hyperopia requires neuroimaging to rule out any underlying neurological disorder. The age of the patient is older than that seen with congenital, acquired, or accommodative esotropia. The refraction is normal, so this does not fit with accommodative esotropia. Diplopia also suggests acute onset. Further workup is therefore necessary. "A" is incorrect because this is a classic history for congenital esotropia. "B" is incorrect because it is consistent with accommodative esotropia. Fixing uncorrected refractive error would be the appropriate first step here. Note that farsightedness (hyperopia) is a much more common cause of accommodative esotropia than is nearsightedness (myopia). "D" is incorrect because we have reason for the esotropia—a congenital cataract is causing poor binocular fusion and coordination.

HELPFUL TIP:
Acute acquired strabismus **always** requires a rapid and complete evaluation. It can be due to trauma, vasculopathic factors, tumor, intracranial hemorrhage, botulism, lead poisoning, etc. Any child (or adult, for that matter) with new onset strabismus requires a full ophthalmologic examination.

▶ **Objectives: Did you learn to …**
· Describe the nomenclature of strabismus?
· Determine the underlying causes of esotropia?
· Recognize some unusual cases of strabismus that require further workup?
· Describe the risk and treatment of amblyopia?

▶ CASE 19.2

A 50-year-old Asian female presents to the emergency department (ED) with severe nausea, vomiting, right eye pain, and blurry vision. She reports the symptoms began only a few hours earlier. She has no significant past medical history. On gross examination, her visual acuity is OD 20/200, her right eye is injected, and her right pupil is larger than her left. There does NOT appear to be a relative afferent pupillary defect (RAPD).

Question 19.2.1 With regard to this patient's presentation, which of the following would NOT be considered in the differential diagnosis?
A) Trauma secondary to blunt injury from a softball
B) Central retinal artery occlusion
C) Contact lens–associated bacterial keratitis
D) Acute-angle closure glaucoma
E) Anterior uveitis

Answer 19.2.1 The correct answer is "B." Among these choices, central retinal artery occlusion would be painless and also associated with a RAPD (from diffuse retinal ischemia). All of the

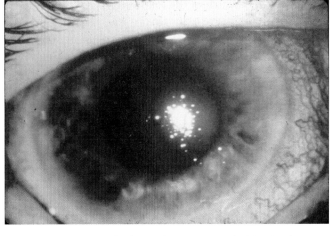

FIGURE 19-3 Acute-angle closure glaucoma. Note the injection, hazy cornea, and mid-dilated pupil.

others will present with pain or irritation and **WITHOUT a RAPD.** "A," blunt injuries, may result in decreased vision secondary to corneal abrasions or edema, intraocular inflammation, hyphema, or retinal injuries. Injury can also cause injection and a traumatic mydriasis (dilation of the pupil). Direct and consensual pupillary reflexes would be normal (no RAPD) unless there was an associated traumatic optic neuropathy or significant retinal damage. "D," acute-angle closure glaucoma, would cause diffuse injection with a hazy cornea and mid-dilated pupil and no RAPD. "E," anterior uveitis, would also cause injection and no RAPD. There is often asymmetry of the pupils in chronic anterior uveitis secondary to central posterior synechiae (adhesions between the iris and lens).

Question 19.2.2 Which of the following is *helpful* in order to diagnose acute-angle closure glaucoma?
A) Slit lamp
B) Tonometer
C) Fluorescein and appropriate UV light
D) Snellen eye chart
E) A and B

Answer 19.2.2 The correct answer is "E." An important examination technique used to diagnose acute glaucoma is intraocular pressure measurement, which could be achieved by Tonopen, Goldmann applanation tonometry at the slit lamp, assessed via digital palpation (a gross measure at best. If the eye is rock-hard, there is a problem), etc. A slit lamp is useful for diagnosing acute-angle closure, and one may see a closed angle, corneal edema, conjunctival injection, and a mid-dilated pupil (see Fig. 19-3). "C," fluorescein, is used to diagnose corneal injuries (de-epithelized cornea will take up fluorescein). "D," a Snellen eye chart, is used to determine visual acuity but is not necessary for diagnosing glaucoma. It is always a good idea to check vision in each eye in every patient with eye complaints; think of checking visual acuity as taking a "vital sign" ("vital signs" of the eye include visual acuity, intraocular pressure, pupil examination).

Question 19.2.3 Which of the following is NOT a risk factor for acute-angle closure glaucoma?
A) Hyperopia (farsightedness)
B) Asian descent
C) Male gender
D) Pharmacologic dilation
E) Advanced cataract

Answer 19.2.3 The correct answer is "C." Associated risk factors for acute-angle closure glaucoma are hyperopia, Asian ancestry, *female* gender, and older age. Patients with hyperopia have smaller eyes and more shallow anterior chambers. Females and people of Asian descent also tend to have smaller eyes. As people age, cataracts may develop, become thicker, and crowd the anterior chamber, increasing the likelihood of developing pupillary block leading to glaucoma. A dimly illuminated environment, which leads to physiologic dilation, may precipitate attacks of acute-angle closure. Think of an older Asian female developing eye pain, blurry vision, nausea, and vomiting after sitting in a dark theater… it could be that she ate too much delicious buttery popcorn, but it is more likely acute-angle closure. Of note, medications, such as topical adrenergics or anticholinergics, sulfa medications, or oral topiramate may also precipitate attacks of acute-angle closure.

HELPFUL TIP:
Pharmacologic dilation may result in an attack of acute-angle closure glaucoma. But where better a place for it to show up than in your office or the ED? Neovascularization of the eye (such as from diabetes or retinal hypoxia) can lead to "neovascular glaucoma" from neovascularization of the iris and angle. Hyphema can cause glaucoma from a clot obstructing the outflow of aqueous humor.

Question 19.2.4 Which of the following is NOT a presentation of acute closed-angle glaucoma?
A) Headache
B) Abdominal pain
C) Vomiting
D) Limitation of extraocular motion
E) Halos around light

Answer 19.2.4 The correct answer is "D." Patients with acute closed-angle glaucoma can present with all of the above findings except for the limitation of extraocular motion. Severe eye pain and blurred vision are commonly noted due to corneal edema and clouding secondary to the increased intraocular pressure. "B" and "C" deserve special mention. A sudden increase in intraocular pressure and angle closure can cause abdominal symptoms including pain and nausea and vomiting. Remember your review of systems? Ask about the eye with abdominal pain in order to not miss this potential sign of eye pathology.

You call your local ophthalmologist or optometrist to see this patient with suspected acute-angle glaucoma. She is going to be delayed because of traffic—it's Iowa, so she's likely stuck behind a big tractor … we don't have "rush hour," only "rush minute."

Question 19.2.5 Which of the following drugs is NOT appropriate to use as a temporizing measure?
A) Topical carbonic anhydrase inhibitors
B) Topical β-blockers
C) Topical glycerin
D) Topical atropine drops
E) Topical prostaglandin analog drops

Answer 19.2.5 The correct answer is "D." Atropine is **contraindicated** in acute glaucoma, since it will dilate the eye, exacerbating the problem. Topical β-blockers ("B") and topical ("A") or oral carbonic anhydrase inhibitors (e.g., acetazolamide) reduce aqueous production and thereby reduce intraocular pressure. In addition to the medications noted above, a topical α-adrenergic agonist (e.g., brimonidine, apraclonidine) lowers eye pressure by selectively affecting the α-2 receptors decreasing aqueous production and increasing aqueous outflow. Prostaglandin analogs ("E," e.g., latanoprost) increase aqueous outflow decreasing intraocular pressure. One suggested regimen includes: timolol 0.5%, apraclonidine 1%, and pilocarpine 2%, one drop of each 1 minute apart followed by IV acetazolamide.

HELPFUL TIP:
In general, eye drops that dilate the eye have a red cap on them, so if you are in a panic and you've forgotten all the good advice from this awesome book, a good rule of thumb is to NOT to *use any eye drop WITH a red cap for glaucoma*. See Table 19-1 for details on glaucoma medications.

TABLE 19-1 DRUGS USED FOR ACUTE GLAUCOMA AND HOW THEY WORK

Drug	Mechanism of Action
Topical β-blockers (e.g., timolol)	Decreases aqueous humor production
Topical α-adrenergic agonists (e.g., brimonidine)	Decreases aqueous humor production
Prostaglandin analogs (e.g., latanoprost, bimatoprost, travoprost)	Increases aqueous humor outflow through uveoscleral channels
Topical carbonic anhydrase inhibitors (e.g., dorzolamide, brinzolamide)	Decreases aqueous humor production
Oral carbonic anhydrase inhibitor (e.g., acetazolamide)	Diuretic and, more importantly, decreases the production of aqueous humor
Mannitol (rarely used now for acute glaucoma, mostly OR cases only)	Osmotic diuretic draws aqueous humor from the eye

HELPFUL TIP:
If the cornea is edematous and cloudy due to the elevated intraocular pressure, topical agents will less effectively penetrate the eye and will be less effective in the reduction of intraocular pressure. In such a case, systemic medications will be indicated. If using acetazolamide, renal function should be tested prior to administration.

An ophthalmologist makes it to the hospital and recommends surgery.

Question 19.2.6 **What is the definitive *treatment of choice* for acute-angle closure glaucoma?**
A) Laser peripheral iridotomy
B) Tapping of the anterior chamber to lower intraocular pressure
C) Aqueous suppressant therapy
D) Surgical iridectomy
E) Chiropractic manipulation

Answer 19.2.6 **The correct answer is "A."** The treatment goal is to allow the free flow of aqueous so that it does not accumulate behind the iris to push it forward to obstruct the trabecular meshwork. A laser peripheral iridotomy creates a small hole in the peripheral iris that allows aqueous flow to improve and thereby decreases intraocular pressure. As long as this hole remains patent, the patient is no longer at risk for an attack of angle closure glaucoma, and it is unusual for the hole to close unless there is a history of intraocular inflammation. "B," tapping the anterior chamber, can be used before laser therapy in order to clear the cornea so that visualization is better for the procedure. However, this is controversial and not the definitive treatment of choice. "C," aqueous suppressant therapy, is discussed in the previous question. "D," a surgical iridectomy, is performed for patients who are unable to sit still for the laser procedure (i.e., children, intellectually disabled). As to "E," this might not be the right choice at this time.

Question 19.2.7 **Which is FALSE regarding closed- and open-angle glaucoma?**
A) The main difference is that the drainage angle (trabecular meshwork) is closed in angle closure glaucoma and open in open-angle glaucoma
B) Scopolamine and other agents with anticholinergic properties are contraindicated in open-angle glaucoma but not in closed angle
C) Acute-angle closure glaucoma usually occurs in hyperopic individuals while myopia is associated with open-angle glaucoma
D) The majority of people diagnosed with glaucoma have primary open-angle glaucoma

Answer 19.2.7 **The correct answer (and false statement) is "B."** Agents with anticholinergic properties, which would cause dilation of the pupil, are actually **contraindicated** in those with

closed-angle glaucoma (and those with **narrow** angles who may not yet have obstructed). Once peripheral iridotomy is performed, anticholinergics are no longer an issue, since the patient is no longer at risk. All of the rest of the statements are correct.

Question 19.2.8 **Which of the following does NOT increase a patient's risk for primary *open-angle* glaucoma?**
A) Family history
B) Caucasian race
C) Elevated intraocular pressure (>21 mm Hg)
D) Age >40

Answer 19.2.8 **The correct answer is "B."** Patients of African heritage are much more likely to develop open-angle glaucoma than are Caucasians and are also more likely to suffer vision loss from glaucoma. Family history, high intraocular pressures, and thin corneas are all risk factors for the development of open-angle glaucoma. High intraocular pressures lead to optic nerve damage. Minor risk factors include diabetes and myopia (near-sightedness). All patients should be screened for glaucoma as part of their routine eye examination. This is usually done by assessing intraocular pressure, examining the optic nerve and corneal thickness, and performing any ancillary diagnostic tests such as visual field analysis.

Question 19.2.9 **Which of the following is typical of early open-angle glaucoma?**
A) Central vision loss
B) Peripheral vision loss
C) Lack of symptoms
D) Decreased contrast
E) Blurring of vision

Answer 19.2.9 **The correct answer is "C."** Most people with early open-angle glaucoma are asymptomatic. This is why screening is important. A significant number of the approximately one million axons of the optic nerve may be damaged before it manifests itself as visual field loss. Screening by examination of the optic nerve for abnormalities is the best way to diagnose *early glaucoma* (as opposed to increased ocular pressure which may result in optic nerve damage and thus glaucoma). Later symptoms involve loss of peripheral or central vision.

Question 19.2.10 **Which of the following is necessary to diagnose a patient with *open*-angle glaucoma?**
A) Optic nerve head cupping or irregularity with corresponding visual field loss
B) Thin corneas
C) Elevated intraocular pressure
D) Narrow but open drainage angle

Answer 19.2.10 **The correct answer is "A."** Cupping of the optic nerve head is caused by thinning of the neural rim. There should be a corresponding visual field defect consistent with the appearance of optic nerve cupping in a patient with glaucoma.

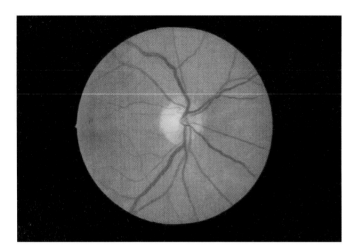

FIGURE 19-4 Normal optic nerve.

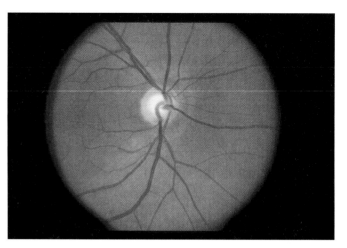

FIGURE 19-5 Glaucomatous optic nerve. Observe the cupping of the optic nerve head. The cup (central depression, seen as the bright part of the disc) of the optic nerve, which represents the axons diving down into the optic nerve, is larger compared with normal. A cup >50% of the disc width may be suggestive of glaucoma. Cupping represents damage to the optic nerve and fewer axons are present.

Note **that elevated intraocular pressure is not diagnostic of open-angle glaucoma.** Elevated intraocular pressure by itself is considered a risk factor for glaucoma and is the only modifiable risk factor to date. When **not** accompanied by cupping or visual field loss, it is considered ocular hypertension. Patients with ocular hypertension still need to be monitored and treated to prevent the development of open-angle glaucoma. Conversely, some patients with glaucoma never develop high intraocular pressure, indicating that glaucoma may, in fact, be due to optic nerve damage arising from a variety of etiologies. Thinner corneas ("B") increase the risk of glaucoma but are not required for diagnosis. "D" is incorrect. The drainage angle must be widely open—thus the name "open-angle glaucoma."

Question 19.2.11 Which of the following statements regarding glaucoma is true?
A) If treated early enough, normalizing the intraocular pressure can reverse the process of glaucoma and restore sight
B) The funduscopic examination in patients with glaucoma will generally show small retinal hemorrhages in addition to optic nerve cupping
C) Papilledema is seen with glaucoma as a result of increased pressure on the optic nerve
D) There are no identified genetic markers that correlate to development of glaucoma
E) None of the above

Answer 19.2.11 **The correct answer is "E."** So, wrong, wrong, wrong ... and wrong. Once there is visual loss, it cannot be restored ("A"). *Optic nerve hemorrhages*, and not retinal hemorrhages, are seen in glaucoma ("B"). Retinal hemorrhages can typically be seen with diabetic or hypertensive retinopathies. Papilledema results from increased **intracranial**—not intraocular—pressure ("C"). There are multiple genes that have been identified that contribute to the development of glaucoma ("D"). See Figure 19-4 for images of normal-appearing optic nerves, and compare these with Figure 19-5, which shows optic nerve findings in patients with glaucoma.

▶ **Objectives: Did you learn to ...**
· Recognize the signs and symptoms of acute-angle closure glaucoma?
· Identify risk factors associated with acute-angle closure glaucoma?
· Describe the pathology and basis for treatment for glaucoma?
· Differentiate between angle closure and open-angle glaucoma?
· Describe optic nerve findings in glaucoma?

 QUICK QUIZ: GLAUCOMA AGENTS

Topical β-blockers lower intraocular pressure by decreasing aqueous production.

Which of the following is NOT considered a systemic side effect of these medications?
A) Bronchospasm
B) Bradycardia
C) Worsening of congestive heart failure
D) Increased low-density lipoprotein (LDL)

The correct answer is "D." β-Blockers do not increase LDL. The take-home message here is that **topical β-blockers can have systemic effects including effects on congestive heart failure, bradycardia, or airway disease such as asthma or COPD.** Be aware of this, especially in the elderly.

 QUICK QUIZ: VISION LOSS

A 70-year-old white female presents with sudden loss of the upper half of her vision in the left eye. *She reports no pain.* Her past medical history is significant for hypertension and type 2 diabetes.

Which of the following is the LEAST likely diagnosis given this history?
A) Retinal detachment
B) Branch retinal artery/vein occlusion
C) Optic neuritis
D) Anterior ischemic optic neuropathy

The correct answer is "C." Retinal detachment, branch retinal artery/vein occlusion, and anterior ischemic optic neuropathy all cause **painless** sectorial loss of vision in this age group. Optic neuritis usually occurs in a younger age group and is associated **with pain**, especially with eye movement, color vision changes, and central, cecocentral, altitudinal, or arcuate scotomas (blind spots).

HELPFUL TIP:
Many patients complain of pain when they move their eyes. Diagnoses to consider include optic neuritis, intraorbital infection/inflammation, sinusitis, and orbital myositis of multiple etiologies such as orbital cellulitis, thyroid eye disease, orbital pseudotumor, sarcoidosis, polyarteritis nodosum, systemic lupus erythematosus, dermatomyositis, rheumatoid arthritis, and Wegener granulomatosis (now known as granulomatosis with polyangiitis).

 QUICK QUIZ: ANTERIOR ISCHEMIC OPTIC NEUROPATHY

Ischemic optic neuropathy is the most common cause of optic nerve pathology causing visual loss in patients older than 50 years. It is referred to as "anterior" when it affects the optic nerve head. It generally results from ischemia of the optic disc (sort of makes sense since it is called "anterior *ischemic* optic neuropathy").

Which of the following is CORRECT regarding nonarteritic (not related to temporal arteritis) anterior ischemic optic neuropathy (NA-AION)?
A) It is not associated with diabetes
B) Women are affected five times as often as men
C) As with giant cell arteritis, it responds quickly and dramatically to systemic corticosteroids
D) Avoiding nocturnal hypotension is an important aspect of treatment

The correct answer is "D." It is important to *avoid* nocturnal hypotension. In higher risk patients, it should be recommended to avoid anti-hypertensive administration at bedtime.

Midodrine can be used to support the blood pressure at night. The remaining statements are incorrect. NA-AION usually presents as painless, sudden unilateral vision loss,

which may become bilateral. As far as risk factors, think of NA-AION risk factors as being equivalent to those of peripheral vascular disease. It is associated with atherosclerosis, hypertension, hyperlipidemia, diabetes, anemia, and sleep apnea. Males and females are equally affected. While the age of patients with NA-AION overlaps with that of patients with giant cell arteritis, the patients with NA-AION tend to be younger. On exam, there may be an afferent pupillary defect, decreased visual acuity, or a visual field defect. There may be a pale disc with swelling, which is often segmental, and disc hemorrhages. In the contralateral eye, there may be a crowded disc with an absent cup (also known as a "disc at risk"), which has also been associated with NA-AION.

HELPFUL TIP:
Surgical intervention for NA-AION is not helpful and may lead to worsening blindness. In fact, there is no known effective therapy. Treatment of risk factors is paramount. Phosphodiesterase-5 inhibitors (e.g., sildenafil), which are often used for erectile dysfunction, can cause hypotension and may be associated with NA-AION, so though it may be a sensitive subject, do not shy away from asking about the use of such medications and advise against their use for patients at risk for NA-AION.

▶ **CASE 19.3**

A 65-year-old white male complains of "seeing wavy lines" when looking at the doorway with his right eye. He has no pain or other ocular symptoms. His past medical history is significant only for hypertension. He has a 40-pack-year smoking history. On examination, his visual acuity is 20/400 in the right eye. He has no RAPD and slit-lamp examination reveals that his anterior segment is normal. Examination of his right fundus reveals a subretinal hemorrhage involving his fovea.

Question 19.3.1 Which of the following is the most likely cause of this patient's vision loss?
A) Age-related macular degeneration (AMD)
B) Acute-angle closure glaucoma
C) Cataract
D) Diabetic retinopathy
E) Malingering

Answer 19.3.1 The correct answer is "A." This is a typical presentation for AMD (continue to the next question for more information). "B" is incorrect because acute-angle closure glaucoma presents with pain. "C" is incorrect since cataracts cause slowly progressive vision loss. "D" is incorrect as the patient has no known history of diabetes. Save "E" for the psychiatry chapter.

Question 19.3.2 Which of the following statements is FALSE?

A) AMD is the leading cause of vision loss in persons older than 60 years in the United States

B) Smoking has been shown to be a risk factor in the development of wet AMD

C) AMD is less common in Caucasians when compared with other populations

D) The Age-Related Eye Disease Study Part 2 (AREDS2) has shown a beneficial effect of vitamin E, vitamin C, lutein, zeaxanthin, zinc, and copper in delaying the progression to advanced AMD

E) A common complaint of wet AMD is metamorphopsia, which is distortion or waviness centrally in the visual field

Answer 19.3.2 The correct answer is "C." AMD occurs more commonly in Caucasian populations. "A" is correct as AMD is the leading cause of vision loss, primarily central vision, in patients older than 60 years. "B" is correct. Smoking is a significant risk factor in the progression to wet AMD; therefore, smoking cessation is highly recommended in any individual with early AMD findings or with a family history of AMD (and anyone, really). As to "D," the listed micronutrients are beneficial in delaying the progression from dry to wet AMD according to the AREDS2 results. "E" is also correct. Patients with AMD complain of distortion and/or waviness in the central visual field.

HELPFUL TIP:
Dry AMD is the non-neovascular form of AMD. It is characterized by drusen (yellow-white lesions in the outer retinal layers of the macula) or atrophy within the macula. Dry AMD may lead to wet (neovascular) AMD, which is associated with a choroidal neovascular membrane (CNVM). The CNVM is an abnormal growth of subretinal blood vessels, which grow in the macula or fovea and affects vision due to fluid leakage.

HELPFUL (BUT UNFORTUNATE) TIP:
Micronutrients (AREDS2 vitamins) for the general population do not seem to prevent the development of AMD. However, they do seem to work to prevent progression to advanced AMD once the patient has early AMD.

HELPFUL TIP:
The primary treatment of wet AMD is intravitreal injection of vascular endothelial growth factor inhibitor (VEGF inhibitor) medications (e.g., bevacizumab, ranibizumab, or aflibercept). You may remember "photodynamic therapy," the injection of verteporfrin (a photoactive dye) followed by laser treatment to occlude the neovascular vessels. This has fallen out of favor with VEGF inhibitors being the first-line

treatment. Early detection of wet AMD and initiation of treatment with a VEGF inhibitor increases the likelihood of obtaining the best results. To help with early detection, patients with early AMD may monitor for metamorphopsia at home with an Amsler grid. In addition, all patients should be encouraged to cease smoking.

▶ **Objectives: Did you learn to …**
- Recognize the signs and symptoms of AMD?
- Differentiate between dry and wet AMD?
- Recognize treatment modalities for wet AMD?

▶ **CASE 19.4**

A 55-year-old white male with a history of newly diagnosed type 2 diabetes mellitus presents for routine evaluation. He has no complaints, including vision. On non-dilated direct ophthalmoscopic examination, both fundi appear to be normal.

Question 19.4.1 When should this patient be referred for formal ophthalmologic examination?

A) At the time of diagnosis

B) Within 3 months

C) Within 6 months

D) Within 1 year

E) When he develops visual symptoms, maybe 2 days before he goes blind

Answer 19.4.1 The correct answer is "A." Patient with type 2 diabetes should be referred for a dilated examination immediately upon diagnosis, since they may have been undiagnosed for a long time period and may already have a degree of retinopathy. **For type 1 diabetic patients**, the recommendation is to refer within 3 to 5 years of disease onset and that they be evaluated annually thereafter.

Question 19.4.2 What are the common findings seen on direct ophthalmoscopic examination in nonproliferative diabetic retinopathy?

A) Exudates

B) Cotton wool spots

C) Dot-blot hemorrhages

D) Microaneurysms

E) All of the above

Answer 19.4.2 The correct answer is "E." Direct ophthalmoscopic examination may reveal all these findings in nonproliferative diabetic retinopathy. These are caused by the increased fragility of capillaries and arterioles of the retina with diabetes. While hemorrhages and microaneurysms appear red, exudates and cotton-wool spots are white and fluffy in appearance.

Question 19.4.3 **What is the main cause of vision loss in** *nonproliferative* **diabetic retinopathy?**
A) Dot-blot hemorrhages
B) Macular edema
C) Cataract
D) Neovascularization

Answer 19.4.3 **The correct answer is "B."** Nonproliferative diabetic retinopathy by definition has no neovascularization (new, fragile blood vessel growth secondary to microvascular disease). The main source of decreased vision is macular edema. Treatment of focal non-center-involving macular edema consists of focal laser photocoagulation to leaking microaneurysms. VEGF-inhibitor intravitreal injections (e.g., bevacizumab, ranibizumab, or aflibercept) may also be used to treat diabetic macular edema.

Question 19.4.4 **What is the main cause of vision loss in** *proliferative* **diabetic retinopathy?**
A) Cataract
B) Macular edema
C) Vitreous hemorrhage
D) Neovascular glaucoma

Answer 19.4.4 **The correct answer is "C."** Vision loss in proliferative diabetic retinopathy occurs when friable neovascular vessels break open and bleed (vitreous hemorrhage). Vision loss can also occur if the neovascular vessels grow over the drainage angle of the eye, causing neovascular glaucoma, although this is far less common than vitreous hemorrhage. See Figure 19-6 for an image of neovascularization.

The treatment of proliferative diabetic retinopathy consists of panretinal photocoagulation, which involves lasering the peripheral retina, thereby decreasing the ischemic drive for neovascularization. Treatment of vitreous hemorrhage includes observation with the head of bed elevated until the hemorrhage settles out and clears enough for laser treatment. Vitreous hemorrhages may be caused by other things, such as retinal detachments, so ultrasound is usually performed acutely, since one will not be able to adequately examine the retina after a significant hemorrhage.

HELPFUL TIP:
Aspirin is safe in patients with neovascularization. The risk of bleeding does not increase significantly, and the cardiovascular benefit outweighs the risk of bleeding in the eye.

▶ **Objectives: Did you learn to …**
· Identify when to refer patients for formal ophthalmologic examination in type 1 and type 2 diabetes?
· Recognize the signs of diabetic retinopathy on direct ophthalmoscopic examination?
· Understand the causes of vision loss in those with nonproliferative and proliferative diabetic retinopathy?
· Describe the basis for treatment of both nonproliferative and proliferative diabetic retinopathy?

▶ **CASE 19.5**

A 20-year-old male presents to the ED, complaining of a "bloody eye." He was in a fight earlier in the evening and was hit in the eye ("… but you should see the other guy!" … and with your luck, you probably will). You examine him and discover the findings in Figure 19-7. His visual acuity in the affected eye is hand motions only. He also has moderate edema of the lids but is able to open his eyes. On slit-lamp examination, the pupil appears normal. His motility is full and there is no diplopia.

Question 19.5.1 **What is the single *most* important first step in evaluation of this patient?**
A) Detection of a RAPD
B) Patching until the heme clears
C) Evaluation for possible open globe
D) Immediate CT scanning to evaluate for an orbital fracture
E) Surgical anterior chamber washout of the heme

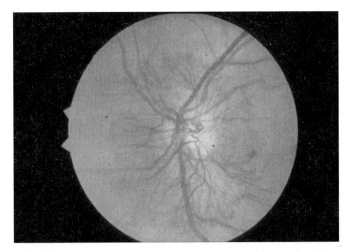

FIGURE 19-6 Proliferative diabetic retinopathy. Neovascularization of the optic nerve.

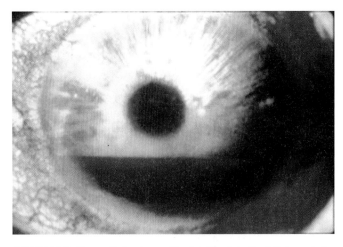

FIGURE 19-7 Traumatic hyphema. Blood settles into the inferior anterior chamber.

Answer 19.5.1 The correct answer is "C." This is a hyphema, with blood filling about one-third of the anterior chamber in Figure 19-7. More important is the history of trauma. The first, and most important, step in ocular trauma is to look for evidence of an open or ruptured globe. **There should be no pressure placed on the eye until an open globe is ruled out.** Signs of ruptured globe would be 360 degrees of subconjunctival hemorrhage, a shallow anterior chamber, an irregular or "peaked" pupil, or low intraocular pressure. *However, a normal globe pressure does not rule out a ruptured globe.* The leak may be small or may be plugged with choroid. **NOTE: Intraocular pressure measurements should not be taken until an open globe is ruled out. If there is any doubt about whether there is an open globe, consult an ophthalmologist or optometrist.** "D" is incorrect and deserves special mention: CT is not sensitive enough to rule out an open globe, even with thin cuts through the globe.

HELPFUL TIP:
When evaluating for a ruptured globe, remember that the most common areas of rupture are the limbus (the margin of the cornea where it meets the sclera) and sclera behind the insertion of rectus muscles. This is where the sclera is thinnest.

HELPFUL TIP:
A "Seidel test" can be used to look for an open globe. A moistened fluorescein strip is gently placed at the site of injury. Slit-lamp examination is done with Cobalt blue light. If a rupture is present, the fluorescein dye will be diluted by the aqueous, which will appear as a dark stream through the green fluorescein.

Question 19.5.2 Which is NOT a complication of hyphema (bleeding into the anterior chamber)?
A) Corneal blood staining
B) Glaucoma
C) Rebleeding
D) Iris neovascularization

Answer 19.5.2 The correct answer is "D." Complications of hyphema include rebleeding, which is most common in the first 3 to 5 days after injury. The hyphema may also stain the corneal endothelium, which may take months to clear. Glaucoma may also occur because of clogging of the trabecular meshwork by red blood cells, leading to a rise in intraocular pressure. "D," iris neovascularization, which may be present in a diabetic patient, may be present in a patient with hyphema but is not a complication of hyphema.

You rule out ruptured globe and orbital fracture. He's seen by the ophthalmologist on call who recommends treatment.

Question 19.5.3 Which of the following is the most appropriate treatment for this patient?
A) Treat at home with bed rest and a cycloplegic agent
B) Hospital admission and IV steroids
C) Hospital admission and IV antibiotics
D) Hospital admission and topical antibiotics
E) Treat at home with topical antibiotics

Answer 19.5.3 The correct answer is "A." This patient has a hyphema, which is blood in the anterior chamber, usually due to direct trauma. The goal of treatment is to prevent further bleeding into the anterior chamber and allow the blood to settle and resorb. While the party line in the past was that all of these patients require admission, sending a patient home with instructions for strict bed rest and avoiding strenuous activity is sufficient in **reliable** patients with limited disease. However, **an ophthalmologist or optometrist should be involved in this decision**. In addition, a cycloplegic agent, such as cyclopentolate or atropine, may be used to induce paralysis of the ciliary muscle and reduce movement of the iris. Patients should avoid antiplatelet or anticoagulant medications unless medically necessary. Topical steroids can be used if there are any signs of iritis, in which patients complain of an "eye ache" or photophobia or when inflammation with white blood cells or protein is present in the anterior chamber. You should check intraocular pressure and treat increased intraocular pressure if needed.

HELPFUL TIP:
If an African-American patient presents with a hyphema, one should inquire about sickle cell disease or trait, as ocular hypertension in patients with sickle cell disease is treated more aggressively and multiple agents *used to treat ocular hypertension* may induce sickling.

OK. Time for a joke. What is the definition of a double-blind study? Two orthopedic surgeons reading an electrocardiogram.

▶ **Objectives: Did you learn to …**
- Recognize the complications of ocular trauma?
- Examine a patient at risk for open globe?
- Identify the complications of hyphema?
- Initiate management of a patient with hyphema?

▶ **CASE 19.6**

A 27-year-old male presents with irritation and redness of his right eye after hammering on an old iron fence. He was not wearing safety glasses at the time (they aren't very cool looking, and he was hoping his attractive neighbor would see his big muscles!). He's now 4 hours out from his injury. On examination, his visual acuity is 20/200. His right eye is injected, and his pupil is irregularly peaked to one side upon gross inspection. Slit-lamp examination reveals a laceration of his cornea extending to the limbus with a wick of iris occluding the laceration site. You place a Fox shield on the eye to prevent any pressure on the globe, update the patient's tetanus vaccine, and start antibiotics.

Question 19.6.1 What would be the next step in the evaluation and treatment of this patient?
A) Imaging for an intraocular foreign body by orbital CT scanning
B) Evaluation for an intraocular foreign body by orbital ultrasound
C) Try to remove the foreign body from the posterior chamber with a magnet
D) Complete ocular examination, including intraocular pressure and dilated funduscopic examination

Answer 19.6.1 **The correct answer is "A."** Given his history, the patient needs to be evaluated for a possible intraocular foreign body. The best imaging modality is with orbital CT scanning. Orbital ultrasound ("B") would also be appropriate, but for surgical planning, CT scanning is preferred. Plus we do not want to put pressure on the eye with an open globe. "C" is incorrect because it is likely to cause more damage. This type of foreign-body removal is best left to a specialist in the operating room. Finally, it would be best to defer intraocular pressure measurements until the extent of the laceration is evaluated since no pressure should ever be placed on a potential open globe.

The patient undergoes an orbital CT. There appears to be a piece of metal within his vitreous cavity.

Question 19.6.2 Which of the following are inert intraocular foreign bodies?
A) Iron
B) Copper
C) Glass
D) Aluminum
E) C and D

Answer 19.6.2 **The correct answer is "C."** Iron, copper, and aluminum are all reactive species and **must** be removed from the eye. Glass is inert and may be left in place, depending on the situation and the risk of surgery.

Question 19.6.3 Which is NOT a sign of a retained *iron* intraocular foreign body?
A) Iris heterochromia
B) Mydriasis
C) Glaucoma
D) Retinal degeneration
E) High refractive error

Answer 19.6.3 **The correct answer is "E,"** also known as severe myopia or nearsightedness, which has nothing to do with the retained iron foreign body. Although, the patient in this case

may have been *extremely nearsighted, metaphorically speaking,* in his decision to not wear safety glasses. All of the rest are signs of siderosis caused by a retained iron intraocular foreign body. Given the toxicity to the eye, the foreign body must be removed surgically.

HELPFUL TIP:
Corneal foreign bodies may be removed using a needle after the administration of topical anesthetic. Metallic foreign bodies in the cornea may leave a rust ring around the area of the foreign body, which can be removed using an ocular burr or an Alger brush. The rust ring may also be left in place if it is out of the visual axis since it does not cause any long-lasting problems.

▶ **Objectives: Did you learn to …**
- Recognize the signs of a corneoscleral laceration?
- Manage a corneoscleral laceration in the emergency setting?
- Appreciate the effects of intraocular foreign bodies?
- Manage an intraocular foreign body in the emergency setting?

▶ CASE 19.7

A 55-year-old farmer presents to the ED complaining of ocular pain and irritation. He reports accidentally splashing ammonia in both eyes. (This is commonly due to cooking methamphetamine or farmers legitimately using ammonia as a fertilizer [both popular pastimes in Iowa].) He attempted to rinse his eyes with water prior to coming to the ED. His visual acuity is OD 20/100 and OS 20/80. Both eyes are injected with corneal edema.

Question 19.7.1 What is the immediate first step in the treatment of chemical injuries to the eye?
A) Complete ocular examination, including dilated funduscopic examination
B) Manual removal of particulate material followed immediately by irrigation with water or saline until the pH is 7
C) Application of topical glycerin to clear the corneal edema
D) Topical anesthetic with debridement of surface epithelium
E) Build rapport by making small talk, asking about his tractor, etc.

Answer 19.7.1 **The correct answer is "B."** Step one: Immediately irrigate! Remove any particulate matter. The upper lid should be everted to check for any particulate matter. A moistened cotton swab may be used to sweep the superior and inferior fornices to remove any residual debris. Irrigation is extremely important and should be completed **before** the examination. Irrigation may be performed at an eyewash station, administered through IV tubing with an irrigation lens (Morgan Lens), or administered through pouring water or saline on the eyes. We have even had patients irrigate at the scene with beer (really…). To check the pH, wait 5 minutes after discontinuing irrigation and use a pH strip in the superior or inferior fornix. Irrigation can be discontinued when you reach a neutral (7–7.4), but it may require multiple liters of irrigation. (To determine the correct pH, it can be helpful to compare patient's pH paper to pH paper used on a normal eye. Your eye!) A topical anesthesia can be applied to alleviate pain. After neutralizing the pH, you can complete the examination.

HELPFUL TIP:
Never try to treat an alkali burn with an acid or an acid burn with a base!

Question 19.7.2 Which of the following is a complication of chemical injuries to the eye?
A) Corneal ulceration
B) Inflammation
C) De-epithelialization of the cornea
D) All of the above
E) None of the above

Answer 19.7.2 **The correct answer is "D."** All of these are complications of chemical injuries to the eye. If you chose "E," you should take a break now! You are tired.

HELPFUL TIP:
Alkali burns tend to be more severe than acid burns. Alkali burns cause ocular surface damage by saponifying fatty acids in cell membranes. Alkaline agents readily penetrate the cornea causing degradation. Acids cause protein denaturation, which creates a barrier to penetration. Therefore, acids cause less tissue destruction. Nerve destruction may cause a decrease in sensitivity to the eye, so absence of pain is not adequate to determine whether further irrigation is needed. **Check the pH as noted above.**

▶ **Objectives: Did you learn to …**
• Describe the difference between acid and alkali injuries to the eye?
• Treat a chemical eye exposure in the emergency setting?
• Recognize the complications of chemical eye injuries?

▶ **CASE 19.8**

A 25-year-old college student complains of redness, sensitivity to light, and tearing of her right eye for the past day. She lives in the dorm but reports no exposure to others with a red eye. For the past few days, she has had a sore throat and slight cough. You suspect she may have the dreaded "pink eye" (conjunctivitis).

Question 19.8.1 Regarding conjunctivitis, which of the following is FALSE?
A) Gonococcal conjunctivitis presents with severe, hyperacute, purulent discharge
B) Adenoviral conjunctivitis generally begins in one eye and spreads to the other eye
C) An enlarged preauricular node is a sign of allergic conjunctivitis
D) Toxic conjunctivitis has been associated with the use of topical antibiotics, antivirals, and preservatives

Answer 19.8.1 **The correct answer (and FALSE one) is "C."** There is no enlargement of preauricular nodes with allergic conjunctivitis. **An enlarged preauricular node is a prominent feature of adenoviral conjunctivitis**—which is extremely contagious (and no matter what the school says, does not respond to antibiotic eye drops). Allergic conjunctivitis tends to itch and affect both eyes. All other statements are true.

....

Your patient has no purulent drainage. On examination, her visual acuity is 20/40. Her right eye is diffusely injected and tearing; the left eye appears normal to inspection. She has a slightly tender right preauricular lymph node about 1 cm in size.

Question 19.8.2 What do you recommend as the initial treatment of this patient's conjunctivitis?
A) Symptomatic treatment with artificial tears four to eight times per day, cool compresses, and strict hygiene to prevent spread to the other eye or to other individuals
B) Treatment with topical vasoconstrictors/antihistamines four times daily for 1 to 2 weeks
C) Topical antibiotic treatment for 1 week so she can go back to class
D) Administration of topical steroids, artificial tears, and cool compresses

Answer 19.8.2 **The correct answer is "A."** This patient appears to have viral conjunctivitis, which is treated symptomatically. There is no need to treat with topical vasoconstrictors and/or antihistamines unless there is a significant itching component. *It's NOT bacterial, so antibiotics are NOT needed.* Additionally, *prophylactic* antibiotics are not necessary, since there is rarely a secondary bacterial infection. See Figure 19-8 for an image of hemorrhagic viral conjunctivitis generally from adenovirus, enterovirus, and coxsackie virus. It is highly contagious.

HELPFUL TIP:
Do antibiotics have magical powers in viral conjunctivitis? How else can you explain the fact that a single dose of topical antibiotics is enough to get a child back into school or day care? Most schools and day care policies require the child to be on some sort of drops (of any sort) in order to return. In reality, children should be kept

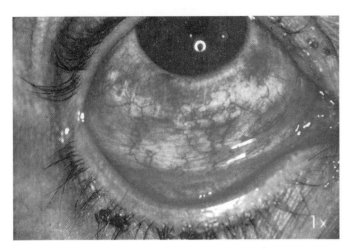

FIGURE 19-8 Viral conjunctivitis. Note the follicles that are round collection of lymphocytes in the inferior fornix.

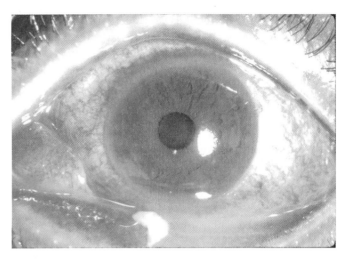

FIGURE 19-9 Bacterial conjunctivitis. Note the mucopurulent discharge.

out of school until the conjunctivitis symptoms resolve. Children may start yelling, "We don't need no education," but it will only last a few days as viral conjunctivitis is self-limiting and will resolve without antibiotics.

Question 19.8.3 If your patient is a part-time nursing assistant at a care facility, how long should she stay away from patient care?
A) Two days
B) Two weeks
C) Until her eyes are clear
D) Until she has taken antibiotics for 24 hours

Answer 19.8.3 The correct answer is "C." Viral conjunctivitis is *highly* contagious and is thought to be infectious as long as the eye is red and producing discharge. Promote good hand hygiene and avoidance of contact with others until the eye clears. In many instances, complete removal from school and/or work is not feasible, but patient education regarding the highly contagious nature of viral and bacterial conjunctivitis remains important.

Question 19.8.4 Which of the following is appropriate in the management of acute gonococcal conjunctivitis?
A) Conjunctival Gram stain and PCR/NAAT
B) Ceftriaxone IM/IV
C) Saline irrigation
D) All of the above
E) None of the above

Answer 19.8.4 The correct answer is "D." The hallmark of acute gonococcal conjunctivitis is severe purulent discharge (lots of pus!), which occurs within 12 to 24 hours of infection. Preauricular adenopathy may also be seen. Management of gonococcal conjunctivitis consists of Gram stain and PCR/NAAT to document infection and the administration of ceftriaxone

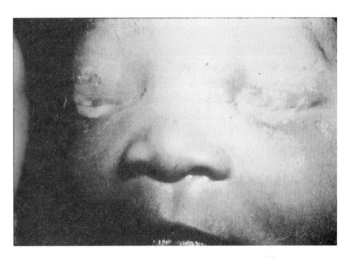

FIGURE 19-10 Ophthalmia neonatorum. Note the severe mucopurulent discharge.

(or spectinomycin if cephalosporin allergic) IM/IV **plus** azithromycin 2 g (for possible concurrent chlamydia infection). Alternative, *second line*, regimens include gentamicin + azithromycin (2 g) or Gemifloxacin + azithromycin (2 g) though there is much less data supporting these regimens. Irrigation is needed initially to remove discharge and regularly until discharge resolves. One should examine the cornea to rule out involvement. Topical fluoroquinolone drops should be started if there is corneal involvement (though resistance rates are high). See Figure 19-9 for an image of bacterial conjunctivitis and Figure 19-10 for an image of Gonococcal ophthalmia neonatorum.

Question 19.8.5 Which of the following is NOT indicated in the treatment of allergic conjunctivitis?
A) Cool compresses
B) Artificial tears
C) Chronic topical vasoconstrictors/antihistamines
D) Short-term topical steroids
E) Diphenhydramine

Answer 19.8.5 The correct answer is "C." Given the possibility of rebound hyperemia with prolonged use, chronic vasoconstrictors/antihistamines are never indicated. Topical steroids should be reserved for severe cases and tapered over 1 to 2 weeks. Topical NSAIDs (ketorolac) and antihistamines or mast cell stabilizers (levocabastine or olopatadine) may be used to alleviate intense itching but can be expensive. Ketotifen is an effective and less expensive OTC mast cell stabilizer and H1-antihistamine that, when used routinely, decreases allergic conjunctivitis symptoms.

▶ **Objectives: Did you learn to …**
- Differentiate among viral, bacterial, and allergic conjunctivitis?
- Not prescribe ophthalmic antibiotics for viral conjunctivitis— you got that, right?
- Choose appropriate treatments modalities for the various causes of conjunctivitis?

▶ **CASE 19.9**

A patient complains of possible foreign body in her eye. She was scraping barnacles off the bottom of her multi-million dollar yacht currently dry-docked right next to one of Donald Trump's yachts (Could she be a radiologist? Maybe a plastic surgeon?). She felt something fly into her eye and had immediate pain.

Question 19.9.1 Which of the following is FALSE regarding the use of topical fluorescein, which is used to highlight epithelial defects of the cornea?
A) Fluorescein is a nontoxic, water-soluble dye
B) It fluoresces under a cobalt blue filter
C) It exhibits positive staining of epithelial defects
D) Fluorescein does not penetrate the corneal stroma

Answer 19.9.1 The correct answer is "D." Fluorescein **does** diffuse through and stain the corneal stroma if there is an epithelial defect. (The first layer of the cornea is epithelium, like on the rest of our skin, and an epithelial defect can be thought of as a scratch or gash on the skin.)

HELPFUL TIP:
Always evert the upper eyelid when there is concern for a foreign body. These can be removed using a cotton-tipped swab. Irrigation may also be useful.

During your complete examination, you notice a small fleck of what looks like paint on the cornea. After successfully removing the piece of paint, you plan to discharge the patient.

Question 19.9.2 Which of the following is NOT an appropriate treatment for corneal abrasions?
A) Observation alone
B) Topical antibiotics
C) Cycloplegics
D) Topical steroids
E) Patching

Answer 19.9.2 The correct answer is "D." In uncomplicated corneal abrasions in non-contact lens wearers, observation alone ("A") is often adequate. Antibiotics ("B") should be used for all contact lens–related abrasions or in non-contact lens–related abrasions which are large, involve the visual axis, or involve vegetative matter. Topical broad-spectrum antibiotics, such as polymyxin B/trimethoprim or erythromycin ointment, are good first-line choices in those without contact lenses. A topical fluoroquinolone can be used in contact lens wearers or for abrasions involving vegetative matter. The patients should also be advised to withhold contact lens use until the abrasion is healed and should be evaluated by their contact lens prescribing provider. Generally, bandage contact lenses and patching ("E") are rarely needed and may increase risk of infection or cause further abrasion. Patching may also be used for patient comfort, but is unnecessary and may actually increase pain and prolong healing time. Topical steroids ("D") may inhibit epithelial healing and promote infection and should be avoided. "C" deserves special mention. Use of a long-acting cycloplegic is acceptable for discomfort related to severe photophobia and blepharospasm secondary to corneal abrasions. However, the cycloplegic agents can be expensive and *do not help in healing.*

HELPFUL TIP:
Multiple vertical corneal abrasions suggest a foreign body under the upper lid (foreign-body "tracking"). Blinking and closing the eye will leave an abrasion on the cornea. Evert the eyelid and sweep the fornices with a moistened cotton swab to remove any residual foreign body.

As you already know, most corneal abrasion should heal within 24 to 48 hours. You ask the patient to follow up in 2 days to make sure that things are going well. On arrival, she notes increased ache in the eye with increased injection and photosensitivity. You place anesthetic drops in her eye, but the pain does not resolve. The corneal abrasion appears to be healing.

Question 19.9.3 What do you expect to see on slit-lamp examination in her anterior chamber?
A) Cells and flare
B) Opacity of the lens
C) Foreign bodies of Schlemm
D) A tear of the anterior lens capsule

Answer 19.9.3 The correct answer is "A." This patient is presenting with typical posttraumatic iritis. Findings would be "cell and flare" in the anterior chamber. "B" and "D" are obviously not going to be a result of a superficial corneal abrasion. "C" is something we made up, but "Canal of Schlemm" is part of the eye and one of our favorite names in medicine—it is just humorous (aqueous humorous, get it? … ah, poor Schlemm).

HELPFUL TIP:
Iritis, also called anterior uveitis, characteristically presents with pain, photophobia, increased redness, or excessive tearing. On slit-lamp examination, the "cell and flare" are due to individual inflammatory cells and protein, respectively. Cell and flare can be viewed in the anterior chamber with a small, bright light beam at the slit lamp.

Question 19.9.4 Appropriate treatment for this patient with post-traumatic iritis includes which of the following?
A) Topical antibiotics
B) Cycloplegic agents
C) Topical steroids
D) A, B, and C
E) B and C only

Answer 19.9.4 The correct answer is "E." Post-traumatic iritis is generally treated with topical steroids and cycloplegic agents. Again, we usually do this in consultation with an eye care provider. While we all worry about the risk of infection with topical steroids, they can also increase intraocular pressure, and when used chronically, it can cause glaucoma. So, these patients require close follow-up.

Assume that this patient was presenting de novo with iritis, and it is not post-traumatic.

Question 19.9.5 Which of the following do you NOT have to worry about as an etiology of iritis?
A) Rheumatoid arthritis
B) Diabetes mellitus
C) Syphilis
D) Sarcoid
E) Lyme disease

Answer 19.9.5 The correct answer is "B." Iritis is an inflammatory process that can be caused by multiple underlying illnesses including ankylosing spondylitis, lupus (rarely), Behcet's disease, syphilis, sarcoid, tuberculosis, Reiter syndrome, toxoplasmosis (common, even in non-immunosuppressed), juvenile idiopathic arthritis, and many others.

▶ **Objectives: Did you learn to …**
· Remove a corneal foreign body?
· Use topical fluorescein in corneal abrasions?
· Manage uncomplicated corneal abrasions?
· Recognize iritis and its causes?

▶ CASE 19.10

A 65-year-old white male with a history of hypertension, adult-onset diabetes, rheumatoid arthritis, and rosacea presents with chronic complaints of redness, tearing, and irritation in both eyes. He sometimes also has "a film over his vision" that comes and goes. His ocular examination appears normal. He does, however, have an oily tear film with rapid breakup of his tears over his ocular surface. There is evidence of capped ("plugged") Meibomian glands (oil glands along the lid margins), but the eyelids are otherwise normal in appearance.

Question 19.10.1 Which of the following is the most likely diagnosis?
A) Meibomian gland dysfunction
B) Conjunctivitis
C) Hordeolum
D) Chalazion
E) Steven–Johnson syndrome

Answer 19.10.1 The correct answer is "A." Meibomian glands are the oil glands of the upper and lower eyelids, which are located along the posterior lid margin behind the lashes. These are punctate openings along the lid margin, which can become clogged with thick solid secretions. When coupled with chronic inflammation of the lid margin, this eventually leads to an unstable tear film, creating symptoms of burning, redness, foreign-body sensation, and filmy vision. It is considered blepharitis (inflammation of the eyelids). "B" and "E" are incorrect and typically have predominant signs of crusting or mattering. "B," "C," and "D" are more focal inflammatory processes, which can occur in conjunction with Meibomian gland dysfunction. A hordeolum affects the anterior lid margin glands, which become acutely plugged and inflamed. A chalazion affects the posterior lid margin glands, which become plugged and chronically inflamed. Of note, a "stye" is typically synonymous with hordeolum; however, both hordeolum and chalazion may grossly appear similar on examination.

Question 19.10.2 What part of his past medical history is associated with Meibomian gland dysfunction?
A) Hypertension
B) Diabetes
C) Rheumatoid arthritis
D) Rosacea

Answer 19.10.2 The correct answer is "D." Meibomian gland dysfunction is associated with rosacea. Typical findings of rosacea include: facial papules, pustules, telangiectasia, erythema, edema, and rhinophyma.

Question 19.10.3 What treatment do you prescribe for this patient?
A) Observation and reassurance
B) Daily warm compresses, lid scrubs with dilute baby shampoo, preservative-free artificial tears, and oral antibiotic if needed
C) Erythromycin ophthalmic ointment PRN
D) Daily warm compresses, topical steroids, and frequent use of artificial tears

Answer 19.10.3 The correct answer is "B." The treatment of Meibomian gland dysfunction consists of lid hygiene, lubrication, and doxycycline or minocycline 50 to 100 mg daily to

BID for 3 to 6 weeks (which will also help treat the rosacea). The dosage may then be tapered according to symptoms. Gastrointestinal upset and photosensitivity are common side effects of doxycycline.

Question 19.10.4 Which of the following is a common complication of Meibomian gland dysfunction?
A) Bacterial keratitis
B) Preseptal cellulitis
C) Chalazion
D) Scleritis
E) Chronic conjunctivitis

Answer 19.10.4 The correct answer is "C." Meibomian gland dysfunction can cause a chronic granuloma to form at the plugged Meibomian gland, which is called a chalazion. The inflammation is sterile—unlike a hordeolum ("stye"), which is a painful purulent abscess. Treatment of a chalazion involves frequent warm compresses and massage. Topical antibiotics are of little value, since it is sterile. If these measures fail, an intralesional injection of steroids or incision and drainage is warranted. Hordeola ("styes") often resolve spontaneously, but warm compresses and massage are often helpful. If there is any evidence of cellulitis, systemic oral antibiotics are indicated. Drainage using a needle may also be helpful. Topical antibiotics are often not effective.

▶ **Objectives: Did you learn to …**
- Recognize the signs and symptoms of blepharitis and Meibomian gland dysfunction?
- Describe the etiologies of blepharitis and Meibomian gland dysfunction?
- Determine appropriate treatment for blepharitis and Meibomian gland dysfunction and the complications of hordeola and chalazion?

▶ CASE 19.11

A 7-year-old female presents with painful swelling and redness of upper and lower lids of her right eye. She reports having a bug bite near her right eye a week ago, and it's been very itchy. Now, it has become more erythematous and painful (infected, one might even say). On examination, her right eyelids are extremely edematous with a well-demarcated area of erythema. Her ocular examination is normal, including normal vision. She has no RAPD, proptosis, or motility deficit.

Question 19.11.1 This presentation is most consistent with:
A) Orbital cellulitis
B) Preseptal cellulitis
C) Anaphylactoid reaction to the insect bite
D) Blepharitis
E) None of the above

Answer 19.11.1 The correct answer is "B." The presentation of this patient is consistent with preseptal cellulitis, which is defined as inflammation/infection **anterior** to the orbital

septum. "A" is incorrect. Infection occurring **posterior** to the orbital septum is called orbital cellulitis. This is characterized by fever, proptosis, restriction of globe motility, chemosis, and pain on eye movements. Orbital cellulitis is considered more dangerous than preseptal cellulitis as it can be complicated by spread to adjacent structures and result in: subperiosteal abscess, cavernous sinus thrombosis, meningitis, or intracranial abscesses. "C" is incorrect since an anaphylactoid reaction is systemic.

Question 19.11.2 Which of the following is TRUE?
A) The most common cause of preseptal cellulitis in children is sinusitis
B) The most common cause of preseptal cellulitis in teens and adults is sinusitis
C) Orbital cellulitis is most commonly caused by bacteremia from a secondary source, as opposed to direct spread from an adjacent structure
D) The most common secondary source for orbital cellulitis is otitis media

Answer 19.11.2 The correct answer is "A." The most common cause of preseptal cellulitis in children is sinusitis. In contrast, teens and adults usually have preseptal cellulitis from a superficial source, such as skin trauma with inoculation. As a rule of thumb, preseptal cellulitis should always have a source or cause. (So put on your detective cap and ask about and look for the bugs, bites, bumps, abrasions, and sinus symptoms!)

 HELPFUL TIP:
Both orbital cellulitis and preseptal cellulitis are commonly secondary to sinusitis. Both preseptal and orbital cellulitis may also occur from direct inoculation or bacteremia from a distant source.

Question 19.11.3 The most common pathogen causing preseptal cellulitis from a skin trauma with inoculation is which of the following?
A) *Staphylococcus epidermidis*
B) *Haemophilus influenzae*
C) *Staphylococcus aureus*
D) *Streptococcus pneumoniae*

Answer 19.11.3 The correct answer is "C." *S. aureus* is the most common pathogen of preseptal cellulitis from skin trauma. Some may have chosen "B." Prior to the introduction of the HIB vaccine, children younger than 5 years often had preseptal cellulitis secondary to *H. influenzae*. However, this is no longer the most common pathogen. Most cases of preseptal and orbital cellulitis in children are caused by Gram-positive cocci. Orbital cellulitis in children may be caused by *H. influenzae*, but again this is rare in vaccinated children. In contrast, adults with orbital cellulitis frequently have infections due to Gram-positive cocci and *Bacteroides species*. Gram-negative rods may be the culprit after trauma. *Mucor* and *Aspergillus* should be suspected in diabetic patients and immunocompromised individuals.

HELPFUL TIP:
Orbital cellulitis is an ophthalmologic emergency. In addition to spread to other structures (e.g., cavernous sinus thrombosis), orbital cellulitis may cause an orbital compartment syndrome, compromising blood flow and leading to blindness. Orbital compartment syndrome can also be due to trauma and secondary to intraorbital (postseptal) bleeding or retrobulbar hematoma leading to proptosis. Signs of orbital compartment syndrome include: elevated intraocular pressure (>35 mm Hg), decreased vision, relative afferent pupillary defect or a fixed, dilated pupil, restricted extraocular motility (ophthalmoplegia), or proptosis with taut lids. The treatment is emergent lateral canthotomy and cantholysis. Time equals vision in these cases and you can find instructions online. One good source is from EyeRounds available through the University of Iowa (https://webeye .ophth.uiowa.edu/eyeforum/tutorials/lateral-canthotomy-cantholysis.htm). It is easy and should be done as quickly as possible.

▸ **Objectives: Did you learn to …**
- Differentiate between orbital and preseptal cellulitis?
- Recognize conditions that predispose patients to these processes?
- Recognize orbital compartment syndrome?

▶ CASE 19.12

A 67-year-old white man with a history of coronary artery disease, hypertension, and peripheral vascular disease presents with the sudden onset of painless loss of vision OD several hours ago. He states he was watching TV when "things went black" in his right eye. He notes that this happened a few times before, but his vision always returned to normal after a couple of minutes. On examination, he has light perception vision, the presence of a RAPD, and a normal anterior segment of the eye. Upon funduscopic examination, the fundus appears diffusely white with a reddish hue within the macula (cherry-red spot) (see Fig. 19-11).

Question 19.12.1 The patient's history and examination are most consistent with which of the following?
A) Central retinal vein occlusion
B) Anterior ischemic optic neuropathy
C) Central retinal artery occlusion
D) Choroidal ischemia

Answer 19.12.1 **The correct answer is "C."** A central retinal artery occlusion is characterized by acute painless loss of vision. The ischemia and edema of the retina causes diffuse whitening. There is a cherry-red spot in the macula, which is the normal choroidal circulation amidst the ischemic retina (see Fig. 19-11). The extensive ischemia causes a RAPD and significant visual loss. His previous history of recurrent

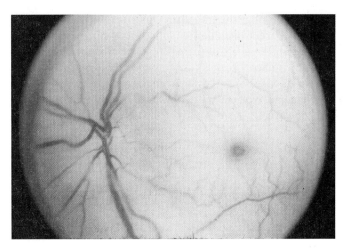

FIGURE 19-11 A central retinal artery occlusion. Note the cherry-red spot in the macula, which is due to the choroidal circulation amid the ischemic retina.

episodes of loss of vision that returned to normal is consistent with amaurosis fugax.

Question 19.12.2 In a patient with this history, irreversible retinal damage occurs after what time frame?
A) 10–15 minutes
B) 30–60 minutes
C) 90–120 minutes
D) 6 hours

Answer 19.12.2 **The correct answer is "C."** If central retinal artery occlusion is complete for more than 120 minutes, irreversible retinal damage and visual loss ensue. Patients should seek medical care immediately. Amaurosis fugax, or transient monocular blindness, is typically caused by carotid, vascular, or heart disease. It is often described as a curtain or shade coming over the vision. It lasts from a few seconds to 15 minutes or longer. The vision always returns back to normal in amaurosis fugax episodes. Patients with a history of amaurosis fugax should be evaluated for carotid and cardiac disease.

Question 19.12.3 Treatment for central retinal artery occlusion includes all of the following EXCEPT:
A) Thrombolytics
B) Digital compression/decompression of the globe
C) Anterior chamber paracentesis
D) Acetazolamide
E) Oxygen

Answer 19.12.3 **The correct answer is "A."** Therapy for central retinal artery occlusion is entirely aimed at dislodging the embolism, maintaining retinal viability, and reducing intraocular pressure (to increase the pressure gradient between the artery and the eye). This can be accomplished by digitally compressing (press hard!) then decompressing the eye with a finger (to dislodge the embolism), and anterior chamber paracentesis or acetazolamide (to reduce intraocular pressure). To accomplish the goals of increasing oxygen and carbon dioxide (which dilates vessels) use carbogen (95% oxygen and 5% carbon dioxide) or try using a nonrebreather facemask with supplemental oxygen; neither have good support in the literature, however.

Question 19.12.4 Comparing central retinal *artery* occlusion to central retinal *vein* occlusion, which of the following is TRUE?

A) Central retinal artery occlusion is more likely to be associated with giant cell arteritis
B) The main feature of both is retinal whitening with a cherry red spot
C) Central retinal vein occlusion usually results from atherosclerotic thrombosis, while central retinal artery occlusion results from hyperviscosity syndromes and hypercoagulable states
D) A RAPD is characteristic of central retinal artery occlusion, but is not seen with central retinal vein occlusion

Answer 19.12.4 The correct answer is "A." If a patient presents with symptoms of central retinal artery occlusion, but no embolus is visualized, he/she should be asked about symptoms of giant cell arteritis. "B" is incorrect because only central retinal artery occlusion is associated with retinal whitening and a cherry red spot. The appearance of a central retinal **vein** occlusion is one of tortuous dilated veins, optic nerve edema, and intraretinal hemorrhages/edema (the so-called "blood and thunder" appearance of the fundus—although since thunder is a sound, having something look like thunder does not make sense). "C" is incorrect because central retinal **artery** occlusion is usually caused by atherosclerotic thrombosis or emboli, while central retinal **vein** occlusion is associated more with hyperviscosity syndromes (e.g., polycythemia) and hypercoagulable states (e.g., protein C deficiency). In older patients with central retinal vein occlusion, the main risk factors include vasculopathic states such as hypertension and diabetes. "D" is incorrect because a RAPD can be seen with either syndrome. There will be a RAPD with a central retinal artery occlusion due to the diffuse distribution of ischemia. A RAPD may or may not be seen with a central retinal vein occlusion depending on the level of ischemia.

 HELPFUL TIP:
Other causes of central retinal artery occlusion include vasculitides and blood dyscrasias. Other causes of central retinal vein occlusions include increased intraorbital or intraocular pressure, glaucoma, blood dyscrasias, lupus anticoagulant, antiphospholipid antibody, oral contraceptives, and protein C deficiency. See Figure 19-12 for an image of the retina in central retinal vein occlusion.

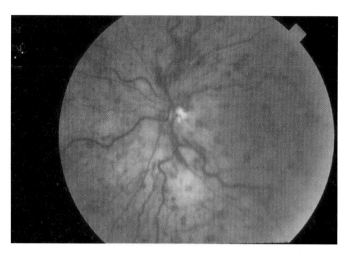
FIGURE 19-12 Central retinal vein occlusion. Note the dilated tortuous veins, optic disc edema, and retinal hemorrhage/edema.

Question 19.12.5 Further evaluation and treatment of a central retinal artery occlusion includes all of the following EXCEPT:

A) Topical timolol
B) ESR/CRP
C) Carotid Doppler
D) Orbital MRI/MRA
E) Echocardiogram

Answer 19.12.5 The correct answer is "D." There is no need for orbital imaging in the management of a central retinal artery occlusion. All of the other choices are important management steps. In addition, blood pressure, fasting blood sugar or glycosylated hemoglobin, CBC, and PT/PTT should be done. If there is a suspicion of giant cell arteritis, an ESR/CRP should be checked. Other tests might include a rheumatoid factor, syphilis serology, serum protein electrophoresis, and antiphospholipid antibodies. A similar workup is warranted in central retinal vein occlusion, except there is no need to search for an embolic source with a carotid Doppler and echocardiogram.

▸ **Objectives: Did you learn to …**
· Recognize the symptoms of vascular disorders of the eye?
· Differentiate between central retinal artery and vein occlusions?
· Describe some causes of ocular vascular occlusions?
· Determine the appropriate systemic workup for artery and vein occlusions?

▶ **CASE 19.13**

A 40-year-old white female presents to your ED complaining of seeing "little floating black spots" in her vision in the left eye. She also notes little sparks of light in the temporal periphery of the left eye. She noted this while shopping today at Wal-Mart. (First, you think this may be the revenge of the gods for shopping at Wal-Mart instead of buying locally. But then, you gather your wits about you.) On examination, her vision is 20/20 in both eyes, and there is no RAPD (she has normal direct and consensual pupillary reflexes). Confrontation visual fields demonstrate peripheral vision loss in the left eye. Dilated peripheral retinal examination reveals billowing gray folds. The macula appears normal.

Question 19.13.1 Which of the following is the most appropriate step in the management of this patient?
A) Place a patch over the left eye
B) Refer to an ophthalmologist immediately
C) Lower blood pressure acutely with IV labetalol
D) Apply timolol solution to the affected eye
E) Offer reassurance

Answer 19.13.1 The correct answer is "B." This patient is presenting with a macula-on retinal detachment, which requires urgent ophthalmology consult. She has classic symptoms of retinal detachment—flashing lights, floaters, visual field disruption, and corrugated retinal folds. The majority of her visual field, including her central vision, is still intact. In her current state, she has a high likelihood of retaining good vision if the macula remains attached. To decrease the changes of the macula detaching, patients should be on bedrest and positioned to decrease the extension of the retinal detachment toward the macula. None of the other treatments offered do anything for retinal detachment. Specifically, "A" does nothing, "C" is treatment for hypertensive emergency, "D" is for glaucoma, and "E" is just plain nuts in this case.

Question 19.13.2 Risk factors for retinal detachment include all of the following EXCEPT:
A) Glaucoma
B) Aphakia (surgical removal of the lens, such as in cataract surgery)
C) Myopia
D) Trauma
E) Prior ocular surgery

Answer 19.13.2 The correct answer is "A." Glaucoma is not a risk factor for retinal detachment. Both myopia (nearsightedness) and aphakia (surgical removal of lens) are risk factors. Trauma and previous surgery also predispose to retinal detachments. Most persons with retinal detachment are older than 50 years. As patients age, the vitreous liquefies and contracts, and this vitreoretinal traction or tugging can cause a tear, detaching the retina from the posterior wall of the eye.

▶ **Objectives: Did you learn to …**
- Suspect retinal detachment in patients presenting with "floaters" and "flashes?"
- Identify patients who are at risk for retinal detachment?

▶ **CASE 19.14**

A 55-year-old white male complains of a gradual decrease in vision in both eyes. He notes glare with oncoming headlights while night driving. Despite this, he feels that he is able to read better without his bifocals.

Question 19.14.1 Based on the history given, which of the following is the most likely cause of this patient's complaints?
A) Retinal detachment
B) Cataracts
C) Glaucoma
D) Diabetic retinopathy
E) Presbyopia

Answer 19.14.1 The correct answer is "B." Progressive visual loss and glare from oncoming headlights while driving at night are common complaints caused by cataracts. Patients may be able to read without bifocals, because cataracts cause a myopic shift and increases the power of the lens. The eye examination can confirm the diagnosis, as most significant cataracts are easily visualized. The red reflex is diminished bilaterally, and a haze of gray is observed over the lens. Symptoms of retinal detachment ("A") are more acute. Glaucoma ("C") and diabetic retinopathy ("D") are less likely but could also be present. Intraocular pressures and a dilated eye examination should be completed to adequately assess and diagnose the patient's condition.

Question 19.14.2 All of the following conditions/ medications are risk factors for cataract formation EXCEPT:
A) Corticosteroids
B) Trauma
C) Radiation
D) Calcium channel blockers
E) Diabetes mellitus

Answer 19.14.2 The correct answer is "D." All of the other choices are associated with cataract formation. Other risk factors include: age, tobacco, alcohol, myotonic dystrophy, Down syndrome, or Wilson disease. Unfortunately, despite what we have been taught, UV blocking sun glasses do not seem to help.

Question 19.14.3 Of all of the patients with cataracts below, which is the best indication for cataract surgery?
A) A patient with no visual complaints with a visual acuity of 20/50
B) A patient with complaints of glare and inability to drive at night with a visual acuity of 20/40
C) An older patient with a history of monocular congenital cataract and best-corrected visual acuity of 20/100 in that eye
D) A patient with right monocular diplopia that resolves with new spectacle correction

Answer 19.14.3 The correct answer is "B." There is no strict visual acuity that determines the appropriate timing of cataract surgery. It is really a functional definition. If there are significant lifestyle limitations secondary to visual disability from a cataract, then cataract surgery may be indicated. "C" is incorrect. An older person with a history of congenital cataracts and poor best-corrected visual acuity most likely suffered from amblyopia; therefore, cataract surgery is unlikely to benefit such a patient. "D" is incorrect. Monocular diplopia (double vision from one eye only) should be evaluated to rule out other causes such as dry eye or irregular corneal surface.

Question 19.14.4 Complications of cataract surgery include all of the following EXCEPT:
A) Endophthalmitis
B) Retinal detachment
C) Glaucoma
D) Hemorrhage
E) Meibomian gland dysfunction

Answer 19.14.4 **The correct answer is "E."** Meibomian gland dysfunction is a chronic condition as discussed previously in this chapter. Modern day cataract surgery is typically done by phacoemulsification (ultrasound fragmentation) of the cataract with implantation of an intraocular lens. Although cataract surgery techniques have been advanced over the years to become a safe surgery with relatively low risks, risks and potential complications still exist. Additional complications include: wound leaks, uveitis, macular edema, dislocation of lens, retained lens material, corneal edema, vitreous loss, and retinal detachment.

 HELPFUL TIP (AND ONE THAT MAY BE ON THE BOARDS):
One of our favorite disease names (besides "exploding head syndrome" … really, look it up) is "floppy iris syndrome." This occurs when patients on alpha-blockers (usually men for BPH) go for cataract surgery. The result is a poorly dilating iris that is irreversibly floppy and may prolapse during cataract surgery. This effect of alpha-blockers may last years after last usage, so be careful when suggesting surgery to these patients.

▶ **Objectives: Did you learn to …**
- Identify patients at risk for cataract development?
- Describe indications for cataract surgery?
- Recognize the symptoms and visual disability in those with progressive cataracts?

 QUICK QUIZ: SOMETHING ON THE EYE

A patient presents to your clinic without vision symptoms, but complains of a growth from the white onto the colored part of his eye (Fig. 19-13). The growth is painless and has been present for several years but is now getting to the point that it is pretty obvious. Strangers tend to stare. Children run the other way when they see him coming. He cries himself to sleep every night because of this.

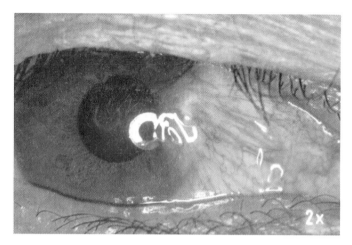
FIGURE 19-13 Pterygium. Note the fleshy, pink conjunctival tissue crosses onto the cornea.

This growth is most likely due to:
A) Systemic inflammatory illness
B) Exposure to UV light and dust
C) Foreign-body granuloma
D) Trauma to the sclera and cornea with scarring
E) Any of the above can lead to this finding

The correct answer is "B." This is a pterygium, an overgrowth of conjunctival tissue, which is a result of recurrent exposure to UV light and high winds with dust. It is of no clinical significance unless it encroaches on the visual field or causes cosmetic distress. It is characterized by involvement of the cornea nasally or temporally as opposed to a pinguecula, which has a similar appearance but does not infringe upon the cornea. Careful history taking often uncovers a patient history of outdoor lifestyle (farming, construction, boating, etc.) or whether they are snowbirds who travel south in the winter. Another name for pterygium is "surfer's eye" (really), not only because surfers are in the sun and are prone to pterygium, but it is a pretty gnarly looking growth!

 QUICK QUIZ: PAINFUL EYE

A 40-year-old patient presents with a painful, red area on the eye (Fig. 19-14). He notes the gradual onset of severe pain of a boring nature with pain in the periocular area as well. He has a history of rheumatoid arthritis.

What is the diagnosis?
A) Episcleritis
B) Pterygium
C) Scleritis
D) Pinguecula
E) Epidemic hemorrhagic conjunctivitis

The correct answer is "C." This is scleritis. Note the erythema and inflammation, which differentiates it from a pterygium. Scleritis may also be nodular in nature or diffuse. Scleritis can be easily

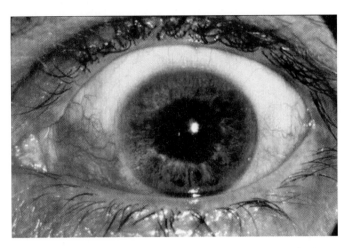

FIGURE 19-14 Scleritis. Note the sectoral inflammation of superficial conjunctival vessels and deep scleral vessels.

mistaken for episcleritis, which may appear similar. Episcleritis is inflammation of the tissues overlying the sclera, the episclera. Although the more superficial conjunctival and episcleral vessels are often inflamed as well the deeper scleral vessels, scleral vessels can be identified because they cannot be moved with a cotton tip and do not blanch with phenylephrine as conjunctival and episcleral vessels do. Another thing that differentiates episcleritis from scleritis is that patients with episcleritis do not have the severity of pain noted with scleritis. Pain of scleritis is typically boring achy pain and is worse with movement of the eye. A pinguecula ("D") appears as yellowish, slightly raised nodule(s) that is found on the conjunctiva nasal or temporal to the cornea. A pinguecula generally appears in middle age, has similar risk factors as pterygium, and removal is rarely indicated.

 HELPFUL TIP:
Episcleritis will generally resolve spontaneously or with a bit of topical steroid. **Scleritis can be serious and result in globe rupture**, and should be referred urgently.

 QUICK QUIZ: SCLERITIS

Which of the following is NOT commonly associated with scleritis?
A) Wegener granulomatosis
B) Lupus
C) Gout
D) Nephrotic syndrome
E) Rheumatoid arthritis

The correct answer is "D." Nephrotic syndrome does not generally represent ongoing inflammation. More than 50% of cases of scleritis have an associated systemic inflammatory disease such as: gout, lupus, rheumatoid arthritis, ankylosing spondylitis, or infectious etiologies such as herpes zoster, syphilis, Pseudomonas, fungi, Nocardia, or atypical mycobacteria.

 QUICK QUIZ: MY IMPLANTED LENS ISN'T WORKING

A 70-year-old female presents for a routine medical evaluation. She reports no problems, but on review of systems she states that she has had a gradual decrease in vision in the right eye over the past several months. She had successful cataract surgery of both eyes 3 years ago. After the surgery, she had 20/20 vision OU. Now on examination, her vision is OD 20/50 and OS 20/20. She has no RAPD. The slit-lamp examination of her anterior segment of both eyes reveals well-positioned bilateral posterior chamber intraocular lens (PCIOL) implants. There seems to be a hazy membrane behind her lens implant in the right eye.

The most likely diagnosis is which of the following?
A) Posterior capsular opacity
B) Endophthalmitis
C) Retinal detachment
D) Posterior uveitis
E) Intraocular lens dislocation

The correct answer is "A." Months to years after successful cataract surgery, patients may experience a gradual decline in their vision due to an opacification of the posterior capsule behind their intraocular lens implant ("secondary cataract"). During cataract surgery, most of the normal capsule of the lens remains and holds the intraocular lens implant. In successful cataract surgery, only the anterior portion of the capsule is removed. The posterior portion of this capsule may become hazy over time due to the proliferation of residual lens epithelial cells. The patient does not have any symptoms of infection or inflammation and reports no flashes or floaters that would eliminate most of the other choices. An intraocular lens dislocation is rare and is usually seen in the setting of trauma. Treatment for capsular opacification is YAG laser capsulotomy, which is a simple procedure performed in an outpatient setting at a slit lamp.

▶ **CASE 19.15**

A 56-year-old white male with a history of hypertension and diabetes complains of double vision and pain for the past 2 days. On examination, his vision is OD 20/50 and OS 20/25. He has a larger pupil with a RAPD OD. The lid of his right eye is slightly lower than the left. His right eye is deviated slightly temporally and inferiorly, and he has difficulty adducting and elevating the eye.

Question 19.15.1 **The most likely diagnosis is which of the following?**
A) Graves' disease
B) Horner syndrome
C) Third nerve palsy
D) Myasthenia gravis

Answer 19.15.1 **The correct answer is "C."** The case presented is a typical scenario of a third nerve palsy. Patients with a third nerve palsy present with diplopia (from ocular muscle paralysis), ptosis, and a dilated pupil with or without pain. Recall that the ocular muscles are innervated by CN3 except for the lateral rectus (CN6) and the superior oblique (CN4), so the eye will be "down and out" when the lateral rectus and superior oblique act unopposed in a third nerve palsy. A third nerve palsy may also present as an incomplete picture as an incomplete palsy may depend on whether the superior or inferior division of the third cranial nerve is involved. **Often the pupil is spared in diabetic patients. Pupil involvement should prompt an investigation for an intracranial aneurysm.** "A," Graves' disease, may present with motility deficits and compression of the optic nerve resulting in a RAPD. However, Graves' disease is less likely in this patient because it should present with gradual onset with lid retraction and proptosis, not ptosis. Graves' disease also may cause restriction of the medial and inferior rectus muscles, which causes difficulty abducting and elevating the eye. "B," Horner syndrome, may present with ptosis, but the affected side would have miosis (not mydriasis as in this patient), and it does not present with motility deficits. "D," myasthenia gravis, may present with fluctuating ptosis and motility deficit, but these findings are usually elicited with fatigue. The pupil is never involved in myasthenia gravis.

Question 19.15.2 The workup of this patient should involve:
A) Cerebral angiography
B) CT/CTA
C) MRI/MRA
D) Orbital ultrasonography

Answer 19.15.2 **The correct answer is "C."** Although cerebral angiography has long been the gold standard in detecting cerebral aneurysms, the first line and less invasive diagnostic test is MRI/MRA. Obtain CBC and ESR/CRP if there is concern for GCA.

▶ **Objective: Did you learn to …**
- Diagnose a third cranial nerve palsy and initiate management?

Clinical Pearls

- Always evert the eyelids in any patient who may have a foreign body in the eye.
- Do not delay urgent consultation with an ophthalmologist in a patient suspected of having a retinal detachment.
- In the case of chemical burn injuries to the eye, irrigate, irrigate, irrigate!
- The vital signs of the eye are visual acuity, pupils, and intraocular pressure. (It is similar to temperature, heart rate, blood pressure, and if you have these three pieces of information when you talk to an ophthalmologist, they will be impressed!)
- Do not prescribe antibiotics for viral conjunctivitis.
- Perform a complete and thorough ophthalmologic examination and consider imaging for any patient presenting with new onset strabismus.

- Refer patients with type 2 diabetes for dilated eye examination at initial diagnosis. Patients with type 1 diabetes should have a dilated funduscopic examination within 3 to 5 years of diagnosis.
- Proptosis and ocular hypertension associated with trauma should be immediately evaluated for possible lateral canthotomy and cantholysis.

ACKNOWLEDGMENTS

Photographs were provided by the Department of Ophthalmology, University of Iowa. Special thanks to Dr. Greenlee, Dr. James Folk, and Dr. Young Kwon for their photograph contributions.

BIBLIOGRAPHY

American Academy of Ophthalmology. *Basic and Clinical Science Course. 2017–2018*. San Francisco, CA: American Academy of Ophthalmology; 2017.

Dickersin K, et al. Surgery for nonarteritic anterior ischemic optic neuropathy. *Cochrane Database Syst Rev*. 2006;1:CD001538.

Evans JR. Antioxidant vitamin and mineral supplements for slowing the progression of age-related macular degeneration. *Cochrane Database Syst Rev*. 2006;2:CD000254.

Fingert JH. Primary open-angle glaucoma genes. *Eye (Lond)*. 2011;25(5):587–595.

Liu Y, Allingham RR. Molecular genetics in glaucoma. *Exp Eye Res*. 2011;93:331–339.

Nicholson BP, Schachat AP. A review of clinical trials of anti-VEGF agents for diabetic retinopathy. *Graefes Arch Clin Exp Ophthalmol*. 2010;248:915–930.

Ozcura F, et al. Effects of central corneal thickness, central corneal power, and axial length on intraocular pressure measurement assessed with Goldmann applanation tonometry. *Jpn J Ophthalmol*. 2008;52:353–356.

Pediatric Eye Disease Investigator Group. The clinical spectrum of early-onset esotropia: experience of the Congenital Esotropia Observational Study. *Am J Ophthalmol*. 2002;133:102–108.

Rixen J, et al. Lateral canthotomy and cantholysis. University of Iowa Department of Ophthalmological and Visual Sciences. March 12, 2013. Available at: https://webeye.ophth.uiowa.edu/eyeforum/tutorials/lateral-canthotomy-cantholysis.htm. Accessed April 22, 2019.

Sheikh A, Hurwitz B. Antibiotics versus placebo for acute bacterial conjunctivitis. *Cochrane Database Syst Rev*. 2006;2:CD001211.

Shields MB. *Textbook of Glaucoma*. 5th ed. Philadelphia, PA: Lippincott Williams & Wilkins; 2005.

Sowka J, et al. *Handbook of Ocular Disease Management*. Supplement to Review of Optometry. 19th ed. 2018. Available at: https://www.reviewofoptometry.com/CMSDocuments/2018/06/hod0618i.pdf. Accessed April 22, 2019.

Wormald R, et al. Photodynamic therapy for neovascular age-related macular degeneration. *Cochrane Database Syst Rev*. 2007;3:CD002030.

Otolaryngology

20

C. Blake Sullivan and Scott R. Owen

▶ CASE 20.1

A 2-year-old is brought to your office by her mother who is concerned that she has been pulling at her left ear since late last night and has a fever of 101.3°F. She has had recurrent bouts of these symptoms, the last of which was 9 months ago. Each time, the symptoms resolved with one "shot of medicine." She is alert and interactive. She has some evidence of mucoid discharge from her nares bilaterally.

Question 20.1.1 Each of the following findings is diagnostic of acute otitis media (AOM) EXCEPT:
A) Profuse, purulent ear discharge without other evidence of otitis externa
B) Air–fluid level behind the tympanic membrane (TM) with marked redness of the TM and poor movement with pneumatic otoscopy
C) Bulging, thickened yellow, and red TM that does not move well with pneumatic otoscopy
D) Bubbles in fluid behind the TM with impaired mobility of the TM on pneumatic otoscopy
E) Yellow, opaque TM, poor movement with pneumatic otoscopy, and substantial ear pain

Answer 20.1.1 **The correct answer is "D."** Suspected ear infections drive many parents to bring their children to a family physician. There may be fluid in the middle ear that is not infected (otitis media with effusion [OME]). In order to diagnose AOM, you need evidence of fluid in the middle ear **and** inflammation, and the symptoms should be acute (starting in the last few days and lasting less than 3 weeks). A middle ear effusion is diagnosed by bubbles and/or air–fluid level behind the TM OR **two or more of the following:** decreased or absent TM movement with pneumatic otoscopy, opacification of the TM, and discoloration of the TM (yellow, white, blue). These findings describe OME, but not AOM. To diagnose AOM, you will need to meet criteria for OME with evidence of acute inflammation such as: marked pain, thickened and/or bulging TM, and erythematous TM. For these reasons, "B," "C," and "E" are examples of AOM.

"A," purulent otorrhea without evidence of otitis externa, would be the one exception where you can diagnose AOM without even seeing the TM. "D" describes OME without inflammation.

HELPFUL TIP:
Don't believe a red eardrum. By itself, erythema of the TM has a 15% positive predictive value for diagnosing AOM. **Use pneumatic otoscopy,** which is the standard of care for diagnosing AOM. **Tympanometry** (testing volume of middle ear and mobility of TM) is an alternative to pneumatic otoscopy. Of course, you still need to look in the ear.

Your patient's left TM is opaque, erythematous, and immobile upon pneumatic otoscopy.

Question 20.1.2 Each of the following factors increases her risk for developing otitis media EXCEPT:
A) She attends day care
B) Her mother smokes inside the house
C) The patient is a female
D) Patient still uses a pacifier
E) She was exclusively breastfed as an infant

Answer 20.1.2 **The correct answer is "C."** The following are known risk factors for the development of AOM: day care attendance, smoking inside the home, **male gender**, pacifier use, children in developing countries, age between 6 and 18 months, lack of breastfeeding, and going to bed with a bottle.

Question 20.1.3 Which of the following findings is reliably found in patients with AOM?
A) Fever
B) Ear pulling
C) Irritability
D) Rhinitis
E) None of the above

Answer 20.1.3 **The correct answer is "E."** None of the above is reliably found in patients with AOM. Other unreliable factors include vomiting, diarrhea, and cough. The presence or absence of any of these findings is **NOT** helpful in making the diagnosis of otitis media. Note that while ear pain is a symptom of inflammation, it is a relatively weak predictor of AOM and must be accompanied by other findings as listed previously. However, **pneumatic otoscopy or otoscopy plus tympanometry is the way to make the diagnosis**; but always make sure that you have a good seal or you run the risk of a "false-positive" finding.

HELPFUL TIP:
All children <6 months of age with otitis media should be treated with antibiotics. Patients from 6 months to 2 years should receive antibiotics if **the diagnosis is suspected and the patient meets high-risk criteria** (moderate-to-severe ear pain, fever >39°C, immunosuppressed). In patients 6 months to 2 years, observation is an option if they meet low-risk criteria (fever <39°C, mild otalgia, immunocompetent, unilateral AOM, parental education, and shared-decision provided **and** follow-up assured within 48–72 hours). Patients with proven AOM who are older than 2 years may be observed rather than treated with antibiotics as long as they meet low-risk criteria. Analgesics should be given to all patients. There's also the option of providing a "backup" antibiotic prescription (endorsed by the American Academy of Pediatrics) for the patient to start if the symptoms are persisting longer than 2 to 3 days.

This patient has not had any problems with otitis media for at least 9 months, has not been on antibiotics during that time, is not in day care, and has no allergies. You opt to treat her with an antibiotic.

Question 20.1.4 **What is the most appropriate treatment for this patient?**
A) Amoxicillin 40 mg/kg/day divided TID
B) Amoxicillin 80 to 90 mg/kg/day divided BID
C) Ceftriaxone 50 mg/kg IM once
D) Azithromycin 10 mg/kg for 1 day then 5 mg/kg for days 2 to 5
E) Amoxicillin/clavulanate 40 to 80 mg/kg/day divided BID

Answer 20.1.4 **The correct answer is "B."** Amoxicillin is the first-line treatment of AOM. The dose is 80 to 90 mg/kg/day in all patients whether antibiotic-naive or not. More broad-spectrum drugs such as ceftriaxone and amoxicillin/clavulanate should be reserved for patients who fail initial therapy with a first-line drug or have a penicillin allergy.

HELPFUL TIP:
Remember that you can treat children older than 6 years with a 5-day course of amoxicillin. Amoxicillin/

clavulanate should be reserved for treatment failures. Cefdinir, cefuroxime, or clindamycin are backups in case of penicillin allergy.

HELPFUL TIP:
No antibiotic has been proven superior to amoxicillin in the treatment of otitis media. Other antibiotics will work but are more expensive and/or have greater side effects. This is likely secondary to the fact that most OM is viral and will get better regardless of what we do.

Question 20.1.5 **Which of the following statements best characterizes the role of antibiotics in the treatment of AOM?**
A) Antibiotics have been shown to reduce suppurative complications of AOM, such as mastoiditis, in developed countries.
B) The majority of patients with AOM benefit from the use of antibiotics.
C) The use of antibiotics for AOM reduces hearing loss and benefits language development.
D) With or without antibiotics, about 75% of children have resolution of AOM symptoms after 7 days.
E) All of the above are true.

Answer 20.1.5 **The correct answer is "D."** The benefit of antibiotics for most children with AOM is marginal and the number needed to treat (NNT) is about 12; thus, the option exists to observe and not even give antibiotics in children ≥2 years who have mild symptoms, are immunocompetent, and have good follow-up (and, as stated above, observation can even be extended to kids as young as 6 months). The rest of the statements are incorrect. Antibiotics do **not** reduce suppurative complications in **developed** countries, but they do seem to prevent suppurative complications in developing countries where sanitation and healthcare access are not optimal. "B" is incorrect. The benefit is limited to a 5% absolute reduction in those who have pain at days 2 to 3 (11.6% without antibiotics vs. 15.9% with antibiotics). "C" is incorrect as well, since treating with antibiotics does not impact these outcomes in any way.

HELPFUL TIP:
AOM is usually caused by *Streptococcus pneumoniae*, *Haemophilus influenzae*, *Moraxella catarrhalis*, and various viruses. Most are viral, and the majority of cases—bacterial or viral—will resolve spontaneously.

You prescribe amoxicillin for 10 days and suggest acetaminophen for comfort. A few days later, the patient's mother calls to say that she is no better. You ask her to come in to clinic for evaluation.

Question 20.1.6 When treating AOM, which of these individuals should be considered a treatment failure and switched to another antibiotic?

A) A patient with a fever that continues at 24 hours after starting an oral antibiotic
B) A child who is still tugging at his ear 5 days into a course of antibiotics
C) A symptomatic child who still has a bulging, erythematous, immobile TM 3 days after starting antibiotics
D) A child who continues to have rhinorrhea 1 week after starting antibiotics
E) All of the above

Answer 20.1.6 **The correct answer is "C."** You should consider switching to a different antibiotic in patients who remain symptomatic at 3 days **and who continue to have positive findings on pneumatic otoscopy**. Symptoms are not enough; they are unreliable. Remember, since most of these are viral infections, you are not doing a whole lot of good with your antibiotics anyway. "A" is incorrect because 24 hours is not sufficient to determine if a particular antibiotic will be effective. "B" is incorrect because children pull at their ears for a number of reasons besides AOM (such as "Ha! I just discovered I have ears!"). "D" is incorrect. If you chose this one, back to Microbiology 101 for you! Rhinorrhea does not respond to antibiotics and is most likely not bacterial in origin.

HELPFUL TIP:
For treatment failures, amoxicillin/clavulanate is recommended by the AAFP and AAP. Other options include: cefdinir, cefpodoxime, ceftriaxone, and cefuroxime. Macrolides and TMP/SMX are less effective as second-line therapy because of bacterial resistance (this includes the ever-popular azithromycin, folks). Remember the number needed to harm is about 8 with amoxicillin/clavulanate; the diarrhea and resultant diaper rash are often more distressing than the otitis.

She returns with persistent pain and fever after taking amoxicillin for 3 days. On examination, you find evidence of persistent AOM. You switch the patient to your favorite second-line antibiotic. You see her back in 2 weeks for an ear check and find complete resolution. The mother asks what she could do to avoid these troublesome infections in the future.

Question 20.1.7 All of the following have been shown to reduce the incidence of recurrent otitis media EXCEPT:

A) Antibiotic prophylaxis
B) Conjugate pneumococcal vaccine
C) Tympanostomy tubes
D) Tonsillectomy
E) Influenza vaccine

Answer 20.1.7 **The correct answer is "D."** Primary tonsillectomy has not been shown to reduce the recurrence of otitis media. However, *adenoidectomy* (due to obstruction of the Eustachian tube, or harboring otitis-causing bacteria) with or without tonsillectomy may reduce the rate of recurrent otitis media in patients *who already have tympanostomy tubes*. "A," the use of antibiotic prophylaxis, will reduce recurrent otitis media. Antibiotic prophylaxis should be considered in the patient who has had ≥3 episodes of otitis media in 6 months or ≥4 episodes in 12 months. Reasonable choices for antibiotics include amoxicillin and trimethoprim/sulfamethoxazole. Give half of the usual daily dose. This is generally given at bedtime. Often, antibiotics can be stopped during the summer since an upper respiratory infection (URI) is the precipitant of most cases of otitis media. Pneumococcal vaccine (e.g., Prevnar) will reduce the risk of recurrence in children with severe and recurrent AOM. The same is true of influenza vaccine. Also recommended to reduce the frequency of AOM: avoid pacifier use, avoid bottle propping at night, avoid smoke exposure, and encourage breast feeding for at least the first 6 months of life.

HELPFUL TIP:
Although it is traditionally done, there is no reason to follow up AOM in patients >15 months of age who are asymptomatic. Clearly, if they are still symptomatic, follow-up is warranted.

HELPFUL TIP:
Adding Cortisporin **suspension** (the solution burns) or ciprofloxacin otic suspension is appropriate if there is AOM with a ruptured TM (manifested by purulent ear drainage). Other antibiotic/steroid combination drops (e.g., Ciprodex) can be used as well but are more expensive. No … Cortisporin won't cause hearing loss.

The patient returns 4 weeks later with the mother saying, "She is still pulling at her left ear." There are no other complaints. On examination, you find the left TM is without erythema or opacity but there is still a fluid level. The right ear examination is unremarkable.

Question 20.1.8 What is your next diagnostic step?

A) Pneumatic otoscopy
B) Hearing test
C) Tympanostomy
D) No further diagnosis needed—treat with antibiotic

Answer 20.1.8 **The correct answer is "A."** Even though we all think we can do it well, the diagnosis of otitis media is fraught with problems. Pneumatic otoscopy should be done in essentially all patients but especially in those in whom long-term therapy is being considered. Remember that fluid can persist for a month or more after an otitis media.

On your examination, the TM does not move with insufflation. The patient's mother asks you if the child should have tubes placed.

Question 20.1.9 Which of the following is NOT a criterion for tympanostomy tubes?
A) Chronic bilateral effusions for more than 3 months with unilateral hearing loss
B) Failure of antibiotic therapy to prevent recurrent otitis media
C) Language delay secondary to otitis media
D) Greater than 20 dB hearing loss bilaterally

Answer 20.1.9 The correct answer is "A." Patients should meet the criteria listed above before being considered for tympanostomy tubes. Note that this requires that patients **also** meet the criteria for prophylactic antibiotic therapy (≥3 episodes of AOM in 6 months or ≥4 episodes in 12 months). A modification of "A" is also a criterion: chronic bilateral effusions for more than 3 months with **bilateral** hearing loss. Although included as a criterion, there is no evidence that tympanostomy tubes improve language development in the short or long term.

....

If fluid persists in the middle ear after AOM, it is termed "otitis media with effusion," (OME) aka "serous otitis media."

Question 20.1.10 Which of the following interventions has proven benefit in patients with OME?
A) Oral decongestants
B) Oral antihistamines
C) Prolonged treatment (≥1 month) with oral antibiotics
D) Oral corticosteroids
E) None of the above

Answer 20.1.10 The correct answer is "E." For persistent OME (the most common cause of pediatric hearing loss), there are no useful medical interventions. Autoinflation ("Eustachian tube exercises" or forced exhalation with closed nose and mouth) is often recommended, but has not shown a benefit (and try explaining how to do this to a 6-month-old). Patients may benefit from surgical intervention with tympanostomy tube placement ... and then there's always the good, old-fashioned "tincture of time."

▶ **Objectives: Did you learn to ...**
   · Diagnose otitis media appropriately?
   · Initiate treatment in a patient with otitis media?
   · Recognize failed antibiotic therapy and choose a new antibiotic for otitis media?
   · Describe prevention strategies for recurrent otitis media?
   · Recognize indications for tympanostomy tube placement?

 QUICK QUIZ: EAR PAIN

Which of the following can cause ear pain?
A) Temporomandibular joint (TMJ) syndrome
B) Cervical spine degenerative arthritis
C) Cranial nerve lesions (5, 7, 9, or 10)
D) Bell's palsy
E) All of the above can cause ear pain

The correct answer is "E." All of the above can cause ear pain. A more complete list is given in Table 20-1. The main point here is that not all ear pain is otitis media—or even originating from the ear.

▶ **CASE 20.2**

A 23-year-old female college student presents to your clinic complaining of ear pain. She is on the swimming team and notes that this pain occurs during swimming season. The pain is increased by motion of the pinnae. The external auditory canal is erythematous, edematous, and exquisitely tender when you try to use the otoscope to examine her TM. There is whitish debris in the external auditory canal.

Question 20.2.1 The most likely organism involved in this patient's disease is:
A) *Streptococcus*
B) *Haemophilus*
C) *Moraxella*
D) *Pseudomonas*
E) *Parainfluenza*

Answer 20.2.1 The correct answer is "D." This patient likely has otitis externa. The most common pathogenic organism isolated in cases of otitis externa is *Pseudomonas* (20–60%) followed closely by *Staphylococcus aureus*. However, up to one-third of cases of otitis externa are polymicrobial.

Question 20.2.2 Which of the following is/are considered first-line treatment for otitis externa?
A) Oral ciprofloxacin
B) Acetic acid ear drops
C) Polymyxin and neomycin combination ear drops
D) A and C
E) B and C

TABLE 20-1 CAUSES OF EAR PAIN
- Auricular disease
- Canal disease
  - Otitis externa
  - Foreign body
  - Trauma
  - Eczema
  - Ramsay–Hunt syndrome
- Middle ear disease
  - Otitis media
  - Mastoiditis
  - Ménière disease
- Referred pain
  - Dental disease (e.g., abscess)
  - Temporomandibular joint syndrome
  - Carotidynia
  - Pharyngeal disease (e.g., pharyngitis)
  - Cranial nerve lesions (CN V, VII, IX, X)
  - Upper cervical nerve disease, any causes (e.g., disk disease)
  - Bell's palsy and other neurologic diseases (e.g., trigeminal neuralgia)

Answer 20.2.2 The correct answer is "E." Otitis externa can be treated with a wide array of topical agents. One option is to acidify the external ear canal. Neither *Pseudomonas* nor *Staphylococcus* species can thrive at an acidic pH. Thus, acetic acid drops (e.g., VoSol®) can be used: they are cheap and effective. Another approach is to use a topical antibiotic. Polymyxin/neomycin combinations (e.g., Cortisporin) are safe and effective. A number of other antibiotic preparations are available as well. Alcohol-based solutions are another alternative. "A" is incorrect because oral treatment is not indicated for simple otitis externa. However, topical ciprofloxacin may be used but is more expensive. Avoid aminoglycoside drops in patients with tympanostomy tubes due to risk of ototoxicity.

HELPFUL TIP:
There are a number of much more expensive treatments for otitis externa on the market, including fluoroquinolone otic drops. These have no advantage and are very expensive. In fact, there is no treatment advantage to using antibiotics at all. Topical drying agents, alcohols and acetic acid, have just as good an outcome as antibiotics.

Question 20.2.3 This patient is concerned about recurrences of her otitis externa. What advice can you give her?
A) Avoid exposure by putting a petroleum jelly (e.g., Vaseline) impregnated cotton plug in her ear before swimming
B) Use a blow dryer on her ear after swimming
C) Instill a 50/50 mixture of alcohol and vinegar in her ears after swimming
D) Avoid swimming when she has active disease
E) All of the above

Answer 20.2.3 The correct answer is "E." All of the above can be used to minimize disease recurrence. The benefit of "C" is less certain.

HELPFUL TIP:
Remember that **necrotizing (malignant) otitis externa** is a different creature altogether that occurs primarily in diabetic patients, but also in those with HIV and other immunosuppressing diseases/meds. It is an invasive pseudomonal (95%) cellulitis that causes erythema and tenderness around the ear. Complications include osteomyelitis, meningitis, abscess formation, and cranial nerve palsies. It is a true emergency requiring IV antibiotics and surgical consultation.

You treat the patient with neomycin/polymyxin drops, and the symptoms persist and possibly worsen a little after 5 days. The patient has no fever and no signs of cellulitis around the ear.

Question 20.2.4 Of the following possibilities, which is the LEAST likely to explain her persistent symptoms?
A) Resistant organisms
B) Noncompliance with medical recommendations
C) Misdiagnosis of otomycosis
D) Development of contact dermatitis

Answer 20.2.4 The correct answer is "A." Several things could explain her persistent symptoms. First, the patient should be questioned regarding compliance. Is she still swimming despite advice to the contrary? Is she using the drops at least TID and letting them soak into her ear? Another issue is the development of an allergic reaction, especially in response to neomycin (up to 35% of patients treated chronically with topical neomycin develop a dermatitis). Patients may also "fail" treatment for otitis externa due to misdiagnosis. Otomycosis, a fungal infection of the auditory canal, causes erythema, discharge, itching, and sometimes pain. With respect to "A," treatment failures due to antibiotic resistance are uncommon, and as noted above, antibiotics are not even necessary in the treatment of most cases of otitis externa.

On examination, you notice fine, white, cotton-like fibers filling the ear canal along with the other debris. The examination is otherwise unchanged.

Question 20.2.5 What is your next step?
A) Admit for intravenous (IV) antibiotic and antifungal therapy
B) Clean the ear canal under direct otoscopy and add oral amoxicillin/clavulanate to her medication regimen
C) Clean the ear canal under direct otoscopy and add topical clotrimazole 1% to her medication regimen
D) Order CT or MRI of the head and neck to rule out abscess
E) Refer to an otolaryngologist

Answer 20.2.5 The correct answer is "C." On examination, you have identified signs of otomycosis. It could be that the otomycosis was present initially or developed in the interval with antibiotic administration. Otomycosis is usually due to *Aspergillosis; Candida* only represents 10% to 20% of cases. Thorough debridement of the external ear canal is an important part of therapy. A topical antifungal that is active against *Aspergillosis* is recommended (e.g., clotrimazole, miconazole, and nystatin).

HELPFUL TIP:
Ear wicks can be a helpful tool to aide in delivery of medication and to prevent canal stenosis, but they must be removed/changed 3 to 5 days after placement.

▶ **Objectives: Did you learn to …**
· Identify bacterial pathogens implicated in otitis externa?
· Diagnose and treat a patient with otitis externa?
· Recommend prevention strategies for otitis externa?
· Determine why treatment for otitis externa may fail?

▶ CASE 20.3

A 59-year-old male presents with a 3-week history of hoarseness. He denies sore throat or heartburn. He has had no fevers, night sweats, or weight loss. When he initially presented a week ago, your partner treated him empirically for postnasal drainage. He smokes two packs of cigarettes per day and drinks alcohol daily. On examination, his vital signs are normal. His voice sounds husky. You find no other abnormalities (besides the burn holes in his shirt and the pint of whisky in his back pocket).

Question 20.3.1 The best next step in the management of this patient is:
A) Empiric antibiotic treatment
B) Empiric proton pump inhibitor treatment
C) Laryngoscopy
D) Esophagogastroduodenoscopy (EGD)
E) Neck MRI

Answer 20.3.1 The correct answer is "C." The first concern is to rule out malignancy, and a thorough head-and-neck examination is warranted. Laryngoscopy is a straightforward office procedure frequently performed within a few minutes using a flexible laryngoscope or mirror. If the equipment and expertise are not available in your office, the patient should be referred to an otolaryngologist. Although there are no firm guidelines, some authors recommend laryngoscopy after 2 weeks of hoarseness in patients who are at risk (older patients and those who have a history of tobacco and alcohol use). Since laryngoscopy is such an available, low-cost, low-risk procedure, it is hard to justify postponing it for any patient at risk for malignancy. Therefore, "A" and "B" are incorrect, as further empiric medication trials will only delay laryngoscopy. Besides, antibiotics are not indicated for the lone symptom of hoarseness. In other instances (e.g., low-risk patient with heartburn and hoarseness), empiric proton pump inhibitor therapy may be more practical, since gastroesophageal reflux is a common cause of hoarseness. "D" is incorrect. In this case, laryngoscopy is preferred to EGD. Finally, "E" is incorrect. Neck MRI is not indicated in the initial evaluation of hoarseness, but it might be used for follow-up after laryngoscopy or to investigate a neck mass.

Question 20.3.2 All of the following are potential causes of hoarseness EXCEPT:
A) Vocal cord mass
B) Infectious laryngitis
C) Hypothyroidism
D) Lung malignancy
E) A vow of silence

Answer 20.3.2 The correct answer is "E." Far from being a cause of hoarseness, voice rest is often recommended for patients with hoarseness due to overuse (e.g., singers). All of the other options are known to cause hoarseness. Of particular note is "C": hypothyroidism can result in an accumulation of connective tissue

elements, basically myxedema, in the vocal cords. Intrathoracic processes such as lung cancer can present with hoarseness (see "Helpful Tip" below).

Characterizing the nature of the patient's hoarseness can narrow the differential diagnosis. The voice changes may be further characterized as breathy, low-pitched, strained, tremulous, or hoarse. A "breathy" voice may be seen with vocal cord paralysis, abductor spasm, or functional dysphonia. "Low-pitched" voice changes might be due to edema (seen in smokers), vocal abuse, reflux laryngitis, vocal cord paralysis, or muscle tension dysphonia. A "strained" voice may occur with adductor spasm, muscle tension dysphonia, or reflux laryngitis. A "tremulous" voice occurs in parkinsonism, essential tremor, spasmodic dysphonia, or muscle tension dysphonia. A "hoarse" voice may be due to vocal cord lesions, muscle tension dysphonia, and reflux laryngitis. Vocal fatigue (loss of volume over time) may also be noted (especially during presidential campaigns) and is often caused by muscle tension dysphonia, vocal cord paralysis, reflux laryngitis, or vocal abuse. However, one cannot eliminate a cause of hoarseness based on these characteristics.

HELPFUL TIP:
The intrinsic muscles of the larynx (the muscles that make the vocal cords move) are innervated by the recurrent laryngeal nerve, a branch of the vagus nerve (cranial nerve X). The cricopharyngeus muscle, essential to changing vocal pitch (i.e., necessary for singing), is the exception as this is innervated by the superior laryngeal nerve (another branch of CN X). The superior laryngeal nerve also provides sensation to the glottis. In addition to being fun and interesting medical trivia, knowing the innervation of the laryngeal muscles is important because chest malignancy, aneurysms, complications of thoracic surgery, etc., can potentially present with hoarseness.

On laryngoscopy, you notice a mass lesion on the right vocal cord. You refer the patient to an otolaryngologist. The patient asks if you think that the mass is cancer. Because you are compassionate and also not entirely certain, you avoid saying, "Oh, heck yeah. That's cancer all right." You try to be more optimistic.

Question 20.3.3 However, you want to remind him of risk factors for laryngeal cancer, which include all of the following EXCEPT:
A) Tobacco smoking
B) Alcohol use
C) Epstein–Barr virus (EBV)
D) Family history of head-and-neck cancers
E) Male sex

Answer 20.3.3 The correct answer is "C." EBV infection is associated with the development of nasopharyngeal cancer, not laryngeal cancer. Additionally, EBV infection has been associated with Burkitt lymphoma (children in Africa), Hodgkin disease, and non-Hodgkin lymphoma. Tobacco and alcohol use are independent risk factors for the development of most types of head-and-neck cancers (oral, laryngeal, etc.), and the two substances may act synergistically in the promotion of these cancers. A family history of head-and-neck cancer has a weaker association, but the association is still present. Males are two to four times more likely to have head-and-neck cancers compared with females. These risk factors sound a lot like our patient.

Question 20.3.4 If this patient is found to have cancer, what pathologic variant is most likely?
A) Adenocarcinoma
B) Squamous cell carcinoma
C) Schneiderian papilloma
D) Neuroblastoma

Answer 20.3.4 **The correct answer is "B."** Upon pathologic examination, the great majority of head-and-neck cancers are found to be squamous cell carcinomas. Adenocarcinoma may arise from the gastrointestinal tract and could be seen on laryngoscopy but would rarely occur on the vocal cords. Schneiderian papillomas ("C") are polyps that arise from the nasal and sinus mucosae, are associated with HPV, and may transform into carcinomas. Neuroblastomas ("D"), which arise from the sympathetic nervous system, rarely occur in the head-and-neck region.

During your examination of the oral cavity, you also encountered a small, white, indurated plaque on the lateral and ventral surfaces of the tongue. The plaque was not able to be scraped off with a tongue blade (see Fig. 20-1).

Question 20.3.5 This lesion is most appropriately described as:
A) Squamous cell carcinoma
B) *Candida albicans*
C) Leukoplakia
D) Geographic tongue
E) Aphthous ulcer

Answer 20.3.5 **The correct answer is "C."** Primary leukoplakia is a premalignant lesion of the oral cavity and oropharynx (about 10–30% will progress to cancer over 10 years). It occurs in response to trauma and/or exposure to irritants and carcinogens, having an especially strong association with smokeless tobacco (e.g., "snuff," "chew") use. In fact, the lesion **could** be squamous cell carcinoma ("A"), and it should be biopsied. However, it would be premature to diagnose the patient with squamous cell carcinoma, and the lesion is more accurately described as leukoplakia. "B," *C. albicans* lesions, may look just like leukoplakia (white plaques on oral mucosa with an erythematous base and bleeding once scraped), but you should be able to scrape the plaques off with a tongue blade (although thrush can be remarkably adherent and may cause some bleeding). A trial of antifungal therapy may be appropriate if the lesion is low-risk and you suspect thrush but cannot scrape it

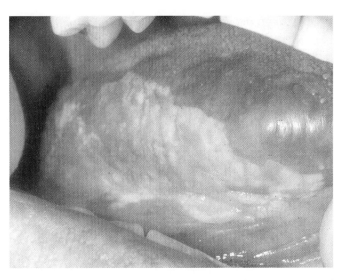

FIGURE 20-1. From Usatine RP et al., eds. *Color Atlas of Family Medicine*. 2nd ed. New York: McGraw-Hill; 2013. Courtesy of Richard P. Usatine, MD.

off; but the patient needs close follow-up for serial monitoring. "D," geographic tongue, is so named because of the meandering white-bordered patches that occur on the dorsum of the tongue. It is most often asymptomatic, and the lesions vary in shape (or completely resolve) over time. Finally, "E," an aphthous ulcer, is just that—an ulcer, not a plaque. You should not confuse leukoplakia for an aphthous ulcer.

HELPFUL TIP:
No interventions have been shown to be useful in promoting the regression of leukoplakia.

HELPFUL TIP:
Increasingly, a history of human papilloma virus (HPV) infection is being recognized in oropharyngeal cancers (tonsils and base of tongue). As much as 70% of these cancers, usually squamous cell carcinomas, may be caused by HPV infection. HPV type 16 and 18 carries the strongest association with head-and-neck cancers and are covered by modern vaccines. These tumors generally present in younger patients without common risk factors for head-and-neck cancer (heavy tobacco/alcohol use), typically as a neck mass and possible tonsil/tongue base ulcer. HPV vaccination is expected to reduce the incidence of oropharyngeal cancers in future generations—just one more reason to call the HPV vaccine an "anticancer" vaccine and not a "safer sex" vaccine.

You receive a letter from the otolaryngologist stating the patient does indeed have squamous cell carcinoma of the larynx. The patient will be seen in consultation with an oncologist and presented at tumor board. His treatment may consist of surgery, chemotherapy, and/or radiation. Unfortunately, he lost the roll of the cosmic dice.

▶ **Objectives: Did you learn to ...**
  - Generate a differential diagnosis for hoarseness of voice?
  - Evaluate a patient with a voice complaint?
  - Identify oral lesions, particularly leukoplakia?
  - Recognize important issues in the prevention and treatment of head-and-neck cancers?

▶ **CASE 20.4**

A 61-year-old man presents to your office complaining that over the past few months he cannot seem to understand what people are saying when they are standing to his left side. He also has episodes of "dizziness," that last hours, unchanged with position change. He denies nausea and vomiting. He worked for 30 years in a factory and has had bilateral tinnitus for the last 10 years. He has had no previous hearing problems or evaluation. His past medical history is significant for CAD and hypertension. He takes atenolol, atorvastatin, chlorthalidone, and aspirin. There is no family history of ear disease. On examination, both ears are normal in appearance. Weber test is best heard by the patient on his right side (remember that his hearing loss is on the left). Rinne test on both sides was negative (air conduction was greater than bone conduction).

Question 20.4.1 These findings are consistent with which type of hearing loss on the *left*?
A) Conductive
B) Sensorineural
C) Mixed
D) Selective
E) Unable to tell

Answer 20.4.1 The correct answer is "B." Hearing can be assessed in the office using the Weber and Rinne tests. The Weber test is performed by putting the tuning fork on the forehead and seeing if the sound lateralizes to one side or the other. In conductive hearing loss ("A"), the sound will be **louder** (i.e., the test will lateralize) to the "bad" side (e.g., the side with wax occluding the canal, middle ear effusion, otosclerosis). However, in sensorineural hearing loss, the sound will lateralize to the "good" side (e.g., the side not affected by a hearing problem).

The Rinne test is performed by comparing bone conduction (on the mastoid) to air conduction. Patients will notice poor air conduction versus bone conduction if there is a conductive hearing loss. Normal Rinne tests in both ears suggest that neither ear has **conductive** loss. Our patient (or more likely his family) complains about decreased hearing on the **left** and the Weber test lateralizes to the **right**, and these findings point to a problem with sensorineural hearing loss in the **left** ear.

Question 20.4.2 Which of the following is LEAST likely to be responsible for this patient's hearing loss?
A) Ménière disease
B) Vestibular schwannoma (acoustic neuroma)
C) Presbycusis

D) Otosclerosis
E) Noise exposure

Answer 20.4.2 The correct answer is "D." Otosclerosis is a bony remodeling that involves the stapes and leads to a **conductive** loss. Your patient has a sensorineural hearing loss. Ménière disease ("A") presents with the classic triad of fluctuating low-frequency hearing loss, tinnitus, and vertigo. These manifestations may be temporally separated with hearing loss, tinnitus, and vertigo occurring at different times. Patients with Ménière disease will note aural fullness, which resolves with the onset of vertigo. Typically, the vertigo will last for minutes (at least 20 minutes by definition) to hours. "B" is true. Sensorineural hearing loss can also be caused by a vestibular schwannoma (a benign tumor that arises from cranial nerve VIII), and symptoms include unilateral hearing loss, tinnitus, imbalance, and vertigo. "C," presbycusis, is one of the most common causes of sensorineural hearing loss and is often thought of as the "normal" age-related hearing loss. Presbycusis manifests as an inability to hear high frequencies. This leads to problems with speech discrimination, especially in noisy environments. It is typically symmetrical and may be associated with tinnitus. However, it may be unilateral, especially in those who have one ear turned toward noisy equipment in their job (e.g., farmers driving tractors and having one ear closer to the engine, hunters with one ear cocked toward the gun). See Table 20-2 for some causes of conductive and sensorineural hearing loss.

Question 20.4.3 What is the next step in the evaluation of this patient?
A) Audiogram
B) Brainstem evoked responses
C) MRI
D) Tympanogram

Answer 20.4.3 The correct answer is "A." An audiogram can further define the air versus bone conductance relationship, word understanding scores, and define the frequency pattern of hearing loss. Brainstem-evoked responses evaluate the neural pathways of hearing and, along with MRI, could be useful if a tumor or retrocochlear lesion was suspected. A tympanogram,

TABLE 20-2 CAUSES OF CONDUCTIVE AND SENSORINEURAL HEARING LOSS

Conductive Hearing Loss	Sensorineural Hearing Loss
Trauma: ossicle disruption, TM perforation	Presbycusis
Cerumen in the canal	Ménière disease
Otosclerosis	
Barotrauma	Stroke
Otitis media	Tumor (e.g., acoustic neuroma)
Middle ear effusion	Infection (e.g., syphilis, CMV, etc.)

which evaluates mobility of the TM, might be useful if a conductive hearing loss were suspected.

HELPFUL TIP:
Brainstem-evoked potentials measure how long it takes an auditory signal to reach the brain stem. If a vestibular schwannoma (acoustic neuroma) is present, the brainstem-evoked potential will be prolonged. However, the false-negative rate is up to 30%, and brainstem-evoked potentials have been all but replaced by high-resolution MRI in the diagnosis of vestibular schwannoma.

The audiogram confirms sensorineural hearing loss in the left ear. Because of the associated symptoms of vertigo, you order an MRI brain to rule out a vestibular schwannoma, and the results are negative. The patient continues to have episodes of vertigo, and the hearing loss on his left side persists. When probed further, he does in fact have an increase in tinnitus during his vertiginous episodes.

Question 20.4.4 You should consider all of the following treatments for this condition EXCEPT:
A) Salt, caffeine, and tobacco restriction
B) Diuretics (e.g., hydrochlorothiazide)
C) Intracochlear injection of gentamicin
D) Labyrinthectomy or endolymphatic sac shunt
E) H₂-blockers (e.g., cimetidine)

Answer 20.4.4 **The correct answer is "E."** The clinical picture now looks most like Ménière disease—a disease for which only symptom control is possible. Luckily not all patients with Ménière disease will experience worsening of their condition over time, and up to 90% are able to maintain normal daily activities with optimal medical management. Few patients progress to debilitating disease. The mainstays of therapy include diet/lifestyle modification and diuretics. Outside the United States, betahistine, an **H₁-blocker**, is commonly used (to theoretically reduce endolymphatic hydrops), but H₂-blockers have no role in therapy. A more aggressive approach is indicated in patients with more severe disease, and this might include intracochlear gentamicin (to kill the nerve and reduce vertigo), labyrinthectomy, vestibular neurectomy, or endolymphatic sac shunt.

HELPFUL TIP:
Treating Ménière disease can be problematic. Studies of this condition are frequently of poor quality with a significant placebo effect (including the studies of diuretics and betahistine). This, along with spontaneous remissions and exacerbations, limits the usefulness of data about treatment.

HELPFUL TIP:
Things to remember about tinnitus: It can be caused by a number of medications including NSAIDs, calcium

channel blockers, diuretics, etc. It can rarely be caused by a vascular lesion (bruits, A-V shunts, etc.). Other causes include TMJ syndrome, Eustachian tube dysfunction, and—most commonly—sensorineural hearing loss (especially presbycusis).

▶ **Objectives: Did you learn to …**
· Evaluate a patient with hearing loss?
· Describe differences between conductive and sensorineural hearing loss?
· Generate a differential diagnosis for hearing loss?
· Diagnose and treat a patient with Ménière disease?

 QUICK QUIZ: PERIPHARYNGEAL INFECTION

A 7-year-old female is brought to your office by her concerned parents. Over the last 24 hours, the patient has developed pain in her mouth, drooling, and fever. She refuses to eat. On examination, she is febrile and slightly tachycardic. The sublingual, submandibular, and submental spaces are swollen, tender, and are "woody" bilaterally. The tongue is elevated in the mouth. There are no ulcerations. Her respirations are normal, and her lung sounds are clear.

What is the next step in the evaluation and management of this patient?
A) Reassurance, oral rehydration, and analgesics
B) Oral antibiotics
C) MRI of the head and neck
D) IV antibiotics
E) Intubation and mechanical ventilation

The correct answer is "D." This patient is presenting with classic signs and symptoms of Ludwig's angina (related neither to angina nor to Ludwig von Beethoven). These include brawny edema, tenderness, and warmth in the submandibular region along with elevation of the tongue. Ludwig's angina is a rare cellulitis of the bilateral submandibular, sublingual, and submental spaces. The most common cause is from an abscessed tooth, but may also occur from a piercing, mandible fracture or salivary stone. **The status of the patient's airway needs urgent attention** as the infection of the submandibular space may rapidly spread to the parapharyngeal space resulting in airway compromise. Consideration of emergent intubation is important, but this patient is stable, and her airway appears patent; therefore, "E" is incorrect. Even so, patients should be monitored closely for airway issues. "A" and "B" are incorrect because patients with Ludwig's angina may experience rapid progression of symptoms and should be treated with IV antibiotics and admitted to the hospital. Finally, "C" is incorrect because Ludwig's angina is a clinical diagnosis. Also, MRI may delay antibiotic treatment and is unlikely to be of any value, unless you suspect the presence of an abscess, but even then, CT would be the examination of choice. Surgical intervention may be necessary.

HELPFUL TIP:
Trismus is usually absent in Ludwig's angina as opposed to peritonsillar abscess, etc.

▶ CASE 20.5

A 30-year-old man comes to your office complaining of a swollen neck. He noticed it after a bee sting 3 weeks ago on the right side of his anterior neck. The area has continued to enlarge. It is no longer tender. It was erythematous after the nick, but the redness has resolved. He notes no other symptoms. On examination, you find a 2-cm firm, somewhat tender, enlarged lymph node in the right anterior cervical chain. The node is mobile, non-fluctuant, and without surrounding erythema. There is shotty anterior and posterior cervical adenopathy in addition to the larger lymph node described. You find neither splenomegaly nor lymphadenopathy of the supraclavicular, axillary, and inguinal regions.

Question 20.5.1 What elements of the presentation make malignancy LESS likely?
A) The node is freely mobile
B) The node is only 2 cm
C) The node is associated with trauma (bee sting 3 weeks ago)
D) The node is tender
E) All of the above help to rule out malignancy

Answer 20.5.1 The correct answer is "A." Non-malignant nodes are generally *less than* 1 cm in size, freely mobile, and rubbery in consistency. Malignant nodes tend to be larger, rock-hard in consistency, and fixed to adjacent structures. Remember that pain in a node, "D," is not always indicative of an inflammatory or benign process. Hemorrhage into, or necrosis of, a malignant node can cause capsular distention leading to pain. "C" is of particular note. This patient's bee sting was quite a while ago and is unlikely to be a useful part of the history unless there is infection or ongoing inflammation. Patients will often attribute a physical malady to something in their lives whether or not it makes sense from a biological and medical perspective (one of us had a patient who swore that his purulent sputum was because his lungs were connected to his gallbladder). Of course, lymphadenopathy is not the only source of neck masses. See Table 20-3 for the differential diagnosis of neck masses in adults.

Question 20.5.2 What is the most appropriate next step in the management of this patient?
A) Empiric antibiotics
B) Observation for 2 weeks
C) Open biopsy of the node
D) Fine needle aspiration of the node
E) Incision and drainage

Answer 20.5.2 The correct answer is "B." According to the Clinical Practice Guidelines published in 2017 (*Journal of*

Otolaryngology—Head and Neck Surgery, Vol. 157), patients with lymphadenopathy and without symptoms of malignancy (e.g., fever, night sweats, and weight loss) can be observed for 2 weeks. The patient should be reassessed at 2 weeks, and if the lymphadenopathy is not resolved, the patient should be referred for neck CT or open biopsy or fine needle aspiration (FNA). "A," empiric therapy with antibiotics, is possibly correct if you suspect a lymphadenitis or a bacterial infection causing secondary lymphadenopathy. However, in our patient, there are no signs of infection, arguing against lymphadenitis.

Question 20.5.3 Which of the following tests is NOT helpful in arriving at a diagnosis in a patient with GENERALIZED lymphadenopathy?
A) CBC
B) Chest radiograph
C) Glucose, BUN, creatinine
D) HIV
E) Heterophile antibody

Answer 20.5.3 The correct answer is "C." Glucose, BUN, and creatinine are not likely to help you with the diagnosis of generalized lymphadenopathy. Generalized lymphadenopathy in primary care is malignant approximately 1% of the time. After a period of observation, the workup should proceed in stages. First step: CBC, chest radiograph. Second step: PPD, HIV, syphilis test (RPR or other), ANA, heterophile antibody. Final step:

TABLE 20-3 DIFFERENTIAL DIAGNOSIS OF NECK MASS IN ADULTS

Congenital Anomalies
- Lateral neck: branchial cysts and fistulae, cystic hygromas, dermoids
- Central neck: thyroglossal duct cyst, thyroid masses, thymic rests, dermoids

Infection/Inflammation
- Mononucleosis
- Tuberculosis
- Toxoplasmosis
- Cat-scratch disease (*Bartonella henselae*)
- Staphylococcus
- Streptococcus
- Other viral, bacterial, and fungal infections
- Sialadenitis
- Abscess
- Inflammatory or reactive lymphadenopathy

Neoplasm
- Benign masses: lipoma, hemangioma, neuroma, fibroma
- Malignant masses: mucosal head-and-neck cancers, lymphoma, thyroid cancer, salivary gland cancer, sarcoma, distant metastases

Trauma
- Hematoma (acute or fibrosed)
- Pseudoaneurysm
- AV fistula

Idiopathic and Others
- Metabolic: gout, CPPD (pseudogout)
- Inflammatory pseudotumor
- Castleman disease (a benign lymphoproliferative disorder)
- Kimura disease (a chronic subcutaneous inflammatory condition, cause unknown)

biopsy. Use your clinical judgment to determine the extent of testing necessary in any individual case.

HELPFUL TIP:
Just like in real estate, lymph nodes are all about location, location, location. Supraclavicular nodes are malignant up to 50% of the time in those older than 40 years.

HELPFUL TIP:
Benign lymphadenopathy is common in young children. In patients younger than 5 years presenting for a health maintenance examination, up to 44% have palpable lymph nodes. Occipital and posterior auricular nodes are common in infants but not in children older than 2 years of age.

▶ Objectives: Did you learn to …
- Describe features of malignant and non-malignant lymph nodes?
- Evaluate a patient with lymphadenopathy?

▶ **CASE 20.6**

A 42-year-old businesswoman presents to your office with the chief complaint of 2 days of headache, sore throat, and nasal congestion productive of green mucus. She denies any fever, contact with ill persons, and gastrointestinal symptoms, but she does have a history of seasonal allergies. On examination, she has completely normal vital signs. Her posterior oropharynx has mild erythema and postnasal drainage but no exudates. There is nasal mucosal erythema and swelling with clear rhinorrhea. Her neck is supple with no adenopathy. Respirations are clear.

Question 20.6.1 The most likely agent causing her symptoms and the most common cause of acute rhinosinusitis is:
A) Rhinovirus
B) *S. pneumoniae*
C) *H. influenzae*
D) *M. catarrhalis*
E) Norwalk virus

Answer 20.6.1 **The correct answer is "A."** Viruses are the most common cause of URIs (colds or rhinosinusitis). Up to 50% of colds are caused by the 100 different serotypes of rhinoviruses. Other viruses that commonly cause "colds" include: coronaviruses, RSV, parainfluenza, and influenza. Norwalk virus typically causes an intestinal illness. The bacteria listed ("B"–"D") are also associated with infections of the upper respiratory tract, particularly otitis, and sinusitis, but are much less common than viruses.

HELPFUL TIP:
Resident bacteria in the nasopharynx include *S. pneumoniae, H. influenzae,* and *M. catarrhalis.* While most causes of sinusitis are viral, these bacteria make up the great majority of organisms causing bacterial sinusitis. Sinusitis may also result from extension of dental root infection into the sinus cavity. These infections are caused by microaerophilic and anaerobic bacteria.

Question 20.6.2 Initial treatment for this patient includes:
A) Oral decongestants
B) NSAIDs
C) Oral antibiotics
D) A and B
E) A and C

Answer 20.6.2 **The correct answer is "D."** Most cases of rhinosinusitis are viral and need only symptomatic treatment. Analgesics and systemic and nasal decongestants are reasonable options. Other treatment options include nasal saline irrigations, ipratropium nasal spray (which will also help to decrease mucus production), nasal steroids (should be administered on a daily basis for several weeks to see improvement … of course by then the cold is better anyway), and first-generation antihistamines with anticholinergic activity (e.g., diphenhydramine).

HELPFUL TIP:
Yeah, yeah … we know. The party line is that first-generation antihistamines are not useful for rhinorrhea from a URI. However, this is technically incorrect. A Cochrane review showed some benefit of first-generation antihistamines and some effect of combination products (*Cochrane Database Systematic Rev.* 2003;3; 2012;2.)

Question 20.6.3 Which of the following does NOT increase the likelihood that a patient has a bacterial sinusitis?
A) Persistence of symptoms for greater than 7 days
B) Thickened nasal mucosa or effusion on CT scan
C) Maxillary tooth pain
D) Unilateral maxillary sinus pain

Answer 20.6.3 **The correct answer is "B."** Radiography is particularly poor at differentiating bacterial sinusitis from a simple URI. Thickened nasal mucosa is only 40% to 50% specific for sinusitis (flip a coin, it's cheaper). The other problem with imaging is that essentially all patients with a URI will have fluid in the sinuses. Clinical criteria are more helpful in predicting the presence of bacterial sinusitis; thus, "A," "C," and "D" are correct. Additionally, a biphasic course, sometimes referred to as "double sickening," is a helpful predictor of bacterial sinusitis—if the patient initially improves and then gets worse, consider a secondary infection. The color of nasal drainage is meaningless. **Thick, green, nasal drainage does not necessarily mean**

that bacteria are present. Secretions will turn green with a viral illness, as with anything else that concentrates protein in the mucous (e.g., anticholinergics).

HELPFUL TIP:
A viral URI can last up to a month. In fact, 25% of patients with a URI are still symptomatic at 14 days, so duration of symptoms **alone** is not diagnostic of bacterial sinusitis. So, don't tell your patient that she will be better in 4 to 5 days. Give your patients realistic expectations: 10 to 14 days.

The patient is initially convinced that only antibiotics will make her better. Through skillful negotiation (and a hefty dose of haloperidol), you manage to avoid prescribing antibiotics for what you strongly suspect is a viral infection. Two weeks later, the patient returns. Initially, she improved, but then she developed subjective fever, facial pressure, maxillary tooth pain, and copious green nasal drainage. You now suspect that a bacterial sinusitis has developed. The look on her face says, "I told you so … and I am not taking any more of that haloperidol stuff." She has no drug allergies.

Question 20.6.4 Which of the following treatments do you offer as first-line therapy?
A) Azithromycin
B) Trimethoprim/sulfamethoxazole
C) Prednisone
D) Ceftriaxone
E) Amoxicillin/clavulanate

Answer 20.6.4 **The correct answer is "E."** According to 2012 Infectious Diseases Society of America guidelines addressing the treatment of acute bacterial sinusitis, amoxicillin/clavulanate should be used as first-line treatment for adults and children—although the evidence is weak versus simple amoxicillin. Of note, in 2015 the AAFP endorsed the American Academy of Otolaryngology—Head and Neck Surgery guidelines that promote amoxicillin with or without clavulanate as first-line therapy in suspected bacterial sinusitis. Previously trimethoprim/sulfamethoxazole ("B") would have been the best choice, but there is increasing resistance. Azithromycin ("A") is not recommended due to resistance patterns and poor penetration into the sinuses. "C" is incorrect. There is no reason to prescribe steroids here. "D," ceftriaxone, might be considered in cases of treatment failure, but oral antibiotics are generally preferred. Per guidelines, doxycycline is recommended as second-line therapy, followed by cefixime or cefpodoxime +/− clindamycin. Respiratory fluoroquinolones will work but use at your own peril; there are several FDA warnings advising not to use these for simple sinusitis. Of course, you should continue to recommend that the patient use decongestants and other symptom-oriented therapies.

HELPFUL TIP:
Even with bacterial sinusitis, the NNT for antibiotics to benefit one patient is 9. Most patients are getting no

benefit from your careful ministrations—or knee-jerk reaction to prescribe antibiotics (whichever applies …).

HELPFUL TIP:
Remember that when treating sinusitis you are basically treating an abscess. Draining it is the key: use topical oxymetazoline (Afrin) for limited periods, systemic decongestants, and saline irrigation.

HELPFUL TIP:
All noses that run are not infectious. Remember allergic rhinitis, vasomotor rhinitis (now termed idiopathic rhinitis), etc. Idiopathic rhinitis is an exaggerated response to stimuli such as cold, recumbency, and air pollution. It can be differentiated from allergic rhinitis by the absence of other allergic symptoms (itching, eye involvement, perhaps asthma, etc.) and the absence of eosinophils on Hansel stain of mucus (who looks at snot under a microscope anyway?). Other considerations include rhinitis medicamentosa as a result of withdrawal from topical vasoconstrictors (e.g., oxymetazoline (Afrin), cocaine).

▶ **Objectives: Did you learn to …**
- Describe the most common pathogens involved in rhinosinusitis?
- Recognize clinical signs and symptoms that are more consistent with bacterial sinusitis than viral rhinosinusitis?
- Prescribe treatment for viral and bacterial sinusitis?

▶ **CASE 20.7**

A 65-year-old male presents with dizziness that started a few days ago. He reports that he is otherwise healthy and takes no medications.

Question 20.7.1 Which of the following is the best question to ask him in order to elicit a better characterization of his dizziness complaint?
A) "Is the room spinning round and round?"
B) "Do you feel that you are going to faint?"
C) "Can you describe the dizziness using any other words?"
D) "Do you feel as though you are drunk?"
E) "Are you really just drunk right now?"

Answer 20.7.1 **The correct answer is "C."** When exploring a complaint of dizziness, insist that the patient characterizes the nature of the dizziness further without using the word "dizzy." Is the room spinning? Do they feel light headed? Faint? Weak? This is a good time for that old technique learned in medical school but rarely used in practice: the open-ended question. There are essentially four types of dizziness: vertigo, presyncope, imbalance (disequilibrium), and undifferentiated dizziness. Patients will usually come up with their own terminology that will allow you to categorize their dizziness into one of these four types. Issues with the vestibular system will result in a true vertigo. Vertigo is a hallucination of movement: something seems to be moving that isn't. It doesn't matter if the room is spinning, the patient is spinning, or the floor seems to be coming up toward the patient. It should be associated with nystagmus.

The patient describes a sensation of the room spinning, usually lasting less than a minute. Further, this sensation comes on in different positions and has led to a fall, which resulted in minor injuries. He denies any upper respiratory symptoms, fevers, hearing loss, or tinnitus. He sometimes feels nauseated with the dizziness but has not vomited. He first noticed the dizziness while in bed and rolling over, but it now occurs more frequently and in various positions. Sudden turning of the head definitely exacerbates his symptoms. It tends to be worse in the morning and better in the evening. You are comfortable calling this type of dizziness vertigo.

Question 20.7.2 Which of the following is LEAST likely to cause vertigo (in a general sense ... not in this particular patient)?
A) Labyrinthitis
B) Ménière disease
C) Migraine aura
D) Otitis media
E) Perilymphatic fistula

Answer 20.7.2 The correct answer is "D." There are many causes of vertigo, but otitis media should not generally be thought of as one of them (or at least should be a diagnosis of exclusion). Labyrinthitis ("A") is usually caused by viral infection and results in severe vertigo that lasts for days. That said, in our experience, dizzy patients always expect an otoscopic exam, so looking in the ear may at least serve as a patient satisfier. Ménière disease ("B") results in episodic vertigo that lasts for minutes (at least 20 by definition) to hours. Migraine aura ("C") can present with vertigo as well as many other symptoms (e.g., scotoma, diplopia, blindness, and paresthesias). Perilymphatic fistula ("E") occurs when perilymph leaks through a tear in the oval window (secondary to a fall or barotrauma—including sneezing). It typically resolves on its own. Although a perilymphatic fistula often results in vertigo, it is a relatively uncommon cause of vertigo.

Question 20.7.3 Which of the following is the best next step in the diagnosis of this patient?
A) Dix–Hallpike maneuvers
B) Obtain blood for CBC, electrolytes, BUN, and creatinine
C) MRI brain and brainstem
D) CT brain
E) Audiometry

Answer 20.7.3 The correct answer is "A." A complete evaluation of the patient with vertigo includes examination of the neurological and cardiovascular systems as well as the ears, eyes, nose, and throat. On physical exam, look for nystagmus. The Dix–Hallpike maneuver is designed to differentiate central from peripheral vertigo and can be a useful tool (more on this later ...). In order to perform the maneuver, quickly move the patient from a seated to a supine position, turning the head to the left or right, and observe for nystagmus. The patient is helped into a seated position, and the maneuver is repeated, turning the head to the other side. If nystagmus occurs within 30 seconds of performing the maneuver, it is considered a positive test. "B" is incorrect. Laboratory tests are rarely helpful. "C" and "D" are not correct because neuroimaging should only be performed if the history and/or examination indicate the need for it. In this case, the examination is not even complete yet! Likewise, audiometry (although helpful in the diagnosis of Ménière disease) is premature.

Dix–Hallpike maneuver is positive with rotation of the head to the left. The rest of the physical examination is unremarkable. The patient gets vertiginous and then it resolves in less than 1 minute.

Question 20.7.4 Given the history and examination, the most likely diagnosis in this patient is:
A) Labyrinthitis
B) Benign paroxysmal positional vertigo (BPPV)
C) Vertebrobasilar stroke
D) Motion sickness
E) Cerebellar stroke

Answer 20.7.4 The correct answer is "B." The history of episodic, positional vertigo and the positive Dix–Hallpike maneuver makes BPPV the most likely diagnosis. Note that the Dix–Hallpike maneuver is not specific for BPPV. The Dix–Hallpike maneuver is designed to differentiate central from peripheral vertigo. In this case, the history is probably the most important aspect in making the diagnosis. BPPV is more common in older patients but can occur at any age. Women, especially peri-menopausal, are more commonly affected than men. BPPV is caused by calcium stone deposition in the posterior semicircular canal. BPPV tends to be worse in the morning and better toward evening because, being of peripheral origin, the vertigo response fatigues as the day goes on (see Table 20-4). The other diagnoses listed are less likely. However, "C" and "E" deserve special mention. Stroke should be considered in any patient presenting with sudden onset, persistent vertigo, and risk factors (e.g., hypertension and atrial fibrillation, age, etc.). In general, there should be other findings such as diplopia, dysmetria, and ataxia; only 1% of patients with a stroke have vertigo (*Neurol Clin.* 2012;30(1):61–74). However, not every elderly patient with vertigo needs an MRI. If the history is consistent with BPPV, then neuroimaging is not necessary.

HELPFUL TIP:

"Past pointing" on finger-to-nose testing usually indicates a peripheral lesion. And, patients generally fall toward the side of peripheral dysfunction.

Question 20.7.5 For this patient with BPPV, the LEAST appropriate treatment at this time is:

A) Prednisone
B) Lorazepam
C) Meclizine (Antivert)
D) Rehabilitation exercises
E) Dimenhydrinate (Dramamine)

Answer 20.7.5 The correct answer is "A." Steroids are not likely to improve symptoms in BPPV. Benzodiazepines, anticholinergics, and antihistamines have all been employed in treating the symptoms of BPPV but *should all be second-line therapies after rehabilitation and repositioning exercises.* Vestibular rehabilitation exercises, physical therapy, and physician-directed head positioning (e.g., Epley maneuvers to help reposition stones out of the posterior semicircular canal) may be successful. Most patients will improve with time, although many will have relapses and can complete the Epley maneuver at home.

HELPFUL TIP:

Simply treating the patient with medications to suppress the vertigo *can actually prolong the course of the disease.* The brain needs to learn to adapt to the signal causing vertigo. If your brain were talking (a scary prospect), it would say, "OK, I am not falling. I can ignore that input." Suppressing the vertigo delays this adaptation. However, medications may be necessary for symptom control in some patients. That said, your editors implore you to recommend or prescribe medications as a second- or third-line therapy, especially in the elderly patient who is at risk from the anticholinergic and sedative effects of these drugs.

Here are some easy associations with very common causes of vertigo:

- **Benign paroxysmal positional vertigo**: Frequently happens after trauma but can be spontaneous. Symptoms are brought on by rapid head movement, lasting **seconds to about a minute**, and are **fatigable** (repeat movement immediately afterward results in less severe symptoms). This is caused by displaced

TABLE 20-4 DIX–HALLPIKE MANEUVER

Suggestive of Peripheral Vertigo
- Delayed onset of nystagmus and symptoms
- Nystagmus always in same direction
- Vertigo reflex fatigable after multiple maneuvers
- Nystagmus suppressible by patient

Suggestive of Central Vertigo
- Nystagmus in multiple directions
- No latency to onset of nystagmus
- Reflex not fatigable

otoliths most commonly into the posterior semi-circular canal from its home in the utricle. Clinical test: Dix–Hallpike maneuver. Treatment: Epley repositioning maneuvers. These can be performed in clinic or at home and may require multiple maneuvers. However, they may cure patient immediately.

- **Meniere disease**: Recurrent episodes of vertigo lasting minutes (at least 20) to hours, but not typically longer than 24 hours. **Vertigo is associated with sensorineural hearing loss**. Patient will describe decreased hearing at the time of the event in one ear. Hearing improves as the episode resolves, but over time/repeat episodes patients typically progressively lose low-frequency hearing. Pathophysiology is somewhat poorly understood, but described as endolymphatic hydrops, with a pressure imbalance between perilymph and endolymph in the inner ear. The thought is that as the pressure differential increases, it results in a small tear in the delicate membranes separating the compartments, and loss of the ion differential that allows the balance organ to function, which makes the ear think that it is spinning. Treatment: prevention involves salt restriction and diuretic therapy, acute episodic relief frequently with benzodiazepines. Ultimately in severe cases it may warrant referral to otolaryngologist for surgical intervention. Hearing aids and ultimately cochlear implants may be indicated.

- **Superior semi-circular canal dehiscence**: Fistula formed between the superior semi-circular canal and the intracranial space. Patients frequently experience seconds of vertigo with loud noise or pressure change in the ear. Nystagmus can be produced in clinic with pneumatoscopy. Associated commonly with obesity. Treatment: Referral to neuro-otologist for surgical repair.

- **Vestibular neuritis/labyrinthitis**: Most commonly viral but can be suppurative with a bacterial infection of the vestibule. Patients complain of debilitating vertigo lasting **days**. May be associated with purulent otitis media, but can have a normal ear exam/no hearing loss with viral labyrinthitis. Bacterial cases should be treated aggressively with myringotomy and antibiotic drops and otolaryngology involvement. Viral neuritis is frequently managed symptomatically.

- **Vestibular migraines**: Generally these have recurrent episodes of vertigo lasting hours, and may also have other typical migraine features such as aura and headache with photophobia. Generally these are treated with preventative/abortive migraine therapy.

- **See** Table 20-5 for a summary of causes of vertigo.

▶ **Objectives: Did you learn to …**
- Describe types of dizziness?
- Generate a differential diagnosis for vertigo?
- Diagnose and treat a patient with BPPV?

▶ **CASE 20.8**

A 15-year-old male wrestler presents to the ED with a nosebleed and a swollen ear. He clearly did not win this round. Prior to coming to the ED, he held pressure to his nose for

TABLE 20-5 VERTIGO BY DURATION AND ASSOCIATED FINDINGS[A]

Disease State	Duration of Vertigo	Timing of vertigo	Antecedent Event	Fatigable	Treatment	Notes
Barotrauma/ ruptured oval window	Variable	Worse in evening (from perilymph leak while upright, better in AM after recumbency)	Fall, diving	No	Referral to otolaryngology if not spontaneously resolving	Can make worse with pneumo-otoscopy (pump the eardrum to change pressure and will get perilymph leak)
BPPV	Seconds to minutes	Worst in morning (fatigues on repetition)	Perhaps mild trauma, often nothing	Yes	Epley maneuvers	
Drug related/ Alcohol	Variable	Related to time of ingestion	Ingestion	n/a	Remove offending agent	
Labyrinthitis	Days	Continuous or waxing/waning	Often URI but history of viral infection not always present	No	Steroids (variable effectiveness), antibiotics if bacterial	Debilitating vertigo, severe nausea and vomiting
Meniere disease	Minutes to hours (less than 24 hours)	Variable	None	No	Diuretics, low salt diet	Associated tinnitus, ear fullness, hearing loss
Posterior circulation stroke/TIA	Generally > 10–15 minutes (differentiate from BPPV which is seconds to a minute)	Variable	DM2, HTN, other risk factors for vascular disease	No	See Chapter 18	Only 1% of posterior strokes present with isolated vertigo
Vestibular migraine	Hours	Variable	Variable triggers (menstruation, stress, fatigue, acute illness, etc.)	No	As for migraine (Chapter 18)	May have migraine aura, headache, photophobia, etc.

[a]All should also have nystagmus.

30 minutes. He has had nosebleeds before, but none were this bad. When asked how much blood he lost, his father shrugs and says it was "all over the mat." On examination, you see blood oozing slowly from the anterior nasal septum.

Question 20.8.1 Which of the following is a source of anterior epistaxis?
A) Ethmoid artery
B) Sphenopalatine artery
C) Kiesselbach arterial plexus
D) Palpatine artery

Answer 20.8.1 The correct answer is "C." Kiesselbach plexus is a collection system involving several terminal arteries (anterior ethmoidal, greater palatine, and superior labial arteries) in the anterior nose. It is the most common site of nasal bleeding. Don gloves, retract the patient's nasal tip, shine a light, and you will see it. The ethmoid and sphenopalatine arteries supply the posterior area of the nose, and bleeding from these sites is more difficult to control. Of special note is "D." Emperor Palpatine, also known as "Darth Sidious," converted Anakin Skywalker to the

Dark Side using hatred, anger, and lies (sounds like a contemporaneous political figure)—not epistaxis caused by an eponymous artery. Also, don't confuse the Kiesselbach plexus with the Kessel Run, which the Millennium Falcon allegedly completed in under 12 parsecs.

Question 20.8.2 What is the best next step in managing this patient's nosebleed?
A) Continue to hold pressure against the septum
B) Gently pack the anterior naris with gauze
C) Spray the mucosal surface with oxymetazoline (Afrin)
D) Chemical cautery with silver nitrate
E) Any of the above can be used

Answer 20.8.2 The correct answer is "E." Any of the options listed could be used alone or in combination to try to stop the bleeding. Generally speaking, over 90% of nosebleeds in healthy patients can be stopped by spraying oxymetazoline (Afrin) along the septum bilaterally and holding firm pressure along the soft/cartilaginous portion of the nose for 15 solid minutes (with no peeking!). If these methods are not successful, consider chemical cautery (silver nitrate), topical tranexamic acid (*Acad Emerg Med.* 2017 Nov 10) or packing ("Rhino rocket," etc.). A coagulopathy workup (e.g., CBC, PT/PTT) and otolaryngology consultation can be considered in select cases. Laboratory studies will rarely be helpful, though.

HELPFUL TIP:
If you pack a patient's nose, plan on leaving the packing in place for 3 to 5 days. Also, prescribe anti-staphylococcal/streptococcal antibiotics to prevent a bacterial super infection/toxic shock syndrome while packing is in place.

With oxymetazoline and direct pressure, you were able to stop the bleeding. You now turn your attention to his left ear. You find a purplish, tender, fluctuant swelling at the left pinna.

Question 20.8.3 The best treatment for this condition is:
A) Analgesics, protection, and observation
B) Compressive dressing, using a headband (preferably that sweatband in your gym bag)
C) Oral antibiotics
D) Incision and drainage, leaving the wound open to drain and heal by secondary intention
E) Needle drainage followed by compressive dressing sutured into the pinna

Answer 20.8.3 **The correct answer is "E."** With a traumatic auricular hematoma/seroma, fluid collects between the perichondrium and underlying cartilage, predisposing the cartilage to loss of vascular supply and necrosis. In order to avoid "cauliflower ear" deformity, the hematoma or seroma must be evacuated via incision or needle drainage. However, you cannot stop there: a compressive dressing must then be sutured into the pinna, or the fluid is likely to re-accumulate. "B" is incorrect because compressive dressing alone is insufficient. "D" is incorrect only because it does not include compressive dressing. "A" and "C" are incorrect because taking these actions will delay definitive treatment—and antibiotics are not needed anyway. If the patient were to present late (10 days or more after the injury), he will not benefit from incision or needle drainage, and instead should be referred for otoplasty.

HELPFUL TIP:
Repeat after me, "The nose is not the release valve of the cardiovascular system." Most nasal bleeding is venous and not directly related to elevated blood pressure, though long-term hypertension may cause vasculopathy predisposing to epistaxis.

▶ **Objectives: Did you learn to …**
• Evaluate and treat a patient with epistaxis?
• Treat a patient with auricular trauma?

 QUICK QUIZ: MOUTH SORES

A 20-year-old female presents with three painful ulcerations on her inner lip and tongue. She has no other symptoms. Although she has never had such sores before, everyone else in her family has had similar mouth sores. She only smokes when drinking cheap wine coolers, which occurs about once per week. When asked about sexual activity, she shrugs and says, "My sex life is DOA. I'm the original Jane the Virgin." She is afebrile, and her examination is otherwise unremarkable.

The most likely diagnosis is:
A) Aphthous ulcers
B) Behcet disease
C) Crohn disease
D) Gluten enteropathy
E) Squamous cell carcinoma

The correct answer is "A." This otherwise healthy young woman with a family history of "similar sores" most likely has aphthous ulcers or "canker sores." The etiology of aphthous ulcers is not well understood, and they are alternatively explained as viral, autoimmune, genetic, traumatic, or due to chemical irritants or other processes (also, karmic retribution, divine punishment for sin, etc.). "B," Behcet disease, is uncommon in the United States. It is thought to be an autoimmune disease, and it presents with recurrent oral and genital ulcerations and skin and eye lesions among other findings. "C" and "D" can both present with isolated oral ulcers but are less common than idiopathic aphthous ulcers, and one would also expect other GI symptoms. "E" is incorrect because it is highly unlikely that this young, healthy person has developed cancer … in three places … simultaneously. Finally, lupus pemphigoid, pemphigus, and multiple infections (e.g., Hand-Foot-Mouth, HIV, herpes, and syphilis) may present with oral ulcers.

▶ **CASE 20.9**

A 34-year-old male dentist presents to your office with a 1-week history of right facial weakness and a bit of tongue numbness. He states that he "just woke up this way one morning." He would have come in sooner, but he was busy with his practice and he has felt fine. He has not noticed any other neurological symptoms. He denies pain, fever, or upper respiratory symptoms. He reports being healthy and taking no medications. On examination, his vital signs are normal. You note that his right eyebrow sags, as does the right corner of his mouth. He cannot close the right eye completely or raise his right eyebrow, and the right nasolabial fold is less prominent than the left. The remainder of the neurological examination is normal.

Question 20.9.1 The neurological finding in this patient that most suggests a cranial nerve process (as opposed to a central brain lesion) is:
A) Normal strength in the upper extremities
B) Inability to smile on the right

C) Inability to wrinkle the forehead
D) Normal blood pressure
E) Normal speech rate and rhythm

Answer 20.9.1 The correct answer is "C." Partial sparing of the forehead muscles suggests a brain lesion because innervation of the forehead contains crossed fibers from both sides of the brain; a bilateral brain lesion is possible but unlikely. Thus, a dense paralysis is more likely to be peripheral (CN7) since all innervation is knocked out when this is involved. This patient's entire right face, including the forehead, is paralyzed, which suggests a lower motor neuron (CN7) palsy. While "A" and "E" are found in a normal neurologic examination and are reassuring, they are not as helpful in isolating the location of the lesion to a lower motor neuron source. "B," lower facial muscle weakness or paralysis, can occur with upper or lower motor neuron disease. "D," normal blood pressure, is not helpful.

HELPFUL TIP:
Of note, taste alterations are not unusual in Bell's palsy. The seventh nerve is involved in taste sensation on the anterior two-thirds of the tongue (chorda tympani nerve runs through the middle ear space). Patients may note a headache in the retroauricular area before the onset of weakness symptoms.

You tell the patient that you suspect he has Bell's palsy. He asks what causes this problem.

Question 20.9.2 Which of the following is the most likely cause of this patient's Bell's palsy?
A) Herpes virus
B) Tick-borne illness
C) Diabetes
D) Adenovirus
E) Idiopathic

Answer 20.9.2 The correct answer is "E." Bell's palsy is by definition idiopathic, with unknown causes. We know that it can be associated with diabetes or a recent upper respiratory tract infection, but an actual cause is still unknown. Most experts believe it may be caused by a viral infection or other inflammatory insult that results in swelling of the nerve and compression/vascular compromise in the narrow bony canal as it leaves the skull through the stylomastoid foramen. Lyme disease is occasionally implicated, but most commonly presents as a bilateral facial nerve weakness. Ramsay–Hunt Syndrome is a similar condition that is caused by activation of geniculate varicella zoster. Ramsey–Hunt, while similar to Bell's palsy, is much more inflammatory and is associated with severe otalgia, a vesicular rash (usually in the ear canal/concha) and sensorineural hearing loss/vertigo. While the vast majority of Bell's palsy patients will have a complete recovery, prognosis for facial function after Ramsay–Hunt syndrome is worse (45% chance of facial nerve synkinesis after Ramsay–Hunt).

HELPFUL TIP:
Bell's palsy is more likely to occur in pregnancy, especially the last trimester and the first week postpartum.

Question 20.9.3 Which of the following treatments is most likely to benefit this patient?
A) Acyclovir
B) Prednisone
C) Artificial tears and eye patching at night
D) B and C
E) None of the above

Answer 20.9.3 The correct answer is "D." In a patient with Bell's palsy and weakness to eye closure, good eye care and protection from trauma must be employed to prevent corneal damage (remember that this patient cannot close his right eye). There is strong evidence for starting high-dose oral steroids in Bell's palsy. These are most efficacious if started in the first 72 hours but may still improve outcomes if started later. Antiviral therapy is recommended if a viral etiology is suspected (e.g., Ramsay–Hunt). In true Bell's palsy, antiviral therapy alone is not helpful with several double-blind studies failing to show benefit. However, benefit has been demonstrated with combination therapy (corticosteroids PLUS antiviral therapy) if the patient has severe disease (cannot entirely close eye, disfiguring asymmetry). The bottom line is that steroids should always be used, and adding antivirals for *severe disease* is low-risk and may improve patient outcomes.

Question 20.9.4 The patient can expect which of the following?
A) Complete resolution (~100% likelihood) with nearly zero risk of recurrence
B) Likely resolution (>50% likelihood) with nearly zero risk of recurrence
C) Likely resolution (>50% likelihood) with about 10% risk of recurrence
D) High probability (~95% likelihood) of persistent paralysis

Answer 20.9.4 The correct answer is "C." Most patients will recover (71% complete, 13% minor impairment with the rest having significant sequelae), but it may take months. If a patient with suspected Bell's palsy has no improvement in symptoms after a few months, reconsider the diagnosis. Patients with complete paralysis are more likely to have persistent symptoms, whereas those with partial paralysis usually recover more quickly and completely. Surgical decompression is an option for *some* patients with Bell's palsy. If a patient's facial nerve is completely paralyzed (no discernible movement), they should be referred for electroneurography (ENoG)/EMG and otolaryngology consultation. If degeneration of nerve is greater than 90% on ENoG, there is evidence that surgical decompression will improve outcomes if performed within the first 2 weeks.

HELPFUL TIP:
Ramsay–Hunt syndrome is the name given to zoster oticus complicated by hemifacial paralysis. If identified early, antivirals may help the patient with Ramsay–Hunt syndrome. You may see blisters in the ear canal, in conjunction with sensorineural hearing loss/vertigo. These patients should be treated aggressively with corticosteroids and antivirals and should have an audiogram.

▶ **Objectives: Did you learn to …**
· Differentiate Bell's palsy from a central lesion?
· Describe causes of Bell's palsy?
· Manage a patient with hemifacial paresis?

 QUICK QUIZ: OH, MY ACHING JAW

A 30-year-old female presents with several months of pain and stiffness in her jaw. When asked to localize the pain, she points to the temporomandibular joints (TMJ) bilaterally. She notes that the pain is worse with stressful situations, driving, and chewing. Her husband complains that she grinds her teeth at night. She is otherwise healthy. On physical examination, you find palpable popping in the TMJs bilaterally, and the remainder of her examination is unremarkable.

You make all of the following recommendations EXCEPT:
A) Start chewing gum daily
B) Use ibuprofen as needed
C) Use a bite block at night
D) Learn relaxation techniques

The correct answer is "A." This patient's history is consistent with TMJ syndrome. In addition to those described in the case, symptoms of TMJ may include ear pain, headache, "sinus" headache, limited jaw mobility, and crepitus and tenderness on palpation of the joint. TMJ syndrome may occur unilaterally or bilaterally. No single therapy appears to have greater efficacy than any other, and many different interventions have been tried, although poorly studied. "A," increased use of the joint by chewing gum, is the exact opposite of what the patient should be doing. Jaw rest is important. All of the other interventions are reasonable. Also, you might recommend a softer diet, hot packs, and TMJ massage.

HELPFUL TIP:
The headache of TMJ may be felt in the midfacial region, retro-orbitally, or as an earache. Check for TMJ when patients present with these types of symptoms.

▶ **CASE 20.10**

A 22-year-old female presents to your office complaining of severe facial pain for the past 3 days. She has poor dentition and you find that on examination, there is mandibular swelling and tenderness.

Question 20.10.1 All of the following are causes of mandibular area swelling EXCEPT:
A) Submandibular duct stone
B) Dental abscess
C) Retropharyngeal abscess
D) Ludwig angina
E) Branchial cleft cyst

Answer 20.10.1 The correct answer is "C." Retropharyngeal abscesses generally are not visible but present with fever, throat pain, and symptoms due to swelling of the retropharyngeal space (dysphagia, drooling, odynophagia, and airway obstruction). All of the other options can cause swelling around the mandible.

Question 20.10.2 One of the diagnoses you are considering is parotitis. Which of the following is true regarding parotitis?
A) You will only see mumps in science-denying, anti-vaccine, whack jobs
B) Mumps can be associated with pain and inflammation of the meninges, pancreas, and gonads as well as the parotid glands
C) Bacterial parotitis is mostly caused by pan-sensitive streptococcus and can be treated with penicillin
D) Mumps is usually treated with IVIG

Answer 20.10.2 The correct answer is "B." Mumps can lead to inflammation of other tissues including the meninges, pancreas, and gonads (possibly leading to decreased fertility in males but not in females) and will occasionally require hospitalization. Thankfully, most people recover spontaneously with good supportive care, including NSAIDs and warm compresses. IVIG would be reserved for those with severe complications. "A" is incorrect. While the MMR vaccine is about 88% effective after two doses, this still leaves over 10% of the population susceptible to outbreaks. Therefore, you may see mumps in immunosuppressed patients as well as anyone who is more than 10 years out from their last vaccination. Bacterial parotitis ("C") is usually caused by *Staphylococcus aureus* and anaerobes. In the hospital setting, approximately 40% of the *Staphylococcus aureus* is methicillin resistant, so first-line therapy is usually IV vancomycin pending culture results. Parotitis secondary to stones is often treated with cephalexin, dicloxacillin, or amoxicillin/sulbactam. Use clinical judgment and assure good follow-up.

Question 20.10.3 Which of the following is NOT typical of sialolithiasis (salivary duct stones)?
A) Intermittent swelling of the salivary gland
B) More than 80% of stones involve the parotid gland
C) The majority resolve with conservative, nonoperative treatment
D) Anti-staphylococcal antibiotics should be used in their treatment
E) Sialogogues (e.g., lemon drops) should be used as part of the treatment

Answer 20.10.3 The correct answer is "B." In actuality, more than 80% of cases of sialolithiasis involve the submandibular gland. Saliva in the submandibular gland is more viscous and contains more mucous and dissolved salts than the parotid glands. Additionally, these glands rely more on muscular contraction in the ducts to function as they need to express saliva against gravity. "A" is true. Swelling tends to occur when patients eat and tends to resolve between meals as saliva slowly makes its way through the duct. "C" is true. Most salivary duct stones pass spontaneously. "D" is true. Think of this as an abscess. If there is any sign of infection, anti-staphylococcal antibiotics should be used until the stone passes. Finally, sialogogues such as lemon drops promote saliva formation. The effectiveness is questionable, but it is worth a try and it gives the patient something to do.

Question 20.10.4 Which of the following is considered good practice with regard to salivary duct stones?
A) Patients should be counseled to drink lots of water, use hot compresses/salivary gland massage, use sialogogues such as lemon drops and be followed closely
B) Stones can be removed using sialolithotomy (using a probe and/or scalpel to nick the outlet)
C) Patients should be referred for sialography/sialendoscopy if stones do not pass within 4 days
D) Surgical excision of the duct/gland may be performed with multiply recurrent or complicated cases
E) All of the above

Answer 20.10.4 The correct answer is "E." First line for sialadenitis/sialolithiasis is to encourage passing of the stone conservatively. This is performed by increasing the amount of saliva passing through the duct. Hydration, massage, warm compresses, and sialogogues will help wash out pus in either a gland or a stone. A probe can be used to "dilate" the duct. Occasionally, the outlet needs to be nicked using a scalpel blade to allow the stone to egress. In other cases, sialography may help visualize the stone and may therapeutically dilate the duct by cannulation/injection of contrast dye. Sialendoscopy may be used to perform lithotripsy and remove the stone in a minimally invasive manner. In recurrent or complicated cases, removal/marsupialization of the duct, or even salivary gland excision may be necessary.

You check the patient's mouth and decide that there is likely a dental abscess, not a salivary duct stone, so you wasted a lot of energy thinking about stones. She needs to have her tooth extracted, but the dentist will not be able to see the patient until the morning…of the first Tuesday…of next month. She requires antibiotics but is penicillin-allergic.

Question 20.10.5 The antibiotic of choice for this patient is:
A) Erythromycin
B) Clindamycin
C) Azithromycin
D) Levofloxacin
E) Trimethoprim/sulfamethoxazole

Answer 20.10.5 The correct answer is "B." Clindamycin is the drug of choice as an alternative to penicillin. The drug used for a dental abscess should cover anaerobes. There is resistance to erythromycin and azithromycin. Neither levofloxacin nor trimethoprim/sulfamethoxazole covers anaerobes.

During your examination, you also noticed a firm nodule in the submental area in the midline (definitely not this patient's day!). It moves up and down when she swallows. She says that it has been there for years—as long as she can remember.

Question 20.10.6 The most likely cause of this midline nodule is:
A) Submandibular gland infection
B) Thyroglossal duct cyst
C) Infected frenulum
D) Branchial cleft cyst
E) An accumulation of midi-chlorians

Answer 20.10.6 The correct answer is "B." This is likely a thyroglossal duct cyst. The rest are not likely. Submandibular glands ("A") and branchial cleft cysts ("D") are lateral to the midline. "C" is incorrect. The frenulum is under the tongue. As for "E," another *Star Wars* reference—midi-chlorian levels are high in Force-wielding beings. Maybe there will be a Wookie at the end of the chapter. Keep reading.

You start the patient on clindamycin, but she returns in the morning with severe submandibular swelling. The tongue is elevated in the mouth and there is brawny edema; she is having trouble talking. You make the diagnosis of Ludwig's angina. ("Didn't we just do this?" you ask. "Yes, we are going to do it again," we reply.)

Question 20.10.7 At this time, the most appropriate treatment for this patient is:
A) Continue PO clindamycin and add saltwater gargles
B) Continue PO clindamycin and add PO metronidazole
C) Incise and drain the swollen area under the tongue
D) Refer immediately for surgical evaluation for I&D, securing of the airway with intubation vs. possible tracheostomy
E) Administer IV fluids and ceftriaxone in the office and follow up tomorrow

Answer 20.10.7 The correct answer is "D." This patient's situation has become fairly desperate overnight even while on an appropriate antibiotic. Securing an airway should be your first concern. Unfortunately, these patients do not respond to local incision and drainage, as the swelling is usually diffuse, quickly spreading, and does not result in discrete pus pocket formation until late in the course. She should be admitted for IV fluids, appropriate IV antibiotics (not levofloxacin), and possible securing of her airway. Patients with advancing Ludwig's angina may be challenging to intubate; thus, an alternative airway is sometimes provided with tracheostomy.

▶ **Objectives:** Did you learn to …
- Diagnose salivary stones?
- Treat salivary stones?
- Recognize the presentation of submandibular masses?

▶ CASE 20.11

A 21-year-old male presents for a sore throat. His symptoms started 3 days ago. He has had subjective fevers, sweats, fatigue, and mild nausea. He has no cough or rhinorrhea. His temperature is 38.5°C. His vital signs are normal otherwise. He has symmetrically enlarged tonsils with exudates present and tender anterior cervical lymphadenopathy.

Question 20.11.1 **At this point, you:**
A) Reassure and recommend saltwater gargles
B) Obtain a routine aerobic culture of the oropharynx
C) Prescribe penicillin 500 mg BID for 10 days
D) Prescribe levofloxacin 500 mg daily for 7 days

Answer 20.11.1 **The correct answer is "C."** This patient has four of four signs/symptoms suggestive of streptococcal (group A strep or *Streptococcus pyogenes*) pharyngitis. These are the Centor criteria: (1) fever, (2) tender cervical adenopathy, (3) exudative pharyngitis, and (4) lack of other URI symptoms (especially cough). In this case, the most appropriate step would be empiric antimicrobial treatment. "B," performing a culture, will take a few days and does not add much, given the strength of the clinical argument for strep throat. Furthermore, the oropharynx is colonized by many kinds of flora that do not cause disease, and we only really care about group A streptococcus, so a routine aerobic culture is of no value. Alternatively, a rapid assay or a specific "rule-out" culture for group A strep could be done rather than treating based on clinical grounds (the rapid strep has a 5% false-negative rate). While saltwater gargles seem to help reduce the pain of pharyngitis, "A" is incorrect because you would want to do more than that for this patient who likely has strep throat. "D" is incorrect because levofloxacin and other fluoroquinolones are not indicated for treatment of strep throat.

Here are three strategies for the patient you think might have strep throat:

Strategy 1: No testing (or minimal testing)

In this strategy, one treats based on clinical symptoms. You are looking for four things: fever, exudate, absence of other URI symptoms, and tender anterior cervical adenopathy. Treat patients with 3 or 4 criteria, and do not treat others. Another approach is to treat patients with 4 criteria, do a rapid strep test on those with 3 (and maybe 2) criteria, and avoid treatment and testing of others. The CDC has recommended this for non-immunosuppressed patients in the absence of an outbreak of rheumatic fever in the community.

Strategy 2: Testing

Test all patients and treat those with a positive strep screen. Do not culture others.

Strategy 3: Test +/– Culture and Treat (For Children)

The majority of group A strep pharyngitis occurs in children between ages 5 and 15 years. In this age group, 15% to 30% of acute pharyngitis is caused by group A strep. In children, doing a rapid strep test is considered the standard (although many argue convincingly that it is not even necessary here in the older child). Cultures are again optional depending on the reliability of your rapid antigen test. Many would culture *all* rapid strep test *negative* patients, and this is certainly an acceptable strategy as well.

So, now you are quite confused. So is everyone else …

Question 20.11.2 **Which of the following is true about antibiotic therapy of streptococcal pharyngitis?**
A) Azithromycin is the drug of choice because of resistant streptococci
B) There is no significant resistance seen in Group A β-hemolytic streptococci, and penicillin is still the drug of choice
C) Cephalexin is the preferred drug because it covers *H. influenzae*, which is a frequent co-infector with streptococci
D) Amoxicillin is preferred for strep throat because it does not cause a rash if the patient happens to have mononucleosis

Answer 20.11.2 **The correct answer is "B."** There is no significant resistance among group A β-hemolytic streptococci to penicillin. Thus, penicillin remains the drug of choice despite drug detailing. There is no reason to use **anything else**, except in the case of allergy where **erythromycin or cephalexin** can be used. Remember that there is now resistance to erythromycin, azithromycin, and clarithromycin. "D" is important. Amoxicillin can cause an uncomfortable rash should your patient turn out to have mononucleosis rather than strep throat.

 HELPFUL TIP:
Penicillin VK can be used BID in streptococcal pharyngitis, and this administration frequency increases compliance.

Question 20.11.3 **Antibiotics should be started within what time period to reduce the risk of rheumatic fever from streptococcal pharyngitis?**
A) Less than 2 days after presentation
B) 2 to 4 days after presentation
C) 4 to 6 days after presentation
D) 6 to 8 days after presentation
E) 8 to 10 days after presentation

Answer 20.11.3 **The correct answer is "E."** Antibiotics should be started within 9 days after presentation in order to prevent rheumatic fever, which is really our goal when we treat streptococcal pharyngitis. Thus, there really is no reason to hurry treatment.

Your patient is a student teacher and wants to know how long to stay out of the classroom.

Question 20.11.4 A patient with streptococcal pharyngitis should be considered infectious and kept out of school for what period after beginning antibiotics?
A) 12 hours
B) 24 hours
C) 36 hours
D) 48 hours

Answer 20.11.4 The correct answer is "B." Patients should be considered infectious for 24 hours after the initiation of therapy for streptococcal pharyngitis. The risk of transmission goes down markedly after this point. Unfortunately, the patient is actually infectious for the 3 to 5 days before they become symptomatic, so removing the patient for 24 hours after treatment is closing the barn door after the horses have left. There is some preliminary data that it is OK to return to work/school 12 hours after starting treatment but this is not yet the standard of care (*Pediatr Infect Dis J.* 2015;34(12):1302).

You see the same patient 3 weeks later. He took all of his penicillin even though he felt fine a few days after he left your office. (Wow! A compliant patient!) However, he now has the same symptoms, starting 2 days ago. His examination is the same.

Question 20.11.5 Which of the following is the most likely cause for his current symptoms?
A) Gonococcal pharyngitis
B) Infection with a resistant *streptococcal* organism
C) Mononucleosis
D) Staphylococcal pharyngitis
E) None of the above

Answer 20.11.5 The correct answer is "E." Since his symptoms resolved, you either got the diagnosis and treatment right or he had some other self-limited infection. Therefore, it would be unlikely that he had gonococcal pharyngitis or resistant *streptococcal* organisms. Besides, "B," penicillin-resistant Group A *Streptococcus* organisms causing pharyngitis, like the Tooth Fairy, are nonexistent. Nonetheless, sexual history is important—even when confronted with pharyngitis; if a patient with exudative pharyngitis is not improving, think about gonococcal disease. Remember that gonococcal disease will be missed for two reasons in this scenario: the history is never obtained regarding oral sex and gonococcus requires Thayer–Martin agar to grow, so it will not show up on routine culture, and there are a lot of false-negative cultures; obtain a swab for PCR if you are considering gonococcal pharyngitis. "C" is unlikely in this case because his symptoms resolved, but mononucleosis can cause prolonged symptoms of sore throat and fatigue and can be confused with strep throat. In this case, *recurrent* strep throat is most likely, and he should be advised appropriately: retreat with penicillin, not a more broad-spectrum antibiotic; consider testing and/or treating cohabitants; have the patient replace his toothbrush.

HELPFUL TIP:
Many causes of throat pain are acute infections (strep throat, other bacterial infections, viral pharyngitis, mononucleosis), but consider other noninfectious causes as well—carotidynia, viral thyroiditis, mouth-breathing, peritonsillar abscess. Non-group A streptococci (especially *Streptococcus agalactiae*, a group B strep) are increasingly being cultured from the pharynx. *S. agalactiae* can cause invasive disease and is probably worth treating if found. It will respond to cephalexin or clindamycin (among others).

It's a "two for Tuesday" at your clinic. The next patient comes in for a sore throat and tender anterior and posterior cervical adenopathy. He is febrile and relatively stoic. He has been sick for 2 weeks with significant fatigue and just isn't getting better. In addition to the adenopathy, you notice left-sided abdominal tenderness with minimal guarding but no rebound tenderness. You believe that you feel a spleen edge. However, the patient's heterophile antibody (monospot) is negative. You decide to get anti-EBV (Epstein–Barr virus) antibodies. The results of the anti-EBV antibody test are as follows (VCA is against the capsid): IgM-VCA positive, IgG-VCA negative, anti-EBV nuclear antigen antibody negative.

Question 20.11.6 How do you interpret these results?
A) The patient has acute EBV infection
B) The patient has had EBV at least 6 weeks ago
C) The absence of anti-EBV nuclear antigen antibody makes acute infection highly unlikely
D) The patient has never been infected with EBV

Answer 20.11.6 The correct answer is "A." The patient has an EBV infection, starting in the last few weeks. Here is why. IgM-VCA is produced acutely and is elevated in the acute infection for 2 to 4 weeks. Since this patient's IgM-VCA is positive, he has had an acute EBV infection within the past month. IgG-VCA is measurable 3 to 4 weeks after acute infection and persists for life. Thus, it gives no information about when infection occurred. The absence of IgG-VCA means either (1) the patient has no history of EBV infection or (2) the patient has had a recent EBV infection. Antibodies against the EBV nuclear antigen show up at 6 to 12 weeks after infection. If this antibody is present in the blood, it suggests that there has not been an acute infection; the infection had to have been at least 6 weeks ago.

Question 20.11.7 Of the following, which DOES NOT cause a mononucleosis-like syndrome?
A) Human immunodeficiency virus (HIV)
B) Cytomegalovirus (CMV)
C) Toxoplasmosis
D) West Nile virus (WNV)
E) Leptospirosis

Answer 20.11.7 The correct answer is "D." WNV is characterized by fever, headache, myalgias, back pain, and anorexia lasting 3 to 6 days. Much less common manifestations are nausea, vomiting, diarrhea, encephalitis, etc. Thus, WNV does not cause a mononucleosis-like syndrome because it does not last as long and rarely includes pharyngitis. One thing to note is that WNV may include lymphadenopathy. All the other answers can cause a mononucleosis-like syndrome. Other causes of mononucleosis-like syndromes include adenovirus, parvovirus B19 (erythema infectiosum), herpes virus 6 (roseola infantum), Zika, and ehrlichiosis (Asian form only). Remember these diagnoses in heterophile-negative mono-like illness.

HELPFUL TIP:
Depending on what population is studied, 1% to 2% of patients with a mononucleosis-like syndrome who are **heterophile negative** are HIV positive.

Question 20.11.8 There is some concern of splenic rupture in patients with mononucleosis who have splenomegaly. If splenomegaly were confirmed in this patient, what would be the generally accepted recommendation with regard to athletic participation (e.g., cage fighting)?
A) No participation until negative acute titers for EBV
B) No participation for 2 weeks after the diagnosis is made, assuming complete resolution of symptoms, and then full participation
C) No participation until 3 weeks after the diagnosis is made, assuming complete resolution of symptoms, and then only noncontact training for another week
D) Full practice and competition allowed immediately unless abdominal pain occurs
E) Full practice and competition immediately with body armor (e.g., Kevlar vest)

Answer 20.11.8 The correct answer is "C." It is generally thought that return to practice or **noncontact training** is safe 3 weeks after the diagnosis of mononucleosis, provided that all other symptoms have also resolved. If there are no clinical concerns for splenic enlargement at 4 weeks, then the athlete may be cleared to return to full competition. This recommendation is based on the observation that most cases of splenic rupture in athletes have occurred when those athletes returned to competition in less than 4 weeks from the time of diagnosis.

....

The patient returns 2 days later and is noting increased pharyngeal swelling and difficulty swallowing. You look into his throat and note "kissing tonsils." There is no stridor, but he feels as though there is something in his throat.

Question 20.11.9 What is the best treatment for this patient at this time?
A) Observation
B) Amoxicillin
C) Clindamycin
D) Prednisone
E) Tonsillectomy

Answer 20.11.9 The correct answer is "A." You may want to give steroids ("D"), but you will find little data to back you up. A Cochrane Collaboration Review updated in 2015 found insufficient evidence for steroids for symptom control in patients with mononucleosis (and other causes of "glandular fever" and sore throat). However, many physicians still prescribe steroids for patients with significant symptoms. Antibiotics are not indicated for mononucleosis. Tonsillectomy is also not indicated. The patient likely has paratracheal node swelling, as well. In this patient, hospital admission may be indicated if there is concern for airway obstruction.

Question 20.11.10 What is the approximate sensitivity of the heterophile antibody test ("monospot") for mononucleosis within the first 2 weeks of symptoms?
A) 10%
B) 30%
C) 50%
D) 70%
E) >90%

Answer 20.11.10 The correct answer is "D." The sensitivity of the monospot ranges from 60% to 80% about 2 weeks into the illness. The point here is not the number per se but the fact that there are heterophile-negative mononucleosis syndromes **and** not everyone with EBV mononucleosis will have a positive monospot when tested. However, they should have atypical lymphocytes on WBC differential.

HELPFUL TIP:
Consider peritonsillar abscess in a patient with a sore throat. There will generally be a muffled, "hot potato," voice, deviation of the uvula away from the side of the abscess, and protrusion of a tonsil toward midline. This may be an extension of a prior pharyngitis but may also arise de novo. Treatment is antibiotics and drainage (needling it is OK—no need for surgical involvement in all cases). It is also important to pay attention to the airway since there is the possibility of obstruction.

HELPFUL TIP:
The monospot is not as sensitive in children. It will become positive in less than 40% of children younger than 5 years when they are infected with EBV. However, anti-EBV antibodies will be positive.

HELPFUL TIP:
Arcanobacterium haemolyticum is a bacterium that causes pharyngitis especially in young adults (teens, early

twenties). It clinically looks like strep throat but often has an associated rash especially on the arms (50% only). It does not cause long-term sequelae, so testing for it is not necessarily indicated (but it is cool to identify when the patient comes in with the appropriate rash!). If you choose to treat (which some practitioners do), it is generally sensitive to penicillins, cephalosporins, and tetracyclines.

▶ **Objectives: Did you learn to …**
- Describe different strategies to approaching the patient with symptoms of *streptococcal* pharyngitis?
- Treat a patient with *streptococcal* pharyngitis and recurrent pharyngitis?
- Develop a broad differential for sore throat?
- Diagnose and treat mononucleosis?

⧗ QUICK QUIZ: IN THE SAME VEIN …

Uh, oh. You have treated a 19-year-old college student for presumed streptococcal pharyngitis with azithromycin (didn't we say not to do this?!). In your defense, he wanted to get better fast because he landed the lead role in the new musical *You Had Me at Arrrgh: A Wookie Love Story*. He returns 1 week later with high fever and a cough, looking quite ill. Chest radiograph shows small pulmonary abscesses and he is tender over a swollen carotid sheath. His throat looks awful ….

The most likely diagnosis is:
A) Lemierre syndrome
B) Complication of EBV mononucleosis
C) Cardiac valvular disease from rheumatic fever
D) Aspiration pneumonitis from his pharyngitis
E) Scarlet fever

The correct answer is "A." This is a classic case of Lemierre syndrome, or septic thrombophlebitis of the jugular vein from (generally) *Fusobacterium necrophorum*. This is an anaerobic infection of the posterior pharynx that may be misdiagnosed as streptococcal disease. Generally, patients look ill with a temperature of >39°C, have tenderness in the neck, and have septic emboli in the lungs. The basic problem is a septic thrombophlebitis of the jugular vein. It is being increasingly recognized especially in young adults (teens–early twenties). This patient must be admitted for IV antibiotics and may require anticoagulation and/or surgical intervention. In the pharyngitis stage, it is sensitive to penicillin. See, if you would have listened to us and used penicillin in the first place you wouldn't be in this bind!

Clinical Pearls

- *Arcanobacterium* and *Fusobacterium* pharyngitis can look just like Strep throat although the rapid Strep will be negative. *Arcanobacterium* is often associated with a rash. *Fusobacterium* can lead to a septic thrombophlebitis of the jugular vein (Lemierre syndrome).

- Consider mumps in a patient with salivary gland swelling even in patients who have had both MMR vaccinations; immunity wanes with time and there are yearly outbreaks in the United States.

- Do not suggest ear tubes for patients with unilateral serous otitis. The main function of ear tubes in this situation is to assist with language development. This is not an issue with unilateral serous otitis.

- Infections of the cartilaginous ear pinnae from piercings are often from *Pseudomonas*. This is an emergency.

- Most nasal trauma need not be addressed at a first visit: you can get a better cosmetic result in 3 to 5 days once the swelling has subsided. However, a septal hematoma is an emergency that requires prompt attention to prevent septal cartilage necrosis.

- Penicillin is still the drug of choice for Strep throat. There is no resistance and if the patient has mononucleosis you haven't fated them to 6 weeks of a rash, which might occur with amoxicillin.

- A wick can be used when treating otitis externa with topical drops. This will help assure that the medication gets to where it is needed.

BIBLIOGRAPHY

American Academy of Pediatrics Subcommittee on Management of Acute Otitis Media. Diagnosis and management of acute otitis media. *Pediatrics*. 2013;131(3):E964–E969.

Aring AM, Chan MM. Acute rhinosinusitis in adults. *Am Fam Physician*. 2011;83(9):1057–1063.

Buescher JJ. Temporomandibular joint disorders. *Am Fam Physician*. 2007;76(10):1477–1482.

Centor RM, Samlowski R. Avoiding sore throat morbidity and mortality: when is it not "just a sore throat?". *Am Fam Physician*. 2011;83(1):26, 28.

Chow AW, et al. Executive summary: IDSA clinical practice guideline for acute bacterial rhinosinusitis in children and adults. *Clin Infect Dis*. 2012;54(8):1041–1045.

Ely JE, et al. Diagnosis of ear pain. *Am Fam Physician*. 2008;77(5):621.

House SA, Fisher EL. Hoarseness in adults. *Am Fam Physician*. 2017;80(4):363–370.

Lockhart P, et al. Antiviral treatment for Bell's palsy (idiopathic facial paralysis). *Cochrane Database Syst Rev*. 2009;4:CD001869.

Lodi G, et al. Interventions for treating oral leukoplakia. *Cochrane Database Syst Rev*. 2006;4:CD001829.

McAllister K, et al. Surgical interventions for the early management of Bell's palsy. Cochrane *Database Syst Rev*. 2011;2:CD007468.

Paradise JL, et al. Developmental outcomes after early or delayed insertion of tympanostomy tubes. *N Engl J Med*. 2005;353:576–586.

Parnes LS, et al. Diagnosis and management of benign paroxysmal positional vertigo (BPPV). *CMAJ*. 2003;169(7):681.

Pynnonen MA, Gillespie MB, Roman B, et al. Clinical practice guideline: evaluation of the neck mass in adults. *Otolaryngol Head Neck Surg.* 2017; 157(2S) S1-S30.

Rosenfeld RM, et al. Clinical practice guideline: acute otitis externa. *Otolaryngol Head Neck Surg.* 2014;150(1S):S1–S24.

Salinas RA, et al. Corticosteroids for Bell's palsy (idiopathic facial paralysis). *Cochrane Database Syst Rev.* 2010;3:CD001942.

Care of the Older Patient

21

Victoria Linares and Nicholas R. Butler

An 83-year-old female patient whom you have followed for many years has just been admitted to a nursing home following a short hospitalization. Because of a steady decline in function and lack of family and social support, you and the patient have come to the realization that she can no longer safely live alone in her home and her needs were too great for assisted living. Her medical problems include: heart failure, chronic atrial fibrillation, osteoarthritis, and depression. Her current medications are: warfarin, furosemide, acetaminophen, calcium carbonate, lisinopril, metoprolol, and fluoxetine. Both the patient and the nursing staff report poor sleep and depressed mood for the last 2 weeks, and the nurses are asking for a sleep aid.

Question 21.1.1 What is the best next step in the management of her insomnia?
A) Add diphenhydramine 50 mg PO nightly
B) Add diazepam 5 mg PO nightly as needed
C) Add amitriptyline 25 mg PO nightly
D) Recommend increased activity during the day, avoidance of naps, warm milk before bed, and waking at the same time each morning
E) Add 2 shots of bourbon PO nightly

Answer 21.1.1 The correct answer is "D." There are no great medicines for promoting sleep in elderly nursing home residents. Given the lack of efficacy data of most hypnotics coupled with the known adverse effects, a trial of good sleep hygiene should be undertaken first. "Good sleep hygiene" generally consists of the following: eliminate or reduce daytime naps, add daily activities, maintain a set waking time, increase aerobic exercise (but not within a few hours of bedtime), and maintain a quiet, comfortable sleeping environment. Nighttime rituals, such as meditation and warm milk, may help insomnia and are unlikely to cause any harm, but avoid the bourbon as alcohol interferes with normal sleep architecture. If these initial efforts fail, a low dose of a hypnotic (e.g., zolpidem, zaleplon) or

trazodone is an appropriate choice. Trazodone has fewer anticholinergic and blood pressure effects than other options, such as tricyclics and benzodiazepines, but should still be used with caution while monitoring for adverse effects. Diphenhydramine ("A") has powerful antihistaminic and anticholinergic properties that may result in increased confusion and falls. Diazepam ("B") has an exceptionally long half-life in elderly patients and may cause daytime somnolence. Amitriptyline ("C") is listed by the Centers for Medicare and Medicaid Services (CMS) as a medication to be avoided in nursing home patients due to high potential for severe adverse drug reactions (falls, confusion, constipation, etc.).

HELPFUL TIP:
Melatonin receptor agonists (e.g., ramelteon) are another option for insomnia but are not great. Patients sleep about 7 minutes more per night compared to placebo (let's talk about statistically significant vs. clinically significant now!). They are relatively safe and do not lead to a "hangover" as with many hypnotics. The use of ramelteon and melatonin has also been shown to be beneficial in preventing the onset of delirium in acutely ill elderly patients. Melatonin has poor evidence for primary insomnia treatment but low chance of harm, so some physicians will try it first. And then there are orexin receptor antagonists, such as suvorexant (Belsomra), which possess a side effect profile that is not favorable for older patients (e.g., suicidal ideation, "sleep driving," daytime somnolence). Suvorexant *has a 12-hour half-life* in the non-elderly, leading to significant dysfunction the day after taking the drug.

HELPFUL TIP:
There are many potential causes of sleep disturbance in the nursing home. The following are sources of sleep problems that you may want to investigate or treat

empirically: pain, anxiety, depression, delirium, dementia, primary sleep disorders (e.g., sleep apnea, restless leg syndrome), environmental issues (e.g., alarms and lights).

....

The nurses grudgingly accept your recommendation to try sleep hygiene ("Can't we just give her a pill?"), and over the next month your patient's sleep improves, as does her mood. There's one in the win column for the doctor! Unfortunately, she experiences two falls with minor injuries while ambulating in her room. When you see her one week later, she recalls the falls and can describe what happened with each—essentially, she tripped. Upon examination, you find normal vital signs, no orthostatic hypotension, and no focal neurological deficits.

Question 21.1.2 Which of the following is the most appropriate next step?
A) Discontinue warfarin
B) Employ bed and chair alarms
C) Obtain a computerized tomography (CT) scan of the head
D) Reduce or discontinue fluoxetine
E) Restrict activities and prescribe a wheelchair

Answer 21.1.2 The correct answer is "D." As often happens in life, there is no great answer here. Falls are usually multifactorial in origin, so simple interventions do not generally solve the problem. SSRIs have been shown (in imperfect studies) to increase the risk of falls in the elderly, so reducing or discontinuing fluoxetine is prudent, but you will have to watch for mood and anxiety symptoms. "A," discontinuing warfarin, may be appropriate if she continues to fall but this action is not likely to reduce her fall risk. "B," the use of bed and chair alarms, is helpful when patients have cognitive impairment and cannot remember to ask for help when getting up; however, these devices can act as tethers to further restrict a patient's movement. Likewise, further restriction of activities and mandatory wheelchair use ("E") may lead to deconditioning, loss of muscle strength, and an increased risk of falls. A CT scan of the head may be warranted if the patient sustained a head injury or had an abnormal neurological examination, but it's unlikely to determine the cause of her falls.

....

Over the next year, you observe a steady decline in your patient's function, with a series of falls despite interventions. Ultimately, your patient has a devastating thromboembolic stroke, which results in right hemiparesis and dysphagia. After a short hospital stay, she returns to the nursing home and undergoes therapy. You order a swallow study (as you do for all stroke patients). She continues to have difficulty with her swallowing but is able to tolerate thickened liquids without aspirating. She has a 5% weight loss over the next 2 months, and her nurse reports poor oral intake. Her medications are now warfarin, furosemide, acetaminophen, calcium carbonate, and lisinopril.

Question 21.1.3 In this malnourished, elderly nursing home patient, which of the following interventions or diagnostic studies will most likely lead to improvement in her condition?
A) Admit to the hospital and initiate parenteral feeding
B) Refer for esophagogastroduodenoscopy (EGD)
C) Screen for depression
D) Add megestrol acetate
E) Add marijuana

Answer 21.1.3 The correct answer is "C." Depression is one of the most common causes of weight loss in the nursing home, and stroke survivors are at high risk for depression. Also, this patient has a history of depression with no current treatment (since we stopped the fluoxetine earlier). Consider using a screening tool, such as the Geriatric Depression Scale. A positive screen requires further investigation. Now that she is bedridden, falls are not as much of an issue, so an antidepressant may be appropriate. "A" is incorrect. We are not sure of the patient's wishes regarding intravenous (IV) nutrition, and more conservative measures should be instituted before considering parenteral nutrition. "B" is incorrect. While an EGD may be important at some point, proceeding to EGD immediately is premature. "D," megestrol acetate, has been reported to improve food intake in patients with cancer cachexia, but its value in the nursing home is questionable, and it may be associated with an increased risk of mortality. "E" is also incorrect. Even if you practice in one of the tokin' states, we cannot have her lighting up in the nursing home.

HELPFUL TIP:
The initial evaluation of a nursing home patient with weight loss should focus on medication review, gastrointestinal symptoms, dental and mouth problems, swallowing dysfunction, ability to feed one-self, and neuropsychiatric disorders (e.g., depression, dementia, psychosis). Hyperthyroidism, hyperparathyroidism, malignancy, and chronic infection should be considered as causes of weight loss, albeit less likely. Factors associated with aging, such as decreased olfaction, taste, and salivation (and nursing home food), may decrease the enjoyment of eating. Patients with dementia commonly develop apathy and lose interest in eating in latter stages.

....

You diagnose depression and initiate treatment. You also encourage the nursing staff to observe your patient while eating and assist her if necessary. You add a daily multivitamin. Her mood improves slightly and her weight stabilizes. However, over the next 6 months, your patient becomes more withdrawn and spends most of her time in bed. Because of her stroke, she is not very mobile, and she requires assistance with transfers and movement in bed. Ultimately, she develops a skin ulcer on her sacrum. Nursing staff reports a sacral pressure ulcer measuring 3 × 2 cm. There is interruption of the epidermis, like an abrasion.

TABLE 21-1 PRESSURE ULCER STAGES

Stage I	Stage II	Stage III	Stage IV	Unstageable
Nonblanchable erythema	Partial-thickness skin loss	Full-thickness skin loss	Full-thickness skin loss	Ulcer covered in eschar and depth unknown
Intact skin	Epidermis and/or dermis	Damage or necrosis of subcutaneous tissues, extending to underlying fascia	Extensive destruction, tissue necrosis, or damage to muscle, bone or supporting structures	
Changes in skin temperature, consistency, or sensation	Presents as abrasion, blister, or shallow crater	Presents as deep crater		

Question 21.1.4 **According to conventional staging criteria, what stage is this pressure ulcer?**
A) Stage I
B) Stage II
C) Stage III
D) Stage IV
E) Unstageable

Answer 21.1.4 **The correct answer is "B."** Pressure ulcers (in older parlance, decubitus ulcers, pressure sores, or bed sores) are caused by unrelieved pressure resulting in ischemic damage to underlying tissue. Stage II ulcers are partial thickness injuries that are shallow and appear as open ulcers. Anatomic areas of concern in bed-bound patients include sacrum, coccyx, heels, and occiput. Chair-bound patients are more likely to develop ulcers over the ischial tuberosities. Risk factors for pressure ulcers include advancing age, immobility, moisture (e.g., urinary or fecal incontinence), malnutrition, and decreased sensory perception. Ulcers are staged by clinical appearance (see Table 21-1).

Because of miscommunication within the nursing home staff, the ulcer goes untended over the weekend. An alarmed nurse calls you to report full thickness skin loss. You arrange to visit the patient in the evening … here comes another "above and beyond" award.

Question 21.1.5 **In the meantime, you prescribe what treatment?**
A) Foam pad with occluding dressing (e.g., Allevyn, Mepilex)
B) Wet-to-dry dressing
C) Topical antibiotics
D) Transparent, occlusive dressing (e.g., Tegaderm)
E) Chemical enzyme debridement (e.g., Accuzyme)

Answer 21.1.5 **The correct answer is "A."** In treating pressure ulcers, there are several principles to follow: relieve pressure, protect the wound and surrounding skin from further trauma, maintain a clean wound bed, provide a moist wound environment, eliminate dead space, control exudates, ensure adequate nutrition, and diagnose and treat infection. Your patient's ulcer has worsened and is now at least stage III. Without further information, foam dressing is a safe choice for initial treatment of a stage III ulcer. Foam pads are useful for deeper wounds with moderate exudate and may also protect the wound from further pressure. In most cases, the wound should be kept moist, so wet-to-dry dressings are not appropriate (they debride the wound of **both** necrotic and healthy tissues—ouch, and are not helpful). If moist gauze packing is used, it should be kept moist with intermittent reapplication of saline or changed before drying. Wet-to-dry dressings ("B") have fallen out of favor due to tissue trauma secondary to removing the dry dressing. From the nurse's report, there is no evidence of necrosis, excessive drainage or infection, so antibiotics ("C") and debridement ("E") would not be helpful at this time. A transparent, occlusive dressing ("D") is used for stage II ulcers, but is insufficient for stage III or IV. In addition to dressing the wound, you should employ the following measures: repositioning every 1 to 2 hours, use pressure-relieving mattress and cushions, and optimizing nutrition. Consultation with a wound care specialist or a surgeon may be necessary if these measures fail.

HELPFUL TIP:
There is minimal evidence of benefit for the use of most adjunctive therapies for pressure ulcers (electrical stimulation, ultrasound, hyperbaric oxygen, ultraviolet light, vasodilators, vacuum devices, etc.). In general, stick with pressure relief, good wound care, and nutrition.

HELPFUL TIP:
To prevent pressure ulcers, schedule regular and frequent repositioning for bed- and chair-bound individuals. Turn at least every 2 to 4 hours on a pressure-reducing mattress or every 2 hours on a non-pressure-reducing mattress. Also, maintain the head of the bed ≤30 degrees if possible to reduce pressure and shear forces on the sacral area. See Figures 21-1 and 21-2 to better understand how positioning and shear forces lead to the development of pressure ulcers.

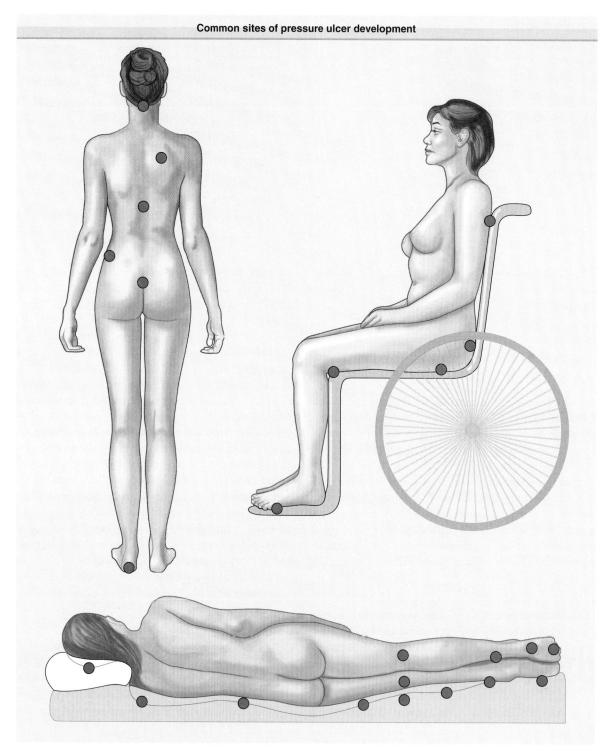

Common sites of pressure ulcer development

FIGURE 21-1. Common sites of pressure ulcer development for patients in supine (left upper figure), seated (right upper figure), and lateral decubitus (lower figure) positions. (From *Preventing Pressure Ulcers: A Patient's Guide*. Washington, DC, US Department of Health and Human Services, USGPO 617-025/68298, 1992.)

Question 21.1.6 Which of the following statements is NOT true about the evaluation and treatment of pressure ulcers?

A) A pressure ulcer covered by eschar cannot be staged until the eschar is removed.

B) If a pressure ulcer shows no signs of healing over 2 weeks, one should reevaluate wound management strategies and reexamine factors affecting the wound.

C) One should consider osteomyelitis or deep soft-tissue infection in a wound that is not healing.

D) Wound cultures should be obtained routinely to target antibiotics toward the organisms found.

E) In an otherwise clean wound that is not healing as expected, one should consider empiric therapy with topical antibiotics.

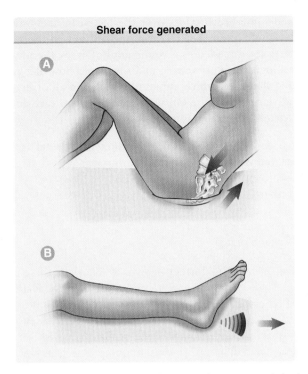

Shear force generated

FIGURE 21-2. The effects of shear forces on the sacrum and the heel. (From Grey JE, Harding KG, Enoch S: Pressure ulcers. *BMJ* **332**:472, 2006, with permission of Blackwell Publishing.)

Answer 21.1.6 The correct answer is "D." The routine culturing of pressure ulcers is not recommended. Antibiotics are generally not useful since the organisms found are polymicrobial colonizers and not responsible for infection. Obviously, this does not hold true for patients with a true infection, and empiric therapy with topical antibiotics is indicated if a wound shows no improvement with good wound care. Remember that a flap cannot be used to repair the ulcer until infection is resolved.

▶ **Objectives: Did you learn to …**
- Manage insomnia in elderly nursing home residents?
- Develop an approach to the problem of falls in nursing home residents?
- Identify nursing home residents at risk for malnutrition?
- Develop a treatment plan for malnutrition in the institutionalized elderly?
- Diagnose, evaluate, and manage pressure ulcers in the nursing home setting?

 QUICK QUIZ: VACCINES

A 65-year-old healthy male presents for a routine visit and asks about pneumococcal vaccination. You correctly tell the patient:
A) "The CDC recommends that you receive Pneumovax (23-valent pneumococcal polysaccharide vaccine) at your age."
B) "Pneumococcal vaccines are proven to reduce your risk of all causes of pneumonia."

C) "According to the CDC, you are due to receive Prevnar (13-valent pneumococcal protein-conjugate vaccine) at your age."
D) "Pneumococcal vaccines have a high rate of serious adverse effects"
E) "Pneumococcal vaccines basically make you invincible, unless they give you autism"

The correct answer is "A," the 23-valent vaccine (Pneumovax) is recommended at age 65. This recommendation has changed. The 13-valent vaccine (Prevnar) is now optional; the elderly are protected by herd immunity secondary to the vaccination of children. For those immunosuppressed, give the 13-valent (Prevnar) followed in 23 valent (Pneumovax) in 8 weeks. For others who might want both, give the 23 valent first followed by the 13 valent in one year. While the PPSV has clearly demonstrated efficacy in reducing the risk of invasive pneumococcal disease (e.g., bacteremia, meningitis), PCV has been shown to reduce pneumonia due to the serotypes against which the vaccine is directed in addition to invasive disease. Neither of the vaccines reduce the risk of all-cause pneumonia. The vaccines are well-tolerated.

 QUICK QUIZ: VACCINES, AGAIN

A 67-year-old healthy male presents as a new patient and brings his immunization records with him (and you physically stop yourself from slapping your forehead in disbelief at this patient's foresight). He has received both pneumococcal vaccines (Prevnar and Pneumovax) at age 65 and 66, respectively, following the old guidelines. He had Tdap (tetanus, diphtheria, and pertussis) and Zostavax (shingles) vaccines at age 60. In accordance with CDC recommendations, you tell him he is due for:
A) Shingrix (recombinant zoster vaccine)
B) Prevnar (pneumococcal protein conjugate vaccine)
C) Tenivac (Td or tetanus/diphtheria vaccine)
D) Zostavax (live, attenuated zoster vaccine)
E) All of the above

The correct answer is "A." The recombinant zoster vaccine (Shingrix) is currently recommended for all immunocompetent patients over the age of 50 years, whether or not they have received the attenuated live virus vaccine (Zostavax), had a case of shingles, or recall having chicken pox. Since early 2018, the CDC has recommended Shingrix over Zostavax due to markedly superior efficacy. Studies have shown that Shingrix is 91% effective in preventing shingles in patients age 70 and older who received both doses. It is a two-dose vaccine, and doses should be separated by 2 to 6 months. The other vaccines in the foils are not indicated for the following reasons: the patient already received both recommended doses of pneumococcal vaccines ("B"); the patient received Tdap 7 years ago and tetanus vaccine ("C") boosters are due every 10 years; and there is no indication for re-dosing Zostavax ("D").

QUICK QUIZ: HORMONES AND AGING

Noticing advertisements for testosterone treatment to "make you a vital man again," one of your vivacious older female patients asks about testosterone for her husband wondering if it can make him 50 years old again.

Regarding sex hormone changes associated with aging, which of the following is true?
A) Leydig cells in the testes increase with aging
B) Total testosterone levels increase with aging
C) Sex hormone–binding globulin levels increase with aging
D) Follicle-stimulating hormone levels are unchanged with aging
E) Luteinizing hormone levels decrease with aging

The correct answer is "C." Sex hormones in males over age 40 demonstrate declining total testosterone at a rate of 1% to 2% per year. Simultaneously, sex hormone–binding globulin increases, resulting in a sharper decline in bioavailable testosterone. In response to low testosterone, follicle-stimulating and luteinizing hormone levels increase. Leydig cells (responsible for producing testosterone) decrease in number. Older males with subphysiologic testosterone levels are at increased risk of sexual dysfunction, osteoporosis, diminished lean body mass, depression, and inability to kill a mountain lion with their bare hands. Although controversial, some experts recommend testosterone supplementation in symptomatic males with low-serum testosterone. Testosterone supplementation may (notice the word "may") improve strength, lean body mass, depressed mood, bone mineral density, and sexual function in aging males with documented low testosterone levels. Side effects of testosterone supplementation in older males include: cardiac disease, liver dysfunction, dyslipidemia, erythrocytosis, prostate tissue growth, acne, gynecomastia, and edema. If your patient is baleful and pushes the request for "T," point out that testosterone adds nothing to the treatment of erectile dysfunction beyond that benefit which is offered by tadalafil (Cialis), sildenafil (Viagra), etc. You can reassure him that he will be just as virile at age 98 without testosterone and will avoid the risk of worsening heart disease. A consensus statement does recommend testosterone **For Postmenopausal Women** with hypoactive sexual desire disorder (J Clin Endocrinol Metab 2019 Oct 1; 104:4660). This a "disease" probably invented by men.

HELPFUL TIP:
Any time you see the word "may," think "may not." They are logical equivalents.

▶ CASE 21.2

A 79-year-old female patient, well known to you from 5 years of treating her hypertension, presents to your office for an "annual examination" and "medication refill." Her medications are lisinopril, amlodipine, and acetaminophen. She's noticed some hearing loss over the last year, and wonders if she should blame her medications and not all those rock concerts she attended as a young adult. Oh, by the way, her gynecologist recently retired and she would now like you to assume that care, which apparently included all of her preventative care (because OB/GYNs are "primary care doctors for women"— sarcasm intended).

Question 21.2.1 Which of the following drugs is NOT associated with sensorineural hearing loss?
A) Ibuprofen
B) Aminoglycosides
C) Furosemide
D) Magnesium salicylate
E) Acetaminophen

Answer 21.2.1 **The correct answer is "E."** All of these drugs except for acetaminophen can cause hearing loss. Platinum-based chemotherapeutics, aminoglycoside antibiotics, and loop diuretics have been associated with hearing loss, as have salicylates (e.g., aspirin) and some of the other NSAIDs (e.g., ibuprofen and diflunisal) and chloroquine. This list is obviously not exhaustive.

HELPFUL TIP:
Hearing loss, and sensory impairments in general, can be confused with cognitive impairment or an affective disorder. Hearing aids are useful for most cases of presbycusis, but if speech discrimination is <50%, results with hearing aids may be poor.

Your patient then asks, "Do I have to keep getting mammograms and Pap smears?" She relates a history of normal annual mammograms and Pap smears for the last 20 years, as her previous physician hadn't changed her practice since the Backstreet Boys were popular. She had a hysterectomy for uterine fibromas and has been monogamous with her husband for 55 years. Her sister died of breast cancer. Using your magic crystal ball, you estimate her life expectancy at 10 years or greater.

Question 21.2.2 Consistent with current guidelines, you recommend:
A) Continue Pap smears and pelvic examinations yearly
B) Discontinue mammography but perform clinical breast examinations every 2 years
C) Discontinue pelvic examinations but continue Pap smears
D) Discontinue Pap smears but offer mammography at 1- to 2-year intervals

Answer 21.2.2 **The correct answer is "D."** Tricky question. Screening decisions in the elderly should be individualized, and the patient's overall health status must be considered. This patient has very little risk of cervical, endometrial, or vaginal cancer (status posthysterectomy for a benign condition, low-risk sexual behavior, and a history of normal examinations);

therefore, she has no indication for continuing Pap smears. Annual pelvic examination is more controversial, with the American Cancer Society (ACS) recommending physicians discuss this ovarian cancer screening measure with patients and reach a shared decision while the US Preventive Services Task Force (USPSTF) recommends against it.

Screening for breast cancer continues to be recommended for women with a 5- to 10-year life expectancy, but the optimal interval in older women is unknown: The American College of Physicians and USPSTF recommend screening of asymptomatic women **aged 50 to 74** years every other year. But our patient is 79. Whether this patient will benefit from mammography is unknown. There is a significant question of the "overdiagnosis" of breast cancer—in other words a cancer diagnosed by mammogram that would not ever have caused a problem for the patient (think of it as the equivalent of the diagnosis of prostate cancer in men … they may die *with* the cancer and not *of* the cancer). Before ordering a mammogram, we need to have a discussion with our patients about what types of intervention they would want should a positive mammogram be noted.

HELPFUL TIP:
The 2012 consensus guidelines on screening for cervical cancer recommend discontinuing screening at age 65 if the previous three Pap smears prior to age 65 were completely normal and there were no findings of CIN2 or higher in the previous 20 years. Once stopped, screening should not be resumed for any reason, including a new sexual partner. Note that this is consistent with the 2018 USPSTF guidelines.

Your patient is an overweight white female with no history of bone fracture. She has never had a bone mineral density test and asks if she should have one. You are unaware of any risk factors in her other than Caucasian race and postmenopausal status.

Question 21.2.3 **What do you tell her?**
A) "You are not at risk for osteoporosis and should not be screened"
B) "All women over age 65 should be screened for osteoporosis regardless of risk"
C) "Take 1,000 mg of calcium per day to prevent osteoporosis. You'll be unbreakable—like Wolverine…in an Iron Man suit… surrounded by marshmallows"
D) "Due to your risk factors, you should start a bisphosphonate, vitamin D, and calcium supplementation"

Answer 21.2.3 **The correct answer is "B."** The USPSTF recommends bone densitometry screening for all women of age 65 years and older. The National Osteoporosis Foundation recommends bone densitometry for postmenopausal females with one or more of the following risk factors: family history of osteoporosis, personal history of low trauma fracture, current smoking, or low body weight (<127 lb). Additional risk

factors for osteoporosis include: female sex, Caucasian or Asian races, alcohol abuse (thus, "E" is wrong), sedentary lifestyle, and poor intake or absorption of calcium and vitamin D. Smoking is associated with osteoporosis. Diabetes, once thought to protect against osteoporosis, may actually increase the risk of falls and fractures in older adults. The preferred method for measuring bone density is dual-energy x-ray absorptiometry (DEXA). All postmenopausal women should consume 1,200 mg of elemental calcium per day in divided doses (either in food or as supplements or both). The optimal amount of vitamin D is 400 to 800 IU/day. Weight-bearing exercises strengthen bone and should be encouraged. Bisphosphonates are indicated for treatment of osteoporosis and should not be used without a diagnosis (so "D" is incorrect).

HELPFUL TIP:
Supplementing vitamin D is probably more important than supplementing calcium. Calcium supplementation has not consistently demonstrated fracture risk reduction. However, many elderly Americans are vitamin D deficient, and correction of the deficiency results in reduced fracture risk. Given the low risk of adverse effects with daily vitamin D (up to 1,000 IU/day), empiric supplementation is justifiable. Finally, 1,000 to 1,200 mg (not 1,500 mg) of calcium is probably plenty. Additional calcium has been linked to an elevated risk of coronary artery disease and no change in fracture risk. Calcium and vitamin D are clearly beneficial in those with osteoporosis, however. These recommendations change frequently. What is clear is that high dose (>4000IU/day reduces bone density and has no benefit on overall mortality (JAMA 2019 Aug 27; 322:736, JAMA 2019 Aug 27; 322:7360.

You could also use the FRAX Fracture Risk Assessment Tool to provide your patient with some idea of her risk of future fracture and to plan preventive strategies accordingly.

Question 21.2.4 **All of the following data elements are required to use the FRAX calculator EXCEPT:**
A) Sex
B) Weight
C) Age
D) Bone Mineral Density
E) Smoking status

Answer 21.2.4 **The correct answer is "D."** The FRAX tool is a validated calculator for assessing the 10-year probability of developing a major osteoporotic fracture. The tool requires numerous demographic and medical history elements and can be made more accurate by including the bone mineral density (BMD), but it does not require the use of BMD. Required elements include: age, sex, weight, height, previous fracture, parental hip fracture, smoking status, alcohol use, glucocorticoid use, history of rheumatoid arthritis, and history of secondary osteoporosis. It can be located free of charge online at https://www.sheffield.ac.uk/FRAX/. We are pretty sure that "The FRAX" is also a Dr. Seuss character (or should be).

Next, your patient asks whether any of her medications put her at risk for osteoporosis.

Question 21.2.5 Which of the following is LEAST likely to increase the risk of osteoporosis?

A) Glucocorticoids
B) Anticonvulsants
C) Sulfonylureas
D) Loop diuretics
E) Proton-pump inhibitors

Answer 21.2.5 **The correct answer is "C."** Sulfonylureas do not have a direct effect on bone mineralization. Glucocorticoids ("A") and anticonvulsants ("B") are known to increase bone turnover, resulting in increased risk of osteoporosis. Loop diuretics ("D") cause renal calcium wasting. There is an association between proton-pump inhibitor ("E") use and osteoporosis, possibly through reduced calcium absorption or direct effects on bone metabolism. There does not appear to be this same association with H_2-blockers such as famotidine. Additionally, heparin, methotrexate, cyclosporine, and gonadotropin-releasing hormone agonists may increase the risk of osteoporosis. Excessive amounts of levothyroxine can cause increased bone turnover. Thiazide diuretics are protective.

Your patient asks what causes osteoporosis.

Question 21.2.6 Although most osteoporosis in women is primary (idiopathic), which of the following causes secondary osteoporosis?

A) Hypoparathyroidism
B) Multiple myeloma
C) Estrogen use
D) Hyperlipidemia
E) Overly ambitious, or perhaps calcium-addicted, Tooth Fairies

Answer 21.2.6 **The correct answer is "B."** About 70% of women have no identifiable cause for osteoporosis and therefore are diagnosed with primary (idiopathic) osteoporosis. Common causes of secondary osteoporosis include chronic corticosteroid use, alcoholism, GI disorders, hyperthyroidism, **hyper**parathyroidism (so, "A" is wrong), multiple myeloma, and primary renal diseases. Estrogen ("C") increases bone mineral density. Hyperlipidemia ("D") is not known to be associated with osteoporosis.

You encourage appropriate vitamin D and calcium intake as well as weight-bearing exercises. You plan to obtain a DEXA scan.

Question 21.2.7 Using DEXA scan results, osteoporosis is defined as:

A) A T-score of 2.5 standard deviations or more below the mean of a healthy young adult (T-score ≤ -2.5)
B) A T-score from 1.0 up to 2.5 standard deviations below the mean of a healthy young adult (-1.0 up to -2.5)
C) A Z-score of 2.5 standard deviations or more below the mean for same-aged females (≤ -2.5)
D) A Z-score from 1.0 up to 2.5 standard deviations below the mean for same-aged females (-1.0 up to -2.5)

Answer 21.2.7 **The correct answer is "A."** The T-score compares the patient's bone mineral density to that of young, healthy women (for female patients; male normative data is used for males). Osteoporosis is defined as a T-score of 2.5 standard deviations or more below the mean (≤ -2.5). Osteopenia is defined as a T-score from 1.0 up to 2.5 standard deviations below the mean (-1.0 to -2.5). "C" is incorrect. The Z-score compares bone mineral density to that of age-matched controls. Therefore, it does not reflect the bone loss from baseline in a young healthy female, and it is not used for diagnosis. "D" is incorrect for the same reason.

Question 21.2.8 If you find that your patient has osteoporosis, you may consider using all of the following drugs to treat her osteoporosis EXCEPT:

A) Bisphosphonates (e.g., alendronate and risedronate)
B) Estrogens
C) Progestins (e.g., Provera and Depo-Provera)
D) Vitamin D and calcium
E) Calcitonin

Answer 21.2.8 **The correct answer is "C."** Progestins are not indicated for the treatment or prevention of osteoporosis. In fact, in young, healthy, premenopausal women, they have been associated with decreased bone mineral density due to suppression of estrogen production (such as with Depo-Provera). All of the other options are acceptable choices in the treatment of osteoporosis although some are better than others (keep reading).

She returns to discuss her test results, and her bone density is very low with her hip T-score 3.2 standard deviations below the mean (-3.2). You diagnose her with osteoporosis. "Are my bones like Swiss cheese?" she asks. No, you think. *Swiss cheese has more calcium.*

Question 21.2.9 Given that she is otherwise relatively healthy, what is the most appropriate initial therapy for her osteoporosis?

A) Alendronate (Fosamax) 70 mg PO weekly
B) Estrogen (e.g., Premarin) 0.625 mg PO daily
C) Teriparatide (Forteo) 20 g SC daily for 5 years
D) Zoledronic acid (Reclast) 5 mg IV every 3 months
E) Denosumab (Prolia) 60 mg SC every 6 months

Answer 21.2.9 **The correct answer is "A."** Bisphosphonates are the treatment of choice for osteoporosis. Alendronate, risedronate, and zoledronic acid have all been shown to reduce the risk of vertebral and hip fractures in persons with osteoporosis. Ibandronate only appears to lower vertebral fracture risk; therefore, it should not be the first choice. Side effects of bisphosphonates include hypocalcemia (more likely with IV administration, as with zoledronic acid, and in patients with vitamin D deficiency), nausea, esophagitis, osteonecrosis of the jaw (usually at higher doses, such as those used to treat cancer), and atypical femur fractures. Although you might be tempted to choose "D," zoledronic acid due to this patient's more severe osteoporosis, there is no clear evidence that zoledronic acid is more effective than oral bisphosphonates. The IV route should be reserved for when the patient has failed oral bisphosphonate therapy for some reason—usually due to upper gastrointestinal side effects. Zoledronic acid can cause "flu-like" symptoms, with diffuse myalgia and arthralgia for days after the infusion. "B" is incorrect as the safety data for bisphosphonates is superior to that for estrogen. "C" is incorrect. Teriparatide, a recombinant parathyroid hormone carries a risk of osteosarcoma, and its use is limited to 2 years, not 5. Teriparatide is effective at increasing bone density and reducing fracture risk, but the data are not nearly as robust as the data for bisphosphonates. It is not a first-line drug. Similarly, denosumab should be reserved as a second- or third-line agent. Denosumab (Prolia) is a RANKL inhibitor approved by the FDA for treatment of postmenopausal osteoporosis. It is effective in reducing fracture risk (vertebral and hip) and also appears to be well tolerated. However, it inhibits RANKL in the immune system, which acts similar to TNF, and the long-term effects on infection and carcinogenesis risks are uncertain.

HELPFUL (MAYBE) TIP:

It seems as though more than 5 years of a bisphosphonate may increase atypical femur fracture risk (thought to be due to the suppression of osteoclast activity and reduced ability of bone to remodel). Therefore, a drug holiday is likely warranted. Additionally, many patients maintain bone density after stopping a bisphosphonate after 5 years of therapy—at least for a few years. There are no clear guidelines on this yet. Consider getting a DEXA scan a couple of years after stopping the bisphosphonate. If it shows bone loss, consider restarting the bisphosphonate or starting another agent, such as denosumab.

HELPFUL TIP:

Always check serum calcium, 25-hydroxy vitamin D and creatinine levels prior to starting therapy for osteoporosis. All pharmacologic treatments for osteoporosis may cause hypocalcemia, and low-serum calcium and/or vitamin D levels should be corrected prior to initiating therapy. Patients with chronic kidney disease (glomerular filtration rate < 30 mL/min) and osteoporosis present a therapeutic challenge and should be managed in consultation with an endocrinologist and/or nephrologist.

Before she leaves the office, you present your patient with literature on living wills and durable power of attorney for healthcare (DPOA-HC).

Question 21.2.10 **Which of the following is CORRECT regarding advance healthcare planning?**
A) The Joint Commission requires that patients be asked about their advance directives on admission to the hospital
B) A DPOA-HC can override a patient's decision regarding treatment; this is known as the "gotcha rule"
C) Once the patient has signed a living will, no further changes can be made regarding treatment decisions
D) A DPOA-HC must be a family member or blood relative
E) A DPOA-HC must be prepared by an attorney with a special certification

Answer 21.2.10 **The correct answer is "A."** The Joint Commission requires that patients be asked about their advance directives on admission to the hospital. Advance directives can take many forms but are usually manifest in one of two ways: through a living will or a DPOA-HC. The purpose of a living will is to instruct healthcare decision-making in future events when the patient may not be able to communicate his or her wishes. These documents often contain brief clinical scenarios with patient preferences for life-sustaining measures. In contrast, a DPOA-HC is not as limited and can address situations not foreseen in a living will. If the patient becomes unable to participate in healthcare decision-making, then the DPOA-HC is instructed to exercise substituted judgment, using the patient's previously stated healthcare preferences, to help direct future care. The DPOA-HC is appointed by the patient and can be a family member or another adult. The DPOA-HC cannot override a patient's decision in healthcare matters, as such an action would violate patient autonomy.

HELPFUL TIP:

Although advance directives should be addressed with all patients, it is of particular importance to discuss them in the setting of chronic illness, life-threatening illness, advancing age, and with any deterioration in health status. A patient can change advance care plans whenever he or she wishes, as these decisions may change over time depending on goals of care. While a living will is often quite general in nature, a physician order for life-sustaining treatment form (which takes slightly different form in each state that has this legislation) may be even more helpful for patients with advanced illness. These forms go into greater detail regarding patient/family wishes for various kinds of treatment, including hospitalization, ICU care, artificial nutrition, etc.

▶ **Objectives: Did you learn to ...**
- Identify and implement appropriate preventive health services for older females?
- Discuss issues related to breast and gynecologic cancer screening?

- Define appropriate criteria for osteoporosis screening and identify risk factors?
- Initiate treatment in a patient with osteoporosis?
- Recognize the important and complementary roles of DPOA and advance directives?

 QUICK QUIZ: GERIATRIC PREVENTIVE CARE

Which of the following statements is INCORRECT regarding preventive health in older adults?

A) Although the optimal interval for vision screening is undetermined, many professional organizations recommend vision and glaucoma screening every 1 to 2 years in persons over age 65
B) In women at high risk for breast cancer, prophylactic tamoxifen reduces the relative risk of *estrogen receptor positive* cancer by 35% to 50% (absolute reduction of seven cases in 1,000 women treated for 5 years)
C) The American Cancer Society (ACS) and American College of Obstetrics and Gynecology (ACOG) recommend screening ultrasound for ovarian cancer in all women over the age of 60
D) Although Pap smears are not generally recommended for elderly women, in many countries, the distribution of cervical cancer cases is bimodal, with peaks in the thirties and sixties

The correct answer is "C." In fact, ACOG, the USPSTF, and the American College of Physicians specifically recommend against ultrasound screening for ovarian cancer in asymptomatic women. All other statements are correct. In many countries, there are two age peaks for the incidence of cervical cancer ("D"); however, the median age of cervical cancer diagnosis in the United States is 50, and most new cases are diagnosed between women aged 35 and 65 years. As to "B," nothing is free. The reduction in estrogen receptor–positive breast cancer comes at the cost of an increase of 4 in 1,000 having a thromboembolic event and 4 in 1,000 having an endometrial cancer *and* no change in overall or cancer mortality.

 HELPFUL (AND ENCOURAGING) TIP:
The incidence of cervical cancer in the United States has declined by more than 50% since 1975. Talk about a screening program that works!

▶ **CASE 21.3**

An 82-year-old male patient presents to your office for confusion. His wife reports that he was in his usual state of health until 3 days ago. At that time, he developed abdominal pain and felt feverish. He then began to have a dry, hacking cough. On examination, his temperature is 100.3°F and blood pressure is 118/56 mm Hg. He is pale and lethargic but

in no acute distress. He is oriented to person only. Other than mild upper abdominal tenderness, there are no additional findings on examination. This patient appears to have a new onset of confusion. You suspect delirium.

Question 21.3.1 Which of the following is true with regard to delirium and dementia?
A) In delirium it is rare to find an underlying medical cause
B) A primary feature of delirium is inattention
C) Dementia is characterized by an acutely fluctuating course
D) Delirium only occurs in patients with dementia
E) They are the same. After all, memory is but an ephemeral light in the long shadow of time

Answer 21.3.1 **The correct answer is "B."** The *Diagnostic and Statistical Manual of Mental Disorders* (DSM-V) provides the diagnostic criteria for delirium. A diagnosis of delirium requires the following criteria: disturbance of attention and awareness (previously termed "consciousness" in DSM-IV); disorientation, memory deficit, or another change in cognition that cannot be accounted for by a pre-existing dementia; acute onset with fluctuating course (often changing throughout the day); and evidence that the disturbance is caused by an underlying medical condition or drug use (so "A" is incorrect). Not all signs and symptoms of delirium are present in every patient with delirium, nor will they be present at the same time. Delirium can be confused with dementia, depression, or psychosis. Patients with delirium may present as agitated, psychotic, somnolent, or withdrawn (these are the tough ones to recognize). Dementia is more chronic in nature with an insidious onset (making "C" incorrect). Dementia progresses over time and usually cannot be reversed. Often delirium is treatable or reversible if the underlying medical condition is identified and treated. Patients with dementia usually have intact attention, whereas patients with delirium have markedly impaired attention. Patients with dementia have "poverty of thought," which implies decreased content of their thoughts. Patients with delirium may have a rich content in their thoughts, but the thoughts are disordered. Patients with dementia are at higher risk for developing delirium, but dementia is not a pre-requisite for delirium, and "D" is incorrect.

 HELPFUL TIP:
Delirium may be either hypoactive or hyperactive or both, all in the same patient. Many patients with delirium are not even identified due to their hypoactive state (these aren't the ones screaming obscenities and yanking out inflated bladder catheters—ouch!). Elderly patients are more susceptible to delirium, and delirium is sometimes the only identifiable symptom in an elder with an acute illness.

With further history from the patient's wife, you find that he has coronary artery disease, diabetes mellitus type 2, hypertension, and benign prostatic hyperplasia.

Question 21.3.2 **Which of the following is the most useful question to elicit risk factors for delirium?**
A) "Does the patient have any drug allergies?"
B) "Does the patient use tobacco?"
C) "Does the patient use alcohol?"
D) "Does the patient have edema?"
E) "Does the patient use acetaminophen?"

Answer 21.3.2 **The correct answer is "C."** Studies have consistently identified the following risk factors for delirium: advancing age, pre-existing dementia, underlying structural brain disease other than dementia, uncorrected impairment in vision or hearing, multiple chronic illnesses, polypharmacy, the use of physical restraints, history of alcohol abuse, male gender, and functional impairment.

While hypoxia (due to myocardial infarction, pulmonary embolus, or any other source) may lead to delirium, tobacco use ("B") alone does not predispose a patient to develop delirium. In isolation, knowledge about edema ("D"), acetaminophen use ("E"), or drug allergies ("A") is less helpful. Questioning about alcohol use ("C") will help to identify patients who have a tendency to overuse alcohol, putting themselves at risk for delirium. Also, delirium may result from alcohol withdrawal.

HELPFUL TIP:
Pre-existing dementia greatly increases the risk of delirium, and simply moving a patient with dementia to a new environment can precipitate delirium.

Question 21.3.3 **The appropriate evaluation of the patient with delirium includes which of the following?**
A) Evaluation of metabolic causes such as electrolytes and glucose
B) Evaluation for infection such as pneumonia
C) Evaluation of a patient's medications
D) Evaluation of oxygen saturation
E) All of the above

Answer 21.3.3 **The correct answer is "E."** There are many causes of delirium, often acting together in a multifactorial manner, and are best considered by a systematic approach. Metabolic causes include electrolyte disturbances (especially disturbances in serum calcium and sodium levels), hypoglycemia, and hypoxia. Numerous infections may lead to delirium. Neurologic causes include head trauma, meningitis, and vasculitis. Many medications cause delirium including anticholinergics, antidepressants, sedative–hypnotics, and steroids. Dehydration and prerenal azotemia may lead to delirium. See Table 21-2.

You reach for the "shotgun" (metaphorically, we hope) and order a bunch of tests. The chest radiograph shows a left lower lobe consolidation. The abdominal film shows a nonspecific bowel gas pattern. The white blood cell (WBC) count is 12,700/mm³, blood urea nitrogen 36 mg/dL, creatinine 1.5 mg/dL, and glucose 150 mg/dL. The remainder of the blood counts and chemistries are normal. With the exception of trace ketones, the urinalysis is within normal limits.

TABLE 21-2 CAUSES OF DELIRIUM, "WHHHHIMP" MNEMONIC

Wernicke encephalopathy
Hypoperfusion
Hypoglycemia and other metabolic abnormalities
Hypertensive encephalopathy
Hypoxia
Infection or intracranial bleed
Meningitis or encephalitis
Poisons or medications

Cultures will not be available for at least 24 hours. The ECG shows normal sinus rhythm. With the available information, you decide to admit this patient for treatment of delirium due to pneumonia and dehydration.

You are called in the middle of the night for agitated behavior and noncompliance with nursing care. The patient has pulled out his IV and struck a nurse.

Question 21.3.4 **You appropriately prescribe which of the following interventions?**
A) Haloperidol 0.5 mg PO once
B) Haloperidol 1 mg IV once
C) Physical restraints for the next 24 hours
D) Morphine 5 mg IV every 4 hours as needed
E) Lorazepam 1 mg PO for the patient, 0.5 mg for the nurse

Answer 21.3.4 **The correct answer is "A."** Most of the time, delirium DOES NOT require any pharmacologic treatment. However, this patient is at risk of harming himself and others due to his agitated delirium, so some action must be taken. Agitated delirium causes physiologic and psychologic stress on the patient, results in interference with medical care, and portends a poorer prognosis. The incidence of delirium in hospitalized patients of all ages is 30%, and the incidence in postoperative patients may approach 50%. Agitated delirium with high risk of physical harm to patient or staff should be treated quickly, and haloperidol is the treatment of choice. In older patients, drug clearance decreases, so low doses of antipsychotic medication should be administered initially. As the geriatricians say, "Start low and go slow." Increasing doses of oral haloperidol can be given every 30 minutes if the patient continues to have agitation. "B" is incorrect because IV haloperidol is associated with a greater degree of QT prolongation; PO or IM haloperidol is preferred. "C" is incorrect; physical restraints may lead to patient injury and may worsen delirium, but they may be needed if other methods fail. Restraints should only be applied when absolutely necessary and for as short a duration as possible. "D" is incorrect because we have no reason to believe the patient is in pain, and administering narcotics could worsen his delirium. However, pain can certainly result in agitation, so keep it in mind. Finally, "E" is wrong for at least two reasons: there is a substantial risk of paradoxical agitation with benzodiazepine administration in demented elders, and you should not prescribe controlled substances to staff nurses or it's "Good-bye medical license." **The most recent data suggests that treatment of delirium with antipsychotics does NOT reduce the severity of delirium nor cognitive functioning.**

About the best you can hope for is sedation, which has its own problems (Ann Intern Med 2019 Sep 3;)

....

You reflect on the fact that primary prevention of delirium is probably more effective than treatment. For this patient, delirium must now be treated, but you try to avoid this complication in your hospitalized older patients.

Question 21.3.5 You know that research has shown a reduction in delirium in hospitalized older patients when which of the following strategies is employed?
A) Increased sedative medication use for sleep-deprived patients
B) Early mobilization for immobilized patients
C) Cholinesterase inhibitor (e.g., donepezil) therapy for cognitively impaired patients
D) Physical restraints for combative patients
E) Music therapy for depressed patients

Answer 21.3.5 The correct answer is "B." Identifying risk factors and targeting interventions to reduce or eliminate risk factors can prevent delirium. Because one patient may have numerous risk factors for delirium and because delirium is usually a multifactorial syndrome, a multicomponent intervention strategy is warranted.

An often-cited study by Inouye et al. (1999) demonstrated the effectiveness of a multicomponent strategy. In the study, sleep-deprived patients received a warm drink, relaxing music, and back massage at bedtime. Unit-wide noise reduction was implemented. Early ambulation and active range-of-motion exercises were employed for bed-bound patients. All patients were encouraged to ambulate. Cognitively impaired patients received orienting stimuli and cognitively stimulating activities. Patients with hearing and visual impairments received portable amplifying devices and visual aids, respectively. Investigators used a protocol for early recognition and treatment of dehydration. There was no specific therapy for depression or combativeness. As you can see, the preventative strategies for delirium must also be broad as no one treatment has been singularly effective.

If not prevention, how about early detection? The Delirium Observation Screening Scale (DOSS) is an evidence-based tool that could have helped you identify delirium sooner in your patient, it has been validated in several populations, and it is freely available online. It takes into account consciousness, attention, thinking, memory/orientation, psychomotor activity, sleep/wake cycle, mood, and perception. Using DOSS takes just a few minutes and is, of course, easier and much safer than waiting to find him walking his imaginary dragon through the hospital ward while carrying a half-filled bedpan. See https://igec.uiowa.edu/delirium/delirium-resources for more resources on delirium.

Question 21.3.6 Which of the following statements about delirium is true?
A) Bed rails and restraints are effective in preventing injury in the patient with delirium
B) Atypical antipsychotics (e.g., olanzapine and risperidone) can be used to treat delirium
C) Diphenhydramine is a good choice for a sleep aid in patients who are prone to developing delirium
D) A feeding tube (e.g., Dobhoff tube) should be used in the patient who is not eating in order to prevent delirium
E) Shouting, "You don't have a dragon! They aren't real!" helps to prevent complications of delirium

Answer 21.3.6 The correct answer is "B." Atypical antipsychotics can be used in the treatment of delirium, but nonpharmacologic methods (e.g., bedside sitter and redirection) should be used first. "A" is incorrect because bed rails and restraints actually increase the risk and severity of injury in patients with delirium. Repeat after us: *restraints are used as a last resort.* "C" is incorrect. Diphenhydramine ("C") is a particularly poor choice because of its anticholinergic side effects, which can exacerbate delirium. Melatonin and the melatonin agonist ramelteon have shown some ability to reduce the risk of delirium, but only when started prior to the onset of symptoms and only in small trials. "D" is incorrect, as anyone who has done inpatient work knows: the feeding tube and the Foley are often the first to get yanked! "E" is also no good. Never argue with a patient about his delusion. You will not win. ***See note above regarding antipsychotics in delirium in the hospitalized patient.***

HELPFUL TIP:
Ethical dilemmas abound in the treatment of delirium. Atypical antipsychotic use in patients with dementia is associated with increased mortality. Older antipsychotics pose a greater risk for extrapyramidal symptoms when compared with atypicals and also pose the same mortality risk. By definition, agitated patients with delirium cannot provide informed consent, so "implied consent" is usually substituted to use drug therapy for patients with delirium at risk for self-injury.

▶ **Objectives: Did you learn to …**
- Define delirium?
- Describe the signs and symptoms of delirium?
- Distinguish delirium from dementia?
- Identify causes and risk factors for delirium?
- Treat and prevent delirium?

▶ **CASE 21.4**

In the early morning hours, a 78-year-old female presents to the emergency department complaining of right buttock and hip pain. Several hours before her arrival, she fell in the bathroom of her daughter's home. She recalls standing on a floor mat, leaning her head back to drink a glass of water, and then hitting the ground. She denies loss of consciousness. Her daughter was at the scene quickly and found the patient awake, alert, and moving all extremities. Her vital signs are normal. Other than right hip tenderness, her examination is unremarkable.

Question 21.4.1 Which of the following is most likely to assist you in determining the cause of her fall?
A) CT scan of the head
B) ECG
C) Additional history
D) Serum chemistry profile
E) CBC

Answer 21.4.1 The correct answer is "C." If there's an option for "more history," it's usually the right answer. History is one of the most important factors in determining the etiology of a fall. Ten percent of falls in older persons can result in serious injury, such as a hip fracture or subdural hematoma. Falls in elderly patients are typically multifactorial in nature. Randomized clinical trials demonstrate a reduction in the occurrence of falls in community-dwelling elders when healthcare personnel engage in a multifactorial risk assessment with targeted management. Such an approach requires a thorough history.

Question 21.4.2 All of the following are risk factors for falls in elderly EXCEPT:
A) Use of four or more medications
B) Orthostatic hypotension
C) Attempting tai chi, for which good balance is required
D) Environmental hazards (e.g., poor lighting or uneven walking surfaces)

Answer 21.4.2 The correct answer is "C." In fact, balance exercises such as tai chi and yoga have been shown to reduce the risk of falls in the elderly. All of the others listed increase the risk of falling. Additional risk factors for falls include history of a fall in the last year, impaired balance and gait, poor vision (acuity <20/60), decreased muscle strength, and syncope or arrhythmia. Still more risk factors: poor lighting, lack of grab bars and handrails, cluttered floor, restraint use, and improper bed height.

Question 21.4.3 During your examination, which of the following physical maneuvers is most likely to assist you in evaluating the risk of future falls?
A) Get-up-and-go test
B) Test for pulsus paradoxus
C) Osler maneuver
D) Lumbar spine flexibility test
E) Test for nystagmus

Answer 21.4.3 The correct answer is "A." The "timed get-up-and-go-test" is a commonly used method of assessing disability and fall risk in geriatric assessment. From a seated position, the patient is instructed to stand up, walk 3 m (approximately 10 ft), turn around, and return to their chair. An adult with no disability should be able to complete this test in <10 seconds. Increasingly longer time to perform the test is associated with increasing fall risk. While performing the test, assess the patient's sitting balance, transition from sitting to standing, gait and steadiness, and quickness with turning. While potentially useful in the evaluation, the other tests listed are not directly associated with fall risk. The Osler maneuver may be helpful in finding cases of pseudohypertension and should be checked in patients who are having falls associated with position changes despite normal or even high blood pressures as measure by sphygmomanometer. The Osler maneuver is performed by blowing up the blood pressure cuff until the radial pulse is absent. Then see if you can palpate a sclerotic, noncompressible, radial artery. If so, the Osler test is positive and the patient may have pseudohypertension.

....

After a thorough history, you perform a complete workup, including ECG, radiology studies, and appropriate laboratory tests. You find that the fall was caused by environmental factors (poor lighting and a loose throw rug) rather than an organic cause intrinsic to the patient. Fortunately, x-ray of her hip is negative for fracture. The patient asks how exercise might help her avoid future falls.

Question 21.4.4 Which of the following is the best answer?
A) Physical therapist supervision is essential to have an effective fall prevention program
B) In elderly patients, the effect of exercise on falling is unknown
C) Strength training has a greater effect than balance training on reducing fall risk
D) Unsupervised balance and strength training is effective in reducing fall risk
E) Group exercise is more effective than exercising alone to prevent falls

Answer 21.4.4 The correct answer is "D." There is no particular type of exercise that seems to prevent falls to a greater degree than any other type of exercise. Strength, balance, and gait training all appear to be important. Exercise programs have been shown to benefit elders at risk for falls. Although initial instruction by a therapist may be helpful, a physical therapist need not supervise all exercises. Patients are able to perform exercises targeted toward fall prevention at home, and they do not need to be part of an exercise group. A meta-analysis of the Frailty and Injuries: Cooperative Studies of Intervention Techniques (FICSIT) trials found that combined balance and strength training reduces the risk of falls in community-dwelling elders.

HELPFUL TIP:
Peripheral sensory disturbance is a common finding in the elderly and increases the risk of falling. A common cause of peripheral neuropathy is vitamin B12 deficiency. Check vitamin B12 levels. If they are low, great; treat with oral B12, 1,000 to 2,000 mcg/day. Alternatively, you can treat with 1,000 mcg/month IM. If the B12 level is borderline and you still have a high suspicion, check serum methylmalonic acid and homocysteine levels. These should both be high in B12 deficiency.

You recommend strength and balance exercises to the patient, but she is worried and says, "My heart's too old for exercise."

Question 21.4.5 You assure her that light exercises are safe and then review normal age-related cardiovascular changes, which include:
A) Reduced ventricular compliance
B) Reduced maximal heart rate
C) Reduced response to sympathetic nervous stimulation
D) Increased atrial filling
E) All of the above

Answer 21.4.5 **The correct answer is "E."** Even in the healthy elderly without signs of vascular disease, there are important changes in the cardiovascular system. Maximum cardiac output is reduced, mostly through reduced maximal heart rate; thus the equation:

$$\text{Estimated maximal heart rate} = 220 - \text{age}.$$

Additionally, there is reduced response to sympathetic stimulation, with less chronotropic and inotropic response to stress. Reduced ventricular compliance results in increased atrial filling volume and pressure, increased left atrial size, and increased dependence on atrial contraction for ventricular filling. However, endurance training may improve cardiac output, and active older adults have a higher cardiac output compared with sedentary persons of the same age.

HELPFUL TIP:
Hip fractures in the elderly are often caused by falls. In general, the sooner that a fractured hip is repaired, the better the outcome. Ideally, a hip should be repaired within the first 24 hours after the injury. Also, don't just fix the break. Look for the underlying issues, like osteoporosis and the reasons the patient fell in the first place.

Because of her right hip pain, you consider giving the patient an ambulatory device for temporary use. She has good upper extremity strength, can bear some weight on the right, but needs improved stability.

Question 21.4.6 Which of the following devices would be most appropriate in this setting?
A) Wheeled walker
B) Forearm crutches
C) Walk cane (hemi-walker)
D) Imperial walker
E) Multiple-legged cane (quad cane)

Answer 21.4.6 **The correct answer is "E."** Ambulatory devices are employed with the following goals: improve mobility, decrease the risk of falling, and relieve discomfort associated with acute or chronic musculoskeletal and neurologic conditions. An inappropriately selected device can increase energy expenditure and the risk for falls. Canes widen a patient's base,

resulting in increased stability. They are typically used for balance, not weight bearing. Multiple-legged canes—called "quad canes" because of the presence of four tips—provide a more stable base and some weight bearing, when compared with standard, single-tipped canes. Walk canes are useful for patients who require full weight bearing on one arm, as in a stroke survivor with loss of lower extremity function. Crutches, either forearm or axillary, are used for patients who cannot bear any weight on one leg.

Walkers can support a patient's weight, provide lateral stability, and expand a patient's support base. Standard walkers, those with four rubber tips, provide the greatest support and are helpful in cases of ataxia. Front-wheeled walkers are useful for patients with a fast gait, such as a festinating gait in parkinsonism. Also, a front-wheeled walker is easier to manipulate than a standard walker. Four-wheeled walkers should be used when the patient requires some increased stability but does not need as much weight-bearing as a standard walker would provide. Patients with mild-to-moderate Parkinson disease may benefit from four-wheeled walkers. In this case, the patient requires only improved stability and slight assistance with bearing weight. Of the available choices, the multiple-legged cane is the best option. A single-tipped cane may have been a reasonable choice as well. "D" is incorrect because the Imperial Walkers in *Star Wars* are infamously unstable and can be felled by a simple harpoon cable shot from the back of a snowspeeder.

The nurse brings you a quad cane from your supply closet.

Question 21.4.7 What method do you use to fit the cane?
A) Allow the patient to fit the cane length to her comfort level
B) Select a device with a length equal to the distance from the floor to the greater trochanter of the femur
C) Fit the cane length so that the handle comes to rest at the patient's waist
D) Select a device with a length equal to the distance from the floor to the fingertips with the arm relaxed
E) Extend the cane to its maximum length, giving it the appearance of a shepherd's crook or wizard's staff

Answer 21.4.7 **The correct answer is "B."** You should fit a cane for a patient by selecting a device that reaches from the floor to the greater trochanter of the femur. Another option is to fit the cane so that it reaches the flexor crease of the wrist when the arm is extended to the side. A properly fitted ambulatory device should be comfortable, allowing the patient to stand erect without excessive forward flexion of the spine. Excessive forward flexion occurs when the device is too short and can result in increased risk of falling. To obtain maximum efficiency from the upper extremities, the device should not be too long. The usual recommendation is to have a device fitted so that the elbow is flexed at 15% to 30% when the cane is in use. This is done by measuring as noted above.

▶ **Objectives: Did you learn to …**
- Recognize the morbidity associated with falls in older people?
- Evaluate causes and risks of falls in this population?
- Implement appropriate interventions for falling patients?
- Assess gait abnormalities that may lead to falls?
- Select ambulatory devices for appropriate patients?

 QUICK QUIZ: ASSISTIVE DEVICES

If a patient is having difficulty walking due to left-sided hip pain from osteoarthritis of the hip, in which hand should a cane be used?
A) Left hand
B) Right hand
C) Either hand
D) Both hands simultaneously
E) No cane should be prescribed; a wheelchair is preferred

The correct answer is "B." Whenever a cane is used to support lower leg function limited by weakness or pain, the cane should be used in the hand *contralateral* to the affected side (left side weak, right hand gets the cane). This enables the patient to maintain normal arm swing while advancing the cane and the affected leg at the same time to reduce the weight-bearing forces on the affected limb during the step.

▶ **CASE 21.5**

A 69-year-old female with no complaints presents to your office with her two daughters. Further history from her daughters reveals that the patient was widowed 4 years ago, now lives alone, and has experienced memory loss over the last 2 years. One daughter has taken over the patient's finances. The daughters report that their mother often wears the same clothes and bathes infrequently—new and unfortunate habits for her. The past medical history includes hypothyroidism and hypertension. Family history is significant for depression and memory problems in the patient's mother prior to her death from "old age." The patient takes chlorthalidone, levothyroxine, and acetaminophen as needed.

Physical examination reveals a thin, elderly female in no distress. She is alert but does not correctly identify the year. She describes her mood as "happy" most of the time. The remainder of the examination is unremarkable. You suspect that she has a "major neurocognitive disorder," previously termed "dementia." (Note: we don't make this stuff up…. the name has been changed. However, the term "dementia" is so commonly used and well understood that we will continue to use this term here.)

Question 21.5.1 According to the DSM-V, which of the following is true regarding the diagnosis of major neurocognitive disorder (NCD, formerly dementia)?
A) The diagnosis is rarely missed in the primary-care setting
B) To diagnose a major NCD, impairment in executive function *must* be present
C) To diagnose a major NCD, impairment in cognition *must* be present
D) Alzheimer disease (AD) is a diagnosis of exclusion
E) Neuroimaging is essential in the diagnosis of any major NCD

Answer 21.5.1 The correct answer is "C." The DSM-V has redefined the diagnostic criteria for dementia and in fact renamed it "major neurocognitive disorder." *In one of the most significant revisions, there is no longer a requirement for memory impairment to diagnose dementia.* Rather, major neurocognitive disorder is a deficit in any of the following six cognitive domains: learning/memory, language, executive function, complex attention, perceptual-motor function, and social cognition. The deficit must be acquired and not be due to other medical conditions, mental health issues, or substance abuse. *Finally, it is referred to as major neurocognitive disorder because it interferes with a patient's independence.* Mild cognitive disorder, on the other hand, is the term for patients with some cognitive decline but who remain independent. "A" is incorrect. In contrast to delirium and depression, the onset of dementia is insidious. Symptoms often go unrecognized for months to years prior to diagnosis. Although the patient may complain of confusion or memory loss, family members are more likely to provide the chief complaint and history. During the initial phases of a dementing illness, patients and family members may attribute cognitive changes to normal aging. In early cognitive impairment, memory symptoms may wax and wane. However, symptoms of dementia can be differentiated from occasional normal lapses based on their increasing severity. For example, it is normal to forget an acquaintance's name, but clearly abnormal to forget a spouse's name. "B" is incorrect. Many patients with dementia have impaired executive functioning (e.g., judgment, reasoning, and planning), but the presence of impaired executive functioning is not a requirement. "D" is incorrect, as AD is diagnosed by a specific set of clinical criteria. DSM-V provides diagnostic criteria for dementia and AD, making AD a diagnosis of inclusion rather than exclusion. "E" is incorrect. Dementia is a clinical diagnosis and does not require neuroimaging for confirmation. Experts and professional medical associations differ in their recommendations regarding the use of neuroimaging in dementia. In general, neuroimaging is recommended if dementia occurs in the following scenarios: onset before age 65, sudden onset, presence of focal neurologic signs, and suspicion of normal pressure hydrocephalus.

You use several office assessment tools to further characterize the memory loss. She scores 23/30 on the Folstein Mini-Mental State Exam, missing orientation and recall items. Clock drawing is grossly abnormal. Her geriatric depression scale is 3 positive responses out of 15 (positive screen is 5/15 or greater). She performs all basic activities of daily living (ADLs) independently but has voluntarily given up driving and control of her finances.

Question 21.5.2 Regarding assessment tools used in the evaluation of memory loss, which of the following statements is most accurate?

A) The Mini-Mental State Exam (MMSE) evaluates executive function and visual-spatial skills
B) Formal neuropsychological testing offers no benefit over the MMSE for detecting dementia
C) The use of a screening tool for depression is not helpful in the evaluation of memory loss
D) Clock drawing evaluates executive function and visual-spatial skills
E) The MoCA evaluates the ability to discern a chocolate coffee beverage from regular coffee

Answer 21.5.2 The correct answer is "D." Clock drawing can be used to evaluate executive function as well as visual-spatial skills. **Clock drawing is a simple test that takes 1 minute or less to perform.** The patient is asked to draw a clock face and set the hands to 2:50 or 11:10. This test requires planning and visual-spatial ability on the part of the patient—two areas that are incompletely evaluated by the MMSE. A normal clock does not rule out dementia, but an abnormal clock is suggestive of cognitive impairment. There are several scoring systems, and the sensitivity and specificity for dementia are as high as 87% and 82%, respectively. Of course, in 50 years no one alive will have ever seen a clock with hands, and this test will go the way of the dodo bird.

"A" and "B" are incorrect. The MMSE is a 30-point scale, with the cutoff for dementia between 24 and 26. The MMSE can be performed in a few minutes and tests memory, orientation, language, construction, and concentration. The MMSE does not test prosody (expressive and receptive inflection of vocalization) or executive function and, as a result, has poor sensitivity for early cognitive impairment in some individuals. Performance on the MMSE is strongly correlated with education; therefore, there may be false-positives in undereducated patients and false-negatives in highly educated individuals. Compared with the MMSE, formal neuropsychological testing assesses a broader array of cognitive functions, identifies behavioral abnormalities and assesses mood disorders. It can also help to differentiate between types of dementia. In general, neuropsychological testing is the most sensitive and specific cognitive assessment tool, but it is time-consuming and requires a high level of expertise to administer and interpret. "C" is incorrect because depression may cause memory problems, especially in the elderly, and depression screening should be included in the workup of memory concerns. Depression often coexists with dementia, and treatment of depression may improve memory problems. *It is also important to keep in mind that depression commonly is the first presenting sign of memory problems.* "E" is incorrect. See the related Helpful Tip for more on the MoCA.

HELPFUL TIP:
The Montreal Cognitive Assessment (MoCA) is a cognitive assessment tool freely available online, published in multiple languages, and validated in the diagnosis of dementia. Like the MMSE, it is a 30-point scale, but the MoCA tests a wider range of cognitive domains with less emphasis on orientation. Compared to the MMSE for the diagnosis of dementia, the MoCA has greater sensitivity (94% compared to 87% for MMSE), but takes a few minutes longer to administer and has a higher false-positive rate (around 40%).

So far, you have collected the following information on this patient: MMSE score 23/30, inability to properly draw a clock, impairment in driving and managing finances, disorientation to time, but intact abilities to cook, clean, and care for herself.

Question 21.5.3 Using conventional staging for Alzheimer disease (AD), how would you categorize this patient's dementia?

A) Mild
B) Moderate
C) Severe
D) Terminal
E) Insufficient information to determine the stage

Answer 21.5.3 The correct answer is "A."

- Mild AD symptoms include impaired memory, mild personality changes, and mild disorientation (MMSE 19–24)
- Moderate AD symptoms include aphasia, apraxia, insomnia, and increasing confusion (MMSE 10–19)
- Severe AD symptoms include severe memory loss, motor impairment, and loss of some basic ADLs (MMSE <10)
- Symptoms of terminal AD include immobility, dysphagia, weight loss, and increasing susceptibility to infections

Question 21.5.4 Which of the following findings would most likely cause you to search for a diagnosis other than AD in a patient presenting with moderate cognitive impairment?

A) Paranoid behavior
B) Apraxia
C) Poor judgment
D) Aphasia and personality changes
E) Bradykinesia and rigidity

Answer 21.5.4 The correct answer is "E." Bradykinesia and rigidity are features of parkinsonism, which, in the setting of memory loss, should prompt consideration of Lewy body dementia or Parkinson disease. Paranoid behavior, delusions, and hallucinations can all occur with more severe AD. Aphasia, apraxia, and personality changes typically occur later in AD but can be initial complaints in atypical presentations of AD.

Although you strongly suspect AD in this patient, you consider other types of dementia as well. Suppose this patient presented with urinary incontinence and ataxia in addition to her current findings.

Question 21.5.5 **Which of the following diagnoses would be most likely?**
A) Creutzfeldt–Jakob disease
B) Lewy body dementia
C) Normal pressure hydrocephalus (NPH)
D) Pick disease
E) Walking corpse syndrome

Answer 21.5.5 **The correct answer is "C."** NPH classically presents with dementia, gait ataxia, and urinary incontinence. When detected early, it responds to ventriculoperitoneal shunting and is thus a reversible cause of dementia. However, the dementia is rarely fully reversible. Gait abnormalities typically occur first and are the most likely to improve with removal of cerebrospinal fluid (CSF). The diagnosis of NPH is supported by findings on brain MRI, and it is confirmed by symptom improvement after CSF removal. Incidentally, NPH is a misnomer since intermittent CSF pressure elevations have a pathophysiologic role in the disease. "E" is a real thing, but not the right answer. Walking corpse syndrome is a rare psychiatric illness in which the patient is under the delusion that he is dead. Keep reading to learn why the other foils are wrong.

In discussing this case with one of your colleagues he wonders if you have missed a diagnosis of frontotemporal dementia (FTD).

Question 21.5.6 **You think it is unlikely that your patient has FTD because she does not have:**
A) Depression
B) Disinhibition
C) Hemiplegia
D) Rapidly progressing dementia
E) Tremors and hallucinations

Answer 21.5.6 **The correct answer is "B."** FTDs (including Pick disease) constitute a heterogeneous group of neurodegenerative disorders that have the common pathologic finding of cortical degeneration in frontal and temporal areas of the brain. Typical features of these dementias include an insidious onset and a slowly progressive course. Patients have impairments in judgment and insight. They are disinhibited and socially inappropriate. Patients may present with anxiety, depression, delusions, or emotional indifference. "A" is incorrect. Depression frequently coexists with many types of dementia but does not define one particular type. "C" is incorrect; the presence of hemiplegia in a patient with dementia should bring to mind vascular causes. "D" is incorrect because rapidly progressing dementia is the hallmark of prion disease, such as Creutzfeldt–Jakob disease. "E" is incorrect as tremors, hallucinations, and memory loss are consistent with Lewy body dementia (named

for its characteristic pathological finding—the presence of Lewy bodies in the brain stem and cortex). Clinical features consist of cognitive impairment, detailed visual hallucinations, fluctuation in alertness, and motor symptoms of parkinsonism.

HELPFUL TIP:
Alzheimer disease (AD) is the most common form of dementia, encompassing about 60% of patients with dementia. Vascular and Lewy body dementias account for about 15% to 30%. In many cases, dementia has more than a single cause. AD and vascular dementias frequently coexist—an entity commonly referred to as "mixed dementia."

The elevator gets stuck on your way back from making your morning rounds and your phone's battery is dead, giving you more time to contemplate dementia.

Question 21.5.7 **Which of the following is NOT consistent with the diagnosis of vascular dementia?**
A) Diabetes
B) Tobacco use
C) Diffuse slowing or normal electroencephalogram (EEG)
D) Normal brain MRI
E) History of carotid endarterectomy

Answer 21.5.7 **The correct answer is "D."** A normal MRI essentially rules out vascular dementia. Features suggestive of vascular dementia include a stepwise deterioration in cognitive function, onset of cognitive impairment with stroke, infarcts and white matter changes on neuroimaging, and focal neurologic findings on examination. There are no well-defined criteria for clinically diagnosing vascular dementia, and available rating scales have poor predictive value when compared with autopsy as the diagnostic standard (of course by then it is too late). Known vascular disease (like carotid artery disease) and vascular risk factors, such as diabetes, hypertension, and smoking, support the diagnosis.

Finally back in your office with coffee in hand, you decide to evaluate for reversible causes for this patient's dementia, and you consider ordering laboratory tests.

Question 21.5.8 **Which of the following laboratory tests is NOT indicated in the initial evaluation for reversible causes of dementia?**
A) Cyanocobalamin (vitamin B12)
B) Liver enzymes
C) CBC
D) CSF analysis
E) Thyroid function tests

Answer 21.5.8 **The correct answer is "D."** When evaluating a newly diagnosed case of dementia, one must consider infectious, metabolic, toxic, and inflammatory etiologies. Therefore, the

TABLE 21-3 LABORATORY EVALUATION OF DEMENTIA

Required Minimum Testing
- Complete blood count
- Serum glucose and electrolytes
- Vitamin B12
- Renal function tests
- Liver function tests
- Thyroid function tests

Testing Based on Clinical Suspicion
- Neuroimaging (recommended for all patients by some societies)
- Urinalysis
- Urine toxicology screen
- HIV antigen/antibody assay
- CSF analysis
- Syphilis

minimal required laboratory tests should include CBC, serum glucose and electrolytes, vitamin B12, and renal, liver, and thyroid function tests. Further laboratory tests should be obtained as clinical suspicion indicates. In the appropriate patient, one might obtain urinalysis, urine toxicology screen, HIV antibody assay, syphilis serology, and CSF analysis. Because of the extremely low incidence of neurosyphilis in modern times, routine testing for syphilis is no longer required but should be considered in the appropriate setting. Neuroimaging is not a required part of every workup but may be helpful in some patients. See Table 21-3.

....

Blood chemistries, blood counts, thyroid hormone levels, vitamin B12 level, and liver enzymes are in the normal range. A noncontrast CT scan of the brain shows nonspecific "age-related" changes (that was helpful!). The patient and her family return to discuss the test results. You begin to educate them about AD and dementia in general. The two daughters are concerned that other family members may be at risk for developing AD.

Question 21.5.9 Which of the following is the strongest risk factor for developing AD?
A) Age
B) Apolipoprotein E 4 (*APOE 4*) allele
C) Family history
D) Head trauma
E) Low educational level

Answer 21.5.9 **The correct answer is "A."** As with many diseases, age is the greatest risk factor for developing AD. Among persons 65 to 69 years old, the incidence of AD is 1%. In persons 85 years and older, the incidence rises to 8%. All of the other answer options are associated with an increased risk of AD but not to the same degree as age.

Family history is another factor strongly associated with developing AD. By age 90, almost half of persons with first-degree relatives with AD develop the disease. There are genetic risk factors as well. Mutations on chromosomes 1, 14, and 21 are known risk factors for AD. Trisomy 21 is a risk factor for developing AD at

an earlier age (often by age 50). *APOE 4* allele increases risk and decreases age-of-onset of AD in a dose-related fashion, with the greatest risk present in persons homozygous for *APOE 4*.

Other potential risk factors include a history of head trauma, lower educational achievement, female gender, and depression. Postmenopausal estrogens may actually increase the risk of dementia. Hypertension, diabetes, and hyperlipidemia are associated with dementia, and controlling these diseases might reduce the risk of developing dementia in the future, but the evidence is not strong. Increased physical, mental, and social activities may reduce cognitive decline in later years.

Question 21.5.10 The patient and family ask about medications to treat AD. Which of the following statements is TRUE?
A) Studies show that vitamin E supplementation improves cognition and prevents further neuron loss in AD
B) Ginkgo biloba and cholinesterase inhibitors have a synergistic effect, improving cognition in AD
C) Cholinesterase inhibitors do not prevent neuron loss in AD
D) Cholinesterase inhibitors maintain cognition at baseline levels for 2 years after initiation of therapy; after that time, patients decline slowly
E) Memantine is considered first-line therapy for mild cognitive impairment and early dementia

Answer 21.5.10 **The correct answer is "C."** Cholinesterase inhibitors do not prevent neuron loss. Results with vitamin E have been inconsistent, and some studies have found a slightly **higher** risk of death in those on high-dose vitamin E ($>/=400$ IU/day), primarily in those with coronary artery disease. Given the low cost and potential benefits of vitamin E, it may still be reasonable to use in combination with a cholinesterase inhibitor in AD at a dose of <400 IU/day if the patient or family is so inclined. There is no evidence to support the use of ginkgo biloba in AD. As of 2019, there are just two classes of FDA-approved drugs for AD. Cholinesterase inhibitors (e.g., donepezil, rivastigmine, galantamine) represent the larger class of available pharmacotherapy used to treat mild-to-moderate AD. Studies suggest that cognitive decline may stabilize for 3 to 6 months after which there is steady loss of cognition. By 9 to 12 months, there is no difference in the rate of decline between those on therapy and those on placebo. The other class has only one medication, memantine, which is an *N*-methyl D-aspartate (NMDA) antagonist used to treat moderate-to-severe AD. NMDA antagonists and cholinesterase inhibitors are often prescribed in combination; however, there seems to be little or no clinical benefit to combining these drugs. Memantine appears to do nothing for mild dementia and has shown very minimal (some might say clinically insignificant) difference in moderate-to-severe dementia.

HELPFUL TIP:
All of the cholinesterase inhibitors have similar efficacy. Tacrine is known to cause hepatotoxicity and is rarely used. The choice of cholinesterase inhibitor depends on cost, patient acceptance, and physician experience.

Using your favorite clinical decision aid, the Ouija board, you decide to start the patient on a cholinesterase inhibitor.

Question 21.5.11 In your discussion about the medication, you tell the patient and her family:
A) "These drugs are indicated for treating all types of dementia"
B) "These drugs offer no benefit in moderate Alzheimer dementia"
C) "These drugs are proven to reverse memory loss"
D) "These drugs are proven to reduce mortality"
E) "Gastrointestinal intolerance is one of the most common side effects of these drugs"

Answer 21.5.11 The correct answer is "E." There is no shortage of controversy when it comes to medications for dementia. However, the side effects are indisputable. Gastrointestinal intolerance—with nausea, anorexia, and diarrhea—is the most common. Also, cholinesterase inhibitors have a "vagotonic" action, which can cause bradycardia and syncope and worsen cardiac conduction abnormalities. To minimize adverse events, the dose of cholinesterase inhibitor should be increased only after the patient has been on a stable dose for 4 to 6 weeks.

There are statistical differences in the outcomes measured for AD patients on cholinesterase inhibitors, but are these changes clinically significant? There is no difference in performance of ADLs, time to nursing home placement, etc. "A" is incorrect. Mostly, these drugs are used in AD. Their use in Lewy body and vascular dementia is off-label but may be worth a try; there is some data to support cholinesterase inhibitors for these patients. However, there is no evidence to support their use in FTDs (e.g., Pick disease). "B" is not true. Most studies of cognitive effects of cholinesterase inhibitors have occurred in mild-to-moderate AD (MMSE 10–24). "C" and "D" are incorrect. Compared with placebo, cholinesterase inhibitors delay further cognitive and functional decline but neither reverse dementia nor affect mortality. In cholinesterase inhibitor studies of mild-to-moderate dementia, there is typically a three-point difference on the MMSE between treatment and placebo groups at 6 months. This finding is due to a loss of thinking abilities in the placebo group and a delay in that loss in the treatment group.

 HELPFUL TIP:
Not every confused elderly person should be put on a cholinesterase inhibitor. Consider the diagnosis, severity of disease, and the goals for the patient and family. Determine why you are starting the drug and be clear on the goals you hope to achieve. Then be willing to discontinue it if your patient is not reaching those goals. The side effects of cholinesterase inhibitors are symptoms often seen in nursing home patients (e.g., falls due to bradycardia and weight loss from anorexia). If your patient is losing weight and/or falling, consider discontinuing the cholinesterase inhibitor.

One year later, the patient returns with her daughter, with whom she now lives. The daughter reports disturbing symptoms that occur nightly. The patient wakes up in the middle of the night and wanders the house, becoming confused and agitated. With a subtle nod toward her mother, the daughter states, "I just can't take much more of this."

Question 21.5.12 After inquiring about pain and any changes in health status and finding none, your initial recommendation is to:
A) Employ soft restraints only during the night
B) Consider environmental changes including more daytime structured activities through an adult day care center
C) Initiate an antipsychotic before bedtime
D) Initiate a sedative–hypnotic before bedtime

Answer 21.5.12 The correct answer is "B." Treating behavioral issues in patients with AD can be very challenging. Further history must explore the possibility of pain-related agitation, decline in comorbid conditions or new health conditions, such as occult infection, and any medication changes that may be playing a role. If a treatable cause is not identified, then environmental change is the best initial recommendation. Adding structured daytime activities may facilitate a better sleep–wake cycle. Adult day care can provide structured activities during the day, along with respite for the daughter who is obviously asking for extra support. Although medications are sometimes needed, "C" and "D" are incorrect for initial treatment in this case. Once environmental changes have failed or there are other immediate health risks involved, then medications may be necessary. Antipsychotics currently offer the only drug treatment for behavioral symptoms in **dementia**; as opposed to delirium, which was discussed above however, there are no great choices. Haloperidol, risperidone, and olanzapine are used most often. See Table 21-4 for selected medications used to treat behavioral symptoms in dementia. Sedatives, such as benzodiazepines, often result in paradoxical agitation in elderly patients with dementia. "A" is incorrect. Restraints should be avoided in most cases, even soft restraints. Although they are sometimes required to prevent harm to the patient or caretakers, restraints are known to result in worsened agitation and an increased risk of fall, injury, and rhabdomyolysis.

 HELPFUL TIP:
When patients with Lewy body dementia receive antipsychotic medication for hallucinations, parkinsonian features become much more pronounced. If possible, avoid antipsychotics in these patients. If needed, use a second generation ("atypical") antipsychotic. Zonisimide (an antiepileptic) can improve motor symptoms without worsening cognition (*Neurology*. 2018 Feb;90(8):e664–e672).

Despite the addition of adult day programming, medication becomes necessary. Haloperidol, or "vitamin H," nightly has resolved the agitation. Although you may have increased your

650 FAMILY MEDICINE EXAMINATION & BOARD REVIEW

TABLE 21-4 MEDICATION MANAGEMENT FOR BEHAVIORAL SYMPTOMS OF DEMENTIA

Behavioral Subtype	Acute Management	Long-Term Management
Psychosis	Conventional high potency Antipsychotic (CHAP)[a]	Risperidone, CHAP
Anxiety	Benzodiazepines	Buspirone
Insomnia	Trazodone	Trazodone
Sundowning	Trazodone; consider CHAP, risperidone, olanzapine	Trazodone; consider CHAP, risperidone, olanzapine
Aggression, severe	CHAP, risperidone	Divalproex, risperidone, CHAP
Aggression, mild	Trazodone	Divalproex, SSRIs, trazodone, buspirone

[a]CHAP includes haloperidol, perphenazine, and fluphenazine. For elderly patients with dementia, typical doses should be about one-quarter of the usual dose (e.g., risperidone 0.25 mg, olanzapine 2.5 mg, or quetiapine 25 mg, and haloperidol 0.25–0.5 mg).

Note: Recent data suggests that quetiapine is the safest option for an antipsychotic in this group with haloperidol being associated with the greatest increase in stroke and mortality risk (*JAMA Psych* 2015, March 18).

patient's risk of dying (as seems to occur when antipsychotics are used in dementia), her daughter is thrilled with the result. Three months later she returns with concerns about depression. The patient spontaneously cries several times per day, her appetite is poor, and she has no desire to leave the house or even get dressed most days.

Question 21.5.13 Since a pill worked last time, her daughter wants to know what antidepressant is most effective for depression in patients with dementia?
A) Citalopram
B) Mirtazapine
C) Sertraline
D) None of the above

Answer 21.5.13 The correct answer is "D." There are very few quality studies available to guide treatment of depression in patients with dementia. The available evidence shows no difference between antidepressant therapy and placebo. The diagnosis of depression in a patient with dementia is complicated, since dementia causes apathy, sleep disturbance, appetite loss, and social withdrawal. If depression is suspected in a patient with dementia, a prudent approach would be to employ nonpharmacologic therapy and then provide an empiric trial of an antidepressant.

HELPFUL TIP:
There is some support for using stimulant medication (e.g., methylphenidate) to treat apathy in patients with dementia. The potential benefit must be weighed

against the known adverse effects of stimulants, such as appetite suppression, hypertension, and cardiac arrhythmia.

Over time, as the patient's dementia progresses, you reevaluate end-of-life issues and advance directives. With the support of her family, the patient decides not to have cardiopulmonary resuscitation.

Question 21.5.14 In end-stage AD, which of the following is correct?
A) Malnutrition is the most common cause of death in patients with severe dementia
B) Hospitalization for pneumonia in patients with severe dementia improves morbidity and mortality
C) In severe dementia, gastrostomy tube feeding prevents aspiration
D) To increase comfort, dehydrated patients with severe dementia should receive IV hydration
E) In advanced AD, treatment of infections with oral and IV antibiotics is equally efficacious

Answer 21.5.14 The correct answer is "E." Hospitalization for demented patients with pneumonia is a wash. The number of patients saved by the use of IV antibiotics is offset by an increase in death and functional deterioration as a result of the hospitalization. Thus, on balance, oral and IV antibiotics are equally efficacious in the treatment of infections in these patients; therefore, severely homebound patients with dementia or nursing home residents should be treated in their usual environment rather than hospitalized (if consistent with their healthcare goals). "A" is incorrect. The majority of patients with dementia die of infection, not malnutrition. "B" is incorrect as noted above. "C" is incorrect. Even in moderate-to-severe AD, feeding tubes can be useful in the *acute* setting. But the tube should be removed and natural feeding resumed as soon as the acute event passes. **Permanent gastrostomy tube feeding is not recommended in patients with severe or terminal dementia. Tube feeding does not prolong life, prevent aspiration, or promote weight gain in advanced dementia.** Although many patients with advanced dementia are malnourished and dehydrated, these conditions do not appear to cause discomfort. Hand feeding is as effective as any other means for providing nutrition and can lead to rewarding interactions for both the patient and the caregiver.

HELPFUL TIP:
Remember the caregivers! Ask about their health and mood. Twenty-five percent of caregivers to the elderly are depressed, while older people caring for their disabled spouses have a 63% higher chance of dying than non-caregivers of the same age. Consider screening caregivers using a validated tool like the short form of Zarit Burden Interview.

▶ **Objectives: Did you learn to …**
- Identify symptoms, signs, and diagnostic criteria for dementia?
- Describe different types of dementia and how they are diagnosed?
- Evaluate the patient with dementia, considering the potential causes of dementia?
- Describe potential benefits and limitations of current pharmacologic therapy for AD?
- Describe the natural course of AD?
- Manage a patient with end-stage AD?

▶ CASE 21.6

A 71-year-old male whom you have known since starting your practice recently suffered a stroke, resulting in language deficits and right hemiparesis. His medical history is significant for hypertension, hyperlipidemia, ulcer requiring partial gastrectomy (remote), and coronary artery disease. He quit tobacco and alcohol 5 years ago. He is retired and widowed. After a 3-day hospitalization, he appears stable enough for discharge. His medications include aspirin, metoprolol, lisinopril, and atorvastatin. Prior to entering a care center to receive skilled nursing care and therapies, the patient wants to know who will pay for the services. He has Medicare parts A and B.

Question 21.6.1 You are able to assure him:
A) Medicare will cover all expenses indefinitely regardless of personal financial resources
B) Medicaid will cover all of the expenses for the first 100 days of skilled care regardless of personal financial resources
C) Medicare will cover part of the expenses for the first 100 days of skilled care regardless of personal financial resources
D) Medicare requires a hospital stay of 7 days or longer prior to entering a nursing home for skilled care
E) Medicaid and Medicare do not cover nursing home expenses under any circumstances

Answer 21.6.1 The correct answer is "C." Medicare Part A, which provides some healthcare for patients 65 years and older if they qualify for Social Security benefits, will pay all costs for skilled care for the first **20 days** and part of the costs thereafter up to a total of 100 days per calendar year. This Medicare benefit includes rehabilitation (e.g., physical therapy, occupational therapy, and speech therapy) and skilled nursing care (e.g., nursing home, skilled care facility, and rehabilitation hospital) after a hospital stay of at least 3 days. (Note that the 3-day rule is considered antiquated by many providers and, as of 2019, Medicare has begun piloting programs that do not require three nights in a hospital.) The skilled care benefit is contingent upon the patient having an appropriate diagnosis, rehabilitation potential, and continuing to show improvement during the time the benefit is in place. Medicaid will provide extended nursing home care if a person's assets and income are below a certain threshold, which varies from state to state. Although Medicare Part B will pay for physician visits to nursing home patients, Medicare does not pay for nursing or other care directly related to permanently living in a nursing home.

Although he received fairly intensive physical, occupational, and speech therapies, your patient does not regain much function. He has only minimal movement in the right arm and complains of pain in the right shoulder. A radiograph of the right shoulder shows degenerative changes. The nursing staff administers acetaminophen 650 mg PO when the pain is severe, yet he continues to complain of shoulder pain. You involve physical therapists in his care to reduce the risk of chronic dislocation of the shoulder.

Question 21.6.2 In order to control his pain, which of the following is the most appropriate to add as a *scheduled,* and presumably chronic, medication?
A) Acetaminophen
B) Oxycodone
C) Gabapentin
D) Aspirin
E) Naproxen

Answer 21.6.2 The correct answer is "A." The point here is that scheduled acetaminophen is more appropriate for around-the-clock pain than PRN dosing. Acetaminophen is the safest analgesic of those listed. It may provide sufficient pain relief—if given scheduled (e.g., 1,000 mg PO TID). If it does not, then another medication may be added. "B" is incorrect as a first step as narcotics can cause confusion, sedation, urinary retention, and falls, and they have been associated with an increased mortality risk in the elderly. However, this patient has a history of an ulcer, and a narcotic analgesic may be a reasonable medication to add after acetaminophen (hydrocodone). Use clinical judgment. We have farmers who have been on the same dose of hydrocodone for years and years. "C" is incorrect. Gabapentin is indicated for postherpetic neuralgia and is more useful for neuropathic pain (although not very useful there either; tricyclics are better). "D" and "E" are incorrect. Aspirin and NSAIDs must be used with caution in the elderly due to increased risks of silent GI bleeding, fatal GI bleeding, and kidney injury. NSAIDs are typically not first-line agents for arthritis pain in this age group and probably offer no greater pain relief than acetaminophen. Also, consider topical therapies for pain, including capsaicin and lidocaine. Nonpharmacologic modalities should be employed as well, including massage, exercises, and physical therapy.

A nurse calls to report that your patient has developed lethargy, decreased appetite, and a temperature of 37.8°C. Your first thought is, "So? That's not a fever."

Question 21.6.3 And then you realize that:
A) An elevated temperature in older persons is most often due to changes in basal body temperature regulation
B) Oral antibiotics will not be sufficient to treat this infection
C) Antibiotics will not be necessary to treat this condition
D) Absence of significant fever in the elderly does not rule out serious bacterial infections

Answer 21.6.3 The correct answer is "D." Older persons, especially frail elders and nursing home patients, often have lower basal body temperatures compared with younger persons and may not mount as great a febrile reaction to infection. Recall that the "normal" body temperature of 37°C was determined in the 19th century as a mean temperature in a series of children. The mean healthy adult temperature is actually about a quarter degree lower. While a temperature >38.1°C in a frail elder is most likely associated with a serious bacterial or viral infection, absence of significant fever does not rule out serious bacterial infections. In fact, hypothermia is also an important sign of significant illness in older, frail patients. "C" is incorrect. With the available information, it is difficult to say with any certainty if the patient has an infection treatable with antibiotics. If he did, oral antibiotics are often appropriate in the nursing home setting, even when treating pneumonia.

....

With a decline in his function and a mildly elevated temperature, you plan to evaluate this patient for infection. According to the nursing staff, there are no other residents with apparent infections. Your patient has not developed any focal symptoms (e.g., cough, dysuria, diarrhea, or site-specific pain).

Question 21.6.4 Which of the following tests will be LEAST helpful?
A) CBC
B) Urinalysis with microscopic examination
C) Stool culture
D) Chest radiograph
E) Blood oxygen saturation (pulse oximetry)

Answer 21.6.4 The correct answer is "C." He is not having diarrhea so a stool culture is not likely to be of benefit. This is not a black-or-white area, but there are some principles and expert opinions to follow. Patient and family wishes regarding care must be known prior to initiating an evaluation, therapy, or hospital transfer. While the elderly may have a serious infection with only slight or even no leukocytosis, a normal WBC count on CBC ("A") will reduce suspicion for serious bacterial infection. Even without specific urinary symptoms, urinalysis ("B") is recommended because of the high incidence of UTI in this population. Remember, however, that asymptomatic bacteriuria can occur in up to 50% of women and 40% of men living in long-term care facilities and treating this confers no benefit. Blood oxygen saturation ("E") below the normal range (<90% on room air) may indicate serious respiratory illness; in the setting of hypoxia, a chest radiograph ("D") is recommended.

Question 21.6.5 Regarding infectious diseases in nursing home settings, which of the following is correct?
A) If the influenza vaccine is administered within 24 hours of an outbreak, patients require no further prophylaxis
B) All residents who are carriers of methicillin-resistant *Staphylococcus aureus* (MRSA) must undergo an MRSA eradication program with appropriate antibiotics
C) Most cases of bacteremia are caused by infected skin ulcers

D) New residents should receive a two-step tuberculin skin test, unless positive on the first test
E) All residents who are carriers of *Clostridium difficile* must undergo an eradication program with appropriate antibiotics

Answer 21.6.5 The correct answer is "D." The incidence of tuberculosis is relatively high in the older population, as is mortality from the disease. Institutionalized elders should be screened for tuberculosis with the two-step tuberculin skin test. A two-step test involves repeating the tuberculin skin test 1 to 3 weeks after an initial negative test (<10 mm induration). Anergy testing is no longer recommended. The test is positive if the induration is 10 mm or more.

"A" is incorrect. In a nursing home, an influenza outbreak can have devastating results, with a mortality rate up to 30%. In the event of an outbreak, even residents who received the vaccine should receive antiviral prophylaxis (see Chapter 8 for more). Only about 30% to 50% of nursing home residents will develop an adequate antibody response to the influenza vaccine, and that response takes up to 2 weeks after administration to develop. "B" and "E" are incorrect. Residents who are *carriers* of MRSA or *C. difficile* will not benefit from eradication if they are not infected. In addition, they may return to a carrier state quickly after antibiotic treatment; therefore, antibiotic treatment of these carrier states is not recommended. "C" is incorrect because UTIs are the most common cause of bacteremia in nursing home residents.

HELPFUL TIP:
In elderly nursing home residents, a positive response to tuberculin skin testing is most often due to a reaction to latent disease. Risk factors associated with reactivation of tuberculosis include chronic steroid use, diabetes, malignancy, HIV, malnutrition, renal failure, and chronic institutionalization.

HELPFUL TIP:
The high-dose influenza vaccine (e.g., Fluzone-HD) has four times the usual dose of antigen and is approved for adults 65 years of age or older. Seroconversion rates are higher for patients receiving the higher dose vaccine, and influenza-like illness rates are modestly lower in recipients. However, it has not shown a benefit for more serious morbidity or mortality. The cost is higher than that of the other options, side effects are similar, and its role is not well established.

....

Over the next year, the patient has increasing difficulty with cognition. He begins to experience urinary incontinence several times per day, necessitating the use of a pad. A midstream clean-catch urinalysis shows bacteria and WBCs (2–4 WBC/hpf) but is negative for glucose and nitrites. His postvoid residual bladder volume is 80 cc.

Question 21.6.6 Which of the following is true regarding the potential cause of and therapeutic intervention for urinary incontinence in this patient?
A) The most likely cause is obstruction from the benign prostate hyperplasia, and an alpha-blocker is indicated
B) The most likely cause is immobility, and scheduled voiding is indicated
C) The most likely cause is detrusor hyperactivity, and an indwelling catheter is indicated
D) The most likely cause is stress incontinence, and pelvic floor muscle strengthening (Kegel exercises) is indicated
E) The most likely cause is bacteriuria, and antibiotics will improve the incontinence

Answer 21.6.6 **The correct answer is "B."** Urinary incontinence is incredibly frequent in nursing home residents, with a rate of up to 50%. As with many other geriatric syndromes, incontinence is often multifactorial or the result of decreased physical and/or cognitive functions. A frequent cause of urinary incontinence in nursing home residents is immobility due to severe physical impairment, dementia, or both. In this setting, the initial treatment of choice is prompted voiding every 2 hours when the patient is awake. Also, fluid and caffeine intake should be monitored and adjusted to reduce urine output without causing dehydration.

"A" is incorrect. Although there is no information about the patient's prostate size, he has a relatively normal postvoid residual volume, making overflow incontinence from outlet obstruction less likely. A postvoid residual volume greater than 300 mL would be more concerning for urinary retention. "C" is incorrect—or at least the diagnosis of detrusor hyperactivity cannot be made on the basis of current information. The patient has not been fully evaluated with urodynamic tests, so it is difficult to determine whether his incontinence is stress-type or urge-type. If he has urge-type incontinence due to detrusor hyperactivity, an indwelling bladder catheter is not appropriate. Detrusor hyperactivity can often be treated successfully with pharmacotherapy (anticholinergic medications). It is important to be mindful of the anticholinergic side effects, which include falls, confusion, constipation, dry mouth, and urinary retention and could ultimately be more detrimental than the incontinence.

"D" is also not likely. Stress incontinence is less common in men than women, and urine loss is typically associated with increased abdominal pressure (e.g., coughing, sneezing, and lifting). Finally, "E" is incorrect. The presence of bacteria in the urine is a common finding in nursing home patients. In general, bacteriuria without symptoms (the main symptoms of infection being fever, new dysuria, suprapubic pain, CVA tenderness, worsening urgency and frequency, rather than incontinence (JAMA. 2014 Feb;311(8):844–54.) should not be treated. Studies have demonstrated little or no improvement in incontinence after treating asymptomatic bacteriuria in elderly nursing home patients.

HELPFUL TIP:
When urinary incontinence is due to obstruction or detrusor **hypo**reflexia, intermittent bladder catheterization should be employed and chronic indwelling catheters avoided. Appropriate indications for chronic indwelling bladder catheters in the nursing home include comfort care of the terminally ill, presence of skin wounds contaminated by incontinent urine, and urine retention not practically managed with intermittent catheterization.

Although his urinary incontinence improves, your patient develops difficulty with loose stools and occasional fecal incontinence. The stools are quite watery with no blood or melena. Aside from occasional abdominal cramping, he feels well. He has no new neurologic symptoms.

Question 21.6.7 Which of the following is the most likely cause of fecal incontinence in this situation?
A) Infectious diarrhea
B) Ulcerative colitis
C) Decreased anal sphincter tone
D) Fecal impaction

Answer 21.6.7 **The correct answer is "D."** In nursing home residents with limited physical mobility, overflow incontinence due to fecal impaction is most likely. Nursing home patients are often taking medications that contribute to constipation as well. Even with a stool softener and/or a laxative, constipation may still result. Fecal impaction can be treated with an enema, stool softeners, laxatives, and dietary changes, but sometimes requires manual disimpaction (where's a medical student when you need one?). Decreased sphincter tone may occur as a result of neurologic insult, but this patient was previously continent of stool. Although infection might be causing incontinence, there are no other symptoms of infection. The onset of inflammatory bowel disease is usually seen in younger populations, often with blood in the stools, making ulcerative colitis less likely.

As a result of your patient reporting physical abuse of another patient by the nursing staff, an investigation is under way in the nursing home.

Question 21.6.8 Reflecting on elder abuse and neglect, you realize which of the following is true?
A) Up to 75% of nursing aides in nursing homes have seen or heard of a resident being abused or neglected
B) A "dependent elder" is defined as anyone living in a nursing home
C) Approximately 70% of elder abuse and neglect occurs in nursing homes
D) There is a universally accepted definition of elder abuse and neglect, which is codified in federal law
E) Elder abuse is widely defined as "purposeful physical harm of anyone over the age of 65 years"

Answer 21.6.8 **The correct answer is "A."** In some studies, high rates of mistreatment have been found in nursing homes, with up to 75% of nursing aides witnessing or hearing about acts of abuse. However, it is not known whether nursing home residents are at greater risk than community-dwelling dependent elders. "B" is incorrect. The definition of "dependent elder" is not consistent, and may apply to elders who are cognitively impaired, physically debilitated, or financially dependent. Nursing home residents are frequently dependent; however, living in a nursing home itself is not sufficient to establish that a person is a dependent elder. "C" and "D" are incorrect. The study of elder abuse and neglect (also referred to as elder mistreatment) suffers from lack of a universally accepted definition, variations in laws between states, and inherent difficulties in obtaining accurate reports of abuse. Therefore, attempts to determine the incidence of elder abuse and neglect have resulted in wide variations. "E" is incorrect. Elder abuse may include physical harm, sexual abuse, psychological abuse, neglect, or financial exploitation. Although all states now have laws addressing elder mistreatment, those laws vary between states, and healthcare providers are encouraged to know the laws in their area.

HELPFUL TIP:
Risk factors for elder mistreatment include older age, cognitive impairment, substance abuse, low socioeconomic standing, minority status, and caregiver stress (probably the most important).

As your patient's cognitive impairment progresses, he becomes more withdrawn and uncooperative with nursing care, such as bathing. A nurse calls to ask, "Shouldn't he be on risperidone or something to improve his behavior?"

Question 21.6.9 According to the Omnibus Budget Reconciliation Act of 1987 (OBRA '87), antipsychotic medication is indicated for demented patients with:
A) Repetitive, bothersome behavior (e.g., name calling)
B) Continuous crying out and screaming
C) Uncooperative behavior (e.g., refusing to eat and bath)
D) All of the above

Answer 21.6.9 The correct answer is "B." One goal of OBRA '87 was to decrease the inappropriate use of antipsychotic medications in nursing home residents. In patients with dementia, antipsychotic medications may be appropriately administered in the following settings: agitated, belligerent acts that present a danger to the patient or other residents; psychotic symptoms (delusions, hallucinations, paranoia); and continuous crying out and screaming (lasting 24 hours or longer). Attempts to redirect the patient should always be employed first. You should also attempt to uncover occult causes of agitation, such as infection or pain (keep a log). Once behavior control is attained, assess whether the antipsychotic can be reduced in dose or discontinued. According to OBRA '87, **inappropriate** indications for antipsychotic medication include restlessness, uncooperative behavior, poor self-care, or repetitive and bothersome actions.

 Objectives: Did you learn to ...
· Describe some common Medicare/Medicaid reimbursement issues for nursing home care?
· Manage chronic pain in the nursing home?
· Describe an appropriate evaluation for the nursing home resident with fever?
· Recognize infectious disease issues commonly presenting in the nursing home?
· Develop an appropriate strategy for the evaluation and management of urinary and fecal incontinence in nursing home residents?
· Recognize the impact of elder abuse and neglect? Implement appropriate measures for agitated behavior in the nursing home?

 QUICK QUIZ: GERIATRIC PHARMACOTHERAPY

Which of the following is true about drug therapy in the elderly?
A) GI absorption is substantially decreased in the elderly
B) Sedative–hypnotic drugs should be given an 8-week trial without interruption for anxiety in the elderly
C) Mirtazapine (Remeron) causes anorexia and weight loss in the elderly
D) Compared with young adults, the volume of distribution of fat-soluble drugs is increased in the elderly

The correct answer is "D." The volume of distribution of fat-soluble drugs is relatively increased in the elderly due to a loss of muscle mass and proportionately more fat mass. Therefore, fat-soluble drugs, like diazepam, have a greater relative volume of distribution, while water-soluble drugs, like alcohols, will have a relatively smaller volume of distribution. "A" is incorrect because drug absorption does not change substantially with aging. "B" is incorrect. Sedative–hypnotic drugs should be used only for short-term therapy of 2 to 4 weeks because of the risk of falls and other adverse effects; this is true for both community-dwelling elders and those in nursing homes. "C" is incorrect because mirtazapine can actually increase appetite and lead to weight gain in the elderly. For this reason, it can be useful in patients who are depressed and not eating well.

HELPFUL TIP:
Although hepatic drug metabolism does not change substantially with age, drugs tend to have decreased elimination in the elderly as a result of decreased renal function. For these reasons, the half-life of many sedative–hypnotic drugs is substantially increased in the elderly.

QUICK QUIZ: ELDER MISTREATMENT

An elderly patient with moderate dementia presents for routine follow-up with a visibly fatigued spouse who complains,

"He's always up at night, bumping into things and taking stuff out of drawers." You notice several scratches and bruises on the patient.

Which of the following physical exam findings would be most concerning for physical abuse?
A) Ecchymosis on the forearms
B) Excoriations on the forearms
C) Ecchymoses on the back of the neck
D) Excoriations on the face

The correct answer is "C." Older, frail patients with cognitive impairment simultaneously are at risk of mistreatment from caregivers and are likely to show signs of self-inflicted injuries due to skin fragility and behaviors associated with dementia. For these reasons, bruises and scratches are common in older patients. However, signs of injury in an unusual location for accidental trauma (e.g., back, plantar feet, palmar hands, oral mucosa) may be due to mistreatment and warrant further investigation.

▶ CASE 21.7

Your next patient is an 83-year-old male familiar to your clinic, who presents for routine care. He has hypertension, hyperlipidemia, and osteoarthritis. He has been widowed for 10 years and continues to live independently in an apartment in the same town as his daughter. He stopped smoking 30 years ago, but continues to drink alcohol. He denies any problems related to his drinking, but reports that his routine includes three shots of whiskey per day. He says he likes drinking one shot before his daily walk and the other two shots after he returns. He finds the routine very motivating and keeps him in shape.

Question 21.7.1 **In regard to his drinking behavior, you are aware that:**
A) Older adults accumulate significantly lower blood alcohol levels than younger adults due to decreased absorption
B) Drinking three shots per day should not be any concern as long as his liver function tests are normal
C) Alcohol consumption can reduce the availability of nutrients such as zinc, vitamins A, B1, B2, B6, B12, and folate
D) The lifetime prevalence of alcoholism for men age ≥65 is less than 5%, but should still be screened for routinely
E) The standard screening CAGE questionnaire for drinking problem behavior has not been validated in older adults

Answer 21.7.1 **The correct answer is "C."** Alcohol consumption can reduce the availability of nutrients such as vitamins A, B1, B2, B6, B12, zinc, and folate. Alcoholic patients often present with malnutrition, poor self-care, and alcohol-related illnesses such as anemia, peptic ulcer disease, diabetes, hypertension, liver disease, neuropathy, and cognitive impairment. Checking for deficiencies may be warranted in this situation

depending on your patient's other dietary intake. "A" is incorrect. Older adults accumulate significantly **higher** blood alcohol levels than younger adults. A young adult's blood alcohol level will be approximately 0.03% after "one drink" (1.5 oz of distilled liquor, 5 oz of wine, or 12 oz of beer); whereas in a 75-year-old, the level may rise as high as 0.08%, which is the legal limit for intoxication in many states. "B" is incorrect. **Drinking behavior should be questioned regardless of liver function tests.**

The National Institute on Alcohol Abuse and Alcoholism has identified drinking **more than one** alcoholic beverage per day as potential problem drinking in older adults. "D" is incorrect. The lifetime prevalence of alcoholism for men aged ≥65 is higher, at approximately 14%; while women aged ≥65 have a prevalence of 1.5%. Denial of the problem is common in older patients, and impairments in functioning related to alcohol use may not be recognized until serious complications arise. "E" is incorrect. Diagnosis of alcohol abuse and dependence in older adults is challenging. Brief screening tools such as the CAGE questionnaire (see Chapter 21) have been validated in the older population and could be used in this situation.

In this case, your patient denies any drinking problems and his CAGE screen is negative. Still, you advise him to cut back to one drink per day or less and plan to follow up. He is independent with all basic ADLs and instrumental activities of daily living (IADLs). He walks daily, eats three small meals per day, and maintains a steady weight around 180 lb (BMI = 25 kg/m²). He manages his own finances, prepares his own meals, but usually has his daughter do the grocery shopping for his convenience. When you ask about transportation, he reports that he mostly drives to get around town to the golf club (not Mar-a-Lago), social events, and the post office when needed. He denies any vision or hearing problems.

Just as a review (this is a review book, after all) …

Basic activities of daily living (ADLs) include: bathing, dressing, toileting, grooming, feeding, and functional mobility (transferring or ambulating).

Instrumental activities of daily living (IADLs) include: shopping for groceries, driving or using public transport, using the telephone, performing housework, doing home repairs (not climbing on the roof but changing light bulbs and such), preparing meals, doing laundry, taking medications, handling finances.

HELPFUL TIP:
If you are concerned about driving safety, ask direct questions about any recent driving problems, such as minor accidents, traffic violations, or getting lost. The legal requirements about physician reporting of unsafe older drivers vary from state to state, but the AMA has published a useful guide, available online and updated in 2010, called "Physician's Guide to Assessing and Counseling Older Drivers" (http://www.nhtsa.gov/people/injury/olddrive/OlderDriversBook/pages/Contents.html)

One month later, your patient's daughter calls to inform you that he fell and broke his left hip while vacationing with the family in California. He had total hip arthroplasty (THA) and is still in the hospital recovering. Now they are trying to make arrangements to bring him home. The discharge planner has identified a local nursing home that can provide rehabilitation, but some of the family would like for him to return to his apartment.

Question 21.7.2 In regard to recovery after hip surgery, you inform the daughter that:
A) Rehabilitation after hospital discharge results in better outcomes for patients with hip fracture
B) Rehabilitation can only be provided inpatient at a hospital or nursing home, not at home
C) Surgical repair in elderly patients should be delayed if possible (>72 hours after injury) to reduce 1-year mortality and other complications
D) Early mobilization after hip surgery is recommended in younger patients, but in older patients weight bearing is usually delayed at least 5 days after surgery to allow proper healing

Answer 21.7.2 The correct answer is "A." Studies show that rehabilitation immediately after hospital discharge appears to result in superior outcomes for patients with hip fracture or stroke. "B" is incorrect. Rehabilitation can be provided in either inpatient (i.e., hospital or skilled nursing facility) or outpatient settings (clinic, day hospital, or home). For inpatient care, patients must be able to participate in rehabilitation that includes a minimum of 3 hours of therapy 5 days per week. Care usually involves an interdisciplinary team including nurses and various therapists. Home-based services can provide part-time or intermittent therapy as prescribed by a physician. "C" is incorrect. Early surgical repair (<24 hours after fracture) is ideal and has been shown to reduce 1-year mortality and complications such as pressure ulcers and delirium. Delay for medically unstable patients may be necessary. "D" is incorrect. Early mobilization is the standard of care for both hip and knee arthroplasty in younger and older adults. Weight bearing often begins on the second postoperative day.

Your patient and his daughter agree that rehabilitation locally sounds like the best plan.

Question 21.7.3 The goals of rehabilitation include:
A) Restore function
B) Help patients compensate for and adapt to functional losses
C) Prevent secondary complications
D) Maximize potential for participation in social, leisure, or work roles
E) All of the above

Answer 21.7.3 The correct answer is "E." These are all goals of rehabilitation.

The patient returns to the local nursing home for inpatient rehabilitation. Despite wonderful progress with physical therapy, he is unable to ambulate without using a cane. He is frustrated that he cannot walk on his own, and is concerned that all this walking and exercise is going to damage the recently surgically repaired hip joint.

Question 21.7.4 You can tell him that:
A) He does not need to restrict his activity because the hip prosthesis is well designed for bending, walking, and climbing stairs
B) His frustration is likely a major depressive disorder and will require medication treatment
C) He should continue the exercises because the advantages outweigh the low risks of surgical failure
D) He should not expect full recovery even with exercise, because nearly every patient requires an assistive device to walk after total hip replacement

Answer 21.7.4 The correct answer is "C." Whether correction is with screws, partial repair, or complete joint replacement, early weight bearing is usually tolerable with low rates of surgical failure and helps to counteract the poor outcomes clearly associated with prolonged inactivity. As noted in a previous question, early mobilization and continued exercise are the keys to preventing further decline and loss of function. "A" is incorrect. After total hip replacement, patients should avoid certain motions such as bending over to tie shoes and crossing legs when seated. Oftentimes a raised toilet seat is also recommended to reduce the load placed on the hip prosthesis in extreme flexion. Walking and general range of motion exercises should be encouraged as tolerated. "B" is incorrect. Depression is not uncommon after a disabling injury such as hip fracture. However, this patient's frustration may or may not reflect clinical depression and should be further evaluated before starting medication. "D" is incorrect. Although hip fractures carry approximately 5% in-hospital mortality and a mortality of approximately 25% in the year following fracture, about 75% of survivors recover to prior level of function. Up to 50% of these patients require an assistive device, but certainly not everyone.

HELPFUL (AND REALLY IMPORTANT) TIP:
For hip fractures or replacement, repair using an anterior approach as opposed to the traditional posterior/lateral approach reduces recovery time and is associated with a lower risk of dislocation.

After 2 more weeks, your patient is now functioning well enough to return home. He can transfer independently and ambulates with a cane for support. Prior to discharge, the rehabilitation team would like to assess his home environment.

Question 21.7.5 The occupational therapy practitioner on the team:

A) Provides a comprehensive assessment wherever the patient is employed based on his/her occupation, which does not typically include the home environment

B) May provide training for specific adaptive equipment for patients to enhance performance in everyday activities and promote independence

C) Is a skilled professional who has completed an occupational therapy training program after completion of high school

D) Is licensed to write prescriptions in most states, primarily for pain control

Answer 21.7.5 The correct answer is "B." Occupational therapists (OTs) provide training for specific adaptive equipment to enhance performance in everyday activities and promote independence. They also provide guidance to family members and caregivers if needed. "A" is incorrect. OTs provide home or job-site assessment, regardless of employment status or occupation. "C" is incorrect. OTs are skilled professionals whose education includes the study of human growth and development with an emphasis on the social, emotional, and physiological effects of illness and injury. One must have earned a bachelor degree or beyond to enter the field of occupational therapy. There are also occupational therapy assistants who generally earn an associate degree and practice under the supervision of a trained OT. "D" is incorrect since OTs do not have license to prescribe medications.

▶ **Objectives: Did you learn to …**
  · Identify and screen for drinking problem in the older patient?
  · Promote early rehabilitation after hip fracture repair?
  · Describe some aspects of rehabilitative services?

▶ CASE 21.8

A 68-year-old male arrives at your clinic to establish care. He admits that he does not visit the doctor regularly, but he feels his health has been pretty good since he changed his "bad habits." He did not bring any records, but he knows he has heart disease and high blood pressure. His bad habits included smoking about 1 pack per day for 40 years, but he proudly states he quit "cold turkey" after a heart attack at age 63. As far as healthcare maintenance, he did have a colonoscopy 5 years ago at his wife's request, and he remembers his last PSA was normal, but he does not recall any type of screening for abdominal aortic aneurysm (AAA).

Question 21.8.1 The USPSTF recommends one-time AAA screening:

A) For all men aged 65 to 74 years

B) For all men aged 65 to 74 years who have smoked >100 cigarettes in their lifetime

C) For all men aged 55 to 64 years who have smoked ≥1 pack of cigarettes per day for 10 years or more

D) For all men aged ≥75 if life expectancy >10 years

E) All smokers ≥55, regardless of gender

Answer 21.8.1 The correct answer is "B." The USPSTF recommends one-time AAA screening with abdominal ultrasonography for all men aged 65 to 74 years who have ever smoked (defined as >100 lifetime cigarettes). "A" and "C" are incorrect. The USPTF currently does NOT recommend screening men who have never smoked (<100 cigarettes in a lifetime). The American College of Cardiology/American Heart Association (ACC/AHA) guidelines advise screening men older than 60 years who have a strong family history (parents or siblings) of AAA, but family history is not explicitly considered in the USPSTF guidelines. "D" and "E" are incorrect. The evidence in men older than age 75 years and in women does not support AAA screening, and neither of the above guidelines recommends routine screening in those groups. One of several imaging modalities can be used for screening, including ultrasound and CT scan.

. . . .

You recommend a screening ultrasound for AAA, but then he questions why screening for AAA is necessary (guess you need to work on your rapport-building).

Question 21.8.2 You inform him that:

A) AAA occurs in approximately 1 in 20 older men who have ever smoked

B) Rupture of an AAA has a morality rate of 50%

C) AAA ruptures cause approximately 1,000 deaths per year in the United States

D) Treatment for AAA includes open surgical repair, endovascular repair, or surveillance once the aneurysm reaches 6 cm but not before this

Answer 21.8.2 The correct answer is "A." AAA is a common condition, occurring in approximately 1 in 20 older men who have ever smoked. "B" is incorrect. Rupture of an AAA is associated with an even higher mortality rate of 80%, hence the importance of screening. "C" is incorrect. Epidemiologic studies indicate that AAA ruptures are responsible for 10,000 to 20,000 deaths per year in the United States. "D" is incorrect. Treatment of AAA is based on the aneurysm size, rate of expansion, and symptoms. Asymptomatic patients with aneurysms ≥5.5 cm in diameter should undergo repair, not surveillance. Surveillance for medium-sized aneurysms (4–5.4 cm) is by ultrasound or CT every 6 to 12 months and every 2 to 3 years for aneurysms 3 to 4 cm. Earlier repair in men with AAA ≥5 cm or women with AAA ≥4.5 cm may be indicated if rate of increase is ≥0.5 cm in 6 months. AAA repair options include open surgical repair or endovascular repair. Endovascular repair has lower 30-day mortality rate, but overall mortality is identical after 3 to 4 years. In 2011, the ACC/AHA updated their guidelines regarding AAA repair, recommending either surgical or endovascular repair for most patients.

The ultrasound shows minimal atherosclerotic disease of the abdominal aorta and no aneurysm. Two years later, the patient returns for follow-up at the prompting of his daughter who has been noticing that he complains about his knees hurting all the time. He has never been interested in surgery, but he would like to try something different. When asked about his pain on a scale of 0 to 10 (0 meaning no pain and 10 meaning the worst pain possible), he reports pain around 2/10 most days, and up to 6/10 after moderate activity. He uses acetaminophen sometimes but does not want to get addicted to pain medicine.

Question 21.8.3 In addition to increasing his dose of acetaminophen, you suggest a topical analgesic such as:

A) The 5% lidocaine patch because it can be applied conveniently anywhere on the body to provide additional knee pain control

B) The 5% lidocaine patch because it acts locally where applied without achieving clinically significant serum drug levels

C) Capsaicin cream because it can be applied topically once per day as needed for effective pain control

D) Capsaicin cream because it only takes 1 to 2 days to achieve a clinical effect

E) Diclofenac 1% gel because it can provide anti-inflammatory effect with lesser GI toxicity compared with systemic NSAIDs

Answer 21.8.3 The correct answer is "E." Older adults are less likely to be adequately treated for pain compared with younger adults. Acetaminophen remains the best choice for first-line therapy of mild-to-moderate pain due to its tolerability. Topical agents such as the lidocaine, capsaicin, or diclofenac can also provide localized pain control. Topical agents can be very useful pain therapy because they penetrate the skin to act on peripheral nerves and soft tissue directly underlying the application site. These topical agents have minimal systemic absorption and thus limited potential for any clinically significant systemic effect or drug–drug interactions. Diclofenac 1% gel is a topical NSAID well-suited for treatment of osteoarthritis. Adverse GI events are less common compared to oral NSAID therapy.

"A" is incorrect. The lidocaine patch must be applied directly over the painful area for best results, but it is not effective in arthritis. Topical lidocaine seems to work for neuropathic pain (e.g., post-zoster) or for local, superficial, skin irritation. "B" is wrong for the same reason. "C" and "D" are incorrect. Capsaicin cream is dosed on a regular schedule every 6 hours to achieve maximal effect, which generally takes 2 to 4 weeks.

He tries acetaminophen 1,000 mg TID and capsaicin three to four times per day, and reports improved pain control. You see him 1 month later for a follow-up visit. Today he picked up a coupon at the local drug store for an arthritis pill that contains chondroitin. He wants to know if this might help his knee pain.

Question 21.8.4 You discuss the current evidence and inform him that:

A) Large-scale trials indicate significant symptomatic benefit in osteoarthritis with the use of chondroitin supplements

B) For patients with severe osteoarthritis only, a clinically relevant benefit is likely and the use of chondroitin should be encouraged

C) Chondroitin is a large macromolecule that is poorly digested and is potentially unsafe in older patients with any stomach problems

D) The combination of chondroitin and glucosamine is no better than placebo for knee arthritis

Answer 21.8.4 The correct answer is "D." The combination of chondroitin and glucosamine remains an extremely popular supplement sold over-the-counter for joint pain. However, scientific evidence is lacking to support the use of chondroitin to prevent or reduce joint pain associated with osteoarthritis. The largest randomized-controlled trial of chondroitin and glucosamine for osteoarthritis of the knee showed no improvement in pain versus placebo. Most studies are negative or show very modest improvement, although a systematic review in 2015 concluded that chondroitin may have minimal short-term benefits versus placebo. Therefore, "A" is incorrect. Similarly, "B" is incorrect. For patients with advanced osteoarthritis, a clinically relevant benefit is unlikely. "C" is incorrect. Chondroitin is a large macromolecule, and only 12% to 13% of ingested chondroitin is absorbed into the blood stream. However, multiple studies have found no evidence to suggest that chondroitin is unsafe (except to the sharks that provide the cartilage to make the supplement—they are rapidly becoming extinct).

Now that your patient has seen you for a few years, he feels more comfortable in discussing other health concerns … like constipation (hey, you've built some rapport!). He usually has a bowel movement (BM) every 2 to 3 days, but sometimes he gets hard stools that require excessive straining. His wife tells him to eat more fiber, but he wants to know what else he can do to help "keep regular."

Question 21.8.5 Which of the following statements is true about constipation?

A) The prevalence of self-reported constipation decreases with aging

B) Patients should be encouraged to defecate before meals when the colonic activity is the greatest

C) Fiber is a safe, inexpensive approach to improve stool consistency and accelerate colon transit time

D) Increased caloric intake correlates well with constipation in the elderly

Answer 21.8.5 The correct answer is "C." Fiber is a safe, inexpensive approach to improve stool consistency and accelerate colon transit time. Increasing fiber is a good first-line approach and should be encouraged. The daily

TABLE 21-5 ROME CRITERIA FOR FUNCTIONAL CONSTIPATION

Two or more of the following should be present for at least 12 weeks out of the preceding 12 months:
- Straining for greater than 25% of defecations
- Lumpy or hard stools for greater than 25% of defecations
- Sensation of incomplete evacuation for greater than 25% of defecations
- Less than three defecations per week
- Manual evacuation or assistance to facilitate defecation

recommended fiber intake is 20 to 35 grams. "A" is incorrect because the prevalence of self-reported constipation increases with aging—up to 45% of frail elderly individuals report constipation as a health issue. It is not uncommon for patients and physicians to have different clinical definitions of constipation, so further history is helpful to clarify what the patient means by "constipation." The Rome Criteria offers a consensus definition of constipation used in clinical trials as outlined in Table 21-5 and may be helpful to further characterize constipation. "B" is incorrect. Patients should be encouraged to defecate first thing in the morning or 30 minutes **after** meals when colonic activity is the greatest, and to take advantage of the gastrocolic reflex. "D" is incorrect. Decreased (not increased) caloric intake is more likely to be associated with constipation in the elderly.

You rule out secondary causes of constipation and decide that your patient likely has primary transit constipation. You first provide nonpharmacologic recommendations to promote regular bowel habits, including dietary changes and increased exercise.

Question 21.8.6 Which of the following options would be the best pharmacologic approach to use on a daily basis in order to help this patient with his constipation?
A) Fiber: psyllium (Metamucil), oat bran, or methylcellulose (Citrucel)
B) Stool softener: docusate calcium (Surfak) or docusate sodium (Colace)
C) Stimulant laxative: senna (Senokot), castor oil, or bisacodyl (Dulcolax)
D) Enema: tap water, sodium bisphosphonate, or soap enema
E) Any of the above would be equally valid choices

Answer 21.8.6 **The correct answer is "A."** Primary causes of constipation fall into three categories: (1) normal transit constipation, (2) slow transit constipation, and (3) anorectal dysfunction. There is no evidence-based guideline for the preferred order of using different types of laxatives. Supplemental fiber helps improve stool form and frequency and is a good first step. Psyllium also has the benefit of reducing lipids and improving glucose control in diabetics. Adequate fluid intake is necessary when using psyllium since it may exacerbate constipation when fluid intake is insufficient. "B" is incorrect.

While stool softeners are commonly prescribed and may be helpful, they are less effective than other options including psyllium. "C" is incorrect. Stimulant laxatives, when used in recommended doses, are unlikely to harm the colon. However, stimulant laxatives may cause electrolyte imbalance or abdominal pain and are not the first-line therapy. "D" is incorrect. Enemas should only be used in acute situations and with caution due to the risk of colonic perforation. Large-volume enemas can result in hyponatremia, while enemas containing phosphate can lead to hyperphosphatemia and renal failure, especially in patients with renal insufficiency.

HELPFUL TIP:
There are many causes of secondary constipation, including numerous medications (e.g., anticholinergics, calcium channel blockers, opiates) and coexistent medical conditions such as diabetes, hypothyroidism, scleroderma, and amyloidosis.

▶ **Objectives: Did you learn to …**
- Screen for AAA?
- Provide the safe and effective treatment for osteoarthritis pain?
- Identify and treat constipation in the older patient?

 QUICK QUIZ: DIABETES TARGET

A 73-year-old male patient returns to see you for further management of diabetes mellitus type 2. He has had diabetes for decades and he has been generally well controlled on oral medications of metformin and glipizide. He also has hypertension and hypercholesterolemia for which he is treated. He thinks he is in otherwise fair health and is active in his community and lives independently with his wife.

What is his target hemoglobin A_{1C}?
A) <5.5%
B) <6.5%
C) <7.5%
D) <8.5%

The correct answer is "C." The American Diabetes Association and the American Geriatrics Society recommend a goal of hemoglobin A_{1C} less than 7.5% for older adult patients who are otherwise healthy and have good functional performance. The benefits versus the risks of intensive diabetic control start to shift as the medical complexity and functional impairments of the patient increase. Therefore, older patients with multiple chronic medical conditions, cognitive impairment, or functional impairments have a less stringent goal A_{1C} between 8.0% and 8.5%. For older patients with limited life expectancy such as these, the goals of diabetes care are to reduce the risks associated with hyperglycemia and hypoglycemia rather than prevent long-term complications of diabetes.

Clinical Pearls

○ Avoid antipsychotics in the demented elderly with behavioral and psychological disturbances. First, explore and treat potential underlying causes, modify the environment, and educate caregivers.

○ Conduct a complete drug review regularly, looking for drug–drug interactions, drug–disease interactions, ineffective drugs, and symptoms attributable to medications.

○ Do not perform cervical cancer screening on women over the age of 65 years if the previous three Pap smears prior to age 65 years were completely normal and there were no findings of CIN2 or higher in the previous 20 years.

○ Do not treat asymptomatic bacteriuria in older adults. Cystitis does not cause confusion (J Am Geriatr Soc 2019 Mar; 67:484).

○ Do not treat insomnia in older adults with sedative drugs, including diphenhydramine. First, employ good sleep hygiene, cognitive behavioral therapy, and melatonin.

○ Do not use medical interventions, such as appetite stimulants and gastric tube feedings, for demented older adults who are losing weight. Provide appealing and calorically dense foods, feeding assistance, and a social context for eating.

○ Estimate longevity and determine patient preferences prior to initiating screenings and preventative interventions.

○ Older patients who sustain a hip fracture have better clinical outcomes with early repair (within the first 24 hours).

○ Periodically reassess cholinesterase inhibitors for dementia; taper and discontinue the drug if there is no perceived benefit or if adverse events occur (e.g., weight loss, bradycardia).

○ Pressure ulcers should be treated primarily with pressure relief, good wound care, and good nutrition. Minimal benefit is attributable to dressing type or advanced wound care treatments (e.g., electrical stimulation, ultrasound).

BIBLIOGRAPHY

Allman RM, et al. Pressure ulcer risk factors among hospitalized patients with activity limitation. *JAMA.* 1995;273(11):856–870.

American College of Physicians/American Academy of Family Physicians. Current pharmacologic treatment of dementia: a clinical practice guideline from the ACP/AAFP. *Ann Intern Med.* 2008;148(5):370–378.

American Medical Association/National Highway Traffic Administration/US Department of Transportation; 2010. Physician's guide to assessing and counseling older drivers. Available at: http://www.nhtsa.gov/people/injury/olddrive/OlderDriversBook/pages/Contents.html. Accessed June 17, 2015.

American Occupational Therapy Association. Available at: http://www.aota.org/featured/area6/index.asp. Accessed November 22, 2007.

American Psychiatric Association. *Diagnostic and Statistical Manual of Mental Disorders (DSM-V).* 5th ed. Washington, DC: American Psychiatric Association; 2013.

Barnes A. Legal issues in geriatric medicine and gerontology. In: Hazzard WR, Blass JP, Ettinger WH Jr, et al. eds. *Principles of Geriatric Medicine and Gerontology.* 4th ed. New York, NY: McGraw-Hill; 1999:545–556.

Bentley DW, et al. Practice guidelines for evaluation of fever and infection in long-term care facilities. *Clin Infect Dis.* 2000;31:640–653.

Bergstrom N, et al. Treatment of pressure ulcers. Clinical Practice guidelines No. 15. Rockville (MD): US Department of Health and Human Services, Public Health Service, Agency for Health Care Policy and Research. *Dec. AHCPR Pub. No*; 1994:95–0653. (At press time, a new guideline was under review but not yet published.)

Bradley SM, Hernandez CR. Geriatric assistive devices. *Am Fam Physician.* 2011;84(4):405–411.

FDA Drug Safety Communication: New restrictions, contraindications, and dose limitations of Zocor (simvastatin) to reduce the risk of muscle injury. Available at: http://www.fda.gov/Drugs/DrugSafety/ucm256581.htm. Accessed June 2015.

Girard TD, et al. Haloperidol and ziprasidone for treatment of delirium in critical illness. *N Engl J Med.* 2018;379:2506–2516.

Hatta K, et al. Preventative effects of Ramelteon on delirium: a randomized placebo-controlled trial. *JAMA Psychiatry.* 2014;397–403.

Inouye SK, et al. Clarifying confusion: the confusion assessment method. *Ann Intern Med.* 1990;113:941–948.

Inouye SK, et al. A multicomponent intervention to prevent delirium in hospitalized older patients. *N Engl J Med.* 1999;340:669–676.

Kirkman S, et al. Diabetes in older adults: a consensus report. *J Am Geriatr Soc.* 2012;60(12):2342–2356.

Loue S. Elder abuse and neglect in medicine and law: the need for reform. *J Leg Med.* 2001;22:159–209.

Mehr DR, Tatum PE. Primary prevention of diseases in old age. *Clin Geriatr Med.* 2002;18(3):407–430.

Murata M, et al. Adjunct zonisamide to levodopa for DLB parkinsonism. *Neurology.* 2018; 90(8):e664–e672.

Panel on Prevention of Falls in Older Persons, American Geriatrics Society and British Geriatrics Society. Updated AGS/BGS clinical practice guideline for prevention of falls in older persons. *J Am Geriatr Soc.* 2011;59(1):148–157.

Pergolizzi J, et al. Opioids and the management of chronic severe pain in the elderly. *Pain Pract.* 2008;8(4):287–313.

Pham CB, Dickman RL. Minimizing adverse drug events in older patients. *Am Fam Physician.* 2007;76(12):1837–1844.

Podsiadlo D, Richardson S. The timed "Up & Go": a test of basic functional mobility for frail elderly persons. *J Am Geriatr Soc.* 1991;39(2):142–148.

Ross GW, Bowen JD. The diagnosis and differential diagnosis of dementia. *Med Clin North Am.* 2002;86(3):455–476.

Schwartz RS, Buchner DM. Exercise in the elderly: physiologic and functional effects. In: *Hazzard's Geriatric Medicine and Gerontology.* 6th ed. New York, NY: McGraw-Hill; 2009:1381–1395.

Tariot PN. Medical management of advanced dementia. *J Am Geriatr Soc.* 2003;51(5):S305–S313.

Thom TW, et al. 2011 ACCF/AHA focused update of the guideline for the management of patients with peripheral artery disease. *J Am Coll Cardiol*. 2011;58:2020–2045.

Tomcyk S, et al. Use of 13-valent pneumococcal conjugate vaccine and 23-valent pneumococcal polysaccharide vaccine among adults aged ≥65: recommendations of the advisory committee on immunization practices. *MMWR Morb Mortal Wkly Rep*. 2014;63:822–85.

US Preventive Services Task Force. Screening for abdominal aortic aneurysm: recommendation statement. *Ann Intern Med*. 2005;142:198–202.

Watson YI, et al. Clock completion: an objective screening test for dementia. *J Am Geriatr Soc*. 1993;41(11):1235–1240.

Wuillen DA. Common causes of vision loss in elderly patients. *Am Fam Physician*. 1999;60(1):99–108.

Care of the Surgical Patient 22

Alka Walter, Erin Hayward, and Brigit E. Ray

▶ CASE 22.1

A 40–year-old male patient with type 2 diabetes, taking a "flozin" (SGLT2 inhibitor), calls your office because he is having difficulty urinating and quite a bit of pain in the perineal area. He has not felt well for several days and was running a low-grade fever. He went to his chiropractor 2 days ago when he only had pain and swelling in the scrotum and the chiropractor adjusted his … well, we won't go there… . He is now noting that his temperature is higher (he doesn't have a thermometer and is reading his temperature via his old mood ring from the 1990s). You suggest that he present to your office.

Examination reveals an obese male who is waddling into the office because of pain in his scrotal area. Vitals: blood pressure 150/100 mm Hg, pulse 112 bpm, respirations 20 bpm, and temperature 39.0°C. Other significant findings include a swollen scrotum that is dusky red, exquisitely tender to touch, and without crepitus. You do not have extended laboratory access in your office, but a urine dipstick is negative for blood and leukocyte esterase. His blood sugar, which is usually fairly well controlled, is elevated at 320 mg/dL.

Question 22.1.1 Your next step for this patient will be which of the following?
A) Start the patient on cephalexin (Keflex) for methicillin-sensitive *Staphylococcus aureus* and *Streptococcus* coverage and follow-up with the patient in the morning
B) Emergent surgical referral
C) Begin trimethoprim/sulfamethoxazole (Bactrim) for methicillin-resistant *S. aureus* (MRSA) coverage and follow-up with the patient in the morning
D) Admit the patient and start him on IV vancomycin, piperacillin/tazobactam, and metronidazole for coverage of MRSA, *Streptococcus*, *Pseudomonas*, anaerobes

Answer 22.1.1 The correct answer is "B." This presentation likely represents Fournier gangrene (and remember that SGLT2 inhibitors, such as this patient is on, increase the risk of

Fournier). The erythematous, swollen scrotum with pain out of proportion to examination and associated signs of fever, tachycardia, and elevated blood sugar make Fournier gangrene the most likely diagnosis. While crepitus is common with Fournier gangrene due to presence of gas-forming anaerobic bacteria, its absence does not rule out gangrene. Without early surgical debridement and IV antibiotics, infection can progress rapidly to sepsis and multiorgan failure. Therefore, "B," emergent surgical referral, is the best option for this patient. Antibiotics, particularly oral (options "A" and "B"), are inappropriate as a sole therapy. Broad-spectrum IV antibiotics may be part of initial management, but "D" is incorrect because the patient emergently needs surgical debridement to remove the necrotic tissue.

Question 22.1.2 Fournier gangrene can best be described as:
A) Necrotizing fasciitis
B) Necrotizing cellulitis
C) Caused by aerobic bacteria
D) Secondary to streptococcus
E) A mathematical function that can be written as an infinite sum of harmonics

Answer 22.1.2 The correct answer is "A." Fournier gangrene is a form of necrotizing fasciitis. This is termed "Type I" necrotizing fasciitis and is caused by mixed aerobic and anaerobic bacteria. This subset is typically seen in individuals with a "weakened" immune system such as the elderly or patients with diabetes. There are two other subtypes of necrotizing fasciitis: types II and III. Type II necrotizing fasciitis is caused by hemolytic Group A *Streptococcus* and *staphylococci* (including MRSA) and is frequently referred to in the media as "flesh-eating bacteria." This subset can occur in *any* individual. Type III necrotizing fasciitis is typically caused by *Clostridia* infection and is typically referred to as "gas gangrene." This subset typically can occur after significant injury or surgery. "B" is incorrect. Necrotizing cellulitis is isolated to the superficial skin. Fournier gangrene involves deep tissues including the fascia. "C" and "D" are incorrect because, as noted above, Fournier gangrene is caused by mixed aerobic and anaerobic bacteria. Common pathogens involved include coliforms, *Clostridia*, *Bacteroides*, *Klebsiella*, *Staphylococcus*, and *Streptococcus*. If you used "the-longest-answer-is-always-right" method and chose "E," you are way off base and possibly a musician; "E" describes Fourier's transform (look it up).

Question 22.1.3 Which of the following is NOT a risk factor for Fournier gangrene?
A) Diabetes
B) Immunosuppression
C) Varicella infection
D) End-stage renal disease
E) Advanced age

Answer 22.1.3 The correct answer is "C." Varicella infection is a risk factor for Type II necrotizing fasciitis. All the other options are risk factors for Fournier gangrene (Type I necrotizing fasciitis).

The surgeon evaluates the patient and asks for your opinion on the antibiotic regimen. You nearly fall over in shock that your advice was solicited.

Question 22.1.4 What do you recommend for this patient with necrotizing fasciitis?
A) Penicillin and clindamycin
B) Clindamycin and metronidazole
C) Meropenem, vancomycin, and clindamycin
D) Piperacillin/tazobactam (Zosyn), vancomycin, and metronidazole
E) C or D

Answer 22.1.4 The correct answer is "E." As noted above, a mixture of aerobic and anaerobic bacteria causes Fournier gangrene. The first two choices ("A" and "B") will cover anaerobes and some Gram-positive organisms. However, Gram-negative coverage is lacking. More broad-spectrum antimicrobial coverage is needed in this situation. Most experts and guidelines recommend a broad-spectrum antibiotic with anaerobic and Gram-negative coverage (e.g., piperacillin/tazobactam, ampicillin/sulbactam, or a carbapenem) **plus** MRSA coverage (usually vancomycin) **plus** anaerobic coverage (e.g., clindamycin, metronidazole). Although MRSA is not usually the causative agent, these infections are polymicrobial, and empiric MRSA coverage is required. Clindamycin deserves a special mention. *Clindamycin targets toxin production, so it is especially helpful in invasive Streptococcal disease and Staphylococcal and Streptococcal toxic shock syndromes.*

HELPFUL TIP:
IVIG has been used in necrotizing fasciitis caused by *Clostridium* species as well as in those with streptococcal fasciitis. While there is a suggestion of benefit, the data are incomplete and more study is warranted. Hyperbaric oxygen has also been used, but suffers from the same lack of data. These treatments are potential adjunct therapies. The definitive treatment is early, aggressive, surgical debridement!

The patient has a wide excision of necrotic tissue. After surgery, he becomes hypotensive and tachycardic (blood pressure 85/50 mm Hg, pulse 128 bpm), and his serum lactate is 8 mg/dL (high).

Question 22.1.5 What is the most appropriate next step in his management?
A) Start IV dopamine to stabilize his blood pressure
B) Start IV norepinephrine to stabilize his blood pressure
C) Start IV 0.9% normal saline (NS) boluses to stabilize his blood pressure (30 mL/kg)
D) Start IV albumin boluses to stabilize his blood pressure
E) Read him the hospital charges he has accumulated thus far. The epinephrine release will improve his blood pressure

Answer 22.1.5 The correct answer is "C." This patient is likely hypovolemic secondary to third spacing and/or is in septic shock and needs volume resuscitation. The lactate of 8 mg/dL suggests that he has hypoperfusion with poor tissue oxygenation (although it could also be secondary to necrotic tissue). Just giving dopamine (or other vasopressors) will not increase peripheral circulation and, in fact, may decrease tissue oxygenation by increasing vascular tone and decreasing perfusion. For patients with sepsis who remain hypotensive in spite of volume resuscitation (0.9% NS boluses at 30 mL/kg), the preferred initial vasopressor is norepinephrine. Albumin has not been shown to have any advantage over crystalloids in almost any circumstance— following large-volume paracentesis (>5 L) and perhaps dengue being the notable exception. Mortality of necrotizing fasciitis approaches 30% even with appropriate management. You may have heard that Lactated Ringers (LR) may be superior to NS in critically ill patients (*N Engl J Med.* 2018 Mar 1;378(9):829–839). This did not appear to be the case in *non-critically ill* patients being cared for outside the ICU setting (*N Engl J Med.* 2018:378(9):819–828). These recommendations are not definitive; either LR or NS is reasonable for fluid resuscitation.

HELPFUL TIP:
The thinking about sepsis has changed in the past few years with the Surviving Sepsis Campaign (*Crit Care Med.* 2017 Mar;45(3):486–552) and several subsequent studies. Successful treatment of sepsis requires early recognition, early aggressive fluid resuscitation (boluses of 30 mL/kg) within the first 3 hours, and broad-spectrum antibiotics within 1 hour of recognition of severe sepsis or septic shock. Monitor closely including ultrasound assessment of IVC pressure, urine output, etc. More recent studies indicate that early goal-directed therapy (e.g., aggressive use of central lines, vasopressors with central venous pressure and hematocrit goals) and

early renal replacement therapy do not result in better outcomes (*N Engl J Med.* 2017 Jun 8;376(23):2223–2234; *N Engl J Med.* 2014;371(16):1496–1506; *N Engl J Med.* 2018 Oct 11; 379:1431–1442).

Take home point: Recognize sepsis, promptly treat with fluids and control infection (antibiotics, surgery if appropriate), and continually re-evaluate your patient.

▶ **Objectives: Did you learn to …**
- Diagnose and treat Fournier gangrene?
- Differentiate between types of necrotizing fasciitis?
- Prescribe fluids and vasopressors as appropriate to treat sepsis and septic shock?

 QUICK QUIZ: PAIN CONTROL

Which of the following drugs will give you the most rapid pain control when given intravenously?
A) Fentanyl (Sublimaze)
B) Hydromorphone (Dilaudid)
C) Meperidine (Demerol)
D) Morphine

The correct answer is "A." Fentanyl has a peak effect at 3 to 5 minutes. This is followed by meperidine at 5 to 7 minutes, morphine at 20 minutes, and hydromorphone at 15 to 30 minutes. For rapid control of pain, fentanyl is the preferred agent. Meperidine is the least preferred agent because of drug interactions (MAO inhibitors, SSRIs) and toxic metabolites (normeperidine, which can cause agitation and seizures).

 HELPFUL TIP:
Vancomycin is not a great drug for treating *Staphylococcus*. In fact, inpatient mortality rates are higher in patients with **methicillin-sensitive** *Staphylococcal (MSSA)* infections treated with vancomycin than with other antibiotics. So, if you are treating MSSA, change antibiotics to something other than vancomycin, such as nafcillin or ampicillin/sulbactam—or whatever the susceptibilities indicate.

 QUICK QUIZ: ANTIBIOTIC COVERAGE

Which of the following organisms is/are not generally covered by trimethoprim/sulfamethoxazole (TMP/SMX)?
A) *S. aureus*
B) Streptococcal species
C) *Escherichia coli*
D) *Enterococcus*
E) B and D

The correct answer is "E." Neither *Streptococcus* nor *Enterococcus* species are sensitive to TMP/SMX. This has implications for the treatment of MRSA. Cellulitis (one of the manifestations of MRSA) can be from either staphylococcal or streptococcal species. If there is an abscess, treat for MRSA (incision and drainage with TMP/SMX or doxycycline). If there is a superficial cellulitis, treat for *Streptococcus* (cephalexin or amoxicillin/clavulanate). If you are not sure, one option would be clindamycin as long as local resistance rates are only 10% to 15%; clindamycin resistance rates are on the rise.

 HELPFUL HINT:
The IDSA 2014 guidelines on skin and soft-tissue infections recommend no additional antibiotic therapy following the incision and drainage of a simple skin abscess. However, two large trials have subsequently shown that treatment failure occurred at a lower rate in patients who were given antibiotics. Antibiotics used in these trials were TMP/SMX and clindamycin (*Ann Emerg Med.* 2019;73:8–16).

▶ **CASE 22.2**

You are working in a rural ED when you get a call that a 62-year-old farmer has been trapped between a tractor and a silo while loading silage. It seems to have pinned his legs and pelvis, but from the waist up he is fine. The ambulance crew places the patient in a collar and on a backboard, per protocol, and transports him to the ED.

The patient is in significant pain in his lower extremities and pelvis (of course, since he is a stoic farmer, he denies this and insists he wants to go back to and finish his chores). His blood pressure is initially 100/65 mm Hg with a pulse of 118 bpm. Primary survey is unremarkable, although he is still "boarded and collared."

Question 22.2.1 Which of the following most clearly reflects the best approach to this patient's pain?
A) Use IV meperidine (Demerol) for pain control
B) Use IV morphine for pain control
C) Use IV fentanyl (Sublimaze) for pain control
D) Pain medications are contraindicated at this point given the patient's overall condition
E) Since he's so tough, just offer him some useless platitudes like "no pain, no gain"

Answer 22.2.1 The correct answer is "C." Fentanyl generally has a negligible effect on blood pressure (although one should never say "never"). Both morphine and meperidine tend to drop a patient's blood pressure, so they are relatively contraindicated in this patient with a marginal blood pressure or hypotension. Those who chose "D" or "E" have been hanging around old-time surgeons too long. It is unconscionable to withhold pain medication in this case.

Further examination, by gentle inward pressure on the anterior superior iliac spines bilaterally, shows that the patient's pelvis is unstable. As you recall, a fractured pelvis can lead to significant blood loss into the retroperitoneal space.

Question 22.2.2 *In the short term*, what is the best way to temporize the underlying pathology?
A) Vasopressors (e.g., dopamine) plus fluids
B) Pelvic binder
C) Fluids (normal saline)
D) Activated factor VIIa (NovoSeven)
E) Embolization by interventional radiology (45-minute delay)

Answer 22.2.2 The correct answer is "B." A pelvic binder will significantly reduce bleeding in most unstable pelvis fractures. In 2018, ATLS also added the option to treat pelvic hemorrhage from pelvic fractures with preperitoneal packing as this has shown success. This is a more invasive procedure and thus it is reasonable to start with the more conservative pelvic binder before moving to this action; particularly in a relatively stable patient. "A" is incorrect. Dopamine is not indicated when the problem is hypovolemia. In fact, vasopressors increase mortality in hypovolemic shock. "C" is incorrect. While normal saline is a good choice for resuscitation fluids, we want to tamponade the bleeding and not just chase our tails with fluids. "D" is incorrect. Recombinant activated factor VIIa has not been shown to improve outcomes after trauma (*J Trauma.* 2010;69:353–359). Additionally, it has a number of adverse effects including increased thromboembolic phenomenon (pulmonary embolism, deep venous thrombosis, etc.). Finally, interventional radiology will likely play a role in his management. Those folks are quite skillful at stopping bleeding vessels, but you'll have to call them in from home. While you're waiting, a pelvic binder should be placed.

HELPFUL TIP:
Tranexamic acid, a drug that prevents fibrinolysis, has been shown to (marginally) reduce mortality from bleeding in trauma patients and is now recommended in the 2018 ATLS guidelines. The dose is 1 g IV over 10 minutes followed by 1 g over the next 8 hours. It should be started *within the first hour*. If started after 3 hours, it increases mortality (*Lancet.* 2010 Jul 3;376(9734):23–32). Additionally, tourniquets placed above the area of injury are now back in favor and are supported by the 2018 ATLS guidelines to treat uncontrolled hemorrhage. Consider tranexamic acid and placement of tourniquet as temporizing measures if you have an actively bleeding patient.

You appropriately place a pelvic binder to tamponade the bleeding. The patient's blood pressure stabilizes. You now turn to other issues. This patient will clearly need a Foley catheter.

Question 22.2.3 Relative contraindications to placement of a Foley catheter include which of the following?
A) Blood at the urethral meatus
B) Gross hematuria
C) High-riding prostate
D) Gross blood from the rectum
E) A and C

Answer 22.2.3 The correct answer is "E." Both blood at the meatus and a "high-riding prostate" (ever wonder what it is riding on?) signify the possible disruption of the urethra. You don't want to place the catheter in the wrong place, like the peritoneal space, so catheterization is relatively contraindicated with these findings. Of note, a "high riding prostate" has been found to be a relatively unreliable indicator for injury. The 2018 ATLS guidelines no longer recommend routine palpation of the prostate to evaluate for urethral injury. "B," gross hematuria, can be from the kidney and is not a contraindication to catheterization.

You find blood at the urethral meatus. The patient complains that he really needs to void.

Question 22.2.4 Your options at this point include which of the following?
A) Urethrogram to document an intact urethra
B) Suprapubic cystostomy under ultrasound guidance
C) Use of a Coudé catheter to catheterize the urethra
D) Placement of a bladder catheter via the urethra
E) A and B

Answer 22.2.4 The correct answer is "E." One could perform a urethrogram using a water-soluble dye (e.g., Gastrografin) to document that the urethra is intact and if so place a standard Foley. One could also do a suprapubic cystostomy using ultrasound guidance. "C" and "D" are both incorrect. A Coudé catheter is used to bypass a stricture (prostate or otherwise) and would be no safer than a regular catheter in this patient. Likewise, a wire could end up anywhere and should not be used in this case.

HELPFUL TIP:
If you feel uncomfortable doing a formal cystostomy, a central line with balloon placed into the bladder can be used as a temporizing solution.

▶ **Objectives: Did you learn to …**
· Treat acute traumatic pain?
· Recognize and treat pelvic trauma and intrapelvic hemorrhage?
· Describe contraindications to bladder catheter placement?

▶ **CASE 22.3**

A 55-year-old gentleman with history of smoking and type 2 diabetes presents to your office after finding a mass in his right groin. He works as a night stocker in a local supermarket. He first noticed the mass after lifting a 60 lb box from the floor to the shelf several nights ago. Since then, he notices that the mass is painful and "pulses" when he coughs. He has not been able to work due to the pain. In fact, he wonders if you should just fill out disability papers for him now (never happens, right?). He endorses a history of chronic constipation for which he takes over-the-counter medications. He denies weight loss, nausea, vomiting, and urinary symptoms.

On examination, the patient is afebrile with a blood pressure of 135/86 mm Hg and a pulse of 84 bpm. Abdominal examination demonstrates a mildly obese gentleman with no scars of prior surgeries. Bowel sounds are normal. He denies tenderness with palpation of all four quadrants. There is no guarding. Upon standing, exam of the groin demonstrates an enlarged scrotum on the right side. You have him cough. The mass becomes more prominent and you can feel something protruding from the inguinal canal.

Question 22.3.1 Based on the information above, what is the next step in this patient's overall care?

A) Get CT scan of the abdomen to evaluate for etiology of the mass
B) Refer the patient to a surgeon
C) Have the patient monitor the mass over the next couple of months for changes
D) Have the patient cut back on his constipation medication
E) Place the patient in an inguinal binder

Answer 22.3.1 **The correct answer is "B."** The patient has an inguinal hernia. "A" and "C" are incorrect. History and physical examination are typically sufficient to make the diagnosis of a hernia. The hernia is relatively large and affecting his ability to work, so surgical repair is recommended rather than watchful waiting. Expectant management is an option for small, asymptomatic, or mildly symptomatic hernias, and surgical repair can be deferred. The patient should be provided with counseling on signs and symptoms of strangulation that would warrant emergent evaluation. "D" is incorrect. Constipation is a risk factor for hernias, so advising him to cut back on his constipation medication is not recommended. Have him eat more fiber, though. Finally, "E" sounds like a medieval torture device rather than a therapeutic intervention.

 HELPFUL TIP: STUFF THE GUTS BACK IN OR NOT? Observation of asymptomatic or minimally symptomatic hernias is acceptable—the "watchful waiting" strategy. However, over 7 to 10 years, two-third will elect to go on to repair, with 2% needing emergency repair (*Ann Surg.* 2018 Jan; 267(1):42–49). Tension-free mesh repair is recommended as first choice (don't listen to those late-night TV lawyers!) either by an open or a laparoscopic repair technique (*Hernia.* 2018 Feb;22(1):1–165). Laparoscopic repair has faster recovery times and results in less groin numbness and pain

in the long term. However, open repair has been shown to have lower rates of hernia recurrence (*Ann Surg.* 2012;255(5):846–853).

You refer the patient to a general surgeon within the month and he undergoes a laparoscopic hernia repair with mesh placement. He is discharged the following day. He is relieved that he doesn't need that disability paperwork filled out after all (Phew! You are too!). On postoperative day 2, he is wondering when he can go back to work. He is unable to reach his surgeon, who is in the OR (or maybe on the golf course), and calls your office asking when he can return to work … lifting 60 lb boxes.

Question 22.3.2 How do you counsel him about when he can return to work?

A) He may return to work once he is no longer requiring any pain medications and can drive a car
B) Return to work is typically permitted within 2 to 4 weeks for laborers and within 1 to 2 weeks for those in sedentary jobs
C) Return to work at his current job is not recommended, as it requires too much heavy lifting. He should seek another line of work
D) Return to work is typically permitted within 6 weeks for all professions

Answer 22.3.2 **The correct answer is "B."** Hernia repair patients are typically able to return to work within 2 to 4 weeks, primarily based on their surgeon's recommendations. For workers with more sedentary jobs, return may be as early as a few days. "A" is not correct. Being off pain medications is not a condition for returning to work. "C" is not correct. He should be able to resume his prior activities once the surgical wound heals completely. However, the patient should be counseled on safe lifting techniques and the possibility of recurrence of his hernia.

The patient is able to successfully return to work about 4 weeks postoperatively. He is feeling so well that he no-shows his follow-up appointments. Two years later, he returns after starting a running regimen to lose weight. Unfortunately, he is now having groin pain on the left after he runs, and he is worried that he has an inguinal hernia on the left (his prior hernia was on the right). He denies any nausea, vomiting, constipation, urinary symptoms, or masses in the groin area. Pain is an aching sensation and worsened with changing positions from sitting to standing or going up stairs. He denies any injury.

The patient is afebrile with a blood pressure of 120/78 mm Hg and a pulse of 84 bpm. Abdominal examination demonstrates a normal-weight gentleman with well-healed laparoscopic incisions. Bowel sounds are normal. He denies tenderness with palpation of all four quadrants. There is no guarding or rebound. Pain is reproducible with palpation of the inguinal ligament on the left. There is no inguinal lymphadenopathy.

Upon standing, examination of the groin reveals normal symmetric scrotum without any abnormal findings. There is no mass when the patient coughs.

Question 22.3.3 What is the most likely diagnosis for this patient's symptoms?
A) Osteoarthritis of the left hip
B) Femoral adenitis
C) Left direct inguinal hernia
D) Osteitis pubis
E) Ligamentous strain

Answer 22.3.3 **The correct answer is "E."** All of the above should be considered in the differential for groin pain, but the most likely diagnosis for this patient's symptoms with his new running regimen is a ligamentous strain. Without a bulge detected on Valsalva maneuver (coughing) or a palpable abdominal wall defect, a hernia is unlikely ("C"). There are no palpable inguinal lymph nodes and patient does not have clinical signs of a fever, so "B" is unlikely. Hip osteoarthritis ("A") can be a cause of groin pain, particularly in people with good old wear-and-tear. However, the type of pain with hip osteoarthritis tends to be a deep and aching sensation within the groin area that is not reproducible on palpation. Of particular note is "D." Osteitis pubis, an inflammatory process of the symphysis pubis, is a very common overuse syndrome causing groin pain in athletes; it manifests as pain over the pubic symphysis, not the inguinal ligament. Other causes of osteitis pubis include childbirth, urologic or gynecologic surgery, and rheumatologic conditions. Treatment includes rest, NSAIDs, and, in rare cases, injection of the symphysis pubis with a steroid mixture (for athletes). Other causes of groin pain that should be considered within the differential and should be based on your clinical history and findings include epididymitis, referred pain, ectopic testes, stress fractures, and tendinopathies. If the pain had been localized to the right, adhesions and mesh complications from prior hernia repair must also be considered.

You treat your patient conservatively and he goes on to complete his first half-marathon a year later.

▶ Objectives: Did you learn to …
 · Diagnose a hernia based on clinical history and physical examination?
 · Appropriately manage treatment for hernias?
 · Counsel patients on recommended return to activities postoperatively?
 · Identify other potential causes of groin pain?

▶ CASE 22.4

A 60-year-old female presents to your office for abdominal pain … at 4:45 PM … on a Friday … on Christmas eve. Two months prior, she underwent a partial colon resection and primary re-anastomosis following a perforated bowel, most likely secondary to a perforated diverticulum. The pain is crampy and intermittent. Further history reveals a 24-hour history of vomiting, abdominal bloating, and malaise. She reports her last bowel movement was 2 days ago and denies any flatus over the last 24 hours. On examination, her temperature is 37.1°C, pulse 105 bpm, respirations 12 bpm, and blood pressure 158/60 mm Hg. Her abdomen is slightly distended, diffusely tender to palpation without rebound or guarding, and has hyperactive bowel sounds. On flat plate and upright views of the abdomen, there are dilated loops of small bowel and multiple air fluid levels.

Question 22.4.1 Which of the following is true regarding this patient's current disease process?
A) She most likely has a closed-loop small bowel obstruction (SBO)
B) She most likely has an extramural source of obstruction
C) Dilated loops of small bowel are defined as being >5 cm in diameter on plain film
D) Both partial and complete bowel obstructions reveal no colonic gas on plain film

Answer 22.4.1 **The correct answer is "B."** This patient most likely has an external source of obstruction. Bowel obstructions are divided into two classes: mechanical and functional (the latter also known as pseudo-obstruction, ileus, or neurogenic obstruction). Mechanical obstructions are further classified by both their location—small versus large bowel—and etiology. Possible etiologies include intraluminal bodies (e.g., gallstone ileus or foreign body), intramural lesions (e.g., tumor, stricture, or intussusception), and extramural lesions (e.g., adhesions). Obstructions can further be divided into open and closed loop. Open-loop obstructions have an outlet for gas and secretion relief (e.g., vomiting) whereas closed-loop obstructions block both inflow and outflow to an area. Closed-loop obstructions, like bowel torsion or volvulus, cause acute, severe abdominal pain, and generally require urgent surgical intervention.

Bowel obstruction presents with crampy, intermittent abdominal pain, vomiting, distension, and obstipation. History often includes previous abdominal surgery. Depending on the degree of obstruction and its duration, there may be hyperactive bowel sounds, high-pitched bowel sounds, or decreased/absent bowel sounds. An upright abdominal plain film or lateral recumbent abdominal film confirms diagnosis with findings of dilated loops of small bowel (bowel >3 cm in diameter) on the flat plate and air fluid levels on the upright or decubitus film. However, plain radiographs, only have a sensitivity and specificity of 79% to 83% and 67% to 83% respectively. **CT scan is more sensitive and specific (93% and 100%) for obstruction than are plain films and will often reveal the source of the obstruction.** CT abdomen and pelvis has become the primary imaging modality to guide management (American College of Radiology Appropriateness Criteria, 2018). Patients with a complete SBO will lack air in the colon on plain film; but remember that air can be introduced into the rectum during a rectal examination. Of note, ultrasonography performed at the bedside is both less invasive and less expensive and is 75% sensitive and 75% specific *in the hands of an experienced operator*. It is a safe alternative to CT/x-ray especially in children and pregnant women.

Question 22.4.2 Which of the following cause ileus?
A) Burns
B) Spinal cord injury
C) Hypokalemia
D) Pneumonia
E) All of the above can cause an ileus

Answer 22.4.2 The correct answer is "E." All of the above can cause an ileus. Additional causes include peritonitis, pancreatitis, retroperitoneal inflammation or hematomas, uremia, surgery, and medications like narcotics and anticholinergics.

You diagnose an SBO, which you believe is most likely related to adhesion formation after her hemicolectomy.

Question 22.4.3 Which of the following is INCORRECT regarding the management of bowel obstruction?
A) Initial treatment orders should include NPO, IV fluid resuscitation, and electrolyte replacement as needed
B) This patient should undergo emergent surgical intervention
C) If she has fever or leukocytosis, she should undergo surgical intervention
D) If she requires surgery, broad-spectrum antibiotics to cover anaerobes and Gram-negative aerobes should be administered perioperatively

Answer 22.4.3 The correct answer is "B." Uncomplicated small bowel obstruction is not an indication for emergent surgery. Peritoneal adhesions account for more than half of all SBOs, and 80% of these resolve without surgical intervention. Answer "A" is true. Initial treatment includes restricting oral intake, IV fluid resuscitation, and electrolyte correction.

Answers "C" and "D" are also true. Patients can be safely observed if there is no evidence of strangulation. Evidence of strangulation includes rapidly progressing abdominal pain or distension, development of peritoneal findings, fever, diminished urine output, leukocytosis, hyperamylasemia, metabolic acidosis, and persistent obstruction. Closed-loop obstructions should always be treated surgically and *patients with a transition point often go on to have surgery*. Patients with de novo obstruction (e.g., no history of laparotomy) usually require surgical intervention to determine etiology. If surgery is necessary, broad-spectrum antibiotics that cover anaerobes and Gram-negative aerobes should be administered perioperatively to reduce wound infection and abdominal sepsis rates.

HELPFUL TIP:
Although an NG tube is traditionally used in the treatment of SBO, its use is optional. An NG tube may help alleviate vomiting and distension but does not hasten the resolution of the SBO.

▶ **Objectives: Did you learn to …**
• Assess abdominal pain and recognize an acute abdomen?
• Provide appropriate perioperative management for gastrointestinal (GI) surgery?

• Identify and treat small bowel obstruction after abdominal surgery?

▶ CASE 22.5

Mr. and Mrs. Biggs have always been "big boned." They have decided that weight reduction surgery is the thing for them. However, they are concerned that, for the first time in their lives, they may not be big enough.

Question 22.5.1 Which of the following is NOT a necessary condition for weight loss surgery?
A) BMI $\geq$40 kg/m^2 regardless of the presence of weight-related disease
B) BMI $\geq$35 kg/m^2 without the presence of weight-related disease
C) BMI $\geq$35 kg/m^2 with at least one serious comorbidity like sleep apnea, diabetes, severe joint disease, nonalcoholic fatty liver disease (NAFLD), or weight-related cardiomyopathy
D) Failure to control weight with diet and other medical interventions

Answer 22.5.1 The correct answer is "B." A BMI of $\geq$40 kg/m^2 (not $\geq$35 kg/m^2) alone is considered an appropriate weight for surgical intervention **in the absence of other comorbidities**. As noted above in "C," BMI of $\geq$35 kg/m^2 with weight-related comorbidities is considered an indication for bariatric surgery. "D," failure of medical therapy, is surgeon dependent. Some won't consider weight loss surgery until the patient has demonstrated lifestyle changes. Others do not require such a trial.

A BMI between 30 and 34.9 kg/m^2 and either uncontrollable type 2 diabetes or metabolic syndrome may be an acceptable indication for bariatric surgery, although there is not currently enough evidence to support this in routine practice.

To their delight (and chagrin), Mr. and Mrs. Biggs remain above 40 kg/m^2. There are several surgeons in town who perform different techniques, including a Roux-en-Y and laparoscopic banding.

Question 22.5.2 Which of the following is NOT true?
A) Roux-en-Y is associated with greater weight loss at 1 year
B) Laparoscopic adjustable gastric banding (LAGB) is associated with a greater need for repeat surgery compared with Roux-en-Y
C) Mortality is higher with Roux-en-Y than LAGB and there are more hospital admissions for complications
D) Vertical banded gastroplasty leads to sustained weight loss and few complications

Answer 22.5.2 The correct answer is "D." Vertical banded gastroplasty ("stomach stapling") does not lead to sustained weight loss and has many complications including disruption of the staple line, GERD, vomiting, and erosion of the band into the stomach. For this reason, it has (or should have) fallen out of favor. The rest are true. Laparoscopic Roux-en-Y gastric bypass (LRYGB) results in the best long-term weight loss and requires fewer repeat surgeries when compared with LAGB. However, the mortality rate is higher (0.14 vs. 0.09%) for Roux-en-Y and there are more perioperative complications. It also requires longer hospital stays.

HELPFUL TIP:
Bariatric surgeries help with weight loss by decreasing the storage capacity of the stomach and/or creating conditions for malabsorption. Often, a combination of techniques is performed in a patient. Restrictive surgeries include sleeve gastrectomy and adjustable gastric bandings (vertical or horizontal gastroplasty is not performed these days). Surgeries that promote malabsorption are Roux-en-Y gastric bypass and biliopancreatic diversion with duodenal switch. Most surgeries are performed laparoscopically. Newer procedures include endoscopic bariatric procedures with intragastric balloon placement and vagal nerve blockage device implantation (see "Helpful Tip(s): An Orchestra Conductor for Weight Loss?" for more information) (Fig. 22-1).

Mr. and Mrs. Biggs learn more about the procedures and are wondering if this is worth all the trouble.

Question 22.5.3 You can tell them that:
A) Although they may lose weight, weight loss surgery does nothing for their underlying diabetes, hypercholesterolemia, and coronary artery disease (CAD)
B) There is no psychological or quality-of-life benefit to weight loss surgery: they will have the same existential crises before and after the surgery
C) NSAIDs are relatively contraindicated after weight loss surgery
D) Dumping syndrome is more common after laparoscopic banding than with Roux-en-Y
E) There is rarely a need for supplemental vitamins after bariatric surgery

Answer 22.5.3 **The correct answer is "C."** The rate of gastric ulcers from NSAIDs is higher after bariatric surgery. The rest are not true. Weight loss does improve lipid profiles, decreases mortality due to cardiovascular events, and promotes glycemic control. Therefore "A" is incorrect. There are well-demonstrated psychological and quality-of-life benefits from bariatric surgery ("B"). Dumping syndrome is commonly seen after a Roux-en-Y but not with laparoscopic banding ("D"). Most patients will need supplemental vitamins ("E"). Vitamin deficiencies, especially folic acid, are common after bariatric surgery. Although deficiencies are more of a concern with malabsorptive procedures, supplementation is recommended for all post-bariatric surgery patients.

HELPFUL TIP:
Cholelithiasis is common after bariatric surgery, especially Roux-en-Y, and occurs as a result of rapid weight loss.

After their operations, Mr. and Mrs. Biggs return to see you. Mr. Biggs (who opted for the Roux-en-Y procedure and who is changing his name to Mr. Little) complains of recurrent postprandial colicky abdominal pain, diaphoresis, nausea, diarrhea, and tachycardia. His wife, who went for the laparoscopic banding, has no such symptoms. You make the diagnosis of "dumping syndrome."

Question 22.5.4 Your advice is to:
A) Start an anticholinergic to reduce stomach emptying
B) Increase the content of simple sugars to quickly raise the blood sugar with meals
C) Increase the size of feedings a bit in order to increase the amount of food available for digestion
D) Separate solid from liquid intake for at least 30 minutes (no beer with that pizza!)
E) None of the above

Answer 22.5.4 **The correct answer is "D."** Separating liquid from solid intake by 30 minutes may help to reduce dumping syndrome. The others are incorrect. While theoretically plausible, anticholinergics have not been shown to be of benefit in dumping syndrome. However, drug therapy with octreotide may be considered if there is no response to dietary modifications after 3 to 4 weeks. Small and frequent meals **devoid of simple sugars** are the way to go. The symptoms seem to be related to the rapid transit of simple sugars into the bowel. Smaller volume meals without simple sugars are an effective treatment for most patients with mild symptoms.

While we're on the subject, there is another component of dumping syndrome—"late dumping." This occurs as a result of hypoglycemia secondary to an insulin surge during a meal and presents a few hours after eating. As you might expect with hypoglycemia, vasomotor symptoms are present with fewer GI symptoms.

HELPFUL TIP:
Nutritional deficiencies following bariatric surgery can result from not only decreased absorption, but also low food intake, food intolerances, or excessive vomiting. Consider the following labs at 3, 6, and 12 months, and then annually: CBC, basic metabolic panel with calcium, iron studies, vitamin B1 (thiamine), vitamin B12, folate, liver enzymes, albumin, lipid profile, zinc, and copper.

HELPFUL TIP(S): AN ORCHESTRA CONDUCTOR FOR WEIGHT LOSS?
"Maestro" (yes, that is the name) is a surgically implanted vagus nerve stimulator that interrupts the signal of the vagus to the brain, thus reducing hunger. It has the

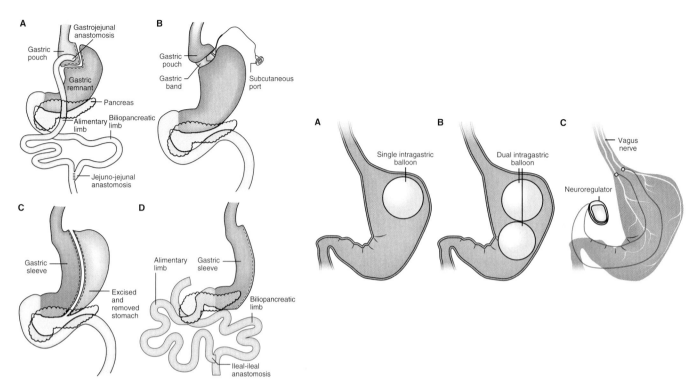

FIGURE 22-1. Common and newer bariatric surgery procedures to induce weight loss.
From Nguyen NT, et al. Bariatric surgery for obesity and metabolic disorders: state of the art. Figures 1 and 2. *Nat Rev Gastroenterol Hepatol.* 2017 Mar; 14(3): 160–169.

same indications as other surgical techniques and leads to 8% more weight loss than those in the sham group.

Finally, in some instances a gastrostomy tube ("feeding tube" … e.g., AspireAssist) can be placed. The patient can eat all they want and then empty the stomach via the gastrostomy tube after a meal (really).

▶ **Objectives: Did you learn to …**
- Recognize the indications for bariatric surgery?
- Describe some different techniques for bariatric surgery and their pros and cons?
- Provide long-term management of the bariatric surgery patient and dumping syndrome?

▶ CASE 22.6

A 24-year-old male presents to your clinic with a 5-day history of rectal bleeding. For several years, he has had hard stools but has developed rectal bleeding in the last few days. In addition, he has severe, intermittent, and crampy abdominal pain that he thinks is due to constipation. He reports a mild fever.

On examination, temperature is 37.9°C, pulse 95 bpm, respirations 12 bpm, and blood pressure 108/78 mm Hg. His abdomen is nontender and without guarding or rebound tenderness. Anoscopy reveals gross blood and two internal hemorrhoids.

Question 22.6.1 Regarding hemorrhoids in general, which of the following is TRUE?
A) Patients with hemorrhoids most commonly present for perianal burning, swelling, and pain
B) A grade III hemorrhoid can be reduced manually
C) If a patient under the age of 50 with rectal bleeding is found to have hemorrhoid on examination, further studies are not indicated
D) Because they are above the dentate line, strangulated internal hemorrhoids are not painful

Answer 22.6.1 The correct answer is "B." Grade III hemorrhoids can be reduced manually. Hemorrhoids are normal vascular structures in the anal canal; however, "hemorrhoids" (the occurrence our patients complain about) arise when the vessels become engorged. Symptoms such as painless bleeding and itching may result. Two types of hemorrhoids exist: external hemorrhoids, from the inferior hemorrhoidal plexus below the dentate line, and internal hemorrhoids from the anal cushions above the dentate line. Internal hemorrhoids occur on the left lateral, right anterior, and right posterior anal walls and are classified into grades I to IV. Grade I hemorrhoids slide below the dentate with straining but not through the anus. Grade II hemorrhoids protrude the anus but spontaneously reduce, whereas Grade III hemorrhoids must be manually reduced. Grade IV internal hemorrhoids cannot be reduced and are at risk for strangulation. "A" is incorrect because most patients with symptomatic hemorrhoids present with painless rectal bleeding. "C" is incorrect. You should consider further evaluation (e.g., flexible sigmoidoscopy and colonoscopy) in patients under the age of 50 presenting with rectal bleeding, even if hemorrhoids are present and are the likely source of bleeding. In patients older than 50 with rectal bleeding, a full colonoscopy is routinely recommended to rule out any cancerous process. "D" is incorrect. Although most internal hemorrhoids do not cause pain, **strangulated** internal hemorrhoids are very painful and can become necrotic and gangrenous, requiring emergent surgery. Note that *strangulated* (when blood supply is cut off) is different from *thrombosed* (when clot forms within the hemorrhoid).

Question 22.6.2 Which of the following would you NOT consider as a treatment of this patient's hemorrhoids?
A) Psyllium
B) Dicyclomine
C) Warm sitz baths
D) Short course of topical hydrocortisone
E) Increased water intake

Answer 22.6.2 **The correct answer is "B."** Dicyclomine (Bentyl, Antispas) is not indicated. Dicyclomine is an anticholinergic and will contribute to constipation—exactly what you want to avoid in hemorrhoids. "A" and "E" are the primary modes of treatment. Psyllium, as well as a diet high in fiber and water, will reduce straining and thus reduces intra-abdominal pressure. "C," warm baths or showers (40°C), have been shown to reduce anal canal pressures. "D," a short course of topical hydrocortisone (e.g., Anusol HC), may be of benefit, although strong evidence is lacking. Long-term topical steroids are contraindicated as they can cause thinning of the anal mucosa. Finally, good hygiene and analgesia should be prescribed as needed.

 HELPFUL TIP:
Most symptomatic hemorrhoids respond to conservative measures. Surgery should not be performed unless conservative measures fail or other indications exist (e.g., strangulation).

Question 22.6.3 Which of the following is true about managing hemorrhoids in an office setting?
A) Irritable bowel syndrome is a relative contraindication to excising hemorrhoids
B) It is best to ligate all hemorrhoids in a single office visit
C) Band ligation results in sloughing of hemorrhoid in about 1 to 2 weeks
D) Following excision, thrombosed external hemorrhoids should be closed to prevent bleeding

Answer 22.6.3 **The correct answer is "C."** Rubber-band ligation generally results in the sloughing of the hemorrhoid in 1 to 2 weeks. "A" is incorrect. Inflammatory bowel disease (IBD)—not irritable bowel syndrome (IBS)—is a relative contraindication to the management of hemorrhoids in an office setting. Other contraindications to office-based hemorrhoid procedures include

coagulopathy, pregnancy and postpartum period, anorectal fissures, perirectal abscess, anorectal tumors, immunocompromised states, portal hypertension, and patients on anticoagulant/antiplatelet medications. It is preferable to treat hemorrhoids in the latter three conditions with sclerotherapy. A formal hemorrhoidectomy can be safely performed in pregnancy. Common complications following the excision of internal hemorrhoids are bleeding and urinary retention. Other rare ones include rectal perforation, recto-vaginal fistula, and pelvic abscess. "B" is incorrect. Although evidence is scarce, standard of care dictates that only one hemorrhoid be ligated in a single office visit (due to concerns about excessive tissue necrosis). "D" is incorrect. Patients who present with external hemorrhoids that are painful, tender, swollen, with bluish discoloration have thrombosis. If the patient presents within 48 hours of thrombosis, the thrombosed hemorrhoid should be excised. However, if a surgical evaluation is not available and the provider is not comfortable with excision of the hemorrhoid, an incision and evacuation of the clot can be performed. It is important **not** to close the hemorrhoid once the clot is evacuated. In fact, a small ellipse of the hemorrhoid should be removed to facilitate continued drainage and prevent re-accumulation of clot.

You prescribe conservative treatment for your patient's hemorrhoids, and since he does not return for his next scheduled appointment, you assume he is doing well. You see him again 6 months later. He reports that he had indeed healed—he is back for a new problem. Although he still takes psyllium, he began having painful bowel movements with blood-streaked stool 2 days ago. Upon examination of the anus, you find a fissure.

Question 22.6.4 All of the following findings would lead you to consider Crohn disease EXCEPT:
A) Posterior midline fissure
B) Painless fissure
C) Multiple fissures
D) Nonhealing fissure

Answer 22.6.4 **The correct answer is "A."** The posterior (dorsal) midline is where solitary fissures, unrelated to IBD, are typically located. Fissures in any other location should raise suspicion for Crohn disease. "B," "C," and "D" are also suggestive of Crohn disease. See Chapter 7 for more on Crohn Disease and IBD.

Question 22.6.5 In a patient with an uncomplicated, initial anal fissure, what do you recommend for *first-line* therapy?
A) Lord dilation
B) Botulinum toxin injections
C) Topical nitroglycerin
D) Oral psyllium
E) Oral nifedipine

Answer 22.6.5 **The correct answer is "D."** All of the options are employed for treating anal fissures. However, in patients with an uncomplicated, initial anal fissure, it is always prudent to initiate conservative therapy (e.g., psyllium, dietary fiber, water, and warm soaks) prior to proceeding to more invasive measures. Most fissures will respond to conservative measures. Generally, healing takes 2 to 4 weeks. In addition to the treatments listed, topical diltiazem and topical nifedipine are also useful as are various surgical approaches like lateral anal sphincterotomy. Lord dilation ("A") deserves special mention as a relatively arcane procedure for stretching the anal sphincter muscle (under anesthesia, we hope!). One note about Botulinum toxin injection ("B") for rectal fissures: It also gets rid of those unsightly wrinkles!

▶ **Objectives: Did you learn to …**
- Characterize hemorrhoids based on location?
- Grade internal hemorrhoids based on severity?
- Manage hemorrhoids with conservative and surgical treatments?
- Treat an uncomplicated anal fissure?
- Recognize anal fissures as potential signs of Crohn disease?

▶ CASE 22.7

A 58-year-old female presents to your clinic for a lump found on routine breast self-examination. Her older sister died from breast cancer, and she is very concerned about the possibility of breast cancer in herself. She never misses her monthly breast examination and notes she has never felt this lump before. She first noticed the lump 2 weeks ago, and it has not changed in size or consistency since that time. Consistent with her personal healthcare goals but totally inconsistent with any current guidelines, she has had yearly mammograms since age 40 that have always been normal. She denies any weight loss or fatigue and reports being postmenopausal for the last 5 years. She previously took combination hormone replacement therapy, which she discontinued last year.

On examination, her breasts appear symmetrical with no skin abnormalities. The nipples are symmetric in size, shape, and color without retraction or discharge. You palpate a small, pea-sized thickening in upper outer quadrant of the right breast. This is the lump that she noticed 2 weeks ago. It is fixed to the deep aspect of the chest wall, so you have a hard time delineating whether the borders are smooth.

Question 22.7.1 Regarding breast lumps, which one of the following is FALSE?
A) Abnormal screening mammography is the most common presentation of breast carcinoma
B) Cysts are more common in premenopausal women than postmenopausal women
C) A history of fibroadenoma is associated with an increased risk of breast cancer
D) A radiographic oil cyst is pathognomonic for fat necrosis

Answer 22.7.1 The correct answer is "A." The most common presentation of breast carcinoma is a breast lump felt by the patient, although screening mammography makes up a large

percentage of diagnosed breast cancers as well. Breast masses can be benign—including fibroadenomas (most commonly), lipomas, fat necrosis, soft-tissue inflammation or infection—or malignant. "B" is true. Cysts primarily present when women are premenopausal and are uncommon in the postmenopausal state, unless the woman is taking hormone replacement. Cysts are typically well-demarcated, mobile, and firm. The diagnosis is confirmed with aspiration of non-bloody fluid followed by complete resolution of the mass. Fibroadenomas occur between the ages of 20 and 50 and are described as firm, rubbery, and mobile. They can be confirmed by characteristic findings on ultrasound and tissue biopsy if necessary. "C" is also true. While historically believed to be entirely benign, fibroadenomas are associated with a small but significant increased risk for breast cancer. "D" is true. A radiographic oil cyst (a circumscribed mass of mixed soft-tissue density and fat with a rim that is often calcified) is due to fat necrosis, which occurs in areas of the breast that have been subject to trauma, surgery, infection, or radiation therapy. About half of the time, fat necrosis has no precipitant. Oil cysts are most common in the superficial aspects of pendulous breasts of obese women. When an oil cyst is seen radiographically, no further evaluation is needed.

When making diagnostic decisions regarding breast masses, age matters. In women under 30, if there is low suspicion for cancer based on history and exam, a palpable breast mass can be observed for one to two menstrual cycles, and further evaluation only pursued if the mass persists. For this age group, ultrasound is the imaging modality of choice, but mammogram may be added to workup if there is high clinical suspicion for malignancy. *For women 30–39, observation is not recommended, and you should proceed with mammogram or ultrasound, or both.* Ultrasound is still probably more sensitive in this age range. For women over 40, obtain a diagnostic mammogram and ultrasound.

. . . .

Your patient is concerned about her family history of breast cancer. She asks about genetic testing.

Question 22.7.2 You are able to tell her that the BRCA genes are associated with which of the following?
A) Breast cancer
B) Uterine cancer
C) Ovarian cancer
D) A and B
E) A and C

Answer 22.7.2 The correct answer is "E." Approximately 7% of breast cancers and 15% of ovarian cancers are associated with mutations to the BRCA (**BR**east **CA**ncer) 1 and 2 tumor suppressor genes. These mutations increase risk of familial breast cancer and ovarian cancer. They are not associated with uterine cancer. Specific criteria from the National Comprehensive Cancer Network (NCCN) exist to determine who should undergo testing for BRCA 1/2 and other gene mutations that put patients at risk for hereditary breast and ovarian cancers.

Patients with a particularly concerning family history may benefit from seeing a genetic counselor.

....

For your patient, you decide to use one of many risk assessment tools (i.e., Gail score... below for more) and find that this patient's 5-year breast cancer risk, even before she came to you with a concerning lump, is estimated to be higher than that of the average 58-year-old woman. You are suspicious that this patient's mass may be cancer, and you order diagnostic mammography and ultrasound. However, these studies show no mass. When your patient returns to discuss her test results, you examine her again. The mass is still palpable and essentially unchanged.

Question 22.7.3 **The next best step in management of this patient is:**
A) Breast examination and mammogram every 6 months
B) Breast examination and mammogram every 3 months
C) Referral to a surgeon to consider excisional biopsy
D) Ultrasound-guided needle biopsy
E) Return to normal screening

Answer 22.7.3 **The correct answer is "C."** A palpable mass that is suspicious for cancer cannot be ignored even in the presence of negative radiologic studies. No other option is acceptable, nor would any other option be defensible if this patient were to develop overt breast cancer. *"D" would be an option if a mass had been identified on ultrasound (see below).*

Question 22.7.4 **But let's suppose for a moment that a mass was detected on your patient's imaging. You would now turn to the "Breast Imaging Reporting and Data System" (BI-RADS®) criteria which score radiologic findings and the probability of cancer. These designations should be included on any mammography report. For more information, please go to https://www.acr.org/-/media/ACR/Files/RADS/BI-RADS/BIRADS-Reference-Card.pdf or Google "BI-RADS." Which of the following is NOT TRUE about how a diagnostic evaluation should proceed?**
A) In women <30 years of age, lesions that are BI-RADS® 3 (probably benign) on ultrasound may be followed by a repeat examination in 6 to 12 months, then every 1 to 2 years if clinical suspicion for malignancy remains low
B) In women >40 years of age, lesions that are BI-RADS® 3 (probably benign) on ultrasound need no follow-up
C) In women >40 years of age who have a palpable mass that is not seen on mammogram or ultrasound, BI-RADS® 1 (negative), excisional biopsy should be performed if clinical suspicion dictates
D) In women >40 years of age who have breast imaging rated as BI-RADS® 4 or 5 should have a core needle biopsy of the area in question

Answer 22.7.4 **The correct (incorrect) answer is "B."** Women over the age 40 absolutely need follow-up for anything other than a specific benign finding (e.g., lymph node), and even with

that finding, a correlative ultrasound may be indicated. "A" is true. If this young woman had a "likely benign," BI-RADS® 3 ultrasound, this is an appropriate approach. If the mass were a simple cyst, or BI-RADS® 2 (benign), diagnostic evaluation could stop following the ultrasound. With an ultrasound more concerning than BI-RADS® 3, she should have a mammogram and a core needle biopsy for further diagnosis. "C" is true. If the palpable mass cannot be identified radiographically, and clinical suspicion remains high, the mass should be removed by excision. "D" is also true; core needle biopsy is recommended for BI-RADS® 4 and 5 findings, and should be considered versus short-term follow-up for BI-RADS® 3 findings. The American College of Radiology (ACR) and the NCCN are less directive for women aged 30 to 39, with subsequent workup based on whether initial imaging was mammogram or ultrasound.

A needle biopsy either by core needle biopsy or fine needle aspiration (FNA) is the next step after imaging in evaluation of solid tumor masses requiring further diagnosis. Needle diagnosis offers the advantages of being simple, quick, inexpensive, relatively noninvasive, highly available, and an accurate way of diagnosing atypical cells. **Core needle biopsy is the way to go if you have a choice.**

....

You perform an FNA because you are practicing in a low resource setting without a surgeon. The cytopathologist reads this as "probable malignancy." You recall from previous visits that the patient's older sister had breast cancer. Additionally, your patient went through menopause at age 56, and used hormone replacement therapy for 5 years. You obtain further history, including a history of menarche at 14 years of age and the fact that the patient has never been pregnant.

Question 22.7.5 **Which of these factors DOES NOT contribute to an increased risk of breast cancer in THIS patient?**
A) Her nulliparity
B) Her age at menarche
C) Her family history
D) Her age at menopause
E) Her history of hormone replacement

Answer 22.7.5 **The correct answer is "B."** The risk of breast cancer is roughly associated with the lifetime exposure to estrogen. This patient's age at menarche is in the mid-to-late age range and is thus **not** a risk factor for breast cancer. Younger age at menarche (e.g., 10 years old) is associated with an increased risk of breast cancer. Nulliparity and greater age at first pregnancy (over 30 years) are associated with an increased risk, as is older age of menopause. A history of a first-degree relative with breast cancer is a strong risk factor. Modifiable risk factors for breast cancer appear to be increased BMI, sedentary lifestyle, and increased alcohol intake. Exposure to thoracic radiation prior to age 30 is something you should remember to ask your patients about. Women who are identified as having dense breasts on mammogram are at increased risk for breast cancer, at least partially due to difficulty in interpreting their mammograms (an ultrasound or MRI may be recommended for these women if they are already at increased risk of breast cancer). Finally, as demonstrated in the Women's Health Initiative, estrogen/progesterone replacement therapy (HRT) is associated with an increased risk of breast cancer (an excess of about 8 breast cancers per 10,000 women treated with HRT).

. . . .

While you wait for definitive pathology results, you consider the different types of breast cancer that this patient might have.

Question 22.7.6 Regarding various types of breast cancer, all of the following are true EXCEPT:
A) Phyllodes tumors are not always malignant
B) Infiltrating lobular carcinoma is the most common histological type of invasive breast carcinoma
C) Paget disease of the breast clinically appears eczematous
D) Sarcomas, lymphomas, melanomas, and angiosarcomas are all possible causes of cancer in the breast

Answer 22.7.6 The correct answer is "B." Infiltrating **ductal** (not lobular) carcinoma is the most common histological type of invasive breast cancer. Invasive breast carcinoma includes a wide variety of histological diseases. Infiltrating **ductal** carcinoma accounts for 65% to 80% of breast cancers, whereas infiltrating **lobular** carcinoma is the second most frequent, accounting for about 10% of breast cancers. "A" is true. The more rare phyllodes tumors, which often have a clinical presentation similar to fibroadenomas, may be either malignant or benign. The malignant nature of phyllodes tumors is sometimes difficult to determine on FNA or core needle biopsy, and wide local excision may be required. "C," Paget disease of the breast, is a rare form of breast cancer with eczematous changes of the nipple, including itching, erythema, and nipple discharge. "D" is true as well. Many other malignancies may occur in the breast, including sarcomas, lymphomas, melanomas, and angiosarcomas.

. . . .

The pathology results are final and show infiltrating ductal carcinoma. Your patient will see a breast surgeon next week. As you await the results of surgery, you consider her prognosis.

Question 22.7.7 All of the following are favorable prognostic indicators in breast cancer EXCEPT:
A) Hormone receptor negative
B) Absence of axillary nodal involvement
C) Low-grade tumor
D) Pure tubular, mucinous, or medullary histological types
E) Tumor size <1 cm

Answer 22.7.7 The correct answer is "A." Patients whose tumors are hormone receptor negative have worse outcomes than do patients whose tumors are hormone receptor positive. "B," absence of axillary nodal involvement, is obviously a better prognostic factor than the presence of nodal involvement. In fact, axillary lymph node status is the single most important

predictor of overall survival in breast cancer. "C," low tumor grade, is also a good prognostic factor. "D," patients with a single cell type have a better prognosis as well. "E" is true. A very useful predictor of tumor behavior is tumor size, and tumor size <1 cm is a positive prognostic sign.

HELPFUL TIP:
Tumors can be either estrogen or progesterone receptor positive or negative and Her2/neu (tyrosine-protein kinase receptor) positive or negative. Tumors that are positive for estrogen and/or progesterone receptors are the most likely to respond to hormonal therapy (e.g., tamoxifen). Tumors that are positive for Her2/neu are most likely to respond to tyrosine kinase inhibitors (e.g., Herceptin).

HELPFUL (BUT DISTURBING) TIP:
It turns out that approximately 16% to 20% of women who undergo breast-conserving surgery for breast cancer need repeat surgery. Some never go for re-excision (15% in one study). Disturbing with major implications for informed consent (*Ann Surg Oncol.* 2017 Jan;24(1):52–58.

A second issue with breast cancer is the matter of "overdiagnosis." Up to 20% or more of the cancers we diagnose on mammogram would never cause problems (*BMJ.* 2009;339:b2587). We are subjecting women to unnecessary chemotherapy/surgery/radiation. What to do about this is a matter of debate.

▶ **Objectives: Did you learn to …**
· Generate a differential diagnoses for breast masses?
· Evaluate a patient with a breast mass?
· Identify risk factors for breast cancer?
· Describe several types of breast cancers?
· Describe factors that are used to establish prognosis in breast cancer?

 QUICK QUIZ: BREAST CANCER RISK

A 50-year-old female presents for a routine physical. She wants to know her risk of developing breast cancer. You want to give her a more accurate picture, and you decide to use the Gail model.

When taking her history, you must ask about all of the following EXCEPT:
A) Number of first-degree relatives with breast cancer
B) Age at first menstrual period
C) Number of breast biopsies
D) Age at first live birth
E) Number of live births

The correct answer is "E." The Gail model is a statistical model that estimates a woman's chance of developing breast cancer. Factors that affect the score include the number of first-degree relatives with breast cancer, current age, age of first menstrual period, number of breast biopsies, BRCA gene status, age at first live birth, race, and history of atypia in a biopsy. This tool may be useful in determining which patients are high risk or even candidates for hormonal therapy for breast cancer prophylaxis. **However, the Gail score is much better at predicting the likelihood of breast cancer in populations than in any individual.** The National Cancer Institute maintains a website for the Gail model calculation, located at http://bcra.nci.nih.gov/brc/q1.htm.

▶ CASE 22.8

An orthopedic colleague asks you to consult on a 64-year-old male prior to an elective total hip replacement. The surgery is scheduled for 5 weeks from now. The patient is a smoker with hypertension, diabetes mellitus type 2, and coronary artery disease. He is currently asymptomatic and is able to walk stairs without dyspnea or chest pain. The surgeon would like some perioperative recommendations.

Question 22.8.1 You would recommend all of the following EXCEPT:
A) The patient should stop smoking TODAY
B) The patient should have preoperative and postoperative β-blockers started on the day of surgery
C) The patient should have an ECG done
D) The patient should have his hemoglobin/hematocrit drawn
E) The patient should have his creatinine measured

Answer 22.8.1 **The correct answer is "B."** If a patient has a medical indication for a chronic β-blocker, it should be continued perioperatively as long as the dose has been stable well in advance of the day of surgery. While the β-blocker offers some protection against myocardial infarction, there is also increased risk of stroke, hypotension, and overall mortality. **A β-blocker should NOT be started on the day of surgery.** "A" is true. Nonsmokers have better surgical outcomes than smokers, in addition to longer lives and better breath. A few small studies have raised concerns about quitting smoking too close to the date of surgery. Sooner is definitely better (at least 30 days out), but the quitting at any time is better than continuing. Answers "C," "D," and "E" are probably true for this patient who has known cardiac disease and an increased risk of acute kidney injury due to his other medical conditions. Many other "routine" preoperative assessments are not supported in the literature. See Tables 22-1 and 22-2 for the appropriate evaluation of the preoperative patient.

Question 22.8.2 You inform your patient that a hip replacement surgery is among the procedures with the highest rates of deep venous thrombosis. Which of the following is effective for the prevention of postoperative DVT?
A) Sequential compression devices for in-hospital recovery
B) Enoxaparin 30 mg subcutaneously every 12 hours
C) Therapeutic warfarin
D) Unfractionated heparin 5,000 Units subcutaneously every 12 hours
E) All of the above

Answer 22.8.2 **The correct answer is "E."** All of the modalities listed above can be used to prevent the development of DVT. The non-warfarin direct oral anticoagulants are also increasingly being used at prophylactic doses if patients refuse injectable medications, but careful—DOACS are not to be used following hip *fracture* repair, where there is an increased risk of bleeding compared to hip arthroplasty (replacement). Aspirin is also commonly used though the data is poor. Subcutaneous heparin may require TID dosing in larger patients, and don't forget that enoxaparin requires renal adjustment for creatinine clearance <30 mL/min. The minimum time frame for prophylaxis is 10 to 14 days, but usually should be continued longer—up to 35 days. Early mobility is always a goal, so encourage your patient to make good use of that new hip as soon as possible.

TABLE 22-1 PREOPERATIVE STUDIES AND THEIR INDICATIONS

Tests	Indications
BUN/creatinine	Over 60; history of renal, cardiac, or vascular disease
CBC/H&H	Possible hematologic or infectious process; significant blood loss predicted
Coagulation studies	Stigmata liver disease, history of coagulopathy, possible DIC, anticoagulation, alcohol abuse
ECG/CXR	As indicated by history and physical (e.g., exacerbation of pulmonary disease with cough)
Electrolytes	Diuretic use, history of renal or cardiac disease, possible dehydration by history or physical
Glucose	Diabetics, obese patients, undergoing vascular procedures, other reason for increased glucose (e.g., steroids)
Liver enzymes	History of liver disease or stigmata of liver disease
Urine β-hCG	If indicated by history or female of child-bearing age
Urinalysis	Pregnancy, diabetes, urologic surgery, symptomatic patients

Adapted from Feely MA, Collins CS, et al. Preoperative testing before noncardiac surgery: guidelines and recommendations. *Am Fam Physician.* 2013;87(6): 414–418.

TABLE 22-2 NATIONAL INSTITUTE FOR HEALTHCARE AND CARE EXCELLENCE (NICE) GUIDELINES FOR PERIOPERATIVE TESTING[a,b]

	ASA Class		
Surgery Grade	1 (Normal Healthy Patient)	2 (Mild Systemic Disease)	3 or 4 (Severe Systemic Disease OR Severe Systemic Disease That is a Constant Threat to Life)
Minor (i.e., excising skin lesion, draining abscess, cataract surgery)	• No routine perioperative testing	• No routine perioperative testing	• Creatinine (at risk of acute kidney injury (AKI)) • ECG (if none in past 12 months)
Intermediate (i.e., inguinal hernia repair, arthroscopy, tonsillectomy)	• No routine perioperative testing	• Creatinine (at risk of AKI) • ECG (CV, DM, Renal disease)	• Creatinine • CBC (renal or CV disease without test) • Coagulation studies (chronic anticoagulation or chronic liver disease) • ECG
Complex (i.e., total abdominal hysterectomy, prostatectomy, joint replacement, GI surgery, back surgery, lung surgery)	• CBC • Creatinine (at risk of AKI) • ECG (> 65 if none in past 12 months)	• CBC • Serum creatinine • ECG	• CBC • Creatinine • Coagulation studies (chronic anticoagulation or chronic liver disease) • ECG

[a]Do NOT routinely offer testing for sickle cell disease. Do not obtain a urinalysis in anyone or an A1c in those without diabetes.
[b]Be sure to obtain a pregnancy test in *all women of childbearing potential*.
Adapted from National Institute for Healthcare and Care Excellence (NICE). Routine preoperative tests for elective surgery: NICE Guideline [NG45]. London, UK: NICE; 2016 Apr 5. Available at: https://www.nice.org.uk/guidance/ng45. Accessed 23 April 2019.

HELPFUL TIP:
Graduated compression stockings are marginally beneficial at best for DVT prevention and lead to increased skin breakdown, etc. For this reason, intermittent pneumatic compression with sequential compression devices (SCDs) is preferred (*Ann Surg.* 2010;251(3):393–396 and *Lancet.* 2009;373:1958–1965).

The patient undergoes his hip replacement, and his postoperative ECG is normal. **Four hours after surgery, he develops mild respiratory distress, a fever, and cough. On chest x-ray, there is a right lower lobe infiltrate. There is no evidence of fluid overload.**

Question 22.8.3 Which of the following is the most likely cause of this patient's fever and infiltrate?
A) *Pneumococcus*
B) Gram-negative organisms
C) Atelectasis
D) Chemical pneumonitis
E) Aspiration pneumonia

Answer 22.8.3 The correct answer is "D." In the hours after surgery, a chemical *pneumonitis* would be the most likely cause of this patient's current findings. This requires aspirating gastric

contents with a pH of less than 2.5 and at least 25 mL of stomach contents. Aspiration pneumonitis develops over a matter of hours after aspiration. In contrast, pneumococcal and Gram-negative pneumonias generally develop *several days* after surgery (unless a subclinical pneumonia was present at the time of surgery). Aspiration *pneumonia* is caused by anaerobes and mixed flora and develops slowly over days to a week. Atelectasis warrants special mention. **Atelectasis does not cause fever.** Both atelectasis and fever occur frequently in the postoperative period, but their occurrence together is most likely due to chance. In the postsurgical patient with fever, look for another cause besides atelectasis.

Question 22.8.4 Of the following, which typically IS NOT a cause of postoperative fever in the first 48 hours?
A) Malignant hyperthermia
B) Surgical "trauma" (e.g., cutting through muscle)
C) Wound infection
D) Hyperthyroidism
E) Drug fever

Answer 22.8.4 The correct answer is "C." Wound infections generally are not found in the first 48 hours after surgery, although any fever should prompt a physical exam, including inspection of the surgical site. All of the rest can be found either immediately after surgery (malignant hyperthermia, hyperthyroidism, drug fever, etc.) or soon thereafter (fever from surgical trauma secondary to the release of cytokines). Table 22-3 summarizes the time course and causes of postoperative fever.

The patient's chest radiograph is consistent with aspiration (for our patient, who was presumably supine in the OR at the time of aspiration, the dependent lobes were probably the superior segments of the lower lobes and the posterior segments of the upper lobes. If he'd been upright, which is not the typical positioning for hip arthroplasty, we would expect him to aspirate exclusively into his lower lobes).

Question 22.8.5 Which of the following is NOT TRUE with regard to chemical pneumonitis?

A) It can progress to ARDS
B) Patients with chemical pneumonitis can present with fever, dyspnea, bronchospasm, and hypoxia
C) It should be treated immediately with antibiotics that cover for anaerobes
D) It tends to resolve within 2 to 3 days (unless it progresses—see option A!)

Answer 22.8.5 **The correct answer is "C."** Chemical *pneumonitis* is a process that is unrelated to infection. Therefore, chemical pneumonitis does not need to be treated with antibiotics at all (although as a practical matter they are often given anyway). The rest of the options are true. Supportive care is the best initial therapy for those poor acid-burned lungs. Chemical pneumonitis can, however, progress to pneumonia via secondary bacterial infection—new fever or worsening symptoms should prompt re-evaluation and re-imaging, and possible ICU transfer.

HELPFUL TIP:
The term "aspiration pneumonia" is used differently in different parts of the literature. This leads to some confusion. Some use the term to include all pneumonias caused by aspiration. Many of the cases included in this definition are caused by many of the same organisms that cause community-acquired pneumonia, including *pneumococcus* and *Haemophilus influenzae*. These patients tend to have a fever and infiltrate, etc., which develop within 2 days of the aspiration. For these patients, the appropriate antibiotics should include agents to cover hospital-acquired organisms, especially Gram-negative organisms, including *Pseudomonas*.

Other groups may define aspiration pneumonia as anaerobic infections that result from aspiration. Predisposing factors include intoxication, poor dentition, stroke with swallowing difficulties, weak cough, etc. These patients have a more indolent course, with onset of symptoms over days to weeks. Generally, these patients have purulent sputum, with lower lobe involvement most common. The upper lobes may be involved if the patient aspirates while recumbent. These patients may have a polymicrobial infection including *Peptostreptococcus*, *Fusobacterium*, *Bacteroides*, and *Prevotella*. These patients should be treated with antibiotics such as clindamycin, ampicillin/sulbactam (Unasyn), or amoxicillin/clavulanate (Augmentin); avoid metronidazole as a single agent due to high failure rate.

So, when you read the literature about aspiration pneumonia, be sure you know which definition the authors are using, because the description of the disease and the treatments vary.

HELPFUL TIP:
Drugs that raise the gastric pH (H$_2$-blockers, proton pump inhibitors), commonly used in critically ill patients, can increase the risk of postoperative pneumonia (and *Clostridium difficile*). They don't change mortality but do reduce the risk of GI bleed (*N Engl J Med*. 2018:379:2199–2208). Just make sure to stop them upon discharge.

You treat the patient with fluids and tracheal suction. However, he remains febrile and tachycardic at about 128 bpm; ECG shows a sinus tachycardia. There is no evidence of dehydration at this point and he seems euvolemic, including by IVC ultrasound.

Question 22.8.6 Which of the following would be an appropriate first step in the treatment of tachycardia in *this* postsurgical patient?

A) Oral or rectal aspirin
B) Oral or rectal acetaminophen
C) IV β-blockers
D) IV fluids

TABLE 22-3 CAUSES OF POSTOPERATIVE FEVER

Immediate (within first 48 hours following surgery):
- Drug (including malignant hyperthermia) or blood product reactions
- Tissue trauma either intraoperative or preoperative
- Chemical pneumonitis
- Preexisting subclinical infection (consider any infectious cause)
- Thrombophlebitis, DVT, MI, gout, pancreatitis, alcohol withdrawal, hyperthyroidism (these noninfectious causes typically result in fevers <39°C)

Acute (48 hours to 1 week after surgery):
- Pneumonia (aspiration, hospital or ventilator associated, or other)
- Abscess or surgical site infection (typically after 1 week, but Group A Strep and Clostridium infections may manifest within 1–3 days)
- UTI or GI infections including *C. difficile*
- Also: Pancreatitis, alcohol withdrawal, PE, MI, thrombophlebitis, gout

Subacute (1–4 weeks after surgery):
- IV and central catheter site infections
- Antibiotic associated diarrhea, including *C. difficile* infection
- Drug fever: β-lactams, sulfa, heparin, etc.
- DVT, PE, fat emboli from long bones, acute chest syndrome (SSA)

Answer 22.8.6 The correct answer is "B." The **initial** treatment of this patient is acetaminophen. Reducing the fever and metabolic stress should result in a reduction of the heart rate. "A" is not the best choice since this patient is postsurgical. Giving aspirin, an antiplatelet agent, may result in increased postoperative bleeding. "C," IV β-blockers, might be appropriate if the patient were having ischemic symptoms and needed an immediate reduction in pulse. Beta blockers would not impact the underlying cause of his tachycardia—sinus tachycardia is usually not a problem in the heart. "D," IV fluid—okay, debatable, but take our word for it that he was euvolemic. IV fluids **are** appropriate in postoperative tachycardia if the patient is dehydrated.

The patient's pulmonary status has improved. The surgeon notices that the patient has hyperkalemia and thrombocytopenia. The patient is on a number of meds postoperatively. She is wondering if one of these drugs is to blame.

Question 22.8.7 You let her know that the most likely cause is:
A) β-Blockers
B) Albuterol
C) Aspirin
D) Morphine
E) Heparin

Answer 22.8.7 The correct answer is "E." Heparin can cause both thrombocytopenia and hyperkalemia. Hyperkalemia is caused by heparin's action against adrenal cells that produce aldosterone—this is typically only clinically important if the patient has renal failure, or is on an ACE-I, ARB, or spironolactone. Thrombocytopenia secondary to heparin use comes in two flavors. The more common, mild form (sometimes called heparin-induced thrombocytopenia (HIT) type 1) is a non–immune-mediated thrombocytopenia that occurs in up to 20% of individuals who receive heparin. This mild thrombocytopenia occurs within the first 4 days of heparin administration, typically has a platelet nadir of greater than 100,000/μL and no significant clinical consequences. Continue the heparin for these patients.

The more rare and serious form of heparin-induced thrombocytopenia is immune-mediated (aka HIT type 2), caused by the development of IgG antibodies to the heparin/platelet factor 4 complex. This typically occurs 5 to 10 days after the start of heparin therapy and is associated with a high risk of venous or arterial thrombosis. Stop the heparin if you suspect HIT type 2 (including heparin flushes and low-molecular-weight heparin) and anticoagulate with a nonheparin agent.

"A," β-blockers, may result in hyperkalemia at high doses (via a β1-receptor effect inhibiting renin release) but do not cause thrombocytopenia, and remember, we didn't start these on the day of surgery! "B," albuterol, can cause *hypokalemia* (as can other catecholamines) by driving potassium into the intracellular space. "D" is incorrect because morphine is not associated with hyperkalemia or thrombocytopenia.

HELPFUL TIP:
Heparin can also cause a postoperative fever, as can β-lactams, sulfa drugs, H2 blockers, phenytoin, procainamide, and others.

You leisurely sip your coffee as you review the labs and notice that your patient's platelets have dropped from 250,000/μL to 100,000/μL and is now down to 30,000/μL. Your patient has been waiting around in the hospital for placement in a rehabilitation facility, and it is already post-op day 6. You are concerned for the immune-mediated form of HIT, so you go through the 4Ts to assess his risk: Degree of Thrombocytopenia, Timing of the platelet count dropping, Thrombosis, other causes of thrombocytopenia (see MDCalc.com for a calculator).

Question 22.8.8 Which of the following would increase the pretest probability that our patient will test positive for antibodies to the PF4-heparin complex (HIT antibodies)?
A) A fall of greater than 50 percent in his platelet count to a nadir greater than 20,000 platelets/μL
B) Occurrence of this drop between days 5 and 10 since the start of his heparin dosing
C) New venous thrombosis, arterial thrombosis, or skin necrosis following heparin use
D) All of the above

Answer 22.8.8 The correct answer is "D", all of the above. All of these factors increase our patient's likelihood of testing positive for HIT. Other factors that increase our patient's pretest probability for HIT antibody positivity include the fact that he was a surgical rather than a medical patient, and that he received unfractionated heparin following his surgery rather than low-molecular-weight heparin (HIT can occur secondary to LMW heparin use, but it is less common).

You immediately stop the patient's heparin, and the thrombocytopenia begins to resolve. As he continues to wait for a rehabilitation bed, you get the results of your antibody testing, which confirm the diagnosis of HIT. Fortunately, you have started him on an alternative anticoagulant (the risk of thrombosis in HIT can be up to 50 percent in patients who are not started on alternative therapy).

Question 22.8.9 Which of the following is TRUE about the use of heparin in patients with a history of heparin-induced thrombocytopenia (HIT)?
A) A low-molecular-weight heparin (LMWH) should be used in patients with a history of HIT
B) Warfarin may be started immediately at time of diagnosing HIT
C) The use of bivalirudin and argatroban is contraindicated in the treatment of HIT

D) A direct oral anticoagulant (DOAC) such as apixaban or rivaroxaban may be used in patients diagnosed with HIT

E) None of the above

Answer 22.8.9 **The correct answer is "D."** The DOACs are increasingly used to reduce the risk of thrombosis in HIT. "A" is incorrect. LMWH should be avoided in patients with strongly suspected (or confirmed) HIT, as should heparin flushes and heparin-coated catheters. "B" is incorrect—although warfarin may eventually be used in these patients, it should not be used immediately following diagnosis. Remember that there is a transient hypercoagulability at the onset of warfarin use, and combining this effect with florid HIT can have bad outcomes (like tissue necrosis). "C" is incorrect. In fact, these medications are often first-line treatment for patients with HIT who need continued parenteral anticoagulation.

▶ **Objectives: Did you learn to …**
- Perform a preoperative medical evaluation?
- Generate a differential diagnosis for postoperative fever?
- Diagnose and treat aspiration pneumonitis?
- Recognize some complications of heparin use?
- Employ appropriate DVT prophylaxis measures?
- Manage a patient with heparin-induced thrombocytopenia?

 QUICK QUIZ: GENERAL ANESTHESIA FOR SURGERY

Regarding anesthesia evaluation both preoperatively and intraoperatively, which one of the following is FALSE?

A) Minimum potassium before proceeding with elective coronary artery bypass graft (CABG) surgery should be 3.5 mEq/L

B) Patients with obstructive sleep apnea (OSA) have higher rates of pre-, intra-, and postoperative complications than patients without OSA

C) American Society of Anesthesiologists (ASA) Class IV designation includes patients who have well-controlled major systemic disease

D) Risks of anesthesia include allergic drug reactions, failure to intubate and provide adequate oxygenation and ventilation, nerve damage, and malignant hyperthermia

The correct answer is "C." ASA Class IV includes patients who have a systemic disease that is life threatening and NOT well controlled. All the other options are true. "B" is a correct statement. Patients with OSA are more difficult to intubate and are more likely to have pulmonary complications before and during surgery. OSA is also strongly associated with hypertension, pulmonary hypertension, and heart failure. "D" is also a correct statement. Anesthesia risks include allergic drug reactions, failure to intubate and provide adequate oxygenation and ventilation, nerve damage (from unrelieved pressure on the nerve), and malignant hyperthermia, among others. Mortality rate from anesthesia is surmised to be about 1 to 2 per 10,000

patients. The American Society of Anesthesiologists Physical Classification System is outlined in Table 22-4. The higher your class, the higher your risk of perioperative mortality.

 QUICK QUIZ: THE RHYTHM IS GONNA GET YOU

A 60-year-old male patient of yours is planning to undergo coronary artery bypass grafting (CABG). After you perform a physical examination and laboratory tests, you discuss his case with the surgeon. He asks if you will help to manage him postoperatively, and you agree. He quizzes you on the risk of arrhythmia during the postoperative period.

You correctly reply:

A) "His risk for atrial fibrillation is less than it would be if he were undergoing valve replacement simultaneously with CABG"

B) "Of the potential arrhythmias, he is most likely to experience bradycardia"

C) "Nonsustained ventricular tachycardia is highly unlikely in this setting"

D) "Keep his potassium low, around 3 mEq/L, and he will be less likely to experience tachyarrhythmias"

The correct answer is "A." With CABG, the risk of postoperative atrial flutter or fibrillation is around 30%. That risk almost doubles when valve replacement is accomplished simultaneously with CABG. "B" is incorrect because brady-arrhythmias occur much less frequently than tachyarrhythmias. "C" is incorrect. Nonsustained ventricular tachycardia is extremely common in the immediate postoperative period. "D" is also incorrect. Plasma potassium levels <3.5 mEq/L are strongly associated with an increased risk of tachyarrhythmias.

TABLE 22-4 ASA PHYSICAL STATUS CLASSIFICATION

Class	Description
Class I	Healthy person
Class II	Patient with mild systemic disease
Class III	Patient with severe systemic disease that is controlled
Class IV	Patient with severe systemic disease that is uncontrolled and a threat to life
Class V	Patient who is unlikely to survive for 24 hours, with or without surgery

▶ **CASE 22.9**

A 15-year-old male presents to your office with a 3-day history of diarrhea and right lower quadrant abdominal pain. He has tenderness in the right lower quadrant with guarding

and rebound. He remains afebrile and has been hungry, scarfing down five bacon-wrapped waffles for breakfast (but less than his usual 6 …). The patient has no other significant history. You consider that this patient might have appendicitis, so you draw some labs. The white blood cell count is normal (7,500/mm³), as is the urinalysis.

Question 22.9.1 Which of the following is true about the diagnosis of appendicitis?
A) A normal white count effectively rules out the diagnosis of appendicitis
B) The majority of patients with appendicitis present with fever
C) The absence of anorexia effectively rules out appendicitis
D) A fecalith is found on radiograph in the majority of patients with appendicitis
E) None of the above

Answer 22.9.1 **The correct answer is "E."** None of the above is true. Taking these in order, 10% of patients with appendicitis have a normal white count, a minority of patients with appendicitis present with fever (15% in one study), only 75% of patients with appendicitis complain of anorexia, and a radiographic fecalith is found in only a minority of patients.

Question 22.9.2 Which of the following is *specific* for appendicitis?
A) Obturator sign
B) Psoas sign
C) Rovsing sign
D) Tenderness at McBurney's point
E) None of the above is specific for appendicitis

Answer 22.9.2 **The correct answer is "E."** None of the above is specific for appendicitis. An obturator sign ("A") is present if there is pain on internal and external rotation of the hip. The obturator sign can be seen with any pelvic abscess that is in contact with the hip area, but is more commonly seen with a retrocecal abscess. The psoas sign ("B") is pain on use of the psoas muscle (e.g., lifting the leg at the hip), and it can be seen with any inflammatory process that is in contact with the psoas muscle, including a psoas abscess. Rovsing sign ("C") is when pain increases in an area of peritonitis when the abdomen is palpated elsewhere. For example, in a patient with appendicitis, right lower quadrant pain will be increased with palpation of the *left* lower quadrant. This is indicative of peritonitis in the area that has increased pain, but it is not specific for appendicitis. Tenderness at McBurney's point ("D") can be seen in a number of processes including appendicitis, ileitis, any process in the cecum, and urinary tract infection.

Question 22.9.3 Which of the following is true about the treatment of pain in the acute abdomen?
A) Early treatment with morphine will obscure the proper diagnosis
B) Treatment with pain medication invalidates informed consent
C) Codeine can be used in the treatment of pediatric abdominal pain
D) Ketorolac is preferred for patients who may undergo a surgical procedure
E) None of the above is true

Answer 22.9.3 **The correct answer is "E."** None of the above is correct. Early treatment of pain in the acute abdomen does not affect diagnostic accuracy in children or adults ("A"). "C" is not true. Although codeine was used commonly in the treatment of pediatric pain, it is now contraindicated in children due to highly variable metabolism that can result in dangerous levels of opioids in the system. Ketorolac ("D") is not a good choice because of its antiplatelet effects, which increase the risk of bleeding intraoperatively, should your patient go to surgery. Pain medication does not necessarily invalidate informed consent ("B") if your patient remains oriented—but your patient is 15, so he can't consent for himself anyway.

....

Although you have thought a lot about the top item on your differential, you have not actually done anything more to evaluate this 15-year-old with abdominal pain.

Question 22.9.4 The test most likely to help you arrive at a diagnosis in this patient is:
A) Erythrocyte sedimentation rate (ESR)
B) C-reactive protein (CRP)
C) Abdominal ultrasound
D) Abdominal CT scan
E) Colonoscopy

Answer 22.9.4 **The correct answer is "D."** The test most likely to arrive at a diagnosis in this patient is a CT scan of the abdomen looking at the appendix. "A" and "B" are incorrect. Both the CRP and the ESR are nonspecific markers of inflammation and are not helpful in the diagnosis of appendicitis. "C," an ultrasound, can be used and is *often recommended as the first test in pediatric patients* to avoid the ionizing radiation associated with CT. The specificity for ultrasound is high (95–99%). However, it is not as sensitive as a CT scan (as varied as 60–85% depending on the study) and is very operator dependent. *If you can see the appendix*, sensitivity is 98% with a specificity of 92%. Although "D" is the textbook answer, it would be reasonable to start with an ultrasound, and if equivocal, one can then move on to CT or surgical consultation for serial abdominal examinations depending on institutional preference. Finally, ultrasound can also be useful in the female patient in whom other diagnoses need to be ruled out, such as ovarian pathology. "E," colonoscopy, is not particularly useful in the diagnosis of appendicitis, but could be used for other purposes such as looking for IBD once appendicitis is ruled out by CT.

HELPFUL TIP:
Not all patients with potential appendicitis need a CT scan. Those with obvious appendicitis may need to go

directly to the OR. CT is best used in patients in whom the clinical diagnosis is equivocal. There are long-term risks from radiation exposure, so CT should not be done without a good indication. Be aware of the standard practice in your location as many surgeons now insist upon a CT scan prior to going to the OR.

Question 22.9.5 If this patient's CT scan is positive for appendicitis, the likelihood that he will have a normal appendix removed at appendectomy is:
A) 0%
B) 10%
C) 20%
D) 30%
E) 50%

Answer 22.9.5 The correct answer is "B." With the advent of CT scanning, the false-positive rate (of taking normal patients to the OR) has improved, but perhaps not as much as you would think. The negative laparotomy rate is still about 10% in boys and men and up to 20% in women of reproductive age, where other pathology may mimic appendicitis. Overall, those who did not undergo CT were more than three times more likely to have a negative appendectomy. The negative laparotomy rate has gone down in men and the young but has increased in the elderly and in women. There is evidence that CT scanning changes the treatment plan in more than half cases of suspected appendicitis. The sensitivity of CT for appendicitis is 91% to 98%, but the specificity is as low as 75% depending on the radiologist and the population tested (range 75–93%).

HELPFUL TIP:
There is growing evidence that antibiotic therapy alone may adequately treat **uncomplicated** appendicitis. In a recent large trial, approximately 60% of patients who were randomized to the antibiotics-only arm for treating appendicitis did not have recurrent appendicitis, or require appendectomy, within 5 years of their initial event (which means that 40% still ended up with surgery, most within the first year) (*JAMA.* 2018;320(12):1259–1265 and *JAMA Surg.* 2019;154(2):149). The antibiotic regimen used was: IV ertapenem for 3 days followed by PO levofloxacin and metronidazole for an additional 7 days.

Question 22.9.6 In general, which of the following is TRUE about appendicitis?
A) Pain is in the right upper quadrant in the majority of pregnant women with appendicitis
B) Atypical presentations are more common in the elderly than in nonelderly adults
C) Patients with a retrocecal appendix generally present with well-localized tenderness and signs of peritoneal irritation
D) An appendicitis episode is great way to postpone your board examination—get one soon!

Answer 22.9.6 The correct answer is "B." Symptoms tend to be atypical in the elderly. In fact, elderly patients may have appendicitis with a normal white count, poorly localized pain, and absence of fever. So, maintain a high index of suspicion. The same is true of children, who may have abdominal pain and vomiting, accompanied by refusal to walk. Neonates also have a hard time describing their symptoms—they are the group most likely to present with perforation. "A" is incorrect. Despite classic teaching, patients who are pregnant tend to have "typical" symptoms with right lower quadrant pain. This is especially true in the first half of pregnancy. Certainly the appendix can be displaced cephalad, but the majority will still have right lower quadrant pain. "C" is incorrect. Patients with retrocecal appendicitis will commonly complain of a dull ache on the right side but peritoneal irritation may be minimal or absent.

HELPFUL TIP:
Some patients have recurrent appendicitis. These patients will present with multiple times with "typical" appendicitis that resolves during observation. When the appendix is finally removed, it is frequently scarred down.

HELPFUL HINT:
Appendicitis can occur at *any* age. Individual lifetime risk is 7% to 14% and it is more common in males than females until the age of 30, when the rates equalize. The younger the patient (especially <5 years), the more likely they are to present with a perforated appendix.

▶ **Objectives: Did you learn to …**
- Describe the findings in acute appendicitis?
- Diagnose appendicitis and determine how diagnostic tests are best used in the patient presenting with signs and symptoms of appendicitis?
- Manage a patient with appendicitis?

▶ **CASE 22.10**

A 72-year-old male presents to your office for a 3-month history of episodic abdominal pain. It is primarily located in the epigastric region and radiates to the back. It occurs both during the night and day and lasts about 1 hour. His past medical history is significant for a 5-year history of diabetes. He takes glyburide, atorvastatin, and aspirin (he clearly isn't your patient … he is not on metformin, the drug of choice in type 2 diabetes). He has no previous surgical history. You order an ultrasound. The ultrasound reveals a normal aorta, but the technician notes several stones in the gallbladder.

You are concerned that this patient may have symptomatic cholelithiasis.

Question 22.10.1 Which of the following is true of his risk for gallstones?
A) This patient has an increased risk of cholesterol stones because he is diabetic
B) This patient's risk of gallstones would have peaked in his fourth decade of life
C) This patient's risk of gallstones is increased because of his atorvastatin use
D) This patient's risk of gallstones is increased because he is male

Answer 22.10.1 **The correct answer is "A."** Patients with diabetes have an increased risk of gallstones when compared with the general population. Other associations include female gender (not male, so "D" is wrong), family history, obesity, and certain medical illnesses including hyperlipidemia, cystic fibrosis, short bowel syndrome, parenteral nutrition, hemolytic anemia (e.g., sickle cell), and history of terminal ileum resection. "B" is incorrect because the risk of gallstones increases linearly with age. "C" is incorrect. Atorvastatin and other statins are not associated with an increased risk of gallstone formation, but clofibrate and other fibrates are. It is good to remember that estrogen therapy also has an association with gallstones and that ceftriaxone can cause biliary sludge as well as cholestasis.

Question 22.10.2 Which of the following statements is FALSE regarding the evaluation of the gallbladder?
A) Ultrasound will find pericolic fluid in only 50% of patients with cholecystitis
B) An HIDA scan can be abnormal/positive (e.g., no tracer in the duodenum) in patients with common bile duct obstruction and/or cholecystitis
C) Endoscopic retrograde cholangiopancreatography (ERCP) has an attendant risk of pancreatitis
D) The absence of disease on ultrasound effectively rules out gallbladder disease

Answer 22.10.2 **The correct answer is "D."** While ultrasound is highly sensitive for stones (95% or greater), it might miss some. "A" is a correct statement as are "B" and "C." A HIDA (hepatic iminodiacetic acid) scan can be abnormal (e.g., no tracer in the duodenum) not only in cholecystitis but also in other conditions in which the common bile duct (CBD) is blocked including a CBD stone or tumor. Additionally, false positives may occur if there is liver disease (which may prevent the uptake of HIDA into the liver and subsequent secretion into the CBD), patients on total parenteral nutrition (where the gall bladder has no stimulus to contract and thus gets distended with mucus, preventing tracer entry), spasm of the sphincter of Oddi or biliary sphincterotomy. MRCP (magnetic resonance cholangiopancreatography) can be used to identify stones in the common duct prior to surgery.

HELPFUL TIP:
CT is not a very sensitive study for gallstones. Ultrasound is the study of choice (sensitivity is 25% for CT vs. 96% for ultrasound). However, a CT is useful in detecting complications that arise secondary to acute cholecystitis (e.g., pericholic abscess, perforation, emphysematous gallbladder, gangrene and gallstone ileus).

Question 22.10.3 Regarding different types of gallstones, all of the following are true EXCEPT:
A) Cholesterol stones are associated with obesity and hyperlipidemia
B) Black pigment stones are associated with cirrhosis
C) Brown pigment stones are associated with liver fluke infection
D) Blue pigment stones are associated with being an avid fan of the St. Louis Blues hockey team and/or the Blue Man Group

Answer 22.10.3 **The correct answer is "D."** While it may seem like beer-swilling hockey fans might be more prone to developing gallstones, there are no studies to support this. Besides, blue pigment stones do not exist. All the other options are true. Stone types include cholesterol, black pigment, and brown pigment stones. Cholesterol stones ("A") are associated with advancing age (due to decreased synthesis of bile salts from cholesterol), hyperlipidemia, diabetes, obesity, and living in the Western Hemisphere (thank you, fast food industry and corn subsidies!). Black pigment stones ("B") contain calcium bilirubinate, calcium carbonate, and calcium phosphonate. They are associated with hemolytic diseases, Crohn disease, ileal resection, cirrhosis, and total parental nutrition (TPN). Brown stones ("C") are observed more often in East Asia and are associated with liver fluke infection.

. . . .

You refer the patient to your favorite surgical consultant, Dr. Hugh Jeego (or his partner, I. M. Agodd), for evaluation of cholecystectomy. However, before his surgery appointment, you see him again in the ED. He presents with fever, nausea, vomiting, and anorexia for the last 48 hours. His examination is significant for temperature 38.9°C, mild tachycardia and tachypnea, and a normal blood pressure. He is tender in the right upper quadrant and has a positive Murphy sign. He has no jaundice or palpable right upper quadrant mass. Laboratory values include WBC 14,800/mm³, ALT 58 IU/L, AST 64 IU/L, alkaline phosphatase 45 IU/L, total bilirubin 1.5 mg/dL (mildly elevated liver enzymes and bilirubin), amylase 95 IU/L, and lipase 52 IU/L (normal amylase and lipase).

Question 22.10.4 At this point in time, your working diagnosis is:
A) Acalculous cholecystitis
B) Acute calculous cholecystitis
C) Pancreatitis
D) Ascending cholangitis
E) Myocardial infarction

Answer 22.10.4 The correct answer is "B." The clinical presentation, examination, and laboratory data point toward acute cholecystitis. "A" is incorrect because acalculous cholecystitis occurs more often in critically ill hospitalized patients, and you already know that this patient has stones, so his cholecystitis is by definition *calculous* in nature. There must be no gallstones detected on ultrasound to diagnose acalculous cholecystitis (hence the name). "C" is incorrect. His pancreatic enzymes are normal; and although one can certainly have pancreatitis with a normal amylase and lipase, you have a better explanation with cholecystitis. "D" is incorrect. Patients with ascending cholangitis usually have markedly elevated transaminases and an obstructive laboratory pattern (e.g., elevated bilirubin, alkaline phosphatase, and pancreatic enzymes). "E" is very unlikely in this patient who has findings more consistent with intra-abdominal pathology, but you should always consider cardiac (and other thoracic organ) etiologies in older patients presenting with abdominal complaints.

Question 22.10.5 Regarding the differential diagnosis of complicated cholelithiasis, which of the following is true?
A) Empyema of the gallbladder is primarily a disease of the elderly and carries a high mortality rate due to associated Gram-positive sepsis
B) Emphysematous cholecystitis occurs primarily in elderly diabetics as a late complication of miliary tuberculosis (TB)
C) The most common consequence of gallbladder perforation is generalized peritonitis
D) Charcot's triad (jaundice, fever, and right upper quadrant pain) is associated with cholangitis

Answer 22.10.5 The correct answer is "D." The classic Charcot's triad (jaundice, fever, and right upper quadrant pain) is associated with cholangitis, but it is **not** seen in the majority of cases, probably due to early detection of cholangitis. Nonetheless, it can be helpful if present. "A" is incorrect because patients generally develop a Gram-*negative* sepsis. "B" is incorrect because emphysematous cholecystitis is not a complication of miliary TB. Emphysematous cholecystitis occurs primarily in elderly male diabetics: gas-producing bacteria, most commonly *C. perfringens*, result in gas in the gallbladder and can cause a severe sepsis. Miliary TB rarely affects the gallbladder. "C" is incorrect. The most common consequence of gallbladder perforation is a localized, walled-off abscess. Additionally, a cholecystoenteric fistula may form between the gallbladder and the duodenum or jejunum. Stones can then pass into the bowel. Stones larger than 2 cm in diameter are likely to lodge in the terminal ileum giving rise to symptoms of small bowel obstruction—a condition termed "gallstone ileus."

Generally, patients with symptomatic cholecystitis have a prior history of biliary colic. Pain with acute cholecystitis is similar to that of biliary colic except that it is more often severe, longer lasting (>24 hours), and associated with anorexia, nausea, vomiting, fever, elevated white count (12,000–15,000/mm³), right upper quadrant guarding, and a positive Murphy sign (arresting inspiration when palpating the gallbladder). **However, Murphy sign is only about 65% sensitive (even less in the elderly).** An ultrasonographic Murphy's sign has an improved sensitivity and specificity of about 90%. Of note, about 30% of patients will have neither a fever nor an elevated white cell count. An elevated bilirubin or alkaline phosphatase level is not typically seen in acute cholecystitis and, if present, should prompt an evaluation for biliary obstruction. However, mild increases in aminotransferases, amylase, and hyperbilirubinemia may occasionally be found in acute cholecystitis due to the passage of sludge or a stone through the CBD without causing an actual obstruction.

Biliary pancreatitis can occur when there is blockage of the ampulla of Vater, and cholangitis occurs when there is ductal stone obstruction and biliary infection. If you think there is obstruction, the patient may need an ERCP to remove the obstruction. Consider an MRCP to document obstruction before referral for ERCP.

Given our patient's physical findings, leukocytosis, and mild elevation of transaminases, you conclude that this patient has acute calculous cholecystitis.

Question 22.10.6 Which of the following should NOT be considered in the management of this disease?
A) Initial treatment includes hospitalization with IV fluid resuscitation
B) Consider an antibiotic regimen to include a third- or fourth-generation cephalosporin plus metronidazole or ertapenem or ticarcillin/clavulanate
C) Choose a narrow-spectrum antibiotic to treat *Enterococcus* (e.g., vancomycin)
D) If early cholecystectomy is not chosen as treatment, it should be performed late (at least 6 weeks after diagnosis)

Answer 22.10.6 The correct answer (and what you don't want to do) is "C." This answer is incorrect for two reasons. First, just over 50% of episodes of cholecystitis are sterile; as a matter of course, they are treated with antibiotics because of our inability to initially determine which are infected. Second, while you may encounter *Enterococcus*, it is rarely found in isolation, making "C" incorrect. The initial treatment of cholecystitis includes hospitalization, broad-spectrum IV antibiotics, and IV fluid resuscitation ("A"). In addition to the antibiotics mentioned in "B," other agents like imipenem, meropenem, or piperacillin/tazobactam may also be used with metronidazole. Definitive therapy for cholecystitis is cholecystectomy. Option "D" is correct. It is generally accepted that early cholecystectomy is associated with better outcomes and lower costs and should be completed during the same hospitalization for acute cholecystitis. If this is not possible, cholecystectomy should be delayed for 6 weeks to allow inflammation to subside.

▶ **Objectives: Did you learn to …**
- Identify risk factors for gallstones?
- Recognize complications of gallbladder disease?
- Manage a patient with symptomatic gallstones and cholecystitis?

▶ CASE 22.11

A 68-year-old male who was the restrained front passenger of a vehicle traveling in excess of 60 mph is brought to the ED via ambulance. The driver of the vehicle was found dead at the scene. Ambulance personnel report it took 5 to 10 minutes to extricate the patient. On arrival, he is mumbling incoherently. He is initially able to give his name, but he is slurring his words. He denies any medical problems, medications, or allergies. Vitals signs include temperature 35.5°C, pulse 148 bpm, respirations 35 bpm, blood pressure 65/30 mm Hg, and oxygen saturation 81% on 100% FiO2 by facemask. On examination, he is in severe respiratory distress. Lung sounds are absent on the right and diminished on the left. Heart sounds are muffled. You determine that this patient needs immediate treatment of a tension pneumothorax.

Question 22.11.1 Which of the following is most appropriate at this time?
A) Perform needle decompression on the left
B) Perform needle decompression on the right
C) Place a chest tube on the left
D) Place a chest tube on the right
E) Perform a chest radiograph and act on the basis of the results

Answer 22.11.1 The correct answer is "B." The combination of hypotension, hypoxia, and absent breath sounds suggests a tension pneumothorax. **Immediate decompression of the affected hemithorax should be performed by placing a large-bore (14- or 16-gauge) needle through the chest wall to relieve intrathoracic pressure.** Most of us were taught to aim our needles at the second intercostal space at the mid-clavicular line. The 2018 Advanced Trauma Life Support (ATLS) recommendations have changed and the preferred placement of the thoracostomy needle is now in the fourth or fifth intercostal space at the mid-axillary line. Either site is acceptable if the pleural space can be reached (it may be more difficult in the mid-axillary line, given increased subcutaneous tissue). Of particular note is "E." If tension pneumothorax is suspected, you **should never** wait for confirmation of the diagnosis by a chest radiograph. It is a true emergency that requires treatment on the basis of clinical examination.

HELPFUL (AND UNFORTUNATE) TIP:
Given the epidemic of obesity in the United States, a simple needle may not be long enough to reach the pleura (yes, really, it has been studied). Have a backup option, such as a longer, pigtail catheter.

His vital signs and oxygen saturation improve with needle decompression. You place a chest tube and give boluses of normal saline through two peripheral IVs. Then the patient is placed in an external fixation device for his femur fracture. Operating room fixation is deferred secondary to unstable medical status. He is ultimately intubated for increased work of breathing. He is admitted to the intensive care unit

(ICU) on a ventilator with a cervical collar following negative FAST examination (focused assessment with sonography for trauma—a sonographic evaluation to rule out fluid in perihepatic, perisplenic, pelvic, and pericardial spaces).

Repeat chest x-ray in the ICU shows the endotracheal (ET) tube and chest tube in appropriate positions. Several rib fractures are noted. There are "fluffy infiltrates" in the left chest that were not present on initial trauma chest series.

Question 22.11.2 Which of the following is true of pulmonary contusions?
A) They most commonly occur with penetrating rather than blunt trauma
B) Treatment includes aggressive IV steroid and fluid administration
C) The condition can resolve over the course of 1 to 2 weeks
D) Treatment includes appropriate antibiotics

Answer 22.11.2 The correct answer is "C." Pulmonary contusions develop over the first 24 to 48 hours following a blunt chest trauma and resolve over the course of weeks if not complicated by pneumonia or ARDS. "A" is incorrect. Pulmonary contusion is the most common injury associated with blunt chest trauma. Seventy percent of these injuries result from motor vehicle collisions. Pulmonary contusions are usually, but not always, associated with fractured ribs or flail chest. Chest x-ray changes are usually evident within 1 hour post-trauma but may not appear for up to 24 hours as hemorrhage and edema develop. Pulmonary contusions result in a ventilation–perfusion mismatch, hypoxia, and an increased A-a gradient. If a patient is able to maintain oxygenation and ventilation, intubation is not always required. "B" and "D" are incorrect. Treatment consists of respiratory support as needed, pain control, and pulmonary hygiene (suction and incentive spirometry).

You elect to proceed with pulmonary artery catheter (Swan–Ganz catheter) placement due to the severity of this patient's condition. Overnight, he begins to decompensate. The nurse pages you with his vital signs and Swan–Ganz readings: temperature 37°C, pulse 100 bpm, respirations 20 bpm (ventilator set at 14 bpm), blood pressure 82/30 mm Hg, PCWP 24 mm Hg (normal 5–15), cardiac index 2 L/min/m² (normal 2.5–3.5), systemic vascular resistance 2,000 dyne-sec/cm² (normal 1,000–1,500), and decreased mixed venous oxygen saturation (about 60%).

Question 22.11.3 What is the cause of shock at this time?
A) Hypovolemic shock
B) Neurogenic shock
C) Cardiogenic shock
D) Septic shock

Answer 22.11.3 The correct answer is "C." Based on these numbers and the choices above, this patient appears to be in cardiogenic shock (elevated pulmonary capillary wedge pressure, decreased cardiac output). **Cardiogenic shock** may be caused by myocardial infarction, valve failure, or malignant dysrhythmias. Similar physiology may occur with another class of shock, **obstructive shock**, which affects the heart function but etiology is extracardiac (pulmonary embolism, tamponade, or tension pneumothorax). Hypovolemic shock, answer "A," is caused by hemorrhage or other fluid losses. Answer "B," neurogenic shock, is a type of distributive shock, where classic features are hypotension and relative bradycardia. Answer "D," septic shock, is also a type of distributive shock. Treatment is directed at the underlying disorder. See Table 22-5 for more on the categories of shock.

HELPFUL TIP … OR NOTE OF CAUTION:
The routine use of Swan–Ganz catheters in seriously ill patients is no longer recommended and may worsen outcomes. Resist your reflexive urge to "float a Swan." Bedside echocardiography is a noninvasive way to assess cardiac function and volume status.

A passenger from a second car involved in this accident is brought to the ED with burns to the abdomen and back.

Question 22.11.4 Which of the following is FALSE regarding burn wound management in general?

A) The Modified Brooke formula for fluid resuscitation in burns calls for 2 mL/kg to be given for each percent of total body surface area (TBSA) burned (2 mL/kg × weight (kg) × TBSA burned)

B) Escharotomy should be performed on all partial-thickness burns

C) Patients with chemical burns should be treated first with tap water irrigation

D) A nonadherent gauze should be applied to most burns following gentle cleansing and application of a topical antimicrobial agent

Answer 22.11.4 The correct answer is "B." Remember that any time you see "all," it is probably the wrong answer because medicine is never that easy. Escharotomy is usually not necessary unless there is a *full-thickness* wound. However, escharotomy is often done early in chest and abdomen burns even if noncircumferential; these burns often compromise respiration. It *should be done* if it is circumferential and compromising vascular supply to a limb or the trunk (e.g., abdominal compartment syndrome). Regarding answer "A," some clinicians prefer the modified Brooke formula to the more familiar Parkland formula (4 mL/kg × weight (kg) × % TBSA burned, with the first half of the volume given in the first 8 hours, second half over the next 16 hours) because Parkland has frequently resulted in overresuscitation. **Any resuscitation strategy should rely heavily on hourly reassessment of fluid status including urine output (0.5 mL/kg/hr for adults).** "C" is also correct with the addendum that any particulate matter should be brushed off prior to irrigation. Water may activate some substances such as sodium hydroxide. "D" is also a correct statement. **There is broad consensus that patients with extensive burns should be transferred to a specialty burn center.**

HELPFUL TIP:
Fluids are required for adults with >15% TBSA burns (second degree or higher) and >10% for children aged 10 years and younger. For **adults** the "Rule of 9's" is used to determine TBSA affected. Body surface area is estimated as follows: 9% TBSA to each of the following body parts: the head, each arm, front of each leg, and back of each leg; 18% TBSA for the anterior trunk, 18% TBSA for the posterior trunk; the remaining 1% TBSA is accounted for by the genitalia. TBSA affected in children and adolescents should be based on age-specific charts. Both affected and unaffected BSA should be calculated to assure accurate estimation.

TABLE 22-5 SHOCK CATEGORIZED BY HEMODYNAMIC PARAMETERS

Type of Shock	Pulmonary Capillary Wedge Pressure (Preload)	Cardiac Output	Systemic Vascular Resistance (Afterload)	Central Venous Oxygen Saturation
Hypovolemic (Late)	Decreased	Normal, then Decreased	Increased	Normal, then Decreased
Cardiogenic	Increased	Decreased	Increased	Decreased
Distributive (sepsis, neurogenic)	Normal, then Decreased	Increased	Decreased	Normal
Obstructive (PE, tension pneumothorax)	Normal, then Decreased	Normal, then Decreased	Increased	Normal or Decreased

The cutoff for mixed venous oxygen saturation on PAC is 65%.
Adapted from "Hemodynamics in shock." In: Gaieski DF and Mikkelsen ME. Definition, Classification, Etiology, and Pathophysiology of Shock in Adults. Uptodate.com. Accessed 2 May 2019.

Question 22.11.5 Which of the following is TRUE regarding fluid resuscitation?

A) A peripheral line will deliver fluid more rapidly than a central line of an equivalent gauge
B) Albumin is the fluid of choice in the treatment of burns and should be considered for all patients with significant fluid deficits
C) D5W-½ NS (D5W-0.45%NS) is the preferred fluid for resuscitation in all nonburn patients
D) All of the above are true

Answer 22.11.5 **The correct answer is "A."** A peripheral line will deliver fluid more rapidly than a central line of an equivalent gauge, according to Poiseuille's law (flow is directly proportional to tube radius and inversely proportional to tube length). The **shorter** the catheter, the more quickly fluid is delivered. The largest port on a traditional triple lumen catheter will give the same flow rates as a 20 gauge peripheral IV. Consider a larger diameter, shorter central line if placing a central line in a patient who may require rapid fluid resuscitation. **You can also consider an intraosseus line for rapid volume resuscitation, especially in children.** "B" is incorrect. Albumin is not helpful and may be harmful in the initial management of burns and trauma. "C" is also incorrect. Normal saline (0.9% NS), or Lactated Ringer's are the fluids of choice for resuscitation. In the age-old battle of NS versus LR, the jury is still out. Remember, though, that LR cannot be given in the same IV as blood.

▶ **Objectives: Did you learn to …**
- Identify and manage a patient with a tension pneumothorax?
- Describe various types of shock and how they are differentiated?
- Treat a patient in shock?
- Manage a patient with significant burns?

 QUICK QUIZ: INHALATION INJURY

Carbonized particles in the nasal cavity and/or posterior pharynx in a burn patient should suggest:

A) The need for excision of the perichondrium in the nose to prevent underlying cartilage injury from avascular necrosis
B) Inhalational injury to the lungs
C) Ingestion of a large amount of particulate matter
D) The need to check carboxyhemoglobin levels
E) B and D

The correct answer is "E." Carbonaceous material or blistering in the nares or oropharynx should suggest the possibility of an inhalation injury. Consider intubating these patients early, especially if there will be prolonged transfer time to a burn center. A carboxyhemoglobin level and CXR should be obtained in all patients with moderate-to-severe burns from an appropriate source (not so much with scald burns). Monitor frequently and have a low threshold for intubation.

▶ **CASE 22.12**

A 48-year-old female arrives at the ED via ambulance after witnesses saw her vomiting large volumes of blood in a local convenience store before collapsing to the floor—obviously, not her best day. She is barely communicating and cannot provide any history. Ambulance personnel placed two large-bore IVs and started fluid boluses. Just as you start your initial evaluation, she has another episode of large volume hematemesis. You are concerned about her depressed mental status and the severity of her illness and decide to intubate her. After intubation, the chest wall rises symmetrically and the lungs sound clear. Her heart sounds are distant, and she is tachycardic (pulse 120 bpm). Her blood pressure is 80/40 mm Hg. Her oxygen saturation is 78%.

Question 22.12.1 The standard of care in detecting esophageal intubation is:

A) Auscultation
B) Radiograph
C) End-tidal CO_2
D) Oxygen saturation
E) Direct laryngoscopy

Answer 22.12.1 **The correct answer is "C."** The standard of care is the end-tidal CO_2. All of the others are notoriously unreliable. However, they all should be done. If you think you hear breath sounds but the oxygen saturation is not rising and end-tidal CO_2 is low, the ET tube is probably in the esophagus.

Question 22.12.2 The end-tidal CO2 can be falsely negative (detecting no CO2) in which of the following situations?

A) Ingestion of carbonated soft drinks ("pop" as we call it in the Midwest)
B) Intubation in the posterior pharynx above the cords
C) Nasotracheal intubation
D) During cardiac arrest

Answer 22.12.2 **The correct answer is "D."** The end-tidal CO_2 requires that there is gas exchange in the lungs. If there is no gas exchange, the CO_2 will be low. This may be the case during cardiac arrest. "A" can actually cause a **false positive**. Carbon dioxide in the stomach will give a positive end-tidal CO_2 with an esophageal intubation. The same is true of "B." If the patient is breathing spontaneously, the CO_2 will be elevated even when the ET tube is above the cords. "C," nasotracheal intubation, should have no effect on end-tidal CO_2.

You order laboratory studies that include a CBC, basic metabolic profile, liver chemistries, amylase, lipase, and coagulation studies. In addition, you type and cross for six units of packed red blood cells. The nurses have already contacted the gastroenterologist on call, and she is on her way. You consider whether or not to perform nasogastric (NG) lavage.

Question 22.12.3 Which of the following is FALSE regarding NG lavage?

A) NG lavage may be negative even in the presence of an upper GI bleed
B) NG lavage should not be attempted in obtunded patients until they are intubated
C) Iced fluid is best for lavage in patients with an upper GI bleed
D) The placement of an NG tube is contraindicated in patients who may have variceal bleeding

Answer 22.12.3 The correct answer is "C." Iced lavage fluid should NOT be used in patients with a GI bleed. The cooler temperature inhibits hemostasis and can increase bleeding. Both "A" and "B" are true statements, and "D" is controversial. False-negative NG aspirates occur with intermittent bleeding and bleeding beyond the ligament of Treitz. Lavage **should not** be done in patients who are obtunded or otherwise unable to protect their own airway unless they are intubated. It isn't helpful in treatment/stopping bleeding anyway. Regarding answer "D," varices are typically considered a contraindication to the use of an NG tube due to theoretical increased risk of bleeding. If the patient has obvious blood in the vomitus, **NG lavage does not contribute to the diagnosis or management except to maybe clear the stomach before endoscopy.**

HELPFUL TIP:
Other contraindications to gastric lavage include known ingestion of hydrocarbons and caustic agents, such as alkalis and acids.

One of the other ED workers recognizes her as a chronic alcoholic who has a history of liver disease. You now notice her marked jaundice, previously missed as you were so focused on your "ABCs." Other pertinent findings include a 6-cm scalp laceration, which continues to actively bleed, moderate ascites, and lower extremity edema. After lavage with nearly 5 L of isotonic fluid, the patient's aspirate continues to be bloody. At this point, her vitals are somewhat stable but have shown no sign of improvement. Initial emergent labs have returned: Na 142 mEq/L, K 3.2 mEq/L, Cl 106 mEq/L, CO_2 18 mEq/L, BUN 40 mg/dL, Cr 0.8 mg/dL, glucose 110 mg/dL, WBC 7,000/mm³, Hgb 9.8 g/dL, Hct 29%, Plt 62,000/mm³, INR 3, PTT 48, albumin 2.4 g/dL, AST 76 IU/L, ALT 39 IU/L, Bili 6.2 mg/dL, amylase 210 IU/L, and lipase 24 IU/dL. The gastroenterologist is still 5 to 10 minutes away.

Question 22.12.4 Which of the following would be the most appropriate next step?

A) Address the presence of platelet dysfunction by transfusing with a 6-pack of platelets
B) Central line placement should be priority at this time because fluid resuscitation is the primary concern
C) Emergent gastric tamponade should be attempted with a Foley catheter
D) None of the above

Answer 22.12.4 The correct answer is "D." None of the above is a particularly good idea at this juncture. "A" is not necessary since a platelet count of 62,000 is adequate for hemostasis. A platelet count of <50,000 is considered an indication for platelet transfusion in an actively bleeding patient. Hold off on "B"—coagulopathy (INR 3) is a **relative** contraindication to central line placement but if you have to use a central line, remember that the femoral vein can be compressed in the event of bleeding and infection rates are comparable to other central line sites (*Crit Care Med.* 2012 Aug; 40(8):2479–2485). Recall too that peripheral catheters will deliver more fluid more rapidly when compared with central catheters. "C" is incorrect because gastric tamponade with a Foley is just silly. A Blakemore tube (or its variants) require that the patient is intubated and are temporizing measures *only* until you can get endoscopy. What you could do while you're waiting for your GI colleague to park her Jaguar is start the patient on octreotide (50 mcg IV bolus followed by an infusion) to decrease the portal blood flow. *Note that octreotide does not change outcomes in and of itself (see below) and is very short-acting.* Vitamin K should also be given, as well as fresh frozen plasma or cryoprecipitate if she continues to bleed. See chapter 7 for more on treating an elevated INR in the face of cirrhosis.

Question 22.12.5 Effective methods for controlling upper GI variceal bleeding that improve outcomes include all of the following EXCEPT:

A) Variceal ligation
B) Sclerotherapy
C) Transjugular intrahepatic portosystemic shunt (TIPS) procedure
D) Vasopressin

Answer 22.12.5 The correct answer is "D." Vasopressin, while achieving initial control of bleeding in up to 60% of patients, has essentially **no effect on rebleeding and may cause ischemia elsewhere due to vasoconstriction**. Octreotide has fewer adverse effects and has utility *when combined with variceal ligation*. Octreotide *does not* by itself reduce rebleeding or mortality. Variceal ligation and sclerotherapy both reduce mortality. The TIPS procedure has been shown to effectively stop bleeding by reducing portal pressures. It also reduces **acute** mortality. New data makes a strong case for placing a TIPS to improve mortality *even before a first* variceal bleed (*Hepatology.* 2019 Jan;69(1):282–293) though it is not yet standard of care. *Antibiotics (ceftriaxone or a fluoroquinolone) should be given and reduce rebleeding (Hepatology. 2004 Mar; 39(3):746–753).* See Chapter 7 for more on variceal bleeding.

HELPFUL TIP:
Indirect evidence of a GI bleed in patients with liver disease includes an elevated BUN, which results from the digestion of blood.

Despite Dr. Graber's warning to the contrary, you consider placing a central line.

Question 22.12.6 Which of the following locations of central line placement is associated with the lowest rate of infection?
A) Internal jugular
B) Femoral vein
C) Subclavian vein
D) They all have similar infection rates

Answer 22.12.6 The correct answer is "D." With new infection control techniques, infection rates are pretty much the same for all central line locations (*Crit Care Med.* 2012 Aug; 40(8):2479–2485). Subclavian lines have higher risks of complications such as arterial injury, hemothorax, pneumothorax, and lung injury. **Note that ultrasound-guided central line insertion is the standard of care.**

The gastroenterologist arrives and you explain the situation. Vitals at this time include a temperature of 36.8°C, pulse 105 bpm, respirations 14 (ventilator dependent), blood pressure 85/40 mm Hg, and oxygen saturation of 92%. The gastroenterologist plans to attempt endoscopy with sclerotherapy, but would like to have the general surgeons available for backup in case emergent operative intervention becomes necessary.

As you prepare to contact the surgeon, you consider the patient's surgical risk. You quickly recall that there are several prognostic scoring systems including, among others, the Model for End-stage Liver Disease (MELD) scoring system and the Child–Pugh score.

Question 22.12.7 Which of the following is TRUE regarding the MELD scoring system?
A) The MELD score can be used to predict 3-month survival following TIPS
B) The three components of the MELD score are bilirubin, INR, and creatinine
C) The MELD score assesses mortality risk for prioritizing patients on the waitlist for liver transplant
D) All of the above

Answer 22.12.7 The correct answer is "D." The MELD score was originally used to predict the 3-month mortality after TIPS ("A"). However, the MELD score has also been validated as a tool to estimate overall mortality related to liver disease and to prioritize patients on the transplant wait list ("C"). The MELD score is computed using creatinine, INR, and bilirubin levels. There are handy online calculators readily available (MDCalc… no we don't have any commercial interest).

The MELD score is interpreted as follows: **score ≥40,** 71.3% mortality in 3 months; **30–39,** 52.6% mortality in 3 months; **20–29,** 19.6% mortality in 3 months; **10–19,** 6% mortality in 3 months; **<9,** 1.9% mortality in 3 months.

The Child–Pugh classification also assesses prognosis in liver disease, need for transplant (minimum score of 7), predicted

TABLE 22-6 CHILD–PUGH CLASSIFICATION

Points assigned	1	2	3
Encephalopathy	None	Low grade	High grade
Ascites	None	Slight	Moderate-large
Bilirubin	1–2 mg/dL	2–3 mg/dL	>3 mg/dL
Albumin	>3.5 g/dL	2.8–3.5 g/dL	<2.8 g/dL
INR	<1.7	1.8–2.3	>2.3

mortality rate from variceal bleed, and outcomes after surgery or TIPS (Table 22-6).

Child–Pugh Class A is defined as having **5 to 6 points** (well-compensated cirrhosis, operative mortality for abdominal surgery 10%), Class B is **7 to 9 points** (significant functional compromise, operative mortality 30%), and Class C is **10 to 15** points (decompensated cirrhosis, operative mortality 82%).

▶ **Objectives: Did you learn to …**
- Manage a patient with a massive upper GI bleed?
- Determine if an ET tube has been placed correctly?
- Recognize the uses and limitations of gastric lavage?
- Recognize the uses and limitations of central line placement and Swan–Ganz catheter placement?
- Evaluate a patient with liver disease, using the Child–Pugh and MELD classification systems?

 QUICK QUIZ: INTUBATION

Which of the following IS NOT a contraindication to a blind nasotracheal intubation?
A) Patient is not breathing
B) Patient is anticoagulated or has had TPA
C) Midface trauma
D) History of a septoplasty

The correct answer is "D." All of the rest are contraindications to a blind nasotracheal intubation. Specifically, it is not possible to do a blind nasotracheal intubation in a nonbreathing patient. Patients who are anticoagulated may bleed profusely after a nasotracheal intubation, and midface trauma suggests the possibility that the tube could end up in the brain, never a good idea. Avoid nasotracheal intubation in midface trauma, except as a last resort.

▶ **CASE 22.13**

You are seeing a 33-year-old resident at a large university hospital setting where medical care is provided freely to him. He is about to complete his Internal Medicine residency and wants to "get his money's worth" of free procedures before he leaves. He has scheduled a full afternoon of procedures with you, including toenail removal, excision of a mole on his neck, and a stylish new cartilage ear piercing for his new job as a cruise ship doctor.

He has had trouble with recurrent pain and inflammation on the lateral side of his left great toe. On examination you identify onychocryptosis (ingrown nail). He has tried soaks, growing the nail plate past the skin, and regular paring—all without success.

Question 22.13.1 Regarding nail removal in this patient, which one of the following is FALSE?
A) The great toe is the most commonly affected toe for onychocryptosis
B) If the patient chooses partial nail removal, about 25% of the nail should be removed on the affected side
C) Phenol should be placed for no longer than 10 seconds to the germinal tissue to prevent necrosis
D) When removing the nail, an upward twist of the hand to the medial side should be performed

Answer 22.13.1 **The correct answer is "C."** Phenol can be left in place for 3 minutes. Options "A," "B," and "D" are all true. Ingrown toenails almost exclusively affect the great toe on the lateral side, occasionally on the medial side. Partial or full nail removal should be implemented when conservative measures have failed. Besides ingrown nails (onychocryptosis), onychomycosis (fungal infection of the nail), recurrent paronychia (nail fold inflammation), and onychogryphosis (deformed, curved nail) are all indications for partial or full nail removal. If recurrent ingrown nails have occurred, germinal tissue can be ablated with phenol on a cotton swab held in place for 3 minutes, and afterward the phenol should be neutralized with alcohol. Other approaches to matrixectomy include electrosurgical and laser techniques and application of sodium hydroxide.

Next, he complains about a small regular mole on his neck that he repeatedly cuts while shaving. He would like to have it removed in whatever way you deem best. The lesion is raised above the skin. Although it is mildly irregular in appearance from the repeated trauma of shaving, there is no other worrying feature of malignancy.

Question 22.13.2 Which of the following is NOT a correct statement regarding removal of this lesion?
A) Curettage with cautery or shave biopsy would be ideal for this sort of lesion
B) If sutures are required, 6-0 nylon would be ideal in this location
C) If a punch biopsy is performed, skin should be held taut perpendicular to the angle of the mandible (the natural skin lines of the neck)

D) In this location, both shave and punch techniques require closure by suture approximation

Answer 22.13.2 **The correct answer is "D."** Various types of skin lesion removal exist: punch biopsy, shave biopsy, curettage, and elliptical excisional biopsy. Punch biopsy involves taking a full-thickness sample in skin areas (except for the eyelids, lips, or penis). Skin should be held taught perpendicular to the natural skin tension lines, and punch instrument is rotated through the skin. The site is closed with either a single interrupted or vertical mattress suture. Shave biopsy is indicated for removal of elevated skin lesions where complete thickness removal is unnecessary. Shave should be made from both lateral edges into center to avoid cutting too deep. No suturing is necessary. Curettage entails a method of removing lesions that also does not require full-thickness sampling. A Fox dermal curettage is used to scrape away unwanted tissue followed by electrical or chemical cautery for hemostasis. Finally, elliptical excision is used when full dermal thickness excision is necessary. Contraindications to skin biopsy include infection at the site and coagulopathy.

Finally, your patient is a little embarrassed to be seen at the mall getting his ear pierced, and asks if you could pierce it for him. He is considering a standard lobe pierce versus an auricular cartilage piercing.

Question 22.13.3 Which of the following is true in regard to counseling and technique?
A) Eczema at the site is a contraindication to piercing
B) Auricular cartilage piercing should only be performed by a trained physician
C) Ears should be pierced from the posterior to anterior site
D) Ear piercing involves boring a 20-gauge needle into the marked site
E) Ear piercing is contraindicated in nerds

Answer 22.13.3 **The correct answer is "A."** Eczema in the area is a contraindication to piercing. Other contraindications include: infection, previous keloid formation, immunodeficiency, and coagulopathy. All of the other options are incorrect. Auricular cartilage piercing is prone to infection and destruction of the cartilage. *Pseudomonas* is a common pathogen and oral fluoroquinolones are indicated as treatment. "E" deserves special mention, as "nerds" can be converted to "hipsters" simply by piercing their ears. However, there is a corollary to this axiom: any aging male with a gray ponytail should avoid piercings; a pony tail and piercing don't make you young and attractive and mostly look silly.

▶ **Objectives: Did you learn to …**
  · Describe techniques and indications for toenail removal?
  · Describe various skin biopsy techniques?
  · Identify contraindications to ear piercing?

QUICK QUIZ: DOC, IS THAT A HOSE IN MY CHEST?

What statement represents correct chest tube management?

A) A tube that shows no water fluctuations when placed on "water seal" should have wall suction increased in an attempt to re-open

B) Initial postoperative setting of a chest tube is most often −100 cm H_2O

C) Unless there is major injury to the lung, continuous bubbling of the water seal chamber most likely represents an apparatus leakage

D) If a purse string was placed during initial placement of the chest tube, tightly tying the purse string when pulling the chest tube is enough to prevent pneumothorax

The correct answer is "C." Continued bubbling in the water seal chamber suggests that there is a leak in the system. Theoretically, once the pleural space is drained of air, there should be no further bubbling. Air leakage is seen as air bubbles that increase with increased intrathoracic pressure (e.g., cough, Valsalva maneuver, and positive pressure ventilation). Continuous air leakage may be due to a large tear in the lung parenchyma, bronchopleural fistula, or an apparatus leak. "A" is incorrect. A tube that is nonfunctional should first be evaluated by a clinician familiar with the management of chest tubes—preferably by the person who placed it. An attempt to clear debris or clot can be made by various maneuvers, e.g., stripping the tube. If this is not successful, the tube should be replaced. Increasing the suction will not reopen it. "B" is incorrect as well. Initial suction should be −20 cm H_2O. "D" is incorrect because an occlusive dressing, such as petrolatum gauze, should be placed over the former chest tube site once the tube is removed. **Note that "purse string" sutures are passé. They increase pain and have no advantage over placement of appropriate anchoring sutures**.

A chest tube can be removed when the following criteria are met: fluid drainage is less than 150 cc/day, the lung is fully expanded on chest x-ray, and no air leak is present. Many clinicians perform a "clamping trial" of 4 to 6 hours followed by a chest x-ray to ensure lung expansion prior to removing a chest tube.

Clinical Pearls

- An elevated lactate can indicate tissue ischemia from hypoperfusion (shock, vascular compromise—the so-called "type A" lactic acidosis). Be aware that other causes of a lactic acidosis include ingestions such as methanol or ethanol, liver disease, diabetes, metformin, diabetes, etc. ("type B" lactic acidosis).

- Consider use of tranexamic acid and tourniquet above the injury to help stabilize uncontrolled bleeding.

- An NG tube is not necessary in the treatment of a small bowel obstruction. However, it can be helpful in preventing vomiting. The trade-off is that an NG tube is uncomfortable.

- Compression stockings do nothing to prevent postoperative DVTs and may cause skin breakdown: don't use them. Use subcutaneous heparins or intermittent pneumatic compression along with early mobilization.

- Do not get "baseline" labs such as a CBC, PT/PTT/INR, or electrolytes preoperatively without an indication in patients who do not have significant systemic disease. They are not helpful. Target your preoperative workup based on the patient's comorbidities.

- Do not use colloids for fluid resuscitation unless there is a specific indication (e.g., albumin after large volume paracentesis). The outcomes are generally worse than with crystalloid and the colloids are more expensive.

- Only about 65% of patients with cholecystitis will have a positive Murphy's sign and 30% will have neither a fever nor an elevated white count.

- Patients who have had bariatric surgery can be vitamin-deficient including vitamins D, thiamine, B12, and folate. A multivitamin should be suggested in these patients.

- Prophylactic antibiotics should be given *before* surgery and *not* continued after surgery.

- Ten percent of patients with appendicitis will have a normal white count. Only 75% will have anorexia.

- When categorizing liver disease, the MELD score is less subjective than the Child–Pugh score and requires only creatinine, INR, and bilirubin.

BIBLIOGRAPHY

American College of Surgeons Committee on Trauma. *Advanced Trauma Life Support for Doctors: Student Course Manual.* 10th ed. Chicago, IL: American College of Surgeons; 2018.

ARISE Investigators, et al. Goal-directed resuscitation for patients with early septic shock. *N Engl J Med.* 2014;371(16):1496–1506.

Barbar SD, et al. Timing of renal-replacement therapy in patients with acute kidney injury and sepsis. *N Engl J Med.* 2018; 379:1431–1442.

Bilehjani, et al. Using central venous catheter for suprapubic catheterization in cardiac surgery. *Res Rep Urol.* 2017;9:1–4.

Burgess BE. Anorectal disorders. In: Tintinalli J, Stapczynski JS, Cline DM, et al., eds. *Tintinalli's Emergency Medicine.* 7th ed. New York, NY: McGraw-Hill Medical; 2011:587–601.

Cameron JL, Cameron AM. *Current Surgical Therapy.* 12th ed. Philadelphia, PA: Elsevier Saunders; 2016.

Cannon JW, et al. Damage control resuscitation in patients with severe traumatic hemorrhage: a practice management guideline from the Eastern Association for the Surgery of Trauma. *J Trauma Acute Care Surg.* 2017;82(3):605–617.

Carroll PJ, et al. Surgeon-performed ultrasound at the bedside for the detection of appendicitis and gallstones: systematic review and meta-analysis. *Am J Surg.* 2013;205(1):102–108.

The CLOTS Trial Collaboration. Effectiveness of thigh-length graduated compression stockings to reduce the risk of deep vein thrombosis after stroke (CLOTS Trial 1): a multicentre, randomised controlled trial. *Lancet.* 2009;373:1958–1965.

CRASH-2 trial collaborators, et al. Effects of tranexamic acid on death, vascular occlusive events, and blood transfusion in trauma patients with significant haemorrhage (CRASH-2): a randomised, placebo-controlled trial. *Lancet.* 2010;376(9734):23–32.

de Goede B, et al. Watchful waiting versus surgery of mildly symptomatic or asymptomatic inguinal hernia in men aged 50 years and older: a randomized control trial. *Ann Surg.* 2018; 267(1):42–49.

Dellinger RP, et al. Surviving sepsis campaign: international guidelines for management of severe sepsis and septic shock: 2012. *Crit Care Med.* 2013;41(2):581–637.

Dennis M, The CLOTS Trials Collaboration. Effectiveness of thigh-length graduated compression stockings to reduce the risk of deep vein thrombosis after stroke (CLOTS Trial 1): a multicenter, randomized controlled trial. *Lancet.* 2009;373:1958–1965.

Drake FT, et al. Progress in the diagnosis of appendicitis: a report from Washington State's Surgical Care and Outcomes Assessment Program. *Ann Surg.* 2012;256(4):586–594.

Expert Panel on Gastrointestinal Imaging:, Scheirey CD, et al. *ACR Appropriateness Criteria: Acute Non-localized Abdominal Pain.* Revised 2018. Reston, VA: American College of Radiology; 2019. Available at: https://acsearch.acr.org/docs/69467/Narrative/. Accessed 23 April 2019.

Feely MA, et al. Preoperative testing before noncardiac surgery: guidelines and recommendations. *Am Fam Physician.* 2013;87(6):414–418.

Gottlieb M. et al. Systemic antibiotics for the treatment of skin and soft tissue abscesses: a systematic review and meta-analysis. *Ann Emerg Med.* 2019;73:8–16.

Graber MA, et al. *University of Iowa: The Family Practice Handbook.* 5th ed. Philadelphia, PA: Elsevier Saunders; 2006.

Gruber PJ, et al. Presence of fever and leukocytosis in acute cholecystitis. *Ann Emerg Med.* 1996;28(3):273–277.

Hayden GE, et al. Triage sepsis alert and sepsis protocol lower times to fluids and antibiotics in the ED. *Am J Emerg Med.* 2016;34(1):1–9.

Hernández-Gea V, et al. Preemptive TIPS improves outcomes in high-risk variceal bleeding: an observational study. *Hepatology.* 2019;69(1):282–293.

HerniaSurge Group. International guidelines for groin hernia management. *Hernia.* 2018;22(1):1–165.

Hou MC, et al. Antibiotic prophylaxis after endoscopic therapy prevents rebleeding in acute variceal hemorrhage: a randomized trial. *Hepatology.* 2004; 39(3):746–753.

Jan TB et al. Bedside ultrasonography for the detection of small bowel obstruction in the emergency department. *Emerg Med J.* 2011; 28(8):676–678.

Jain A, et al. History, physical examination, laboratory testing, and emergency department ultrasonography for the diagnosis of acute cholecystitis. *Acad Emerg Med.* 2017;24(3):281–297.

Jørgensen KJ, et al. Overdiagnosis in publicly organized mammography screening programmes: a systematic review of incidence trends. *BMJ.* 2009;339:b2587.

Krag M, et al. Pantoprazole in patients at risk for gastrointestinal bleeding in the ICU. *N Engl J Med.* 2018:379:2199–2208.

LeBlanc KE, et al. Inguinal hernias: diagnosis and management. *Am Fam Physician.* 2013;87(12):844–848.

Linkins LA, et al. Treatment and prevention of heparin-induced thrombocytopenia: antithrombotic therapy and prevention of thrombosis. 9th ed. American College of Chest Physicians Evidence-Based Clinical Practice Guidelines. *Chest.* 2012;141(2 Suppl):e495S–e530S.

Lo GK et al. Evaluation of a pre-test clinical score (4T's) for the diagnosis of heparin-induced thrombocytopenia in two clinical settings. *J Thromb Haemost.* 2006;4(4):759.

Maglinte DD, et al. Reliability and role of plain film radiography and CT in the diagnosis of small-bowel obstruction. *Am J Roentgenol.* 1996;167:1451–1455.

Marik PE, et al. The risk of catheter-related bloodstream infection with femoral venous catheters as compared to subclavian and internal jugular venous catheters: a systemic review of the literature and meta-analysis. *Crit Care Med.* 2012;40(8):2479–2485.

Marino PL. *Marino's The ICU Book.* 4th ed. Philadelphia, PA: Wolters Kluwer Health/Lippincott Williams & Wilkins; 2014.

Maung AA, et al. Evaluation and management of small-bowel obstruction: an Eastern Association for the Surgery of Trauma practice management guideline. *J Trauma Acute Care Surg.* 2012;73(5 Suppl 4):S362–S369.

Mechanick JI, et al. Clinical practice guidelines for the perioperative nutritional, metabolic, and nonsurgical support of the bariatric surgery patient—2013 update: Cosponsored by American Association of Clinical Endocrinologists, The Obesity Society, and American Society for Metabolic & Bariatric Surgery. *Obesity.* 2013;21(S1):S1–S27.

Mersch J, et al. Cancers associated with BRCA1 and BRCA2 mutations other than breast and ovarian. *Cancer.* 2015;121(2):269–275.

Mittal MK, et al. Performance of ultrasound in the diagnosis of pediatric appendicitis in a multicenter cohort. *Acad Emerg Med.* 2013;20(7):697–702.

Morris RJ, et al. Intermittent pneumatic compression or graduated compression stockings for deep vein thrombosis prophylaxis? A systematic review of direct clinical comparisons. *Ann Surg.* 2010;251(3):393–396.

National Institute for Healthcare and Care Excellence (NICE). Routine preoperative tests for elective surgery: NICE Guideline [NG45]. London, UK: NICE; 2016 Apr 5. Available at: https://www.nice.org.uk/guidance/ng45. Accessed 23 April 2019.

Nguyen NT, et al. Bariatric surgery for obesity and metabolic disorders: state of the art. *Nat Rev Gastroenterol Hepatol.* 2017;14(3):160–169.

O'Reilly EA, et al. A meta-analysis of surgical morbidity and recurrence after laparoscopic and open repair of primary unilateral inguinal hernia. *Ann Surg.* 2012;255(5):846–853.

Pfenninger JL, Fowler GC. *Pfenninger and Fowler's Procedures for Primary Care*. 3rd ed. Philadelphia, PA: Elsevier Mosby; 2011.

PRISM Investigators, et al. Early, goal-directed therapy for septic shock: a patient-level meta-analysis. *N Engl J Med*. 2017;376(23):2223–2234.

Reitz KM, et al. Treating patients with appendicitis, not just the appendicitis. *JAMA Surg*. 2019;154(2):149.

Rhodes A, et al. Surviving Sepsis campaign: international guidelines for management of sepsis and septic shock: 2016. *Crit Care Med*. 2017; 45(3):486–552.

Roberts et al. Tranexamic acid in bleeding trauma patients: an exploration of benefits and harms. *Trials*. 2017:18(1):48.

Salminen P, et al. Five-year follow-up of antibiotic therapy for uncomplicated acute appendicitis in the APPAC randomized clinic trial. *JAMA*. 2018;320(12):1259–1265.

Sauret JM, et al. Rhabdmyolysis. *Am Fam Physician*. 2002;65(5):907–913.

Schulman AM, et al. Reexcision surgery for breast cancer: an analysis of the American Society of Breast Surgeons (ASBrS) Mastery^SM Database following the SSO-ASTRO "no ink on tumor" guidelines. *Ann Surg Oncol*. 2017;24(1):52–58.

Self WH, et al. Balanced crystalloids versus saline in non-critically ill adults. *N Engl J Med*. 2018;378(9):819–828.

Semler MW, et al. Balanced crystalloids versus saline in critically ill adults. *N Engl J Med*. 2018;378(9): 829–839.

Stevens DL, et al. Practice guidelines for the diagnosis and management of skin and soft tissue infections: 2014 update by the Infectious Diseases Society of America. *Clin Infect Dis*. 2014;59(2):e10–e52.

Suri S, et al. Comparative evaluation of plain films, ultrasound and CT in the diagnosis of intestinal obstruction. *Acta Radiol*. 1999;40(4):422–428.

Svensson JF, et al. Nonoperative treatment with antibiotics versus surgery for acute nonperforated appendicitis in children: a pilot randomized controlled trial. *Ann Surg*. 2015;261(1):67–71.

Thwaini A, et al. Fournier's gangrene and its emergency management. *Postgrad Med J*. 2006;82(970):516–519.

Townsend CM, et al. *Sabiston's Textbook of Surgery: The Biological Basis of Modern Surgical Practice*. 19th ed. Philadelphia, PA: Elsevier Saunders; 2012.

Wade CE, et al. Use of recombinant factor VIIa in US military casualties for a five-year period. *J Trauma*. 2010;69:353–359.

Psychiatry

23

Monika Jindal

You are seeing a 48-year-old female who presents with a 3-month history of low mood, low energy, poor concentration, and irritability. She has lost interest in most things she had enjoyed and has also noticed a 20-lb weight gain. She has been having frequent headaches, has been short-tempered, and has noticed that it is hard to wake up in the morning. She reports no thoughts of suicide but has wondered if death would be a relief. She says she has felt restless for a while and feels that she is a bad person. Her mother suffered from depression. She does not consume alcohol or any other substances. She is divorced and has no children.

You think that this patient may meet criteria for a depressive disorder.

Question 23.1.1 Which of the following is NOT a criterion for the diagnosis of major depressive disorder (MDD)?
A) Low mood
B) Presence of suicidal ideation
C) Decreased appetite
D) Anhedonia or loss of interest
E) Mood fluctuations

Answer 23.1.1 **The correct answer is "E."** While low mood is a criterion, the presence of mood fluctuation is not used to make the diagnosis of depression. The other options listed are part of the criteria set forth in the *Diagnostic and Statistical Manual of Mental Disorders,* 5th ed. (DSM-5). Special emphasis is placed on the presence of depressed mood and decreased interest, **one of which must be present** in order to diagnose MDD. Instead of depressed mood, patients may report somatic complaints or irritability.

Per DSM-5, in order to diagnose MDD, five or more of the following nine criteria must be present for at least two weeks or more. At least ONE must be depressed mood OR loss of interest/anhedonia:

- Depressed mood
- Loss of interest/anhedonia

- Significant change in weight or appetite
- Insomnia or hypersomnia
- Psychomotor agitation or retardation
- Fatigue or loss of energy
- Feeling worthless or excessive guilt
- Poor concentration
- Recurrent thoughts of death, suicidal ideation, attempt, or plan

 HELPFUL TIP:
Several mnemonics have been developed to help clinicians remember the DSM-5 criteria and two of these are "SIG E CAPS" (**S**leep, **I**nterest, **G**uilt, **E**nergy, **C**oncentration, **A**ppetite, **P**sychomotor changes, **S**uicidality) and "SPACE DIGS" (same but add **D**epression).

Question 23.1.2 Which one of this patient's symptoms is considered a symptom of *"atypical* depression" or major depressive disorder (MDD) with atypical features?
A) Hypersomnia
B) Low mood
C) Anhedonia
D) Psychomotor retardation
E) Irritability

Answer 23.1.2 **The correct answer is "A."** The typical somatic symptoms of depression include poor sleep or insomnia, decreased appetite, and decreased libido. Patients with *atypical depression* may have hyperphagia, hypersomnolence, leaden paralysis, and mood reactivity.

You begin to explain the nature of depression to this patient.

Question 23.1.3 **Which of the following epidemiological statements is NOT true?**
A) The average American has about a 16% chance of developing depression over his or her lifetime
B) About 7% of Americans suffer depression each year
C) Women are five times as likely to suffer depression as are men
D) The incidence of depression is higher in younger cohorts than the elderly
E) Divorced people are more likely to be depressed

Answer 23.1.3 **The correct answer is "C."** The lifetime prevalence of MDD is 16% with 6.9% of adults suffering from MDD in any given year. Depression may be recurrent throughout one's lifetime. Women are **twice** (not five times) as likely to experience depression as are men. Rates of depression are similar across all age groups, though elderly men are at a higher risk of suicide than elderly women. Being divorced is a risk factor for depression.

HELPFUL TIP:
Anxiety, not meeting the level of an anxiety disorder, frequently accompanies depression (70%). However, 60% of people with a lifetime diagnosis of MDD have had a diagnosable anxiety disorder.

This patient's situation is not unusual for your practice.

Question 23.1.4 **What is the prevalence of MDD in primary care patients?**
A) 1% to 2%
B) 5% to 15%
C) 30% to 35%
D) 45% to 50%
E) 100% (seems like everyone … even the clinic staff)

Answer 23.1.4 **The correct answer is "B."** About 5% to 10% of primary care patients meet criteria for MDD and about twice of that (10–20%) many have "minor" depression. If you answered "E," you work in a sad, sad place. Hire a clown to work the front desk—but not one of those scary, murderous clowns.

HELPFUL TIP:
One reason for lack of diagnosis of depression in primary care is that depression often presents with a wide variety of somatic complaints. Another is that the spectrum of disease in primary care offices is less severe, leading to fewer diagnoses.

Question 23.1.5 **Which of these epidemiological statements about depression in primary care is true?**
A) Most depressed patients (about 80%) seek mental health care from primary care physicians
B) About 50% of patients suffering from depression are clinically recognized by their primary care physician

C) Only about 50% of the patients diagnosed with MDD receive adequate treatment
D) The 2015 United States Preventive Services Task Force (USPSTF) recommends screening for depression and having adequate systems for treatment, follow-up, and/or referral
E) All of the above

Answer 23.1.5 **The correct answer is "E."** All are correct. "D" requires special mention. The previous (2009) recommendation suggested screening *contingent* upon having adequate services for patients diagnosed with depression.

HELPFUL TIP:
There are several brief self-rating depression scales that can be used for screening (e.g., Beck Depression Inventory, Primary Care Evaluation of Mental Disorders, Patient Health Questionnaire, and Zung Depression Scale). A two-question screen (PHQ-2) may be as effective for screening as these more extensive scales. Simply ask:

- Over the past 2 weeks, have you often felt down, blue, or in the dumps?
- Over the past 2 weeks, have you lost interest in most activities or things that used to bring you pleasure?

A positive answer to **either** of those two questions should prompt a more thorough evaluation of depression with one of the more extensive self-rating depression scales. A negative answer to both questions likely rules out depression in most patients.

You realize that it is also important to focus on the social history in patients with depression.

Question 23.1.6 **Which of the following is associated with a DECREASED risk of depression?**
A) Unemployment
B) Poverty
C) Being unmarried
D) Family history of depression
E) Asian race

Answer 23.1.6 **The correct answer is "E."** Factors associated with an increased risk of depression include having a family history of depression, being unmarried (single, divorced, or widowed), a recent childbirth or pregnancy, medical comorbidities, lack of social support, female gender, unemployment, poverty, and substance use. There is a lower prevalence of depression among people of Asian ancestry when compared to the Caucasian populations. Protective factors include: marriage, having children, and being retired (so, retirement is when we are supposed to have fun?).

You believe that your patient is suffering from an episode of major depression, and you decide to initiate treatment with an antidepressant.

Question 23.1.7 Following the first episode of depression, what is her risk of relapse?
A) <1%
B) 25%
C) 50%
D) 75%
E) >99%

Answer 23.1.7 The correct answer is "C." About 50% of patients relapse following the first episode of depression. Following the second episode, the risk of relapse is roughly 75%, and climbs to about 90% after the third episode. In order to reduce the risk of relapse, most authorities recommend antidepressant therapy for 6 to 12 months after remission in patients with their first episode of depression. Approximately two-thirds of relapses can be prevented by continuation of antidepressant medications indefinitely. Patients who might benefit from indefinite medical therapy include: those with a severe first episode (e.g., significant suicide attempt), patients diagnosed with MDD with psychotic features, patients with three or more episodes of MDD, elderly patients with their first episode of depression, and possibly those with a strong family history of depression.

You choose to treat your patient with a serotonin reuptake inhibitor (SSRI) and tell your patient to contact you if she suffers from adverse effects.

Question 23.1.8 Which of the following is NOT a typical adverse effect of SSRIs?
A) Nausea
B) Headaches
C) Restlessness
D) Insomnia
E) Urinary retention

Answer 23.1.8 The correct answer is "E." Urinary retention is not seen with SSRIs, but the other four options are typical SSRI side effects. The anticholinergic effect of urinary retention is typical of the tricyclic antidepressants (TCAs). Sexual and GI problems are commonly seen with SSRIs including loss of libido. Akathisia and dystonic reactions can (rarely) be seen with SSRIs as well. To be complete, paroxetine (Paxil) does have anticholinergic effects and can cause urinary retention.

Your patient returns to see you 2 weeks after starting her SSRI and reports that she has not noticed any benefit from the medication.

Question 23.1.9 Which of the following statements is most accurate?
A) The antidepressant is not going to work, so she should switch to another antidepressant of the same class
B) The antidepressant is not going to work, so she should switch to another antidepressant from a different class
C) It is too early to judge the efficacy of the antidepressant at this point

D) She's probably suffering a paradoxical reaction of increased depression with her medication
E) Going up on the dose is not an option at this time

Answer 23.1.9 The correct answer is "C." The benefit of antidepressant medication usually takes about 3–4 weeks (although side effects may occur upon initiation). Thus, it is premature to abandon this medication. Most authorities recommend trying an antidepressant for 6 weeks at an adequate dose before considering that medication a "treatment failure." Increasing the dose **or** giving it at least 4 to 6 weeks total at the current dose would both be valid options.

You increase the medication dose, and the patient returns to see you in another 2 weeks. This time, she is feeling better and more energetic. People at work are beginning to notice her improved attitude, and her sleep has become more refreshing. She wants to know how long she should stay on the medication.

Question 23.1.10 The correct answer is:
A) At least 1 month
B) At least 2 months
C) At least 4 to 6 months
D) At least 2 years
E) Forever

Answer 23.1.10 The correct answer is "C." Different organizations recommend different durations of treatment, but the shortest recommended course is 4 to 6 months, with most authorities recommending treatment for 6 to 12 months after remission.

▶ **Objectives: Did you learn to …**
· Diagnose MDD?
· Describe the epidemiology and natural history of depression?
· Recognize features of depression with atypical features?
· Initiate treatment of depression?
· Identify adverse effects of SSRIs?

▶ **CASE 23.2**

You are assessing a 45-year-old professional male who has a history of MDD in his early twenties but has fully recovered since. He recently suffered an uncomplicated anterior wall myocardial infarction (MI). His wife mentions that she thinks he is depressed. He is tired all the time, has poor sleep, a poor appetite, and he has been irritable. He has also been tearful and blames himself for his MI (too many "pounder" burgers … with cheese … and bacon). He is willing to consider the diagnosis of depression because he remembers having suffered from it before. He also knows a history of MDD puts him at risk for medical illnesses.

Question 23.2.1 **Which of the following illnesses is more prevalent in patients with MDD?**
A) Coronary heart disease
B) Cerebrovascular disease
C) Diabetes mellitus
D) Osteoporosis
E) All of the above

Answer 23.2.1 The correct answer is "E." It is unclear if patients with depression are more likely to have these illnesses as a result of the depression or the reverse: patients with these illnesses are more likely to be depressed. Depressed patients have an average of 3.4 more chronic medical conditions than nondepressed patients. At least two studies have now linked a lifetime history of MDD to an increased risk (1.2–3 times) of early menopause (of course that would be a bit strange in this patient, a male).

You know that some of this patient's symptoms could be secondary to his medical illness.

Question 23.2.2 **Which one of the following symptoms, if present, is the *most specific* for depression?**
A) Sleep problems
B) Appetite difficulties
C) Psychomotor agitation
D) Low energy
E) Excessive preoccupation with death

Answer 23.2.2 The correct answer is "E." In the mnemonic "SPACE DIGS," the last four letters stand for symptoms that are more specific for depression and more independent of somatic illnesses. These symptoms are **D**epressed mood, loss of **I**nterests, inappropriate **G**uilt, and thoughts of **S**uicide ("DIGS"). The presence of any of these symptoms should lead you to suspect depression.

HELPFUL TIP:
While a stressor can often precipitate onset of depression, depression can also arise with no precipitating factor, and the response to treatment is independent of whether it is "reactive" (identifiable stressor present) or "endogenous" (no identifiable stressor).

Question 23.2.3 **Which of the following statements is NOT true about depression post-MI?**
A) Major depression is an independent risk factor for post-MI mortality
B) Minor depression is an independent risk factor for post-MI mortality
C) Minor depression is more prevalent than major depression post-MI
D) Treating depression improves cardiac outcomes in post-MI patients
E) Approximately half of the people who sustain an MI have symptoms of depression afterward

Answer 23.2.3 The correct answer is "D." In the post-MI period, major depression occurs in almost 20%, and minor depression in another 27%. Concurrent major depression elevates mortality risk after MI by a factor of 3.5, which is the same degree of risk as heart failure. Patients with a mood disturbance (e.g., minor depression) also have a higher mortality rate. While treatment of depression has been shown to improve some medical outcomes (e.g., HbA1C levels in diabetics), this is not the case in cardiovascular disease. Treatment of depression does not change mortality or morbidity after an MI (but may improve quality of life).

HELPFUL TIP:
Patients suffering strokes also have an elevated risk of depression with approximately one-third of post-stroke patients meeting criteria for MDD; there is a similar correlation of depressive symptoms with stroke mortality.

You decide to recommend treatment to this patient.

Question 23.2.4 **Which of the following therapies is the LEAST desirable choice for treating his depression?**
A) Bupropion (Wellbutrin)
B) Cognitive behavioral therapy
C) Nortriptyline (Pamelor)
D) Fluoxetine (Prozac)
E) Sertraline (Zoloft)

Answer 23.2.4 The correct answer is "C." TCAs should be avoided in patients with cardiovascular disease because of their arrhythmogenic potential (e.g., torsades de pointes). Remember that the SNRIs as well as some SSRIs (citalopram [Celexa] and escitalopram [Lexapro]) can also prolong the QT interval. Generally, SSRI therapy ("D" and "E") would be the preferred drug for the majority of patients who are candidates for pharmacotherapy. Bupropion ("A") and cognitive behavioral therapy ("B") are also reasonable choices.

HELPFUL TIP:
Consider a baseline ECG in all patients for whom you are initiating TCAs and citalopram to evaluate the QT interval, particularly if the patient is on other medications that prolong the QT interval. If the QT is prolonged at baseline, it predisposes patients to arrhythmias.

▸ **Objectives: Did you learn to …**
· Diagnose depression occurring with an acute medical illness?
· Recognize the impact of depression on other medical conditions?
· Treat a post-MI patient with depression?

QUICK QUIZ: SAD ALL THE TIME

A 44-year-old patient of yours has come to see you multiple times for low mood. She does not have trouble with energy or sleep, but with prompting reports occasional problems with concentration and appetite. Basically, she tells you, "I've been depressed for as long as I can remember." You have tried treating her with two different SSRIs, but she had trouble with side effects and did not notice much improvement in her mood.

Which of the following is the best diagnosis for this patient?
A) Adjustment disorder
B) Bipolar affective disorder
C) Persistent depressive disorder (previously called dysthymia)
D) MDD
E) Premenstrual dysphoric disorder

The correct answer is "C." Persistent depressive disorder (formerly dysthymia in DSM-IV) is best thought of as long-term, low-level depressive symptoms that do not meet criteria for MDD. Symptoms include depressed mood most days for at least 2 years and two or more of the following: low energy, hopelessness, concentration difficulties, sleep disturbance, appetite change, fatigue, and low self-esteem. In order to diagnose persistent depressive disorder, the person cannot be free of the symptoms for more than 2 months during the first 2 years. The treatment is the same as for depression—SSRIs and psychotherapy. Many people with persistent depressive disorder may also experience one or more episodes of MDD in their lifetime.

▶ CASE 23.3

A 34-year-old female presents to your clinic for treatment of depression. She reports a lifelong history of low-level depressive symptoms that have worsened over the past 6 months since she lost her job (don't worry—this is a different case than the previous one). She also suffers from inadequately controlled diabetes mellitus (HbA1c 9%) and has been diagnosed with a personality disorder in the past. She drinks three to four beers everyday (hmm . . . multiply by 2 just to be safe) and has been arrested for driving while intoxicated twice. On questioning, you realize she has a moderately severe level of depression. She is not suicidal, so you decide to initiate treatment as an outpatient with close follow-up.

Question 23.3.1 **Which of these factors does NOT contribute to a poor outcome when treating depression?**
A) Chronic depressive symptoms
B) Female gender
C) Personality disorder
D) Comorbid medical conditions
E) Alcoholism

Answer 23.3.1 **The correct answer is "B."** Even though females are twice as likely to be diagnosed with MDD as males, gender does not seem to influence treatment response. The presence of any of the other factors listed reduces the chance of a successful response to treatment.

In choosing an antidepressant for this patient, you would like to use one with a high success rate (whereas, sometimes you choose the least efficacious drug—what?!). However, you know that the success rates for most antidepressants are fairly similar.

Question 23.3.2 **What are the chances of this patient failing to respond to the first antidepressant chosen?**
A) <1%
B) 10% to 20%
C) 30% to 40%
D) 60% to 70%
E) 90% to 95%

Answer 23.3.2 **The correct answer is "C."** Studies have consistently shown an antidepressant response rate of somewhere between 60% and 70% with 30% to 40% failing to respond, regardless of what antidepressant is tried. When unpublished studies are included, the failure rate for SSRIs approaches 50%. Despite this, SSRIs are still the first-line recommended therapy for treatment of depression.

 HELPFUL TIP:
Fifty percent of patients who do not respond to an initial SSRI will respond to another drug in the same class. So, changing to another SSRI is reasonable in a patient who has failed one SSRI. Is this observed effect due to differences between drugs, pharmacodynamics, pharmacogenetics, or longer treatment? No one knows.

When you spin your Random Depression Therapy Wheel that your occultist friend gave you during the last blue moon, it lands on escitalopram (Lexapro). So, you start your patient on that drug. Ten days later, she calls you just to say that the new medicine seems no better and her sleep is even worse. She started taking the medication in the morning because she thought it might be interfering with her sleep. She tends to lie in bed for 2 hours before falling asleep.

Question 23.3.3 **In addition to recommending good sleep hygiene and increased exercise, you prescribe:**
A) Trazodone
B) Zolpidem
C) Lorazepam
D) Phenobarbital
E) Two shots of whiskey QHS, preferably a classic like Basil Hayden

Answer 23.3.3 The correct answer is "A." Trazodone may be helpful with insomnia and can boost serotonergic activity. For depression with disordered sleep, it is preferred to benzodiazepines unless anxiety is a significant issue. Additionally, given this patient's daily alcohol use, neither benzodiazepines (nor more alcohol) are advised. Phenobarbital should be avoided. Zolpidem might be a consideration but is often associated with considerable side effects (Gee, Doc, I don't remember driving the car in my underwear and baking two pans of lasagna last night, but oh well) particularly in women who tend to be slower metabolizers. Due to this, the FDA recommended maximum dosage of zolpidem be lower in women, 5 mg compared to 10 mg in men. Obviously avoid alcohol for treatment of insomnia in this and other patients as it can actually disrupt sleep cycles.

HELPFUL TIP:
Indications for psychiatric referral for depression include:
*   Failure of medical treatment
*   Imminent suicidality
*   Severe depression for which hospitalization is thought to be necessary
*   Diagnostic clarification or treatment recommendation
*   Comorbidities that make treatment response less likely
*   Patient requests referral

You add trazodone 50 mg HS PRN and titrate up to the maximum dose of escitalopram, and your patient's symptoms are now coming under control. When you see her next, she describes a 20-minute episode of chest tightness, dyspnea, diaphoresis, and extreme anxiety. You believe that she suffered a panic attack. You wonder if you should alter your diagnosis.

Question 23.3.4 In which of the following disorders might panic attacks occur?
A) Panic disorder
B) MDD
C) Generalized anxiety disorder
D) Social phobia
E) All of the above

Answer 23.3.4 The correct answer is "E." Panic attacks consist of a cluster of symptoms signifying anxiety and are not a disorder by themselves. As such, they can be part of any affective syndrome including depression, social phobia, generalized anxiety disorder, and panic disorder. The presence of a single panic attack in a person with a depressive disorder should not necessarily lead to a new diagnosis.

► **Objectives: Did you learn to …**
*   Identify risk factors for a poor outcome when treating depression?
*   Assess the likelihood of a successful outcome in a patient with depression?
*   Generate alternative methods for treating resistant depression?

► **CASE 23.4**

A 41-year-old female comes to your office complaining of difficulty trusting people, irritability, low mood, and recurrent nightmares. Her symptoms started when she was a teenager following the death of her parents in one of the mass shootings in _____(insert your state here). She has never been able to forgive herself for surviving while her parents died. She has not been able to form close relationships, and she is seeking help because of renewed nightmares. They were common in the first 2 years following the incident but had faded away until recently. Now, when she hears news stories of gun violence and school shootings, the memories come flooding back in a very real and visceral manner. She sometimes wakes up in a fright after dreaming that her own house is on fire. She avoids going near any bright lights or fireworks displays. When she is forced to be in the presence of fires, she frequently notices palpitations, dyspnea, and a sense of doom.

Question 23.4.1 What is the patient's primary diagnosis?
A) MDD
B) Generalized anxiety disorder
C) Panic disorder
D) Post-traumatic stress disorder (PTSD)
E) Acute stress disorder

Answer 23.4.1 The correct answer is "D." The patient's symptoms are characteristic of PTSD. This may occur after being exposed to a situation in which one's life or "physical integrity" (or that of another person) is in danger. Some such events are cancer, combat, rape, or other sexual or nonsexual assault; an intensive care unit stay (or, one could hypothesize, taking the boards, perhaps?) may also result in PTSD. Keep reading for further explanation of why this is the best choice.

HELPFUL TIP:
A mass shooting is defined either as at least four victims killed in a single shooting event or at least four victims injured. Hundreds of these incidents occur each year in the United States—only the really big ones make national headlines.

Question 23.4.2 Which of the following is NOT necessary for a diagnosis of PTSD?
A) The patient needs to experience, witness, or be confronted by a potentially life-threatening event, or an event threatening the physical integrity of self or others
B) The patient must respond with intense fear, horror, or helplessness
C) Symptoms have to be present for more than a month
D) The patient must be involved in combat
E) The patient must meet a specified number of symptoms

Answer 23.4.2 The correct answer is "D." Although PTSD is common among military veterans (and was previously known by terms like "shell shock" and "battle fatigue"), there is no requirement that the patient has been in combat. To meet criteria for PTSD, the patient must have been exposed to an event that is threatening to the integrity or life of self or others. The patient then must have symptoms of recurrent intense fear, helplessness, or horror that lasts for >1 month. Symptoms occurring within 4 weeks of the event and lasting for at least 2 days but less than a month are characteristic of acute stress disorder.

Question 23.4.3 Which of the following is *NOT* a part of PTSD?

A) Nightmares
B) Flashbacks
C) Hypervigilance
D) Fear of death
E) Difficulty maintaining relationships

Answer 23.4.3 The correct answer is "D." Fear of death is not a criterion. Symptoms of PTSD are divided into four clusters. To meet the symptom criteria for PTSD, the patient needs at least one symptom from the first cluster, one from the second, two or more from the third, and two or more from the fourth.

The **first cluster (one required)** involves intrusive symptoms regarding the traumatic experience. Examples of symptoms include: flashbacks, nightmares, intrusive memories, and psychological distress in response to triggers that evoke the experience.

The **second cluster (one required)** involves avoidance of stimuli associated with the trauma (people, places, events) and avoidance of distressing memories, thoughts, or feelings related to the trauma.

The **third cluster (two or more required)** relates to negative mood and negative changes in cognition after the traumatic event. Patients may report a numbing of general responsiveness such as markedly diminished interest or participation in significant activities, feeling of detachment or estrangement from others, inability to experience positive emotions, or being in a negative emotional state. They may have negative thoughts distortions toward themselves (negative beliefs about themselves or the causes of the traumatic event).

The **fourth cluster (two or more required)** involves persistent symptoms of increased arousal, such as difficulty falling or staying asleep, irritability or outbursts of anger, difficulty concentrating, hypervigilance, or an exaggerated startle response.

Question 23.4.4 Which of the following is true of treatment for PTSD?

A) There is no effective treatment
B) There are no FDA-approved medications
C) Most patients experience spontaneous remission
D) Although treatment is often effective, most patients do not achieve cure
E) Atypical antipsychotics have no role in treatment

Answer 23.4.4 The correct answer is "D." Symptom improvement, but not cure, is the norm. Cognitive behavioral therapy (if available) is the first-line therapy followed by SSRIs, then SNRIs, particularly venlafaxine. Mediation (specifically transcendental meditation) is effective and can be easily taught (*Lancet Psych.* 2018 Dec; 5:975). Interestingly, "critical incident debriefing" (essentially talking through the incident or reliving the event to try to minimize symptoms, such as with emotive journaling) actually seems to make things worse. CBT and "objective, non-emotive" journaling seem to help (*Soc Sci Med.* 2011;7: 316–326; *Ann Behav Med.* 2002;24:244–250). There is lack of good efficacy data for TCAs, atypical antipsychotics, monoamine oxidase inhibitors (MAOIs), or other drugs. Prazosin may help with sleep and nightmares, but the studies are small and results are mixed. Still, it may be worth a trial added to other pharmacotherapy if the patient is not responding in an adequate manner. Psychotherapy can be helpful and benzodiazepine use should be limited because of the high risk of dependency in this population and the lack of efficacy as monotherapy.

▶ **Objectives: Did you learn to …**
- Recognize risk factors for PTSD?
- Diagnose PTSD?
- Treat PTSD?

▶ **CASE 23.5**

A 29-year-old female presents to you for a second opinion, bringing a large stack of medical records with her. In fact, she says that this is more like a "fourth or fifth opinion" (lucky you). She heard from a friend of a friend that you are the smartest doctor around and could determine what is wrong with her. In fact, she notes, "None of those other doctors understand my symptoms at all. But you will. They say you're the best."

Although you find many negative diagnostic studies in her record, she is sure that her many symptoms must have some physical cause. Over the past few years, she has had chronic headaches, multiple joint pains, diarrhea, fatigue, and intermittent abdominal and chest pains. Her symptoms have prevented her from working. Upper endoscopy, colonoscopy, CT scans, and numerous other studies have not revealed an etiology. Nothing she does improves any of these symptoms. She has spent hours each day researching her symptoms and would like yet another referral to a number of specialists.

Question 23.5.1 Which of the following is the most likely primary diagnosis?

A) Illness anxiety disorder (formerly hypochondriasis)
B) Somatic symptom disorder (formerly somatization disorder)
C) Generalized anxiety disorder
D) Factitious disorder
E) Conversion disorder

Answer 23.5.1 The correct answer is "B." Typically, patients with unexplained symptoms see many doctors, have numerous tests, and often undergo a variety of procedures. Though it is important to consider a primary psychiatric disorder, a thorough and appropriate evaluation into possible organic causes should be completed before a psychiatric diagnosis is decided upon. Many times, patients with unexplained symptoms will ultimately be diagnosed with a somatic symptom disorder as well as a related disorder (of which "A," "D," and "E" are all types).

This patient presents with probable somatic symptom disorder, which by definition must have:

- One or more somatic symptoms that is distressing or disruptive of daily life;
- Excessive thoughts, behaviors, or feelings associated with the somatic symptoms which are exhibited by disproportionate thoughts about the seriousness of symptoms, high anxiety about symptoms, or large amounts of time and energy spent on the health concerns;
- Symptoms are persistent, generally at least 6 months.

"A" is incorrect. **Illness anxiety disorder** is characterized by a preoccupation that one has some sort of serious disease, but somatic symptoms are absent or less pronounced. "C" is incorrect because anxiety is present but totally overshadowed by the somatic complaints. "D," **factitious disorder**, is diagnosed in patients who intentionally produce symptoms (e.g., overdosing on insulin or injecting feces into the bloodstream) to assume the "sick role." "E" is incorrect. With **conversion disorder**, patients present with sudden onset of anatomically implausible neurological symptoms (e.g., whole-body numbness and bilateral deafness). **Conversion disorder** is, by definition, not under conscious control. Remember that conversion disorder is a diagnosis of exclusion. You need to make sure there is not an organic basis for the patient's symptoms. If the symptoms are under conscious control, the diagnosis is "malingering" (really … that is a diagnosis).

....

You believe that this patient has somatic symptom disorder.

Question 23.5.2 **You begin by saying:**
A) "Relax. This is all in your head"
B) "Your pain isn't real. But your psychiatric illness is. It's called somatic symptom disorder"
C) "You have a number of symptoms that are very real but cannot be explained by our investigations. The evidence suggests that you do not have any life-threatening illnesses. You have a well-defined disorder, and other patients have similar problems"
D) "You have a lot of very serious symptoms. But my physical exam is inconsistent with your complaints. Basically, I don't believe a word your saying. The sooner that you admit to falsifying these symptoms, the sooner I can start helping you"
E) "I have a specialist to refer you to in Outer Mongolia … take your time getting back"

Answer 23.5.2 **The correct answer is "C."** In patients with somatic symptom disorder, it is best to use an honest but gentle approach. Most patients feel better if they have a name for an illness, but using the term "somatic symptom disorder" may

actually be detrimental. It is important to affirm the patient's symptoms (these are real problems causing real distress) and to try to find some common language to use to describe what he or she is feeling. Patients may not be receptive to your interpretation initially, but repeating the discussion at subsequent visits and focusing on normal diagnostic tests may help them accept the diagnosis.

....

Next, you discuss a plan of action with this patient.

Question 23.5.3 **You initially recommend:**
A) A multidisciplinary approach, utilizing many different specialty services
B) Starting an SSRI
C) Starting electroconvulsive therapy (ECT)
D) Monthly visits with you and limited diagnostic testing and specialty consultation
E) Referral for exploratory laparotomy

Answer 23.5.3 **The correct answer is "D."** It is best to have patients with somatic symptom disorder establish regular clinic visits, ideally with one provider. Unscheduled visits to the emergency department should be discouraged unless first discussed with the primary provider. Patients should be allowed to discuss all of their complaints, and a physical examination should be performed at every office visit. These measures will let the patients know that their concerns are being taken seriously. Laboratory tests, radiographs, and consultations should be limited; use your best judgment as to when such diagnostic tests are indicated. "B" and "C" are incorrect as SSRIs and ECT are not primary therapy for somatic symptom disorder, though an SSRI may help with related anxiety symptoms.

 HELPFUL TIP:
In patients with somatic symptom disorder who are willing to be referred to mental health providers, individual psychotherapy, CBT, and group therapy may be beneficial.

▶ **Objectives: Did you learn to …**
- Recognize and describe somatic symptom disorder?
- Generate an appropriate plan for a patient with somatic symptom disorder?

▶ **CASE 23.6**

A 21-year-old college student presents to your office for evaluation. She is complaining of feeling stressed out. She is taking classes full-time and is also in one of the military reserve units at the college. One weekend a month, she must attend drill that involves handling weapons. Although she did not have problems handling the weapons initially, she now gets very emotional and upset when she thinks about having to use them at the next drill weekend. She is nervous and is afraid that she might accidentally fire a weapon. She knows that her fears are silly, and she has been telling herself to "just get over it." Last weekend, while in class, she suddenly felt that she was going to have a heart attack. She developed tightness in her chest, her heart was racing, and she felt unable to breathe. Although the symptoms eventually abated, the episode made her even more alarmed, and now she is worried that it will happen again, and she will have a heart attack. She comes to see if you can help.

Question 23.6.1 Which of the following is UNNECESSARY for the initial workup?
A) Take more medical, psychiatric, and family history
B) Order an echocardiogram
C) Perform a physical examination
D) Order thyroid function tests
E) Perform a mental status examination

Answer 23.6.1 The correct answer is "B." Given the information you have so far, an echocardiogram is not indicated and is rarely used as part of a primary workup. When it comes to test questions, never say no to more history (unless you are supposed to be managing a patient's airway). A complete history and physical examination, including mental status examination, is essential in the evaluation of this new patient. Thyroid abnormalities can be a cause of some of these symptoms, including palpitations and chest tightness.

She has no prior psychiatric history, but her mother is taking medication for depression. While taking her social history, you ask questions regarding substance abuse.

Question 23.6.2 Use of which of the following substances might explain her symptoms?
A) Nicotine
B) Alcohol
C) Caffeine
D) Herbal weight loss medication
E) Any of the above

Answer 23.6.2 The correct answer is "E." Potential causes of this patient's symptoms include stimulants, such as caffeine, nicotine (including cigarettes and vaping), amphetamines, ADHD stimulant drugs, pseudoephedrine, some herbal weight loss products containing ephedra (*Ma Huang*), etc. Marijuana can also cause similar symptoms, as can withdrawal from sedatives such as alcohol and benzodiazepines.

She does not smoke, doesn't use recreational drugs, and doesn't drink alcohol; she drinks 1 cup of coffee on weekday mornings before class. Her physical examination is normal. Her mental status examination is remarkable for a neutral mood, a restricted and anxious affect, but no suicidal thoughts, and no psychotic symptoms. The

laboratory tests you order are normal. You are leaning toward a psychiatric diagnosis at this point, specifically an anxiety disorder.

Question 23.6.3 Which of the following is NOT an anxiety disorder?
A) Panic disorder
B) Social anxiety disorder
C) Agoraphobia
D) Generalized anxiety disorder
E) Delirium

Answer 23.6.3 The correct answer is "E." Delirium, while it may present with features similar to an anxiety disorder, is a cognitive disorder. Anxiety disorders are the most common form of mental illness in the United States, with a lifetime prevalence of approximately 30%. They include options "A" through "D" as well as separation anxiety disorder, specific phobias, selective mutism, unspecified anxiety disorder, and anxiety disorders that are judged to be secondary to a medical condition or a substance.

Of the listed anxiety disorders, you think she has developed panic disorder and that she has been having panic attacks.

Question 23.6.4 Which of the following is NOT a typical symptom of a panic attack?
A) Palpitations
B) Diaphoresis
C) Syncope
D) Dyspnea
E) Dizziness

Answer 23.6.4 The correct answer is "C." The symptoms of a panic attack are those associated with an activation of the "fight-or-flight" response referable to the sympathetic nervous system. Typical symptoms include chest pain, fear of dying, paresthesias, dyspnea, a sense of smothering or "impending doom," nausea, dizziness, numbness, palpitations, sweating, trembling, and derealization or depersonalization. (At this point, we'd like to ask Mother Nature how chest pain helps us when facing a saber-toothed tiger.) It would be rare for a patient to actually lose consciousness from a panic attack (though they may feel they might); and if the patient has true syncope, other diagnoses should be entertained.

 HELPFUL TIP:
Hyperventilation can cause cerebral vasoconstriction and secondary cerebral hypoxia resulting in syncope. This *can* occur with panic disorder. However, this is pretty unusual. Syncope should still prompt one to rule out alternative diagnoses.

To make your diagnosis of panic disorder, the patient needs to meet certain criteria.

Question 23.6.5 Which of these is NOT a criterion for panic disorder?

A) Recurrent and unexpected panic attacks
B) At least 1 month of worry about having more attacks
C) Worry about the implication of the attack or its consequences (dying, "going crazy," etc.)
D) Change in behavior related to the attacks
E) Predictable panic attacks that occur in response to cues

Answer 23.6.5 The correct answer is "E." The criteria for panic disorder do not include predictable panic attacks in response to cues. After patients have had repeated panic attacks, they often develop phobic avoidance of places, objects, or events associated with their symptoms (e.g., agoraphobia). Agoraphobia is a separate diagnosis in DSM-5. Patients often scout out routes of escape before going to places that might provoke a panic attack.

HELPFUL TIP:
The vast majority of patients with panic disorder present with somatic complaints rather than cognitive or mood symptoms. Patients are often misdiagnosed initially. Consider panic attacks in patients presenting with the appropriate somatic symptoms. But never rule out a physical diagnosis (e.g., PSVT, MI) without an appropriate workup.

Your patient is worried that these attacks will keep occurring.

Question 23.6.6 How would you best describe the prognosis for panic disorder?

A) It is easily curable in most patients
B) There is no effective drug treatment beyond benzodiazepines, especially alprazolam (Xanax)—lots of alprazolam
C) Most patients do not improve over time
D) It is a recurrent or chronic illness
E) It almost always progresses to total disability

Answer 23.6.6 The correct answer is "D." Panic disorder is a recurrent or chronic disease in most patients. "A," "C," and "E" are incorrect. Although panic disorder is not easily curable, almost all patients will improve over time. However, very few attain complete remission even with medical treatment. Relapse is common (see more about treatment below).

The patient is, of course, very concerned about future panic attacks. She asks what to do when another occurs.

Question 23.6.7 You advise her to do all of the following EXCEPT:

A) Move to a quiet area
B) Slow down her breathing
C) Reassure herself that she is not dying
D) Breathe into a brown paper bag
E) Avoid stimulants like caffeine or nicotine

Answer 23.6.7 The correct answer is "D." All of the other options are reasonable recommendations for a patient suffering from panic attacks. Although commonly observed in popular lore, breathing into a paper bag is not recommended. Breathing into a brown paper bag can have the opposite effect of that intended—the patient may continue hyperventilating with CO_2 building up, which may contribute to more panic symptoms. Hyperventilating (blowing off CO_2) does not produce a panic attack nor relieve it. It's just a symptom of one. However, educating the patient on consciously slowing her breathing—using slow, deep breaths—may help abort the panic attack. In fact, there's an app for that. Refer patients to Breathe2Relax (or similar apps). Quiet rooms and reassurance can also help.

You begin to discuss treatment options with this patient.

Question 23.6.8 Which of the following is NOT an effective treatment of panic disorder?

A) Benzodiazepines such as clonazepam (Klonopin)
B) Bupropion (Wellbutrin)
C) Psychotherapy such as CBT
D) SSRIs such as fluoxetine (Prozac)
E) TCAs such as imipramine

Answer 23.6.8 The correct answer is "B." Bupropion is not the best choice for anxiety disorders as it can exacerbate anxiety in many patients. More effective medications include SSRIs, SNRIs, and TCAs; no class has proven superior, and medication choice is based on safety, comorbid illnesses, tolerability, adverse effect profile, history of substance use, cost, etc. SSRIs are frequently considered first line. Psychotherapy has been found to be as effective as medications for the treatment of mild-to-moderate panic disorder and can be used in combination with medications for more severe cases.

As you decide on the medication and dosage, you remember an article you just read in a journal on common mistakes made by physicians treating panic disorder in the community.

Question 23.6.9 Which of these is NOT one of the common mistakes made in the treatment of panic disorder?

A) Starting the SSRI too high
B) Not achieving a high-enough target dose
C) Underutilization of benzodiazepines
D) Too slow a titration
E) Often using medications not proven to work with panic disorder

Answer 23.6.9 The correct answer is "C." Far from being underutilized, **benzodiazepines are often overprescribed**. While effective for panic disorder, problems with tolerance, dependence, and abuse limit benzodiazepines as long-term agents for panic disorder. Patients with panic disorder are extremely sensitive to medication side effects and are likely to suffer from jitteriness and restlessness if started at a high dose of an SSRI. In order to reduce the chances of precipitating jitteriness and restlessness, a lower dose of SSRI (about half the starting dose used to treat depression) is usually recommended. The same problems can occur with rapidly increasing doses of SSRIs, so "start low and go slow," increasing the dose every 2 to 4 weeks to reach the maximum allowable dose. Benzodiazepines are at least third line (after CBT and SSRIs). *A plea: avoid alprazolam (Xanax) like the plague.* It is addictive, short-acting, and has a rebound effect which may be indistinguishable from a panic attack/anxiety disorder even after missing or being late for **one** dose. Short-acting drugs such as alprazolam often lead to withdrawal symptoms and subsequent abuse. If you are going to choose a benzodiazepine, choose one that is longer acting such as clonazepam or diazepam. Taper benzodiazepines as soon as possible. Avoid them in patients with severe personality disorders and substance abuse.

Your patient says, "I know another female in the reserve who has something similar, but I've never noticed the guys to have a problem. Is this just something that happens to women?" You tell her a bit about gender differences in anxiety disorders.

Question 23.6.10 Which of these is NOT true about the gender ratio of the following disorders?
A) Generalized anxiety disorder affects more women than men in a 2:1 ratio
B) Panic disorder affects more women than men in a 2:1 ratio
C) PTSD affects more men than women in a 2:1 ratio
D) Social anxiety disorder affects slightly more women than men

Answer 23.6.10 The correct answer is "C." Many affective illnesses (mood and anxiety disorders) including depression and some anxiety disorders are socially determined sexist: women are more likely to be affected than men. All of the options listed are correct except "C," which inverts the true ratio.

▶ **Objectives: Did you learn to …**
  · Evaluate patients with anxiety symptoms?
  · Recognize panic attacks and diagnose panic disorder?
  · Initiate treatment of panic disorder?
  · Describe some epidemiologic issues with anxiety disorders?

▶ CASE 23.7

You have a 34-year-old male patient who has started sustained-release bupropion (Wellbutrin SR) 150 mg BID for depression. He reports partial but not total resolution in his symptoms. He also thinks that the medication is causing some side effects.

Question 23.7.1 Which of the following is the most likely adverse effect attributable to this medication?
A) Insomnia
B) Sexual dysfunction
C) Weight gain
D) QT prolongation
E) Nicotine cravings

Answer 23.7.1 The correct answer is "A." Bupropion is associated with vivid dreams and insomnia. Taking the second dose no later than 4 PM can help reduce this of this side effect (or use a long-acting bupropion preparation). Unlike most other antidepressants, bupropion is not associated with sexual dysfunction or weight gain. In fact, it has been associated with weight loss in the short term, and patients who quit smoking are less likely to gain weight if they are taking it. Bupropion can cause dry mouth and nausea, which are usually self-limited. It does not cause QT prolongation, unlike TCAs, some SNRIs, and citalopram/escitalopram. Bupropion appears to curb the cravings for nicotine. It lowers the seizure threshold and should be avoided in patients with epilepsy.

This patient is relatively healthy and takes no other medications, giving you a wide number of options for treatment. In other words, you did not have to think too hard before starting bupropion. However, sometimes you have to use your brain, so let's think about when not to use bupropion.

Question 23.7.2 In which of the following disease states would bupropion be contraindicated?
A) Hypertension
B) Severe depression
C) Bulimia nervosa (BN)
D) Bipolar depression
E) Borderline personality disorder

Answer 23.7.2 The correct answer is "C." Bupropion is contraindicated in patients with anorexia nervosa (AN) or BN (an increased risk of seizures is found in both diseases) or a current or past seizure disorder. Don't use bupropion in patients taking an MAOI because of the risk of hypertension. Bupropion is as effective as the other antidepressants, and it can be used in bipolar depression (with extreme caution) and severe depression.

He makes a change in his dosing to move the second daily dose earlier and works on some sleep hygiene and meditation, but his insomnia persists. You decide to switch his medication from bupropion to citalopram (Celexa).

Question 23.7.3 Which is the best way to accomplish this switch?
A) Stop the bupropion immediately and then wait for 2 weeks before starting citalopram
B) Taper the bupropion over 2 weeks to avoid a discontinuation syndrome, and then start the citalopram
C) Start citalopram immediately, and then taper the bupropion over several days
D) Start citalopram now, then taper off the bupropion a couple of weeks later if he is doing well

Answer 23.7.3 **The correct answer is "C."** Unlike SSRIs, which can cause a serotonin withdrawal syndrome (see below), bupropion can be discontinued with a minimal (if any) taper. A brief taper may avoid a sudden rebound of depressive symptoms, while the new agent is started. "A" is incorrect. Bupropion can be taken with an SSRI. However, "D" is less desirable, as it is preferable to stop the bupropion rather than continuing it indefinitely while taking another medication, especially since the patient is experiencing side effects. A single effective agent is generally preferred if possible.

▶ **Objectives: Did you learn to …**
- Use bupropion appropriately?
- Identify adverse effects of bupropion?
- Recommend strategies to transition from bupropion to another antidepressant?

 QUICK QUIZ: HOMESICK

A 22-year-old college student who moved to your town from Lagos, Nigeria, last month is referred to you by his academic advisor for concerns that he may be depressed. Although he speaks English well, he does not know anyone in town. His family is still in Lagos, and he does not anticipate returning to see them anytime soon. He has not made many friends yet. He enjoys watching soccer in his spare time (which, of course, nobody in the United States appreciates, but that is another matter and it is still more interesting than Cricket). He is not sleeping well and he feels quite homesick.

Which of the following is the most appropriate diagnosis at this time?
A) MDD
B) Adjustment disorder
C) Bipolar affective disorder
D) Dysthymia
E) Footballer's withdrawal syndrome

The correct answer is "B." Adjustment disorder describes a cluster of symptoms that may include emotional or behavioral symptoms that occur in response to identifiable stressor(s). Symptoms must start within 3 months of the onset of the stressor(s) and there should be no other psychological diagnosis that accounts for the symptoms, such as MDD. The patient's distress should be above and beyond that which would be expected from exposure to the stressor. There should be impairment in social or occupational/academic functioning. The patient's symptoms cannot be due to bereavement (a separate diagnosis). Once the stressor is eliminated, the symptoms should resolve within 6 months. Treatment depends on the level of distress and can range from supportive care to active intervention with medications, therapy, or hospitalization. There are several subtypes of adjustment disorder including: with depressed mood, with anxiety, with disturbance of conduct, and mixed episodes.

▶ **CASE 23.8**

An 85-year-old woman is brought to the emergency department by her daughters because she has been acting strangely lately. Her house is a mess, even though for most of her life she has been quite fastidious. She has been calling her daughters at odd hours of the night, upset and insisting that her youngest daughter is stealing her money. During the day, she goes outside of her house in her nightgown and housecoat, again quite unlike her usual customs. Four months ago, her husband of 58 years was diagnosed with a brain tumor. His condition has deteriorated quite rapidly, and he is now in a nursing home and does not recognize his wife or daughters. The daughters have attributed the patient's odd behavior to the stress she is under. But as her symptoms have continued to worsen, they have become quite concerned and decided to bring her in for evaluation.

In the emergency department, the patient is dressed in her housecoat and slippers and appears disheveled. She is lying on a cart, but she keeps trying to get up and leave. She is angry at her two daughters who are with her, and she is uncooperative with the physical examination. When you ask her about what has been happening, she appears distrusting, and her answers do not make sense.

Question 23.8.1 **Which of the following diagnoses is LEAST likely at this point in time?**
A) Delirium
B) Dementia
C) Bereavement
D) Psychotic depression
E) Alcohol abuse

Answer 23.8.1 **The correct answer is "C."** Although your patient's husband is gravely ill and she is grieving, her symptoms are more severe than what is expected for bereavement. Bereavement is a normal process, but it does not include severe impairment in social or occupational functioning, nor does it include paranoid delusions or other psychotic symptoms. All of the other diagnoses listed could result in the severity of symptoms described in this case.

Question 23.8.2 **Which of the following tests is indicated in the evaluation of this patient's behavior changes?**
A) Chest x-ray
B) Urinalysis
C) CBC
D) Vitamin B12 levels
E) All of the above

Answer 23.8.2 **The correct answer is "E."** A thorough medical workup is warranted in the patient with "mental status changes" (e.g., delirium and new-onset psychotic symptoms). Several medical problems—infection, hypoxia, MI, to name a few—can cause the symptoms the patient is experiencing and must be ruled out.

Her workup does not reveal an organic cause for her altered mental state. You are now suspecting that she has psychotic depression.

Question 23.8.3 All of the following are appropriate management options at this time EXCEPT:
A) Discharge with referral for outpatient psychotherapy
B) Admission to a psychiatric unit
C) ECT (electroconvulsive therapy)
D) Psychiatric consultation

Answer 23.8.3 The correct answer is "A." Psychotherapy is not an appropriate single therapy for psychotic depression—especially in this patient, whose symptoms are so severe. "B" is appropriate, as the patient may benefit from hospitalization. "C" is appropriate as well. ECT is effective in treating psychotic depression and is often indicated if safety is of immediate concern or an early response is needed. "D" is appropriate. In general, patients with psychotic depression should be referred to a psychiatrist.

HELPFUL TIP: A STIMULATING THOUGHT
In recent years, there have been some advancements in brain stimulation therapies for mental health disorders. Repetitive Transcranial Magnetic Stimulation (rTMS) was approved by the FDA in 2008, but didn't gain popularity until 2010 when a study by the National Institute for Mental Health found a fourfold greater rate of remission in patients with resistant depression compared to sham therapy (*Arch Gen Psych*. 2010 May;67(5): 507–516). Benefits of rTMS are that it only takes 30 to 60 minutes, does not require anesthesia, and is more targeted than ECT. Subsequent data is less compelling, but it is still a viable alternative.

Vagus nerve stimulation (VNS) was initially improved for treatment of resistant epilepsy, but was found to have beneficial effects in resistant depression. It was approved by the FDA in 2005 to treat resistant depression if the following conditions are met: patients > 18 years old, depressive illness x 2 years or more, severe or recurrent depression, and depression has not eased after trial of four different treatments. The most rigorous data suggests vagus nerve stimulation is not effective for depression.

Stay tuned as Deep Brain Stimulation (DBS) (yes, the one initially developed for treatment of Parkinson's) and Magnetic Seizure Therapy (MST) are also being developed and studied as possible treatments for mental health disorders.

You determine that your patient's symptoms are severe enough for hospitalization. Her daughters agree, but the patient is adamantly opposed and insists on returning to her home. She's sick of you "NSA-types pushing her around (the one government agency that actually listens to you!)," and

"if you don't let her go, she's going call her friend, Donald Trump."

Question 23.8.4 How would you proceed?
A) Call hospital security and make plans to hospitalize her; after all, she appears quite ill and cannot care for herself; when she is well, she will understand that it was the right plan
B) Discharge her home, asking her daughters to take turns staying with her until she is better
C) Follow state-dictated protocol to attempt to obtain a legal order for hospitalization against her will
D) Follow national protocol (New World Order Directive 55.12.A) to attempt to obtain a legal order for hospitalization against her will
E) Make a medical determination that she is not competent, allowing you to hospitalize her despite her objection

Answer 23.8.4 The correct answer is "C." Each state has its own laws that govern how an involuntary hospitalization process is conducted. If the patient poses an imminent threat to herself or others, the law generally allows involuntary hospitalization for a brief period of time until a court hearing is held. Involuntary hospitalization is also allowed if the patient is unable to care for herself and she is suffering from a mental illness that renders her incapable of making healthcare decisions (of course if there are surrogates/durable power of attorney for healthcare, they can help with the decision). "D" is incorrect. There are no national laws governing involuntary hospitalization (and the New World Order is a paranoid delusion of some extremists … or maybe we just want you to believe that). "B" is incorrect. Because of the severity of this patient's symptoms, it would be inappropriate and unsafe to simply discharge her to the care of her daughters.

You have admitted the patient under a 72-hour hold, and you are discussing treatment options with the psychiatrist, who thinks that ECT might be appropriate. You are concerned about cognitive problems in this patient.

Question 23.8.5 All of the following are associated with an increased risk of memory loss with ECT EXCEPT:
A) Bilateral electrode placement
B) High stimulus doses
C) History of seizure disorder
D) Baseline cognitive functioning
E) Type of anesthesia

Answer 23.8.5 The correct answer is "C." A history of seizure disorder is not associated with an increased risk of memory loss with ECT. ECT is known to cause transient problems with memory loss. This usually manifests with the patient having trouble remembering events that occur around the time of the ECT. Most of the memory complaints completely resolve within a few months of completing ECT. However, some situations may increase the risk of memory loss, including bilateral electrode placement (unilateral is safer) and a higher stimulus dose.

In further discussions with the patient and her family, you try to explain ECT and dispel some myths.

Question 23.8.6 All of the following are potential complications or adverse effects of ECT EXCEPT:
A) Delirium
B) Nonsustained ventricular tachycardia
C) Headache
D) Dementia
E) Fatigue

Answer 23.8.6 The correct answer is "D." Although transient memory loss and even delirium can occur after ECT, it does not cause dementia. A number of cardiac rhythm disturbances can occur and are more likely in patients with cardiac disease. However, these are self-limited and generally minor (e.g., premature ventricular contractions, atrial premature complexes, and nonsustained ventricular tachycardia). Headache and fatigue are common after ECT.

▶ **Objectives: Did you learn to …**
- Recognize abnormal behavior and generate an appropriate differential diagnosis?
- Evaluate a patient with new cognitive and behavioral problems?
- Determine when involuntary hospitalization is appropriate and how it might be undertaken?
- Discuss potential adverse effects of ECT?

 QUICK QUIZ: A REALLY BAD WEEK

A 47-year-old female presents to your clinic in tears, requesting your help. She cannot stop crying, her sleep is poor, and she feels terribly lonely. However, she is able to carry out all life functions with little decrement in ability. She tells you that last week her mother had a stroke. Her mother survived, but is now in a nursing home and suffering from Broca's aphasia. Your patient describes her mother as her "best friend." She has not had trouble with depression or other mental illness in the past.

Which of the following is the most likely diagnosis?
A) Bereavement
B) Adjustment disorder
C) MDD
D) Bipolar affective disorder
E) Dysthymia

The correct answer is "A." Bereavement is a natural reaction to a significant loss. Some of the symptoms may mimic those of depression or adjustment disorder, which can throw you off the track of making the proper diagnosis. Unlike bereavement, both depression and adjustment disorder must, by definition, cause *significant impairment*. In bereavement, feelings of emptiness or loss tend to predominate while MDD is associated with more persistent depression. Additionally, in bereavement self-esteem tends to remain intact, while in MDD people often have feelings of worthlessness. Our patient has only a minor decrement in her level of functioning. The duration and expression of bereavement differs among different cultural groups and subgroups, further complicating the diagnostic process.

▶ **CASE 23.9**

You get a call from a patient complaining of "not feeling well and getting worse" over the past 3 days. She has had electrical shock sensations in her upper extremities and head and also complains of dizziness and malaise. She takes no medications since she self-discontinued her paroxetine (Paxil) and bupropion (Wellbutrin) a few days ago.

Question 23.9.1 Which of the following is the most likely diagnosis?
A) Influenza
B) Bupropion discontinuation syndrome
C) SSRI discontinuation syndrome
D) Serotonin syndrome
E) Hypertensive crisis

Answer 23.9.1 The correct answer is "C." OK, so this was a soft pitch. We already told you above that bupropion does not have a discontinuation syndrome. A discontinuation syndrome (also known as withdrawal syndrome) has been associated with SSRIs when they are suddenly stopped or doses are missed or reduced. This is especially common with paroxetine (Paxil) because of its short half-life. The symptoms described above are typical of the discontinuation syndrome, particularly the paresthesias that patients often describe as an "electric shock" (Table 23-1).

TABLE 23-1 SYMPTOMS OF SSRI DISCONTINUATION SYNDROME

Somatic Symptoms
- Disequilibrium (e.g., dizziness, vertigo, ataxia, and tremor)
- Gastrointestinal symptoms (e.g., nausea, vomiting, and anorexia)
- Flu-like symptoms (e.g., fatigue, lethargy, myalgias, chills, and headache)
- Sensory disturbances (e.g., paresthesias and sensations of electric shock)
- Sleep disturbances (e.g., insomnia and vivid dreams)

Psychological Problems
- Anxiety/agitation
- Crying spells
- Irritability
- Overactivity
- Depersonalization
- Decreased concentration/slowed thinking
- Confusion and memory problems

Question 23.9.2 **Which of the options below is INCORRECT information to give the patient over the telephone?**
A) Symptoms usually begin within a few days of stopping the SSRI
B) The symptoms rarely last longer for 2 weeks and are self-limited
C) Restarting the medication takes about 2 weeks to relieve symptoms
D) The longer the patient has been on the medication, the more likely the risk of a discontinuation syndrome

Answer 23.9.2 **The correct answer (or INCORRECT answer) is "C."** Symptoms can be noticeable in some patients with just one missed dose (especially with paroxetine [Paxil]), but typically develop within 2 days of medication discontinuation. The syndrome is uncomfortable but usually self-limited, lasting <2 weeks. Restarting the medication will lead to cessation of symptoms within 24 hours in virtually all cases. The risk of discontinuation increases with length of therapy, particularly when the patient has been on an SSRI longer than 7 weeks.

Question 23.9.3 **Which SSRI is LEAST likely to cause a discontinuation syndrome?**
A) Fluoxetine (Prozac)
B) Sertraline (Zoloft)
C) Paroxetine (Paxil)
D) Citalopram (Celexa)
E) Fluvoxamine (Luvox)

Answer 23.9.3 **The correct answer is "A."** The risk of withdrawal increases with **shorter** half-lives. The half-life of fluoxetine (Prozac) is about 4 to 6 days, while its active metabolite norfluoxetine has a half-life up to 16 days, making it highly unlikely that fluoxetine would cause a discontinuation syndrome in most patients, as it effectively acts as its own taper. Fluvoxamine (Luvox) (with a half-life of 15 hours) and paroxetine (Paxil) (21 hours) have the shortest half-lives and are most likely to cause the discontinuation syndrome. To minimize the risk of withdrawal syndrome, taper off SSRIs when stopping them.

 HELPFUL TIP:
Discontinuation syndrome is likely a hyposerotonergic state; therefore, all serotonergic agents can cause a withdrawal syndrome. These agents include SSRIs, MAOIs, TCAs, serotonin–norepinephrine reuptake inhibitors (SNRIs), and mirtazapine (Remeron) … but not bupropion (is that horse dead or should we beat it some more?).

Your patient restarts her SSRI and feels better. She has questions about antidepressants in general, wondering if she is taking the right one. As you start to discuss benefits and risks of different medications, you remind yourself about some important issues. For example, all SSRIs are not the same.

Question 23.9.4 **Which SSRI has the most anticholinergic activity?**
A) Fluoxetine (Prozac)
B) Paroxetine (Paxil)
C) Sertraline (Zoloft)
D) Citalopram (Celexa)
E) Escitalopram (Lexapro)

Answer 23.9.4 **The correct answer is "B."** With the exception of paroxetine (Paxil), SSRIs do not possess appreciable anticholinergic activity. Do you get the idea we don't like paroxetine?

Question 23.9.5 **Which of the following SSRIs is LEAST likely to have drug–drug interactions via cytochrome P450 enzymes?**
A) Fluoxetine (Prozac)
B) Paroxetine (Paxil)
C) Citalopram (Celexa)
D) Sertraline (Zoloft)
E) Fluvoxamine (Luvox)

Answer 23.9.5 **The correct answer is "C."** Citalopram (Celexa) and its stereoisomer, escitalopram (Lexapro), have relatively clean profiles with no major interactions with any of the cytochrome P450 enzymes. Of course, this benefit of citalopram (Celexa) is tempered by its known problems with QT prolongation, which can be exacerbated by other QT prolonging drugs. Sertraline (Zoloft) is also an attractive option if drug–drug interactions are a concern. The other three have significant inhibition of CYP enzymatic pathways and drug–drug interactions that have clinical importance. Paroxetine and fluoxetine are potent inhibitors of the CYP2D6 enzymatic pathway, while fluvoxamine is a potent inhibitor of the CYPC19 pathway.

Question 23.9.6 **Mirtazapine (Remeron) is commonly associated with all of the following side effects EXCEPT:**
A) Sedation
B) Weight gain
C) Dizziness
D) Lycanthropy
E) Increased triglycerides

Answer 23.9.6 **The correct answer is "D."** Lycanthropy is, of course, the ability to transform into a werewolf. Although close in behavior to antisocial personality disorder, lycanthropy is NOT caused by mirtazapine but rather by the bite of another lycanthrope. Mirtazapine is a potent antihistamine, and an α2-adrenergic antagonist, potentially leading to orthostatic hypotension. Sedation is present in over 50% of patients taking the drug, while weight gain is reported in as many as 12%. It can also lead to increased triglycerides. Paradoxically, the side effect of sedation lessens with increasing doses. It is a great antidepressant for patients who have lost their appetite, lost weight, or have insomnia. Typical doses range from 15 to 60 mg/day, with a starting dose between 7.5 and 15 mg.

Question 23.9.7 Which of the following antidepressants has a black box warning about hepatic failure?

A) Nefazodone (Serzone)
B) Bupropion (Wellbutrin)
C) Paroxetine (Paxil)
D) Nortriptyline (Pamelor)
E) Phenelzine (Nardil)

Answer 23.9.7 **The correct answer is "A."** Nefazodone (Serzone) is a 5HT-2A receptor antagonist and is an effective antidepressant with sedative properties. It has significant inhibitory effects on CYP3A4 and has several significant drug interactions as a result. In the recent past, several cases of hepatic failure have been reported with this drug, leading to a black box warning on the package insert and limiting its clinical use. None of the other antidepressants listed have had such problems.

Question 23.9.8 Venlafaxine (Effexor) has been noted to typically cause all of the following side effects EXCEPT:

A) Increased blood pressure
B) Dizziness
C) Dry mouth
D) Weight gain
E) Sexual disturbance

Answer 23.9.8 **The correct answer is "D."** Venlafaxine (Effexor) and duloxetine (Cymbalta) are both norepinephrine and serotonin reuptake inhibitors and have minimal activity on the cholinergic, histaminergic, and α-receptors. There is a dose-related increase in blood pressure ("A"), with a mean elevation of 10 to 15 mm Hg in diastolic pressure at doses of 300 mg or greater in up to 10% of patients. There is a slight increase in pulse, as well. "D" is not true. In fact, weight loss is a common complaint. Otherwise, venlafaxine (Effexor) and duloxetine (Cymbalta) generally have the same side-effect profile as the SSRIs, potentially causing sexual dysfunction ("E"), dizziness ("B"), and dry mouth ("C"). Patients can have a significant withdrawal from venlafaxine mimicking a "flu-like" illness and should be tapered off it slowly.

 HELPFUL TIP: ANTIDEPRESSANTS AND BIRTH DEFECTS
Fluoxetine (Prozac) and paroxetine (Paxil) are **associated** with birth defects in some studies. Most studies do not control for maternal mental illness, which is likely a confounding variable. This doesn't prove causality and the chance is slight (e.g., anencephaly risk goes from 2 in 10,000 to 7 in 10,000). However, it is worth discussing risks and benefits with the prospective parents. The other SSRIs do not seem to have the same association (*BMJ.* 2015;351:h3190). SSRI *do* predispose to persistent pulmonary hypertension of the newborn. We still don't like paroxetine (Paxil).

 HELPFUL (AND SCARY) TIP:
Venlafaxine (Effexor) and duloxetine (Cymbalta) are toxic in overdose. They cause QT and QRS prolongation in overdose. Treatment is the same as the treatment of TCA overdose (bicarbonate, etc.), although data is limited. Remember that citalopram (Celexa)/escitalopram (Lexapro) can cause a prolonged QT interval with both regular doses and in overdose.

You decide to switch the patient to fluoxetine (Prozac) and she does well.

▶ **Objectives: Did you learn to …**
· Identify SSRI discontinuation syndrome?
· Recognize important antidepressant interactions?
· Describe adverse effects of various antidepressants?

 QUICK QUIZ: MAOIS

You are seeing a new patient with a history of recurrent major depression. Many years ago a different physician put him on phenelzine (Nardil), which you recognize as having potentially serious food and drug interactions. You are considering switching him to an SSRI.

How long after an MAOI is discontinued can an SSRI be started?

A) 1 day
B) 3 days
C) 7 days
D) 14 days
E) SSRIs and MAOIs can be given together

The correct answer is "D." Because of significant drug–drug interactions (see next question), SSRIs should not be started until 2 weeks after discontinuation of an MAOI.

 QUICK QUIZ: MAOI + SSRI = BADNESS

What is the drug–drug interaction of concern with SSRIs and MAOIs?

A) Stevens–Johnson syndrome
B) Serotonin syndrome
C) Anticholinergic crisis
D) Hypertensive crisis
E) Existential crisis

The correct answer is "B." Serotonin syndrome is caused by an excess of serotonin and can be caused by drug–drug interactions involving serotonergic agents including SSRIs, buspirone (Buspar), meperidine (Demerol), dextromethorphan, lithium, tramadol (Ultram), and triptans, among others. MAOIs inhibit monoamine oxidase, which is an enzyme involved in the metabolism of many neurotransmitters, including serotonin. Therefore, MAOIs increase serotonin as well. Serotonin syndrome is characterized by muscle rigidity, hyperreflexia, hyperthermia, confusion, and agitation among other symptoms. It can be fatal. As a result, the concurrent use of an SSRI and MAOI is absolutely CONTRAINDICATED. Stevens–Johnson syndrome ("A") is an autoimmune dermatological disorder that leads to desquamation of mucosal surfaces and is not associated with antidepressant use (although it can be seen with other drugs). Anticholinergic crisis ("C") is not a term used in common medical parlance but does evoke the idea of anticholinergic syndrome, caused by excess anticholinergic drugs, such as TCAs, etc. (see Chapter 1). Hypertensive crisis ("D") occurs when foods containing tyramine (e.g., aged cheese and cured meats) interact with MAOIs to release catecholamines, causing hypertension, headaches, nausea, and diaphoresis. In severe cases, it can lead to strokes or death.

> **HELPFUL TIP(S):**
> Linezolid (Zyvox) is absolutely contraindicated with MAOIs. It is a serotonergic drug. Among the foods that cause a hypertensive crisis with an MAOI are banana peels (but not the banana … we are not sure who figured this one out …), aged meats (best avoided anyway if you think about it), draught beer (boo) but not bottled beer (yes!), and kimchi/sauerkraut.

► CASE 23.10

A 43-year-old man who you started on citalopram (Celexa) for depression 4 weeks ago returns for a follow-up visit. He feels better but complains of delayed ejaculation. You consider changing him to an antidepressant that is less likely to cause sexual dysfunction.

Question 23.10.1 Which of the following would you AVOID?
A) Nefazodone (Serzone)
B) Bupropion (Wellbutrin)
C) Mirtazapine (Remeron)
D) Trazodone (Desyrel, Oleptro)
E) Nortriptyline (Pamelor)

Answer 23.10.1 **The correct answer is "E."** Sexual dysfunction is a common side effect of most psychotropics. There are few controlled data to guide us as to how to approach this issue, but sildenafil (Viagra) and similar drugs are effective in antidepressant-induced erectile dysfunction. Of the options given, nortriptyline (Pamelor)—and other TCAs—are more frequently associated with sexual dysfunction.

> **HELPFUL TIP:**
> St. John's wort may be effective in mild-to-moderate depression. However, it is a known inducer of the CYP450 enzyme, reducing the efficacy of oral contraceptives.

It has also been associated with decreased efficacy of antiretrovirals, cyclosporine, digoxin, theophylline, and warfarin.

This patient is also having sleep difficulties and asks what herbal therapy he might be able to use.

Question 23.10.2 Which of the following is a herbal alternative to benzodiazepines for anxiety and insomnia?
A) Valerian root
B) St. John's wort
C) Saw palmetto
D) Ginseng
E) Ginkgo

Answer 23.10.2 **The correct answer is "A."** Valerian root (*Valeriana officinalis*) has been touted to have anxiolytic properties, similar to benzodiazepines, and its mechanism of action is thought to be similar (e.g., inhibition of GABA). It appears to be safe and has the same drug interactions and contraindications as benzodiazepines. The other options are not known to affect sleep to a significant degree.

> **HELPFUL TIP:**
> Kava-kava is advertised as an anxiolytic but should generally be avoided. Kava-kava (*Piper methysticum*) has been reported to cause liver damage, in some cases leading to liver transplant or eventual death.

► **Objectives: Did you learn to …**
  • Identify which antidepressants are less likely to cause sexual dysfunction?
  • Recognize herbal therapies that might be employed in treating symptoms of depression?

► CASE 23.11

You are seeing a 28-year-old female whose first child you delivered a month ago. She comes to your clinic with her son for his 1-month well-child check. You observe that she seems tired and is less animated than usual. She is gentle with her infant, but her face doesn't seem to light up with the glow that you often see with new mothers. You know … the glow of terror, sleeplessness, and anxiety? That's the one.

Question 23.11.1 Which of the following best explains your observations?
A) Sleep deprivation
B) Marital discord at home
C) Postpartum depression
D) Thyroid dysfunction
E) Any of the above

Answer 23.11.1 **The correct answer is "E."** Your patient's symptoms could be due to any of these problems and more, including difficulty with role adjustment, alcohol or drug abuse, and anemia.

You want to gather more information to see if there is a pathological process underlying her behavior.

Question 23.11.2 You would do all of the following EXCEPT:
A) Ask her to fill out an Edinburgh Postnatal Depression Scale (EPDS)
B) Order thyroid function tests
C) Order a sleep study
D) Ask more questions about how things are at home and how she is coping
E) Ask about a previous history of depression

Answer 23.11.2 **The correct answer is "C."** In this case, there are many other more likely problems than a primary sleep disorder, and a sleep study is unlikely to be helpful (plus as those of us who have had infants know, your sleep is naturally disordered). The EPDS is a validated self-rated scale that is useful for detecting postpartum depression. Hypothyroidism can always mimic depression and might need to be ruled out. A thorough history is always essential.

Question 23.11.3 The incidence of postpartum depression is about:
A) 1%
B) 10%
C) 30%
D) 50%

Answer 23.11.3 **The correct answer is "B."** About 7 in 10 women suffer from "baby blues," postpartum symptoms that can manifest as mood swings, anxiety, fatigue, and sadness occurring within a few days of delivery and lasting only a week or so. However, postpartum depression affects approximately 10% of women, and symptoms can appear anywhere from weeks to months after birth. The diagnosis is often missed because many mothers are ashamed to admit feeling unhappy at a time when they think (and society tells them) that they should be happy. Physicians may focus on the infant's physical health and miss assessing the mother–baby interaction.

In obtaining more history, you realize that this patient was having some troubles with depression even during her pregnancy.

Question 23.11.4 When is the most common time for pregnancy-related depression to occur?
A) At conception
B) First trimester
C) Second trimester
D) Third trimester
E) Postpartum

Answer 23.11.4 **The correct answer is "D."** A large epidemiological study from the United Kingdom followed pregnant women prospectively throughout the course of their pregnancies and found that the **incidence of depression was actually higher in the third trimester than it was in the postpartum period**. This suggests the need for the physician to begin to enquire about symptoms earlier. Updated USPSTF recommendations in 2016 for depression screening included screening pregnant and postpartum women. The EPDS, PHQ-9, or other screening tools can be used to assist with screening.

HELPFUL TIP:
Repeat after us, "Pregnancy does not treat depression." For some reason, it had been assumed in the past that a woman's depression would abate during pregnancy. Studies in the last couple of years have disproved this myth making ongoing treatment for depression crucial.

If you had been aware of her depression earlier and wanted to prescribe an antidepressant during her pregnancy, you would have been cautious, hoping to prescribe a drug with the most robust safety data in pregnancy—you're just that kind of doctor.

Question 23.11.5 Which of the following antidepressants is generally considered safest in pregnancy?
A) Sertraline (Zoloft)
B) Bupropion (Wellbutrin)
C) Nortriptyline (Pamelor)
D) Mirtazapine (Remeron)
E) Paroxetine (Paxil)

Answer 23.11.5 **The correct answer is "A."** There is no antidepressant (or any medication for that matter) that is 100% safe in pregnancy. There is also a growing field of study examining the impact of untreated maternal depression and other mental illness on pregnancy. This is not to say that antidepressants must be avoided in pregnancy, but the benefits and risks should be weighed carefully.

Question 23.11.6 Risks associated with SSRI use during pregnancy include all of the following EXCEPT:
A) Irritability of the neonate
B) Preterm delivery
C) Low birth weight
D) Persistent pulmonary hypertension
E) Tetralogy of Fallot

Answer 23.11.6 **The correct answer is "E."** SSRIs have not been linked to development of Tetralogy of Fallot. However, some studies suggest adverse effects with SSRI use in pregnancy, including neonatal irritability, low birth weight, and preterm labor. In many of the studies, it is difficult to determine whether adverse effects are related to the SSRI, maternal depression, or other factors. Infants exposed to SSRIs during the second half of pregnancy (i.e., after 20 weeks gestation) had an increased risk (approximately 1% absolute risk) of developing **persistent pulmonary hypertension, not a birth defect** but still a potentially life-threatening condition, after birth (*BMJ.* 2012;344:d8012). Other studies have not demonstrated this association, and more information is needed. Shared decision-making, including weighing the risks and benefits, with the patient is crucial. Mothertobaby.org and womensmentalhealth.org have resources to aid this discussion.

Question 23.11.7 If you had decided to prescribe an antidepressant medication for her during pregnancy, which one of the following would have been LEAST desirable?
A) Paroxetine (Paxil)
B) Sertraline (Zoloft)
C) Nortriptyline (Pamelor)
D) Citalopram (Celexa)

Answer 23.11.7 **The correct answer is "A."** Although no antidepressant medication has been shown to be risk-free when used during pregnancy, paroxetine (Paxil) is the only antidepressant with increased incidence of cardiac anomalies (mainly atrial and ventricular septal defects) in infants who were exposed in utero. Do you still think we don't like paroxetine?

You start her on sertraline (Zoloft) and offer to watch her baby for a few days (she's so cute!), and everyone is happy.

▶ **Objectives: Did you learn to …**
- Recognize the high incidence of depression and depressive symptoms in the postpartum period?
- Diagnose postpartum depression?
- Treat depression in the pregnant and postpartum patient?

▶ **CASE 23.12**

A couple, you have known for some time, brings in their 7-year-old son, Jimbo, to your clinic because his behavior has changed over the past month. His school performance has worsened, and he has started to get into fights at school. He is not eating as well and is having frequent nightmares. He now has frequent headaches and stomach aches and clings to his mother when it is time to go to school. The parents cannot understand what is going on and report no antecedent trauma.

Question 23.12.1 Which of the following is the most likely diagnosis?
A) MDD
B) Disruptive mood dysregulation disorder
C) Adjustment disorder
D) Bereavement
E) Normal childhood difficulties

Answer 23.12.1 **The correct answer is "A."** Up to 3% of children and 9% of adolescents suffer from depression. DSM-5 criteria are the same as in the adult, except **irritability can be**

substituted for the depressed mood requirement in children. Disruptive mood dysregulation disorder ("B") is a new addition to DSM-5. It is characterized by severe, persistent irritability. There must be frequent temper outbursts, grossly out of proportion to the inciting event, that occur over the course of at least a year and must be in two different settings. Symptoms are present before age 10. Adjustment disorder ("C") is not likely since there have been no major changes in the child's regimen, and bereavement ("D") is not likely since there have been no losses in the child's life. This patient's symptoms are clearly not part of normal childhood ("E"), even if his name is Jimbo.

HELPFUL TIP:
Of course, bullying at school and other social problems need to be investigated when any child presents with symptoms of depression.

Question 23.12.2 Which of the following is NOT true about depression in children?
A) Abuse or neglect increases the risk of depression
B) Having a depressed parent increases the risk of being a depressed child
C) The clinical course is roughly the same as in adults
D) "Masked" symptoms, such as abdominal pain, are more common in children than the typical symptoms of depression, such as sleep disturbance
E) Male and female children are equally affected by depression

Answer 23.12.2 **The correct answer is "D."** Although clinicians should be aware of age-appropriate manifestations (see Table 23-2), symptoms of depression are similar in children and adults. In fact, typical symptoms of depression are more common in children than are "masked" symptoms such as stomach aches and fear of leaving home.

You tell the family about Jimbo's prognosis.

TABLE 23-2 COMMON MANIFESTATIONS OF DEPRESSION IN CHILDREN

- Being bored
- Reckless behavior
- Outbursts of shouting, complaining, unexplained irritability, or crying
- Poor school performance
- Fear of death
- Alcohol or substance abuse
- Frequent nonspecific physical complaints such as headaches, muscle aches, stomach aches, or fatigue

Depression in Children and Adolescents, National Institutes of Health Publication No. 00-4744. http://www.nimh.nih.gov/publicat/depchildresfact.cfm.

Question 23.12.3 **Which of the following statements regarding prognosis is FALSE?**
A) Childhood MDD confers a two- to fourfold increase in risk for adult MDD
B) About 25% of adolescents with MDD develop substance abuse disorders
C) Almost half of children with MDD will attempt suicide sometime in their life
D) Roughly 20% of adolescents have suffered at least one episode of MDD by age 18, while 65% report transient symptoms of depression
E) After the initial episode, only 10% of children/adolescents will suffer a relapse

Answer 23.12.3 **The correct answer is "E."** Between half and two-thirds (**not** 10%) of children/adolescents will have a recurrence within 5 years after resolution of their first episode. The other options are all true. In children and adolescents, the mean depression episode length is 7 to 9 months with remission typically occurring over 1.5 to 2 years.

HELPFUL TIP:
The risk of suicide is very high among depressed youths. It is the third leading cause of death in the 15- to 24-year age group, and children with MDD have a four- to fivefold higher lifetime incidence of suicide attempts than non-depressed children. Fifteen to twenty percent of adolescents have suicidal ideation each year, and 5% to 8% will attempt suicide each year. Pretty depressing statistics, eh?

You recommend treatment for Jimbo.

Question 23.12.4 **Which of the following therapies has NOT shown efficacy in childhood depression in randomized controlled trials?**
A) Fluoxetine (Prozac)
B) Sertraline (Zoloft)
C) Cognitive Behavioral Therapy (CBT)
D) Venlafaxine (Effexor)
E) Interpersonal therapy (IPT)

Answer 23.12.4 **The correct answer is "D."** Early reports have demonstrated concerns of increased incidence of emotional lability with use of venlafaxine (Effexor) in children. More importantly, venlafaxine (Effexor) lacks efficacy data in children. The bottom line is that fluoxetine (Prozac) is probably the SSRI of choice in children, followed by sertraline (Zoloft). The number needed to treat for SSRIs is 10 to benefit one child; it may be as low as 4 for fluoxetine (Prozac). Avoid paroxetine (Paxil) since it may be associated with a higher suicide risk (there is a pattern developing here …). TCAs should be avoided because of lack of efficacy and potential suicide risk. Cognitive behavioral therapy and interpersonal therapy ("C" and "E") have been shown to be effective in children and adolescents.

HELPFUL TIP:
As you would expect, CBT/counseling/therapy plus an antidepressant are more effective than either modality alone. Adverse effects of medication in children are similar to those in adults and include: insomnia, fatigue, headaches, and nervousness. Suicidal thoughts, but not completed suicide, are more common in children and adolescents with SSRI treatment which has led to a black box warning being placed by the US Food and Drug Association (FDA) on SSRI agents for children and adolescents in 2004. This was further extended to the age of 25 in 2006. Despite this, the benefits of antidepressant therapy and SSRIs are felt to outweigh these risks. Moral of the story: Keep a close eye on adolescents who you start on antidepressants, and warn patients and their parents that depression can worsen in the early phase of treatment. Have them return often in the first few months of treatment.

▶ **Objectives: Did you learn to …**
· Increase your awareness of childhood depression?
· Diagnose depression in children?
· Describe the natural history of depression in children?
· Generate an appropriate treatment plan for children with depression?

▶ **CASE 23.13**

Tommy is a 9-year-old male who has been having difficulty with his behavior since he started first grade. He is often fidgety and squirming in his chair and has difficulty remaining in his seat. He talks out of turn, is often "on the go," and is not liked by the other kids because he intrudes into games and has a hard time waiting his turn. His mom also notes similar problems at home. He is the product of an uncomplicated pregnancy and has no significant past medical history.

Question 23.13.1 **What is the most likely diagnosis?**
A) Attention-deficit/hyperactivity disorder (ADHD)
B) Adjustment disorder
C) Oppositional defiant disorder (ODD)
D) Conduct disorder (CD)
E) Specific learning disorder

Answer 23.13.1 **The correct answer is "A."** The symptoms of ADHD are listed here. "B," adjustment disorder, is unlikely since there is no history of a significant life event. ODD ("C") and CD ("D") are characterized by aggressive behavior and a disregard for rules and adults. These are not given as part of Tommy's history. Specific learning disorders ("E") present with school performance problems and may be associated with ADHD, but would not be directly responsible for this patient's hyperactivity.

For the diagnosis of ADHD, patients must meet one of the following criteria:

1. At least six symptoms of inattention for at least 6 months that is maladaptive and inconsistent with the level of development:

   - Careless mistakes, poor attention to details
   - Cannot sustain attention
   - Does not seem to listen
   - Poor follow through on tasks
   - Difficulties with organization
   - Avoids or dislikes tasks that require sustained attention
   - Often loses things required for a task (notebooks, pens, etc.)
   - Easily distracted from a task
   - Forgetful in daily activities

2. Six or more of the following hyperactive–impulsive symptoms for 6 months, which are maladaptive and inconsistent with the level of development:

   - Hyperactivity symptoms
   - Fidgets or squirms in seat
   - Leaves seat at inappropriate times
   - Hyperactivity in inappropriate settings
   - Cannot play or relax quietly
   - Always in motion
   - Talks too much

   Impulsivity symptoms

   - Blurts out answer before questions completed
   - Trouble waiting for turn in games, school, etc.
   - Interrupts others (verbally, in games, etc.)

3. In addition to fulfilling criteria 1 and/or 2 above, the following are required:

   - Symptoms must be present *before* age of 12 years.
   - Impairment in two settings (home, work, school, worship, etc.)
   - Clinically significant impairment in social, academic, or occupational spheres
   - Symptoms are not due to another problem (developmental delay, personality disorder, mood disorder, etc.)

Question 23.13.2 Which of the following is FALSE about ADHD?

A) It affects 3% to 7% of children
B) There are genetic and environmental influences on the risk of developing ADHD
C) Males are more likely to be diagnosed with ADHD than females
D) The incidence of ADHD has increased over the years
E) Comorbid disorders are not common

Answer 23.13.2 **The correct answer is "E."** ADHD affects 3% to 7% of children. Heritability is 70%, similar to that for schizophrenia and bipolar disorder. Alcohol and tobacco exposure in utero have both been linked to at least a twofold increase in risk. Males are twice as likely to be diagnosed with ADHD as females. Comorbid disorders are very common in ADHD with CD, ODD, depression, anxiety, learning disabilities, and developmental delay being the most frequently seen.

Question 23.13.3 Which of the following is NOT TRUE of the prognosis and treatment of Tommy's ADHD?

A) The natural history of ADHD is that one-third of children will outgrow the symptoms, one-third will have the same frequency and intensity of symptoms, and one-third will have residual symptoms, which are subclinical
B) Tommy has a 70% to 80% chance of responding to stimulants
C) If Tommy is treated with stimulants, his risk of drug abuse is halved
D) Tommy is at increased risk of getting into accidents
E) Behavior therapy is effective for reducing ADHD symptoms

Answer 23.13.3 **The correct answer is "E."** Unfortunately, intensive behavior therapy has been shown to be ineffective. The breakdown of the prognosis for children with ADHD symptoms is that roughly one-third will experience complete symptom resolution, one-third will get some improvement, and one-third will remain ill with the disorder. Stimulants, which are first-line therapy, will work in 70% to 80% of the patients. If a patient does not respond to the first stimulant, there is still a 70% to 80% chance of responding to a second stimulant. Children treated with stimulants are half as likely to abuse substances as those who are not treated. Children with ADHD are at risk for impulsive behavior and risk-taking, which leads to substance abuse, accidents, etc. There are nonstimulant medication options as well. Atomoxetine, (Strattera) guanfacine (Tenex), and clonidine (Catapres) are all FDA approved for the treatment of ADHD.

You decide to start Tommy on methylphenidate.

Question 23.13.4 Which of the following is NOT true about treatment with methylphenidate?

A) It improves handwriting
B) Optimal dosing is 0.6 to 1 mg/kg/day
C) It can cause reduced growth
D) Short-term memory is not affected
E) Tommy might get along better with his classmates

Answer 23.13.4 **The correct answer is "D."** In fact, stimulants improve short-term memory in patients with ADHD. The rest are true. As to "A," do you think this is why doctors have notoriously bad handwriting? Maybe we all need stimulants.... Stimulants have a widespread effect on multiple domains, some of which are listed in Table 23-3.

Tommy's father is happy with his son's response to methylphenidate and wonders if he too would benefit from a similar medication. He recalls being in trouble ever since grade school for talking "out of turn" and always being put in detention. He was always restless and fidgety, but this has improved as he has aged. He has a hard time at work sitting through meetings, as he tends to daydream, and he has numerous fights with his wife because she accuses him of not listening to her. He has been unable to get promoted because he cannot pass the examinations he has to take, but he thinks that he is smart enough. He says that he just cannot concentrate.

TABLE 23-3 STIMULANT EFFECTS ON PATIENTS WITH ADHD

Effects of Stimulants on Motor Response
- Reduce activity to normal
- Decrease excessive talking, noise, and disruption in the classroom
- Improve handwriting
- Improve fine motor control

Effects of Stimulants on Social Skills
- Reduce off-task behavior in classroom
- Improve ability to play and work independently
- Decrease intensity of behavior
- Reduce bossiness with peers
- Reduce verbal and physical aggression
- Improve (but not normalize) peer social status
- Reduce noncompliance, defiance, and oppositional behavior with adults
- Parents and teachers become less controlling and more positive

Effects of Stimulants on Cognitive Ability
- Improve ability to sustain attention, especially in boring tasks (like studying for the FM Board Exam)
- Reduce distractibility
- Improve short-term memory
- Reduce impulsivity
- Increase amount of academic work completed
- Increase accuracy of academic work

Side Effects
- Lack of appetite
- Decreased growth, especially initially
- Insomnia
- Headaches and stomach aches
- Irritability
- Tachycardia or blood pressure increase (rare)
- Muscle tics or switches (rare)
- Psychosis or delirium (rare)

TABLE 23-4 PRESENTATIONS OF ADHD SYMPTOMS IN CHILDREN AND ADULTS

Children	Adults
Hyperactive child: squirms, cannot stay in his seat, and constantly on the go	*Hyperactive adult*: has subjective inner restlessness and trouble relaxing
Impulsive child: blurts out answers, interrupts others, and talks incessantly	*Impulsive adult*: speeding tickets, car crashes, impatient, smokes more, higher divorce rate, higher substance use rate, and overeating
Inattentive child: does not follow through, is forgetful, does not listen Fewer enter college and graduate, compared with children their age without ADHD	*Inattentive adult*: often late for appointments, forgets anniversaries, has difficulty with work meetings; problems with focusing, planning, organizing, and completing tasks at home and at work; advances more slowly at work than peers; misplaces keys, glasses, and other items; may forget to pay bills, pick up the kids on time, etc.

compensate by pursuing careers that reward their intellectual curiosity, endless energy, and desire for change (like family medicine?). Table 23-4 compares adult and child presentations of ADHD.

 HELPFUL TIP:
Remember that an adult who had ADHD as a child may have residual symptoms, which do not meet full criteria for ADHD at the time of evaluation. A clear history of symptoms starting in childhood before age 12 must be present to diagnose an adult with ADHD. **There is no such thing as "Adult-Onset ADHD" in DSM-5 (but there is such thing as adult stimulant abuse).** Confirmation of the history can be obtained from collateral sources, including old school reports and family members. Think about other diagnoses such as anxiety disorder and depression in patients who think they have "adult-onset ADHD."

Question 23.13.5 Which of the statements below is NOT true for an adult presenting with ADHD?
A) Adults present with the same core symptoms as children but in a different fashion
B) Adults are less likely to have overt hyperactivity symptoms compared with children
C) Adults often present when their children are diagnosed
D) Adults are less likely to smoke than same-age persons without ADHD
E) Adults often seek professions that allow them to use their symptoms to their advantage

Answer 23.13.5 The correct answer is "D." Adults with ADHD are more likely to smoke than their same-aged peers (perhaps it's because nicotine is a stimulant?). Adults present differently than children, but have the same core symptoms of hyperactivity, inattention, and impulsivity. Many adults are diagnosed with ADHD only when their children have been diagnosed or when increasing difficulty at work or at home leads them to seek help. Often, comorbidities drive them to seek help, and the primary diagnosis of ADHD is made only incidentally. Adults typically present seeking help for their inattention and concentration difficulties, as overt hyperactivity lessens with age. Some adults

After thorough history and evaluation, you decide to treat Tommy's father with a medication. He would prefer not to have a stimulant, and he asks if there are other options for treatment.

Question 23.13.6 Which of the following medications would you recommend?
A) Fluoxetine (Prozac)
B) Bupropion (Wellbutrin)
C) Mirtazapine (Remeron)
D) Phenelzine (Nardil)
E) Risperidone (Risperdal)

Answer 23.13.6 The correct answer is "B." In addition to stimulants, which are also first-line agents in adults, there are a variety of medications that can be used to treat ADHD, although most studies are undertaken in children and most of these medications are not FDA approved for treating ADHD. Second-line agents include the antidepressants bupropion (Wellbutrin), desipramine (Norpramin), imipramine (Tofranil), and nortriptyline (Pamelor). The α-blockers guanfacine (Tenex) and clonidine (Catapres) are also used, mostly as an adjunct in children with concomitant conduct disorder or sleep problems. Remember that a history of substance abuse or psychotic disorder should be carefully evaluated with cautious consideration of whether to initiate a stimulant vs. nonstimulant in a patient.

HELPFUL TIP:
Stimulants do not cause cardiac problems and seem to be safe in both children and adults (*JAMA.* 2011;306:2673; *JAMA.* 2011;306:2723; *N Engl J Med.* 2011;365: 1896). However, stimulants *can* increase heart rate and blood pressure, and these should be monitored carefully. Use of stimulants in those with underlying cardiac conditions is not well studied and generally avoided in those with serious heart conditions.

HELPFUL TIP:
Atomoxetine (Strattera) is a nonstimulant drug approved for ADHD (it is a selective norepinephrine reuptake inhibitor) and is the only nonstimulant drug approved by the FDA for adult ADHD. It is not a controlled prescription, as it has no apparent abuse potential. Its place in therapy is not yet well defined but might be used in those with a drug abuse history. Maximum efficacy of atomoxetine is achieved in a few weeks, and it has a similar side-effect profile to the stimulants.

▶ **Objectives: Did you learn to …**
- Recognize childhood and adult presentations of ADHD?
- Prescribe efficacious treatments for ADHD?
- Recognize side effects and advantages of various medications for ADHD?

▶ CASE 23.14

A gentleman calls your office because he is concerned that his wife of 2 years is acting strangely. She has not slept for most of the past week, staying up at night cleaning the house and sending multiple texts to friends and family. She even went out and spent $3000 on a dress that left nothing to the imagination and was seen kissing another man (Santa Claus, you hope). You ask him to bring his wife in as soon as possible.

That afternoon you find a provocatively dressed 30-year-old female sitting in your office and laughing giddily as her husband gives most of the intelligible history. She keeps reaching over to touch you on the leg as you interview her. You find her hard to understand because she talks so fast. You manage to catch something about "running for President."

Question 23.14.1 What is the most likely diagnosis?
A) Mania
B) Psychosis
C) Agitated depression
D) Anxiety disorder
E) ADHD

Answer 23.14.1 The correct answer is "A." Mania is the correct diagnosis. None of the other conditions can fully explain the abnormal elevation in mood and the subsequent behavior changes. Patients with **bipolar I disorder** must have had at least one episode of mania: a distinct period of abnormally and persistently elevated, expansive, or irritable mood, lasting at least 1 week (or any duration if hospitalization is necessary). In addition, there must be at least three of the following symptoms concurrently: (1) inflated self-esteem or grandiosity, (2) decreased need for sleep, (3) more talkative than usual, (4) flight of ideas or racing thoughts, (5) distractibility, (6) increased goal-directed activity or psychomotor agitation, and (7) excessive involvement in pleasurable activities that have a high risk for negative consequences/impulsivity (gambling, spending spree, risky sexual behaviors, etc.). The episode must cause impairment in occupational or social functioning and cannot be substance induced.

Patients with **bipolar II disorder** have had at least one episode of depression and one episode of hypomania: a distinct period of persistently elevated, expansive, or irritable mood, lasting for at least 4 days, which is clearly distinct from the usual, nondepressed mood. During the hypomanic episode, at least three of the manic symptoms listed above must be present, although the episode is not severe enough to cause marked impairment in occupational or social functioning, require hospitalization, or include psychotic symptoms.

HELPFUL TIP:
Although patients with bipolar disorders often have depressive episodes as well as manic or hypomanic episodes, depression is not required for the diagnosis of bipolar I disorder. ("So why is it called bipolar," you ask? Well, who are you to question tradition?)

Question 23.14.2 Regarding the epidemiology of bipolar illness, which of the following is FALSE?
A) The prevalence of bipolar I is about 0.6% to 1.5%
B) Many patients are misdiagnosed initially with depression
C) Untreated, the suicide rate is almost 20%
D) Women are twice as likely to be affected as men
E) Suicide risk is highest in the depressed or mixed state

Answer 23.14.2 The correct answer is "D." Unlike depression, bipolar illness affects males and females equally. Bipolar I affects about 0.6% to 1.5% of the population, while bipolar II affects about 0.8% to 3%. Untreated, nearly 20% will commit suicide—a rate about 20 times that of the general population. Risk is highest in depressed states or the mixed states (both mania and depression present at the same time). Bipolar disorder typically has its onset in early adulthood, although it can begin in childhood or adolescence. Depression is present 20% to 30% of the time, even with ongoing maintenance treatment. Over half of bipolar patients are initially misdiagnosed with depression, and the average patient is only accurately diagnosed after 5 years of symptoms.

HELPFUL TIP:
Up to 50% of people with bipolar disorder have concomitant alcohol abuse or dependence.

You want to start a medication for this patient ... or commit her ... or both.

Question 23.14.3 Which of the following would NOT be an appropriate treatment choice for her mania?
A) Lithium
B) Olanzapine (Zyprexa)
C) Divalproex (Depakote)
D) Carbamazepine (Tegretol)
E) Buspirone (Buspar)

Answer 23.14.3 The correct answer, and the medication to avoid, is "E." Buspirone (Buspar) is not effective in the treatment of bipolar disorder. Lithium ("A") was the first medication approved for treatment of bipolar mania and depression. It reduces the incidence of recurrence of mania, hypomania, and depression by about two-thirds. Lithium has a significant anti-suicide effect with an estimated eight- to ninefold reduction in risk. It is dosed at nighttime or twice daily. Lithium has a narrow therapeutic window, and there are numerous drug–drug interactions (including serotonergic drugs).

Both olanzapine (Zyprexa) ("B") and divalproex (Depakote) ("C") have FDA approval for treatment of acute mania and appear to be somewhat effective in the prevention of recurrent episodes. However, only lithium and lamotrigine (Lamictal) are FDA-approved mood stabilizers for bipolar treatment and maintenance. Lamotrigine (Lamictal) should not be used for acute mania, though. Carbamazepine (Tegretol) ("D") is a second-line agent that is also effective, but side effects limit its use. Atypical antipsychotics like olanzapine (Zyprexa), risperidone (Risperdal), ziprasidone (Abilify), and quetiapine (Seroquel) can also be used to treat acute mania. Side effects of atypical antipsychotics include extrapyramidal symptoms, sedation, and weight gain.

You decide to start lithium.

Question 23.14.4 Which of the following is a well-recognized side effect of lithium?
A) Diabetes mellitus
B) Hypothyroidism
C) Immunosuppression
D) Abnormal hair growth
E) The ability to donate an electron

Answer 23.14.4 The correct answer is "B." Patients who take lithium should have their thyroid function monitored. Also, lithium can affect renal function and electrolyte levels, so check serum electrolytes periodically. As lithium has a narrow therapeutic window, serum lithium levels should be measured ideally 12 hours after the last dose, with a goal of 0.6 to 1 mEq/L.

Question 23.14.5 Which of the following drug classes do NOT alter lithium levels?
A) NSAIDs
B) Diuretics
C) ACE inhibitors
D) ARBs
E) Opioids

Answer 23.14.5 The correct answer is "E." Lithium is cleared by the kidney. Anything that can cause a change in renal function can affect lithium levels. NSAIDs, diuretics, ACE inhibitors, and ARBs can all affect renal function.

▶ **Objectives: Did you learn to ...**
• Recognize and diagnose bipolar disorder?
• Initiate treatment of bipolar disorder?
• Describe some potential adverse effects of treatment of bipolar disorder?

▶ **CASE 23.15**

A 20-year-old female gymnast presents to you because she has missed her period for 6 months. She feels cold all the time and has noticed that when she crosses her legs, she gets pins-and-needles sensations down her leg. She had a stress fracture of her right tibia 5 years ago but denies any other medical history. She denies being sexually active and the review of systems is positive for frequent heartburn, constipation, and fatigue.

Question 23.15.1 Which of the following diagnoses would be in your differential?
A) Pregnancy
B) Hyperthyroidism
C) Malignancy
D) Anorexia nervosa (AN)
E) All of the above

Answer 23.15.1 The correct answer is "E." All the answers should be part of a reasonably broad differential diagnosis in this young woman. In patients presenting with weight loss and a possible eating disorder, you should eliminate medical causes of weight loss, using history, physical examination, and appropriate labs. Despite her denial of sexual activity, a pregnancy test is a necessary part of the evaluation, given that pregnancy is the most common cause of amenorrhea in this population. Hyperthyroidism and malignancy can present with vague complaints similar to this patient. Likewise,

AN can give rise to this patient's constellation of symptoms, though amenorrhea is no longer a diagnostic criteria for AN in DSM-5.

As you take more history, you realize that this patient is a very finicky eater. She is a strict vegan (So? What is wrong with that?) and restricts her calories to <1,000 kcal/day in order to stay in shape. She is 5 ft 3 in tall and weighs 100 lb, but she thinks she is overweight.

Question 23.15.2 Which of these additional findings would you expect on physical examination?
A) Bradycardia
B) Hypertension
C) Adnexal mass
D) Clonus
E) Proptosis

Answer 23.15.2 The correct answer is "A." Common physical findings in weight loss, and specifically AN, include emaciation, sunken cheeks, hypotension, bradycardia, lanugo, mottled teeth, and dry or yellow skin. Peripheral edema may develop during weight gain (refeeding syndrome… see below) or when laxative or diuretic abuse is stopped. Murmurs can occasionally be auscultated.

Question 23.15.3 Patients with AN may present with:
A) Paresthesia
B) Cold intolerance
C) Constipation
D) Fatigue
E) All of the above

Answer 23.15.3 The correct answer is "E." All of the above are symptoms of AN. These are common symptoms seen in starvation. "A" is not intuitive but is true. Loss of fat allows for greater exposure of superficial nerves, so the act of crossing the legs or sitting down on a hard chair can cause paresthesia.

HELPFUL TIP:
Patients with AN rarely have insight into the illness and often deny that weight loss is a problem. These patients are often perfectionists and overachievers who are sensitive to criticism and come from families with conflict. Weight loss is a method of control and is seen as a significant achievement.

HELPFUL TIP:
The word "anorexia" in AN is a misnomer, as loss of appetite is exceedingly rare in this illness. Patients are hungry but voluntarily restrict their caloric intake. The initial weight loss may be precipitated by appetite loss caused by depression, medical illness, dieting, or stressful life event.

Question 23.15.4 Which would be an expected laboratory finding in this patient?
A) Leukocytosis
B) Hyperkalemia
C) Increased amylase
D) Decreased cholesterol
E) Erythrocytosis

Answer 23.15.4 The correct answer is "C." Amylase may be increased as a result of purging behavior (and thus salivary stimulation). "A" and "E" are incorrect. Leukopenia, not leukocytosis, with a mild, normochromic, normocytic anemia is a common hematologic finding, although the CBC may be normal. "B" is incorrect. There is usually whole-body depletion of potassium, zinc, magnesium, and phosphate (from vomiting and/or inadequate intake). "D" is also incorrect, as cholesterol is often elevated (as are BUN and liver enzymes). This cholesterol elevation is neither intuitive nor well understood but is observed to occur in patients with AN. See Table 23-5 for more medical complications of AN.

TABLE 23-5 SELECTED MEDICAL COMPLICATIONS OF ANOREXIA NERVOSA

Neurologic	Seizures
	Peripheral neuropathy
	Cortical atrophy
	Cognitive impairment
Cardiovascular	Bradycardia
	Orthostatic hypotension
	Heart failure
	ECG changes: low voltage, nonspecific ST segment changes, QT prolongation
Endocrine	Amenorrhea
	Low T3, T4, and TSH (transient central hypothyroidism, previously called "euthyroid sick syndrome")
	Osteopenia/osteoporosis
	Growth retardation
	Hypoglycemia
	Hypothermia
Fluids and electrolytes	Dehydration
	Metabolic alkalosis
	Hypokalemia
	Hypomagnesemia
	Hypocalcemia
Gastrointestinal	Elevated liver enzymes
	Constipation
	Esophagitis
	Mallory–Weiss tears
	Parotid gland hypertrophy
Dermatologic	Lanugo
	Brittle nails and hair
	Acrocyanosis
	Dry, scaly skin
Hematologic	Bone marrow suppression
	Leukopenia/Neutropenia
	Anemia

In order to increase your patient's motivation to comply with medical recommendations, you describe some of the adverse effects of excessively low weight.

Question 23.15.5 All of the following abnormal findings will resolve when an adequate body weight is regained EXCEPT:
A) Bradycardia
B) Muscle wasting
C) Osteoporosis
D) Infertility

Answer 23.15.5 **The correct answer is "C."** Patients with AN are usually young and therefore experience some of their lowest weights and amenorrhea at the same time they are expected to reach peak bone mass. If a patient becomes osteopenic or osteoporotic when she is young, she will remain so as she ages (sans treatment). Return to good nutrition will not add bone mass that has been lost. Typical treatment for osteoporosis in this group remains combined estrogen–progesterone oral contraceptive agents as there are adverse effects related to bisphosphonates. All of the other physical changes listed should return to normal with return to a normal weight.

Question 23.15.6 **Which of the following is the most appropriate next step in the management of this patient?**
A) Tell her to stop gymnastics, withdraw from classes, and go to live with her mother
B) Start an antidepressant
C) Admit her to the hospital
D) Consult psychiatry and nutrition specialists
E) All of the above are equally valid options at this time

Answer 23.15.6 **The correct answer is "D."** This patient is most likely to benefit from a coordinated plan involving a multidisciplinary team, including primary care, psychiatry, and nutrition. "A" is incorrect, as it is a dramatic reaction that does not address the patient's primary problem, and the patient is unlikely to comply with it. "B" is incorrect. An antidepressant may be helpful in patients with a clearly defined depressive or anxiety disorder. However, the use of antidepressant therapy for AN specifically has not been successful, and certain antidepressants are associated with weight loss. "C," hospitalization, is not likely to be beneficial at this point. The utility of hospitalization has been difficult to determine in AN. Commonly accepted reasons for hospital admission include the following: severe low weight (70–75% of ideal body weight), marked symptomatic acute food refusal, hypotension or syncope, acute psychiatric emergency (threatened suicide), significant dehydration or severe bradycardia (<40 bpm) or cardiac arrhythmia, electrolyte disturbances, and failed intensive outpatient therapy.

While you plan to involve psychiatric and nutritional services, you continue your discussion of eating disorders with this patient.

Question 23.15.7 Which of the following is NOT TRUE about the epidemiology of eating disorders?
A) At least 90% of eating disorder patients are female
B) Rates are higher in industrialized, Western nations
C) A family history of depression increases the risk of females developing eating disorders
D) Male wrestlers have a higher risk of eating disorders than the average male
E) Mortality rates in AN are similar to the general population

Answer 23.15.7 **The correct answer is "E."** AN is characterized by a high mortality, one of the highest of psychiatric illnesses. It must be taken very seriously. Up to 10% of hospitalized patients die from direct effects of starvation, suicide, electrolyte imbalances leading to arrhythmias, or refeeding syndrome. At least 90% of eating disorder patients are female with prevalence rates higher in certain groups, such as models, actresses, athletes, and dancers. Western, industrialized societies endorse thinness and dieting as an ideal for women, resulting in higher rates of eating disorders. Despite having a normal body weight, over 40% of 9- and 10-year-old American girls believe they are overweight and consider dieting as an option! Eating disorders are uncommon in poorer countries where starvation is a potential reality and no cultural endorsement of thinness exists. "C" is true. A family history of depression or obesity increases risk of an eating disorder by two- to fivefold, with a family history of depression alone increasing the risk about fivefold. "D" is also true. In males, wrestlers have a higher prevalence of eating disorders because of weight requirements in their sport. In males, body shape and not necessarily absolute body weight is the typical focus of concern.

HELPFUL TIP:
There are two subtypes of AN: restrictive and binge/purge. Therefore, a patient who binges and purges (through forced emesis, laxatives, etc.) does not necessarily have bulimia.

HELPFUL TIP:
Comorbidities are prevalent in eating disorder patients and include MDD (50–75%), anxiety disorders, obsessive–compulsive disorder, and substance abuse. Personality disorders are also prevalent with the anxious, sensitive, rigid, and perfectionistic types predominating (Cluster C).

In your discussion of eating disorders, your patient asks about bulimia and how you distinguish between AN and bulimia nervosa (BN).

Question 23.15.8 Which of the following is NOT TRUE when comparing patients with AN and BN?
A) BN is more prevalent than AN
B) BN patients are more likely to be of normal weight than AN patients
C) The prognosis for AN is better than that for BN
D) BN patients are more likely to have esophageal tears
E) Medications are effective in BN but less so in AN

Answer 23.15.8 **The correct answer is "C."** BN has a better prognosis than AN, with only 20% of patients still meeting diagnostic criteria 5 to 10 years after initial presentation. BN is more common than AN, but with the prevalence increasing just like it has with AN. "B" is true. Patients with BN are usually close to normal weight. However, they show several stigmata: loss of dental enamel and chipped teeth with cavities; enlarged parotid salivary glands with elevated serum amylase from repeated vomiting episodes; menstrual irregularities; bradycardia, hypotension, and decreased metabolic rate. Rare complications include esophageal tears from frequent vomiting or gastric rupture due to gastric dilatation secondary to binging. "E" is true. Treatment of BN involves the same principles as AN with the caveat that medications can be helpful. Fluoxetine (Prozac) is the first-line drug with a target dose of 60 mg being shown to be effective in trials. Other SSRIs are second line. Third-line agents include TCAs, MAOIs, and trazodone. These agents reduce binge eating and bulimic symptoms whether patients are depressed or not.

HELPFUL TIP:
The mean age of onset of eating disorders is 18 to 21 years, with very rare onset after the age of 40 (although recurrence can occur in this population).

▶ **Objectives: Did you learn to …**
- Evaluate a young person with a suspected eating disorder?
- Diagnose AN?
- Recognize medical complications of eating disorders?
- Distinguish between AN and bulimia?
- Initiate appropriate treatment and referral for a patient with an eating disorder?

 QUICK QUIZ: BINGE AND PURGE

In order to be diagnosed with BN according to DSM-5, a patient must meet all of the following criteria EXCEPT:
A) Recurrent purging via self-induced vomiting
B) Recurrent binge eating
C) Symptoms are present on average at least once per week for at least 3 months
D) Self-evaluation is unduly influenced by body shape and weight

The correct answer is "A." For the diagnosis of BN, self-induced vomiting need not be present. Rather, some sort of compensatory behavior must be present during bulimic episodes. This behavior might include vomiting, but is not limited to vomiting, and may also include laxative or diuretic use, fasting, or excessive exercise. "B," "C," and "D" are required for the diagnosis of BN. BN affects about 1% to 3% females (more common in white females) and 0.1% to 0.3% males. Comorbidities of depression, anxiety, substance abuse, and personality disorders are also common. Dramatic, unstable personality traits (cluster B) predominate in this illness unlike the sensitive, rigid (Cluster C) personality traits in AN.

 QUICK QUIZ: EATING DISORDERS (OR, HOLD THE PIE FOR NOW, PLEASE)

A previously healthy 17-year-old female is hospitalized for AN. She has her weight rapidly restored with intravenous fluids and a 3,000 kcal/day diet. She gains 10 lb in her first 2 days (so gaining 10 lb in 2 days sounds like a good thing?) and seems to be doing well. However, when you round the next morning, she is unresponsive. Physical examination reveals evidence of JVD, pulmonary rales, and lower extremity edema.

What is the most likely cause of this patient's apparent heart failure?
A) Previously undiagnosed heart disease
B) Refeeding syndrome
C) Suicide attempt by SSRI overdose
D) Myocardial infarction
E) Takotsubo cardiomyopathy

The correct answer is "B." The scenario described fits with the clinical picture caused by refeeding syndrome. Refeeding syndrome occurs when rapid expansion of the circulating volume overwhelms the cardiovascular system's ability to adapt, leading to heart failure. It also involves changes in electrolytes and glucose. It typically occurs in malnourished patients. Prevention involves careful monitoring of electrolytes including magnesium, phosphorus, potassium, and calcium, while advancing caloric intake in a small, linear fashion and keeping track of volume status. "A," "D," and "E" are incorrect as the patient is unlikely to have significant heart disease given her age and gender.

HELPFUL TIP:
There is no case for this table but editors hate it when there is no "call out" for a table. So, see Table 23-6 for warning signs that an agitated patient may become violent. See Table 23-7 for ways to calm the agitated patient (although in the editors' experience nothing beats IM haloperidol and IM lorazepam—after other options are exhausted, of course).

TABLE 23-6 WARNING SIGNS THAT AN AGITATED PATIENT MAY BECOME VIOLENT

Hyperactivity: pacing or other increase in psychomotor activity

Loud, angry, or profane speech

Increased muscle tension, manifested by clenched jaw, fist, rigid posture, gripping chair, sitting on chair edge, etc.

Intoxication

Suspicious, angry, or irritable affect

Breathlessness, tachycardia, diaphoresis, pupillary dilation, visibly palpitating temporal arteries

Uncooperativeness with requests

Door slamming, chair toppling, or other form of property destruction

Grabbing objects that could be potential weapons

Verbal or physical threats

The clinician's response to the patient: if you feel anxious, take it seriously and be alert to possible danger

TABLE 23-7 TECHNIQUES TO CALM THE AGITATED PATIENT

Remove the patient to a quiet and nonstimulating environment

Keep a distance from the patient and avoid physical contact

Identify exits and alarms

Maintain nonthreatening demeanor and stance

Keep your hands at your side where they are easily visible

While maintaining steady eye contact, speak in a steady but authoritative voice, using the patient's name with each sentence

Avoid sudden jerky movements and remain calm

Have familiar faces nearby if possible

Show the patient concern but tell him that violence is not acceptable and you are willing to work with him if he calms down

There is strength in numbers; have other personnel nearby to help if necessary

Call for help from police or security if needed; a back-up system, which has been tested, should be in place

Consider antipsychotics, such as haloperidol (available in oral and parenteral forms) and risperidone (available in liquid); a benzodiazepine may be used as an adjunct, but should **not** be used alone

Mechanical restraints may be employed if absolutely necessary

Remember to figure out **why** the patient is agitated (e.g., take history, perform mental status examination, and order appropriate tests)

TABLE 23-8 FACTORS AFFECTING SUICIDE RISK

Risk Factors
- Previous history of suicide attempt
- Family history of suicide attempt or completion
- Substance misuse
- Mood disorders (e.g., depression, bipolar disorder)
- History of trauma or abuse
- Loss of spouse/significant other, separation or end of a relationship
- Having access to a gun or other readily lethal means
- Loss of activity, job, property, academic difficulty, financial difficulty, bullying
- Mild/minimal cognitive impairment
- Exposure to suicidal behavior or others
- Chronic illness including chronic pain

Protective Factors
- Contact with providers (e.g., follow-up phone calls, communications)
- Effective treatment of mental and physical disorders
- Social, community, faith, and familial support with strong connections
- Effective problem solving and conflict resolution skills

Adapted from Parekh R and American Psychiatric Association. Suicide prevention. June 2018. Available at: https://www.psychiatry.org/patients-families/suicide-prevention. Accessed February 2, 2019.

in men and women is equivalent. This occurs despite the fact that female physicians have fewer attempts than the general female population. Physicians have roughly the same rate of depression as the general population, while medical students and residents have higher rates than the general population (15–30% vs. 16% in the general population … if you were ever a medical student or resident, we are sure you got this one right). Other factors affecting suicide risk (in addition to being a physician) are noted in Table 23-8.

 QUICK QUIZ: SUICIDE RISK

You have a colleague who is depressed and has transient thoughts of suicide.

Which of the following would suggest that he should be hospitalized today?
A) He thinks about suicide only infrequently
B) He has not formulated a plan to commit suicide
C) He has updated his will within the past few days
D) He is willing to follow up in clinic tomorrow

The correct answer is "C." If a person admits to suicidal ideation, ask the following questions to assess his level of risk and to determine whether or not he should be hospitalized:

- How often does he think about suicide?
- Does he have a concrete plan? And if so, is it plausible? (Tying oneself to a rocket does not count … for most people.)
- Is he giving away treasured belongings, updating his will, making final plans, etc.?

 QUICK QUIZ: PHYSICIAN HEAL THYSELF?

Which of the following is true about physicians' risk of suicide compared to the general population?
A) Female physicians have a risk of successful suicide equal to male physicians
B) Physicians are more likely to be depressed than the general population
C) Female physicians are more likely to attempt suicide than the general female population
D) Medical students and residents are less likely to be depressed than the general population

The correct answer is "A." In the general population, women have two to four times more suicide attempts than men, while men are four times more likely than women to complete a suicide. However, among physicians, the rate of successful suicide

- Is he in danger of acting on his thoughts?
- Why has he not attempted suicide yet? What keeps him from doing it?
- Does he have access to harmful means (e.g., guns and drugs)?

Asking about suicidal thoughts does not increase the likelihood of suicide. There are evidence-based interventions, developed by the Action Alliance for Suicide Prevention, that can be completed in a clinic or office setting if suicide risk is identified. First, develop a safety plan with the patient, which may include providing the patient with the National Suicide Prevention Lifeline or local crisis resources. Next, evaluate the presence or thoughts of lethal means with mechanisms to remove the lethal means or minimization of its access if possible. Lastly, make a referral to a mental health professional and contact the patient within 48 hours for a caring contact. **Contracting for safety doesn't work. Do not depend on this to prevent a patient from committing suicide.**

 QUICK QUIZ: PSYCHOTROPIC DRUGS

Which of these antidepressants can be administered once weekly?
A) Paroxetine (Paxil)
B) Buspirone (Wellbutrin)
C) Fluoxetine (Prozac)
D) Escitalopram (Lexapro)
E) Venlafaxine (Effexor-SR)

The correct answer is "C." Fluoxetine has a long-enough half-life that it can be administered once a week. You don't need to prescribe the "long-acting" fluoxetine. Any fluoxetine can be dosed once weekly. It is traditionally dosed daily, but if patients are experiencing side effects or Have difficulties adhering to a daily medication, dosing can be adjusted to every other day or weekly.

▶ **CASE 23.16**

You are on call and have been paged to see a 21-year-old female who has just overdosed on a handful of acetaminophen because her boyfriend left her after their most recent fight. She has had similar overdoses three times in the past (they fight a lot). According to a friend, she has a history of tumultuous relationships. In the emergency department, she is combative and yelling, "I'm so angry that I'm still alive!" She has a blood alcohol level of 106 mg/dL. There are scars on her arms, presumably from cutting.

Question 23.16.1 **What is the most likely primary diagnosis?**
A) Antisocial personality disorder
B) Bipolar affective disorder
C) MDD
D) Borderline personality disorder
E) Intermittent explosive disorder

TABLE 23-9 CHARACTERISTICS OF BORDERLINE PERSONALITY DISORDER

- Fears of abandonment
- Unstable and intense relationships
- Unstable sense of self
- Impulsivity
- Suicidal behavior, threats or gestures or self-mutilation (cutting is often a feature of borderline personality disorder)
- Significant mood reactivity
- Chronic feelings of emptiness (Camus or Nietzsche?)
- Intense anger outbursts
- Transient stress-related paranoid ideation or dissociation

Answer 23.16.1 **The correct answer is "D."** This patient's history is consistent with a diagnosis of borderline personality disorder. Persons with borderline personality disorder often have stormy relationships, characterized by extremes of emotional intensity (e.g., "love–hate" relationships). You might also consider depression as a diagnosis here, but the history does not support MDD. However, concomitant depression is common in patients with borderline personality disorder. "A," "B," and "E" are not supported by the clinical presentation. Borderline personality disorder is mostly a diagnosis of females (over 90%). Characteristics are listed in Table 23-9.

 HELPFUL TIP:
A personality disorder is an enduring pattern of relating to the world in ways that are inflexible, ineffective, and markedly different from cultural norms. Personality disorders cause distress or functional impairment and start by adolescence in most people. The prevalence rate of personality disorders varies widely across studies, with borderline personality disorder being the most prevalent of all.

Your patient's boyfriend storms into the emergency department and demands to see her. He has "love" and "hate" tattooed on his knuckles and another less savory symbol tattooed on his arm—although he swears it's just a Tibetan good luck charm. The nurse recognizes him immediately as a frequent visitor. Apparently, he has been in the emergency department on multiple occasions for injuries sustained from fights. Your patient pulls you aside to tell you that she is afraid of him, saying, "I just worry when he gets mad. He went to jail for beating and raping his last girlfriend." The nurse also informs you that he is suspected of stealing narcotics from a pharmacy in town. You call security.

Question 23.16.2 **Which of the following personality disorders is most likely in this man?**
A) Paranoid personality disorder
B) Histrionic personality disorder
C) Schizotypal personality disorder
D) Antisocial personality disorder
E) None. This patient is just a character on MTV's Jersey Shore.

TABLE 23-10 CHARACTERISTICS OF ANTISOCIAL PERSONALITY DISORDER

- Recurrent criminality
- Deceitfulness shown by repeated lying, use of aliases, or conning others
- Impulsivity
- Irritability and aggression
- Reckless disregard for safety
- Consistent irresponsibility, failing to fulfill financial obligations or work
- Lack of remorse
- History of childhood conduct disorder before age 15

Answer 23.16.2 The correct answer is "D." Antisocial personality disorder is primarily seen in males, and of the options given, it is the only personality disorder that really fits. Antisocial personality disorder is quite prevalent in prison populations. "A" and "C" are incorrect because these are Cluster A disorders, which are characterized by strange rather than violent behavior. "B" is incorrect. Histrionic personality disorder shows attention-seeking and seductive behavior. Although patients with antisocial personality disorder can be charming, they also use violence and threats to achieve their purposes. Characteristics of antisocial personality disorder are listed in Table 23-10.

Question 23.16.3 Besides borderline personality disorder, which other personality disorder increases the risk of completed suicide the most?
A) Paranoid personality disorder
B) Histrionic personality disorder
C) Schizotypal personality disorder
D) Avoidant personality disorder
E) Antisocial personality disorder

Answer 23.16.3 The correct answer is "E." Along with borderline personality disorder, antisocial personality disorder is the other personality disorder most likely to be seen in completed suicides.

Question 23.16.4 Borderline personality disorder and antisocial personality disorder fall within what cluster or category of personality disorders?
A) Cluster A
B) Cluster B
C) Cluster C
D) Cluster D

Answer 23.16.4 The correct answer is "B." There are three clusters of personality disorders that are categorized based on their characteristics.

- Cluster A: "the weird cluster"—patients are aloof, act strange, and prefer to be alone. Paranoid, schizoid, and schizotypal personality disorders are included here.
- Cluster B: "the wild cluster"—patients have significant problems with mood lability, impulsivity, or are preoccupied with being admired for their sexuality or intelligence. Borderline, antisocial, histrionic, and narcissistic personality disorders are included here.

- Cluster C: "the whiny or worried cluster"—patients are clingy, sensitive, and rigid. Avoidant, dependent, and obsessive–compulsive personality disorders are included here.

HELPFUL TIP:
You will be happy to know (as are we) that, as of DSM-5, the old "axis" designation system (axis 1, axis 2, etc.) for psychiatric disease has gone the way of the dodo bird (or pick your favorite extinct species).

HELPFUL TIP:
Impulsivity is a risk for completed suicide. Even though patients may not truly intend to die, an impulsively taken overdose or other suicide attempt may inadvertently lead to death. This is why patients with borderline personality disorder and antisocial personality disorder have a high risk of completed suicide.

You have a frank discussion with your female patient about suicide.

Question 23.16.5 Which of the following is NOT TRUE about suicide in the general population?
A) Medical diagnoses can increase the risk of suicide
B) Over 90% of people who commit suicide have a diagnosed mental health disorder
C) Older Americans are at higher risk of suicide than the general population
D) The rate of successful suicides has increased over the years
E) Suicide is one of the top 10 causes of death in the United States

Answer 23.16.5 The correct answer is "B." The rate of successful suicide has increased nationally from 1999 to 2016, with half of states experiencing a greater than 30% increase in suicides during this time. Of those that completed suicide, only 46% had a known mental illness, excluding substance use disorder. "A" is a correct statement. Medical diagnoses can be risk factors for suicide. Particularly problematic are chronic illness, terminal illness, chronic pain, or recent surgery. Older Americans commit suicide at a rate four times than that of the general population with a peak incidence at age 75 for men and 60 for women. "E" is also correct. Suicide is the seventh leading cause of death in the United States and the third leading cause of death in those aged 15 to 24 years. There are two mnemonics that are useful for assessing suicide risk: "NO HOPE" and "SAD PERSONS" (see Table 23-11).

HELPFUL TIP:
Seventy-five percent of older Americans who commit suicide have seen their primary care physician within the preceding 4 weeks and 39% within the same week. Up to half of successful suicides have made a prior attempt.

TABLE 23-11 MNEMONICS FOR SUICIDE RISK ASSESSMENT

NO HOPE	SAD PERSONS
No framework for meaning (Reading Nietzsche?)	**S**ex—male
Overt change in clinical condition	**A**ge—older
Hostile interpersonal environment	**D**epression
Out of hospital recently	**P**revious attempt
Predisposing personality factors	**E**thanol abuse
Excuses for dying to help others	**R**ational thought loss
	Social support lacking
	Organized plan
	No spouse
	Sickness

▶ **Objectives: Did you learn to …**
- Identify borderline and antisocial personality disorders?
- Classify personality disorders?
- Assess suicide risk?

▶ **CASE 23.17**

A 21-year-old man presents to your clinic because his girl-friend dragged him in. He just started his first year in college but quit 2 days ago because he feels that "they are all out to get me." ("If he's talking about the IRS, or New World Order, he's probably right," you think to yourself.) He has not been sleeping because he thinks he might be murdered in his sleep. He tells you that the FBI has bugged your office and that the NSA is tapping your phone (OK, that one's probably right); therefore, he does not want to answer your questions.

Question 23.17.1 Which of the following would you NOT expect to find on mental status examination?
A) Delusions
B) Hallucinations
C) Lack of insight
D) Decreased psychomotor activity
E) Poverty of speech

Answer 23.17.1 **The correct answer is "D."** The patient described is acutely psychotic. You would expect him to have increased psychomotor activity. All of the other options would also be anticipated findings in this patient. Common symptoms of psychosis include delusions, hallucinations, psychomotor agitation, flight of ideas, nonsensical speech and behavior, lack of insight into one's behavior, and lack of judgment. Note that "poverty of speech" refers to brief, empty replies to questions and not to content, which may be quite fanciful.

Question 23.17.2 All of the following are potential causes of this patient's psychosis EXCEPT:
A) Substance abuse
B) Alcohol withdrawal
C) Bipolar disorder
D) Bereavement
E) Schizophrenia

TABLE 23-12 CAUSES OF PSYCHOSIS AND DELIRIUM: A PARTIAL LIST

Potentially Imminently Life-Threatening Causes
- Meningitis or encephalitis
- Hypoxemia
- Hypertensive encephalopathy
- Wernicke encephalopathy
- Intracranial bleed
- Drug withdrawal, intoxication, or reaction to prescribed drugs

Other Medical Causes
- Metabolic disorders (e.g., hyperglycemia and hyponatremia)
- Neurologic disorders
- Nutritional deficiencies (e.g., pellagra, beriberi, and pernicious anemia)
- Industrial exposure to toxins

Psychiatric Causes
- Schizophrenia or schizophreniform disorders
- Brief psychotic disorder
- Mood disorders including bipolar disorder and psychotic depression
- Schizoaffective disorder
- Dementia
- Delirium
- Delusional disorder

Answer 23.17.2 **The correct answer is "D."** Bereavement may result in mild delusions and sometimes hallucinations regarding the bereaved subject (Hey? Is that mom back from the dead?), but it should not cause overt psychosis. Moreover, there is nothing in the history here to support a diagnosis of bereavement. The remaining options are potential cause of psychosis, and they are listed along with other potential causes in Table 23-12.

HELPFUL TIP:
Psychosis is a symptom and not a diagnosis. It should prompt a search for an etiology. Some of the causes are potentially life threatening as listed in Table 23-12.

Hypnotized by your calm and steady voice, the patient relaxes and becomes cooperative, and you are able to obtain a history and perform a physical examination. He denies drug use or medical illnesses. Your patient worries that he is going "crazy" and admits that he has been having these symptoms "for a while" but did not want to tell anybody, for fear of being institutionalized. Your physical examination and labs (TSH, BMP, glucose, urine drug screen) are unremarkable.

Question 23.17.3 Which of the following diagnoses is the most likely cause of this patient's psychosis?
A) Schizophrenia
B) Psychotic depression
C) Delirium
D) Drug intoxication
E) Dementia

Answer 23.17.3 The correct answer is "A." Schizophrenia is a heterogeneous group of disorders characterized by the following: positive symptoms (delusions, hallucinations, disorganized behavior, disorganized speech); negative symptoms (poverty of speech, anhedonia, affective flattening, avolition, withdrawal from social activities); mood symptoms (dysphoria, suicidal thoughts, hopelessness); and cognitive symptoms (attention and memory deficits and difficulty with abstract thinking). It is the most common of the psychotic disorders. A negative laboratory evaluation and physical examination make drug intoxication unlikely, while this patient's ability to converse with you and give a history makes delirium and dementia unlikely. Psychotic depression is unusual in young people, but rather is more commonly seen in older patients with severe depression.

Question 23.17.4 Which of the following is NOT true about schizophrenia?
A) Nearly 50% of patients attempt suicide with a 10% success rate
B) Lifetime prevalence is 1% worldwide, consistent across cultures
C) Schizophrenia is a disease of late adolescence or early adulthood
D) Men are more likely to be affected than women
E) Risk of relapse is at least 50% after successful treatment in patients who do not remain on antipsychotic maintenance therapy

Answer 23.17.4 The correct answer is "D." Schizophrenia has a worldwide prevalence of about 1%, which is true for all cultures, countries, and both genders ("B"). It generally begins in late adolescence or early adulthood, and onset after age 50 is rare and should prompt the search for other etiologies to explain the psychosis ("C"). Men have a slightly earlier age of onset (early twenties) than women (late twenties), but men and women are affected equally by the illness. The course is variable with some patients having exacerbations and remissions (although full remissions are rare), while others remain chronically ill. About half of the patients who develop schizophrenia have a family history of schizophrenia. Suicide attempts are common, usually the result of depression or a response to command hallucinations, paranoid delusions, or agitation. Nearly 50% of patients will attempt suicide, while about 10% will be successful ("A"). After successful treatment of the first episode, about 50% will relapse if not on maintenance medication ("E").

Question 23.17.5 Which of the following medication options is the proper treatment choice?
A) Olanzapine (Zyprexa)
B) Risperidone (Risperdal)
C) Haloperidol (Haldol)
D) Aripiprazole (Abilify)
E) Any of the above

Answer 23.17.5 The correct answer is "E." All of the antipsychotics listed are first-line treatment choices for schizophrenia. Most psychiatrists have replaced older "typical" (now known as "first-generation" agents like haloperidol, chlorpromazine, fluphenazine, thioridazine) with newer "atypical" (now known as

"second-generation" agents, such as risperidone, clozapine, ziprasidone, paliperidone, and olanzapine) because of better tolerability and possibly increased benefit for negative symptoms. Although, the newer agents are significantly more expensive than the older agents, more generics are becoming available. Also, many "atypicals" cause significant weight gain, and some have been linked to new-onset diabetes and metabolic syndrome. Of the newer agents, aripiprazole (Abilify) and ziprasidone (Geodon) are less associated with weight gain and diabetes.

Question 23.17.6 Which of the following is TRUE of the course of schizophrenia?
A) Positive symptoms usually occur first
B) Negative symptoms are easier to treat than positive symptoms
C) Negative symptoms often look like depression
D) Schizophrenia is not typically associated with brain changes
E) Family therapy is not helpful in this illness

Answer 23.17.6 The correct answer is "C." Negative symptoms often precede the development of the positive symptoms by many years, are often nonspecific, and can be mistaken for depression. A typical history is that of a normal young man or woman who begins to fail classes and avoid his old friends as he gets to the end of high school. This is often mistaken for teenage rebellion, depression, or drug use until the onset of positive psychotic symptoms of hallucinations or delusions develop several years later. "B" is incorrect. Negative symptoms are chronic and are resistant to treatment with all currently available antipsychotics. Antipsychotic drugs modulate dopamine and/or serotonin and are much better at treating positive symptoms. "D" is not true, as brain imaging may reveal enlargement of cerebral ventricles and decreased brain volume. However, these findings are neither sensitive nor specific enough to have much value in diagnosis. "E" is incorrect. A large body of literature supports the fact that family therapy, especially directed at support and psychoeducation, reduces the risk of relapse. Recent evidence indicates that individual CBT can also be effective.

HELPFUL TIP: DUAL ANTIPSYCHOTICS
There is almost never an indication for more than one antipsychotic at a time. Don't do it.

▶ **Objectives: Did you learn to …**
• Recognize psychosis and its causative diagnoses?
• Treat psychosis?
• Recognize schizophrenia and understand its epidemiology and prognosis?

▶ **CASE 23.18**

A 33-year-old factory worker comes to your clinic complaining of sleep difficulty since he moved to the "graveyard shift." He complains of falling asleep at work and having difficulty sleeping during the day.

Question 23.18.1 Which of the following is the most likely diagnosis?
A) Narcolepsy
B) Circadian rhythm sleep–wake disorder
C) Obstructive sleep apnea
D) Primary insomnia
E) Fatal familial insomnia

Answer 23.18.1 The correct answer is "B." This patient suffers (as do most residents and a significant number of physicians) from a circadian rhythm sleep–wake disorder, which is defined as a sleep disruption leading to excessive sleepiness when the patient wishes to be awake or insomnia when the patient wishes to be asleep. It occurs as a result of a mismatch between the biological circadian rhythm and the person's environment. He does not give a history consistent with narcolepsy or obstructive sleep apnea, and primary insomnia is a diagnosis of exclusion. Fatal familial insomnia ("E") is a rare genetically determined prion disease resulting in complete inability to sleep, dementia, and death within a few years.

He asks your advice on how to treat his sleeplessness.

Question 23.18.2 What would be the best advice to offer at this time to help adapt to the nighttime schedule?
A) Have him sleep at work
B) Have him take naps throughout the day
C) Tell him to quit his job
D) Recommend bright light at night before going to work
E) Prescribe stimulants for when he is at work

Answer 23.18.2 The correct answer is "D." This patient's circadian rhythm disturbance might also be called a "phase-advance" type sleep disorder (early sleep onset with insomnia at the desired sleep period). Such problems respond best to bright light in the evening to keep one awake during the time the individual would usually be asleep. Light boxes are available commercially and should provide white light at 2,500 lux or more. The light should be fairly close to the patient's eyes, and a bit off to the side. The other options are not likely to be helpful if this patient wants to keep his job.

Question 23.18.3 If this patient wished to use a nutritional or herbal supplement, which of the following would you recommend?
A) Melatonin
B) Kava-kava
C) Ginkgo
D) Ginseng
E) St. John's wort

Answer 23.18.3 The correct answer is "A." There is some evidence to suggest that melatonin can help with circadian rhythm disorders (and may decrease sleep onset latency in insomnia). Melatonin should be taken at the time of day the patient wants to sleep. In this case, you should advise him to take it in the

morning. The doses used for circadian rhythm disturbances are much less than the dose used for primary insomnia, typically 0.5 mg or less, compared with 3 to 5 mg. The other herbal supplements have no evidence for use in sleep disturbances except for kava-kava, which is too dangerous to recommend.

Question 23.18.4 Which of the following is NOT a delayed sleep phase type of circadian rhythm sleep disorder?
A) Re-adaptation to day work from night work
B) West-to-east jet lag
C) East-to-west jet lag
D) All of the above are delayed sleep phase disorders

Answer 23.18.4 The correct answer is "C." Delayed sleep phase involves a persistent pattern of late sleep onset and late morning awakening. This is exemplified by the average teenager during summer vacation (just try to get him to mow the lawn before noon!). West-to-east jet lag and re-adapting to day shift after working night shift also cause similar problems; sleep onset can be late and one wants to sleep longer in the morning. "C" does not cause a delayed sleep phase disturbance. East-to-west jet lag causes the opposite problem, advancing sleep phase so that persons are sleepy early in the evening but then awake early in the morning. A potentially effective treatment of delayed sleep phase would include prescribing a bright light in the morning and melatonin in the afternoon.

▸ **Objectives: Did you learn to …**
 · Recognize circadian rhythm disorders?
 · Recommend treatment of circadian rhythm disorders?

 QUICK QUIZ: LEST YOU FORGET

A 70-year-old man presents with memory loss that has been progressive over the years. He often has fluctuating attention and is rigid with bradykinesia. He frequently experiences visual hallucinations.

Which of the following is the most likely diagnosis?
A) Alzheimer disease
B) Dementia with Lewy bodies (DLB)
C) Parkinson disease
D) Vascular dementia
E) Frontotemporal dementia

The correct answer is "B." DLB shares many features in common with Parkinson disease including parkinsonian motor symptoms, such as rigidity, tremor, and bradykinesia, Both Parkinson disease and DLB are characterized histologically by the presence of Lewy bodies. However, in DLB, Lewy bodies are diffusely spread in the cortical regions and brainstem, whereas in Parkinson disease, Lewy bodies are primarily present in the subcortical nuclei (substantia nigra). Fluctuating cognition that resembles delirium, visual hallucinations, and an exquisite sensitivity to the adverse effects of neuroleptics all characterize

DLB. Cholinesterase inhibitors may have modest benefit on cognitive symptoms, though none are FDA approved, and only rivastigamine is FDA approved for Parkinson's dementia.

 QUICK QUIZ: DEMENTIA

A 65-year-old man with a history of hypertension, diabetes, and peripheral vascular disease has been noted to have abrupt deterioration in his cognitive ability following an episode of disorientation and word-finding difficulty 1 month ago.

Which of the following is the most likely diagnosis?
A) Alzheimer disease
B) Dementia with Lewy bodies
C) Parkinson disease
D) Vascular dementia
E) Frontotemporal dementia

The correct answer is "D." Vascular dementia (previously known as multi-infarct dementia) is caused by vascular disease (Surprise! An illness with a name that makes sense!). After Alzheimer and Lewy body dementias, vascular dementia is one of the most common causes of dementia. It classically presents with an abrupt onset followed by step-wise deterioration of cognitive function. Medical comorbidities are common, including hypertension, diabetes, and obesity. Evidence of vascular disease is usually present on clinical examination with focal neurological signs, such as are seen after a stroke involving motor areas. Imaging typically shows infarctions of periventricular and deep subcortical white matter, presenting as white matter hyperintensities on T2-weighted MRI. Treatment includes modifying vascular risk factors.

▶ CASE 23.19

A 37-year-old female patient returns to see you for follow-up of depression. You last saw her 4 weeks ago, and at that time she was experiencing her third relapse of recurrent major depression. She had been in remission for 3 years before, and until 2 years ago she had been taking sertraline 150 mg daily, a regimen that she had found effective during an 18-month course of treatment. At her visit last month, you assessed her symptoms with the Patient Health Questionnaire-9 (PHQ-9), and her score at that time was 21. You reinstituted sertraline at 50 mg daily for 2 weeks and then 100 mg daily. At her visit today, now on sertraline 100 mg daily for 2 weeks, her PHQ-9 score is 17. She denies having thoughts of death or suicide.

Question 23.19.1 Which of the following statements is NOT true regarding the PHQ-9?
A) The PHQ-9 is a clinician-administered questionnaire to evaluate for symptoms of major depression
B) It takes 3 to 5 minutes to complete the PHQ-9
C) A score of 10 or more on the PHQ-9 is a positive screen
D) The PHQ-9 can be used to screen for depression as well as to monitor symptom severity over time
E) The PHQ-9 does NOT assess for suicide risk

Answer 23.19.1 The correct answer is "A." The PHQ-9 is a *patient*-administered, nine-item questionnaire that takes 3 to 5 minutes to complete. It can be used to screen for major depression as well as to monitor symptom severity over time. A score >10 is considered a positive screen, while a score <5 is considered to be negative or in remission. The maximum score is 30. While the PHQ-9 does ask about the presence of "thoughts of death or dying," it does not assess whether someone is at low or high risk for suicide attempt.

Question 23.19.2 Which of the following options is LEAST appropriate to recommend to your patient at this time?
A) Continue sertraline 100 mg daily and return for follow-up in 1 month
B) Continue sertraline 100 mg daily, add weekly CBT, and return for follow-up in 1 month
C) Increase sertraline to 150 mg daily and return for follow-up in 1 month
D) Stop the sertraline and start citalopram/escitalopram 20 mg daily and return for follow-up in 1 month
E) Continue sertraline 100 mg daily and add bupropion SR 150 mg BID, return for follow-up in 1 month

Answer 23.19.2 The correct answer is "D." At the current visit, the patient has been taking sertraline for 1 month and has been at the present dose for 2 weeks. It can take up to 6 to 8 weeks for an antidepressant medication to reach its full effect, so it is reasonable to maintain the medication at its present dose and reassess in 1 month. However, options "B," "C," and "E" are reasonable as well. Combination treatment with CBT and an antidepressant medication has been shown to be more effective for treating depression than either treatment strategy alone. You can also consider the addition of an augmentation agent (bupropion, liothyronine [T3], or a second-generation antipsychotic). Since she has had a partial response to the current regimen, adding an augmentation agent is a reasonable option. Switching to a new antidepressant at this time is not indicated.

Despite increasing the dose of sertraline, your patient's depression does not improve. She's been watching a lot of TV (no wonder she's depressed) and seen ads for a medication called Happify, which is used to augment traditional antidepressant therapy. She says, "I think I need one of those new wonder drugs, Doc" (the so-called "wonder drugs" because it is a wonder that they ever got FDA approval).

Question 23.19.3 Which of the following have gained FDA approval as therapy for depression?
A) Aripiprazole (Abilify)
B) Haloperidol (Haldol)
C) Olanzapine (Geodon)
D) Quetiapine (Seroquel)
E) A, C, and D

Answer 23.19.3 The correct answer is "E." Aripiprazole (Abilify), quetiapine (Seroquel), and olanzapine (Geodon) are FDA approved as add-on medications to augment antidepressants in monopolar depression. The benefits are marginal, when examining a population with treatment resistant depression. For example, aripiprazole added to a traditional antidepressant in this population improved depression by 3-point difference on a 60-point scale and then only in men. For aripiprazole, the number needed to treat to achieve this small reduction in depressive symptoms is 10. On the bright side, aripiprazole is less associated with weight gain compared with other atypical antipsychotics.

▶ **Objectives: Did you learn to …**
- Develop strategies to treat resistant depression?
- Describe a widely used depression assessment tool, the PHQ-9?

The world of psychiatric drugs is constantly moving (akathisia?). See https://www.ncbi.nlm.nih.gov/books/NBK84656/ OR https://www.empr.com/clinical-charts/psychotropic-drug-indications/article/123832/ for a list of indications of psychiatric medications.

HELPFUL TIP:
Random things to remember for the examination: clozapine (Clozaril) mandates a CBC monthly (and that prescribers be certified in a national registry) because of bone marrow suppression; second-generation antipsychotics can cause diabetes and are not free of neurologic side effects (e.g., extrapyramidal reactions), and patients on them should be monitored with periodic glucose and/or A1c; anticholinergics (e.g., benztropine) should be used with first-generation antipsychotics to prevent parkinsonian side effects.

Clinical Pearls

- Avoid first-line use of antipsychotic medication for indications other than psychotic disorders (e.g., depression in any patient, insomnia in any patient, behavioral disorders in children, or demented elders).
- Do not prescribe benzodiazepines as first-line therapy for the treatment of anxiety disorders.
- Do not diagnose "adult-onset" ADHD. Explore the history and if the patient has had ADHD symptoms since childhood, he/she may have a missed or delayed diagnosis of ADHD.
- Do not prescribe two antipsychotic medications simultaneously.
- Ensure that systems are in place to treat and refer patients diagnosed with depression, and screen for depression in the general adolescent and adult patient population. This includes assessing suicide risk.
- Offer pharmacotherapy and professional counseling services to all patients diagnosed with depressive disorders, as the combination results in better outcomes than either intervention alone.
- Screen for metabolic syndrome periodically in patients taking second-generation antipsychotics (e.g., olanzapine, risperidone, quetiapine).

BIBLIOGRAPHY

Ables AZ, Nagubilli R. Prevention, recognition, and management of serotonin syndrome. *Am Fam Physician.* 2010;8:1139–1142.

American Psychiatric Association. *Diagnostic and Statistical Manual of Mental Disorders.* 5th ed., Text Revision. Washington, DC: American Psychiatric Association; 2013.

Black DW, Andreasen NC. *Introductory Textbook of Psychiatry.* 6th ed., Washington, DC: American Psychiatric Publishing; 2014.

Brody DJ, Pratt LA, Hughes J. Prevalence of depression among adults aged 20 and over: United States, 2013–2016. NCHS Data Brief, no 303. Hyattsville, MD: National Center for Health Statistics; 2018.

Flockhart DA. Drug Interactions: Cytochrome P450 Drug Interaction Table. Indiana University School of Medicine (2007). Available at https://drug-interactions.medicine.iu.edu. Accessed September 1, 2018.

Garland EJ, Kutcher S, Virani A, Elbe D. Update on the use of SSRIs and SNRIs with children and adolescents in clinical practice. *J Can Acad of Child Adolesc Psychiatry.* 2016;25(1):4–10.

Glick ID, et al. Mid-term and long-term efficacy and effectiveness of antipsychotic medications for schizophrenia: a data-driven, personalized clinical approach. *J Clin Psychiatry.* 2011;72:1616–1627.

Harvard Medical School. National Comorbidity Survey (NCS). Data Table 1: Lifetime prevalence DSM-IV/WMH-CIDI disorders by sex and cohort. 2017, August 21. Available at: https://www.hcp.med.harvard.edu/ncs/index.php. Accessed September 1, 2018.

Hendin H, et al. Confronting depression and suicide in physicians: a consensus statement. *JAMA.* 2003;289:3161–3166.

Khan A, et al. Suicide rates in clinical trials of SSRIs, other antidepressants, and placebo: analysis of FDA reports. *Am J Psychiatry.* 2003;160:790–792.

Lynch T, Price A. The effect of cytochrome P450 metabolism on drug response, interactions, and adverse effects. *Am Fam Physician.* 2007;76(3):391–396.

National Action Alliance for Suicide Prevention: Transforming Health Systems Initiative Work Group. *Recommended Standard Care for People with Suicide Risk: Making Health Care Suicide Safe.* Washington, DC: Education Development Center, Inc.; 2018.

National Institute on Mental Health. Major Depression Among Adults. Available at: http://www.nimh.nih.gov/health/statistics/prevalence/major-depression-among-adults.shtml. Accessed September 1, 2018.

National Institute of Mental Health. Brain Stimulation Therapies. June 2016. Available at: https://www.nimh.nih.gov/health/topics/brain-stimulation-therapies/brain-stimulation-therapies.shtml. Accessed February 2, 2019.

Parekh R and American Psychiatric Association. Suicide Prevention. June 2018. Available at: https://www.psychiatry.org/patients-families/suicide-prevention. Accessed February 2, 2019.

Rader R, et al. Current strategies in the diagnosis and treatment of childhood attention-deficit/hyper-activity disorder. *Am Fam Physician*. 2009;79:657–665.

Rush AJ, et al. Acute and longer-term outcomes in depressed outpatients requiring one or several treatment steps: a STAR D report. *Am J Psych*. 2006;163:1905.

Schatzberg AF, et al. Antidepressant discontinuation syndrome: consensus panel recommendations for clinical management and additional research. *J Clin Psych*. 2006;67(suppl 4):27–30.

Stone DM, Simon TR, Fowler KA, et al. *Vital Signs:* trends in state suicide rates—United States, 1999–2016 and circumstances contributing to suicide—27 States, 2015. *MMWR*. 2018;67:617–624.

Wagner KD, et al. Efficacy of sertraline in the treatment of children and adolescents with major depressive disorder: two randomized controlled trials. *JAMA*. 2003;290:1033–1041.

Wheeler BW, et al. The population impact on incidence of suicide and non-fatal self-harm of regulatory action against the use of selective serotonin reuptake inhibitors in under 18s in the United Kingdom: ecological study. *BMJ*. 2008;336:542.

Nutrition and Herbal Medicine

24

Jason K. Wilbur

▶ CASE 24.1

A 59-year-old male presents for follow-up. He is well-known to you, receiving chronic anticoagulation with warfarin for a mechanical aortic valve. His PT and INR have been in the therapeutic range for years. When asked, he denies taking any other medications. He has had no new medical problems and is feeling well. Today his INR is 6.2 (therapeutic range 2.5–3.5). You inquire about dietary changes, focusing on foods rich in vitamin K.

Question 24.1.1 Which of the following is true regarding vitamin K?
A) Vitamin K is a water-soluble vitamin
B) Broccoli and olive oil are good sources of vitamin K
C) Vitamin K deficiency results in a hypercoagulable state
D) Warfarin reduces the absorption of vitamin K
E) Vegetarians are at risk for developing vitamin K deficiency

Answer 24.1.1 The correct answer is "B." Vitamin K is a fat-soluble vitamin present in leafy green vegetables such as spinach and cabbage and in other foods such as milk, butter, bacon, and vegetable oils. Olive oil and broccoli are particularly rich in vitamin K. Therefore, vegetarians who consume these regularly are not at high risk for developing vitamin K deficiency. Vitamin K deficiency causes a **hypo**coagulable state resulting in a reduction in clotting factors and elevated prothrombin time and INR, leading to poor clotting ability and hemorrhage. Warfarin does act on vitamin K, but by reducing conversion of vitamin K to its active form rather than reducing absorption.

Question 24.1.2 You would be more likely to suspect vitamin K deficiency in this patient if he also suffered from which of the following conditions?
A) Crohn disease
B) Irritable bowel syndrome
C) Well compensated hepatitis C with mild fibrosis
D) Coronary artery disease (CAD)
E) All of the above

Answer 24.1.2 The correct answer is "A." Vitamin K deficiency can occur with chronic small bowel disease, after small bowel resection, and with use of broad-spectrum antibiotics. Microorganisms in the bowel synthesize vitamin K, and use of broad-spectrum antibiotics reduces the number of these organisms. The majority of vitamin K is absorbed in the distal small bowel, and any disease affecting this area—including Crohn disease and celiac disease—can reduce the absorption of the vitamin. Irritable bowel syndrome is a functional disease not associated with impaired absorption. "C" is of special note. Patients with cirrhosis and *decompensated* liver disease are often vitamin K deficient. However, the mere presence of hepatitis C does not cause vitamin K deficiency.

....

Upon more direct questioning, the patient denies any changes in his diet but admits to recently starting a vitamin therapy program. He has no clue what he is actually taking and calls his wife to find out what the products contain (it was Miracle Mega Man… something). Meanwhile, you suspect that he is taking excessive doses of vitamins that may affect his INR.

Question 24.1.3 Large doses of which of the following vitamins are most likely to result in an increased INR in patients taking warfarin?
A) Vitamin A
B) Vitamin C
C) Vitamin D
D) Vitamin E
E) Zinc

Answer 24.1.3 The correct answer is "D." Large doses of vitamin E (>400 IU/day) can interfere with vitamin K metabolism and platelet function, resulting in increased prothrombin time and therefore increased INR in some patients. In patients taking warfarin, starting a high-dose vitamin E supplement should be done cautiously. Extra monitoring of INR and/or warfarin dose adjustments may be needed. See Table 24-1 for more on supplements that can affect the INR.

TABLE 24-1 COMMON VITAMINS AND HERBALS THAT INTERACT WITH WARFARIN (PARTIAL LIST)

Warfarin Interaction	Vitamin/Herbal
↑ INR and risk of bleeding	Danshen Dong quai Fish oil Garlic Ginkgo Policosanol Vitamin E
↓ INR and risk of bleeding	Coenzyme Q10 St. John wort Vitamin K

The other options are unlikely to affect the INR. Vitamin A ("A") consumed in quantities exceeding 10 times the *recommended daily allowance* (RDA) for several months may cause alopecia, ataxia, glossitis, and hepatotoxicity. Vitamin C ("B") is usually well tolerated but large doses can cause nausea, diarrhea, and abdominal pain. Excessive intake of vitamin D ("C") may cause hypercalcemia, hypercalciuria, nausea, vomiting, myalgia, and, paradoxically, bone demineralization. Symptoms of zinc ("E") toxicity include nausea, anemia, loss of sense of smell and taste (when administered nasally), and depressed immune function.

 HELPFUL TIP:
Patients with cholestasis (pregnancy, central venous nutrition, sclerosing cholangitis, cystic fibrosis, etc.), including those with postobstructive jaundice, are often vitamin K deficient due to poor absorption of vitamin K (*Nutr Res*. 2009 Sep;29(9):676–683 and others).

 HELPFUL TIP:
Compared with water-soluble vitamins (B and C), fat-soluble vitamins (A, D, E, and K) are more likely to accumulate, resulting in toxicity. In related news, Americans are said to have the most expensive urine in the world due to the numerous water-soluble, and mostly useless mega dose vitamins and supplements we take … simply to pass them through our kidneys.

 (VERY) HELPFUL TIP:
Vitamin K can be useful in patients with a hard to control INR. Start a vitamin K supplement of 100 to 200 μg/day. This will help to eliminate diet-dependent INR fluctuations.

The patient learns that the vitamin therapy he currently takes has large amounts of vitamin E, but no vitamin K. You counsel him to discontinue this supplement, hold a dose of warfarin, and then continue on the same dose. You ask him to come back next week for another PT/INR. Before leaving, he asks about taking a multivitamin, complaining, "Gotta do something to get my mojo back, Doc."

Question 24.1.4 **From available evidence, and regarding his mojo (whatever that is), you are able to tell him:**
A) "Most multivitamins do not contain enough vitamin E to cause a problem"
B) "Multivitamins should be standard preventive medicine and have a well-described role in improving health"
C) "Iron supplements are recommended for middle-aged males"
D) "Folic acid and B vitamins should be taken by everyone with aortic stenosis to reduce homocysteine"

Answer 24.1.4 **The correct answer is "A."** Most multivitamins contain less than 400 IU of vitamin E and usually will not cause a problem. A fairly well-balanced diet based of whole, unprocessed foods provides the necessary nutrients to avoid vitamin deficiency syndromes. Supplementation with multivitamins is *not* necessary unless there are dietary intake deficiencies related to an unbalanced diet or a specific malabsorption issue, such as might occur with Crohn disease or bowel resection.

Taking a multivitamin has **not** been linked to improved health status. Average adult males generally have adequate iron stores and should not receive supplemental iron due to the potential for exacerbating undiagnosed iron storage disease. While folate, vitamin B6, and vitamin B12 lower serum homocysteine levels, there is no evidence that this intervention is helpful in reducing disease burden or improving health in those with known coronary artery disease or venous thromboembolism. While you may be able to lower serum homocysteine levels in patients with hyper-homocysteinemia, doing so *does not* lower risk of atherosclerotic cardiovascular disease or VTE risk.

Question 24.1.5 **Regarding vitamin and mineral supplementation, which of the statements is FALSE?**
A) Folate supplementation during pregnancy is recommended to decrease the risk of neural tube defects
B) Calcium and vitamin D supplementation in postmenopausal females are recommended to reduce the risk of osteoporosis and fractures
C) Vitamin D supplementation is recommended for breastfed infants, starting in the first few days of life
D) Vitamin D supplementation in elderly patients does not reduce the risk of falling
E) Vitamin E supplementation in elderly patients reduces the risk of cardiovascular disease

Answer 24.1.5 **The correct answer (and false statement) is "E."** Vitamin E supplementation has not been shown to reduce the risk of cardiovascular disease and has been associated with an increased risk of all-cause mortality at doses >400 IU/day. Additionally, high-dose (>400 IU/day) vitamin E is associated with an increase in prostate cancer in men and does not improve cognition in those with mild cognitive impairment or dementia. Basically, vitamin E has lost its "mojo." The other answers are true statements. "A" has plenty of evidence to back it up. Folate supplementation is universally recommended during the prenatal period and should be started even before pregnancy actually occurs. "B" is widely recommended, although the evidence for calcium-reducing fracture risk is weak. As for "C," the American Academy of Pediatrics (AA) and the CDC recommend that totally or partially breastfed infants take 400 IU of vitamin D daily, starting in the first few days of life and continue until taking at least 1 liter per day of vitamin D fortified formula or milk. "D", Vitamin D, a mighty force in medicine just a few years ago, has fallen far. In fact, it is no longer recognized as an intervention for fall prevention in the elderly. Several negative studies have been published, and the Cochrane Collaboration concluded, "Overall, vitamin D supplementation does not appear to prevent falls."

 HELPFUL TIP:
In general, daily multivitamins do not contain large enough doses of vitamins to result in toxicity, and any unneeded water-soluble vitamins are excreted in the urine. So, taking a daily multivitamin is a good way for patients to make expensive, vitamin-fortified urine.

▶ **Objectives: Did you learn to …**
- Describe signs and causes of vitamin K deficiency?
- Identify common vitamins and herbals that interact with warfarin?
- Recognize symptoms of fat-soluble vitamin toxicities?
- Identify benefits, risks, and limitations of vitamin supplementation?

 QUICK QUIZ: SUPPLEMENTS TO BREAST MILK

A 6-month-old male infant presents for routine health examination and immunizations. His mother is a strict vegan and has been nursing him exclusively. She has not introduced any foods and she wants to keep breastfeeding him primarily for at least the next 6 months … or until his friends start to tease him, she jokes (you hope). She takes no medicines and no supplements of any kind.

For this mother and her child, you recommend all of the following EXCEPT:
A) Vitamin B12 supplementation for the mother
B) Vitamin C supplementation for the mother
C) Vitamin D supplementation for the infant
D) Iron supplementation for the infant

The correct answer is "B." Children breastfed by strict vegan mothers should have vitamin B12 supplementation for either themselves or their mother. Vitamin C supplementation is not required. As above, vitamin D is recommended for all breastfed infants. According to the AAP and CDC, iron supplementation is recommended in all breastfed infants starting at 4 months of age until iron-containing foods become a routine part of their

diet (supplemental dose is 1 mg/kg/day). There are a variety of liquid multiple vitamins to choose from (e.g., Poly-Vi-Sol®).

▶ **CASE 24.2**

A 34-year-old female presents to your office with concerns about weight gain. She has gained over 100 lb since she graduated from high school. She tearfully reveals that the weight gain has come despite "not eating much." She walks for exercise, but is unable to quantify her walking (the Fitbit battery died).

She denies chronic illnesses. Her only surgery was a tubal ligation after her last child. She smokes 10 cigarettes per day and is unwilling to quit due to fears of further weight gain. She drinks alcohol once or twice per week, never consuming more than three beers. The review of systems is positive for a dry cough, bilateral knee pain, and fatigue.

On physical examination, you find an afebrile female with an elevated blood pressure (142/94 mm Hg). She is 5 ft 3 in tall and weighs 231 lb. Her body mass index (BMI) is 41 kg/m². You find trace pitting edema at the ankles bilaterally. There is increased pigmentation in the folds of the neck and the knuckles. The remainder of the examination is unremarkable.

The patient realizes that she is overweight and asks, "How bad am I?"

Question 24.2.1 Regarding definition and classification of obesity, which of the following is true?
A) Obesity is defined as BMI ≥25 kg/m²
B) Severe obesity is defined as BMI >30 kg/m²
C) Underweight is defined as BMI <20 kg/m²
D) Obesity is defined as BMI ≥30 kg/m²
E) Malnourished supermodel status is defined as BMI <30 kg/m²

Answer 24.2.1 The correct answer is "D." Obesity is defined by BMI ≥ 30 kg/m²; therefore, only "D" is correct. See Table 24-2 for definitions of weight status by BMI. The calculation for BMI is as follows:

$$BMI\,(kg/m^2) = weight\,(kg)\,/\,[height\,(m)]^2.$$

TABLE 24-2 DEFINITION OF WEIGHT STATUS BY BMI

Weight Status		BMI (kg/m²)
Underweight		<18.5
Normal		18.5–24.9
Overweight		25.0–29.9
Obese	Class I	30.0–34.9
	Class II	35.0–39.9
Extremely/Severely obese	Class III	≥40.0

Example: weight $= 110\,\text{lb}\,(50\,\text{kg})$, height $= 59\,\text{in}\,(1.5\,\text{m})$, therefore

$$\text{BMI} = 50/(1.5)^2 = 22.2\,\text{kg/m}^2.$$

HELPFUL TIP:
In American adults in 2016, the CDC estimated that the prevalence of obesity was 39.8%, which does not include people in the "overweight" category. Now that's what we call an epidemic! Prevalence of obesity appears to be somewhat socioeconomically determined, with poorer and less educated populations having higher rates of obesity. There are many reasons for this: epigenetics, "food deserts" where it is hard to find fresh foods, the cost of fresh foods versus high calorie carbohydrates and fats, etc.

HELPFUL TIP:
There has been controversy regarding whether the current BMI cut-offs are applicable across different ethnic populations, as there is evidence that body fat percentage, distribution of body fat (waist-hip ratio), and BMI may differ within different ethnic groups. Further, there is evidence that waist-to-hip ratio correlates more strongly with mortality and obesity-related disease than does BMI (*Ann Intern Med*. 2017;166(12):917–918).

You ask her about medications, focusing on those related to obesity.

Question 24.2.2 All of the following drugs are associated with weight gain and an increased risk of obesity EXCEPT:
A) Olanzapine
B) Topiramate
C) Gabapentin/Pregabalin
D) Valproic acid
E) Glipizide

Answer 24.2.2 The correct answer is "B." Topiramate may actually help patients lose weight. In fact, it is one of the components of the weight loss drug Qsymia® (phentermine/topiramate). Note especially that gabapentin and pregabalin cause weight gain, a bad thing when used in diabetes. See Table 24-3 for a list of medications associated with weight gain.

Question 24.2.3 Which of the following is the most appropriate next step in the evaluation of this patient's weight gain?
A) Refer for a sleep study
B) Check urinary free cortisol level
C) Draw blood for thyroid-stimulating hormone level
D) Evaluation for adrenal adenoma causing Cushing disease
E) Cast your gaze down realizing that affecting behavior change is difficult

TABLE 24-3 DRUGS ASSOCIATED WITH WEIGHT GAIN (NOT AN EXHAUSTIVE LIST)

Class	Specific Agents
Alpha Blockers	Prazosin, doxazosin, terazosin
Anticonvulsants	Valproate, carbamazepine, gabapentin
Antidepressants	Tricyclics (e.g., amitriptyline) and monoamine oxidase inhibitors (MAO-Is), selective serotonin reuptake inhibitors (SSRIs) in some patients
Antihistamines	Cyproheptadine, diphenhydramine
Antipsychotics	Olanzapine, thioridazine, haloperidol, risperidone
Beta blockers	Propranolol, metoprolol, atenolol
Diabetes drugs	Insulin, sulfonylureas, thiazolidinediones
Steroid hormones	Corticosteroids, oral contraceptives, estrogen, progesterone, testosterone

Answer 24.2.3 The correct answer is "C." Because of her obesity, this patient is also at risk for sleep apnea, diabetes, hypertension, and hyperlipidemia. These concerns will need to be addressed. However, her chief complaint is weight gain, which could certainly be due to an underlying disease. Although in most overweight patients a cause for weight gain is not found, the physician is obligated to search for potentially treatable causes of weight gain, including hypothyroidism. The symptoms of hypothyroidism are often nonspecific and include weight gain and fatigue. That said, an exhaustive search for underlying causes of obesity is not required for the vast majority of patients. History, exam, and limited laboratory evaluation should be sufficient for most patients.

HELPFUL TIP:
Complications of obesity include heart disease, type 2 diabetes, hypertension, stroke, hyperlipidemia, gallbladder disease, obstructive sleep apnea, reduced fertility, increased risk of certain cancers (prostate, colon, breast, endometrial), and emotional distress.

Question 24.2.4 On physical examination of this patient, you note velvety patches of hyperpigmentation in her axillary areas and at her posterior neck. This finding raises concern for which of the following diseases?
A) Skin cancer
B) Diabetes
C) Hemochromatosis
D) Colon cancer
E) Hypertriglyceridemia

Answer 24.2.4 The correct answer is "B." Acanthosis nigricans, classically described as velvety hyperpigmentation in skin creases (axilla, back, neck, flexor aspects of arms), is associated with a number of diseases. Acanthosis nigricans occurs in insulin-resistance syndromes, commonly in patients with type 2 diabetes. It is also associated with other endocrine abnormalities, including Cushing disease and hypothyroidism. Acanthosis nigricans can be an external sign of internal malignancy, most commonly gastrointestinal (GI) cancers. However, this patient is at lower risk of colon cancer than diabetes, given her age, weight gain, and lack of other signs and symptoms of cancer. Hemochromatosis, hypertriglyceridemia, and skin cancer are not associated with acanthosis nigricans.

She wonders which popular diet she should use to lose weight.

Question 24.2.5 You let her know that the most effective popular diet is:
A) Low carbohydrate ("Atkins diet")
B) Low fat ("Ornish diet")
C) Low glycemic load diet ("Zone diet")
D) High protein ("Paleo diet")
E) No one particular diet is more effective than others for weight loss. The key to success is choosing a diet that you can maintain

Answer 24.2.5 The correct answer is "E." Any diet you can stick to seems to work. There does not seem to be any advantage to one diet over another for weight loss (except for making the proprietors wealthy). For example, Weight Watchers may have a bit better success because of peer pressure, weekly meetings, and motivational techniques (*BMJ*. 2011;343:d6500). But any diet that you can maintain long-term will work. Of note, the common belief that maintaining a 3,500 calorie weekly deficit will result in 1 lb (0.45 kg) of weight loss per week is a myth. But reducing calorie intake by 100 calories per day may lead to a gradual weight loss of approximately 10 lb over 1 to 3 years (*Am Fam Physician*. 2015;91(9):634–638).

HELPFUL TIP:
If you want to give your patients a more realistic (and, sadly, more complicated) method of determining how much weight they can expect to lose when making lifestyle changes, point them to the evidence-based Body Weight Planner produced by the NIH, available online at www.niddk.nih.gov/bwp. The website links to multiple tools for patient education and self-management.

She is wondering about her level of physical activity and is afraid that her obesity will decrease her ability to become functionally fit with exercise.

Question 24.2.6 Your response to this is that:
A) Gluttony and sloth go together, so give up the exercise
B) One cannot improve one's physical performance without weight loss
C) Dante did not know what he was talking about; it is TV and sloth that go together

D) Exercise is beneficial for fitness regardless of whether or not one loses weight
E) Exercise is useless for weight loss—every cookie you eat is another mile on the treadmill, minimum

Answer 24.2.6 The correct answer is "D." Losing weight is notoriously hard to do. Thankfully, exercise, in and of itself, increases functional capacity regardless of weight loss (*N Engl J Med*. 2011;364(13):1218–1229). Obviously, patients do better if they both exercise and lose weight. But sticking to an exercise regimen is still helpful. With regard to the others, there was no evidence-based medicine or TV during the time of Dante, so we will never know.

HELPFUL TIP:
Aside from weight loss, some of the popular diets have other health benefits. A low-glycemic index diet (vegetables, chicken, fish, whole grains, beans, nuts, etc.) can lower HbA$_{1C}$ in patients with type 2 diabetes when compared with a high whole-grain carbohydrate diet (brown rice, whole wheat foods, etc.). Psyllium (Metamucil and others) can also help reduce HbA$_{1C}$. A Paleolithic diet based on meat, fish, fruits, vegetables, root vegetables, eggs, and nuts also results in lower mean values of HbA$_{1C}$, diastolic blood pressure, weight, BMI, and waist circumference over a 3-month period when compared to an American Diabetes Association diet (*Cardiovasc Diabetol*. 2009;8:35). In a "dose-dependent" fashion, the Mediterranean diet improves glycemic control and reduces cardiovascular risk, including stroke risk (*Stroke*. 2018;0:2415–2420).

You find that the patient's thyroid function is normal. After consultation with a nutritionist and a prescription for exercise, she returns 3 months later. Her weight is 222 lb. Clearly frustrated, she tells you that she barely eats and needs something more to help her lose weight.

Question 24.2.7 According to evidence-based consensus guidelines, which of the following is/are generally accepted criteria that patients must fulfill to be candidates for weight loss pharmacotherapy?
A) BMI of 30 kg/m^2 or greater
B) BMI of 27 to 29.9 kg/m^2 with an obesity-related comorbidity
C) BMI of 25 kg/m^2 or greater and an acting career in jeopardy
D) All of the above
E) None of the above

Answer 24.2.7 The correct answer is "E." Sorry, readers. This fits under the category of "trick question." Here's the issue: there are **no** evidence-based consensus guidelines for weight loss pharmacotherapy. However, expert recommendations and insurance coverage for drugs (if it exists, which often is not the case) generally agree with "A" and "B." Pharmacotherapy may be considered when comprehensive lifestyle modification fails to achieve reasonable weight loss goals (e.g., 5% body weight) for patients with BMI 30 kg/m² or greater or with BMI 27 to 29.9 kg/m² with health complications. "C" is clearly incorrect—hopefully. Don't prescribe weight loss drugs simply for patients whose BMI is in the overweight range (25–29.9 kg/m²) and who are not suffering any obesity-related health effects.

....

As your patient is not meeting with an ounce of success (literally), you engage in a discussion about weight loss pharmacotherapy.

Question 24.2.8 Which of the following medications is indicated by the FDA to treat obesity?
A) Levothyroxine (Synthroid, Levoxyl)
B) Methylphenidate (Ritalin)
C) Orlistat (Xenical, Alli)
D) Paroxetine (Paxil)

Answer 24.2.8 **The correct answer is "C."** Drug therapy is considered appropriate as an add-on to lifestyle management for people with a BMI of 30 kg/m² or greater, or a BMI of 27 kg/m² or more who already have a comorbid condition such as diabetes, hypertension, or hyperlipidemia. Of the choices listed, only orlistat is indicated by the FDA to treat obesity (more below). "A" and "B" are incorrect. Although patients treated with these medications might lose weight as a side effect, obesity alone is not an indication for levothyroxine or methylphenidate. Paroxetine ("D") may be associated with weight gain and is not indicated for obesity.

Question 24.2.9 Which of the following weight loss drugs results in GI side effects in up to 40% of patients using it?
A) Orlistat (Alli, Xenical)
B) Topiramate (Topamax)
C) Phentermine (Adipex-P, Ionamin)
D) Lorcaserin (Belviq)

Answer 24.2.9 **The correct answer is "A."** Orlistat is a lipase inhibitor that functions in the intestines and prevents the absorption of about 30% of dietary fats. Because of its mechanism of action, orlistat is associated with GI side effects in 40% of patients taking the drug. The most bothersome potential adverse effects include fecal incontinence and abdominal pain. Orlistat should be taken with meals. The prescription dose is 120 mg three times per day (Xenical); while an over-the-counter version (Alli) is available at half the dose—and far less than half the cost with relatively similar efficacy. Weight loss is modest: 3 to 4 kg over 1 year compared with placebo. Topiramate ("B") alone is not approved by the FDA for use as a weight loss drug, but the combination phentermine/topiramate (Qsymia) is. Phentermine ("C") is a sympathomimetic and carries adverse effects of hypertension, tachycardia, etc., and is indicated for up to 12 weeks due to concerns about the potential for abuse. Lorcaserin ("D") is a 5HT$_{2c}$ selective serotonin agonist that is FDA-approved for treating obesity, and it is relatively safe. Unlike serotonin agonists that preceded it, lorcaserin has not (yet) been associated with cardiac valvulopathy.

HELPFUL TIP:
Orlistat may result in fat-soluble vitamin deficiencies. If a patient is taking orlistat long-term, advise them to take a multivitamin separated in time from orlistat—experts often recommend this before bedtime since orlistat is taken with meals.

....

Your patient points out that she has a family history of diabetes and wonders about taking a weight loss medication that could help her prevent or treat diabetes.

Question 24.2.10 Which of the following medications is FDA-indicated to treat both obesity and type 2 diabetes (albeit at different doses and under different brand names)?
A) Glipizide
B) Liraglutide
C) Metformin
D) Sitagliptin

Answer 24.2.10 **The correct answer is "B."** Liraglutide is a GLP-1 agonist (also called an incretin mimetic) which is marketed as Saxenda® for obesity and Victoza® for diabetes. Its maximum dose varies depending on the indication: for obesity the maximum daily dose is 3 mg and for diabetes it is 1.8 mg. Compared to placebo, patients taking liraglutide lose 2 to 4 kg of body weight and significantly more patients reach 5% total body weight reduction. GI side effects are the most common adverse events, and cost may be prohibitive for many patients. Glipizide ("A") is associated with weight gain. Although metformin ("C") and sitagliptin ("D," Januvia®) are associated with modest weight loss, they are not FDA-indicated for treating obesity.

....

You initiate a medication to help her lose weight and refer her to a weight loss program that focuses on overall lifestyle modification. When she returns in 3 months, her weight is 235 lb, and she is very frustrated.

Question 24.2.11 You appropriately recommend which of the following?
A) Adding a second drug for weight loss
B) Referral to psychiatry
C) Referral to bariatric surgery
D) Referral to plastic surgery

Answer 24.2.11 **The correct answer is "C."** This patient now meets accepted indications for bariatric surgery. See Chapter 22 for more information about weight loss surgery.

....

HELPFUL TIP:
Drug therapy and surgery are no substitute for basic lifestyle modifications, including appropriate dietary modifications and regular aerobic exercise. These lifestyle approaches should be continued during drug treatment and are absolutely essential after surgery.

▶ **Objectives: Did you learn to …**
- Define normal weight, overweight, and obesity?
- Appropriately evaluate the obese patient?
- Recognize goals and methods of treating obesity?
- Recognize complications that occur as a result of obesity?

 QUICK QUIZ: VITAMIN DEFICIENCIES

A 63-year-old male presents to the office after his daughter came home for the holidays and found him confused. At first she thought he was drunk, but after a few days, the confusion persisted. He has never had problems with complicated alcohol withdrawal before. According to the daughter, the patient drinks about half of a bottle of vodka per day and has done so for years (Hawkeye Vodka is the Iowa favorite …). Although the patient is not able to give much of a coherent history, you are able to determine that he has developed shortness of breath and leg edema. His appetite has been poor for "a long time" and he may have lost some weight although he is not sure.

Physical examination reveals a malnourished, disoriented male who appears older than his stated age and is disheveled. He is mildly tachycardic, but his other vital signs are normal. He has bibasilar crackles on lung examination, 2+ pedal edema, hepatomegaly, and spider telangiectasias.

What is your first action to take with this patient?
A) Administer D50 intravenous (IV)
B) Administer thiamine IV
C) Administer vitamin B12 IM
D) Administer niacin orally
E) Administer folate orally

The correct answer is "B." This patient almost certainly has thiamine (vitamin B1) deficiency and appears to be symptomatic. In the United States, thiamine deficiency is most often seen in malnourished alcoholics. Early symptoms of thiamine deficiency are vague (similar to how the author/editors wrote the case) and include anorexia, fatigue, and irritability. Thiamine-deficient patients may progress to beriberi (wet or dry), possessing symptoms of heart failure and/or neuropathy (motor and sensory). Other possible manifestations of thiamine deficiency include Wernicke encephalopathy (ataxia, ocular-motor abnormalities [e.g., gaze paralysis], mental status changes, dietary deficiency) and Wernicke–Korsakoff syndrome (Wernicke syndrome plus additional memory loss and confabulations). **Note that most patients do not have all of the findings. Most have a partial syndrome.** Treatment is to administer thiamine IV and then to continue oral supplementation. IV carbohydrates, such as D50 ("A"), should be avoided until thiamine is given as they can worsen encephalopathy (although if the patient is neuroglycopenic, treatment is still warranted).

 HELPFUL TIP:
The dosage of thiamine administered for treatment and prevention of Wernicke encephalopathy differs. For prevention of Wernicke encephalopathy, give thiamine

100 mg daily. For treatment of Wernicke encephalopathy, give thiamine 500 mg IV BID–TID for 2 days followed by 500 mg IV daily for 5 more days (although recommendations vary and no randomized trials support one regimen over another).

 HELPFUL TIP:
Other micronutrient deficiencies that occur in alcoholic patients include niacin deficiency resulting in pellagra (dermatitis, diarrhea, and dementia); folate deficiency resulting in macrocytic anemia; vitamin B12 deficiency (generally due to problems with GI absorption rather than as a direct effect of alcoholism) resulting in anemia, neuropathy, and dementia. A multivitamin is certainly reasonable in this patient population.

▶ **CASE 24.3**

A 58-year-old postmenopausal female presents to your office with concerns about osteoporosis. A review of her medical history shows a bone density T-score of –1.8 from 2 years ago, suggesting moderate osteopenia. As you review her medical record, you note that last year she had lipids measured which were: total cholesterol of 210 mg/dL, LDL 140 mg/dL and HDL 45 mg/dL, and triglycerides 125 mg/dL. She had a partial thyroidectomy 15 years ago and currently takes levothyroxine 88 µg/day.

Question 24.3.1 **Based on the evidence, which of the following supplements is most appropriate for this patient?**
A) Calcium alone
B) Calcium and vitamin D
C) Vitamin D alone
D) Ipriflavone

Answer 24.3.1 **The correct answer is "B."** Postmenopausal women should take 1,200 mg/day of **elemental** calcium with total of diet plus supplements not exceeding 2,000 mg of elemental calcium per day. The recommendations for supplemental calcium are muddied a bit by the observation that higher calcium **supplement** intake is associated with greater risk of CAD. Vitamin D is also appropriate, and many women do not get enough. As supplements go, vitamin D may be more important than calcium.

In terms of vitamin D, recommended doses are 400 IU/day for infants, 600 IU/day for ages 1 to 70, and 800 IU/day in those over age 70 (Institute of Medicine, 2011). The guideline also concludes that there is not any good evidence for vitamin D beyond its use for bone health.

Ipriflavone is a semisynthetic isoflavone produced from soy isoflavones. There is evidence that it can prevent bone mineral density loss when used with calcium in postmenopausal women, but it has not been shown to reduce fracture rates. There are also concerns that it might cause lymphocytopenia in some patients.

HELPFUL TIP:
If you are concerned about prevention of osteoporosis, start early, really early. Counsel adolescent females to get at least 1,300 mg of elemental calcium and 600 IU of vitamin D daily.

You counsel her to take 1,200 mg of elemental calcium per day.

Question 24.3.2 In order to improve GI absorption of calcium, you recommend:
A) Taking 1,200 mg at one time with a meal
B) Taking 1,200 mg at one time an hour before eating
C) Taking 1,200 mg in three divided doses with meals
D) Taking 1,200 mg in three divided doses on an empty stomach
E) Taking 1,200 mg with her levothyroxine

Answer 24.3.2 The correct answer is "C." Calcium is best absorbed when taken with food. Theoretically, GI absorption of calcium is limited, and for that reason divided dosing in 500 to 600 mg aliquots or less is recommended. Patients should take levothyroxine separately from their calcium. If taken together, calcium reduces levothyroxine absorption. This is also true of iron and levothyroxine.

She then asks you about her cholesterol levels and whether taking soy would be helpful. A friend told her that older women should take soy to prevent heart disease, breast cancer, osteoporosis—basically, they told her soy will help her to cheat death.

Question 24.3.3 Which of the following is appropriate to tell this patient?
A) Soy isoflavone supplements are preferred for reducing lipid levels
B) Dietary soy protein is not associated with a reduced risk of developing heart disease in Western women
C) Soy protein is as effective as a statin for lowering cholesterol
D) Soy isoflavones are an acceptable alternative to calcium and vitamin D for preventing osteoporosis

Answer 24.3.3 The correct answer is "B." Soy protein can modestly reduce lipid levels in some patients but has been shown not to affect important outcomes such as heart attack or death in Western women. Soy isoflavone supplements have not been shown to reduce lipid levels. Soy protein is not nearly as effective as statin drugs (e.g., atorvastatin and simvastatin) are. Soy protein or soy isoflavone supplements are not an appropriate alternative to calcium and vitamin D.

Your patient is hoping you can settle a bet. She asks about her younger sister who is going through "the change" (quarters, nickels, pennies ...) and started taking black cohosh. Her sister swears the black cohosh helps her hot flashes, but your patient thinks it's "all in her head."

Question 24.3.4 Regarding the use of black cohosh for the treatment of perimenopausal vasomotor symptoms, you tell her:
A) Black cohosh is equivalent to hormone replacement therapy
B) Black cohosh is equivalent to placebo
C) Black cohosh is not good for vasomotor symptoms but does promote liver health
D) Black cohosh is only effective when taken as part of a multi-botanical supplement

Answer 24.3.4 The correct answer is "B." Most studies of black cohosh are not well done. A Cochrane Collaboration review in 2012 found insufficient evidence for black cohosh for menopausal symptoms. The arguments against its use are the *rare* (if any) cases of hepatotoxicity, so "C" is wrong.

HELPFUL TIP:
Soy protein integrated into the diet is generally recognized as safe and is acceptable for women who want to try it. But it should not replace proven therapies. Soy is a common food allergen. See Table 24-4 for an overview of soy benefits.

HELPFUL TIP:
While other herbal products like phytoestrogens, wild yam, primrose oil, and vitamin E claim efficacy in treating menopausal symptoms, rigorously designed clinical trials performed to date have not confirmed their efficacy.

Question 24.3.5 Which of the following natural products could be recommended for lowering LDL cholesterol?
A) Fish oil
B) Psyllium
C) Garlic
D) Policosanol (a drug derived from sugar cane)
E) All of the above

Answer 24.3.5 The correct answer is "B." Taking a psyllium supplement (e.g., Metamucil) 10 to 12 g daily can reduce total cholesterol by up to 14% and LDL by up to 10%. Fish oil ("A") is effective for lowering triglycerides, but not total cholesterol or LDL cholesterol. Clinical outcomes do not seem to change with the use of fish oil and it has fallen by the wayside. Garlic ("C") was long considered effective for modest reduction in cholesterol, but the evidence shows that garlic does not significantly reduce cholesterol in most people. Similarly, policosanol ("D") was once considered effective for reducing cholesterol, but evidence is inconsistent. The most reliable evidence shows that it is ineffective. To be complete, "red yeast rice" does lower LDL and contains lovastatin, though the dose, and thus the response, is inconsistent; it is a poor substitute for a statin.

TABLE 24-4 OVERVIEW OF THE EFFECTIVENESS OF SOY

Condition	Effectiveness Data	Comment/Recommendation
Breast cancer	Higher intake of soy in the diet is associated with decreased risk of breast cancer. But most research limited to Asian populations. May not apply to Western populations. No clinical trials.	Unknown benefits in Western populations. Data are not strong enough to recommend dietary soy for this use.
Hyperlipidemia/cardiovascular disease	Consuming soy protein in place of other protein sources might modestly reduce lipid levels. Does not apply to soy isoflavone supplements. No evidence that eating soy improves outcomes such as death or heart attack. Population research shows no decreased risk of these outcomes in Western women.	Substituting dietary soy for other proteins is acceptable, but only modest benefit expected; not an alternative to mortality or cardiovascular event-reducing therapies such as statins.
Osteoporosis	Consuming dietary soy protein might improve bone mineral density in postmenopausal women and possibly reduce fracture risk; however, not all evidence is consistent.	There is possible benefit to adding soy protein to the diet, but benefit is likely to be modest at best. Soy is not a substitute to calcium and vitamin D.

Question 24.3.6 What percentage of Americans use alternative therapies?

A) 10%
B) 20%
C) 30%
D) 40%
E) 50%

Answer 24.3.6 The correct answer is "D." Thirty-eight percent of adults and 12% of children use complementary or alternative therapy (*Natl Health Stat Report.* 2015;79:1–15). Only 40% of patients informed their physicians. Examples of complimentary therapies used include:

Relaxation	Self-help groups	Homeopathy	Spiritual healing
Chiropractic	Biofeedback	Lifestyle diets	Acupuncture
Massage	Energy healing	Herbal medicine	Exercise
Imagery	Hypnosis	Megavitamins	Prayer

At least 15 million patients take prescription medications along with their alternative medications, sometimes with adverse outcomes.

Question 24.3.7 Which of these is *NOT* a reason that patients might use alternative therapies?

A) They believe they are safer than medications
B) Conventional medicine is too technical or impersonal
C) Prescription medicines are too expensive
D) Cultural practices
E) They didn't like the shark in *Jaws* and therefore use shark cartilage in an attempt to rid the oceans of sharks

Answer 24.3.7 The correct answer is "E." Many patients use alternative therapies including herbal supplements for various reasons, some of which are listed above. Other reasons cited include perceived physician apathy, difficulty with physician access, fear of medication side effects, belief that medications lack efficacy, and the fact that they are not "natural." Many patients do not inform their physicians about their use of these products, mistakenly believing that "natural" means safe. As for "E," unfortunately there is a large demand for shark cartilage including its use as chondroitin sulfate. Shark populations have been severely stressed as a result. Up to 100 *million* sharks per year are killed for their fins and cartilage.

Question 24.3.8 What is the current status of the regulation of "natural" therapies?

A) The FDA does not have a regulatory role with regard to natural therapies
B) Natural products have to be proven safe and effective in order to be marketed in the United States
C) Natural therapies are regulated by the Department of Health and Human Services
D) As long as they contain the ingredients claimed, natural therapies can be marketed in the United States

Answer 24.3.8 The correct answer is "A." The FDA has no regulatory role with regard to natural therapies. They are classified as dietary supplements and not medications. All of the rest are incorrect. "B" is incorrect because natural therapies need **not** be proven safe and effective in order to be marketed. "D" is incorrect. There is no quality control on "natural" therapies in the United States. Products may contain varying amounts of the advertised therapy or, in some cases, none at all. In fact, there are data suggesting that some products for sale do not contain what they advertise and in other cases, contain prescription drugs such as warfarin, steroids, alprazolam, and diethylstilbestrol.

HELPFUL TIP:
The FDA can remove natural therapy products if it can show that they are hazardous. This is a slow and laborious process as evidenced by how long it took to remove ephedra from the US market.

A partial list of unsafe alternative remedies is as follows:

- Hepatotoxic: Chaparral, germander, life root
- Carcinogenic: Borage, calamus, coltsfoot, comfrey, life root, and sassafras
- Miscellaneous toxicity: Ma Huang (ephedra), poke root

HELPFUL TIP: SOMETHING IS A BIT FISHY …
The role of omega 3 fatty acids from fish oil in cardiovascular disease (CVD) is pretty settled. The best studies show no benefit in those with preexisting CVD. Nor is there a benefit in primary prevention (*N Engl J Med.* 2019;380:23–32). Bottom line: save your money.

Question 24.3.9 Grapefruit juice interacts with multiple medications. Which of the following IS NOT affected by grapefruit juice?
A) Tacrolimus
B) Itraconazole/Ketoconazole
C) Benzodiazepines
D) Clopidogrel
E) Aspirin

Answer 24.3.9 **The correct answer is "E."** All of the other drugs interact with grapefruit juice. Grapefruit juice is a potent CYP3A4 inhibitor and can interact with numerous medications including: those listed above, some calcium channel blockers, carbamazepine, benzodiazepines, amiodarone, atorvastatin, lovastatin, simvastatin, and others. This underscores the importance of knowing what "alternative" medications your patient might be using.

Question 24.3.10 Which of the following supplements has been touted as being effective for memory problems and peripheral circulatory problems?
A) Ginkgo biloba
B) S-Adenosylmethionine (SAM-e)
C) Glucosamine
D) None of the above

Answer 24.3.10 **The correct answer is "A."** Ginkgo biloba is one of the most popular herbal products and is promoted for mild memory loss, dementia, and peripheral circulatory disorders. Ginkgo has some antiplatelet effect and is touted for helping with vascular disease and dementia, although proof is lacking. Given its antiplatelet effects, gingko should be used with caution or not at all in patients taking aspirin. Side effects include GI disturbances, headaches, and dizziness. "B," SAM-e, is used for arthritis and depression and has been shown to be "likely effective." "C," glucosamine, has NOT been shown to be effective for osteoarthritis, either alone or in combination with chondroitin—so lay off the sharks!

Question 24.3.11 Which herbal product has aldosterone-like properties and can cause a pseudohyperaldosteronism?
A) Ma Huang
B) Ginseng
C) Licorice
D) Melatonin

Answer 24.3.11 **The correct answer is "C."** Licorice (*Glycyrrhiza* spp.) has aldosterone-like effects and can lead to fluid retention, hypertension, and hypokalemia. Thus, it should not be combined with other potassium-wasting drugs such as thiazides and loop diuretics. It is also contraindicated in patients with severe liver disease and in pregnant patients (may induce premature labor).

Question 24.3.12 For which of the following diseases is SAM-e "likely effective"?
A) Depression
B) Fibromyalgia
C) Cirrhosis
D) Osteoarthritis
E) Both A and D

Answer 24.3.12 **The correct answer is "D."** SAM-e is "likely effective" in treating osteoarthritis and comparable to NSAIDS (though maximum effect takes 14 days versus 7 with NSAIDS). It is "possibly effective" in treating depression and fibromyalgia, and there is insufficient evidence to rate its use in cirrhosis. SAM-e is contraindicated in bipolar patients as it can induce mania. SAM-e can possibly interact with antidepressants, including MAOIs, leading to serotonin syndrome. GI disturbance is the only notable side effect.

Question 24.3.13 Which of these is useful in the treatment of migraine headaches?
A) St. John wort
B) Valerian root
C) Ginger
D) Feverfew
E) Saw palmetto

Answer 24.3.13 **The correct answer is "D."** Feverfew is "possibly effective" in treating migraine headaches, although there is limited moderate-quality evidence for this conclusion. On the bright side, feverfew is deemed safe, so you might consider it as a prophylactic intervention for patients with frequent migraine headaches. "A," St. John wort, is useful for depression. **However, there are major interactions between St. John wort and other multiple drugs including: cyclosporine, nevirapine, and digoxin among others.** "B," valerian root, is useful for insomnia and has been shown to reduce sleep latency. Ginger is used for nausea and seems to be effective; it is likely safe though there are anecdotal reports of miscarriage and bleeding and it *may* interfere with sex hormones in the doses required for its anti-nausea properties. Remember that OTC ginger supplement products are not regulated, so that they might contain other substances that could be unsafe in pregnancy. Recommend ginger supplements with some degree of caution in pregnant patients. On the other hand, dietary ginger is probably safe, and fresh ginger rhizome is efficacious. Saw Palmetto is used for benign prostatic hypertrophy but is ineffective.

Question 24.3.14 Which of these is NOT potentially useful for women with pregnancy-related nausea and vomiting?
A) Acupressure
B) Vitamin B6
C) Doxylamine
D) Black cohosh

Answer 24.3.14 **The correct answer is "D."** Vitamin B6 ("B," pyridoxine) and doxylamine ("C"), an antihistamine, have been shown individually and together to be safe and effective in pregnancy-related nausea and vomiting. Acupressure ("A") has no known adverse effects, and there is some suggestion of efficacy. Black cohosh ("D") can stimulate uterine contractions and has no known efficacy for nausea and vomiting in pregnancy, and so it is contraindicated in pregnancy.

▶ **Objectives: Did you learn to …**
- Describe the prevalence of alternative therapy use?
- Appreciate the various indications for various herbal products and the evidence base for them?
- Recognize herbs considered safe and those considered unsafe?
- Recognize problematic drug interactions with a variety of alternative therapies?

HELPFUL TIP:
Did you know that metformin, PPIs, and H2 blockers can all cause B12 deficiency? Now you do.

QUICK QUIZ: ALTERNATIVE CURE FOR THE COMMON COLD?

One of your patients who often uses complementary and alternative medicine comes into your office with several days of rhinorrhea, sore throat, and ear pain. Your examination reveals a viral upper respiratory infection. He asks you to recommend an alternative cure.

Which of these are touted as alternative remedies for the common cold?
A) Echinacea
B) Zinc
C) Vitamin C
D) All of the above
E) None of the above

The correct answer is "D." The three choices listed above have the reputation of helping alleviate the symptoms of the common cold. The efficacy of all of these is questionable, however. Intranasal zinc has been removed from the market in the United States due to reports of permanent loss of sense of taste and smell after its use.

▶ CASE 24.4

A 17-year-old male patient of yours comes to your office for a sports pre-participation physical. He is a little smaller than most of his classmates and has heard that creatine supplementation can help him increase muscle mass and improve his performance.

Question 24.4.1 Which of the following is NOT true about creatine?
A) Creatine exists primarily in skeletal muscle
B) It causes weight gain by increasing muscle mass
C) It is possibly effective in boosting performance in aerobic exercise
D) It can lead to increased creatinine levels in patients with normal renal function

Answer 24.4.1 **The correct answer is "B."** Creatine monohydrate is a naturally occurring protein in the body that exists primarily in skeletal muscle ("A"). High levels of creatine are thought to enhance the ability to renew ATP for short bursts of energy. It is "possibly effective" for enhancing muscle performance ("C"). Studies in rowers seem to be positive. Studies in cyclists, sprinters, swimmers, and "high intensity training" are inconsistent. It is "possibly effective" in older adults seeking to build muscle mass but only when combined with weight training. *It causes weight gain by increasing water retention and not by effecting muscle mass.* Creatine can cause elevated creatinine levels in patients with normal renal function as creatine is metabolized to creatinine ("D"). Complicating this is the fact that creatine has been linked to renal dysfunction in some cases.

Question 24.4.2 Which of these is NOT a disease that creatine is purported to treat?
A) Heart failure
B) Neuromuscular disease
C) Mitochondrial cytopathies
D) Muscular dystrophies
E) Diabetes

Answer 24.4.2 **The correct answer is "E."** Creatine is also promoted for heart failure, neuromuscular diseases, mitochondrial cytopathies, and various muscular dystrophies. Oral creatine may improve exercise tolerance in patients with heart failure but has no effect on ejection fraction. *IV creatine seems to improve ejection fraction temporarily.* When used orally, it seems to *marginally* improve muscle strength and daily-life activity in adults and children with various muscular dystrophies in the *short term (although data are contradictory)*. There is no evidence of its efficacy in the treatment of diabetes. It appears to be safe when used orally and in appropriate doses, though high doses raise the concern of adverse hepatic, renal, or cardiac function. Side effects include GI pain, nausea, and diarrhea, while college athletes taking it frequently complain of muscle cramping.

Confused about creatine? Given that at best it is "possibly effective" for most indications and is relatively safe in "normal" doses, sure, have patients give it a try if they want to. But give them reasonable expectations; there are both positive and negative studies out there.

▶ **Objective: Did you learn to …**
  · Describe the use and adverse effects of creatine?

 QUICK QUIZ: KRAZY FOR KRATOM

A 51-year-old female patient presents with her adult son for chronic and severe pain due to knee osteoarthritis. Her son is convinced that she needs kratom to treat her pain, and relates stories of multiple friends with chronic pain who were able to stop using opioids with the help of kratom. Since you are a rational human being, you don't recommend a treatment without knowing something about it, so you quickly consult your favorite point-of-care reference to educate yourself.

Which of the following safety concerns is present with kratom?
A) Kratom has been associated with liver toxicity
B) Cessation of kratom results in withdrawal symptoms
C) Kratom use has been associated with depression
D) Some kratom products have been found to contain opioids
E) All of the above

The correct answer is "E." Kratom has emerged as a herbal treatment for pain, opioid addiction, and fatigue. However, evidence for efficacy is lacking. It is derived from the plant *Mitragyna speciosa*, which has been used medicinally for centuries in Asia. Kratom is believed to act at opioid receptors and can have stimulant effects at low doses. Known side effects include: nausea, vomiting, dry mouth, constipation, weight loss, appetite loss, liver damage, and myalgia. In larger doses, it may cause hallucinations, depressed mood, sedation, and respiratory depression. Some products have been removed from the market due to contamination with opioids or Salmonella (really!). Withdrawal phenomena have been described, and there appears to be potential for addiction. In short, we don't recommend it.

 HELPFUL TIP:
Cannabidiol is another product promoted for its effects on pain and potential to help curb the opioid epidemic. While cannabidiol does appear to work to reduce frequency and severity of seizures in certain types of epilepsy (Epidiolex® is FDA-approved as an anticonvulsant), its effectiveness for pain is questionable. Better studies are required.

 QUICK QUIZ: A BLOODY HERB

A 51-year-old patient of yours is about to have a scheduled cholecystectomy. He is in otherwise good health and is taking the following herbs and supplements.

Which would you recommend him to stop before surgery because of association with prolonged bleeding time?
A) Valerian root
B) Ginseng
C) Vitamin B complex
D) Echinacea
E) Ginkgo

The correct answer is "E." Ginkgo is the only one above that has been associated with a prolonged bleeding time. Thus, it should be stopped prior to planned surgery. Other supplements that have antiplatelet effects include garlic, feverfew, vitamin E (at doses of greater than 800 IU/day), and fish oil.

Clinical Pearls

○ All breast-fed infants should receive supplemental vitamin D within the first few days of life and supplemental iron at 4 months of life if not eating iron-containing foods.
○ All women considering becoming pregnant should take a prenatal vitamin or a folate supplement.
○ Do not recommend more than 400 IU per day of vitamin E.
○ Do not routinely recommend multivitamins to patients for general health.
○ Recognize that 40% of patients use complementary and alternative therapies, often in addition to traditional medical treatments, and that the FDA does not regulate natural therapies.
○ Recognize that alcoholics may have multiple nutritional deficiencies, including folate, thiamine, B vitamins, and vitamin K in addition to protein deficiency.

BIBLIOGRAPHY

Barnes PM, Bloom B. Complementary and alternative medicine use among adults and children: United States, 2007. *Natl Health Stat Report.* 2008;12:1–23.

Barry MJ, et al. Effect of increasing doses of saw palmetto extract on lower urinary tract symptoms: a randomized trial. *JAMA.* 2011;306(12):1344–1351.

Bischoff-Ferrari HA, Dawson-Hughes B, Staehlin HB, et al. Fall prevention with supplemental and active forms of vitamin D: a meta-analysis of randomised controlled trials. *BMJ.* 2009;339:b3692.

Bolland MJ, et al. Calcium supplements with or without vitamin D and risk of cardiovascular events: reanalysis of the Women's Health Initiative limited access dataset and meta-analysis. *BMJ.* 2011;342:d2040.

Chaiyakunapruk N, et al. The efficacy of ginger for the prevention of postoperative nausea and vomiting: a meta-analysis. *Am J Obstet Gynecol.* 2006;194(1):95–99.

Clarke TC, et al. Trends in the use of complementary health approaches among adults: United States, 2002–2012. *Natl Health Stat Report.* 2015;79:1–15.

Fisher L, et al. Prevalence of vitamin K and vitamin D deficiency in patients with hepatobiliary and pancreatic disorders. *Nutr Res.* 2009;29(9):676–683.

Ford SK, Moll S. Vitamin K supplementation to decrease variability of international normalized ratios in patients on vitamin K antagonists: a literature review. *Curr Opin Hematol.* 2008;15(5):504–508.

Hamer M, et al. Normal-weight central obesity and risk for mortality. *Ann Intern Med.* 2017;166(12):917–6918.

Holick MF, et al. Evaluation, treatment, and prevention of vitamin D deficiency: an Endocrine Society Clinical Practice guideline. *J Clin Endocrinol Metab.* 2011;96(7):1911–1930.

Institute of Medicine Committee to Review Dietary Reference Intakes for Vitamin D and Calcium, Ross AC, Taylor CL, Yaktine AL, et al, eds. *Dietary Reference Intakes for Calcium and Vitamin D.* Washington, DC: The National Academies Press; 2011.

Jellin JM, Gregory PJ, eds. *Natural Medicines Comprehensive Database.* Stockton, CA: Therapeutic Research Faculty; 2015. Available at http://naturaldatabase. therapeuticresearch.com. Accessed September 25, 2015.

Jenkins DJ, et al. Effect of a low-glycemic index or a high-cereal fiber diet on type 2 diabetes: a randomized trial. *JAMA.* 2008;300(23):2742–2753.

Jolly K, et al. Comparison of range of commercial or primary care led weight reduction programmes with minimal intervention control for weight loss in obesity: lighten Up randomised control trial. *BMJ.* 2011;343:d6500.

Jönsson T, et al. Beneficial effects of a Paleolithic diet on cardiovascular risk factors in type 2 diabetes: a randomized cross-over pilot study. *Cardiovasc Diabetol.* 2009;8:35.

Lesser LI, et al. Nutrition myths and healthy dietary advice in clinical practice. *Am Fam Physician.* 2015;91(9):634–638.

Manson JE, et al. Marine n-3 fatty acids and prevention of cardiovascular disease and cancer. *N Engl J Med.* 2019;380:23–32.

Neuhouser ML, et al. Multivitamin use and risk of cancer and cardiovascular disease in women's health initiative cohorts. *Arch Intern Med.* 2009;169(3):294–304.

Newton KM, et al. Treatment of vasomotor symptoms of menopause with black cohosh, multibotanicals, soy, hormone therapy, or placebo: a randomized trial. *Ann Intern Med.* 2006;145(12):869–879.

Paterson KE, et al. Mediterranean diet reduces risk of incident stroke in a population with varying cardiovascular disease risk profiles. *Stroke.* 2018;0:2415–2420.

Rahman M, Berenson AB. Accuracy of current body mass index obesity classification for white, black, and Hispanic reproductive-age women. *Obstet Gynecol.* 2010;115(5):982–988.

Reed SD, et al. Vaginal, endometrial, and reproductive hormone findings: randomized, placebo-controlled trial of black cohosh, multibotanical herbs, and dietary soy for vasomotor symptoms: the Herbal Alternatives for Menopause (HALT) Study. *Menopause.* 2008;15(1):51–58.

Snitz BE, et al. Ginkgo biloba for preventing cognitive decline in older adults: a randomized trial. *JAMA.* 2009;302(24):2663–2670.

Study of the Effectiveness of Additional Reductions in Cholesterol and Homocysteine (SEARCH) Collaborative Group, Armitage JM, Bowman L, et al. Effects of homocysteine-lowering with folic acid plus vitamin B12 vs placebo on mortality and major morbidity in myocardial infarction survivors: a randomized trial. *JAMA.* 2010;300(24):2486–2494.

Villareal DT, Chode S, Parimi N, et al. Weight loss, exercise, or both and physical function in obese older adults. *N Engl J Med.* 2011;364(13):1218–1229.

World Health Organization. Waist circumference and waist–hip ratio: report of a WHO expert consultation, Geneva, 8–11 December 2008. *Geneva, Switzerland; World Health Organization: 1–39.* Available at: http://whqlibdoc.who. int/publications/2011/9789241501491_eng.pdf. Accessed September 24, 2015.

Substance Use Disorders

25

Dustin Z. DeYoung

CASE 25.1

A 45-year-old male presents to your clinic to establish care for his chronic back and leg pain. He denies any other medical conditions. He reports being injured at work approximately 5 years ago, at which time he was started on oxycodone. He reports being on a stable dose for the past few years. He appears slightly drowsy during the appointment, has small pupils, and is having moderate difficulty describing his injury and previous treatments. He reports his mood as okay but becomes irritable when you begin to ask specifics about his injury. He has not been able to keep a job for the last year because "everyone fires me." He states that he needs the oxycodone to function and that he ran out of his medication one week ago. He does report occasional alcohol use, although he states that he knows not to mix alcohol with his oxycodone.

Question 25.1.1 What is the most likely explanation of the patient's current presentation?
A) Opioid withdrawal
B) Opioid intoxication
C) Uncontrolled pain
D) Alcohol intoxication
E) Alcohol withdrawal

Answer 25.1.1 The correct answer is "B." The patient presents with pupillary constriction, drowsiness, impairment in attention and memory, psychological changes (dysphoria/irritability), and impairment in functioning (not able to keep a job). All of these findings are included in the diagnostic criteria for opioid intoxication. The *Diagnostic and Statistical Manual of Mental Disorders Fifth Edition* (DSM-5) criteria for opioid intoxication include: (1) recent use of an opioid; (2) clinically significant problematic behavioral or psychological changes (euphoria followed by apathy, dysphoria, psychomotor agitation or retardation, impaired judgment, or impaired social or occupational functioning) that develop during, or shortly after, opioid use; (3) pupillary constriction (or pupillary dilation from severe overdose) and one or more of the following signs: drowsiness or

coma, slurred speech, and impairment in attention or memory; (4) and the symptoms are not due to a general medical condition or another mental disorder.

"A" is incorrect and will be discussed later in this case. "C" is incorrect because a patient would not display the above symptoms with significant pain. "D" could be correct because acute alcohol intoxication is characterized by slurred speech and impairments in memory and judgment; however, the patient does not have other findings consistent with alcohol intoxication such as an unsteady gait or nystagmus. "E" is incorrect as the patient was not hypertensive, febrile, diaphoretic, and did not have tremors or vomiting.

You are hesitant to prescribe oxycodone partly because you recently reviewed the CDC report estimating over 72,000 overdose deaths in 2017 (with opioids accounting for almost 50,000), a record number reflecting an increase of approximately 7%. In 2016, there were over 19,000 overdose deaths from opioid pain relievers alone. You offer him alternatives for pain control, including a referral to physical therapy, NSAIDs, and acupuncture.

Question 25.1.2 Which of the following nonopioid treatments has NOT shown to be more effective than placebo in reducing chronic low back pain?
A) Nonsteroidal anti-inflammatories (NSAIDs)
B) Acetaminophen
C) Duloxetine (Cymbalta)
D) Gabapentin
E) B and D

Answer 25.1.2 The correct answers is "E." NSAIDs have been shown to be more effective than placebo in reducing pain in a variety of acute and chronic pain conditions, including back pain. Although frequently recommended, there is little quality clinical evidence to support the efficacy of acetaminophen for chronic back pain. Duloxetine, an SNRI, has been shown to decrease low back pain intensity, but tricyclic antidepressants

(TCAs) and selective serotonin reuptake inhibitors (SSRIs) do not help chronic low back pain. Gabapentin (and pregabalin) are not effective for low back pain (*PLoS Med* 2017;14:1002369, *CMAJ* 2018;190:E786). Acupuncture reduces pain more than sham in nonspecific musculoskeletal pain, including low back pain. According to a Cochrane review of TENS units for low back pain, there is no evidence to support the use of a TENS unit for low back pain.

HELPFUL TIP:
For chronic, noncancer pain, guidelines recommend prioritizing nonopioid medications over opioid analgesics in all patients but particularly in patients with substance use disorders. While evidence for some of the pain medications and modalities we often use is lacking, given the known adverse events and abuse/addiction issues with opioids, it is worth trying the less harmful options (e.g., acetaminophen, TENS unit) prior to considering opioids for chronic, noncancer pain.

He says he has tried them all and none of them work (ever heard that before?). When not offered an opioid, he gets upset and walks out of your office. Two days later, while you are covering an emergency department (ED) shift, the same male presents to the ED for severe, uncontrolled pain. He is vomiting, complains of muscle aches and diarrhea, his pupils are dilated, and he is febrile.

Question 25.1.3 What is the most likely explanation for the patient's current presentation?
A) Opioid withdrawal
B) Opioid intoxication
C) Uncontrolled pain
D) Alcohol intoxication
E) Alcohol withdrawal

Answer 25.1.3 **The correct answer is "A."** The criteria for opioid withdrawal are cessation (or reduction in) opioid use that has been heavy or prolonged (several weeks or longer) or administration of an opioid antagonist after opioid use with three or more of the following developing within minutes to several days after the above: dysphoric mood, nausea or vomiting, muscle aches, lacrimation or rhinorrhea, pupillary dilation, piloerection, sweating, diarrhea, yawning, fever, or insomnia. These signs and symptoms cause clinically significant distress or impairment in social, occupational, or other important areas of functioning and are not due to another medical condition or better accounted for by another mental disorder.

After stabilization, the patient is transferred to a substance abuse treatment center voluntarily. Based on the available resources in your community, you decide on buprenorphine induction and maintenance treatment.

Question 25.1.4 **All of the following are true of buprenorphine EXCEPT:**
A) Buprenorphine should be administered prior to onset of withdrawal symptoms
B) The typical first dose of buprenorphine is 4 mg
C) Combination buprenorphine/naloxone is preferred over buprenorphine monotherapy due to lower abuse potential, unless a patient is pregnant, lactating, or allergic to naloxone
D) After initiation, the buprenorphine dose should be increased if withdrawal symptoms continue
E) Nearly all patients will stabilize on 8 to 16 mg daily, but some patients do require higher doses

Answer 25.1.4 **The correct answer, and false statement, is "A."** Buprenorphine is started when patients are exhibiting early signs of withdrawal. For short-acting opioids (e.g., heroin, oxycodone) this may be 12 hours after the last use; while for longer-acting opioids such as methadone, withdrawal symptoms may not manifest until 48 hours after last use. The first day dose should be 4 mg ("B"), and patients should be monitored for withdrawal symptoms for 2 to 4 hours, with the opportunity to administer an additional dose (up to 8 mg in the first day). The addition of naloxone to buprenorphine ("C") is to deter intravenous buprenorphine use as naloxone is poorly absorbed when administered sublingually but precipitates opioid withdrawal if buprenorphine/naloxone is injected. After initiation, the buprenorphine dose should be titrated to relieve withdrawal symptoms ("D") by doubling the previous total daily dose plus adding 2 to 4 mg. Most patients will stabilize on 8 to 16 mg daily; however, some may require doses up to 32 mg daily, which is the maximum dosage ("E").

HELPFUL TIP:
Advantages of buprenorphine over methadone are that it can be dispensed at a physician's office with an appropriate DEA waiver which requires the ability to provide or refer the patient for counseling, unlike methadone, which can only be dispensed at designated treatment centers. Because of its partial agonist action, buprenorphine has a "ceiling effect" with regard to overdose making it safer than methadone; whereas, methadone produces increasing respiratory suppression with increasing doses. Suboxone is a patented combination of buprenorphine and naloxone that requires a physician to obtain a special "X" DEA number in order to prescribe.

▶ **Objectives: Did you learn to …**
- Define opioid intoxication and withdrawal?
- Describe the use of buprenorphine to manage opioid dependence?

▶ **CASE 25.2**

A 70-year-old female is brought into the clinic by her daughter due to concerns about her mother's sleeplessness, isolation, weight loss, falls, and anxiety over the past year. In addition, since the patient has been staying at her daughter's home the past 3 days, she began vomiting, hallucinating, perspiring profusely, and wanting to return to her own home. The patient has no history of medical problems. She is disheveled, confused, diaphoretic, and tremulous. Her blood pressure is 162/110 mm Hg, pulse is 120 bpm, and temperature is 38.5°C. She blames her symptoms on being unable to have a cigarette. She also blames her daughter's nagging. When asked about alcohol use, the patient says she has had a cocktail every evening since she retired from her job last year, and that this helps her to sleep.

Question 25.2.1 Which of the following best describes the patient's current clinical condition?
A) Alcohol withdrawal
B) Alcohol intoxication
C) Alcohol tolerance
D) Alcohol use disorder

Answer 25.2.1 **The correct answer is "A."** The patient presents tachycardic, hypertensive, and febrile, with diaphoresis, tremors, vomiting, and hallucinations. All of these findings are included in the diagnostic criteria for alcohol withdrawal. "B" is incorrect. Acute intoxication is characterized by slurred speech, unsteady gait, nystagmus, and impaired memory and judgment. "C" and "D" are incorrect and are discussed later in this case.

The criteria for alcohol withdrawal include: (1) cessation or reduction of a previously heavy alcohol intake **and** (2) at least two of the following within hours or days: autonomic hyperactivity (hypertension, sweating, tachycardia, etc.), hand tremor, insomnia, nausea/vomiting, hallucinations, agitation, anxiety, grand mal seizures. In addition, one must have significant distress or impairment in functioning with the withdrawal and no other illness causing the symptoms.

Question 25.2.2 Which class of drugs would you choose to treat the symptoms of alcohol withdrawal?
A) Benzodiazepines
B) Antipsychotics
C) Antibiotics
D) Alcohol
E) Phenytoin

Answer 25.2.2 **The correct answer is "A."** The treatment of choice is metabolic support and the use of benzodiazepines to decrease physical distress and to prevent major withdrawal (e.g., delirium tremens) from occurring. "B" is incorrect. Antipsychotics may control behavior but they do not prevent withdrawal seizures and vasomotor instability. "C" is incorrect as this patient is not displaying signs of infection. "D" is incorrect. Although alcohol will work to prevent withdrawal, it has a fairly short half-life, and you generally do not want to endorse the use of alcohol in a patient with an alcohol use problem. "E" is incorrect. Phenytoin does nothing to prevent alcohol withdrawal seizures.

HELPFUL TIP:
The traditional "banana bag" of IV multivitamins is unnecessary. Oral vitamin supplements are just as effective and less expensive. The only exception is thiamine, which you may want to give IV or IM if you suspect thiamine deficiency.

Question 25.2.3 What would be the best approach to evaluating this patient for alcoholism?
A) Ask her the average amount she drinks
B) Ask her how often she drinks
C) Ask her how frequently she gets drunk
D) Ask what her family and friends say about her drinking

Answer 25.2.3 **The correct answer is "D."** The defense mechanism of denial is so strongly evident in alcoholism that the best approach is to explore how alcohol affects her life, rather than direct questions about drinking behavior. Information from family and friends may provide a more accurate account of the problem. The "CAGE" questionnaire is a very brief and useful screening tool, employed effectively in the primary care setting. A positive answer to two or more questions is very sensitive and specific for an alcohol use disorder. It consists of asking the patient the following four questions:

Have you ever

- **C:** felt that you should **Cut Down** on your drinking?
- **A:** been **Annoyed** that people criticized your drinking?
- **G:** felt bad or **Guilty** about your drinking?
- **E:** taken a drink first thing in the morning (**Eye Opener**) to get rid of a hangover or steady your nerves?

HELPFUL TIP:
Asking the question "How many times in the past year have you had five or more drinks in a day (for men) or four or more drinks (for women) in a day?" is a useful screening question for frequency of heavy drinking. A positive screen is one or more incidents of heavy drinking. If you have a positive screen, ask about usual frequency and quantity of alcohol consumed to help determine the presence or absence of alcohol abuse or dependence. This question alone is about 82% sensitive for detecting an alcohol use disorder. Specificity is comparable at about 79%. Sensitivity for the CAGE ranges from about 75% to 95%, but the CAGE may miss nondependent alcohol use disorders (e.g., binge drinking). Yet another possible screen for alcohol use disorders, and one commonly found in primary care clinics, is the Alcohol Use Disorders Identification Test (AUDIT). This is a 10-question survey that has a sensitivity of 92% and a specificity of 94%.

HELPFUL TIP:
Unfortunately, when it comes to substance use, you cannot always trust the family's history either. They

may be enabling the alcohol addiction or unaware of it. Also, laboratory workups (e.g., liver enzymes) are not sufficiently reliable to make the diagnosis of alcohol abuse/dependence. Although elevated GGT and AST/ALT in a ratio of 2:1 are supportive, their specificity is only 90%. Others that may cause a high AST/ALT ratio are hepatitis C, Wilson's disease, hepatitis-associated cirrhosis.

Upon further questioning, you begin to uncover a long history of heavy drinking—seems that there was more than just a nightcap.

Question 25.2.4 **Which of the following statements about this patient's situation is TRUE?**
A) Cerebellar degeneration is uncommon
B) She is at risk for developing peripheral neuropathy
C) Alcoholic "fatty liver" is irreversible
D) She is at decreased or average risk for heart disease
E) Immune function should remain relatively intact

Answer 25.2.4 **The correct answer is "B."** Peripheral neuropathy can be seen in 10% of heavy drinkers as a result of vitamin deficiencies and the direct impact alcohol has on nerve function. "A" is incorrect because cerebellar degeneration—suggested by ataxia and nystagmus—does occur as a result of alcohol overuse. "C" is incorrect because alcoholic "fatty liver" will reverse with abstinence from alcohol. "D" is incorrect. Heavy drinking raises blood pressure and levels of triglycerides, increasing risk of myocardial infarction. Finally, "E" is incorrect. Heavy drinking lowers the white blood cell count and interferes with specific aspects of the immune system; for example, it compromises T-cell function.

This patient reports to you that she has needed to drink increasing amounts of alcohol to help her fall asleep.

Question 25.2.5 **The need for increasing amounts of alcohol is an example of:**
A) Intoxication
B) Dependence
C) Tolerance
D) Relapse
E) Abuse

Answer 25.2.5 **The correct answer is "C."** Tolerance is defined as the need for increasing amounts of a drug to achieve the same response as initial use of the drug. "A" is incorrect. Intoxication is a characteristic syndrome of maladaptive behavior or psychological changes that occur with substance use, is drug-specific, and reverses when the drug use is discontinued. "D" is incorrect. Relapse involves re-starting use of the drug after being abstinent for a while.

HELPFUL (CLARIFYING) TIP:
DSM-IV divided substance abuse and substance dependence. DSM-5 views these two categories as different points on a spectrum of substance use disorder. The criteria for substance use disorder are at least 2 of the following 11 criteria (clustered in 4 groups):
A. Impaired control: (1) taking more or for longer than intended, (2) unsuccessful efforts to stop or cut down use, (3) spending a great deal of time obtaining, using, or recovering from use, or (4) craving for substance.
B. Social impairment: (5) failure to fulfill major obligations due to use, (6) continued use despite problems caused or exacerbated by use, or (7) important activities given up or reduced because of use.
C. Risky use: (8) recurrent use in hazardous situations and (9) continued use despite physical or psychological problems caused or exacerbated by use.
D. Pharmacologic dependence: (10) developing tolerance or (11) withdrawal.

Question 25.2.6 **Which of the following lab test results are you most likely to find in this patient?**
A) Microcytic anemia
B) Low ferritin
C) Decreased serum triglycerides
D) Hyperglycemia
E) Increased gamma-glutamyltransferase (GGT)

Answer 25.2.6 **The correct answer is "E."** Elevated GGT is considered to be a highly sensitive indicator of alcohol intake and is often present along with elevation of the alanine and aspartate transaminases (ALT and AST). Remember that GGT is not specific, as it is an inducible enzyme and can be induced by a number of medications. The classic AST:ALT ratio in active alcohol abusers is 2:1. Remember, however, that these laboratory findings are **not specific** for alcohol use and have multiple potential causes. The other answers are incorrect. Patients with alcoholism typically have **macrocytic** anemia, **elevated** serum triglycerides, and **hypoglycemia**. Ferritin is often **increased** in active alcohol users in the absence of iron overload. In addition, the transferrin saturation may be elevated because alcohol inhibits transferrin synthesis.

You have ordered liver function tests, but the results will not be available until the next day. The laboratory technician is out getting Botox.

Question 25.2.7 **Which of the following medications would be indicated to prevent delirium tremens (DT) in a patient with hepatic impairment?**
A) Alprazolam (Xanax)
B) Chlordiazepoxide (Librium)
C) Diazepam (Valium)
D) Lorazepam (Ativan)
E) Clonazepam (Klonopin)

Answer 25.2.7 The correct answer is "D." Benzodiazepines that are metabolized by the cytochrome P450 system will build up in the presence of liver disease, so using those with intermediate half-lives and no active metabolites is essential. Only lorazepam, oxazepam, and temazepam meet these criteria. "B" is incorrect. Although chlordiazepoxide ("B") is often used to prevent symptoms of alcohol withdrawal, it is hepatically metabolized and has an exceptionally long half-life and, therefore, should be avoided in patients with liver problems. Conversely, alprazolam ("A") is too short acting to use in this situation.

> **HELPFUL TIP:**
> Carbamazepine has been used extensively in Europe to treat the symptoms of alcohol withdrawal and prevent seizures. Evidence for its use in alcohol withdrawal is somewhat limited, and studies are generally underpowered. But guess what? The same is true for benzodiazepines. Don't go switching all your patients to carbamazepine, but it could serve as an alternative in the rare patient with a benzodiazepine allergy or adverse reaction.

You remember from a lecture that patients without serious comorbidities, either medical or psychiatric, who have mild-to-moderate withdrawal symptoms can safely be withdrawn in an outpatient setting. The tool that has been best validated is the revised "Clinical Institute Withdrawal Assessment for Alcohol" (CIWA-Ar) which involves assessment of the severity of 10 signs and symptoms associated with alcohol withdrawal (see MD-Calc: https://www.mdcalc.com/ciwa-ar-alcohol-withdrawal).

Question 25.2.8 Assessment of the severity of which of the following symptoms is NOT included in that tool?
A) Headache or feelings of fullness in head
B) Palpitations
C) Paroxysmal sweats
D) Tactile disturbances
E) Tremor

Answer 25.2.8 The correct answer is "B." Palpitations are not included in the CIWA-Ar scale. In addition to "A," "C," "D," and "E," the other signs and symptoms are nausea/vomiting, anxiety, agitation, auditory disturbance, visual disturbance, and orientation/clouding of sensorium. Each sign or symptom is given 0 to 7 points according to its severity except for orientation/clouding of sensorium, which is only 0 to 4 points. Withdrawal is considered mild if the score is <15, moderate if 16 to 20, and severe if >20.

You are considering whether or not this patient has delirium tremens (DT).

Question 25.2.9 Which of the following is true of DT?
A) The majority of patients with alcohol withdrawal develop DT if not treated

B) Auditory hallucinations are more common than visual hallucinations in DT
C) Symptoms of DT could easily be confused for dementia
D) DT does not occur until at least 1 week has passed since the last drink of alcohol
E) Autonomic instability is present in DT

Answer 25.2.9 The correct answer is "E." Autonomic instability with elevated pulse, blood pressure, and fever are common in DT. "A" is incorrect. Minor withdrawal symptoms are quite common, but DT develops in only 3% to 5% of patients undergoing alcohol withdrawal. "B" is incorrect. Visual hallucinations are common in DT; auditory hallucinations are less likely. "C" is incorrect. Withdrawal **delirium** typically presents acutely over a matter of hours or days; whereas, in **dementia**, the cognitive decline is over a course of months to years. In addition, autonomic instability is not a feature of early dementia (OK, maybe in Shy–Drager syndrome although cognition is usually well preserved—unlike our patient's liver). Finally, "D" is incorrect because the risk for DT usually peaks 72 hours after the last drink.

Question 25.2.10 Which medication would be the best choice for DT in a patient who is vomiting profusely and who has no IV access?
A) Diazepam (Valium)
B) Alprazolam (Xanax)
C) Chlordiazepoxide (Librium)
D) Lorazepam (Ativan)
E) Clonazepam (Klonopin)

Answer 25.2.10 The correct answer is "D." Lorazepam is absorbed well intramuscularly and can also be provided IV. This makes it a good choice for the vomiting patient. Diazepam **is erratically** absorbed IM and should be administered either orally or IV. One could argue that diazepam given rectally is a reasonable alternative to lorazepam IM/IV. However, for reasons stated earlier in this case, lorazepam is the preferred drug of those listed.

> **HELPFUL TIP:**
> The IV form of lorazepam can also be administered sublingually to speed absorption if you want to use an oral medication. Obviously IV is even faster yet (if you have access).

Question 25.2.11 In 2018, DT carries a fatality rate of:
A) <1%
B) 5%
C) 10%
D) 25%
E) 50%

Answer 25.2.11 The correct answer is "B." Prior to modern treatment, the mortality reached almost 40% per episode. The rest are incorrect.

Question 25.2.12 Which of the following does NOT predispose to developing DT?
A) Prior episodes of DT
B) Pneumonia
C) Gastrointestinal (GI) bleed
D) Female gender
E) Hepatic failure

Answer 25.2.12 The correct answer is "D." Female gender does not predispose an individual to DT but the other options do.

Question 25.2.13 Which of the following is NOT a complication of alcoholism?
A) Dementia
B) Pancreatitis
C) Hypermagnesemia
D) Megaloblastic anemia
E) Marchiafava–Bignami disease

Answer 25.2.13 The correct answer is "C." All of the above, with the exception of hypermagnesemia, are associated with alcohol abuse. **Hypo**magnesemia is a complication of alcoholism and may decrease the response to thiamine administration in patients who also have thiamine deficiency. Alcoholic dementia may be related to direct effects of alcohol on the brain or to nutritional deficiencies. Marchiafava–Bignami disease is demyelination and/or necrosis of the corpus callosum and the adjacent white matter. It presents with dementia, dysarthria, spasticity, and inability to ambulate. It can occasionally be seen in nondrinkers as well.

HELPFUL TIP:
Elderly patients with alcohol problems often go unrecognized. Have a high index of suspicion in patients with signs and symptoms such as labile hypertension, insomnia, legal or marital problems, frequent falls and injuries, headaches or blackouts, and vague GI complaints.

Question 25.2.14 Which of the following is FALSE about alcohol use disorders?
A) Most studies have found the prevalence of alcohol use disorders is highest among older adults
B) The lifetime prevalence of alcohol use disorders is approximately 30%
C) Alcohol use disorders are frequently comorbid with psychiatric and other substance use disorders
D) Rates of current (past year) alcohol use disorders are more than twice as common in males than in females
E) Approximately 25% of men and almost 50% of women with alcohol dependence will meet criteria for major depressive disorder in their lifetime

Answer 25.2.14 The correct answer is "A." Actually, most studies have shown that the highest prevalence of alcohol use disorders is in a younger age group (18–29 years old). The rest are correct statements. Especially noteworthy is "C." Half of all people with alcohol abuse have a comorbid psychiatric diagnosis. For example, about 50% to 60% of people with bipolar illness have problems with alcohol abuse or dependence. Results from the National Epidemiologic Survey on Alcohol and Related Conditions in 2007 and 2015 found that persons with an alcohol use disorder had a lifetime prevalence of mental illness of about 30%. "E" is a correct statement as well. Data from the National Comorbidity Survey estimated lifetime prevalence of major depressive disorder among persons with alcohol dependence to be 24.3% and 48.5% among men and women, respectively. A useful way to approach patients who complain of depression along with their alcohol abuse is to obtain a longitudinal history to see which came first. If it is impossible to tease out, as is often the case, observe for 1 to 3 weeks off alcohol. If depression is still present without alcohol use, it is prudent to treat with an antidepressant. Be careful when treating alcohol abusers with antidepressants: active substance use severely reduces the efficacy of these medications.

HELPFUL TIP:
Substance use rates are highest between ages 18 and 25. A lot of this is experimentation that will end as the individual matures. Some, of course, will go on to chronic use and possible development of a substance use disorder.

HELPFUL (AND IMPORTANT) TIP:
Multiple studies have shown that symptom-triggered protocols for benzodiazepine treatment of alcohol withdrawal are superior to scheduled administration of benzodiazepines. Patients receive less medication, have shorter hospital stays, and experience similar or better outcomes with symptom-triggered administration. Symptom-triggered approaches use the CIWA-Ar scoring system every 4 to 8 hours (or more frequently depending on the severity of symptoms) with benzodiazepines provided for scores >8 up to every hour. Do not use fixed dose regimens. They increase length of stay and benzodiazepine dose. Benzodiazepine regimens utilized include: lorazepam, diazepam, and chlordiazepoxide. Use the smallest effective dose of an oral benzodiazepine as needed to improve symptoms. IV formulations of diazepam and lorazepam may be utilized in the acute setting if the oral route is unavailable. Of note, true DT may require absurdly large doses of benzodiazepines (our personal best is 70 mg of IV diazepam in 1 hour or a lorazepam drip at 8 mg/hour—but not in the same patient!).

▶ **Objectives: Did you learn to …**
- Recognize signs and symptoms of alcohol withdrawal?
- Describe diagnostic criteria for alcohol withdrawal?
- Identify adverse effects of heavy alcohol use?

- Treat alcohol withdrawal?
- Appreciate how denial of the illness plays a role in the assessment of substance abuse?
- Identify laboratory abnormalities observed in alcohol abuse and understand the limitations of laboratory studies?

 QUICK QUIZ: NIGHTMARE IN MARGARITAVILLE

A 50-year-old divorced male presents to your clinic in an agitated state, complaining of nausea, vomiting, and double vision. He smells of alcohol, and reports that his last drink was today... about 15 minutes ago... in your clinic parking lot. He has gross bilateral hand tremors and is disheveled. He is picking at his shirtsleeves and is oriented to name only. On physical examination, you observe lateral nystagmus and an ataxic gait. Vital signs include: blood pressure 160/92 mm Hg, pulse 100 bpm, and respirations 20 bpm. Labs are drawn, and his GGT is moderately elevated.

Which of the following is the most likely cause of his symptoms?
A) Wernicke encephalopathy
B) Normal pressure hydrocephalus
C) Dementia
D) Stroke
E) Alcohol withdrawal

The correct answer is "A." Wernicke encephalopathy is the result of thiamine deficiency and can occur in alcoholics and other patients with poor nutrition. See the next question for a description of the clinical findings. Note that several symptoms of Wernicke encephalopathy can mimic withdrawal (agitation, etc.). However, as noted in the question, this patient is still intoxicated.

 QUICK QUIZ: WERNICKE ENCEPHALOPATHY

The triad of Wernicke encephalopathy includes all of the following EXCEPT:
A) Ataxia
B) Oculomotor dysfunction
C) Incontinence
D) Encephalopathy

The correct answer is "C." Wernicke encephalopathy may present with the classic triad of ataxia, encephalopathy (confusion), and oculomotor dysfunction (nystagmus, lateral rectus palsy, etc.). However, the majority of patients present with an incomplete syndrome and may be missing ophthalmoplegia, ataxia, or encephalopathy. If you choose "B," maybe you were thinking of normal pressure hydrocephalus, which presents with dementia, incontinence, and ataxia. For Wernicke encephalopathy, remember that the treatment is *high-dose* thiamine; 500 mg IV TID over 30 minutes for 2 days and then 250 mg IV (or IM) daily for 5 days.

▶ **CASE 25.3**

A 28-year-old pregnant patient and her mother are presenting for a follow-up appointment. At the appointment today, the patient's mother shares that her daughter has been drinking alcohol during her pregnancy. The daughter is very annoyed when confronted with her use of alcohol and will not give specific information about it, but she does admit to drinking. She does not agree to quit during her pregnancy or to be referred for substance abuse evaluation. You discuss some of the effects alcohol might have on the developing fetus, including fetal alcohol syndrome (FAS).

Question 25.3.1 According to the National Institute on Alcohol Abuse and Alcoholism (NIAAA) consensus guidelines (2016), the diagnosis of FAS requires specific manifestations in three areas, including:
A) At least two facial anomalies, retardation of growth ≤ the 20th percentile, significant structural abnormalities on neuroimaging, and impulse control deficits
B) At least two facial anomalies, retardation of growth ≤ the 10th percentile, head circumference ≤ 10th percentile, and significant global intellectual deficits
C) At least three facial anomalies, retardation of growth ≤ the 10th percentile, specific learning impairment, and confirmed alcohol use during pregnancy
D) At least three facial anomalies, retardation of growth ≤ the 10th percentile, head circumference ≤ 20th percentile, and confirmed alcohol use during pregnancy

Answer 25.3.1 The correct answer is "B." The diagnosis of FAS (which is one form of fetal alcohol spectrum disorder) is a complex medical diagnostic process with no universally accepted set of diagnostic criteria. The NIAAA consensus guidelines, which were updated in 2016, were used for this answer and are abbreviated in "B." Major differences with the Department of Health and Human Services/CDC National Task Force on FAS Guidelines from 2004 will be pointed out. If all criteria are met in both guidelines, documented prenatal alcohol exposure is not needed, as this can be a stigmatizing or difficult answer to achieve at times. The diagnosis requires at least two (three in National Task Force Guidelines) facial anomalies, growth retardation (≤ 10th percentile), and CNS abnormalities (clear evidence of brain involvement and neurobehavioral impairments). For the National Task Force guidelines only one CNS abnormality (structural, neurologic, or functional) needs to be documented. The other options are incorrect. Other facial features and minor congenital abnormalities may occur but are not included in diagnostic criteria. See Figure 25-1.

 HELPFUL (HOPEFULLY CLARIFYING) TIP:
Fetal Alcohol Syndrome Diagnostic Criteria:
A. *Characteristic Facial Anomalies:*
Short palpebral fissures, thin vermillion border, and smooth philtrum

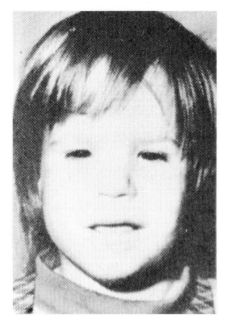
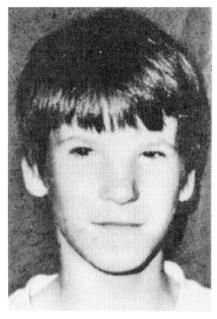
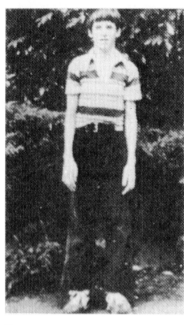

A   **B**   **C**

FIGURE 25-1. Fetal alcohol syndrome. **(A)** At 2 1/2 years. **(B, C)** At 12 years. Note persistence of short palpebral fissures, epicanthal folds, flat midface, hypoplastic philtrum, and thin upper vermilion border. This individual also has the short, lean prepubertal stature characteristic of young males with fetal alcohol syndrome. (Reproduced from Streissguth AP, Clarren SK, Jones KL. Natural history of the fetal alcohol syndrome: A 10-year follow-up of eleven patients. *Lancet.* 1985;326:85–91, with permission from Elsevier.)

B. *Growth Retardation:*
Height and/or weight (adjusted for gestational age) ≤ 10th percentile for age/sex
C. *CNS Involvement:*
1. Clear evidence of brain involvement:
   a. *Structural*—head circumference ≤10th percentile or abnormalities on neuroimaging
   b. *Neurologic*—abnormal reflexes, abnormal tone, cranial nerve deficits, poor coordination or balance, visual-motor deficits, right-left confusion, or difficulty with motor sequencing
2. Neurobehavioral impairment (*Functional*):
   a. Significant global cognitive/intellectual deficits
   b. Significant developmental delay
   c. Functional deficits in one (three for National Task Force guidelines) domain(s):
      - Executive functioning deficits
      - Motor functioning delays
      - Problems with attention or hyperactivity
      - Social skills
      - Other sensory problems, memory deficits, etc.
   d. Significant impairment of self-regulation in at least one domain:
      - Mood or behavioral regulation impairment
      - Attention deficit
      - Impulse control

HELPFUL TIP:
Fetal alcohol spectrum disorders (FASD) is the leading preventable cause of birth defects and developmental disorders in the United States.

Question 25.3.2 Which of the following is the earliest that symptoms and signs of FAS may be detected after birth?
A) Within 12 hours
B) After the first week
C) At 1 month
D) At 3 months
E) After 1 year

Answer 25.3.2 The correct answer is "A." Soon after birth, the neonate may display symptoms of withdrawal, including tremulousness, inconsolability, vomiting, and poor feeding. The characteristic cluster of facial/physical malformations (listed above) is evident within 12 hours of birth, but is usually most pronounced between 8 months and 8 years of age. Other features, such as certain forms of CNS dysfunction, growth deficiency, joint and limb abnormalities, and heart defects, might not be noted until later in the child's life. Given the wide range of disabilities and impairments, many fetal alcohol spectrum disorders are not recognized until later in childhood and are estimated to be underdiagnosed for a variety of reasons.

As you counsel your patient, you describe how FAS is just one form of FASD and even limited alcohol use during pregnancy can contribute to potential problems for her child.

Question 25.3.3 Which of the following conditions are considered a fetal alcohol spectrum disorder (FASD)?
A) Alcohol-related neurodevelopmental disorder
B) Partial fetal alcohol syndrome
C) Neurobehavioral disorder associated with prenatal alcohol exposure (ND-PAE)
D) Alcohol-related birth defects
E) All of the above

Answer 25.3.3 The correct answer is "E." Knowledge continues to grow regarding the subtler effects of maternal drinking, such as that seen with even "social" alcohol use. All of the above listed conditions are considered FASD, with various diagnostic criteria for each (some overlapping).

Question 25.3.4 In which stage of pregnancy does the teratogenic action of alcohol cause facial malformations?
A) During conception
B) During the third week of pregnancy
C) During the late first trimester
D) During the second trimester
E) During the third trimester

Answer 25.3.4 The correct answer is "B." Facial malformations occur with the use of alcohol during the third week. Organs and limbs appear most susceptible to the effects of alcohol during the embryonic phase, which is completed by the eighth week of conception, a time when most women are first confirming pregnancy. Alcohol exposure during any stage of development may affect brain development or function. Thus, there is no "safe time" for pregnant women to use alcohol.

You are able to convince this patient to reduce and eventually eliminate her use of alcohol; she delivers a healthy-appearing newborn who she names "Harley" after the motorcycle.

▶ **Objectives: Did you learn to …**
- Identify problem drinking in a pregnant patient?
- Approach a patient with alcohol use in pregnancy?
- Describe the findings of fetal alcohol spectrum disorders, including fetal alcohol syndrome?

▶ CASE 25.4

A 60-year-old female presents to your office and is determined to stop smoking. She has a history of schizophrenia treated with clozapine (Clozaril) and a 43-year history of smoking up to two packs of cigarettes per day. She asks you what is available to help her stop. You tell her that nicotine replacement therapy (NRT), bupropion (Zyban), and varenicline (Chantix) are currently approved to aid patients who want to stop smoking.

Question 25.4.1 If you want to offer NRT that is easy to use, has few side effects, and provides steady blood levels of nicotine over the whole day, which do you choose?
A) Nicotine patch
B) Nicotine gum
C) Nicotine nasal spray
D) Nicotine inhaler
E) E-cigarettes

Answer 25.4.1 The correct answer is "A." There are benefits and drawbacks to each of the smoking cessation aids with five currently FDA-approved forms of NRT (patch, gum, nasal spray, inhaler, and lozenge). Combining a long-acting (patch) and a short-acting NRT product (e.g., gum) can increase cessation rates. For this question, the nicotine patch ("A") provides the most continuous nicotine delivery among all NRT products and is the simplest NRT to use. The nicotine patch (and gum) are available without a prescription, while nicotine nasal spray and inhaler require a prescription. For a patient with a heavy, long smoking history, begin with the 21 mg patch and taper to the 7 mg patch, generally over a 10 to 12 week time frame, but longer durations can be used and NRT can continue until the patient feels stabilized as a "nonsmoker." Some of the drawbacks of the patch include slower release of nicotine, the potential for skin irritation, insomnia, and vivid dreams. Some of these side effects can be reduced by having the patient rotate application sites daily (to avoid skin irritation) and removing the patch before bedtime. Nicotine gum ("B") is an ion-exchange resin that releases nicotine for absorption through the buccal mucosa with only 30% bioavailability in the rest of the GI tract. Side effects include mouth and throat soreness, jaw fatigue, hiccups, and undesirable taste. There are advantages of nicotine gum: it involves an active coping mechanism (e.g., chewing, placing the gum in one's mouth) and is more likely than the patch to delay weight gain. The nasal spray ("C") delivers 0.5 mg nicotine per dose and is sprayed one to two times per hour for a maximum of 5 sprays per hour and 40 sprays per day. Most of the nicotine nasal spray side effects are attributable to its route of use—nasal and throat irritation, rhinorrhea, sneezing, etc. The oral inhaler ("D") provides an active delivery of nicotine similar to the nasal inhaler, and its side effects are also a consequence of its route of delivery—throat irritation and coughing. E-cigarettes ("E") create a vapor (not smoke) that simulates smoking. Like other nicotine replacement products, the amount of nicotine may be decreased over time.

 HELPFUL TIP:
There are more than 460 different brands of e-cigarettes. Very little is known about their safety. While they don't contain tobacco smoke, they do contain nicotine and other chemicals. E-cigarettes have a checkered track record when it comes to aiding smoking cessation versus being a gateway to nicotine addiction for younger users. There are studies to support their use, but just as many that suggest that they do not aid with smoking cessation.

Question 25.4.2 Which of the following is an absolute contraindication to varenicline (Chantix)?
A) Coronary artery disease
B) Severe psychiatric illness
C) Seizure disorder
D) Urinary incontinence
E) None of the above

Answer 25.4.2 **The correct answer is "E."** Previously, there was an FDA warning about the possibility of suicidal or homicidal ideation with varenicline. In 2016, the FDA removed the boxed warning about this, but the updated labeling still carries a warning of potential psychiatric adverse events. Patients with serious psychiatric illness may have a lower sustained quitting rate compared to those without psychiatric illness when treated with varenicline or bupropion, and the evidence for NRT in this population is unclear. The EAGLES trial demonstrated higher rate of neuropsychiatric symptoms with smokers with a psychiatric comorbidity, but rates were low in both groups and there was no statistically significant difference in neuropsychiatric symptoms among users of nicotine patch, varenicline, and bupropion for patients with and without a psychiatric disorder. A systematic review and meta-analysis in 2015 found no increased risk of suicide, suicidal ideation, depression, or death compared with placebo for those with and without a psychiatric disorder treated with varenicline. Additionally, varenicline is safe to use in CAD and epilepsy. Again, in the EAGLES trial, varenicline, bupropion, and NRT were all shown to be safe in patients with stable CAD.

Although this patient does not mind spending $6 to $7 per day on a pack of cigarettes (or more depending on where you live), she does not want to pay a lot for something to help her quit. You decide not to engage in a philosophical discussion about cognitive dissonance.

Question 25.4.3 Which smoking cessation aid is the most expensive?
A) Nicotine patch
B) Nicotine gum
C) Nicotine nasal spray
D) Nicotine inhaler
E) Varenicline

Answer 25.4.3 **The correct answer is "E."** The cash price of varenicline is approximately $450 per month in 2019, which has increased from a price of about $240 per month in 2013. Even at $10 per pack, it is cheaper to continue smoking a pack per day ($300) than purchasing a month of varenicline. Even if your patient is lucky enough to have this medication covered by her insurance, it is considered a tier 3 drug under many plans, which means high out-of-pocket co-pay costs. The nicotine products are less expensive in the range of $60 to $120 per month (or higher) depending on the product and your daily previous cigarette use. Some health insurance programs will support smoking cessation aids, but coverage and co-pays are variable.

"I tried those things, Doc, and nicotine didn't work and varenicline made me shoot my boyfriend in the leg—but he had it coming. Isn't there something else?"

Question 25.4.4 Which of the following medications might you also prescribe to aid this patient in smoking cessation?
A) Naloxone
B) Metoprolol
C) Haloperidol
D) Bupropion
E) Fluoxetine

Answer 25.4.4 **The correct answer is "D."** Bupropion is marketed as the antidepressant Wellbutrin and the smoking cessation aid Zyban. It reduces the symptoms of nicotine withdrawal by blocking dopamine in the brain's reward center, and this mechanism is thought to result in reduced nicotine craving. Studies have shown that people who use bupropion doubled their chances of quitting smoking. Its effect appears to be additive to that of NRT. Its effect on smoking cessation is independent of its antidepressant effect, as shown by its equal efficacy in depressed and nondepressed patients. Several studies have demonstrated no significant risk of bupropion-induced psychosis in patients with schizophrenia when also treated with an antipsychotic (as our patient is). One of the advantages of bupropion is its ability to prevent the weight gain that occurs in most people when they stop smoking. Bupropion should be started at a dose of 150 mg daily for 3 days then increasing to 150 mg twice daily, if the patient is tolerating the drug. The patient should be advised to stop smoking during the second week of treatment. "E" is incorrect. There is no evidence that SSRIs are effective in smoking cessation.

HELPFUL TIP:
A 2014 Cochrane review found that nortriptyline has essentially the same success rate as bupropion. Nortriptyline is started at 25 mg daily for 3 days, then 50 mg until the 7th day when the dose is increased to 75 mg daily.

The mood in the examination room turns a shade bluer as your patient wonders whether, at age 60 and with an 86-pack-year history, there is even any reason to quit. "It's too late for me," she laments.

Question 25.4.5 How long does it take to reduce the risk of myocardial infarction by 50% after one stops smoking?
A) 24 hours
B) 6 months
C) 1 year
D) 10 years
E) Infinity

Answer 25.4.5 **The correct answer is "C."** Twenty minutes after quitting smoking, blood pressure and heart rate drops, and the temperature of hands and feet increases to normal. After 24 hours, the risk of myocardial infarction (MI) begins to decrease. At 1 year, the chance of having an MI is cut in half. After 5 years, stroke risk is reduced to that of a nonsmoker. After 10 years, the risk of dying from lung cancer is about half that of a person who continues to smoke. After 15 years, the risk of coronary artery disease approaches that of a nonsmoker.

The mood in the examination room is heading into a deeper blue as your patient expresses concern that she will fail in this attempt to quit smoking, as she has in the past. "I'll never do it," she complains.

Question 25.4.6 On average, how many attempts to quit smoking are made before a person succeeds?
A) 1
B) 6
C) 50
D) 365

Answer 25.4.6 **The correct answer is "B."** Historical data had shown that it takes an average of six attempts at quitting before success. A 2016 study published in *BMJ Open* by Chaiton et al. showed that previous data may grossly underestimate the number of attempts. Other organizations provide estimates of the number of quit attempts prior to meeting sustained success (American Cancer Society 8–10 attempts; CDC 8–11 attempts; Australian Cancer Society 12–14 attempts). Here's the moral of the story: if at first your patient doesn't succeed, try again and again and … so on. As with many behavior changes, most patients don't get it to stick on the first try.

HELPFUL (AND UNFORTUNATE) TIP:
None of these cessation aids have a great track record of success, but the significant health benefits of smoking cessation should make us continue to pursue smoking cessation with all of our patients. For quit rates, you can find numbers all over the board. Some studies have shown higher abstinence rates with varenicline than bupropion and NRT (usually shorter duration trials up to 6 months). However, a 2018 meta-analysis showed that NRT, bupropion, and varenicline all had sustained abstinence rates of around 20% at 1 year. Most studies demonstrate that behavioral support (counseling, text messaging, phone apps web-based services) can increase quit rates. Continue to urge all smokers to quit at every appointment since even brief advice has been shown to increase success rates.

This patient has been on clozapine (Clozaril) for control of her psychosis.

Question 25.4.7 The combination of clozapine and bupropion should be used with caution because:
A) Both may lower the seizure threshold
B) Both may cause hypertension

C) Bupropion may interfere with the metabolism of clozapine
D) Severe GI symptoms could occur
E) A psychotic episode could be precipitated

Answer 25.4.7 **The correct answer is "A."** Both drugs may lower the seizure threshold. Hypertension should not be a concern. Bupropion does not interfere with the metabolism of clozapine, cause severe GI symptoms, or precipitate psychotic episodes. There are case reports of bupropion-induced psychosis in patients without a known psychotic disorder, but as noted above, the risk for a psychotic episode for a patient with schizophrenia treated with bupropion and an antipsychotic is very low.

HELPFUL TIP:
Serum levels of clozapine may be decreased by tobacco use. Thus, smoking cessation can cause clozapine levels to rise within 24 hours. Patients should be monitored for adverse events related to higher serum clozapine levels, including sedation, hypersalivation, seizures, hypotension, akathisia, and other neurologic effects. A dose reduction of 30% to 50% may be required.

After all of your discussion, the patient wants to quit "cold turkey." You gently explain that going from 40 cigarettes per day to zero might be hard on her, although quitting cold turkey improves the chance of success (*Ann Intern Med.* 2016;164(9):585–592).

Question 25.4.8 All of the following are symptoms of nicotine withdrawal EXCEPT:
A) Increased appetite
B) Dysphoria
C) Tachycardia
D) Insomnia
E) Irritability

Answer 25.4.8 **The correct answer is "C."** Nicotine withdrawal is actually associated with decreased heart rate. In addition to the above, trouble with concentration and restlessness are common symptoms.

HELPFUL TIP:
Cytisine (not to be confused with cysteine or cystine) is a herbal derivative that is effective in smoking cessation (placebo 2.4% vs. cytisine 8%). It is less expensive than varenicline—which is actually a derivative of cytisine (*N Engl J Med.* 2011;365:1193–1200). A more recent study has shown cytisine to be superior to NRT for continuous abstinence at 1 week, 2 months, and 6 months, but higher self-reported adverse events, primarily nausea/vomiting and sleep issues (*N Engl J Med.* 2014;371(25):2353–2362).

HELPFUL TIP:
Other measures that are effective in helping a patient quit are automated cell phone messages (*Lancet.* 2011;378(9785):49–55), intensive interaction (nurse phone calls, bed-side teaching after an MI, etc., *CMAJ.* 2009;180(13):1297–1303), and paying patients to quit (*N Engl J Med.* 2009;360(7):699–709). In addition, public policies such as taxes on cigarettes and banning smoking indoors have demonstrated effectiveness at increasing quitting rates.

▶ **Objectives: Did you learn to …**
- Employ pharmacotherapy and nonpharmacologic interventions in the treatment of tobacco addiction?
- List the physiological advantages of smoking cessation at any age?
- Recognize signs and symptoms of nicotine withdrawal?

 QUICK QUIZ: ALL IN THE FAMILY

Which of the following characteristics is NOT true of the children of alcoholics?
A) They experience earlier onset of problem drinking
B) They experience earlier pregnancies (well, not the males…)
C) They have less stable family involvement
D) They experience poor academic and social performance in school
E) They have more antisocial behavior

The correct answer is "B." There is no data to suggest early pregnancy as a characteristic. Twin, adoption, and half-sibling studies and studies of familial versus nonfamilial alcoholism indicate that children of alcoholics have four times the risk for developing alcoholism. They also have worse school performance, more antisocial behavior, and less stable family situations.

▶ **CASE 25.5**

A 35-year-old intoxicated female presents to your office requesting to be started on disulfiram (Antabuse). She is otherwise healthy and recently has begun to drink alcohol daily in response to the death of her sister. She wants to decrease her use but has been unsuccessful, has noticed she is needing to drink more to achieve the same effect, has missed a few family functions due to her alcohol use, and has experienced the need to drink in the morning to avoid "feeling bad." Before this, she was a teetotaler (i.e., a nondrinker).

Question 25.5.1 As the patient meets criteria for an alcohol use disorder and is still drinking (as indicated by her intoxicated appearance in clinic today), you suggest an FDA-approved alternative to disulfiram. You recommend:
A) Naltrexone
B) Naloxone (Narcan)

C) Nortriptyline
D) Topiramate

Answer 25.5.1 **The correct answer is "A."** Naltrexone is FDA approved for the treatment of alcohol use disorders. As an opioid antagonist, it blocks the euphoric effects of alcohol. It can be started while a patient is still using alcohol, thus not having to force abstinence (if the patient is not ready for that). Disulfiram (based on its mechanism of action) should only be used in already abstinent patients in order to maintain abstinence. Topiramate ("D," Topamax) has been shown to decrease the craving for alcohol; however, it is not FDA approved for this indication. Nortriptyline ("C") and naloxone ("B") are not used to treat alcohol use disorders.

She agrees to start naltrexone as she is very worried about her continued alcohol use. You start her on 25 mg per day and increase to the FDA-approved usual dose of 50 mg per day.

Question 25.5.2 Which of the following is NOT a common side effect of naltrexone?
A) Nausea
B) Headache
C) Dizziness
D) Insomnia
E) Increased appetite

Answer 25.5.2 **The correct answer is "E."** Nausea, headache, dizziness, and insomnia, along with a *decreased* appetite, syncope, and muscle pain/weakness are some of the more common adverse events with oral naltrexone. However, side effects generally subside with continued use (and should be separated from any alcohol withdrawal symptoms).

HELPFUL TIP:
Higher doses of naltrexone, up to 150 mg per day, have been used in alcohol use disorders, but there is no clear evidence that doses higher than 50 mg per day are more efficacious. Some patients experience liver enzyme elevation when treated with naltrexone—up to fivefold elevation, in fact. Thus, liver enzymes should be checked at baseline and periodically. Elevated liver enzymes can also be due to alcoholic liver injury, hepatitis B or C infection, or use of other hepatotoxic medications.

She returns for follow-up in one week, noting that she has not been able to stop or reduce her drinking. Upon further questioning, she has not been taking the medication consistently and reports she is "not good at taking daily medication."

Question 25.5.3 Given her issues with adherence, you consider other FDA-approved medications and decide to start the patient on:
A) Acamprosate
B) Disulfiram

C) Long-acting naltrexone (Vivitrol)
D) Baclofen

Answer 25.5.3 The correct answer is "C." With any treatment of an alcohol or other substance use disorder, adherence can be a significant barrier to success. A depot preparation of naltrexone (Vivitrol) can be administered at a dose of 380 mg IM every 4 weeks. This can improve adherence with monthly administration and achieve a steady therapeutic medication level. Adverse events of the depot formulation are similar to oral naltrexone, with pain and inflammation at the injection site being unique to this formulation.

At a follow-up appointment 3 months later, she reports a successful reduction in her rate of heavy drinking, but given insurance changes, she is no longer able to afford depot naltrexone. At this point, as an alternative to naltrexone, you decide to prescribe acamprosate (Campral).

Question 25.5.4 Which of the following is/are true about acamprosate?
A) The usual dose of acamprosate is 666 mg three times daily
B) Acamprosate is no better than placebo in reducing heavy drinking days
C) Most prominent adverse events include diarrhea, insomnia, pruritus, and anxiety
D) Acamprosate increases GABA neurotransmission and has complex effects on glutamate neurotransmission at metabotrophic-5 glutamate receptors, which is likely important for its treatment effects
E) All of the above

Answer 25.5.4 The correct answer is "E." All of the above are true. Multiple early meta-analyses had found acamprosate to reduce alcohol consumption, but evidence is mixed. European trials found that acamprosate increased abstinence rates at 6 months (with positive effects seen primarily for maintaining but not initiating abstinence). US and Australia trials have shown no increased alcohol-free days or time to first heavy drinking. As to "A," maybe the drug company is in league with Satan.

Question 25.5.5 Which of the following is/are true about acamprosate?
A) Patients receiving opioid maintenance therapy or opioids for pain will need higher levels of opioid medication
B) It is contraindicated in those with liver impairment/liver failure
C) Patients who require detoxification can be continued safely on acamprosate
D) It is contraindicated in patients who are taking SSRIs
E) All of the above

Answer 25.5.5 The correct answer is "C." Acamprosate does not interact with benzodiazepines or other medications used in medical detoxification and thus can be continued safely

if a patient starts drinking and then requires detoxification. Acamprosate is not metabolized by the liver (excreted unchanged by the kidneys) and can be used safely even in patients with severe liver disease, whereas naltrexone and disulfiram are contraindicated. However, it is contraindicated in those with renal failure and requires dose adjustment for those with chronic kidney disease. Patients receiving opioids for acute or chronic pain or receiving opioid maintenance treatment can use acamprosate because it does not affect these medications. It is safe to take with SSRIs.

Your patient returns to clinic after a month and has not been able to successfully reduce her alcohol use. She feels residential treatment may be needed. She completes a 30-day program and transitions to an intense outpatient program and has achieved initial alcohol abstinence. Now that she has achieved abstinence, she again asks about disulfiram (Antabuse) as she heard people discussing this during her residential program. You discuss the aversive nature of the medication, but given clinical trials suggesting efficacy when taken routinely under supervised conditions, you agree to prescribe it.

Question 25.5.6 Disulfiram should not be administered until the patient has been abstinent from alcohol for how long?
A) 4 hours
B) 12 hours
C) 24 hours
D) 48 hours
E) 72 hours

Answer 25.5.6 The correct answer is "B." A minimum of 12 hours should have elapsed before giving disulfiram to avoid the disulfiram–alcohol reaction. Of course, this depends on how much they were drinking.

 HELPFUL TIP:
Disulfiram is absorbed slowly from the GI tract and is eliminated slowly; therefore, **a patient should wait at least 1 week after stopping disulfiram before returning to drinking.**

Question 25.5.7 If the patient consumes alcohol while taking disulfiram, which of the following is most likely to occur?
A) Respiratory depression
B) Hypertension
C) Nausea and vomiting
D) Cardiovascular collapse
E) The ability to time travel

Answer 25.5.7 The correct answer is "C." Disulfiram inhibits aldehyde dehydrogenase preventing metabolism of acetaldehyde, which accumulates and causes flushing of the skin, nausea, vomiting, palpitations, hypotension, sweating, blurred vision, and dizziness. Rarely, in more severe reactions, respiratory depression, cardiovascular collapse, convulsions, and death may occur. The severity of the reaction is typically dose-related and depends on the amount of alcohol ingested.

Question 25.5.8 Common side effects of disulfiram include which of the following?

A) Hypotension
B) Peripheral neuropathy
C) Insomnia
D) Nausea
E) Depression

Answer 25.5.8 **The correct answer is "B."** Peripheral neuropathy can be seen with disulfiram. Drowsiness, hepatotoxicity, rashes, hypertension, metallic after-taste, and optic neuritis may also occur with disulfiram use. These effects are independent of alcohol ingestion. Additionally, multiple cases of hepatitis have been reported with disulfiram, and baseline liver enzymes should be obtained prior to starting disulfiram and then approximately 2 weeks after initiation of treatment. Occasionally, a rash may occur early on. The rash can be treated with antihistamines and the drug can be continued.

> **HELPFUL TIP:**
> Other medications that have been used to treat alcohol use disorders include topiramate, baclofen, gabapentin, ondansetron, and SSRIs. Topiramate has the best data to support decreased alcohol use in alcohol dependence. Ondansetron has only shown effectiveness in early onset alcoholism (onset of problem drinking prior to 25 years old) or in those who have a specific genetic variant of the serotonin transporter (5-HTT) gene. SSRIs may reduce alcohol intake when alcohol use disorders and depression are both present. Nalmefene, an opioid antagonist, may have advantages over naltrexone, but is not available in the United States.

> **HELPFUL (AND UNFORTUNATE) TIP:**
> None of these drugs are particularly effective, but again the health and cost-related benefits of alcohol abstinence (or even reduced alcohol use) should continue to motivate us to work with our patients. Combining medications (such as naltrexone and acamprosate) had mixed results and did not appear more effective than either medication alone. The number needed to treat (NNT) to prevent a return to any drinking was 12 for acamprosate and 20 for oral naltrexone with a NNT to prevent a return to heavy drinking of 12 for naltrexone (acamprosate did not show reduced days of heavy drinking).

▶ **Objectives: Did you learn to …**
• Describe the mechanisms of action of naltrexone, acamprosate, and disulfiram?
• Recognize side effects of naltrexone, acamprosate, and disulfiram?
• Describe the alcohol–disulfiram reaction?
• Choose between the various pharmacotherapies for alcohol use disorders?

▶ **CASE 25.6**

A 25-year-old comatose female presents to the ED with pinpoint pupils and respiratory depression.

Question 25.6.1 Which of the following is the most likely cause of coma?

A) Blood alcohol level of 200 mg/dL
B) Cocaine overdose
C) Methadone overdose
D) Benzodiazepine withdrawal
E) Phencyclidine (PCP) intoxication

Answer 25.6.1 **The correct answer is "C."** The classic "triad" of opioid overdose consists of respiratory depression, pinpoint pupils (miosis), and coma. Certain patients may have atypical presentations, and the triad may not always be present in opioid overdose. Miosis is particularly variable, often not being seen in those with meperidine overdoses; and co-ingestions, such as with sympathomimetics or anticholinergics, can also prevent miosis. A patient with a blood alcohol level of 200 mg/dL would likely be ataxic; but alcoholic coma typically occurs at blood levels >400 mg/dL and depends on the level of tolerance. Alcohol and PCP intoxication would more likely present with nystagmus and not constricted pupils. Stimulant overdose and benzodiazepine withdrawal would more likely present with psychomotor agitation and autonomic hyperactivity and not likely present with somnolence.

....

You treat her with naloxone and she wakes up (spitting mad, agitated, and in withdrawal).

Question 25.6.2 What is the minimum amount of time that you should observe a patient who has overdosed on methadone?

A) 1 hour
B) 4 hours
C) 12 hours
D) 36 hours
E) 7 days

Answer 25.6.2 **The correct answer is "D."** Methadone has a long half-life (variable, but up to 60 hours), and therefore a patient who has overdosed on methadone should be monitored for at least 36 to 48 hours. Since the half-life of naloxone is 30 to 90 minutes, it may take multiple doses of naloxone to treat a methadone overdose (a naloxone drip is sometimes used).

....

You discover that the patient has been on a methadone maintenance program, and you are not sure why she overdosed, as

her program reports she was stable with no evidence of opioid use. Her urine drug screen returns positive for opioids.

Question 25.6.3 What would be the next most appropriate course of action?
A) Detoxify the patient off methadone as an outpatient
B) Contact the authorities to have the patient arrested
C) Contact the patient's methadone maintenance clinic for dose increase
D) Notify the patient of her positive urine drug screen and let her know you are not surprised by the result, as methadone is metabolized to morphine
E) Have the patient committed to a substance abuse treatment facility

Answer 25.6.3 **The correct answer is "C."** Based on the urine drug screen results, the patient likely overdosed on methadone and another opioid. Methadone does not have any active metabolites (thus, "D" is incorrect). The positive urine drug screen is evidence of other opioid use. Methadone can be detected in urine but requires special testing. Heroin and codeine are metabolized to morphine. It would appear that this patient has relapsed into opioid abuse, and her methadone dose may be too low for maintenance. The rest are incorrect. "A" would be dangerous. "B" is not necessary. "E" would be ineffective for a patient not interested in quitting (but is often used anyway as a desperate measure).

HELPFUL TIP:
High-dose methadone can lead to QT prolongation and torsades de pointes.

Question 25.6.4 Methadone is typically prescribed for opioid maintenance therapy:
A) Once daily
B) Twice daily
C) Three times daily
D) Three times weekly
E) Once monthly

Answer 25.6.4 **The correct answer is "A."** Methadone has an elimination half-life of up to 60 hours (range 15–60 hours). Thus, once daily dosing is appropriate for the treatment of narcotic addiction. The advantage to once daily dosing is that the medication can be given under direct observation. Remember that it is given more frequently (two to three times daily) for pain control.

After regaining consciousness, the patient informs you that she is 20 weeks pregnant.

Question 25.6.5 Regarding pregnancy and usage of opioids, which of the following would most likely have the best outcome?
A) Continuing the patient on methadone

B) Withdrawing the patient from all opioids in the first trimester (too late for this one)
C) Withdrawing the patient from all opioids in the second trimester
D) Withdrawing the patient from all opioids in the third trimester

Answer 25.6.5 **The correct answer is "A."** Opioid withdrawal in a pregnant woman can cause fetal distress and low birth weight. Multiple organizations, including the American College of Obstetricians and Gynecologists, ASAM, and SAMHSA support use of methadone or buprenorphine as potential first-line medications for the treatment of opioid use disorder in pregnant women. Buprenorphine rather than methadone has been associated with a lower risk of pre-term birth, higher birth weight, and possibly less severe neonatal abstinence syndrome. It also can be administered from a physician's office, has a lower risk of overdose, fewer side effects, and fewer potential drug interactions. As successful pharmacotherapy depends on coordinated care, methadone may offer advantages of having to be dispensed daily at a registered opioid treatment center, allowing for more frequent contact for those who may need or want that. Some studies show higher retention rates in treatment for methadone, but others have shown no difference. However, these studies have also shown lower rates of opioid abuse during pregnancy among those on methadone. Whatever you choose, treating opioid use disorder during pregnancy has multiple advantages, including longer durations of maternal drug abstinence, better obstetrical care, reductions in fetal illicit drug exposure, and enhanced neonatal outcomes (e.g., increased fetal growth, reduced fetal mortality, and decreased risk of preeclampsia).

HELPFUL TIP:
Methadone use HAS been associated with greater treatment retention than buprenorphine in men and non-pregnant women. However, the difference was not large. The success of either medication depends on appropriate patient selection.

HELPFUL TIP:
Although it is generally recommended to prescribe buprenorphine with naloxone (Suboxone) in order to reduce intravenous misuse (also reducing risk of diversion), in the past pregnant patients were prescribed buprenorphine alone (without naloxone), given the relative lack of data on safety. This recommendation may be changing as more recent data have been reassuring in regards to using naloxone during pregnancy.

▶ **Objectives: Did you learn to …**
- Recognize symptoms and signs of overdose with opioids and other illicit drugs?
- Use methadone for opioid use disorder?
- Treat a pregnant patient with opioid use disorder?

▶ CASE 25.7

A 40-year-old female is admitted through the ED, arriving via ambulance from a smaller hospital. The local physician called to report that her friends said that she had "shot up a lot of meth." She has been confronted about using her son's Adderall prescription on a regular basis. She appears frightened and anxious. She is uncommunicative, rocking back and forth on the examination table, and picking at her skin trying to remove bugs that only she can see. She becomes angry easily and lashes out at staff in the ED.

Question 25.7.1 A reasonable differential diagnosis for this patient would include which of the following?
A) Schizophrenia
B) Drug-induced psychosis
C) PCP intoxication
D) Hepatic encephalopathy
E) Delirium tremens
F) Methamphetamine intoxication
G) All of the above

Answer 25.7.1 **The correct answer is "G."** Although there is a history of both methamphetamine and amphetamine use, the other options should not be eliminated without further investigation. You do not have the full history and do not know if there is an underlying medical or psychiatric disorder. There also may be more than one substance involved (don't be tricked by the "obvious" substance as polysubstance use is common).

The urine drug screen is positive for both methamphetamine and amphetamine. You admit the patient for further treatment.

Question 25.7.2 Which of the following does NOT address the needs of this patient during withdrawal?
A) Provide a secure environment
B) Provide regular meals and snacks
C) Make sure the patient is awakened if she spends excess time sleeping
D) Consider giving a benzodiazepine if the patient remains anxious
E) Provide education as an intervention toward change

Answer 25.7.2 **The correct answer is "C."** Amphetamine withdrawal requires sleep, adequate hydration, nutritious food, and a safe place until the unstable state of being has diminished. The patient should be allowed to sleep. Stimulant abusers often stay up for a week or more at a time and then "crash," sleeping for days during withdrawal. Antipsychotic medications and benzodiazepines may be administered if needed for control of agitation or violence.

You send off for confirmatory testing which shows only methamphetamine use. Collateral history is obtained from her husband and he is now keeping and dispensing their son's

Adderall. There is no reported psychiatric history, she is not on any other medication, and she does not drink alcohol. After recovering from withdrawal, she is discharged and enters an outpatient treatment program. Success! At least for now…

Question 25.7.3 The following are all symptoms of methamphetamine (and amphetamine) use EXCEPT:
A) Tachycardia
B) Hypertension
C) Perspiration or chills
D) Weight gain
E) Psychomotor agitation

Answer 25.7.3 **The correct answer is "D."** Weight loss, not weight gain, can be anticipated in a methamphetamine user (or amphetamine abuser). All of the other symptoms can be seen as a result of methamphetamine/amphetamine use. Other symptoms include increased energy, disrupted sleep patterns, mood changes, diaphoresis, increased sexuality, confusion, arrhythmia, seizure, tremors/myoclonus, or even coma in severe cases.

HELPFUL TIP:
Stimulant use can cause coronary artery occlusion and severe hypertension. Myocardial infarction with stimulant use should be treated like any other MI. Hypertension from stimulant intoxication is usually well controlled with benzodiazepines, which can also be used to manage any psychomotor agitation or anxiety. If refractory, consider intravenous medications, such as alpha-blockers or nitroprusside. Avoid beta-blockers (unless absolutely necessary) as this may result in unopposed alpha-adrenergic vasoconstriction and worsening of hypertension though outcome data are mixed and some clinicians will use combined alpha/beta blockers such as labetalol and carvedilol.

HELPFUL TIP:
Chronic methamphetamine use is associated with widespread dental caries and gingival disease that can result in loss of many, or even all, teeth. "Meth mouth," as this is commonly called, is probably due to prolonged periods of poor dental hygiene, xerostomia, high calorie food and drink, and tooth grinding. Methamphetamine-induced psychosis is associated with paranoia, auditory/tactile/visual hallucinations (snakes coming out of dashboard), and persecutory delusions and appears to have a relatively long duration of psychosis and can recur even during periods of abstinence.

▶ **Objectives: Did you learn to …**
- Recognize the signs and symptoms of methamphetamine intoxication?
- Appropriately treat a patient with methamphetamine intoxication and withdrawal?

▶ CASE 25.8

A 15-year-old male is brought into the ED by his neighbor who found the boy passed out in his backyard with multiple tubes of glue nearby. He had difficulty rousing the boy. Currently, the patient is lethargic with slurred speech and difficulty walking. When his parents arrive, they are shocked, as their son has been a "good kid." They had no idea he was using any drugs. Of course, he bought lots of tubes of "model glue" but they never did see any completed models.

Question 25.8.1 The signs and symptoms of inhalant intoxication include all of the following EXCEPT:
A) Dizziness
B) Slurred speech
C) Unsteady gait
D) Tremor
E) Dilated pupils

Answer 25.8.1 **The correct answer is "E."** Nystagmus and blurred vision/diplopia can be seen in inhalant intoxication; whereas, dilated pupils are seen in anticholinergic toxicity and other drugs (e.g., sympathomimetics) but not with inhalants. According to DSM-5, other signs and symptoms of inhalant intoxication include: incoordination, lethargy, depressed reflexes, psychomotor retardation, generalized muscle weakness, stupor/coma, and euphoria. Alternatively, patients may also display belligerence and assaultive behavior. Judgment is impaired (probably before and after huffing). The smell of solvents or glue on breath, skin, or clothes, empty containers or rags, and "glue-sniffer's rash" are also suggestive of inhalant use.

Question 25.8.2 Which of the following are considered inhalants used by abusers?
A) Whipped cream aerosol
B) Cleaning solvent
C) Gasoline
D) Spray paint
E) All of the above

Answer 25.8.2 **The correct answer is "E."** All of these products can be used as inhalants. Other products that are known to be inhaled for their intoxicating effects include household products containing hydrocarbons (butane, propane, benzene, toluene, halogenated hydrocarbons), nitrous oxide, and nitrites.

HELPFUL TIP:
The acute intoxicant effect of volatile hydrocarbons and nitrous oxide is produced within seconds of use and generally lasts 15 to 30 minutes. Inhalation of nitrites produces effects within seconds of inhalation, but its effects are very brief, lasting less than 5 minutes.

Question 25.8.3 All of the following can result from chronic solvent or hydrocarbon inhalation EXCEPT:
A) Neurocognitive impairment and cerebellar dysfunction
B) Generalized muscle weakness
C) CNS microhemorrhages and secondary seizures
D) Erythrocytosis
E) Liver and renal damage

Answer 25.8.3 **The correct answer is "D."** Solvents and hydrocarbons can cause all of the effects noted above except for erythrocytosis. In fact, bone marrow suppression can be a result of chronic inhalant use.

Question 25.8.4 Which of the following is FALSE in regard to inhalant use disorders?
A) Male and female adolescents report similar rates of inhalant abuse
B) Use peaks between seventh and ninth grade (age 13 to 15)
C) Those with inhalant use disorders are more likely to have episodes of major depression, conduct disorder, and are at an increased risk of other substance use problems
D) African American adolescents are at higher risk for an inhalant use disorder compared to the general adolescent population
E) Poor school performance (dropping out of school), lower socioeconomic status, and being involved with criminal justice system are risk factors for inhalant use

Answer 25.8.4 **The correct answer is "D."** African American youth have rates of inhalant use about half that of the general population. Unlike other substance use disorder, males and female adolescents report similar rates of inhalant use disorders. Inhalant users tend to be of lower socioeconomic status, younger age (13–15 years old), have difficulty in school, and have mental health and behavioral comorbidities.

HELPFUL TIP:
"Sniffing" is when fumes are inhaled directly from a source container. "Bagging" is when the substance is placed into a bag and then inhaled from the bag by placing over the mouth, nose, or head. "Huffing" is when the substance is placed on a rag and then inhaled with the rag placed over the nose and mouth. You got to know the lingo…

▶ **Objectives: Did you learn to …**
· Identify some types of inhalants abused?
· Recognize the symptoms of inhalant use disorder?
· Describe the demographics of inhalant use disorder?

▶ CASE 25.9

A 40-year-old male who has been smoking marijuana daily for the past 20 years would like to quit his marijuana habit … but he just cannot find the motivation. He wants to apply for

a new job, and a drug screen is part of the application process. He makes an appointment with you to discuss what he can expect when he quits and how long will it be until his drug screen is negative.

Question 25.9.1 All of the following are symptoms of cannabis intoxication EXCEPT:
A) Euphoria
B) Sensation of slowed time
C) Increased mental alertness
D) Increased appetite
E) Dry mouth

Answer 25.9.1 **The correct answer is "C."** Statistically speaking, over 40% of you will know this one from personal experience (you know who you are!). In fact, in 2017 almost 50% of US adults reported using marijuana some time in their lives. Cannabis intoxication decreases mental alertness, although it can reportedly enhance the senses. The DSM-5 criteria for cannabis intoxication include: (1) recent use of cannabis; (2) clinically significant problematic behavioral or psychological changes (impaired motor coordination, euphoria, anxiety, sensation of slowed time, impaired judgment, social withdrawal) that develop during, or shortly after, cannabis use; (3) two or more of the following signs: conjunctival injection, increased appetite, dry mouth, and tachycardia; (4) and the symptoms are not due to a general medical condition or another mental disorder. When inhaled, intoxication peaks after 10 to 30 minutes and lasts about 3 hours (these times vary by person, history of use, and THC content of cannabis). Of note, when ingested, peak effects can be delayed ranging from 30 minutes to 3 hours with effects lasting up to 12 hours.

HELPFUL TIP:
Recent (past year and past month) marijuana use has increased since 2002 among those 18 and older; prevalence among 12 to 17 year olds is actually lower than 2009 to 2014; and use for those older than 50 has significantly increased over the past decade. (Results from the 2016 National Survey on Drug Use and Health.)

Question 25.9.2 How long can marijuana (THC) be detected in the urine?
A) 30 days if used regularly; 2 to 7 days if used occasionally
B) 2 weeks
C) 1 week for females; 2 weeks for males
D) 24 to 48 hours
E) Trick question! It cannot be detected in urine samples

Answer 25.9.2 **The correct answer is "A."** This is the general rule. However, there is no simple answer to this question as detection times in urine are affected by a multitude of factors, including the threshold for the test, potency of marijuana used, frequency of use, route of ingestion (eating can make for slightly longer detection than smoking), and a person's physiological factors (e.g., metabolic rate, level of hydration). This patient will likely have to stop smoking marijuana for a minimum of 30 days before applying for the job, but this may be shorter or longer depending on those factors listed. Waiting longer (one study reported positive urine 77 days after use, which is definitely much longer than average) will assure his urine drug screen will be negative. The drug can be present in hair samples for an extended period of time, anywhere from 1 to 6 months (longer time if using body hair which grows slower than scalp hair). If a positive urine drug screen (for cannabis or any substance) is going to be used for legal or treatment purposes, it should be followed with a confirmatory test (e.g., gas chromatography/mass spectrometry).

Question 25.9.3 Which of these is NOT one of the touted benefits of cannabis?
A) Pain reliever
B) Anticonvulsant
C) Antiemetic
D) Appetite stimulator
E) Antidepressant

Answer 25.9.3 **The correct answer is "E."** In fact, the use of marijuana has a small increased risk for the development of depressive disorders. Cannabis has been used to treat pain, nausea, anorexia, seizures, glaucoma, etc. Despite the fact that nearly half of the states have passed laws allowing some sort of "medical marijuana" use, evidence for many of the touted medical benefits is scant or contradictory. The best evidence of benefit has been seen with chronic neuropathic pain (and these studies are small and of low quality), antiemetics for the treatment of chemotherapy-induced nausea, patient-reported multiple sclerosis spasticity symptoms, and certain pediatric seizure disorders (cannabidiol).

HELPFUL TIP:
There are several FDA-approved cannabinoid-based medications currently on the market and perhaps more to come. **Marinol** (dronabinol) and **Syndros** (liquified dronabinol) are approved for anorexia/weight loss in patients with AIDS and chemotherapy-related nausea/vomiting who have failed other treatments. **Cesamet** (nabilone) is approved for chemotherapy-related nausea/vomiting in patients who have failed other treatments. **Epidiolex** (cannabidiol) is approved for seizures associated with Lennox–Gastaut syndrome and Dravet syndrome. This medication is different than the others as it is the first plant-derived cannabinoid medication. **Sativex** (∆-9-tetrahydrocannibinol and cannabidiol) is an oromucosal spray approved for use in the United Kingdom, Canada, EU, New Zealand, and other countries (but not approved in the United States currently) as a treatment for spasticity due to multiple sclerosis. It is also plant-derived.

HELPFUL TIP:
An association between cannabis use and the development of schizophrenia or another psychotic disorder is supported by data from multiple systematic reviews and appears to be dose-dependent (highest risk among the most frequent users) and moderated by genetic factors.

▸ **Objectives: Did you learn to …**
- Recognize the signs and symptoms of cannabis intoxication?
- Evaluate what positive marijuana urine drug screens mean?
- Recognize possible medicinal benefits of marijuana?

 QUICK QUIZ: DUDE, WHAT WAS IN THAT WEED?

A 20-year-old male is brought by the police into the ED because of severe agitation after smoking what he thought was marijuana. He exhibits tachycardia, vomiting, paranoia, visual hallucinations, and may have had a seizure.

Which of the following substances is most likely causing his symptoms?
A) Marijuana
B) Heroin
C) Methamphetamine
D) Synthetic cannabinoid ("spice")
E) Nicotine

The correct answer is "D." Synthetic cannabinoids (also known as "K2," "spice," "chill x," and many others) are analogs of natural cannabinoids, which have been chemically synthesized. They are typically more potent than natural marijuana. They are often marketed as "incense" or "herbal remedies." They can be added to other herbals and smoked, can be ingested in teas, or insufflated (such as adding to and burning incense). Clinical effects are similar to natural marijuana (tachycardia, conjunctival injection, euphoria, altered perception, sedation, and ataxia). However, there is an increased risk of more serious effects including hypertension, mood dysregulation/agitation, severe anxiety/panic attacks, paranoia, hallucinations, rhabdomyolysis, and seizures. Treatment is typically supportive measures with calming environment and benzodiazepines as needed. Clinical effects occur soon after inhalation/insufflation and can last several hours to days. There are no fatal overdoses linked to marijuana alone, *but overdoses and deaths associated with synthetic cannabinoids are increasing.* Given that chemical analogs used in synthetic cannabinoids are constantly changing and increasing to avoid regulation, additional toxic effects and life-threatening symptoms may result.

HELPFUL TIP:
A few words on other substances, which are becoming increasingly popular and are often difficult to detect on standard urine drug screens.

MDMA (3,4-methylenedioxymethamphetamine; also known as "ecstasy," "molly," "E," and "X") is a synthetic compound with both hallucinogenic (mescaline-like) and stimulant (amphetamine-like) properties. It produces sensations of euphoria, intimacy, and disinhibition. It can cause nausea, diaphoresis, blurry vision, tachycardia, and bruxism (which is why candy pacifiers are popular with MDMA users). MDMA can cause seizures, liver disease, hyponatremia, and hyperthermia among more severe effects. Treatment focuses on supportive care (stabilization of airway, breathing, circulation), treatment with IV benzodiazepines (for hypertension or psychomotor agitation), and cooling techniques if needed for hyperthermia. MDMA is typically ingested orally with peak effects occurring within 2 hours (usually less) after ingestion and lasting 3 to 6 hours. "Molly" refers to drugs that are supposed to be the pure crystal form of MDMA as ecstasy can have other additives, including caffeine, methamphetamine, cocaine, etc.

Synthetic cathinones (also known as "bath salts," "khat," "vanilla sky," "white lightning," "cloud nine," and others) are synthetic stimulant compounds analogous to a naturally occurring substance found in the leaves of *Catha edulis* (khat or qat). Symptoms of intoxication/toxicity are sympathomimetic, similar to amphetamine, including tachycardia, hypertension, mydriasis, hyperthermia, aggression, agitation, memory deficits, hallucination, and paranoia. More severe complications include hepatic failure, acute kidney injury, arrhythmia, rhabdomyolysis, and electrolytic abnormalities. Treatment is typically supportive measures with IV fluids, benzodiazepines for agitation, calming environment, and/or temporary use of low-dose antipsychotics for psychoses. Bath salts can be ingested, smoked, snorted, or injected. Cathinone appears to peak about 1 hour after oral ingestion with effects lasting variable lengths, given widely varying half-lives between different chemicals.

GHB (gamma-hydroxybutyric acid; also known as "grievous bodily harm," "Georgia home boy," "liquid ecstasy," and others) is a short-acting drug that produces both sedation and stimulation (which may cycle rapidly). Patients may be bradycardic and near apneic but when stimulated may become agitated and violent. Confusion, dizziness, and drowsiness are common with low oral doses, but effects are variable (even in the same person at different times). Risks of acute toxicity are high based on abrupt onset of action, narrow safety margin, and unpredictability of effects. Treatment is supportive care, sedation for agitation, monitoring for possible airway support, and treating injuries they may have sustained. GHB is primarily available in a liquid form, which is odorless and clear. Effects with an oral dose typically peak within 30 to 60 minutes and typical effects last 2 to 4 hours. GHB is also known as the "date rape drug" as it has been used in sexual assaults. Sodium oxybate (sodium salt of GHB) is also known as Xyrem, a medication approved for narcolepsy.

Salvia (also known as "magic mint," "diviner's sage," and others) is a naturally occurring herb from the mint family in Mexico (*Salvia divinorum*), structurally unrelated to any other hallucinogen. The herb is typically smoked but can be chewed and absorbed from the buccal mucosa or ingested in a tea. The active ingredient is salvinorin A, which binds as a κ-opioid receptor agonist. Desired effects are similar to ketamine, LSD, and cannabis, including intense, short hallucinations, altered visual perception, and a "modified perception of external reality." Adverse effects include: anxiety, depersonalization, dysphoria, confusion, headaches, drowsiness, tachycardia, and hypertension. Since salvinorin A does not bind to μ-opioid receptors, respiratory depression is not typically seen (unlike with opioids). Treatment for salvia toxicity is supportive with calming environments and benzodiazepines as needed. When smoked, it generally produces a rapid, hallucinogenic effect, altered reality, and mood changes normally appearing within seconds lasting 10 to 30 minutes. Hallucinations and mood changes can be present for more than 2 hours depending on dose and route of administration (shorter when smoked.)

PCP (phencyclidine; also called "angel dust") is a dissociative anesthetic that has hallucinogenic properties. PCP intoxication is characterized by agitation, impulsiveness, nystagmus, hypertension, tachycardia, numbness, ataxia, and perceptual distortions. Intoxication begins 5 minutes after use and peaks in 30 minutes. PCP-induced psychosis is the most common PCP-induced disorder and may mimic a schizophrenic psychotic episode, and antipsychotic medication is sometimes needed (if benzodiazepines are insufficient). PCP may be added to other drugs unbeknownst to the user.

Kratom (*Mitragyna speciose)* is a tropical tree native to Southeast Asia that has stimulant-like effects (at low doses) and opioid-like effects (at higher doses). The FDA has not found any legitimate medical use for kratom, but it is not currently banned in the United States (although certain states have made it illegal). Most users consume kratom as a pill, capsule, or extract, but leaves can be chewed, smoked, or brewed in tea. Effects usually begin within 5 to 10 minutes of ingestion and last for 2 to 5 hours.

Remember the abuse of caffeine (legally available in powder form over the internet) and the toxicity of nicotine (from ingestion of products meant for a vaporizer) when presented with a patient abusing drugs.

 QUICK QUIZ: QUICK COUNSELING

Brief intervention for alcohol problems is one of the most clinically effective and cost-effective preventive services from among those recommended by the USPSTF.

All of the following are components for conducting brief interventions EXCEPT:
A) Ask about use and give feedback on screening results
B) State recommendations about safe drinking levels and offer advice about change
C) Assess the patient's readiness to change
D) Negotiate goals and strategies for change
E) Follow-up in a year or two to see how changes are progressing

The correct answer (and the thing to avoid) is "E." Hopefully, this one wasn't too hard as we wanted to introduce the concept of brief interventions. Follow-up should be arranged much sooner than 1 year. The "5 A's" method for brief interventions has substantial research support for its utility in alcohol use disorders across a variety of settings and can be incorporated with motivational strategies in a step-by-step process. The "5 A's" approach is a brief, goal-directed way to more effectively address substance use with patients. Altogether, the "5 A's" may take 1 to 5 minutes, depending on a provider's clinical setting and roles. These components include **A**sking about use, **A**dvising to cut down/quit, **A**ssessing willingness to quit, **A**ssisting with strategies for abstinence, and **A**rranging follow-up. The 5 A's approach is not the only model for brief interventions for alcohol use disorders with many approaches having been used successfully. Although duration of contact has not been shown to be an important determinant of effectiveness, delivering a clear, consistent message to your patient with whom you have an established relationship is an important part of any method.

 HELPFUL TIP:
As part of any behavioral intervention, it is important to recognize a patient's readiness to change. Tailoring your interventions toward a patient's stage of readiness to change is more effective (and less frustrating) than taking a "one size fits all" approach to counseling. The five stages of change are: precontemplation, contemplation, determination/preparation, action, and maintenance.

Clinical Pearls

- Ask all adults about tobacco use, advise them to stop using tobacco, and provide behavioral interventions and offer pharmacotherapy (if not contraindicated) for tobacco cessation.

- Do not administer intravenous multivitamins to patients with alcohol use disorders and/or withdrawal. Oral multivitamins are sufficient for the majority of patients. IV thiamine may be indicated in those suspected of having Wernicke encephalopathy.

- Provide education and counseling to school-age children and adolescents regarding tobacco, alcohol, and illicit drug use.

- Screen all adults for alcohol misuse and provide persons engaged in risky or hazardous drinking with brief behavioral counseling interventions to reduce alcohol misuse.

- Screen all pregnant women for tobacco use and alcohol misuse. Provide counseling and resources to reduce misuse. Fetal alcohol syndrome is the leading cause of intellectual disability in the United States.

BIBLIOGRAPHY

Ahmad FB, Rossen LM, Spencer MR, Warner M, Sutton P. Provisional drug overdose death counts. National Center for Health Statistics. 2018.

Alpert HR, et al. A prospective cohort study challenging the effectiveness of population-based medical intervention for smoking cessation. *Tob Control.* 2013;22:32–37.

American Academy of Family Physicians. Policies: substance abuse and addiction. 2014. Available at: http://www.aafp.org/about/policies/all/substance-abuse.html.

American Psychiatric Association. Substance-related and addictive disorders. In: *Diagnostic and Statistical Manual of Mental Health Disorders: DSM-5.* 5th ed., Arlington, VA: American Psychiatric Publishing; 2013.

Aoun EG, et al. Emerging drugs of abuse: clinical and legal considerations. *Rhode Island Med J.* 2014;97(6):41–45.

Ballantyne JC. Opioid therapy in chronic pain. *Phys Med Rehabil Clin N Am.* 2015;26(2):201–218.

Barry KL, et al. *Reducing Alcohol-Exposed Pregnancies: A Report of the National Task Force on Fetal Alcohol Syndrome and Fetal Alcohol Effect.* Atlanta, GA: Centers for Disease Control and Prevention; 2009.

Bayard M, et al. Alcohol withdrawal syndrome. *Am Fam Physician.* 2004;69(6):1443–1450.

Bratton RL. Fetal alcohol syndrome: how you can help prevent it. *Postgrad Med.* 1995;98(5):197–200.

Brensilver M, et al. Pharmacotherapy of amphetamine-type stimulant dependence: an update. *Drug Alcohol Rev.* 2013;32:449–460.

Chou R, et al. Systemic pharmacologic therapies for low back pain: a systematic review for an American College of Physicians clinical practice guideline. *Ann Intern Med.* 2017;166(7):480–492.

Daeppen JB, et al. Symptom-triggered vs. fixed schedule doses of benzodiazepine for alcohol withdrawal. *Arch Intern Med.* 2002;162:1117–1121.

Dowell D, Haegerich TM, Chou R. CDC guideline for prescribing opioids for chronic pain—United States, 2016. *JAMA.* 2016;315(15):1624–1645.

Enke O, et al. Anticonvulsants in the treatment of low back pain and lumbar radicular pain: a systematic review and meta-analysis. *CMAJ.* 2018;190:E786–E793.

Free C, et al. Smoking cessation support delivered via mobile phone messaging (txt2stop): a single-blind, randomized trial. *Lancet.* 2011;378(9785):49–55.

Gonzalez D, et al. Pattern of use and subjective effects of *Salvia divinorum* among recreational users. *Drug Alcohol Depend.* 2006;85:157–162.

Howard MO, et al. Inhalant use and inhalant use disorders in the United States. *Addict Sci Clin Pract.* 2011;6(1):18–31.

Hoyme HE, et al. Updated clinical guidelines for diagnosing fetal alcohol spectrum disorders. *Pediatrics.* 2016;138(2):1–18.

Lindson-Hawley N, et al. Gradual versus abrupt smoking cessation: a randomized controlled noninferiority trial. *Ann Intern Med.* 2016; 164(9):585–592.

Moore THM, et al. Cannabis use and risk of psychotic or affective mental health outcomes: a systematic review. *Lancet.* 2007;370:319–328.

Nelson ME, et al. Emerging drugs of abuse. *Emerg Med Clin N Am.* 2014;3(1):1–28.

Rigotti NA. Helping smokers with cardiac disease to abstain from tobacco after a stay in hospital. *CMAJ.* 2009;180(13):1283–1284.

Rosen LJ, et al. Diminishing benefit of smoking cessation medications during the first year: a meta-analysis of randomized controlled trials. *Addiction.* 2018;113(5):805–816.

Shanthanna H, et al. Benefits and safety of gabapentinoids in chronic low back pain: a systematic review and meta-analysis of randomized controlled trials. *PLoS Med.* 2017;14(8):1002369.

Shapiro B, et al. A primary care approach to substance misuse. *Am Fam Physician.* 2013;88(2):113–121.

Smith PM, et al. Smoking cessation initiated during hospital stay for patients with coronary artery disease: a randomized control trial. *CMAJ.* 2009;180(13):1297–1303.

Spithoff S, Kahan M. Primary care management of alcohol use disorder and at-risk drinking part 1: screening and assessment. *Can Fam Physician.* 2015;61:509–514.

Spithoff S, Kahan M. Primary care management of alcohol use disorder and at-risk drinking part 2: counsel, prescribe, connect. *Can Fam Physician.* 2015;61:515–521.

Thomas KH, et al. Risk of neuropsychiatric adverse events associated with varenicline: systematic review and meta-analysis. *The BMJ.* 2015;350:h1109.

Thompson A, et al. Pharmacotherapy for alcohol dependence: a stratified approach. *Pharmacology & Therapeutics.* 2015;153:10–24.

Volpp KG, et al. A randomized, controlled trial of financial incentives for smoking cessation. *N Engl J Med.* 2009;360(7):699–709.

Walker N, et al. Cytisine versus nicotine for smoking cessation. *N Engl J Med.* 2014;371(25):2353–62.

Walley AY. HIV prevention and treatment strategies can help address the overdose crisis. *Prev Med.* 2015;80:37–40.

Waterman EH, et al. Reducing fetal alcohol exposure in the United States. *Obstet Gynecol Surv.* 2013;68(5):367–378.

West R, et al. Placebo-controlled trial of cytisine for smoking cessation. *N Engl J Med.* 2011;365:1193–1200.

Ethics

26

Mark A. Graber and Nicholas H. Kluesner

▶ CASE 26.1

A 54-year-old married female, Charlene, has insulin-dependent diabetes and has seen you for her care for the last 7 years. In the last year, she has developed diabetic retinopathy and neuropathy. To your great frustration, Charlene continues to resist the recommended lifestyle changes required to control her diabetes.

She is a casual, friendly woman known as the "candy lady" in her neighborhood where she lives with her husband of 30 years. She loves children and volunteers at the local elementary school, where she is well known for a quick smile, a reassuring hug, and a piece of candy in her large, full pockets. In fact, she is noted during most of her appointments to be munching on M&M's—her favorite candy. She has had dietary consults and many education-oriented doctor appointments but says, "I know I shouldn't eat the way I do, but I just don't have the heart to change who I am, even if it does help my eyes and legs. Who I am is about what I eat and do."

You wonder about Charlene's capacity for decision-making, given her frank noncompliance with care, even in the setting of serious complications from her diabetes.

Question 26.1.1 All of the following variables are necessary in decision-making capacity (DMC) EXCEPT:
A) Ability to communicate a choice
B) Voluntary choice (e.g., absence of coercion)
C) Understanding of the variables involved in the decision
D) Ability to appreciate the personal impact of choices
E) Family agreement that the patient is competent

Answer 26.1.1 The correct answer is "E." All of the other options are considered important for determining decision-making capacity (DMC). Certainly family concerns need to be addressed, but family agreement has nothing to do with determining a patient's DMC. One additional necessary element for respecting DMC is freedom from coercion or other external threats to a person's right to self-determination (autonomy). In this regard, coordinating family agreement to pressure the patient into changing their decisions could be undermining the patient's autonomy.

Question 26.1.2 Which of the following is TRUE about DMC?
A) Patients who have been found legally incompetent do not have DMC
B) A patient's DMC may vary according to the circumstances of the situation
C) A minor's DMC is not clinically relevant since there is a surrogate who bears the responsibility for decision-making
D) DMC should not be evaluated in cases in which the patient makes a conventional, recommended choice
E) Patients with psychiatric disease, who are involuntarily committed to a treatment facility do not have DMC

Answer 26.1.2 The correct answer is "B." DMC is largely considered on a sliding-scale, rather than an "all-or-none" distinction, since the threshold for reaching DMC can vary widely from case to case or setting to setting. *Even patients who have been declared legally incompetent or who have been legally and involuntarily committed may still have a measure of DMC* (for example, meal choices, etc.). Moral theory typically urges clinicians to consider the wishes and reasoning of their patients as morally and clinically relevant, regardless of the placement of a legal guardian or the state as a surrogate decision-maker. DMC may ultimately be overridden in certain kinds of legal circumstances, but it **should not be done lightly** as it suggests a fundamental denial of patient autonomy.

Just as no legal determination removes our responsibility to respect a patient's autonomy, no particular diagnosis does either. As such, many patients with psychiatric illness still have the right to make choices, even with diagnoses such as schizophrenia. Additionally, making unconventional choices can sometimes be a marker that DMC is not intact, but does not automatically lead to this conclusion (a classic example would be an adult Jehovah's Witness patient who refuses a blood transfusion; while this is an unconventional choice, DMC may be intact). Finally, though minors technically cannot make many healthcare choices, their wishes should be taken into consideration as they are often able to articulate a preference. In minors, this is termed "assent," rather than consent. Children may not be able to understand enough to consent on their own but they can "assent" to (or protest) a particular plan of treatment.

Charlene continues to have a slow decline over time but remains in good spirits despite the complications of her uncontrolled diabetes. One day her husband brings her to the emergency department. He had found her in the bathroom, unconscious, and called an ambulance. She has had a stroke and remains unresponsive and is on a ventilator in the ICU. Her prognosis is poor.

Question 26.1.3 What are appropriate considerations for making a treatment decision about end-of-life care for Charlene?

A) Oral statements to her husband about her end-of-life care
B) Her husband's wishes for her care as designated proxy healthcare decision-maker
C) Written advance directives
D) Oral statements to her physician about her end-of-life care
E) All of the above

Answer 26.1.3 **The correct answer is "E."** Written advance directives are considered the most binding, since they are the patient's own declaration of their preferences, although all of these considerations are relevant in making end-of-life decisions since all of them could inform the family and treating medical team on what the patient would have wanted given her critical illness. Since the family is likely also grieving about her poor prognosis, emotions could cloud their recollection of her previously informally expressed wishes. This underscores why anticipatory discussions and advance directives can be profoundly helpful.

Question 26.1.4 Which of the following statements can be used to describe medical futility?

A) No worthwhile goals of care can be achieved
B) The likelihood of success is negligible (any intervention would be "futile")
C) The patient's quality of life is unacceptably burdensome
D) All of the above

Answer 26.1.4 **The correct answer is "D."** All of the above meanings have been explicitly or implicitly drawn into discussions about medical futility. Because of its variable interpretations and explanations, many theorists have objected to the use of the term "futility" as a justification for decisions and urge clinicians to be precise when "futility" is used as an argument to withhold care (e.g., the patient has metastatic lung cancer including to the brain, has been resuscitated two times already, may be resuscitated for this particular cardiac arrest but will never regain consciousness, will likely arrest again within the next 8 hours due to the underlying disease, and will never be able to be weaned successfully from a ventilator). Another definition of "futility" is trying to make it through this book without vast quantities of caffeine.

After discussion with her husband, you decide to discontinue ventilation. Charlene dies.

Question 26.1.5 This intervention is appropriately considered:

A) Active, involuntary euthanasia
B) Physician-assisted suicide
C) Withholding medical intervention
D) The principle of double effect
E) Withdrawing medical intervention (passive euthanasia)

Answer 26.1.5 **The correct answer is "E."** While the answer might seem intuitive to you, many persons (including physicians) do not recognize the differences between these various interventions. Active euthanasia ("A") is when the physician both supplies the means of death and is the final human agent in the events leading to the patient's death (e.g., the physician administers the lethal drug). Whether or not active euthanasia is voluntary, involuntary, or nonvoluntary depends on the DMC of the patient and their consent to the process. Assisted suicide ("B") occurs when the physician provides the means of death but the patient carries out the act, such as taking an overdose of phenobarbital. Withholding medical intervention ("C") means not initiating care for a disease state so that the disease itself results in death (e.g., not placing a gastric tube for artificial feeding in a patient with end-stage dementia). Withdrawing medical intervention ("E") means discontinuing an intervention that has already been used, although the disease state itself results in death with the intervention's discontinuation. Both of these ("C" and "E") are forms of passive euthanasia, where withdrawing life-sustaining treatment, or not starting it, leads to death. The principle of double effect ("D") is an ethical theory that suggests that if there is an unintended but anticipated bad consequence (e.g., earlier death) while pursuing an intended purpose (e.g., pain relief), there is diminished moral responsibility for the unintended outcome. This principle is sometimes used to justify the use of high-dose opiates or sedatives in patients with intractable pain or dyspnea, even when the unintended effect is respiratory depression and death.

Question 26.1.6 Which of the following is TRUE about the role of law in life-sustaining interventions?

A) Courts must be involved in decisions *after* a patient has been declared to not have capacity
B) Life-sustaining treatment may be withheld only if patients are terminally ill or permanently unconscious
C) Physicians may face criminal charges for providing appropriate palliative care and not treating the underlying disease
D) The most prudent legal advice is to continue treatment in medically futile cases
E) The law presents few barriers to physicians withholding life-sustaining interventions

Answer 26.1.6 **The correct answer is "E."** Sometimes physicians inappropriately provide treatment to patients who have made their end-of-life choices clear and have stated that they do not want prolongation of life. Respecting the patient's prior wishes will **not** result in legal liability for the physician, but the converse is not true; *one can be legally liable for treating a patient who does not want treatment* (e.g., transfusing a Jehovah's Witness patient who refused transfusion). While they are exceedingly rare, there are case reports of "wrongful life" malpractice suits against providers who ignored advanced directives to withhold life-sustaining treatment. There is still a risk-management, and likely professional and moral preference to "err on the side of life" when there is ambiguity about the patient's advance directives. While state laws vary, generally speaking "A" is incorrect, since surrogates for the patient have the authority to make decisions after the patient is declared not to have capacity. This may be a relative, a healthcare provider, or court-appointed surrogate. "B" is also incorrect as treatment may be withheld at any time at the request of a competent patient.

▶ **Objectives: Did you learn to …**
- Evaluate a patient's DMC?
- Recognize how DMC may vary based on the patient and the clinical setting?
- Identify some ethical issues in end-of-life care?
- Describe medical futility and understand its importance in making ethical decisions?

HELPFUL TIP:
Do "noncompliant" patients make you frustrated and angry? Just internalize the principle of patient autonomy. We can make suggestions, but it is up to the patient to decide how to act on our advice. In fact, it is their **right** to do so. Understand this and you will have a lot less heartburn.

QUICK QUIZ: AN ETHICAL DILEMMA

You are seeing George, a 30-year-old, HIV-positive male, for routine care and to assess his HIV status. During your conversation, he mentions that he is in a new relationship—a relationship that he hopes will become long term. They use condoms "some of the time", but have unprotected sex on a regular basis when there is no condom available. When you ask him whether or not he has disclosed his HIV status to his partner, he states that he has not done so and will not do so because of the fear his partner will leave him. He also forbids you to contact his partner to notify her of his HIV status.

Your response in this situation is to:
A) Attempt to convince George to notify his partner of his HIV status
B) Depending on your state, contact the health department and have them follow up on the patient's sexual contacts
C) Contact the partner directly and let him/her know of George's HIV status
D) Maintain strict confidentiality and do not warn George's partner nor report his HIV status regardless of the situation
E) A, B, and C

The correct answer is "E." "A" is clearly correct. Anything we can do to convince George that it is critical he notify his partner of his HIV status (short of coercion) should be done. George should be aware that in some states it is a crime not to disclose known HIV-positive status to a sexual partner. "B" is correct but may vary by state. As of this writing, all 50 states and most territories have confidential, name-based reporting for HIV. However, patients can still be tested anonymously which precludes reporting and can circumvent reporting laws. For this same reason, "D" is incorrect. There are mandatory reporter laws on the books. "C" is also correct. Although this is somewhat controversial and there are conflicting duties (the patient's autonomy and confidentiality vs. the duty to warn the partner), we have a duty to protect the patient's partner. This can be clearly apparent in mental health, as in cases of a direct threat to a known individual, where there is a duty to warn the individual—known as the Tarasoff Rule after a court ruling on such a case. One such clear-cut example would be if George were threatening to shoot his partner and storms out of the office with a gun. While this is a more immediate example, the same principle holds. Clearly, we must not take the breaking of patient confidentiality lightly. And, we must inform the patient of our course of action. You may want to set a time frame for George to notify his partner with the understanding that if he does not do so, you must.

There are clear limits to this duty to protect other individuals. For example, if all we know is that George is HIV positive and have no knowledge of his partner(s), we cannot publicize George's HIV status in the local press in order to "protect the public." This would be too profound of a violation of the patient's confidentiality and privacy, without any concrete, individual benefits. But if we have a specific name of an ongoing sexual partner, we have a duty to warn that individual which competes with our duty to maintain confidentiality with George.

▶ CASE 26.2

Robert, a 27-year-old married nurse from your hospital, is referred to your emergency department for an urgent evaluation by his supervisor. In the past 2 weeks, he has been noted to be increasingly distressed while at work, with occasional tearfulness, distractibility, and irritability.

During the initial assessment, Robert reveals that there is a specific reason that he has been so preoccupied. He indicates that 2 weeks ago he was jailed for operating a vehicle while intoxicated and that he feels ashamed. He is afraid that his coworkers have read about it in the newspaper, although no one on his floor has indicated that this is the case. This is his first legal infraction of any kind and he describes it as humiliating.

On further questioning, Robert indicates that he uses alcohol regularly. While it has not overtly affected his work as far as he can tell, it has caused significant marital strife. He reports that his pattern is to stop by the bar on the way home from work to "relax and let go of the hospital stuff that I worry about." He typically drinks three beers and then drives home,

where he continues to drink beer throughout the evening. He notes that his wife and kids complain that he is emotionally absent and even irritable with them, but he says that his family simply doesn't understand the stress of the workplace and his need to "forget about it for a few hours." He and his wife have started arguing lately about his alcohol use, especially since the driving charge. He takes special exception to her stating that he is an "alcoholic."

As you take the history, Robert begins to be more guarded in his responses and more restricted in his affect. Suddenly, he blurts out, "I don't think I'm an alcoholic, but I don't want you to put anything in my record about any of this stuff! And I want you to tell my supervisor that there are some personal problems going on at home and that I'll be fine in a few days."

Question 26.2.1 Which of the following statements is TRUE about your obligation with regard to documentation in the chart?

A) You are obligated to document the visit as it occurred so far as the medical facts are concerned, including the concern about alcohol abuse

B) You can enter incorrect information into the chart in order to protect the patient

C) You are under no obligation to document anything said and can withhold information from the chart at the patient's request

D) Hospital administration or legal counsel should be involved if information is going to be purposefully left out of the chart

E) You can lie in the medical record … we're pretty sure perjury, liable, and slander don't apply to doctors

Answer 26.2.1 **The correct answer is "A."** The ethical principles of beneficence, nonmaleficence, and justice drive the decision here. A patient may legitimately ask for nonactive medical problems (e.g., distant history of sexual abuse) to be withheld from current documentation of an active problem (e.g., allergic rhinitis—by the way, kudos on your detailed history-taking). However, a patient **cannot** legitimately ask to have information withheld from the record if that information is pertinent to an ongoing condition currently being evaluated and treated. In this case, Robert is receiving care simply by virtue of being seen in the emergency department and disclosing the chief complaint and its associated variables. It is important for you to be forthcoming in explaining why the information may not be withheld from the medical record and also in reassuring him that irrelevant medical information will be omitted from the record if he feels that this is necessary. For example, the specifics of the argument with a wife need not be detailed beyond the comment that there is nonviolent marital conflict over the patient's alcohol use—important because it supports an alcohol abuse disorder. Furthermore, the patient can be reassured that many institutions have specific policies on managing sensitive medical information and there may be a formal mechanism for increasing the security of the patient's medical record.

Question 26.2.2 Why is protection of confidentiality important in medical practice?

A) It shows respect for patient autonomy

B) It helps prevent stigmatization and discrimination against patients based on private medical issues

C) It helps solidify trust within the physician–patient relationship

D) It helps establish a boundary between the physician–patient relationship and the rest of the medical system

E) All of the above

Answer 26.2.2 **The correct answer is "E."** The physician–patient relationship is a long-honored tradition in medicine that is increasingly fragile in a medical system with numerous competing obligations. Nevertheless, it is prudent to remember the aspect of the Hippocratic Oath, which states, "What I may see or hear in the course of the treatment … which on no account one must spread abroad, I will keep to myself, holding such things shameful to be spoken about." This is not only important to the tradition of medicine itself but also to the physician–patient relationship. There is no doubt that loss of confidentiality may cause harm to the patient when others are in possession of confidential medical information. Such harms may be as overt as denying insurance coverage for certain genetic conditions or as subtle as devaluing a person waiting to see the psychiatrist. The Health Insurance Portability and Accountability Act of 1996 (HIPAA) codified confidentiality and disclosure of protected health information to respect individual privacy.

Question 26.2.3 Which of the following are legally protected exceptions to the rule of maintaining patient confidentiality?

A) Reporting tuberculosis to public officials without patient consent

B) Warning a third party at risk of imminent and serious bodily harm from the patient without patient consent

C) Reporting a patient's alcohol abuse to a work supervisor without the patient's consent

D) A and B

E) All of the above

Answer 26.2.3 **The correct answer is "D."** Under current national and state laws, physicians are mandatory reporters of some infectious diseases, of intent to harm another, and of child / dependent-adult abuse. In most other cases, provision of protected health information without the patient's written consent is not legally protected, although there may be cases in which it is felt to be morally justifiable. Physicians need to weigh violations of patient confidentiality very carefully, even when legally sanctioned. Ethicists typically agree that if a physician is going to compromise a patient's confidentiality for an overwhelming moral obligation, the patient needs to be notified out of respect for his/her autonomy. In many situations in which a physician hopes to communicate confidential information to a third party even when the patient is unwilling, a process of education and negotiation with the patient occurs such that respect for autonomy is acknowledged while simultaneously making the patient aware of competing moral obligations.

HELPFUL TIP:
Having a faxed, e-mailed, or mailed report containing a patient's confidential medical information misdirected to an unintended recipient is *not* legally protected. Be cautious about transmission of patient information.

Question 26.2.4 **Which of the following interferes with protecting patient confidentiality in the medical structure?**
A) Involvement of managed care organizations in patient care and medical payments
B) Electronic records and transmissions
C) Group practices and/or teaching hospitals with multiple care providers
D) A and B
E) All of the above

Answer 26.2.4 **The correct answer is "E."** While individual physicians and patients continue to prize the tradition of respect for confidentiality, the multiple players in healthcare make it nearly impossible to restrict all information to the dyad of physician and patient. Insurance companies will not provide payment without, at least, information about the diagnosis, and notably, insurance companies are not legally bound by the same codes of conduct that apply to physicians regarding patient privacy. Electronic records and transmissions by e-mail, cellular phones, faxes, and other means are much more easily accessed by the curious or unintended recipients who have no reason to have confidential information. Open waiting rooms and multiple providers of care mean that larger and larger numbers of the community are aware that a patient is being seen in certain clinics for certain purposes. Once information is in written form, it is more difficult to control who might, either now or in the future, have access to the details of the report. For this reason, some physicians try to err on documenting only that which is considered absolutely necessary to patient care, although the distinction between the "absolutely necessary" and unnecessary can be a difficult line to draw in the sand, especially without the ability to appreciate how multiple variables may play out in the patient's future medical care.

Back to the patient at hand … Robert is asking you to be deliberately deceptive with the supervisor. You disagree with this.

Question 26.2.5 **Which of the following is FALSE?**
A) Trust in the physician–patient relationship depends on allowing the patient to make such a directive about communication with outside persons
B) A physician who establishes a precedent for deception may be expected to practice deception in a future situation in which the harms greatly outweigh the benefits
C) A physician who deceives may undermine general trust in the profession
D) All of the above

Answer 26.2.5 **The correct answer is "A."** Another way of phrasing the question is, "What drives a physician to be honest even when what the patient really wants is not honesty?" Will the patient trust you more if you are deceptive for him? Will this help him (aside from allowing him to keep his job)?

The physician–patient relationship is generally not considered an adequate reason to lie to a third party about the nature of a patient's illness and treatment. There has been concern that a physician who deceives a third party, even in the immediate interest of the patient's confidentiality or other concerns, establishes himself or herself as a physician who may not be trustworthy in other matters. A patient may not consider this at the time a deception is requested. These kinds of ripple effects from the decisions of an individual physician can affect the profession in general, ultimately producing fears that physicians will take the self-serving path rather than the higher moral ground.

You tell Robert that he has alcohol dependence and then provide education about the diagnosis and treatment options. You recommend outpatient treatment in Alcoholics Anonymous (AA) and a chemical dependency program. Robert agrees, more for the sake of his family stability rather than because of any true insight into the severity of his problem. You then arrange for follow-up with one of your partners (you've been selected as a contestant on the next *Survivor* and get to escape to a tropical island).

At the next appointment, Robert meets his new physician, Dr. Pincus. At this appointment, Robert indicates that he did attend two AA meetings but was very uncomfortable with the aspect of the 12-step program that requires acknowledging a "higher power." Robert indicates that he is an atheist and secular humanist, believing that the locus of self-control comes from within the individual human spirit. He has refused to continue in AA due to his rejection of its theistic foundation. He has had no further legal problems and reports that work is still going fine, with diminished irritability once he resolved in his mind that his coworkers were unaware of his previous driving violation. However, he continues to drink six to nine alcoholic beverages per night and admits that he occasionally needs a shot of whisky in the morning to "make sure I don't lose it with all the work stress" (this is where his self-control theory really comes together). He also works a night shift about once per week and does use approximately the same amount of alcohol before beginning the night shift, although he denies being intoxicated while on the job on these nights ("My tolerance is high and six beers are no big deal"). He doesn't think this is a problem because "things are quiet at night and everyone just helps each other keep the patients comfortable." He reports that his family is satisfied with the decrease in consumption and that he considers the matter of alcohol abuse resolved.

Dr. Pincus has had her own problems with alcohol in the past. She has had a rocky course over the past many years but found AA to be very helpful. She has become very active in her Jewish synagogue and community, where she receives support and is accountable to her friends. Her own alcohol history has been marked by difficulty with alcohol bingeing, such that when she starts to drink, she drinks to intoxication. Only with aggressive honesty at a professional-group AA, as well as a substance abuse protocol through the state board of medical examiners, does she feel that she's been able to remain completely abstinent for the last 4 years.

Dr. Pincus is considering revealing to Robert some of her own struggles as a healthcare professional with a substance abuse disorder. She believes that this will help him reevaluate the role of AA in sobriety and the importance of very tight control of alcohol consumption to prevent relapsing illness.

Question 26.2.6 **Self-disclosure is best described as involving the ethical issues of:**
A) Deception and nondisclosure
B) Privacy and boundaries
C) Informed consent
D) Impaired colleagues
E) Autonomy

Answer 26.2.6 **The correct answer is "B."** There are explicit and implicit boundaries that exist between a physician's private experiences and the physician–patient relationship. One of these boundaries has to do with preventing physician needs and private matters from encroaching into the visit in a way that is not therapeutic to the patient and does not respect the physician's boundaries. While it would appear that Dr. Pincus has therapeutic reasons—for Robert, not for herself—for crossing the boundary of self-disclosure, both physician motivation for self-disclosure and the immediate and potential effects of the self-disclosure need to be weighed very seriously before private matters are revealed. If there is even a potential of harm, crossing the boundary in this way should be considered a violation of professional norms.

Question 26.2.7 **How could Dr. Pincus appropriately respond to Robert's refusal to participate in AA on the basis of his religious impulse?**
A) "AA is still shown the best intervention for preventing relapsing alcohol use. I hope you can go and get something out of it without acknowledging your acceptance of the 'higher power' explicitly"
B) "AA has important group support from others who understand how difficult it is to stop using alcohol. It is not meant to be religious, but rather a community of care"
C) "I have found both AA and a theistic world-view to be very helpful in understanding my own powerlessness to control some of my behaviors. Would it be helpful to you to hear more about this?"
D) "I understand how the religious aspect of AA is inconsistent with your own philosophy. Would you be willing to investigate nonreligious group meetings for alcohol abusers?"

Answer 26.2.7 **The correct answer is "D."** AA is an example of a prescribed treatment that involves an active theological component. AA's first step involves acknowledgment of a higher power, traditionally invoking a specific monotheistic conception of the divine as a necessity to surrendering the illusion of control. **In the interest of respecting a patient's religious rights in a diverse community, and of optimizing treatment options, it would be disrespectful and ineffective to have the patient participate in AA, while ignoring the first step of the program and the foundational philosophy of AA.** While there are fewer studies about the efficacy of nonreligious alcohol treatment groups, it is appropriate to respect Robert's beliefs by investigating nonreligious alternatives. As to option "A," the Cochrane database concludes, "No experimental studies unequivocally demonstrated the effectiveness of AA."

Whether or not self-disclosure of one's own religious beliefs is appropriate is an important question. As mentioned in the discussion in the question above, it is very important for the physician to measure the intent of the disclosure. Also, physicians need to be exquisitely sensitive to the power differential that exists between a physician and a patient such that strong individual viewpoints might become threatening or coercive in the physician–patient relationship. In certain religious traditions, sharing one's faith is an important step, demonstrating courage and integrity; nevertheless, physicians should be strongly cautioned to pay heed to the virtue of practical wisdom and the unique circumstances of the medical relationship that makes proselytizing most often inappropriate. A better strategy, if a physician feels that a patient might be seeking additional spiritual or philosophical direction, is to ask open-ended questions and then make an appropriate referral to pastoral care or a spiritual counselor who will be sensitive to the issues the patient has raised as relevant.

Question 26.2.8 **Which of the following is true about intervening with an "impaired colleague," like Robert?**
A) Impairment should be reported only to a state licensing board if the colleague's patients are placed at known and documentable risk
B) Because alcohol abuse is a confidential matter, it is inappropriate for a treating physician to report a colleague's impairment to a licensing board
C) Removing a colleague from direct patient care and increasing supervision during patient care are reasonable first-step interventions for a colleague who is actively engaged in substance **treatment** (e.g., a report has already been made)
D) It is preferable to contact a state licensing board directly as opposed to discussing the matter with the patient or institutional administration. This protects both the reporter and the colleague from unnecessary negative repercussions

Answer 26.2.8 **The correct answer is "C."** Legal statutes on reporting impaired colleagues vary from state to state, with some state laws making physicians mandatory reporters of impaired physician colleagues, while others simply recommend reporting. Furthermore, state laws are even less prescriptive with regard to nonphysician health professionals with impairments. Any impairment should be treated seriously, preferably with support from the institution's administration. It is imperative to protect patients from harm. While reporting the impaired colleague may result in anger and disappointment from the colleague or even supervisors who are reluctant to tackle such a difficult question, physicians should consider the needs of vulnerable patients and the patients' rights to adequate care.

Confidentiality adds an additional ethical dimension when an impaired colleague reveals his or her impairment to his treating physician. In an effort to respect patient autonomy, physicians will often urge impaired colleagues to report themselves as well as voluntarily engage in treatment protocols. Many states have less-restrictive policies for treatment and monitoring for impaired colleagues who self-report. If a physician intends to report her patient's impairment without the consent of the patient, the physician is obligated to be truthful with the colleague about her intentions and rationale for reporting.

Question 26.2.9 A colleague may be impaired in her practice by all of the following EXCEPT:
A) Substance use
B) Major depression
C) Dementia
D) Deficits knowledge
E) Barely passing the board examination

Answer 26.2.9 **The correct answer is "E."** Well, "barely passed," is what is needed to achieve certification. All of the others, whether acute or chronic, may impair a health professional's ability to practice, but none of these automatically imply global impairment in medical practice. Each has its own implications for a colleague's medical practice. Special attention should be given to the colleague's actual and possible consequences in practice, given her specific job requirements and compensatory skills/supports, while assessing the presence and degree of impairment. One might say that dementia is OK in physicians working for insurance companies (or at least it seems so!).

▶ **Objectives: Did you learn to …**
- Identify what items are required for inclusion in the medical record?
- Recognize the importance of patient confidentiality and understand when confidentiality might be broken in order to fulfill other ethical obligations?
- Recognize obstacles to protecting patient confidentiality?
- Describe the importance of individual and societal trust in individual physicians and the medical profession as a whole?
- Describe the ethical principles involved in self-disclosure?
- Identify an impaired colleague and determine how to best intervene?

▶ CASE 26.3

Anne is a 19-year-old single female presenting for her first prenatal visit. She is G1P0, and roughly 10 weeks gestation by last menstrual period. She is new to your practice. Anne has had no medical care at this facility and no physician appointments since childhood. In recollecting the past medical history, Anne reveals that she has had several first-degree female relatives who have been diagnosed with breast and/or ovarian cancer: her mother, two maternal aunts, and a maternal grandmother. A great aunt also died young of unknown causes. Anne is unsure of the workup that they had, but there was significant morbidity and mortality as a result of the illnesses. It was as if God were playing with a cosmic grenade launcher when it accidently went off and blasted her family apart. "Oh, well. Genetic roulette," she says. Anne only recently became aware of this family history when her mother and aunts were diagnosed. When you ask if she has discussed genetic risks for breast cancer, Anne looks at you blankly and replies, "No."

Anne has been in a stable relationship with her boyfriend, Jordan, for 2 years. They cohabitate and are engaged, but have not set a wedding date. Anne has completed high school and works in telemarketing while applying to art schools. The pregnancy was not planned, but she and Jordan are thrilled, even if a little nervous, about having a baby.

Being an extraordinarily astute clinician, you are concerned about BRCA1 and 2 genes. In families with a high incidence of breast and ovarian cancer, mutations in BRCA1 are associated with an 85% lifetime risk of developing breast cancer and a 50% risk of ovarian cancer.

You wonder if this is the best time to bring up genetic concerns with Anne, given Anne's concurrent transition with an unplanned pregnancy.

Question 26.3.1 Which of the following is/are true about disclosure?
A) Nondisclosure is not justifiable due to fears that a patient will be distressed by the information, unless disclosure might cause death (e.g., suicide at hearing a diagnosis of cancer)
B) Regardless of the consequences, nondisclosure could be considered deception and would be morally wrong on the basis of this intrinsic feature
C) Disclosure is important because it respects patient autonomy and optimizes a patient's ability to make an informed choice
D) Nondisclosure may be a sign of paternalism rather than beneficence
E) All of the above

Answer 26.3.1 **The correct answer is "E."** There are a variety of moral theories which comment on whether or not deception or nondisclosure is morally appropriate. Most theorists rely on the principle of respect for patient autonomy, such that a person who has incomplete information is not able to act freely in making a choice for herself. "Consequentialism" is also a commonly used moral theory, suggesting that it is not the intrinsic nature of the act itself but the consequences that follow which determines whether the act is good or evil (as in "the end justifies the means"). In virtue ethics, by comparison, the nature and motivation of the act are very important as a reflection of the physician's character and habits. In virtue ethics, deception is morally blameworthy because it is comparable to lying. In virtue ethics, motivation is also an important issue to judge the goodness of the action.

Question 26.3.2 Which of the following is FALSE about testing for genetic conditions?

A) Informed consent for genetic testing should be taken more seriously and formally than other kinds of blood testing, such as obtaining a CBC

B) Physicians should ask patients what they would do with the different possible outcomes of the genetic test before the test is performed

C) Physicians should make a recommendation regarding genetic testing guided by evidence-based medicine and the patient's specific narrative and values

D) Physicians should urge patients to disclose positive results to relatives or spouses if the information is pertinent medically or emotionally to these third parties

E) Physicians should never disclose genetic information to a third party without the consent of the patient

Answer 26.3.2 The correct answer is "E." Genetic testing differs from other blood tests because of multiple actual and potential risks, including personal effects on the patient and her family, as well as discrimination by employers or insurers. There is a shortage of formally trained genetic counselors, and patients rely on their physicians to not only help guide their decision-making about whether or not to perform the test, but also what to do with the information obtained. Because such testing has profound medical and/or psychosocial effects on the patient and family, a discussion about disclosure should happen both before and after the test is obtained.

Confidentiality is important for many reasons, not only in establishing and maintaining a good physician–patient relationship and respecting patient autonomy but also because of the potential discrimination and misuses of genetic information in today's culture. However, when the risk of harm to another related person is high and the patient refuses to disclose important genetic information, there may be adequate cause to break confidentiality in order to prevent serious harm to the third party; therefore, "E" is a false statement. For example, if a female patient has a genetic test that shows an X-linked trait that is lethal at approximately age 5 years in any male offspring, it would be immoral to withhold this information from the patient's reproductive age sister.

You decide to disclose the possibility of genetic risk factors to Anne at the first prenatal visit and also discuss the risk of passing genes to the fetus. Anne seems overwhelmed and asks to bring Jordan to the next visit to discuss this further. When Anne returns with her fiancé, you discuss your concerns about the BRCA1 and 2 genes and why Anne's family history is suspicious. Jordan says, "I think you should be tested right away, Anne. This would totally change our future." Anne replies: "What are you saying? Will you leave me if I have the gene? I can't raise this baby by myself!"

Question 26.3.3 Which of the following statements are appropriate to consider in promoting the patient's best interests?

A) Patients can be a vulnerable population

B) Physicians have expertise that patients lack

C) Patients rely on their physicians

D) Physicians and patients often agree on what constitutes a patient's best interests, although they may differ in the way they plan to meet those interests

E) All of the above

Answer 26.3.3 The correct answer is "E." The nature of a relationship between a physician and a patient may have as many permutations as there are individuals. However, it is important to appreciate the position of the patient and the need that has pushed her to seek care. Patients are vulnerable in many ways, and the vulnerability is enhanced by limited access to technological and scientific information. When external variables, such as Jordan's comment and Anne's response, come into play, physicians should pay attention to this narrative and take some responsibility for establishing and maintaining a supportive network even outside of the office. This is particularly important as physicians give patients information about difficult choices. While physicians and patients may often be able to negotiate a mutually acceptable alternative, an active dialogue is important. Supporters and advocates who are familiar with the patient's values and wishes can be an important adjunct to medical decision-making, as long as there is no material or psychological conflict of interests. Physicians should not adopt a completely hands-off policy in decision-making; rather, physicians should pay attention to supporting the patient with real options and evidence-based variables in a noncoercive, empowering relationship.

Anne decides not to have the test, but to have an elective abortion "just in case I passed on a gene to the baby." For the sake of argument, you are philosophically opposed to elective abortions in this scenario, but you would consider abortion an appropriate intervention if the fetus tests positive for the gene by chorionic villus sampling.

Question 26.3.4 What is the best ethical option for you at this point?

A) Explain that you are personally uncomfortable with abortion, but in deference to Anne's legal rights, you will make a referral to another physician who is willing to provide the elective abortion

B) Refuse to perform or make a referral for the abortion

C) Refer to a "pro-life" counseling agency

D) Tell Anne, for reasons that you do not feel comfortable disclosing, you will no longer be able to care for her

E) Perform the elective abortion, despite personal convictions, out of respect for the law and patient autonomy

Answer 26.3.4 **The correct answer is "A."** Abortion is a fiercely contentious topic in the United States. Under the 1973 *Roe v. Wade* decision and in subsequent rulings such as *Planned Parenthood v. Casey*, the Supreme Court has affirmed a woman's legal right to abort a fetus. Physicians have responsibilities that should transcend views about a physician's own moral values, such as ensuring that informed consent is practiced and that the patient has medical care available. Informed consent requires a physician to provide the necessary information about the various medical choices available and to assess the patient's emotional needs. Coercion and failure to disclose clinically relevant information is inappropriate; for example, a referral to a pro-life group without informing the patient of the counseling center's perspective (when known) is a form of manipulation and failure to disclose. Abandoning the patient ("D") without a simple explanation is disrespectful, although the physician should be careful not to coerce her in other ways while revealing personal values/beliefs.

Three years later, Anne is seen in a new clinic. She had the abortion. Anne is now an art student and is married to Jordan. Since her last clinic visit, Anne has had a prophylactic mastectomy following a positive test for the BRCA1 gene. She has also had an elective tubal ligation. Anne wants to consider in vitro fertilization (IVF) and has a friend, Jessica, who is willing to donate ova. They put 18 embryos into cold storage, using Jessica's ova and Jordan's sperm. Anne has 6 embryos implanted, with the result of two fetuses that are carried to term. Anne decides that she does not want any more children and contacts the lab to discard the remaining embryos, eliminating storage costs. The lab agrees and sells the embryos to a private lab, where stem cell research is under way.

Question 26.3.5 What is NOT true about stored tissue samples?
A) The embryos are considered Anne's property only as long as she claims them
B) Samples used for research purposes are potentially identifiable by third parties as belonging to Jessica and Jordan
C) Tissue samples may be used only for their initial intended purpose, after which time they must be destroyed
D) Third parties, such as research labs, upon discovering genetic anomalies in tissue samples, have no legal obligation to find and inform Anne, Jordan, and/or Jessica
E) Embryos sold to a private lab may be used to establish germ lines via destruction of the embryo

Answer 26.3.5 **The correct answer is "C."** At the time of publication, there is ongoing discussion about how to regulate use of tissue samples. While it might seem that this is an ethical question far removed from the purview of the family physician, patients in family practice clinics are very frequently targeted for various research protocols due to their regular follow-up and easy accessibility.

Patients donating tissue samples often give little thought to what happens to those tissues after they are obtained. In many cases, tissues are banked indefinitely after the initial research is conducted, with various identifiers linked to the tissue potentially including the donor's gender, geographic location, educational level, family history, or other private information (e.g., *The Immortal Life of Henrietta Lacks*). While efforts are made to respect the privacy of the donor, there are ways to track down the donor using even the limited identification information associated with the stored sample. Such means are especially facilitated by the wide availability of personal information via the Internet.

Tissue samples may be collected for one purpose, but later used for another. Tissue samples are very important in research and are often the limiting factor for studies, but should informed consent include asking donors for permission for each and every lab test run on the tissue sample? At what point, if any, does the tissue sample become the sole property of the lab? In the example of embryos, discarded embryos are sometimes sold to private labs; parents using IVF technology are often unaware that such embryos may be used to establish a stem cell line from which genetically identical embryos can be created using nuclear transfers. Such stem cell lines are highly lucrative for research purposes, and there has been discussion, for example, of whether parents should be compensated in some manner when a lab sells their discarded embryos or a research facility develops a product using the embryonic stem cells.

HELPFUL TIP:
Family physicians should continue to serve as advocates for their patients. You can do so by investigating the policies and procedures of research groups prior to recommending them to patients and by taking some responsibility for the informed consent process when patients are volunteering to participate in research.

▶ **Objectives: Did you learn to …**
- Describe the ethical issues regarding disclosure?
- Appreciate the many competing interests involved in genetic testing?
- Identify patient and physician factors that affect the patient–physician relationship?
- Find an ethical and acceptable way to disagree with a patient and continue to assure that patient's healthcare?

▶ **CASE 26.4**

John is a 32-year-old newly practicing physician in your group. As friends on social media, you see his posts from time to time, typically about his family or sharing the latest current events in medicine. On one occasion, however, you notice a posting to a medical group discussing a "hypothetical" clinical case that clearly seems to be a recent real diagnostic dilemma he faced. He has, of course, de-identified the patient, but the

clinical context (recurrent asthma attacks at public sporting events) is important as he seems to be crowdsourcing input on how to distinguish true bronchoconstriction from social anxiety.

Question 26.4.1 Which of the following could pose problems for your colleague's social media activity?

A) De-identification of the patient's information may not be sufficient to protect the patient's privacy

B) Crowdsourcing can result in unreliable and unverifiable information

C) Any publically available dialogue may be held to a higher standard as a physician in terms of the potential to violate confidentiality

D) There may be relevant guidelines or rules that your partner has broken

E) All of the above

Answer 26.4.1 The correct answer is "E." All of the above are true. In addition to the patient's name and other identifiable demographics, the circumstances, time, location, and other public records (e.g., police or news reports) could converge to threaten a patient's confidentiality. Additional caution and restrictions are needed to respect patient privacy on social media "A." Crowdsourcing, "B," occurs when a question is posed to a large group in hopes of generating more clinical insight, can indeed provide a diversity of opinions and perspectives but with unreliable and unverifiable references. Consensus in this platform can falsely reassure a provider. Physicians are de facto held to a higher standard of public discourse than the general public, with tangible consequences (e.g., state medical board investigations) for inappropriate behavior "C." Most hospitals and healthcare organizations have social media policies which this provider may be inadvertently violating; additionally, many medical societies are generating best practices and recommendations in this regard too.

▶ **Objective: Did you learn to …**
• Describe the ethical issues regarding social media use?

▶ CASE 26.5

Jane is a 30-year-old female, newly married, and not typically a patient of your practice. As your sister, she calls you while at work reporting 3 days of dysuria, typical for her previous experience of UTIs. She expresses frustration about urgent care wait times, ER costs, and unavailability of her primary care provider, which is why she's asking if you will call-in a prescription for treatment.

Question 26.5.1 All of the following would be concerns you respond to your sister with EXCEPT:

A) You do not typically call in prescriptions for patients, so wouldn't want to for her

B) You are concerned that your personal relationship may limit both of your comforts in discussing critical information to treat this case appropriately

C) The guiding AMA ethics strongly discourages this practice

D) Without appropriate testing and follow-up established, starting an empiric treatment could cause her harm

E) All of the above would be concerns to express

Answer 26.5.1 The correct answer is "A." While calling in such prescriptions for your patients may be part of your typical practice, there are several compelling reasons to object to this request of a family member. While state administrative rules governing the Board of Medicine may vary, the guiding principles from the AMA in this regard are clear. ***Treating family members is fraught with problems***. Most notably is the limited comfort and interrogation of potentially sensitive information such as sexual/behavioral history and potentially relevant but previously unknown medical comorbidities. Physical examination is often sorely limited when involving family members for similar reasons. Furthermore, because of the blurring of personal and professional boundaries, this can introduce a slippery slope where one called-in prescription develops into enabling deleterious healthcare utilization (e.g., missing the opportunity for her primary care provider to track health maintenance and screening exams). Of additional legal and logistical concern is the under-documentation of such encounters.

Question 26.5.2 Under what circumstances may it be appropriate to engage in such treatment of family members?

A) When the patient's primary physician refuses to provide a prescription for a medicine your family member requests (e.g., Xanax for anxiety)

B) When no other provider is reasonably available due to the isolated, rural community (e.g., nearest primary clinic is 30 miles away and your aging aunt doesn't drive out of town)

C) The trivially innocuous request on the part of the family member (e.g., left BP medication at home while out of town traveling for the weekend)

D) There is a minor, urgent need of the family member (e.g., needs sutures removed)

E) B, C, and D

Answer 26.5.2 The correct answer is "E." The rural family provider may find himself/herself in a unique circumstance of limited alternative resources for patients in the community to utilize. This can create a legitimate logistical exception to the ethical concerns surrounding treatment of family members "B." It is prudent to anticipate how these relationships should be managed in the healthcare setting, setting up referral alternatives should there be such a conflict.

In addition to this, there may be appropriately innocuous circumstances that can be considered ethically appropriate (Answers "C" and "D"). Documentation of such medical encounters—be them with family or otherwise—should be approached in a consistent way. Particular concern should be paid to controlled substances (e.g., mental health and pain medications) as these often have further legal restrictions. It would also be entirely appropriate, and supported by the AMA Code of Ethics to answer "none of these" as permissable, at least in part because of the risk of such inconsequential encounters escalating to serious problems.

▶ **Objectives: Did you learn to …**
- Describe the ethical issues regarding treatment of family members?
- Identify under which circumstances, if any, it *may* be appropriate to provide care for a family member?

Clinical Pearls

○ An impaired medical professional must not be ignored. Physicians are bound by ethics and state laws to protect patients and society by identifying, assisting, and reporting impaired medical professionals.

○ Ask patients about advanced directives periodically at outpatient visits and with every hospital admission. Discuss living will, durable power of attorney for healthcare, resuscitation wishes, and specific interventions (e.g., feeding tube use) in the appropriate setting.

○ Each patient and each clinical question must be assessed individually to determine if a patient has decision-making capacity in that particular circumstance. The same patient may be able to decide not to follow a medically indicated diet, but be incapable of deciding his own disposition after hospitalization.

○ Engage patients in shared decision-making regarding screening and diagnostic tests as well as medical procedures and treatments.

○ Physicians must act in an ethical manner in order to maintain individual trust in the physician as well as societal trust in the profession.

○ Recognize that patients have a right to noncompliance. While it is the physician's responsibility to provide the best care recommendations for a patient, the patient may refuse to follow the advice if other priorities (e.g., money, comfort, avoidance of drug side effects) out rank health in the patient's determination.

○ Take great care in the transmission of patient information. Having a faxed, e-mailed, or mailed report containing a patient's confidential medical information misdirected to an unintended recipient is *not* legally protected.

○ Use caution when using social media as physicians are de facto held to a higher standard of public discourse than the general public, with tangible consequences for inappropriate behavior.

○ Recognize the multiple problems associated with treatment of family members. Follow the AMA Code of Ethics which highly discourages this practice.

BIBLIOGRAPHY

American Medical Association. Code of Medical Ethics. Available at: https://www.ama-assn.org/delivering-care/ethics. Accessed April 7, 2019.

Applebaum PS. Assessment of patients' competence to consent to treatment. *N Engl J Med.* 2007;357:1834–1840.

Beauchamp TL, Childress JF. *Principles of Biomedical Ethics.* 4th ed. New York, NY: Oxford University Press; 1994.

Campbell A, et al. *Medical Ethics.* 3rd ed. South Melbourne, Australia: Oxford University Press; 2001.

Lo B. *Resolving Ethical Dilemmas: A Guide for Clinicians.* 2nd ed. Philadelphia, PA: Lippincott Williams & Wilkins; 2000.

Smith HL, Churchill LR. *Professional Ethics and Primary Care Medicine.* Durham, NC: Duke University Press; 1986.

End-of-Life Care

Juan R. Pagan-Ferrer

27

▶ CASE 27.1

A 75-year-old man is admitted to the hospital for a heart failure exacerbation. This is his second admission for heart failure within the last 6 months. His nurse asks if he is an appropriate candidate for hospice care.

Question 27.1.1 Which of the following would qualify your patient for the Medicare hospice benefit?
A) His cardiac ejection fraction is 20%, and he is dyspneic with moderate exertion (NYHA class II heart failure)
B) He agrees to a do-not-resuscitate (DNR) status in the event of cardiorespiratory failure
C) He needs assistance with ambulation
D) His implanted cardiac defibrillator (ICD) has fired once in the past year
E) He has experienced escalating cardiac hospitalizations despite optimal medical management

Answer 27.1.1 **The correct answer is "E."** If your patient has a terminal disease with declining function, worsening symptoms, worsening laboratory tests, or escalating hospitalizations, he or she probably qualifies for hospice. "A," a low cardiac ejection fraction (typically <20%), is a recommended criterion for heart disease–related hospice care **but must be accompanied by dyspnea at rest** (class IV heart failure). "B" is incorrect. Despite popular belief, a hospice patient need not agree to a DNR status; however, hospice agencies are permitted to have different admission criteria and some require a DNR status for admission. Check with your local hospice agencies. Regardless, you should have a frank discussion with the patient about the role of aggressive resuscitation and the goals of hospice care. "C" is also incorrect. While a decline in functional status is a strong indication of worsening prognosis, it is not automatically a criterion. Most patients with heart failure need assistance with at least four activities of daily living (ADLs) before having a prognosis of death within 6 months. "D" is incorrect. Patients with ICDs are eligible for hospice, and whether or not it has fired does not impact enrollment decisions. It is important to talk about the ICD, ideally before a patient approaches the final weeks/days of life. Many patients choose to have it disabled once they enroll in hospice. If an ICD is not disabled, it is important that the hospice staff be aware of it and know what to do as it will fire when the patient dies, which can be distressing for both the patient and the family.

HELPFUL TIP:
As opposed to an ICD, a pacemaker does not cause distress (shocks) during the dying process; however, if the patient's usual cardiac rhythm is completely dependent on the pacemaker, then the pacemaker is considered to be life-prolonging.

HELPFUL TIP:
Although prognosis may be the most difficult task a physician faces, an attempt at prognosis in patients with a terminal illness may help them. Asking the simple question, "Would you be surprised if this patient died in the next year?" serves as a good screening tool and has been shown to be a reasonably accurate way to predict who might benefit from a hospice referral.

Your heart failure patient is currently on maximal medical management with an ACE inhibitor, beta-blocker, loop diuretic, aldosterone antagonist, long-acting nitrate, hydralazine, and a dual chamber ICD. He wants to discuss the management of his cardiac therapies in relation to hospice.

Question 27.1.2 Which statement is true about cardiac therapies for patients with heart failure in hospice?
A) Hospice will not enroll patients on intravenous inotropic support (such as dobutamine or milrinone infusions)
B) Oral cardiac medications like beta-blockers and diuretics should be stopped because they are unlikely to provide any benefit to quality of life

C) A fluid restriction is no longer relevant once a patient enrolls in hospice
D) Hospice will not enroll patients who have not deactivated their ICD
E) None of the above

Answer 27.1.2 **The correct answer is "E."** Many of the therapies for patients with advanced heart failure provide symptomatic relief and improve quality of life. Just as you would do with any other advanced illness, a thorough evaluation of each medication and intervention should occur with the goal of determining if that intervention will contribute to your patent's overall goals. Physicians need to negotiate the balance between benefit and burden of each individual therapy. Although often a surprise to physicians, "A" is incorrect. A patient can have continuous inotropic infusion and still be enrolled in hospice. Some heart failure patients are dependent on inotropes and require them to maintain a certain level of quality of life, and they are willing to accept the trade-offs of having a continuous infusion to maintain that quality of life. Be aware that inotrope infusions do not prolong survival (in fact they shorten survival compared to no inotropes). The burden of inotrope infusions includes: cost, risk of line infections, and increased risk for arrhythmia.

Hospice agencies are required to provide treatment to manage symptoms related to the terminal condition and many hospice agencies utilize formularies in order to control cost. Some hospice agencies have formularies that will allow the use of inotropes for management of dyspnea, fatigue, etc., while others will specify that the symptoms be controlled with other agents such as opioids.

"B" is incorrect. There is so much more to palliative care than giving morphine for shortness of breath in heart failure! Continuing cardiac therapies may allow a patient to maintain their cardiac functional status and prevent pulmonary congestion and should never be discontinued just because a patient enrolls in hospice. With that being said, there are times when the patient's goals support the discontinuation of these medications. "C" is incorrect because as noted above, every decision comes with both a benefit and a burden, which need to be weighed. Some level of fluid restriction may help with breathing and pulmonary congestion and should be balanced against the discomfort of restricting intake. On the other hand, there is no evidence that sodium restriction is helpful in CHF (*JAMA Intern Med.* 2018;178(12):1693–1700). Individualize the decision. "D" is incorrect because it is not a requirement for an ICD to be deactivated. However, the incidence of arrhythmia can be high in this population, and ICD shocks near the time of death can be very distressing to the patient and the family and should be discussed.

HELPFUL TIP:
If you've seen one hospice agency, you've seen one hospice agency. Hospices often have different formularies, different available ancillary services (e.g., music therapy, pet therapy, massage), and different policies in what they cover for symptom management (e.g., chemotherapy, radiation, blood transfusions). It can be helpful to know what services your local hospice covers.

You think that your patient may be appropriate for hospice and decide that a palliative medicine consult might be useful to address his goals of care, review symptom management, and discuss hospice.

Question 27.1.3 Which statement accurately reflects how palliative medicine is different from hospice?
A) Only palliative medicine affirms life and attempts to help patients live as fully as possible
B) Palliative medicine offers treatments including aggressive medical treatments such as radiation therapy, intravenous (IV) fluids, or interventional radiologic procedures, while hospice does not
C) Palliative medicine is performed by a physician only, while hospice care involves an entire team of providers
D) Palliative care can be offered at any time during a life-limiting illness, even if a patient is still actively seeking a cure
E) Palliative medicine consults are billed under Medicare Part B while hospice care is reimbursed through the Medicare Part H

Answer 27.1.3 **The correct answer is "D."** Palliative care is specialized medical care for people with serious illnesses that focuses on providing patients with relief from the symptoms, pain, and stress of the serious illness—whatever the diagnosis. The goal is to improve quality of life for both the patient and the family. Palliative care is provided by a team of doctors, nurses, and other specialists who work with a patient's primary team to provide an extra layer of support. Palliative care is appropriate at any time in a serious illness and can be provided together with curative treatment. Hospice care is a type of palliative care, which occurs during the final months of someone's life when cure is no longer possible or no longer consistent with the patient's goals. "A" is incorrect because both hospice and palliative care strive to make life meaningful and comfortable for patients. "B" is incorrect. Since the goal of both hospice and palliative care is to prevent and relieve suffering, any of these modalities may be used if appropriate. In fact, **any intervention** can be considered palliative if the intention is to relieve distressing symptoms associated with the fatal disease (such as a hip-pinning for pain control after a pathologic fracture). There are no restrictions prohibiting a hospice agency from providing "aggressive" interventions designed to relieve pain and suffering. "C" is incorrect because both hospice and palliative medicine are built on the concept of a team providing care to the patient and family. Hospice care usually (but not always) is directed by the primary physician. "E" is incorrect because Medicare Part A covers both palliative medicine services (typically billed as inpatient consult services) **and** hospice benefits, and there is no such thing as Medicare Part H—yet!

Question 27.1.4 Which of the following is TRUE regarding the Medicare hospice benefit?
A) The Medicare hospice benefit requires all care related to the primary admitting illness to be covered by the hospice agency, including physician fees, as long as the hospice program does not employ the physician

B) The hospice benefit, similar to the Medicare home care benefit, requires that the patient be homebound

C) Respite care within an acute hospital setting is provided for up to 5 days every 6 months

D) Hospice entry requires that the patient cannot live alone (must have an on-site primary caregiver)

E) A flat per diem rate is paid to the licensed hospice program regardless of the level of services provided

Answer 27.1.4 **The correct answer is "A."** The Medicare hospice benefit requires all care related to the primary admitting illness to be covered by the hospice agency. Think of it as capitated care. However, Medicare affords individual hospice agencies wide latitude in determining what modalities they use to treat the symptoms of a particular illness. For example, one agency might allow blood transfusions for the relief of dyspnea, while another agency only covers the use of medications such as morphine or lorazepam for dyspnea. If necessary for acute symptom management, Medicare also covers acute hospitalizations related to the primary illness. "B" is incorrect. A hospice patient does not need to be homebound. The Medicare hospice benefit provides respite care which can occur as frequently as needed, making "C" incorrect. Respite admissions can last up to five nights at a time. The respite care needs to be provided in a setting where there is a registered nurse available continuously, and the patient must come from a home setting (including assisted living). This can be used if the caregiver is unable to care for the patient for a variety of reasons. "D" is incorrect because Medicare does not require that the patient have a primary caregiver in the home to receive the hospice benefit; however, an individual hospice agency may require a primary caregiver be identified before enrolling a patient. "E" is incorrect because Medicare pays the hospice organization a stratified per diem rate depending on the level of care the patient requires.

After meeting with the palliative care team, your patient's family inquires more about hospice care. They ask what other services are covered.

Question 27.1.5 **The Medicare hospice benefit includes coverage for all of the following expenses EXCEPT:**
A) Medications related to symptom management
B) Social work visits
C) Home health aide services
D) Room and board for a patient living in a nursing home
E) Bereavement services

Answer 27.1.5 **The correct answer is "D."** All of the other options listed are services covered under the Medicare hospice benefit. A patient living in a nursing home is eligible for hospice care, but the cost of room and board for the nursing home is not paid by the hospice benefit. In some special circumstances, nursing home care will be paid for a short duration (e.g., when a hospice patient uses the five-night respite care benefit or if the patient is admitted to a nursing home for management of a distressing symptom that cannot be controlled in the home setting).

A few months go by and your patient has again been hospitalized. You now believe that he has fewer than 6 months to live. The local hospice medical director reviews the case and agrees. The patient is dyspneic at rest, requires 24-hour oxygen by nasal cannula, and his cardiac ejection fraction has decreased to 15%. He wishes to avoid further hospitalization and has elected to have a DNR status. His family wants to know what you can do when he becomes severely dyspneic.

Question 27.1.6 **Which of the following is appropriate palliative treatment of severe dyspnea in this patient?**
A) Intubation and ventilation
B) Morphine
C) Scopolamine
D) Buspirone
E) Hyperventilating into a paper bag

Answer 27.1.6 **The correct answer is "B."** Morphine and other opioid analgesics are indicated for palliation of dyspnea in cardiac failure. Despite concerns about opioids worsening respiratory function in end-stage heart failure, studies have concluded that oral morphine improves dyspnea in this patient population and does not cause respiratory failure or hasten death. This is supported by recommendations from the American College of Cardiology and the American Heart Association. If morphine or other therapies for shortness of breath were to shorten life, the ethical principle of "double effect" would be applicable. The double effect principle states that as long as the intention of a therapy is to reach a good outcome (such as improve pain and alleviate suffering), then even if the unintended consequences result in a negative outcome (e.g., shortening life), the intervention is permissible. The key here is intention. If you choose "A," your patient's ghost will be back to haunt you. This patient has chosen a far less aggressive stance toward life-prolonging measures, and his wishes should be honored. "C" is incorrect. Scopolamine is used to reduce oropharyngeal secretions (resulting in sonorous respirations) but is not likely to relieve dyspnea in this patient. In addition, scopolamine is highly anticholinergic and crosses the blood–brain barrier, which can result in delirium and should be used with caution in an awake and alert patient. Glycopyrrolate is a better choice to control secretions in a patient who is alert and awake. "D" is incorrect. While anxiety and dyspnea often occur together and exacerbate each other, buspirone (BuSpar) is a weak anxiolytic and has no direct effect on dyspnea. Low-dose lorazepam would be a reasonable alternative if you felt his dyspnea was complicated by anxiety. And "E" is just plain wrong—although still not as bad a choice as "A."

Consider diuretics to relieve dyspnea in heart failure patients in hospice. Oftentimes we are guilty of forgetting to treat the underlying illness when someone is in hospice, reaching for morphine first. Are there signs of volume overload (e.g., elevated JVD, diffuse crackles, profound edema)? Diuretic therapy may reduce pulmonary congestion and relieve dyspnea, and the benefits and burdens should be weighed. The burdens that need to be considered include: patient's bed bound status, risk for incontinence decreasing quality of life, patient's agreement with using a bladder catheter, renal function, etc.

HELPFUL TIP:
Benzodiazepines may be used in combination with opioids for added relief of dyspnea and anxiety. The patient should be monitored for excessive sedation and respiratory depression.

▶ **Objectives: Did you learn to …**
- Identify appropriate patients for end-of-life care, particularly for the Medicare hospice benefit?
- Describe the features of the Medicare hospice benefit?
- Treat patients with dyspnea related to end-stage cardiac disease?

 QUICK QUIZ: MORE THAN A LITTLE HEADACHE

A 30-year-old male patient you have known for several years was diagnosed with metastatic melanoma several months ago. He presents now with intermittent, severe headaches associated with nausea. A head CT scan performed last week showed three metastatic foci with surrounding edema. He currently takes maximum doses of acetaminophen and large doses of morphine.

What is the best initial treatment option to help relieve his headache and nausea?
A) Neurosurgical intervention
B) Dexamethasone
C) Sumatriptan
D) Ibuprofen
E) Increased morphine doses

The correct answer is "B." Corticosteroids are the preferred therapy for headaches due to increased intracranial pressure from edema, as is presumably the case here. Whole brain or stereotactic radiation therapy, alone or in combination with corticosteroids, may also be used as palliative therapy for multiple brain metastases. "A" is incorrect because neurosurgical consultation should be reserved for patients who fail other interventions or who present with rapidly worsening symptoms. "C" and "D" are incorrect. Sumatriptan and ibuprofen should not be used to treat increased intracranial pressure. "E," increased morphine doses, may be required, but corticosteroids are typically used first.

 QUICK QUIZ: EARLY PALLIATIVE CARE

A 74-year-old woman presents to your clinic with a new diagnosis of non-small-cell lung cancer found during an evaluation for hip pain that revealed diffuse bony metastases on x-ray. She inquires about ways to improve her quality of life in addition to the care recommended by her oncologist. You recall reading the landmark study (a study that every primary care and palliative care physician should know—and if you don't know you should read it cover-to-cover several times) by Temel et al., regarding the introduction of early palliative care in patients with metastatic non-small-cell lung cancer.

Which of the following is NOT true about the outcomes for the patients that received early palliative care compared to those that received standard oncologic care?
A) Introduction of early palliative care improved patients' quality of life
B) Introduction of early palliative care improved patients' mood
C) Introduction of early palliative care shortened the median survival
D) Introduction of early palliative care resulted in fewer aggressive therapies at the end-of-life

The correct answer is "C." Introduction of early palliative care was shown to **increase** median survival from 8.9 months to 11.6 months, and this occurred despite the intervention group patients receiving fewer aggressive interventions at the end-of-life. Both "A" and "B" are incorrect answers (but true statements) because this study showed that both quality of life and mood were improved when early palliative care was introduced to the standard oncologic care in this patient population. "D" is incorrect (but again a true statement) because 33% of patients who received early palliative care received "aggressive care" (chemotherapy within 2 weeks of death, no hospice care, and/or admission to hospice 3 days or less before death) as compared to 54% of patients in the standard care group. The Temel study applies to a very specific patient population—patients with metastatic non-small-cell lung cancer; however, multiple studies in other settings (mostly with cancer diagnoses) have now shown that including palliative care earlier in treatment of very serious illness may reduce cost, shorten length of stay, and improve quality of life.

▶ **CASE 27.2**

A 74-year-old female was diagnosed with adenocarcinoma of the colon 3 years prior to beginning hospice care. She has known metastases to her liver and pelvis. She complains of a cramping pain in her abdomen and a "deep pain" in her groin. She is currently receiving morphine 10 mg PO every 4 hours (except when asleep) and acetaminophen 650 mg PO TID. She says that her pain is 4 out of 10 on a numeric pain scale. Her past medical history includes hemorrhage secondary to a gastric ulcer 4 years ago (*Helicobacter pylori* negative on biopsy).

Question 27.2.1 **Which of the following strategies is the best next step for improving this patient's pain control?**
A) Start gabapentin to treat the neuropathic aspect of her pain
B) Add a strong nonsteroidal anti-inflammatory drug (NSAID) such as ketorolac (Toradol) to her current regimen

C) Add scheduled tramadol to try to decrease her morphine use

D) Start a long-acting morphine (e.g., MS Contin) at a dose 20% higher than her current morphine use

E) Maximize the dose of acetaminophen to 1,000 mg every 4 hours

Answer 27.2.1 **The correct answer is "D."** The patient is taking short-acting opioids around the clock, which can lead to "chasing the pain" (not to be confused with "chasing the dragon," which is inhaling heroin smoke, which leads to a leukoencephalopathy … you never know … it could be on the test!). Patients often receive much better pain control when they are maintained on a long-acting opioid. It is common practice to increase the dose of opioids by 15% to 25% when a patient's pain is only partially controlled. It is then recommended to have the breakthrough dose equivalent to 10% of her 24-hour use. "A" is incorrect as her pain is better described as visceral or somatic rather than neuropathic. Gabapentin is an acceptable choice for neuropathic pain but is not likely to be effective for this patient. "B" is incorrect. Ketorolac is the NSAID with the highest rate of renal disease and gastrointestinal (GI) bleeds and is contraindicated in a patient who has had a GI bleed. If you were to add an NSAID, ibuprofen would be a better choice, and GI protection with a proton pump inhibitor would be advisable for this patient. "C" is incorrect. Tramadol is a weak mu-receptor agonist, possessing some norepinephrine and serotonin reuptake inhibition and is much less efficacious than morphine. Tramadol is not likely to benefit a patient with severe pain from cancer and metastases. Tramadol also has a number of troubling side effects such as an increased risk of seizures and serotonin syndrome. "E" is incorrect because the current recommended daily maximum dose of acetaminophen for elderly patients is 3,000 mg (don't blame us … blame the FDA), and the frequency suggested in "E" would far exceed this amount.

When determining what medications are appropriate for treating pain, it helps to know what type of pain the patient has.

Question 27.2.2 **Cancer is known to cause which type(s) of pain?**
A) Neuropathic pain
B) Visceral pain
C) Soft tissue/bony pain
D) Pain from increased intracranial pressure
E) All of the above are types of pain

Answer 27.2.2 **The correct answer is "E."** Physiologic pain is separated into four categories: soft tissue or bony pain (also called somatic pain), neuropathic pain, visceral pain, and the pain of increased intracranial pressure. An example of somatic pain is the musculoskeletal pain (e.g., sports injuries and fractures) that everyone experiences at some point. Neuropathic pain is generally described as burning and results from nerve damage, inflammation, or compression. Visceral pain comes from distention of an organ capsule (e.g., liver enlargement from metastases and colicky pain from the colon). Depending on where a metastasis or primary tumor is located, it may cause somatic pain (e.g., bone tumors), neuropathic pain (e.g., Pancoast tumor), visceral pain (e.g., peritoneal carcinomatosis), or a headache from increased intracranial pressure.

HELPFUL TIP:
Avoid using meperidine (Demerol). It has toxic metabolites that may cause agitation and seizures. Meperidine can also interact with a number of drugs to cause serotonin syndrome.

You decide to increase her morphine dose.

Question 27.2.3 **Which of the following statements is TRUE?**
A) Intravenous morphine is 10 times more potent than oral morphine
B) Naloxone should be given if a hospice patient near death demonstrates confusion, decreased responsiveness, a slowed respiratory rate or cool extremities
C) Patients exhibiting a local rash or intense pruritus at the site of intravenous morphine administration must be considered allergic and given an alternate opioid
D) Tolerance to morphine does not occur in patients with cancer, so any increased analgesic need is due solely to uncontrolled pain
E) Renal and hepatic insufficiency both contribute to the accumulation of morphine and its metabolites

Answer 27.2.3 **The correct answer is "E."** "A" is incorrect. Intravenous (IV) morphine is about three times as potent as oral morphine. "B" is incorrect. Patients who are within several days or hours of death often exhibit pallor, peripheral vasoconstriction, apneic episodes, and obtundation as part of the physiologic process of dying. Counseling the family and patient is preferable to administering naloxone, which can cause abrupt opioid withdrawal and significant distress and discomfort to the patient (again, don't make her ghost haunt you). "C" is also incorrect. Local histamine release is a known effect of IV morphine administration. Histamine-mediated skin changes proximal to the IV infusion site of morphine do not represent a contraindication to future morphine use. In fact, antihistamines (e.g., diphenhydramine) can be used to counter morphine-related histamine effects, such as rash, itching, and hypotension. But again, if you choose to use an antihistamine with anticholinergic activity you need to monitor for delirium, constipation, etc. "D" is incorrect. All patients can develop tolerance to the effects of morphine. Of course, in patients with terminal cancer, increasing opioid requirements are often entirely due to increasing pain. And even if your dying patient develops morphine tolerance, you still need to treat the pain. Finally, "E" is correct. Patients with renal and hepatic insufficiency can accumulate metabolites of morphine, some of which are helpful in pain control and others of which may have an anti-analgesic effect.

These patients often need **lower** doses of opioids. If a patient is actively dying and has evidence of renal failure, opioid doses can often be decreased significantly without a worsening of pain control. Fentanyl and methadone are considered the safest opioids in renal failure although methadone use is complicated by its long half-life.

HELPFUL TIP:
Start patients on a regimen to prevent constipation when initiating opioids. Think about the bowel regimen each time you increase the opioid dose. It will save you and your patient a lot of grief in the long run.

HELPFUL TIP:
For patients whose pain cannot be controlled with typical treatments, consider ketamine or lidocaine infusions, both which have been shown to be beneficial in refractory pain.

Question 27.2.4 Which of the following statements is NOT accurate regarding the appropriate use of opioids in end-of-life situations?
A) At times, delirium can be improved with opioid dosage reduction and/or the addition of opioid-sparing analgesics (e.g., acetaminophen)
B) If oral morphine cannot be swallowed, then either an enteral feeding tube or a parenteral route (IM/IV/subcutaneous) must be used
C) Dosage conversion from one opioid to another is affected by the type of opioid used and the route of administration
D) Transdermal opioid delivery products are expensive, have a slow onset of action, and have erratic absorption
E) There is no pre-established ceiling dosage for opioids, and you may increase the opioid dose until adverse side effects occur

Answer 27.2.4 The correct answer (and the false statement) is "B." Concentrated oral morphine solutions (20 mg/mL) can be given in small amounts to patients who are unable to swallow. While it was previously thought that morphine elixir worked by absorption through the buccal mucosa, it is now believed to trickle down the throat to be absorbed through the gastric mucosa. Fentanyl is the only opioid absorbed via the buccal mucosa (thus, the fentanyl lollipops and lozenges). A secret that drug companies do not want you to know is that you can avoid the expense of fentanyl lollipops by using fentanyl IV solution orally for control of breakthrough pain. "A" is true. Delirium is a common and disturbing finding toward the end of life, and it is sometimes precipitated or exaggerated by opioids. On the flip side, untreated pain can cause delirium, and the delirium may improve when opioid doses are escalated. In these situations, it can be helpful to rotate opioids because the lack of cross-tolerance means that the dose can often be decreased while maintaining the same level of pain control. Acetaminophen is

the safest opioid-sparing analgesic, and its adjuvant action may allow for opioid dosage reduction without a loss of overall analgesia. In the appropriate patient, NSAIDs may also be used. "C" is true. When a patient chronically taking one opioid switches to another, a dose adjustment calculation must be made. You cannot switch milligram for milligram. Also, some authorities recommend that after the calculation, you slightly reduce the dose of the new opioid due to incomplete cross-tolerance (refer to opioid dose conversion charts available in numerous pharmaceutical texts and handbooks). "D" is true. The transdermal fentanyl patches, though convenient, have fluctuating bioavailability over the three days that each patch is worn, and breakthrough doses of an alternative opioid should be available. Fentanyl is also fat-soluble and absorption/bioavailability is decreased in thin and/or cachectic patients. The fentanyl patches are expensive and initially have a slow onset until a steady state is achieved. For this reason, a fentanyl patch should never be used alone as an initial treatment of acute pain. In fact, if you want to avoid a lawsuit, a fentanyl patch should never be used as the first method to treat pain in an "opioid-naïve" patient. "E" is true. Because of the extraordinarily wide dosage range of opioids, the ceiling dosage cannot be calculated or assumed. Rather, analgesic requirements allow for continual increase unless adverse side effects clearly undermine the use of the drug.

HELPFUL TIP:
There is no consistent relationship between blood levels of morphine and analgesic effects. This is because of tolerance, metabolism difference, individual variability in drug effect, etc. Thus, there is no single "right" dose. You should titrate morphine to the desired effect while watching for side effects.

You increase the morphine dose considerably over a 2-week period and your patient begins having escalating pain and muscle twitching.

Question 27.2.5 Which statement is true about opioid-induced hyperalgesia (OIH)?
A) Patients with OIH always become delirious
B) When a patient has OIH, the pain improves when the opioid dose is increased
C) The pain in OIH is described as a worsening of the original pain being treated
D) OIH needs to be differentiated from worsening underlying disease

Answer 27.2.5 The correct answer is "D." Before we presume that a patient has OIH, we need to ensure that the increase in pain is not due to further disease progression. We also need to consider increased pain resulting from increased activity or other exacerbation (such as trips to x-ray or radiation therapy). Additional features that can help distinguish OIH from increased pain include: the development of muscle twitching, presence of allodynia (pain elicited from ordinarily nonpainful stimuli, such as stroking skin with cotton—although this can occur with neuropathic pain syndromes as well), and development of seizures or delirium. However, not all patients with OIH become delirious, making "A" incorrect. The key feature of OIH is that the pain increases as the dose of the opioid is increased and will decrease when the dose is decreased. Hence "B" is incorrect as we would expect the pain to worsen as the opioid dose is increased. We are not certain why OIH occurs, but several mechanisms have been proposed. Switching to a medication with NMDA antagonism could prove helpful (such as methadone or ketamine). However, OIH can still occur in patients new to opioids and on low doses. "C" is incorrect as well. OIH typically produces diffuse pain, less defined in quality and extending beyond the preexisting pain distribution.

You are concerned about OIH and you decide to rotate to methadone.

Question 27.2.6 Which of the following statements is FALSE regarding the use of methadone?
A) Methadone can be legally prescribed for pain and addiction by a physician with a current schedule II DEA license
B) Methadone is more easily absorbed by those with bowel problems than is sustained-release morphine
C) The half-life of methadone is 22 hours
D) Methadone may be used as a long-acting, chronic opioid for pain control, similar to extended-release morphine products.
E) Methadone is primarily excreted in the stool and thus drug dosages do not need to be modified in those with mild-to-moderate renal disease

Answer 27.2.6 **The correct answer (and false statement) is "A."** Methadone **can** be prescribed for pain control by physicians with a schedule II DEA license but **cannot** be prescribed for addiction or opioid withdrawal without a special license. "B," "C," and "D" are true. Methadone has a long half-life, and sustained-release preparations are not needed. Sustained-release morphine may pass unabsorbed in patients with short gut or dysfunctional gut, whereas methadone would be absorbed. "E" is also true. Methadone is primarily excreted into the GI tract. Patients with liver disease should have doses adjusted. However, those with renal disease may tolerate "normal" doses since renal excretion is a minor part of methadone elimination.

HELPFUL TIP:
When it comes to switching or dosing opioids, there are several useful tips: (1) don't forget to account for incomplete cross-tolerance when switching classes of opioids—reduce the dose of the new opioid by 30% to 50%; (2) when opioids are not helping, increase the dose by 50%; essentially, treat opioids like you would treat a loop diuretic—if 60 mg of IV furosemide does not work, you wouldn't try 61 mg (or at least we hope

not!), but rather go to 90 or 120 mg; (3) for an opioid-naive patient who is starting a patient-controlled analgesia (PCA) pump, begin with as-needed (PRN only) dosing frequently, such as every 10 minutes, without a continuous ("basal") infusion.

HELPFUL TIP:
Methadone is the only **long-acting** opioid that comes in a liquid form and can be given buccally or in an enteral tube. Methadone can be dosed every 8 to 12 hours with many patients requiring every 8 hour dosing for pain. Although often touted as a good choice for neuropathic pain, data suggests that methadone is no better for neuropathic pain than are other opioids. Remember that methadone prolongs the QT in high doses and can cause torsades de pointes.

Your nurse calls you about your patient and reports that her pain level has been rising, and despite significant increases in both basal and breakthrough opioid therapy, the patient's pain is uncontrolled. The nurse asks you if there is something else that can be added to the opioids as an adjunctive treatment for pain. For no explicable reason, you cannot get gabapentin out of your head—even though you know it's probably useless for this patient.

Question 27.2.7 Which of the following is TRUE regarding the use of the gabapentin?
A) Gabapentin is hepatically cleared and dose adjustment is needed in patients with liver disease
B) The primary utility of gabapentin is in neuropathic pain
C) Gabapentin primarily works via the μ-opioid receptors
D) The most common side effects of gabapentin are supraventricular arrhythmias (thus limiting its utility in heart failure patients)
E) If a patient does not respond to gabapentin, she will also not respond to pregabalin

Answer 27.2.7 **The correct answer is "B."** Gabapentin has proven to be a marginally effective (NNT = 7) therapy for a number of diseases that manifest with neuropathic pain, including postherpetic neuralgia, diabetic neuropathy, and cancer-related neuropathic pain. "A" is incorrect because gabapentin is excreted unchanged through the kidneys—a plus for patients with working kidneys on multiple drugs. Why do we like drugs that are not hepatically cleared? They do not interact in any of the cytochrome P450 pathways and therefore have few drug–drug interactions. "C" is incorrect. The mechanism of gabapentin is complex and not fully understood, but we are fairly certain that it does not work through the μ-opioid receptors. "D" is incorrect. The most common side effect of gabapentin is its effect on cognition, causing dizziness and somnolence. Gabapentin can also cause edema, which can be problematic for patients with heart failure. "E" is incorrect. Although gabapentin and pregabalin are thought to have the same mechanism of action, it appears that some patients will respond to one but not the other. Another important distinction between gabapentin and pregabalin is the time needed to titrate to an effective dose. With gabapentin we typically start at 100 to 300 mg and escalate the dose over the course of weeks up to 3,600 mg divided three times a day; alternatively, pregabalin starts at 75 mg daily and reaches a max dose of 300 mg BID within a week of initiation.

HELPFUL TIP:
An opioid-naive patient should never be started on a fentanyl patch. A patient needs to be taking an oral morphine equivalent of at least 25 mg in 24 hours before the lowest dose (12.5 mcg) fentanyl patch can be applied.

As time goes on, the patient has other concerns, including constipation, weight loss of 20 pounds over 2 months, sleeplessness, nausea, and anxiety. In addition, she expresses how her loss of functional abilities is a hardship for her and her adult daughter who serves as her primary caregiver. Her guilt for losing her health is a continual source of frustration and anger.

Question 27.2.8 What is true regarding her social and emotional pain?
A) It will not affect the patient's analgesic requirements
B) It will likely complicate treatment adherence
C) Active treatment of emotional sources of pain should only occur after the physical source has been addressed and treated
D) Prophylactic antidepressants in patients within 6 months of death decrease the probability of developing depression

Answer 27.2.8 The correct answer is "B." Adherence, always an issue, is especially compromised in those dying patients whose social, spiritual, and emotional problems are not effectively addressed. Similarly, analgesic control of somatic pain is complicated when social, emotional, and spiritual sources of pain exacerbate the patient's response to and perception of somatic pain. Concurrent treatment of all sources of pain is necessary. Antidepressant therapy in dying patients who do not have clinical depression offers no prophylaxis against the development of depression.

You estimate your patient's life expectancy to be 2 months or less. Her frailty has progressed to the point where she is bedbound and utterly dependent for all of her ADLs. You have made some adjustments, and she is now on stable doses of the following medications:

- **Hydromorphone (Dilaudid) 20 mg PO Q 4 hours**
- **Acetaminophen 1,000 mg PO TID**
- **Sorbitol 30 mL PO TID**
- **Metoclopramide 20 mg PO TID**

You want to optimize her medications.

Question 27.2.9 Which of the following is the most appropriate medication adjustment to make at this time?
A) Hydromorphone → scheduled **controlled**-release morphine
B) Hydromorphone → scheduled **immediate**-release morphine
C) Hydromorphone → scheduled **controlled**-release morphine and **immediate**-release morphine as needed
D) Acetaminophen → **immediate**-release morphine
E) Acetaminophen → nortriptyline

Answer 27.2.9 The correct answer is "C." A patient who has reached a stable dose of short-acting opioid, such as hydromorphone, should subsequently be switched to a long-acting opioid agent. An immediate-release medication should be available for acute "breakthrough" pain. There is no reason to change the acetaminophen. Nortriptyline is sometimes useful as an adjuvant medication and is particularly helpful when treating neuropathic pain.

The hospice nurse calls you. Your patient is at home and has become restless with slow respirations (6/min) along with paroxysmal coughing and gagging with a large amount of secretions.

Question 27.2.10 The following are all appropriate orders for this patient EXCEPT:
A) Obtain subcutaneous access through placement of a subcutaneous button or butterfly needle
B) Lorazepam 1 to 2 mg PO or SL every hour PRN
C) Glycopyrrolate 2 mg PO or SL every 4 hours PRN
D) Midazolam 0.4 to 4 mg SC every hour PRN
E) Naloxone 2 mg SC every 2 hours PRN

Answer 27.2.10 The correct answer is "E." Naloxone is a potent opioid receptor antagonist. Although the sudden change in the patient's status could be partly due to opioid accumulation, the risks of naloxone antagonism are great and include severe pain, cardiac arrhythmias, and seizures (and again, you don't want that ghost haunting you). Withholding or reducing the next dose of opioids is a safer approach. A subcutaneous infusion pump ("A") may allow effective administration of medications and fluids in patients who cannot tolerate oral administration. The use of hydration at the end of life is controversial. Withholding fluids and nutrition has strong merit, but the evidence is not compelling enough to declare that fluid infusion is futile and possibly harmful in this setting. In addition, dehydration is a common cause of delirium at the end of life, and her confusion may improve with gentle hydration. It is more important to review the patient's goals and only administer fluids if consistent with her goals. Glycopyrrolate ("C") has been shown to decrease oral/pulmonary secretions that lead to the "death rattle" in the final days and hours of life. Such treatment benefits the patient and her grieving family and friends. "B" and "D" may also be useful. Benzodiazepines have the potential to reduce anxiety, agitation, and insomnia; however, any benzodiazepine can worsen confusion and cause delirium. Benzodiazepines with an extended half-life (e.g., diazepam and chlordiazepoxide) should generally be avoided because of the potential for toxic accumulation.

▶ **Objectives: Did you learn to …**
- Define major physiologic pain categories?
- Describe the pharmacology of pain control?
- Prescribe opioid pain medications and adjuvant therapies for pain?
- Identify emotional, social, and spiritual symptoms and recognize how they can affect pain management?

 QUICK QUIZ: THE SUBCUTANEOUS ROUTE

Regarding the subcutaneous administration of fluids and medications, which of the following is true?
A) Not more than 500 cc of saline per day can be given by hypodermoclysis (subcutaneous administration)
B) Only medication with low lipid solubility can be delivered via subcutaneous administration
C) Most drugs used in end-of-life care can be given subcutaneously
D) In general, subcutaneous administration dosage conversion is closer to oral dosage than to IV dosage

The correct answer is "C." The subcutaneous route can be quite effective. Adverse events such as local irritation, pulmonary edema, and local edema are less frequent with subcutaneous administration when compared with IV administration. In general, most drugs used in end-of-life care can be given subcutaneously. "A" is incorrect. Evidence demonstrates that up to 3,000 cc of crystalloid solution can be given subcutaneously in a 24-hour period with limited adverse effects. Experience suggests that even greater volumes can be given. "B" is incorrect. Lipid solubility is not a clinically relevant aspect of bioavailability during subcutaneous administration. "D" is also not true. Subcutaneous doses are generally very close to, but lower than, the IV dose of a drug. As with IV administration, the onset of action is more rapid than with enteral dosing.

▶ **CASE 27.3**

You assume care for the 84-year-old father of one of your patients. He has severe dementia, which has caused him to require nursing home care for the last 5 years. He has stable heart failure due to ischemic cardiomyopathy. He requires full assistance to eat, with the staff members spending an hour at each meal. He has lost 20 lbs in the last 6 months (BMI now is 21 kg/m². A facility nurse calls you worried about his weight.

Question 27.3.1 What would be the best intervention for weight gain in this patient?
A) Megestrol
B) Nutritional supplements

C) Dronabinol
D) Mirtazapine
E) Feeding tube

Answer 27.3.1 **The correct answer is "B."** The most effective means to maintain weight in elderly patients with dementia is hand feeding and providing favorite foods (yes, ice cream with every meal is OK!) and frequent offerings. Hand feeding is expensive and often problematic in nursing homes with limited staff. Nutritional supplements have been shown to be modestly effective in promoting weight gain in elderly patients with dementia. Other important considerations related to nutrition in dementia patients is being aware of effective ways to decrease aspiration risk, including sitting upright, eating small portions, use of thickened liquids, and hand feeding. "A," megestrol (Megace), is minimally effective in improving appetite and increasing weight in patients with cancer cachexia and weight loss related to HIV/AIDS, but there is sparse evidence for use in geriatric patients. Trials are of short duration (1–2 months) using widely varying amounts of megestrol (240–1,600 mg/day), and the weight gained is typically fluid and not muscle mass. With such poor evidence for benefit but well-known side effects, there is no role for megestrol in this setting. In fact, there is no role for hormones or steroids in the treatment of weight loss in the elderly patient with dementia. "B," dronabinol, is a synthetic derivative of cannabis (known to cause "the munchies"… we've heard). It increases appetite and improves nausea, but again the studies are small and exploratory in nature and focused mainly on patients with HIV/AIDS and cancer. Additionally, dronabinol has CNS side effects in the elderly. "D" is incorrect. If the patient were depressed and losing weight as a result, mirtazapine might be a reasonable choice since it may stimulate appetite. However, mirtazapine has not been shown to boost appetite in nondepressed subjects (and like the SSRIs, does not improve depression in the demented elderly anyway). Some antidepressants, such as SSRIs and bupropion, are associated with **weight loss**. Finally, a feeding tube ("E") is invasive with numerous side effects (cellulitis, leakage, and increased fecal incontinence which can contribute to bed sores). While enteric tube feeds may improve caloric intake, they do not extend life, increase weight, improve functional status, or reduce the incidence of pressure sores or aspiration in dementia patients (exceptions to this are ALS and gastrointestinal cancers with proximal obstruction with a good functional status). Tube feeding is associated with agitation, greater use of physical and chemical restraints, and also greater healthcare use due to tube-related complications.

 HELPFUL TIP:
Remind and reinforce to families that dementia is a terminal illness and that our current understanding is that tube feeding is unlikely to alter the course of the illness.

Your nutrition shakes are not doing the trick. The patient continues to lose weight. To further stage his dementia, you attempt a Folstein Mini Mental Status Exam, but he cannot

participate. The nurse reports that he needs assistance with all ADLs, he is incontinent, and he is unable to speak more than six intelligible words (and although you remember a couple of post-call days when you were in the same condition, you say nothing). The nursing staff asks you if the patient is appropriate for hospice care.

Question 27.3.2 Which of the following is TRUE?

A) The life trajectory of terminally demented patients is unclear. Wait until his cardiac disease worsens
B) He does not yet meet Medicare hospice benefit criteria for dementia
C) A history from the nursing staff or family regarding the rate of his functional loss is the best predictor of death
D) The nursing home staff can provide all of the end-of-life services provided by hospice, so hospice is not needed
E) Presence of a stage 2 pressure ulcer and aspiration risk is sufficient for referral to hospice

Answer 27.3.2 The correct answer is "C." Predicting death in patients with dementing illness is difficult which is why it is one of most underutilized diagnoses for referral to hospice care. In fact, dementia has the greatest variability among hospice diagnoses when it comes to predicting survival. However, waiting until a more predictable organ system failure occurs is not a reason for delaying a hospice referral, which makes "A" incorrect. "B" is incorrect because he *does* meet criteria for hospice enrollment. The National Hospice and Palliative Care Organization (NHPCO) hospice guidelines for eligibility in dementia include three components: (1) demonstrating severity of dementia (e.g., an inability to walk or dress or bathe without assistance, urinary/fecal incontinence, or inability to speak six different intelligible words per day); (2) evidence of a severe comorbid condition within the past 6 months (e.g., aspiration pneumonia, pyelonephritis, sepsis, stage ≥3 decubitus ulcer, or fever despite antibiotics); (3) inability to maintain fluid/caloric intake (by demonstrating weight loss >10% in 6 months or albumin <2.5 g/dL). "E" is incorrect. Aspiration risk and stage 2 pressure ulcers alone are not sufficient for referral to hospice. If the patient had stage 3 or 4 pressure ulcers, he would likely meet NHPCO hospice criteria for severe dementia. It is the extrapolation of the patient's loss of basic functions over time that best predicts death, as in "C." "D" is incorrect because while most nursing homes routinely care for dying patients without the assistance of hospice, they are typically not able to offer the full range of services or the end-of-life expertise that hospice offers.

Your patient develops nausea and vomiting and on examination you feel a large abdominal mass. He is still having bowel movements, which are positive for occult blood. You inform the family that you suspect he has colon cancer, and they elect for no further evaluation but want his symptoms aggressively managed.

Question 27.3.3 Which of the following drugs is the best initial choice for treatment of this patient's nausea and vomiting?

A) Octreotide
B) Metoclopramide
C) Diphenhydramine
D) Ondansetron (Zofran)
E) Aprepitant (Emend)

Answer 27.3.3 The correct answer is "D." "B" is not correct. Using a pro-peristaltic agent in a patient who may have an obstruction is not a good idea in general. Also, metoclopramide has central antidopaminergic properties and can cause confusion and extrapyramidal side effects. By understanding the pathophysiology of nausea and targeting antiemetics to specific receptors, therapy can be optimized and side effects minimized. An easy way to remember the causes of vomiting is to use the "VOMIT" mnemonic. In Table 27-1, pathophysiologic mechanisms causing nausea are described using the letters of the mnemonic. Blockade of these receptors allows rational, focused therapy.

Using Table 27-1, another reasonable alternative would be promethazine, although promethazine is not a great antiemetic. "A" is incorrect. Octreotide works by slowing the GI track, and its main use is found in patients with nausea and vomiting due to malignancy-related intestinal obstruction. However, it does not rapidly treat nausea and is not easily administered (usually continuous IV infusion, but it can be given subcutaneously or intramuscularly). "C" is incorrect because diphenhydramine alone is a weak antiemetic, mostly used for motion sickness, and it can cause confusion, particularly in the elderly. Aprepitant (Emend) is a neurokinin receptor antagonist that is most effective when used **with** serotonin receptor antagonists such as ondansetron; its primary use is in the management of chemotherapy-induced nausea, and it is very expensive.

HELPFUL TIP:
When treating chemotherapy-induced nausea, add something to their current regimen. Do not just drop one medication and add another. This is counterintuitive but is considered the approach of choice.

The patient's nausea is ultimately controlled with scheduled low-dose promethazine and ondansetron (Hey, look! Two drugs instead of a large dose of one!). He is continuing to lose weight and has been coughing after eating. He spikes a fever and you suspect he has developed aspiration pneumonia.

Question 27.3.4 Which is true regarding the use of antibiotics for pneumonia in patients with end-stage dementia?

A) Antibiotic use is considered the standard of care and should be initiated without discussing with the family
B) Antibiotics might prolong patients' lives but treatment comes with significant risks that need to be weighed

TABLE 27-1 CAUSES AND TREATMENT OF NAUSEA AND EMESIS

Type of Nausea	Receptors Causing Nausea	Useful Drug Classes	Examples of Drugs of Choice
V Vestibular	Cholinergic Histaminic	Anticholinergic Antihistaminic	Scopolamine Promethazine
O Obstruction (caused by constipation)	Cholinergic Histaminic 5-HT$_3$	Stimulate myenteric plexus	Senna products Prunes
M Dys**M**otility	Cholinergic Histaminic 5-HT$_3$	Prokinetics to stimulate 5-HT$_4$ receptors	Metoclopramide
I **I**nfection, **I**nflammation	Cholinergic Histaminic 5-HT$_3$	Anticholinergic Antihistaminic	Promethazine
T Toxins (stimulating the CTZ in the brain, i.e., opioids)	Dopamine 2 5-HT$_3$	Antidopaminergic 5-HT$_3$ antagonist	Prochlorperazine Haloperidol Ondansetron

5-HT$_3$, 5-hydroxytryptamine (serotonin); CTZ, chemoreceptor trigger zone.

C) Antibiotics given in a controlled setting such as a nursing home, where compliance can be ensured, lead to less antibiotic resistance

D) Parenteral antibiotics are more successful at treating aspiration pneumonia in patients with dementia, compared with oral antibiotics

Answer 27.3.4 **The correct answer is "B."** While antibiotics may prolong life in patients with dementia, they do so with the cost of increasing discomfort, making "B" the correct answer. The previous prevailing belief of carte blanche use of antibiotics is being challenged. Currently, antibiotic use is very common in nursing homes, and a majority of nursing home residents will receive antibiotics in the 2 weeks before their death. Most of those antibiotics will be given intravenously, which increases patient discomfort. But more importantly, patients are often admitted to a hospital, placing demented patients at risk for delirium, restraints, and exposure to hospital-acquired organisms. The reason we emphasize "might prolong" patients' lives is that the literature shows that in the extremes of advanced dementia plus another advanced illness (such as bacteremia), antibiotics may not provide improved survival. In fact, in patients with advanced dementia, infections often characterize the final stage of their illness. "A" is incorrect because antibiotic use in patients with dementia (specifically in patients with dementia who are hospice appropriate) should always be discussed with the surrogate decision maker, and antibiotic use should be based on an informed choice and the patient's wishes/goals. "C" is incorrect because nursing homes have been shown to harbor drug-resistant bacteria, likely due in part to the frequent use of antibiotics in these patients. Oral antibiotics have been shown to be as effective as other more invasive administration routes in patients with dementia, making "D" incorrect.

The patient is enrolled in hospice and 3 weeks later you are called by a nurse reporting an acute condition change. You go to see the patient and he is unresponsive, breathing is labored, and his feet are mottled.

Question 27.3.5 **All of the following can be signs of impending death EXCEPT:**
A) Cheyne–Stokes breathing
B) Fever
C) Cyanosis and mottling
D) Aldosterone escape phenomenon with increased urinary output
E) Talking to someone who is already dead (and not via medium at Coney Island)

Answer 27.3.5 **The correct answer is "D."** Most dying patients have a decrease in urinary output prior to death. The other options describe changes that are commonly seen in patients who are actively dying. Respiratory changes in the active dying phase include Cheyne–Stokes breathing, terminal secretions (the "death rattle"), and periods of apnea. Dying is often accompanied by decreased circulation, which can result in cool extremities and mottling (the skin turning blue and patchy particularly in the fingers and toes). It is not uncommon for a dying patient to have a fever in the last 24 to 48 hours of life, typically thought to be secondary to aspiration pneumonia or another serious infection. It is not uncommon for someone who is dying to talk about going on a journey or talk about seeing someone who is dead. This is typically believed to be part of the normal dying process and in the absence of other symptoms should not be confused with delirium or psychosis.

HELPFUL TIP:
Delirium is very common (up to 85%) in the last few days of life. If the symptoms are distressing to the patient or family, it is best treated with an antipsychotic such as haloperidol.

You need to call the son to tell him of his father's decline.

Question 27.3.6 Which of the following should you say when giving the son an update?
A) "There have been some changes in your father's condition. I think you should go to see him. Call me if you have any questions after you have seen your dad"
B) "Good news, your dad will soon be out of his misery and released from this mortal world"
C) "I'm afraid I have some bad news for you regarding your dad. Would you like to talk over the phone or meet at my office later today to discuss it?"
D) "Your dad is dying. If you want to see him alive again you had better go today"
E) Don't call at all. Ask the nurse to inform the son of his father's condition while you duck out quietly

Answer 27.3.6 The correct answer is "C." It gives a "warning shot" and allows the person receiving the bad news some control by allowing him to determine how and where he wants to receive the bad news. "A" avoids giving the bad news at all. "B" is inappropriately flippant and uses euphemisms. "D" is inappropriately blunt and sounds awful—and if it doesn't sound awful to you, it's probably time to take an online psychopathy test. "E" avoids having the discussion at all and is only appropriate if you will be unable to reach the son in a timely fashion. Besides, you will be forever after known to the nurses as "Dr. Wuss." A common format for giving bad news is to use the SPIKES six-step protocol in Table 27-2.

HELPFUL TIP:
When giving bad news, do not use phrases such as, "I'm afraid there is nothing more we can do for you." This leaves patients and family feeling abandoned. It is better to be more specific to say, "I am afraid that I don't have any treatments that will cure your cancer, but there is still a lot I can offer to help improve your quality of life." This assures the patient and the family that there is still something to be done and that you will not abandon them.

Breaking bad news is difficult in person and can be more difficult over the phone.

Question 27.3.7 Which suggestion below is NOT recommended when breaking bad news over the phone?

TABLE 27-2 A MNEMONIC FOR GIVING BAD NEWS
S Setting. An inappropriate setting can make it difficult to give bad news effectively. Make sure the physical setting is as conducive as possible by trying to ensure privacy, involving significant others, sitting down, connecting with the patient (eye contact, hand holding), ensuring enough time, and minimizing interruptions.
P Patient's perception. Ask what the patient's (or family's) knowledge and understanding of the current medical illness is.
I Invitation. Ask what information the patient wants to receive. Some patients do not want to hear bad news themselves, and in this case it can be helpful to ask if there is someone else with whom you should speak.
K Knowledge. Give the medical facts in a straightforward manner using vocabulary and language appropriate to the patient's level. Avoid medical jargon and do not be excessively blunt (i.e., avoid saying things such as "you have very bad cancer and unless you do something, you will die"). Give the information in small chunks and frequently assess what the patient has understood. When possible, start off with a warning shot (i.e., "Unfortunately, I have some bad news for you").
E Exploring/empathy/emotion. A patient's emotional reaction can vary and is often hard for a physician to experience. An empathetic response can be helpful. This can be fostered by allowing silence after breaking the bad news and watching and listening for the emotion. When you have identified the emotion, it can be helpful to name it and determine what caused it. Then make an empathetic statement such as "I'm sorry. I know this isn't what you wanted to hear."
S Strategy/summary. After the emotions have been addressed, it is helpful to review what has been said and agree on a plan. Consider asking the patient if he wants to discuss treatment options at this time or wait until a future meeting. Receiving bad news can be overwhelming, and patients often forget the details of what is said. It is important to have clear, well-defined, timely follow-up such as "Go home and talk with your family, I will see you (and your family) back tomorrow at 9 AM, and we can discuss specific treatment options and answer questions at that time."

Data from Baile WF, et al. SPIKES-A six-step protocol for delivering bad news: application to the patient with cancer. *Oncologist.* 2000;5:302–311.

A) Take time to prepare what you are going to say and find a quiet place to make the call
B) If no one answers the phone, it is acceptable to leave a message or voicemail detailing the bad news
C) Identify yourself and avoid answering any direct questions until you are sure of the identity of the person to whom you are talking
D) Ask if the person is alone
E) Speak clearly and slowly, allow time for questions; be empathetic

Answer 27.3.7 The correct answer is "B." When breaking bad news over the phone, steps similar to breaking bad news in person should be used. You should obtain the full name, address, and phone number(s) of the person(s) you are calling. If you are not calling the patient, try to establish from the chart and nursing staff the relationship of the contact to the patient. In addition, it can be helpful to write down the key information you need and review what you will say and find a quiet area with a phone. Don't delay in making the call. When you do call, clearly identify yourself and ensure you are able to speak with the person closest to the patient (ideally, the healthcare proxy or the contact person indicated in the chart). Avoid responding to any direct question until you have verified the identity of the person to whom you are speaking, in order to avoid violating the patient's right to privacy. Ask if the contact person is alone. Do not give death notification to minor children. If you do not have a prior relationship with the person you are speaking to, ask what they know about the patient's condition. Provide a warning shot. Never deliver the news of death to an answering machine or voicemail. Instead, leave specific contact information. Allow time for questions; be empathetic and ask if you can contact anyone for them. Assess their emotional reaction and arrange follow-up as indicated.

> **HELPFUL TIP:**
> When you need to inform a family that a patient has died, words like "dead" or "died" should be used; avoid euphemisms such as "expired," "passed away," or "didn't make it" (also, "kicked the bucket," "bit the bullet," "bought the farm," and so on), which can be misinterpreted.

▶ **Objectives: Did you learn to …**
- Generate a management plan for a patient with weight loss due to a terminal disease?
- Describe criteria for hospice admission in patients with severe dementia?
- Identify and treat causes of nausea and vomiting at the end of life?
- Identify signs of the active dying process?
- Recognize the proper steps for breaking bad news?

Clinical Pearls

- Avoid meperidine. Other opioid analgesics are preferred.
- Do not delay palliative care assessment in a patient with a serious, life-limiting illness, even if that patient is planning to seek curative therapy. Patients with an early palliative approach live longer and have a higher quality of life.
- Do not leave an implanted cardiac defibrillator (ICD) active without assessing the patient and family's goals of care. In a patient with a terminal illness who is DNR, it is logically consistent to deactivate the ICD, and this option should be discussed with the patient/family.
- Do not start an opioid-naïve patient on a fentanyl patch.
- Opioid analgesics, morphine in particular, relieve respiratory distress in dying patients.
- Start a bowel regimen whenever starting opioid analgesics.
- The addition of a benzodiazepine to an opioid reduces anxiety and breathlessness, but respiratory rate and mental status must be carefully monitored.
- Titrate opioid analgesics to an effect rather than a particular dose or blood level.
- Use equianalgesic reference charts and account for incomplete cross-tolerance when switching from one opioid to another.

BIBLIOGRAPHY

Adler ED, et al. Palliative care in the treatment of advanced heart failure. *Circulation.* 2009;120:2597–2606.

Baile WF, et al. SPIKES-A six-step protocol for delivering bad news: Application to the patient with cancer. *Oncologist.* 2000;5:302–311.

Banerjee S, et al. Sertraline or mirtazapine for depression in dementia (HTA-SADD): a randomized, multicentre, double-blind, placebo-controlled trial. *Lancet.* 2011;378:403–411.

Bennett MI. Gabapentin in the treatment of neuropathic pain. *Palliative Med.* 2004;18:5–11.

Bharadwaj P, Ward KT. Ethical considerations of patients with pacemakers. *Am Fam Physician.* 2008;78(3):398–399.

Blais C, Gabbard J, et al. HIV, dementia, and neurological conditions: UNIPAC 9. *Essential Practices in Hospice and Palliative Medicine.* 2017:69–70.

Bushnaq M, et al. The feasibility of using intravenous fentanyl as sublingual drops in the treatment of incidental pain in patients with cancer. *J Palliat Med.* 2009;12(6):511–514.

Challapalli V, et al. Systemic administration of local anesthetic agents to relieve neuropathic pain. *Cochrane Database Syst Rev.* 2005;(4): Art No. CD003345.

Clemens KE, Klaschik E. Dyspnoea associated with anxiety–symptomatic therapy with opioids in combination with lorazepam and its effect on ventilation in palliative care patients. *Support Care Cancer.* 2011;19:2027–2033.

Coyne PJ, et al. Nebulized fentanyl citrate improves patients' perception of breathing, respiratory rate, and oxygen saturation in dyspnea. *J Pain Symptom Manage.* 2002;23(2):157–160.

Donner B, et al. Direct conversion from oral morphine to transdermal fentanyl: a multicenter study in patients with cancer pain. *Pain.* 1996;(643):527–534.

Flaschner E, Katz D. American Geriatrics Society position statement on feeding tubes in advanced dementia. *J Am Geriatr Soc.* 2015;63:1490–1491.

Fox CB, et al. Megestrol acetate and mirtazapine for the treatment of unplanned weight loss in the elderly. *Pharmacotherapy.* 2009;29:383–397.

Givens JL, et al. Survival and comfort after treatment of pneumonia in advanced dementia. *Arch Intern Med.* 2010;170(13):1102–1107.

Johnson MJ, Oxberry SG. The management of dyspnoea in chronic heart failure. *Curr Opin Support Palliat Care.* 2010;4:63–68.

Kapo J, Adams C, et al. Essentials 4: nonpain symptom management. In: *Essential Practices in Hospice and Palliative Medicine.* 5th ed. Chicago, IL: American Academy of Hospice and Palliative Medicine; 2017: 16–17.

Lampert R, et al. HRS expert consensus statement on the management of Cardiovascular Implantable Electronic Devices (CIEDs) in patients nearing end of life or requesting withdrawal of therapy. *Heart Rhythm.* 2010;7(7):1008–1026.

Mahtani KR, et al. Reduced salt intake for heart failure: a systematic review. *JAMA Intern Med.* 2018;178(12):1693–1700.

Mitchell S, et al. Infection management and multidrug-resistant organisms in nursing home residents with advanced dementia. *JAMA Intern Med.* 2014;174(10):1660–1667.

Murtagh FEM, et al. The use of opioid analgesia in end-stage renal disease patients managed without dialysis: recommendations for practice. *J Pain Palliat Care Pharmacother.* 2007;21(2):5–16.

Pattison M, Romer AL. Improving care through the end of life: launching a primary care clinic-based program. *J Palliat Med.* 2001;4(2):249–254.

Reisfeld S, et al. The effect of empiric antibiotic therapy on mortality in debilitated patients with dementia. *Eur J Clin Microbiol Infect Dis.* 2011;30:813–818.

Sampson EL, et al. Enteral tube feeding for older people with advanced dementia. *Cochrane Database Syst Rev.* 2009;2:Art No. CD007209.

Silverman SM. Opioid induced hyperalgesia: clinical implications for the pain practitioner. *Pain Physician.* 2009;12:679–684.

Temel JS, et al. Early palliative care for patients with metastatic non-small-cell lung cancer. *N Engl J Med.* 2010;363(8):733–742.

Teno JM et al. Survival after multiple hospitalizations for infections and dehydration in nursing home residents with advanced cognitive impairment. *JAMA.* 2013;310:319–320.

Walsh G. Hypodermoclysis: an alternate method for rehydration in long-term care. *J Infus Nurs.* 2005;28(2):123–129.

Yeh SS, et al. Pharmacological treatment of geriatric cachexia: evidence and safety in perspective. *J Am Med Dir Assoc.* 2007;8:363–377.

Evidence-Based Medicine

28

Mark A. Graber

Yeah, we don't like numbers either. But they are at the end of the chapter for those of you who want to learn 2 × 2 tables, etc. We do like evidence-based medicine (EBM) though, and it will be on the examination. So here goes…

Table 28-1 is here for reference. You may want to refer to it as you work your way through the chapter.

> ▶ **CASE 28.1**

Research published in *World's Best Medical Journal* studied screening for lung cancer using a new method. The researchers reported that patients who had lung cancer detected via screening lived longer after diagnosis than people who were diagnosed with lung cancer but not screened.

Question 28.1.1 Which is true?
A) This shows that screening is effective at prolonging survival
B) This may be an example of lead-time bias
C) This may be an example of verification bias
D) Well-respected medical journals (and board review books) are always right

Answer 28.1.1 **The correct answer is "B."** This may be an example of lead-time bias, which is not to be confused with length-time bias (see Table 28-2). Screening is intended to diagnose disease earlier, hopefully allowing for interventions that prevent or slow the progression of the disease. Without screening, the disease may be discovered only after symptoms develop when it may be too late to intervene. Screening, however, can also give the appearance of longer survival even though no additional life has been gained. This is called "lead-time bias." Here's another example. Mr. X has the test, is diagnosed with disease, receives treatment, and dies 5 years later. Mr. Y is in the control group, develops symptoms at year 4 of the study and dies 1 year after that. They have both lived for 5 years after being randomized to screening or no screening. Mr. X and Mr. Y both die at age 65 of the same disease. Did Mr. X have more survival time or just more "disease time"? This lead-time bias may be avoided by

TABLE 28-1 USEFUL EQUATIONS

Sensitivity: True Positives/(true positives + false negatives)

Specificity: True Negatives/(true negatives + false positives)

False Positive Rate: 1 − specificity

False Negative Rate: 1 − sensitivity

Positive Predictive Value: True Positive/(true positive + false positive)

Negative Predictive Value: True Negative/(true negative + false negative)

using age-specific mortality rates rather than survival time from diagnosis. "C," verification bias, occurs when you are looking at a new diagnostic modality, and patients with a negative test result (for the new test) are not evaluated with the gold standard test. For example, verification bias could occur in a study where people with a negative cardiac stress test do not proceed to a cardiac catheterization. This underestimates the prevalence of disease in the population studied (some of those with a negative exercise test will certainly have disease … we just haven't checked for it). It also overestimates the value of the stress test (seemingly, all patients with cardiac disease were picked up by the stress test … but only because we didn't look far enough). See Table 28-2 for more types of bias found in studies.

··

As part of a quality control study, the hemoglobin A_{1c} values of patients with diabetes at two clinics are compared. In a study of 4,000 patients, it is found that the mean hemoglobin A_{1c} value in group 1 is 7.4% and the mean hemoglobin A_{1c} value in group 2 is 7.6%. The authors did the correct statistical test and found a *p*-value of 0.04 for this comparison.

Question 28.1.2 Based on this information, you conclude:
A) Group 1 is significantly different from group 2. Reject the null hypothesis

TABLE 28-2 SOME COMMON TYPES OF BIASES/PROBLEMS SEEN IN STUDIES

Type of Bias	Effect
Confirmation Bias	This occurs when you only look for data that supports your contention and ignore any information to the contrary (i.e., if I believe that the Internet is full of sociopaths, I could confirm that by reading comments under videos posted on related websites and ignoring everything else that would suggest otherwise).
Confounders (Confounding variables)	This occurs when two or more factors are associated with the outcome and only the one being studied is accounted for (i.e., research shows that 9 out of 10 Cubs fans have annoying behavior, but 9 out of 10 Cubs fans are also drunk when the annoying behavior occurs; if we do not account for the confounding variable [drunkenness], we may incorrectly assume that being a Cubs fan *causes* annoying behavior … which can't possibly be true … can it?).
Length time bias (**not** lead time)	This occurs because screening tests are more likely to find slow-growing tumors rather than those that are rapidly growing. This can bias results in favor of screening because more slow-growing cancers with a good prognosis will be found with a screening test.
Selection bias	This occurs when subjects selected for the study do not represent the entire population you might see clinically. For example, they may be sicker or less sick than the patients in your practice or they may be excluded from the study for another reason. For example, let's say we are doing a study on renal failure. If all patients with diabetes are excluded, we will not be able to apply the results to our patients many of whom have renal failure and coexisting diabetes. This is avoided by having large, representative samples with few exclusion criteria.
Spectrum bias	This occurs if a study is skewed toward a particular group of patients, for example, those with an NSTEMI. If you study NSTEMI patients, you cannot apply your results to patients with other related conditions, such as a STEMI or unstable angina. Spectrum bias is common in studies; often the patients studied at a tertiary care institution differ in the severity of illness than those in primary care practices (who in general tend to have less severe disease).
Performance bias	This occurs when one group of subjects in an experiment gets more attention from researchers (e.g., control group gets more frequent visits, more education, etc.) or one group of subjects changes their behavior in response to the experiment (e.g., control group exercises more, eats better, etc.). An example of this is estrogen for heart disease. Case–control studies suggested estrogen was cardioprotective, but it didn't pan out in randomized, controlled trials. Thus, the positive effect was due to something else; maybe the women on estrogen exercised more, maybe they had better diets, maybe they smoked less and were more interested in their health overall. Randomized, blinded trials protect against this bias—especially the blinding part.

B) Group 1 is not significantly different from group 2. Don't reject the null hypothesis
C) Group 1 is not significantly different from group 2. Reject the null hypothesis
D) Group 1 is significantly different from group 2. Don't reject the null hypothesis

Answer 28.1.2 **The correct answer is "A."** To answer this question, you have to know what the usual cutoff for significance is for a *p*-value, and you also have to know what a null hypothesis is. A null hypothesis is the hypothesis that there is no significant difference between two groups being compared or that the observed difference is likely to have occurred by chance alone rather than due to a variable. By setting up null hypotheses in this way, we can then search for proof that the null hypothesis is incorrect. Tests of significance are a method of looking for evidence that a null hypothesis is incorrect. The *p*-value gives you the probability that the results of the study occurred by chance alone. A *p*-value of 0.04 means that if the study results were untrue, we would expect to see these results only 4% of the time by chance alone and not related to the study intervention. By convention, a *p*-value of 0.05 or smaller is considered statistically significant. Thus, when you have a *p*-value $</= 0.05$, you have evidence that the null hypothesis is false and can therefore be rejected.

HELPFUL TIP:
A type I error occurs when a difference is found when in reality the two groups are the same. The *p*-value provides you with the probability of a type I error. For example, a *p*-value of 0.05 is considered statistically significant. But what this means, however, is that 5% of the time, the same conclusion would be produced by chance alone. By contrast, a *p*-value of 0.005 means that there is only a 0.5% chance that the conclusion is mistaken and occurred by chance. The lower the *p*-value, the lower the chance of a type I error.

HELPFUL TIP:
A type II error occurs when a study fails to show a difference where one exists. This may occur because there are not enough subjects in a study or when there is measurement error. For example, in a (real) study of lorazepam versus diazepam for seizures, twice as many patients had their seizures stop with lorazepam. However, the conclusion of the study was that there was no difference between the two drugs. This is only because there were not enough subjects for this to reach statistical significance. Including another 100 subjects may have made this reach statistical significance. Remember this by "Type II error is too few subjects."

▶ **Objectives: Did you learn to …**
- Recognize forms of bias in research studies?
- Define *p*-value and null hypothesis?

• Describe the significance of *p*-value and type I error?
• Recognize a type II error?

▶ CASE 28.2

Being the compulsive physician that you are, you are spending your Saturday morning relaxing by reading your journals (we know who you are; you can't fool us... why else would you be working through the EBM chapter?). You notice a study of particular interest on type 2 diabetes, using a novel drug called Shugabegone (not a real drug), and note that the data were analyzed in two ways. The first method used was an "intention to treat" analysis. The second method was by a "per-protocol" analysis. Hmm, you think. The per-protocol data sure makes you want to start prescribing Shugabegone for your patients with diabetes.

Question 28.2.1 Which of the following applies to a per-protocol analysis?
A) It provides an objective description of how a new therapy will work in our patient population
B) It is more statistically stringent when compared to an intention-to-treat analysis
C) It allows the study authors to manipulate the outcome to make it look better than it is
D) You are wrong, Dr. Graber. I am not reading this chapter

Answer 28.2.1 **The correct answer is "C."** Per-protocol analysis allows the authors to make the outcome look better than it is. To understand why, we must know the difference between an "intention to treat" analysis and a "per-protocol analysis." A per-protocol analysis allows the authors to manipulate the results, usually in favor of the study drug. Here is an example: "Of all of the patients who were enrolled in this study, those who took the drug at least 75% of the time were included in the final analysis." There is a problem here. Many of our patients will not take all of their medicine. Maybe they forgot to take it. Maybe it had side effects that were intolerable. If we only analyze the patients who took all of their medication, the drug will look better in the per-protocol analysis than it will in our clinical practice where adherence to a regimen is less than complete. You will see this in many papers. In some papers, there is a "wash-in period" where everyone is given the medication and only those who tolerate it for 2 weeks (for example) continue to the main trial. The results here will not be representative of our patients, many of whom may not tolerate the medication. In summary, per-protocol analysis = bad.

An intention to treat analysis analyzes *all* study patients in the group to which they were originally assigned. In this case (to continue the hypothetical study above), the authors do not care if the patients took the drug 75% of the time. Even if they *never* took the drug but were assigned to the treatment group, they are analyzed in the treatment group. Many of these patients likely would be treatment failures making the overall results look worse. However, the results will be more applicable to our patient population, many of whom will not take their medications properly. In summary, intention to treat analysis = good.

"OK," you think. "I'll pay attention to the intention to treat analysis." So, you next look at the inclusion and exclusion criteria. In this diabetes drug study, the exclusion criteria include renal disease, a history of heart failure, coronary artery disease, and peripheral vascular disease.

Question 28.2.2 From this we can conclude:
A) The patients in this study are so finely selected that the results *cannot* be applied to our general clinic population
B) The results should be generalizable to our general clinic population given the fact that the medication worked so well in this study
C) This is an example of "selection bias"
D) A and C
E) B and C

Answer 28.2.2 **The correct answer is "D."** We cannot apply these results to our general clinic patients. Think about it: how many of your diabetic patients have no renal disease, no history of CHF, and no history of CAD/PVD? Not too many. Many of our patients with diabetes have at least some renal disease (proteinuria). You always need to look at the inclusion and exclusion criteria of a trial before you can determine if the trial is applicable to your patients. This is called "selection bias"; only select patients are entered into the study.

There is also a phenomenon called "spectrum bias." In the case of spectrum bias, the patients in the study are different than our patients; they may be sicker or not as sick. Case in point: glycoprotein IIB/IIIA inhibitors for acute coronary syndrome (ACS). The initial studies looked at patients going for cardiac catheterization; and it appeared there was a small benefit here. But the drug companies then generalized from these sick patients to say that all patients with ACS should have glycoprotein IIB/IIIA inhibitors. You can't do this. Most of our "ACS" admissions turn out not to have ACS, and they will get better regardless of what we do. They certainly don't need glycoprotein IIB/IIIA inhibitors. And, thankfully, these drugs have fallen out of favor.

HELPFUL TIP:
Subgroup analyses (you know, the "our drug worked in left-handed women over 60" pitch) can only be used to generate a hypothesis. This is called the "derivation set." Before accepting it into practice, a second study of that subgroup, called the "validation set" must be done. This is always true. Don't let them tell you otherwise.

▶ Objectives: Did you learn to ...
• Describe an intention to treat analysis and its value for applying study results?
• Recognize the effect of inclusion and exclusion criteria on the application of study results?

QUICK QUIZ: FEELING SENSITIVE ABOUT SOMETHING SPECIFIC?

Which of the following statements is true?
A) Specificity is the most important test characteristic when trying to find a very dangerous disease
B) As sensitivity increases, specificity decreases
C) Specificity need not be considered as long as a test is sensitive enough
D) As sensitivity increases, specificity increases

The correct answer is "B." As sensitivity increases, specificity decreases. This makes intuitive sense. The more cases you detect, the more false positives you will have. We can have a sensitivity of 100% if, for example, we say that everyone with WBCs in their blood and a cough has pneumonia. We will pick up everyone with the disease (very sensitive), but also a lot of patients without the disease (poor specificity... everyone has at least one, lonely, white cell running around). Ideally, we would like to have a diagnostic test with both high sensitivity and high specificity. In reality, there is an inherent trade-off between sensitivity and specificity—as sensitivity increases, specificity decreases and vice versa. "A" is incorrect. Generally, *when it is very dangerous not to detect a disease, it is important to have a highly sensitive test (one that will find "all" cases)* with an acceptable specificity. "C" is incorrect. This is why both an ELISA and a Western blot may be done when trying to detect HIV. The ELISA is very sensitive (will pick up the great majority of HIV cases), but is not very specific (will categorize a lot of patients who do not have the disease as positive). The Western blot is more specific and will filter the true positives from the false positives found on the screening test (the ELISA).

 QUICK QUIZ: ALL THAT GLITTERS ...

You are having a meaningful discussion with an industry representative (yeah, right). OK, let's recalibrate. You are being sold a package of goods by an industry representative. She says that if their test for Dreaded Disease is positive, the likelihood ratio of the disease being present is 3.

Your response to this is:
A) "Great! The disease is three times more likely to be present if the test is positive"
B) "Not so great! A likelihood ratio of 3 is pretty much worthless in differentiating between those who are ill and those who are not"
C) "What is this likelihood ratio stuff anyway?"
D) "What happened to my free lunch?"

The correct answer is "B." In a situation in which the pretest probability of a disease is between 30% and 70%, a likelihood ratio can meaningfully reduce the possibility of disease presence only if it is <0.1. In a situation in which the pretest probability of

a disease is between 30% and 70%, a likelihood ratio can meaningfully increase the possibility of disease presence only if it is over 10. So, a likelihood ratio of 3 is more or less useless. Draw some lines on this and you will see what we mean (Fig. 28-1).

▶ **CASE 28.3**

One common and debilitating complication of diabetes is neuropathy. In a (fictional) study by Tooth E. Fairie et al., one group had routine therapy and an experimental group had intensive therapy for their diabetic neuropathy. In the first group, those assigned to routine therapy, 10% of patients developed neuropathy. In the second group, those assigned to intensive therapy, 2% of patients developed neuropathy.

Question 28.3.1 **Using the data above, how many patients with diabetes need to be treated with intensive therapy to prevent the development of one case of neuropathy?**
A) 10
B) 11
C) 8
D) 12.5
E) 25.5

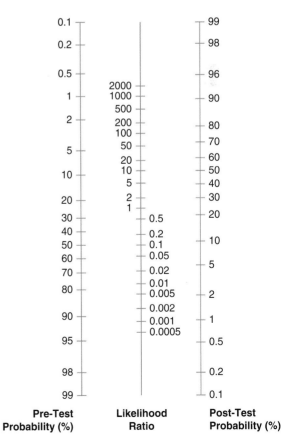

FIGURE 28-1. Reproduced from the Centre for Evidence-Based Medicine. Available at: http://www.cebm.net.

Answer 28.3.1 The correct answer is "D." The question is really asking, "What is the number needed to treat (NNT)"? The NNT is the number of patients who need to be treated to prevent one adverse outcome. In this question, the absolute risk reduction is 8% (10% in control group vs. 2% in the treated group). To calculate this, we need to know a few other terms:

$$ARR = \text{Absolute Risk Reduction}$$
$$= \text{control group event rate (CER)}$$
$$- \text{experimental group event rate (EER).}$$

$$NNT = 1 / ARR \text{ (in percent)}$$

Using the values given above, ARR = 10% − 2% = 8% and NNT = 1/0.08 = 12.5.

....

The anti-clotting properties of aspirin are well described. In a (fictional) trial studying the long-term outcome of stroke patients by Haywood Jabuzzoff et al., 1% of patients on long-term aspirin therapy developed new onset of strokes and 50% of patients without aspirin therapy developed new strokes.

Question 28.3.2 Using the data above, how many stroke patients need to be treated with aspirin therapy to prevent one new stroke (what is the NNT)?
A) 2
B) 8
C) 10
D) 12
E) 25

Answer 28.3.2 The correct answer is "A." Again, the NNT is the number of patients who need to be treated to prevent one adverse outcome. NNT = 1/ARR, where ARR = CER − EER. Using the values given above, 50% − 1% = 49% = ARR and NNT = 1/0.49 = 2 (well, really close to 2).

....

In a (fictional) pharmaceutical study by Anita Hand et al., Group A is the placebo group and Group B is the group that received the actual new drug. Data were gathered on Groups A and B and confidence intervals (CI) were calculated. Side effect rates were calculated as a percentage of each group.

Question 28.3.3 Using the 95% CI, which of the following group comparisons are statistically significantly different?
A) Group A CI 30% to 46% and Group B CI 44% to 88%
B) Group A CI 10% to 30% and Group B CI 44% to 88%
C) Group A CI 0.1% to 0.3% and Group B CI 0.2% to 0.4%
D) Group A CI 88% to 90% and Group B CI 88% to 90%
E) None of the above is statistically significant

Answer 28.3.3 The correct answer is "B." The CI is a range of possible high to low values of data. The true mean is likely to

be in the specified range. In general, the larger the study group, the narrower the CI. When you have a large study, you are more likely to get closer to the true value.

"B" is correct because when comparing the CI between two groups, there is no overlap. When there is an overlap of CI, as in the other options, the groups have no statistically significant difference. For example, in answer "A" the true mean value of Group A could lie anywhere between 30% and 46% (it could be 45%), and the true mean value of Group B could lie anywhere between 44% and 88% (it could also be 45%); therefore, the groups have no statistically significant difference.

> **HELPFUL TIP:**
> Confidence intervals are usually given as "CI 95%," meaning that there is a 95% probability that the true mean value will be within the CI. When looking at CI for relative risk (RR), relative benefit, odds ratio, etc., remember that if the CI 95% crosses "1," there is no difference between the groups. Thus, a RR of 4.2, CI 95% of 0.8 to 10 is consistent with a 0.8 times risk or a 10 times risk. However, since the CI 95% crosses "1," there is no real difference between the groups.

> **HELPFUL TIP:**
> Confidence intervals are useful when determining the magnitude of a treatment effect. For example, if a RR has CI 95% of 1.2 to 1.4, this means there is a small difference (0.2–0.4 times) between the two groups, even though it is statistically significant. Remember, something that is statistically significant may not be clinically significant. On the other hand, if the RR has a CI 95% of 10 to 20, this is a major difference between the groups. This means that one group has a 10 to 20 times greater risk (or benefit depending on what is being studied) than does the other group.

....

In a (fictional) clinical trial testing a new provider order entry (POE) technology at Big Important University Hospital, relative and absolute risk reduction is discussed. A group of family medicine residents at the hospital was allowed to give verbal orders during their intern year and *averaged seven medication errors per year*. In the residents' second year, POE was instituted (in which physicians were required to enter orders, and alerts to medication errors were given before finalization of orders), and the group's *medication errors dropped to an average of four per year*.

Question 28.3.4 Which of the following is true?
A) The RR reduction is 43% and the absolute risk reduction is three in medication errors
B) The RR reduction is 57% and the absolute risk reduction is three in medication errors
C) The RR reduction is 43% and the absolute risk reduction is four in medication errors

D) The RR reduction is 57% and the absolute risk reduction is four in medication errors

E) POE has ruined medicine. I quit! Boo-hoo!

Answer 28.3.4 The correct answer is "A." POE compared with no POE (the control group) resulted in a 43% relative decrease in the risk of a medication error—from seven to four errors per year (3/7 = 43%). The difference in the number of medication errors before and after POE is three errors (7 − 4 = 3), which is the absolute reduction in the risk of a medication error. Now, think about this from a pharmaceutical or medical device representative's point of view. Would you say (a) "We reduced errors by 3 per year," or would you say (b) "We reduced errors by 43% per year!"? That's how you sell a study.

▶ **Objectives: Did you learn to …**
- Calculate number needed to treat?
- Differentiate between absolute and relative risk reduction?
- Use confidence intervals to determine statistical significance?

▶ CASE 28.4

Mr. Handsome Q. Drugrep has come to tell you all about **Happy Lucky Golden Drug (HLGD) that is newly indicated for the treatment of the Dreadful Yucks. As a primary care doctor, you are concerned about better treatment of this disease. Current standard treatment involves ChemoRAdical Pharmacotherapy (CRAP). Cure rates with CRAP are only about 10%. Mr. Drugrep has a study that shows HLGD has a 12% cure rate versus placebo. He's very excited and expects HLGD to be the new standard of care.**

Question 28.4.1 To his argument, you appropriately respond:
A) "Wow. HLGD is clearly superior to CRAP"
B) "Hmm. HLGD is statistically no different from CRAP"
C) "Wow. HLGD is clearly superior to placebo"
D) "Do you have free samples of HLGD? Where's lunch?"
E) "I need more information before I can make an informed decision"

Answer 28.4.1 The correct answer is "E." You need more information. Before coming to market, a drug manufacturer must demonstrate safety and efficacy of a drug. The new drug may or may not be compared with another currently available treatment. Without a study comparing HLGD to CRAP, you cannot say anything about how these drugs compare, even if HLGD looks better versus placebo. In addition, "C" is incorrect because the placebo results have not been given.

You ask Mr. Drugrep for more information. He proudly tells you the drug study involved 10,000 subjects with the Dreadful Yucks, randomly assigned to placebo (5,000) or HLGD (5,000). All of the subjects completed the trial. At the end of 1 year, 400 subjects on placebo (8%) were cured and 600 subjects on HLGD (12%) were cured.

Question 28.4.2 He correctly tells you that:
A) The NNT is 10,000
B) The number needed to harm (NNH) is 10,000
C) The relative benefit of HLGD versus placebo is 50% greater cure rate
D) The absolute benefit of HLGD versus placebo is 50% greater cure rate

Answer 28.4.2 The correct answer is "C." When looking at drug studies, benefit is often stated as "relative benefit" or relative risk reduction. In this question, 600/5,000 patients benefit from HLGD and 400/5,000 benefit from placebo; thus, 200 more patients are cured with HLGD, 200/400 = 0.5 = 50% *relative benefit* of the drug vs. placebo. The *absolute benefit* is only 4% (12% cure with HLGD vs. 8% cure with placebo). For the NNT in this example, think about the previously given equation: NNT = 1/ARR, where ARR = CER − EER. The control group, the placebo, had a risk reduction of 8% (92% still had disease); and the experiment group had a risk reduction of 12% (88% still had disease). So, the ARR = 12% − 8% = 4%, and NNT = 1/0.04 = 25. NNH cannot be calculated with the information available since the adverse event rate is not provided.

In real life, there are often more dramatic examples of how relative and absolute risks differ. It may be stated that there is a 50% reduction in complications of diabetes using Drug A versus placebo. However, when translated into patients, this could be 1/1,000 complications of diabetes in the drug group versus 2/1,000 complications of diabetes in the placebo group. This is a 50% relative decrease in adverse outcomes but in fact may be clinically meaningless. The absolute risk reduction is 1/1,000 or 0.1%! This ploy is often used to make drug studies look good. Thus, anytime you are looking at a new drug, ask for the absolute risk reduction and the NNT and the NNH. Forget the relative risk reduction and the *p*-values.

Mr. Drugrep tells you that the adverse event rate for HLGD is only 1%. Aren't you impressed? But he frowns a little when you want to know the NNH.

Question 28.4.3 To calculate NNH, you ask him for:
A) The types of adverse events that occurred in the treatment group
B) The percentage of adverse events that occurred in the control group
C) The percentage of adverse events with standard treatment
D) The cure rate in the treatment group

Answer 28.4.3 The correct answer is "B." Adverse effects of a drug will often be reported as an absolute number, and here it is given as 1%. So, the conclusion you are given by the pharmaceutical industry may be 50% reduction in disease and only a 1% risk of side effects of the drug. Both of these statements are true, but it's an "apples and oranges" comparison. We prefer comparing apples-to-apples (or corn-to-corn in Iowa). In order to directly compare benefits and harms, we need to know the NNT and the NNH.

Let's say that when you ask Mr. Drugrep, he tells you that the adverse event rate in the placebo group was 0.5%. Here's the calculation: NNH = 1/ARI, where ARI (absolute risk increase) = risk in experiment group − risk in control group.

Using the numbers in this question: ARI = 1 − 0.5 = 0.5; NNH = 1/0.5 = 2.

So, for HLGD, the NNT is 25 and the NNH is 2. By the way, the adverse event in question is disfiguring, painful ear hair growth. You will have to treat 25 patients with HLGD to cure one case of the Dreadful Yucks; but with every two patients you treat, one will have an adverse event. Demand NNT and NNH: how many patients who take the drug will benefit and how many will be harmed?

▶ **Objectives: Did you learn to …**
- Employ CI in the analysis of data?
- Analyze data using risk reduction and relative benefit?
- Understand the importance of absolute risk reduction, NNH, and NNT when clinically applying data from a study?

▶ **CASE 28.5**

Mounting paperwork and electronic medical record hassles have played a role in your decision to make a career change. You have found a nice academic job with a research focus—minimal patient care, 10 weeks of vacation, no paperwork. The only downside is that you get paid peanuts—literally, you get 100 lbs of peanuts per month. Your work centers on reducing the risk of stroke in patients who have survived one stroke.

Question 28.5.1 This is an example of which category of prevention?
A) Primary prevention
B) Secondary prevention
C) Tertiary prevention
D) Quaternary prevention

Answer 28.5.1 The correct answer is "C." The idea behind primary prevention, a big interest in primary care, is to prevent a disease from occurring at all by removing its cause (i.e., influenza vaccine to prevent illness from influenza). Primary prevention may occur in the healthcare setting but is often in the domain of public health. Secondary prevention detects disease at an early stage so that intervention can prevent progression (i.e., Pap smears detecting dysplasia prior to cancer declaring itself or treating elevated cholesterol prior to vascular events). Your new job will be to study tertiary prevention: the reduction in complications and mortality due to disease after it is recognized. The line between secondary and tertiary prevention can be blurry: some would consider preventing another stroke "secondary" prevention and preventing stroke complications (e.g., muscle atrophy and pressure ulcer) "tertiary" prevention. There is no such thing as quaternary prevention.

In between day-trading and coffee breaks, you plan to study two groups of patients (A and B) to see if variable XYZ makes any difference in death or recurrent stroke. There is no randomization and there are no interventions. You are just reviewing records to see how each group did. Subjects in Group A had a stroke and then had another stroke or died a year later. Subjects in Group B had a stroke but were alive with no recurrent stroke at the time of the study. You assess the presence of XYZ in each group.

Question 28.5.2 This type of study is called a:
A) Prospective study
B) Case–control study
C) Cohort study
D) Randomized, controlled study

Answer 28.5.2 The correct answer is "B." A case–control study, like this one, will look at select subjects who are categorized based on outcome and try to find associations with certain variables. Case–control studies do not follow subjects over time and therefore are not prospective (but rather retrospective). Cohort studies ("C") look at groups starting at time zero and following them for a specified amount of time to find an association between a variable and an outcome. The variable in question is not under the researcher's control. An example of a cohort study might be one looking at the association between two different diets (e.g., high-protein vs. high-carbohydrate) and the development of type 2 diabetes. The highest quality evidence is produced by a randomized, double blind, controlled trial ("D"), in which the researcher has control over exposure to a variable and studies its effect on an outcome. In general, the strength of trial design goes: experimental study > cohort study > case–control study > cross-sectional study. Unfortunately, it is not possible to design randomized controlled studies for all conditions. So, a well-done cohort study may be the best we can do.

You are concerned about numerous confounding variables in your study population. Never fear!

Question 28.5.3 Your trusty statistician recommends the following in order to minimize confounding:
A) Multivariate analysis
B) Careful calculation of p-values
C) Matched controls and cases
D) A and B
E) A and C

Answer 28.5.3 The correct answer is "E." Confounders can be a serious threat to any study. Confounders result from extrinsic factors—things that may affect the outcome and are also associated with the variable but are not accounted for in the study. As an example, a study may find an association between long-haul truck driving and lung cancer. Therefore, it is concluded that long-haul trucking is bad for your health. However, some long-haul truckers smoke. If tobacco use was not accounted for in this study, the results of the study would be meaningless. Tobacco is a confounder. It is always advisable to look at a study with an eye for what confounder might be missing. Confounding can be limited by a study design that anticipates confounders and matches controls and cases ("C"). It is important to note that if you match your control and cases on a variable, you can no longer study that variable as a potential cause of the outcome. For example, if you match cases and controls on county of residence among the truck drivers, you can no longer explore county of residence as a risk factor for lung cancer. Also, multivariate analysis ("A") is a statistical method that allows for adjustment of known confounders. "B" is incorrect because *p*-value has nothing to do with confounding but will tell you whether the results should be considered significant or not.

When you review the literature, you find that there are a number of small studies looking at the effect of variable XYZ on stroke victims. You even find a meta-analysis.

Question 28.5.4 If this is a well-done meta-analysis, you should find all of the following EXCEPT:
A) Statistically confirmed heterogeneity between the included studies
B) A thorough search for all valid studies
C) An evaluation of whether estimates change with varying assumptions
D) The exclusion of poor-quality studies
E) The studies included measure the same underlying effect

Answer 28.5.4 **The correct answer is "A."** Hopefully, a meta-analysis would confirm *homogeneity* between studies. For example, if one study measured NIH stroke scale and another measured patient quality of life (the outcomes are heterogeneous), it would be impossible to combine the studies. Although there is controversy regarding the appropriate use of meta-analyses, they are often used to study various outcomes by combining smaller studies. A meta-analysis is a systematic review that combines the results of previous studies to evaluate the magnitude or direction of an effect or to evaluate the effect on a subgroup. All valid studies looking at similar outcomes should be included; poor-quality studies should be excluded. The Jadad score is one common way that studies are judged as to their appropriateness for a meta-analysis (Table 28-3). Other similar scales exist. Meta-analyses should also include a "sensitivity analysis." This may consist of excluding large studies and only analyzing smaller studies. It may consist of changing the economic assumptions in a cost-benefit meta-analysis. If the outcome is the same either way, the result is said to be "robust." If excluding some studies or changing the underlying economic assumption changes the result, one has to wonder about the quality of the studies, etc.

TABLE 28-3 FACTORS IN DETERMINING THE JADAD SCORE FOR META-ANALYSES

Randomization	Withdrawals and dropout numbers	Blinding

▶ **Objectives: Did you learn to …**
- Define different types of prevention?
- Define different study types?
- Identify and account for confounding variables?
- Describe some characteristics of a meta-analysis?

    HELPFUL TIP:
You will see an increasing number of "noninferiority" studies being done. What does "noninferior" mean? Basically, it means that two drugs have *some* overlap in their efficacy. See Figure 28-2. Drugs Y is noninferior to Drug X even though it may not cure as many patients. "Noninferior" does not mean "as good as." "Biocreep" (which is one of our favorite terms and reminds us of zombies) occurs when drug Z is now compared to drug Y. Drug Z is noninferior to Drug Y, although it clearly cures fewer people than Drug X. Thus, the standard against which new drugs are compared becomes progressively less efficacious (Fig. 28-2). In another concern, researchers can define their own "margin" of noninferiority. For example if the margin is "2" (as in some of the new anticoagulant studies), the new drug could allow up to twice as many events (e.g., pulmonary emboli) as the old drug and still be considered "noninferior."

 QUICK QUIZ: ERROR PREVENTION 1

You are seeing a 46-year-old female with complaints of lower abdominal pain. Looking at her chart, you see that the last several notes (from several different doctors) all list the diagnosis as constipation. The patient has tried multiple medications for constipation but is still having the pain. You smartly order an ultrasound which shows ovarian cancer. You are wondering

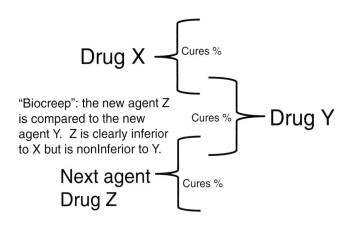

FIGURE 28-2. The Three Major Factors of the Jadad Score.

why the last three providers all put "constipation" without ruling out other illnesses.

This could be an example of:
A) Chronology bias
B) Diagnostic momentum
C) Availability bias
D) Framing bias

The correct answer is "B." Diagnostic momentum occurs when a provider is not sufficiently skeptical of the diagnosis on the chart. It can be a leading source of diagnostic errors. How many times have you seen "migraine" written on the chart and assume it is correct? Always be skeptical of a diagnosis, especially if treatments don't seem to be helping. You may be a better clinician than the last person to see the patient. "A," chronology bias, occurs when a historical cohort is used as the control group in a study. The claim may be made that, "The introduction of fuzzy cookies improves outcomes when compared to historical controls." The problem is that, over time, *other things have changed in medicine besides the introduction of fuzzy cookies* (e.g., sepsis protocols, stroke protocols, early mobilization, other medications for the illness, etc.). If the controls are historical, it may be that one of these other factors is responsible for the improvement in outcomes. "C," availability bias, means that something that happened recently makes you think the same thing is happening again. For example, if you miss a pulmonary embolus (PE), all of a sudden it seems as though patients with marginal symptoms have a PE and thus get a PE workup. Or, if you see something rare, you think the next three patients with similar symptoms also have this rare disease (even though the rate in the population is only 1 in 10,000). That which has recently happened is more "available" in your thought processes, so it tends to be intrusive in your thinking. "D," framing bias, occurs when you try to make symptoms and data fit into your preconceived notion of a diagnosis. For example, a patient presents with fever upon return from Africa, and you assume it is due to malaria, so you specifically look for symptoms and lab data to fit your hypothesis.

 QUICK QUIZ: ERROR PREVENTION 2

You are looking at the patient with ovarian cancer: She is dressed in ripped jeans (not the expensive kind which we don't understand) and a somewhat grubby T-shirt. She has a very annoying, whiny voice. You are thinking that the way she is dressed and speaks may have played a role in the mis-diagnosis.

This is an example of:
A) Affective bias or attribution error
B) Anchoring bias
C) Confirmation bias
D) Probabilistic diagnosis

The correct answer is "A." Ok, be honest now. How many of you like to have other healthcare providers or "VIPs" as a patient?

Probably none of us. If you are like the editors, you treat those patients differently. You might defer painful or embarrassing tests (like a rectal exam or an LP) because you don't want to cause them pain or risk embarrassment. Or, you might do too many tests "just to be sure." Either approach is wrong. These are examples of "affective bias." We let our feelings ("affect") about the patient modify our diagnostic or treatment plan. In the example above, we may (unconsciously) dismiss the patient's complaints because we don't like her, because of the way she dresses, or because she presents as a negative stereotype (strange, unwashed, and somehow slightly dazed—thank you, David Bowie). We tend not to believe patients with whom we don't identify. It is hard to be objective when you really like—or really don't like—the patient. This is one reason we don't treat family members. "Attribution error" is similar. We let negative stereotypes about how the patient looks, etc., change our probability of a diagnosis. For example, we look at the "love and hate" tattoos on the knuckles of a patient who smells strongly of tobacco smoke and has had a couple of beers and assume the patient is not a reliable historian and is (more likely) just looking for narcotics.

"B," anchoring bias, occurs when we hold on too tightly to a piece of information even if other information contradicts it. For example, we may see an infiltrate on x-ray and think, "pneumonia." We may continue to inflate the significance of the positive x-ray as being suggestive of pneumonia even in the presence of other facts (such as eosinophilia… maybe it isn't pneumonia but rather pulmonary filariasis). "D," confirmation bias, occurs when we give excessive weight to data that confirms what we already believe. This is operative in a major way in politics and social media recently. We are in our "bubble" and look only at news sources that confirm our bias. We do the same in medicine: we ignore information that does not fit our hypothesis about the patient's diagnosis. Finally, "D." Essentially, "all" diagnoses and treatments are probabilistic. We make the best guess we can. A good example of this is appendicitis. If you tell a parent that their child has appendicitis, but the surgical pathology is negative, they aren't going to be happy with you. But if you tell them there is a 10% to 15% chance the surgery will yield a normal result, but it is still important to do, they may be more forgiving. *Another way to put this is that there are false-positive and false-negative tests, physical exams, etc.* We can't be sure of a diagnosis until the "gold standard/criterion standard/reference standard" test is done (in the case of appendicitis this is surgery and surgical pathology).

 HELPFUL TIP:
Differential diagnosis checklists have been shown to increase diagnostic accuracy. You can find a set of these at: https://www.healthcare.uiowa.edu/familymedicine/fpinfo/ under "Ely Checklist."

▶ **CASE 28.6**

Uh, oh… Here comes the math. This section is important, especially the concepts of positive and negative predictive values (PPV and NPV) and the concepts of sensitivity and

specificity. We are using cookies as an example in the calculations. Hopefully this will help you visualize and understand it better than if we used a disease. If you don't want to do the math, just get yourself a real cookie. But at least read the summary.

Sensitivity: How often the test will pick up the disease if it is there. Sensitivity = true positives/(true positives + false negatives). Note that the sum of true positives + false negatives represents all of the people **with** disease.

Specificity: Specificity is defined as the proportion of patients **who do not** have the disease and who will test negative for it. Specificity = true negatives/(true negatives + false positives). Note that the sum of true negatives + false positives represents all of the people **who do not** have disease.

Positive predictive value: The probability that someone with a positive test *actually has* the disease. This takes the prevalence of a disease into account. For example, an individual with a positive HIV test who is an IV drug user is more likely to really have the disease than a clean-living nun with a positive HIV test. In the nun, the test is more likely to be a false positive. So for nuns, the number of true positives might be zero but false positives 3 which makes for a PPV of "0." For an IV drug abuser, the number of true positives may be 10 with 1 false positive. The PPV = 90%

$$PPV = \frac{\text{Number of true positives}}{\text{Number of true positive} + \text{Number of false positives}}$$

Negative predictive value: The probability that someone with a negative test actually *does not* have the disease. Again, this takes the prevalence of the disease into account. For example, a negative HIV test in an IV drug user from Sub-Saharan Africa with a CD4 count of 150/mm^3 and PCP is likely to be a false negative. Conversely, a negative HIV test in the risk-averse nun, for example, is likely to be a true negative.

$$NPV = \frac{\text{Number of true negatives}}{\text{Number of true negatives} + \text{Number of false negatives}}$$

 HELPFUL TIP:
A test that has a negative predictive value of 99% may sound good. But if only 1% of the population has the disease, doing no test will have a 99% negative predictive value.

Cookie Monster has a dilemma: He has a stack of cookies in front of him. He would like to eat them but there are also round brownies mixed in. Cookie Monster hates brownies. Sure, he could just take a bite, but he hates brownies so much that this is not an option. Luckily, Cookie Monster has developed a new test called the "cookie-o-meter." It can tell whether a round thing is a cookie or a brownie. When compared with the gold standard of tasting and deciding whether or not it is a brownie or a cookie, the new test has a sensitivity

of 90% (it will detect 90% of the cookies) and a specificity of 95% (thus, 95% of the time when the cookie-o-meter says it is not a cookie [negative test], it will be a brownie).

So, how can you tell if this is a good test or if the Sesame Street Baker is pulling a fast one? You need to know the positive predictive value (PPV) of the test. In order to calculate the PPV, you need three pieces of data: the sensitivity of the test (how often the test will pick up the "disease/cookie" if it is there), the specificity of the test (how often you will get a false positive... that is a brownie is mistakenly called a cookie), and the prevalence of the condition (how many total cookies (vs. brownies) there are in the bowl in front of Cookie Monster).

Let's apply the cookie-o-meter test.

You are currently in Los Angeles, attending a CME course where they really like cookies and the claim is that 99% of the objects in the bowl in front of you are cookies with only 1% brownies. You check your "cookie-o-meter" and it says you have a cookie. But does this mean you have cookie?

In order to answer this question, you can use Bayes theorem or set up 2 × 2 tables. Here's the 2 × 2 table method. Begin by drawing a 2 × 2 table and filling in what you know. See Tables 28-4 and 28-5.

So this makes it easy.

Sensitivity = a/(a + c),
Specificity = d/(b + d),
PPV = a/(a + b),
NPV = d/(c + d)

If we have 100 cookies, the data will look like that above. Now, let's add actual numbers to the table (above). Let's use a total of 10,000 cookies. We multiply by the prevalence of cookies to get the subpopulation totals. Ninety-nine percent of the objects are cookies (99% prevalence). So, 99% prevalence × 10,000 = 9,900 are cookies; 1% × 10,000 = 100 are brownies. Once we have these numbers, we simply multiply by the sensitivity and the specificity to get the exact cell numbers to plug into the table above: 9,900 × 90% sensitivity = 8,910 for cell A ("true positives"); 9,900 − 8,910 = 990 for cell C ("false negatives"); 100 × 95% specificity = 95 for cell D ("true negatives"); 100 − 95 = 5 for cell B ("false positives"). See Table 28-6.

Once the table is filled in, these numbers can then be used to calculate the PPV, using the equation above. In this case, a/(a + b) = 8,910/ (8,910 + 5) = 99.9%.

For those who prefer the Bayes theorem method, here's how this approach is done. Bayes theorem shows the relationships between sensitivity, specificity, prevalence, PPV, and NPV. The

TABLE 28-4 SAMPLE TABLE

Test	Disease	
	+	−
+	a (true positive)	b (false positive)
−	c (false negative)	d (true negative)
Total	a + c	b + d

equation for PPV, derived from Bayes theorem, is shown, as is the calculation based on the numbers from the question:

$$PPV = \frac{Number\ of\ true\ positives}{Number\ of\ true\ positive + Number\ of\ false\ positives}$$

$$PPV = \frac{Sensitivity \times prevalence}{(Sensitivity \times prevalence) + [(1 - specificity) \times (1 - prevalence)]}$$

$$= \frac{0.9 \times 0.99}{(0.9 \times 0.99) + [0.5 \times 0.01]} = 99.9\%$$

Question 28.6.1 What would the likelihood of not having a cookie if the "cookie-o-meter" had said you did not have a cookie (what is the NPV)?
A) 95%
B) 90%
C) 50%
D) 9%
E) None of the above

Answer 28.6.1 The correct answer is "D." The question asks for the NPV, or the likelihood of not having a cookie if the

cookie-o-meter is negative. This also can be derived from Bayes theorem or calculated using a 2 × 2 table.

$$NPV = \frac{True\ negatives}{False\ negatives + True\ negatives}\ or\ \frac{d}{c + d}$$

$$= \frac{95}{990 + 95} = 8.7\%\ (round\ to\ 9\%)$$

You are now in San Francisco where they try to sneak in kale brownies. Cookie Monster hates kale brownies. Here the number of "real" cookies is 10% with 90% kale brownies. You check your "cookie-o-meter" and it says you have a cookie. Do you trust it?

Question 28.6.2 What is the likelihood that you actually have a cookie if the "cookie-o-meter" says you have a cookie (and not the dreaded kale)?
A) 91%
B) 83%
C) 67%
D) 16%
E) None of the above

Answer 28.6.2 The correct answer is "C." You can use the 2 × 2 method or the Bayes theorem methods. Here's what our 2 × 2 table looks like. See Table 28-7.

To convert to 10% prevalence, we start with a large baseline population and multiply by the prevalence to get the subpopulation totals (10% prevalence × 10,000 = 1,000 cookies; 90% × 10,000 = 9,000 kale brownies [yuck!]). Once we have the subpopulation totals, we multiply by the sensitivity and the specificity to get the exact cell numbers (1,000 × 90% sensitivity = 900 for cell "a"; 1,000 − 900 = 100 for cell "c" [or alternately 1,000 × 10% will get the same result for cell "c"]; 9,000 × 95% specificity = 8,550 for cell "d"; 9,000 − 8,550 = 450 for cell "b").

These numbers can then be used to calculate the PPV, using the equation above. In this case, a/(a + b) = 900/(900 + 450) = 66.7% (rounds to 67%). Using Bayes theorem, the equation is as follows:

$$PPV = \frac{Sensitivity \times prevalence}{(Sensitivity \times prevalence) + [(1 - specificity) \times (1 - prevalence)]}$$

$$= \frac{0.9 \times 0.1}{(0.9 \times 0.1) + [0.05 \times 0.9]} = 66.7\%$$

Question 28.6.3 Still in San Francisco, we ask: What would the likelihood of having a cookie be if the "cookie-o-meter" said you did not have a cookie (but rather had a kale brownie)?
A) 50%
B) 40%
C) 30%
D) 1%
E) None of the above

TABLE 28-5 COOKIE-O-METER SENSITIVITY AND SPECIFICITY

		Actual Cookie	
		+	−
Cookie-o-meter Test Result	+	90 (true positive)	5 (false positive)
	−	10 (false negative)	95 (true negative)
Total		100	100

TABLE 28-6 COOKIE-O-METER FOR 99% COOKIE PREVALENCE

After Adding Actual 99% Prevalence

		Actual Cookie	
		+	−
Cookie-o-meter test result	+	8,910	5
	−	990	95
Total		9,900	100
		(99% prevalence)	

TABLE 28-7 EXAMPLE OF A COMPLETED 2 × 2 TABLE FOR QUESTION 28.6.2

		Before Adding Actual Prevalence				After Adding Actual Prevalence	
		Actual Cookie				Actual Cookie	
		+	−			+	−
Cookie-o-meter Test	+	90	5	Cookie-o-meter Test	+	900	450
	−	10	95		−	100	8,550
Total		100	100	Total		1,000	9,000
						(10% prevalence)	

Answer 28.6.3 **The correct answer is "D."** Again, you can use the 2 × 2 method or Bayes theorem. The 2 × 2 table for this question is the same as it was for the previous question (see Table 28-7). However, unlike previously, you are asked for the likelihood of a cookie if the "cookie-o-meter" says it is not a cookie and instead a dreaded kale brownie. In other words, you have been asked to calculate the false negative rate (FNR) for this scenario. The equation for the FNR is below.

$$FNR = \frac{False\ negatives}{False\ negatives + true\ negatives}\ or\ \frac{c}{c+d}$$

$$= \frac{100}{100 + 8,550} = 1\%$$

You were not asked to calculate it, but there is also a false-positive rate (FPR), which is shown below.

$$FPR = \frac{False\ positives}{False\ positives + true\ positives}\ or\ \frac{b}{a+b}$$

$$= \frac{450}{450 + 900} = 33\%$$

Clinical Pearls

- A highly sensitive test helps to rule OUT disease; a highly specific test helps to rule IN disease.

- A treatment that is statistically significantly superior to placebo (or to a comparison drug) may not offer a clinically significant benefit. Use clinical judgment when interpreting study results.

- Compare number needed to treat (NNT) with number needed to harm (NNH) when considering therapies, rather than relying on relative risk reduction. The same calculation can be done for screening tests (e.g., number of women needed to screen to avoid one breast cancer death).

- Do not draw conclusions from subgroup analyses. The only conclusion that can be drawn is, "This must be studied."

- Recognize that the utility of a test is contingent upon the sensitivity and specificity of the test and the prevalence of disease in the population being tested. Therefore, a sensitive and specific test may have a low predictive value in a population with very low disease prevalence.

- When evaluating a noninferiority study, look for the "margin" used by the investigators. This is the maximum extent of clinical difference that will be considered noninferior (e.g., a margin of 2 means twice as many events can occur in the experimental group and still be considered noninferior).

BIBLIOGRAPHY

Centre for Evidence-Based Medicine. Available at: http://www.cebm.net. Accessed June 1, 2015.

Fletcher RH, et al. *Clinical Epidemiology: The Essentials*. 5th ed. Baltimore, MD: Williams & Wilkins; 2012.

Friedland DJ, et al. *Evidence-Based Medicine*. New York, NY: McGraw-Hill; 1998.

Greenhalgh T. *How to Read a Paper: The Basics of Evidence-Based Medicine*. 5th ed. West Sussex, UK: John Wiley and Sons, Ltd, BMJ Books; 2014.

Pagano M, Gauvreau K. *Principles of Biostatistics*. 2nd ed. Australia: Duxbury Thomson Learning; 2000.

Patient-Centered Care 29

Denise A. Martinez

Note: This chapter deals with culturally responsive care and patient safety. Because not all Black patients identify as African-Americans, the authors have elected to use the term Black in this chapter as inclusive of African-Americans as well as those individuals who are of African descent but may be from another country. The authors have also elected to use the term Latinx when referring to individuals of "Hispanic" descent realizing that many individuals identify strongly with their country of origin. We also use the term "race" understanding that this is a social and not biological construct. We understand the sensitivity of this terminology and ask your understanding.

▶ CASE 29.1

You are doing a locum tenens job in Arizona on the Navajo reservation. You are seeing a lot of patients with diabetes, which reminds you that Native Americans, Latinxs, and Blacks all have a greater prevalence of diabetes compared to the general US population.

Question 29.1.1 **Which of the following is TRUE about the age-adjusted prevalence of diabetes in adults?**
A) All Alaska Native and Native American tribes have a higher prevalence of diabetes than non-Hispanic Whites (NHW)
B) Cuban Americans and South Americans have a higher prevalence of diabetes than NHW
C) Mexican Americans and Puerto Ricans have close to 90% higher prevalence of diabetes than NHW
D) Pima Indians in Mexico have the same high prevalence of diabetes as the Pima Indians in Arizona
E) Non-Hispanic Blacks have a lower prevalence of diabetes than Latinxs in the United States

Answer 29.1.1 **The correct answer is "C."** Mexican Americans and Puerto Ricans have a higher prevalence of diabetes compared with NHW ("non-Hispanic White" being the term used by the US Census Bureau). The other statements are false, and

here's how they break down. Although their diabetes prevalence is increasing rapidly, Alaska Natives historically had a 5.5% age-adjusted prevalence of diabetes compared with 7.1% for NHW. Cubans and South Americans actually have the same prevalence as NHW. The Pima Indians in Mexico whose lifestyle is not sedentary and who eat a more traditional diet actually have a diabetes prevalence of about 7%, while those in Arizona have a prevalence of 38%. Non-Hispanic Blacks have a prevalence higher than those of Latinxs and NHW but not quite as high as the Mexican Americans and Puerto Ricans.

HELPFUL TIP:
Ethnic and cultural groups are not uniform from an epidemiological or cultural belief standpoint. Hence, there are often large differences between individuals and subgroups. This is complicated further by the fact that we all belong to, and are influenced by, multiple different cultural groups. Although there are cultural patterns within healthcare, try not to adopt those patterns as stereotypes for the individuals and groups.

You are seeing a 57-year-old Navajo male with poorly controlled type 2 diabetes. You are trying to understand why his hemoglobin A_{1C} is so high since he has access to healthcare, medicines, supplies, and an amazing doctor (if you do say so yourself). You remember a lecture on culturally responsive patient-centered medicine where they talked about investigating a person's health problem using both disease and illness models.

Question 29.1.2 **The difference between disease and illness is:**
A) Disease is the biomedical explanation of the health condition; illness is the patient's experience and understanding of their health condition
B) Disease is chronic; illness is acute
C) Diseases have known causes; illnesses do not

D) Disease is more serious and frequently needs treatment; illness will resolve without medical intervention

E) Disease versus illness ... really? Aren't we just into some phony semantics here?

Answer 29.1.2 The correct answer is "A." Simply put, "disease" is the way that physicians understand a health problem and "illness" is the way the patient experiences it. The culturally responsive patient-centered model looks not only at the pathophysiology of disease, which is the focus of most of our early medical training, but also at what the patient is experiencing, how it impacts him or her, and what is the larger cultural-social-personal context of that health condition. The patient-centered physician weaves back and forth between the disease and illness model, diagnosing and treating both the disease and the illness.

You want to focus on your patient's illness in the larger context of his life and avoid just discussing glucose metabolism, diet, exercise, lab results, and medication adherence. (Your usual approach of explaining diabetes and its complications has not improved his control.) You ask him, "What has your experience with diabetes been like?" And he looks at you strangely and answers that it has been tough.

Question 29.1.3 One way to help get an understanding of his beliefs about diabetes would be to:
A) Ask if family members or tribal medical personnel are willing to share information about the intersection of cultural beliefs and care, specifically diabetes; if they share information on their cultural beliefs, listen with understanding and gratitude
B) Do a literature search on Navajo health beliefs with respect to diabetes to help formulate questions to ask him about his potential cultural beliefs
C) Ask about his experiences and beliefs about diabetes so you can have a greater understanding about his beliefs to communicate with him about care in a way to meet his needs
D) All of the above

Answer 29.1.3 The correct answer is "D." Any of these options may help you understand this patient's health beliefs. Community members can be a good source of cultural patterns. Having a general idea of a cultural belief system makes it easier to ask questions about whether those beliefs apply in this case and how. Asking the right questions will help to get more useful information. There are some canned questions that can be of assistance, including those listed here from a series of questions developed by a psychiatrist–anthropologist named Arthur Kleinman:

- What do you call your problem?
- What do you think caused your problem?
- What do you think is going on with your body?
- How have you treated this?
- What do you think helps?

- Why do you think it started when it did?
- What does your sickness do to you?
- How severe is it?
- What do you fear most about your problem?
- What are the biggest concerns that your sickness has caused for you?
- What kind of treatment do you think would be helpful?
- What are the most important results you hope to receive from the treatment?

HELPFUL TIP:
Don't feel as though you need to memorize all these specific questions. Rather, focus on asking questions that elicit information about the patient's own health beliefs in a nonjudgmental way. Another useful mnemonic that can be applied in many different contexts is "ICE," which stands for **I**deas, **C**oncerns, and **E**xpectations. For "ideas" you might ask what the patient thinks is causing his/her problem. For "concerns" you might ask what he/she is worried is causing the problem. For "expectations" you might ask what they think will happen with their problem and what they are expecting from the visit or healthcare system.

This same patient develops severe osteomyelitis of his right leg and is admitted to your inpatient service. He has not responded to several weeks of appropriate IV antibiotics and debridement. The infection is gradually spreading proximally, and a decision has been made with the patient that you will proceed with a below-the-knee amputation. Although you are confident that this is the right clinical decision, you worry about the fact that Native Americans, Latinxs, Blacks, and people from lower socioeconomic backgrounds all have disproportionally higher rates of limb amputation, even when adjusting for incidence of diabetes (with Navajos having the highest rate of all). The surgeon you are working with asks you to obtain informed consent from the patient. You have heard that Navajos believe that talking about something bad happening (i.e., informing them of the procedural risks) makes those adverse events more likely to occur.

Question 29.1.4 What is the most appropriate approach to gaining informed consent from your patient?
A) Proceed with the informed consent with the full explanation of the benefits and risks of the procedure.
B) Just tell him he needs the surgery and avoid the risk/benefit discussion.
C) Share with him the percentage chance of a good outcome and do not talk about the possible risks and complications.
D) Explain the information to a tribal leader and let the tribal leader decide what to communicate with the patient.
E) Explain the process of informed consent to the patient and allow him to opt out of any part of the process he desires to avoid.

Answer 29.1.4 **The best answer is "E."** This is a challenging situation since this patient's belief system is counter to modern Western medical practices. In order to create a culturally responsive plan of care for the patient, we should try to align our guiding medical principles with the patient's cultural beliefs. Using the four guiding principles of medical ethics (autonomy, beneficence, nonmaleficence, and justice) is one way to work through this dilemma. Some would argue for "A" because the patient cannot make an informed decision without knowing the potential risks and benefits (autonomy), and, "it's the law." However, if the patient has traditional Navajo beliefs, proceeding with the full informed consent may deter the patient from undergoing a beneficial or even life-saving procedure, which presents conflict with the principles of beneficence and nonmaleficence. "B" and "C" rely on stereotypes without making sure of the patient's beliefs. Asking a tribal leader and/or someone from the tribe who works in medicine is an excellent way of obtaining a cross-cultural perspective. However, ultimately, we need to respect the patient's autonomy.

Your patient consents to the surgery but with a request that makes you uneasy—he wants to take the amputated limb home with him after the surgery. He shares with you his cultural belief that his body needs to be buried whole in order to cross over to the next world after he dies (note that this belief is also common among orthodox Jews and others).

Question 29.1.5 **How should you NOT explain to him the potential health hazards of taking an infected limb home?**
A) Explore how other people in the community who have had amputations have managed this
B) Explain to him that you understand his concerns; however, the health risk of him taking the limb home far outweighs any other consideration so the limb will have to be disposed of by standard hospital practice
C) Allow family members and community leaders to participate in the discussion if the patient wishes
D) Negotiate a way where as much as possible his wishes could be met, personal and public health and safety preserved, and community and hospital regulations followed

Answer 29.1.5 **The correct answer is "B."** The underlying concern is that the patient's wishes are in direct conflict with traditional medical practices. Although hospital policy may limit your options, there is usually enough flexibility to allow you to accommodate the patient's wishes at least to some degree. You can use the LEARN mnemonic (**L**isten, **E**xplain, **A**cknowledge, **R**ecommend, **N**egotiate) to help approach this cultural conflict. First, you **L**isten to the patient's perspective. Often you have to probe with nonjudgmental questions to elucidate this. "C" can provide some cultural context for both the **L**istening and **N**egotiating phases. "A" would be part of **E**xplaining your perspective. Next you **A**cknowledge both the differences and similarities between the two perspectives. Then you **R**ecommend a plan hopefully where you and the patient both get what you want. Finally, as in "D," you may need to **N**egotiate.

▶ **Objectives: Did you learn to …**
- Describe some differences in diabetes prevalence among different ethnic groups?
- Define the terms "disease" and "illness"?
- Explore a patient's personal and cultural reasons for nonadherence to traditional medical advice?
- Develop some tools for providing care to patients who have health beliefs that diverge from those of traditional Western medicine?

▶ **CASE 29.2**

A young couple that just immigrated to your town from Bosnia comes to your clinic because they are expecting their first baby. The wife is a healthy 23-year-old woman and in her first trimester of pregnancy.

Your scheduler knows that many Bosnians are of the Muslim faith and has heard that female Muslims are supposed to refrain from care by male physicians.

Question 29.2.1 **When making the appointment for this patient, the scheduler should:**
A) Schedule her with the first available OB provider, regardless if it is male or female
B) Schedule her with the first available female OB provider
C) Schedule her with your only Bosnian-speaking OB provider who is male (this will cut down on the time needed for an interpreter)
D) Ask if she has a preference from whom she would like to receive care and schedule her within her preferred provider
E) Schedule her with the OB provider who has the most experience and interest in working with patients from diverse cultures (maybe Dr. Smith since he eats out at a different ethnic restaurant every night)

Answer 29.2.1 **The correct answer is "D."** Although many Muslim women would find it inappropriate to have a male provider, this is not universally true. Besides, we are not even sure this patient is of Muslim faith (only about 40% of Bosnians are Muslim)! Cultural characteristics and belief systems are generalizations that may accurately describe a population. However, if you extrapolate these generalized beliefs to the individual, you are engaging in stereotyping and may often come to the wrong conclusion.

 HELPFUL TIP:
Use your knowledge of a patient's culture as a starting point. Ask about any assumptions or suspicions in a nonjudgmental way. Make sure you know how the belief applies in the current context.

When she arrives in your clinic, you realize she speaks no English and her husband speaks only a little. Using his limited English and some hand gestures, you feel that you should conduct an interview with them. Because you completed a course entitled "Advanced Life Support for Culturally Responsive Care," you are able to deal with such a situation! Your mind drifts back to that course … ah, CME on the beach!

Question 29.2.2 You recall that "culturally responsive care" is defined as:
A) Learning about multiple cultures
B) Being able to speak multiple languages
C) Taking diversity classes
D) Adopting a set of cultural behaviors and attitudes that enable you to deliver effective medical care to people of different cultures
E) Hiring staff from a variety of different cultures—preferably all good cooks who will provide some excellent ethnic cuisine

Answer 29.2.2 The correct answer is "D." While the other answers are laudable goals, they do not define culturally responsive care. Culturally responsive care is a set of behaviors and attitudes that aims to help healthcare providers deliver better care to patients from many different cultures.

You rack your brain trying to remember why culturally responsive care is important to you. You now regret skipping some of the lectures to go snorkeling in those beautiful Hawaiian waters.

Question 29.2.3 Which of the following is NOT a benefit of providing culturally responsive care?
A) It allows efficient use of time and resources
B) It increases the chance of providing services that are consistent with patient needs
C) It might improve health outcomes for minority patients
D) It might improve patient retention
E) It is less expensive in the long run

Answer 29.2.3 The correct answer is "E." Culturally responsive care allows you to use your time and resources efficiently to increase the likelihood that you will provide the services your patient actually wants and needs. This can lead to improved health outcomes for your patients, increased patient satisfaction and retention of your minority patients (and perhaps increase your patient satisfaction scores!). Unfortunately, no studies so far have shown that it can reduce your practice costs.

HELPFUL TIP:
The National Center for Cultural Competence at Georgetown University has identified six compelling reasons that healthcare providers should incorporate culturally responsive care into their practice. They are as follows:

1. To respond to current and projected demographic changes in the United States.
2. To eliminate long-standing disparities in the health status of people of diverse racial, ethnic, and cultural backgrounds.
3. To improve the quality of services and health outcomes.
4. To meet legislative, regulatory, and accreditation mandates.
5. To gain a competitive edge in the marketplace.
6. To decrease the likelihood of liability/malpractice claims.

Pondering this, you decide to try and provide culturally responsive care to this Bosnian woman.

Question 29.2.4 Which one of the following is NOT a step in providing culturally responsive care?
A) Understanding your own culture
B) Understanding others' cultures
C) Being frustrated with having to work with people different than you
D) Understanding how your patients' cultural beliefs affect their attitude toward healthcare
E) Adapting your way of practicing to provide optimal care

Answer 29.2.4 The correct answer is "C." The goal of culturally responsive care is to provide better healthcare for patients from different cultures. Some of the specific things this goal calls for include:

• Being respectful of *potential* cultural differences
• Learning about other cultures
• Being aware of the health impact of cultural beliefs and practices
• Being sensitive to patients' needs
• Using interpreters when necessary
• Adapting practices to provide optimal care

An easy way to achieve these goals is by using the Berlin and Fowkes' LEARN model described earlier.

HELPFUL TIP:
While learning and respecting patients' different cultural beliefs is vital, *providing good care does not call for accepting practices that are detrimental to your patient's health.* But beware … there are many potential ethical dilemmas that can occur when traditional Western medicine intersects with a culture that has radically different health beliefs. Many cross-cultural medical decisions are not as dichotomous as we would like to think. Western medicine may have to bend a little to accommodate belief systems.

Now that you are ready to proceed with caring for your patient, the question of language comes up. Should you use the husband to interpret (he seems to know a bit of English)?

Question 29.2.5 To help guide you, you call your hospital compliance officer who tells you that:
A) It is Federal Law that you must provide an interpreter for patients who need it, at your own cost if necessary
B) It is Federal Law that patients must provide their own interpreters at their own expense
C) Most insurance companies reimburse for interpreter services
D) Using family and staff to translate rarely reflects current practice standard
E) There are no privacy concerns when using nonprofessional interpreters

Answer 29.2.5 The correct answer is "A." The 2010 census found that more than 60.6 million adults (around 21% of the US population) speak a non-English language at home, while almost 13% of the US population is foreign born. When the healthcare professional does not speak the primary language of the patient, there is potential for loss of important information, misunderstanding of physician instructions, and poor shared decision-making. Title VI of the 1964 Civil Rights Act requires healthcare professionals to provide interpreter services for patients who need them, at the physician's cost if necessary. Failure to do so would qualify as discrimination and could be prosecuted in a court of law. Unfortunately, most insurance companies do not reimburse for these services. Interpreters can be scarce and costly. As a result, many physicians use any help they can get for translation, including staff members and family members who are bilingual (so, "D" is a false statement); but this leaves room for error. Using a family member as an interpreter makes it hard for the patient to disclose private information they do not want known by the family. Professional interpreters have been trained and certified, while ad hoc interpreters often have no formal training and can make translation mistakes.

Question 29.2.6 Regarding provision of healthcare, language barriers may result in:
A) Increased risk of intubation for children with asthma
B) Greater nonadherence to medication regimens
C) Higher resource use in diagnostic testing
D) Increased risk of drug complications
E) All of the above

Answer 29.2.6 The correct answer is "E." Language barriers have been associated with worse health outcomes to include lower likelihood of having a usual source of medical care; lower likelihood follow-up after an emergency room visit; greater nonadherence to medication regimens; increased risk of drug complications; impaired understanding of diagnoses, medications, and need for follow-up; lower patient satisfaction; longer medical visits; higher resource utilization; increased risk of intubation for children with asthma; greater risk of being labeled with psychopathology; and increased risk of leaving the hospital against medical advice.

Question 29.2.7 What is the proper method to use an interpreter?
A) Address all questions to the interpreter while facing the interpreter
B) Address questions to the patient while looking at the interpreter
C) Address questions to the patient while facing the patient
D) Address questions to the interpreter while facing the patient
E) Have the interpreter get you coffee while you muddle through using gestures

Answer 29.2.7 The correct answer is "C." The physician should speak to and look at the patient; in other words, don't speak about the patient in the third person. Remember that nonverbal communication is important even when common languages are not shared. Be aware that seemingly universal gestures such as the "OK" sign and a "thumbs up" may have different meanings in other cultures. The physician should speak clearly and give the interpreter time to translate questions and answers. The physician should periodically pause and ensure that the patient understands the questions that are being asked. Failure to look at the patient while asking questions impairs the establishment of the physician–patient relationship and should be avoided.

You remember from medical school that there was disagreement as to the degree that a medical interpreter should function as a cultural advocate.

Question 29.2.8 Which of the following would be the most effective pre-encounter instructions for your interpreter to facilitate the best possible communication between you and your patient?
A) "Translate word-for-word all that the patient and I say. You may repeat phrases, but do not rephrase anything"
B) "When clarifying, explaining, or culturally translating concepts, make sure that you are transparent (i.e., let both parties know what you are saying and why)"
C) "Be sure to culturally translate whenever you think it is appropriate"
D) "If the patient doesn't seem to understand, go ahead and explain whatever you think that I mean"

Answer 29.2.8 The correct answer is "B." Ideally, an interpreter would do an exact translation. However, many concepts do not translate literally or have very different meanings depending on the context that surrounds them. Good interpreters are often aware when the healthcare provider and the patient do not have the same understanding of an event, concept, or plan. In this case, the translator should be sure to let each party know exactly what has been communicated. This feedback to each party is important so that the interpreter's moral values don't get projected onto the patient and unduly influence decisions made by the patient. Transparency is thus critical.

You remember that low literacy is associated with poor outcomes.

Question 29.2.9 Which of the following is FALSE?
A) Patients with low literacy have a 50% increased risk of hospitalization
B) Only about half of all patients take medications as directed
C) Low literacy is a stronger predictor of a person's health than race
D) Low literacy is only an issue among minorities and immigrants

Answer 29.2.9 The correct answer is "D." Poor health literacy skills are a stronger predictor of health status than a person's race, age, income, socioeconomic status, or employment. This relationship holds across different racial and cultural groups. Unfortunately, up to 90 million people in the United States have low literacy skills and many are ashamed to share this with their physicians. This can lead to "noncompliance" because patients cannot read prescriptions and other instructions. It is not surprising, then, that low-literacy patients have an increased risk of hospitalization. Make sure that patients ask and understand the answers to three simple questions: *What is my main problem? What do I need to do? Why is it important for me to do this?* Other suggestions to improve communication include (1) asking the patient to repeat instructions back to the physician (known as the "teach back"); (2) using basic, nonmedical language when talking to patients; and (3) allowing patients to talk uninterrupted at the beginning of the visit.

HELPFUL TIP:
Between 10% and 40% of low-income children have no books at home. A quarter of college-educated parents do not read to their young children daily. Reach Out and Read is a program designed to increase reading at home. You can employ this program to help with literacy by using the SAFER mnemonic: **S**how the book early in the visit, **S**hare the book with the child yourself (modeling the reading for the parents), **A**sk the parents about reading; **A**ssess the child's development and the parent–child relationship; give **F**eedback about what you've observed the child do and about parents' attitudes and interactions with the child, **E**ncourage the parents to read daily to the child; **E**xplain about literacy development. **R**efer to the library and literacy programs, and **R**ecord in the chart what you did. Other than giving a book and briefly reading to the child, you need not do all the activities at each visit. If your clinic is not involved in the program, you can get started at www.reachoutandread.org.

▶ **Objectives: Did you learn to …**
• Describe ways in which you inquire about a patient's culturally related health beliefs?
• Define culturally responsive care and understand its importance?
• List some complications that can occur as a result of language barriers?

• Use interpreter services effectively and appropriately?
• Describe the state of health literacy in the United States and its impact on population health?

▶ **CASE 29.3**

You are seeing a 67-year-old Black male for the first time in your clinic. He claims to be healthy but has not seen a physician for over three decades. He says, "Doctors … I try to avoid them. My wife made me come today." You tell him you are going to take a history and then perform a physical examination on him. After you are done, you tell him you recommend age-appropriate screening examinations for colon and prostate cancers. The patient politely declines both. You try to explain the importance of screening to him.

Question 29.3.1 Which of the following statements about screening is INCORRECT?
A) Prostate cancer is a leading cause of death among Black men
B) Colon cancer is a leading cause of death among Black men
C) There is clear evidence that screening for colon cancer reduces mortality in Black men
D) There is clear evidence that screening for prostate cancer among Black men saves lives
E) Prostate cancer disproportionately affects Black men

Answer 29.3.1 The correct answer is "D." There is conflicting evidence for screening for prostate cancer and its effect on mortality (see Chapter 16). Prostate cancer is the fourth leading cause of cancer death overall in the United States, and the burden of prostate cancer varies among different racial and ethnic groups. Black men have about a 60% higher incidence and a 2.4-fold higher mortality rate from prostate cancer compared with White men. Compared with White men, mortality from prostate cancer is 17% lower in Latinxs and 55% lower in Asian Americans and Pacific Islanders.

Your patient now agrees to colon cancer screening but still declines prostate cancer screening (which you decide is fine because the evidence is conflicting and especially sparse for Black males). Your examination also revealed an elevated blood pressure (BP) of 160/90 mm Hg with no abnormal cardiac, lung, or other organ system findings.

Question 29.3.2 Assuming you confirm this elevated BP reading at subsequent visits, which of the following antihypertensives would you recommend?
A) Hydrochlorothiazide
B) Ramipril
C) Minoxidil
D) Atenolol
E) Losartan

Answer 29.3.2 The correct answer is "A." While thiazide diuretics are a good choice for most patients with hypertension, they are an especially good choice in Blacks, who tend to have extremely salt-sensitive hypertension. Blacks are more likely than other patients with hypertension to have low renin levels, which make them less likely to respond to ACE inhibitors. β-Blockers also tend to be less effective in Black patients. A reasonable second-line therapy in this patient would be a calcium channel blocker such as amlodipine.

....

Your patient agrees to your medication choice, but he wants to know if the research on which you based your choice included Black people. You can confidently say yes, knowing that the ALLHAT trial specifically addressed the issue of generalizability by making sure that about a third of the 33,357 subjects were Black. However, you know this has not always been true in scientific research. In fact, you know that minorities are very underrepresented in research data on which we base our treatment choices.

Question 29.3.3 Which of the following is NOT a reason why there are few minorities in research studies?
A) Past history of abuse leading to mistrust of the healthcare system
B) Lack of representation of minorities in the medical profession
C) Discrimination
D) Overrepresentation of minorities in lower socioeconomic status
E) Minorities are more likely to volunteer for studies but are generally excluded

Answer 29.3.3 The correct answer is "E." Minorities' contact with the medical system has been fraught with abuse in the past. Possibly the most egregious example of this is the Tuskegee Syphilis Study where Black men with syphilis were recruited for a naturalistic study of the disease in the 1930s. Over 400 Black men with syphilis were recruited with 200 men without syphilis as controls. There was no informed consent, and they were told the lie that spinal taps (done for research) were a form of treatment. It was soon apparent that the death rate among those with syphilis was about twice as high as it was among the controls. When penicillin was found to be effective as a cure for syphilis in the 1940s, the participants were neither informed nor offered treatment, so the naturalistic study could continue.

These and other examples of past mistreatment by the medical community may constitute a significant source of distrust ("A") by minority patients, who are less likely to participate in research. There have also been overt and subtle discriminatory ("C") barriers against minority participation in clinical trials. Minorities are more likely to come from lower socioeconomic groups and have less education ("D"), while research subjects are generally more educated and of higher socioeconomic status. Finally, there is a significant underrepresentation of minorities in the medical profession ("B"). For example, even though Blacks comprise 13% of the population, they are only about 6% of the physician population (and only about 7% of medical students are Black). All these problems lead to difficulties recruiting minority participants for research trials.

Question 29.3.4 As of 2010, what percentage of Americans belong to a minority group?
A) 15%
B) 20%
C) 25%
D) 36%
E) 62%

Answer 29.3.4 The correct answer is "D." According to the 2010 US Census estimates, 36% of Americans are ethnic minorities, up from 31% in 2000 and 24% in 1990. Yet, only 10% of physicians are from underrepresented minority groups. This is problematic. The lack of minority physicians leads to a discrepancy in healthcare access. Data shows that minority physicians are more likely to serve minority patients and are more likely to serve in urban, underserved areas.

HELPFUL TIP:
Patients of all ethnicities consistently rate their relationships with their physician better when their physician is of the same race/ethnic background (*JAMA* 1999;282(6):583–589).

So, everybody's racist? Probably not—this phenomenon appears to be related to patient–physician communication and the patient's perception of participation in their care.

We do need to be aware of "implicit bias", however. We all have unconscious stereotypes and beliefs about groups that effects our patients treatment and relationships.

Question 29.3.5 Which of the following is NOT true?
A) Patients living in a low socioeconomic neighborhood have an increased incidence of coronary artery disease
B) Patients living in low socioeconomic neighborhoods have an increased incidence of asthma
C) Patients of the same minority group with a low socioeconomic status have the same incidence of disease as those with a high socioeconomic status
D) Very low–income Black children have a higher incidence of asthma than White children of the same socioeconomic status
E) Patients from disadvantaged neighborhoods have a higher risk of developing most cancers and are less likely to receive aggressive treatment once diagnosed

Answer 29.3.5 The correct answer is "C." Patients living in low socioeconomic neighborhoods have increased incidences of coronary artery disease, most cancers (lung, colon, cervical), diabetes, arthritis, accidents, adverse birth outcomes, and asthma. They are also likely to obtain overall less care, less aggressive care (except for limb amputations in diabetics), and are less likely to have evidence-based care. Minority patients with higher socioeconomic statuses tend to have better health when compared to their race-matched peers from lower socioeconomic statuses.

Question 29.3.6 **In taking care of Black patients, all of these cultural patterns (not stereotypes) are helpful to keep in mind EXCEPT:**
A) Family relationships are extremely important
B) Religion often has a role in the patient's life
C) It is expected that physicians will call patients by their first name
D) Food has important cultural significance
E) Nonverbal communication is often as important as what is verbally communicated

Answer 29.3.6 **The correct answer is "C."** People in the Black community often maintain extended family ties and view healthcare as a family responsibility ("A"). Therefore, physicians should consider enlisting the family's help in taking care of an ill family member.

Religion ("B") is often an important aspect in Black culture and members of the clergy are highly respected in the community. Churches are often very helpful for community outreach efforts. Evidence exists that the use of churches to conduct preventive care services, such as immunizations and screening programs for illnesses, leads to better patient compliance with preventive guidelines. Some patients may view illness as a test of one's faith, and it is prudent for the physician to acknowledge and respect the patient's beliefs and perception of illness to the extent that it influences their seeking or receiving healthcare. People from lower socioeconomic backgrounds have little choice but to eat what is available at a low cost. This means our advice to patients to eat a well-balanced diet with fresh fruit, lean meat, and fresh vegetables may be met with some challenges due to access to these resources and familial and cultural traditions ("D"). Advising simple changes in diet including substituting fish or chicken for red meat in dishes, eating inexpensive raw vegetables, modifying cooking techniques, and changing to a vegetable-based rather than a meat-based diet may be more likely to be successful.

Communication is important, with individuals in the Black community being particularly attentive to nonverbal aspects of communication such as body language and voice inflection ("E"). Respect is also emphasized in the culture, and patients often like to be addressed by their formal titles and not their first names. Asking patients' permission to call them by their first names can be appreciated.

Information using real-life examples can be a useful communication tool, instead of cold, dry data, or written messages (this actually holds true for most patients of a variety of cultures!). A useful summary of general principles to keep in mind when caring for Black patients is found in an article on Preventive Care for African Americans by Witt et al. (2002). They are as follows:

• Gaining trust and understanding the historical distrust of the healthcare system.
• Understanding and employing the kinship web in decisions regarding screening and treatment.
• Involving the church in developing and delivering prevention and care messages.

• Asking patients about the meaning of words or phrases.
• Asking patients about the use of alternative medicines and herbs.
• Tailoring messages about prevention to depictions of real-life situations.
• Paying attention to body language and other nonverbal communication.

You have learned in medical school about the importance of behavior change in the management of chronic diseases like hypertension, heart disease, and diabetes, yet are frustrated that you have less success in patients who come from low socioeconomic backgrounds or from minority racial or ethnic groups.

Question 29.3.7 **Which of the following behaviors or attributes is most strongly associated with your patient's health status:**
A) Physical activity level
B) Health insurance coverage
C) Dietary choices
D) Socioeconomic status
E) Tobacco use

Answer 29.3.7 **The correct answer is "D."** All of the other choices do have an impact on overall health. However, socioeconomic status has the highest correlation with a patient's overall health. It's like U2 says in their song *God Part II*, "The rich stay healthy; the sick stay poor." Socioeconomic status is a key driver of health status.

HELPFUL TIP:
Fresh produce is often not available or quite expensive in low socioeconomic neighborhoods (and good luck finding sustainably caught Copper River salmon). Predominantly White neighborhoods have four times as many supermarkets as predominantly Black and Latinx neighborhoods. These areas that are relatively devoid of grocery stores and/or stores with healthy foods are called "food deserts." This makes dietary modification especially difficult.

▶ **Objectives: Did you learn to …**
· Identify the impact of race on prevention and management of chronic diseases such as colon cancer screening and hypertension?
· Describe barriers to minority participation in research studies?
· Explain the impact of socioeconomic status on a patient's healthcare?
· Relate cultural patterns to the provision of healthcare education and services?

▶ CASE 29.4

Your next two patients are a couple of Cuban friends who present to your office seeking a family physician to take care of their general health needs. They are both of Cuban descent, but one looks White and the other looks Black.

Question 29.4.1 Which of the following assumptions is correct?
A) Latinx people are of one race
B) Latinx people can all speak English
C) Latinx people come from many different countries and can look different from one another
D) Latinx people are not American
E) Latinx people all like to be called Hispanic

Answer 29.4.1 The correct answer is "C." The term "Latinx" denotes an ethnic group who shares some cultural practices but not necessarily other characteristics. Latinxs comprise a significantly diverse group who may or may not speak Spanish or English, may be of any race, hail from different countries of origin, have differing histories, socioeconomic status, and cultural identities. Further, some feel the term "Hispanic" is derogatory, suggesting European ancestry, and may prefer the term Latinx. Thirteen percent of the overall US population now identifies as Hispanic or Latinx, which makes this population the largest ethnic group in the United States. Latinxs come from a broad spectrum of socioeconomic backgrounds and a variety of living conditions in the United States, which has an enormous impact on immigrant and public health.

Despite the diversity represented within the Latinx culture, there exist shared values such as strong family ties, with families often tending to be large and extended. Families frequently serve as the main source of support and share in decision-making. Physicians with a warm bedside manner who demonstrate appropriate respect (especially to the elderly) are appreciated.

HELPFUL TIP:
Despite alarmist paranoia from some parts of our political spectrum, second-generation Latinx immigrants are as likely to speak English as were prior waves of immigrants from European countries. Don't even get us started on the absurd idea of building a wall. Ever hear of ladders?

Question 29.4.2 Which of the following is FALSE regarding health issues affecting the Latinx community?
A) Infectious diseases are common
B) Fear of deportation prevents some from seeking healthcare
C) Latinxs are less likely to obtain preventative healthcare in comparison to Whites or Blacks
D) Moving to the United States can paradoxically raise the risk for habits that lead to illness such as obesity and diabetes
E) Elderly Latinxs have a higher mortality than their White counterparts

Answer 29.4.2 The correct, and false, answer is "E." Recent immigrants are often prone to infectious diseases ("A") due to inadequate housing, sanitation, and/or immunizations. Many reasons exist why patients may not get vaccinated. These include disbelief in the need for the vaccine, being unaware of the vaccine, lack of patient education by a healthcare provider, lack of transportation, and financial restrictions.

Immigrating to the United States can result in worse nutrition, obesity, a sedentary lifestyle, and an increase in smoking and risky sexual behavior in Latinas (women) ("D"). This translates, in part, into a twofold increased incidence of diabetes in Latinas. For Latinos (males), there is an increased risk of drug abuse, alcohol abuse, tobacco use, and driving under the influence. These risks increase the longer the patient lives in the United States.

Latinxs often fail to get preventive healthcare ("C"). For example, they have a lower rate of screening for diabetes and hypertension than Blacks or Whites. Some avoid presenting for healthcare because they fear being discovered by immigration authorities ("B"). Complementary and alternative practices are also common. Even though they are less likely to access healthcare, older Latinxs seem to have a similar or greater life expectancy than same-age Whites in the United States and enjoy lower mortality rates from cardiovascular diseases, cancer, and chronic illnesses. The risk of diabetes, however, is higher. This phenomenon has been described as "selective immigration" and implies a predilection for healthier individuals to immigrate to this country.

You get into a discussion on race with your new Cuban patients, and they point out several things to you that you had not thought of before.

Question 29.4.3 Which of the following is true about race?
A) It is a valid biological construct
B) It is interchangeable with ethnicity
C) All members of a certain culture are the same race
D) It is a purely social construct

Answer 29.4.3 The correct answer is "D." Race is a much politicized and emotionally charged topic in the history of the United States. Since the late 18th and early 19th centuries, attempts have been made to validate race as being biologically based to justify discriminatory practices. However, the Human Genome Project demonstrated conclusively that there is NO biological basis for race. Humans share over 99.9% of their DNA, and one cannot tell a member of one "race" from another on the basis of genetics alone. To add a wrinkle: commercially available DNA tests can place a patient in an ancestral group and clarify geographic backgrounds of ancestors, but they cannot provide the context required to identify race. "B" is incorrect. While race and ethnicity are often used interchangeably, they are not necessarily equivalent. Race is an arbitrary social construct that is given to people based on visual appearance, while ethnicity refers to people with a common country of origin, a shared ancestry, or a common history. Culture refers to a specific set of values, beliefs, and customs shared by members of a community. "C" is obviously incorrect. People from the same culture can be of different races, so one can see White and Black Latinxs from Cuba, for example.

Question 29.4.4 Which of the following health outcome disparities is FALSE?

A) White Latinxs have a higher incidence of breast and colorectal cancer than Blacks and Non-Hispanic Whites
B) Clinicians may order fewer diagnostic tests if they do not understand a patient's description of symptoms
C) Clinicians may over-compensate by ordering more tests when they do not understand what their patients are saying
D) Minority children are more likely to be evaluated and reported for suspected abuse even after controlling for likelihood of abusive injury
E) Blacks have the highest colorectal cancer mortality rates of any group in the United States

Answer 29.4.4 **The correct answer is "A."** The incidence of colorectal and breast cancer is actually lower in White Latinxs than in other Non-Hispanic Whites and Blacks. However, this does not always translate into less significant disease. There are significant disparities in healthcare quality and outcomes for minorities compared with nonminorities, even when controlling for possible confounding factors, such as income, education, and insurance. So even though Latinxs have a lower incidence of the above-named cancers, they have a similar mortality when compared with non-Latinxs. All of the rest of the statements are correct. Of particular note, Blacks have the highest colorectal cancer mortality rates. Also, of note is the fact that when toddlers of different races present with similar fractures, minority toddlers are significantly more likely to be reported for suspected abuse, even after controlling for age, insurance status, and likelihood of abuse. This is a reflection of biases and stereotyping.

HELPFUL TIP:
Minority patients are significantly less likely to receive appropriate pain medication, even after surgery and for long bone fractures. Additionally, there are often few, if any, pharmacies in poor, inner city areas that have opioids available for patients with a prescription. This adversely affects the pain management of minority patients even further.

In general, mortality rates among racial and ethnic minorities are higher for cancer, heart disease, diabetes, stroke, kidney failure, and HIV/AIDS. Minority groups are also disproportionately affected by asthma, lead poisoning, accidents, homicides, and other environmental health concerns. Some minorities experience higher infant mortality rates and are less likely to receive timely prenatal care. There are numerous other examples of healthcare disparities that exist between majority and minority groups. These include but are not limited to:

- Infant death rates for Blacks are twice that of Whites.
- Heart disease mortality rates are 40% higher in Blacks as compared with Whites.

- Latinxs are almost twice as likely as Whites to die from diabetes and are more likely to be obese and have high blood pressure than are Non-Hispanic Whites.
- Blacks are 13% less likely to undergo coronary angioplasty and one-third less likely to undergo bypass surgery than are Whites.
- Only 7% of Black and 2% of Latinx preschool children hospitalized for asthma are prescribed routine medications to prevent future hospitalizations compared with 21% of White children (not in itself a good reflection on our profession).
- The length of time between an abnormal screening mammogram and follow-up diagnostic testing is more than twice as long for Asian American, Latinxs, and Blacks compared with Whites.
- Minorities are less likely to get immunizations, mammograms, and other preventive care, even when paid for by Medicare.
- There are higher rates of uninsured and lack of physicians in minority communities, leading to reduced access to primary care.
- Minorities are less likely to get heart catheterizations, bypass grafting, dialysis, lung cancer surgery, and organ transplants.
- Blacks have 55% higher mortality rate and 6-year shorter life expectancy than Whites.
- Several studies show the deleterious effect of discrimination on health outcomes, including increasing the risk of diabetes, hypertension, depression, and preterm birth independent of other risk factors.

HELPFUL TIP:
Although perhaps not overtly racist, there is data that suggests that unconscious biases can affect our care of patients. A well-known study in the NEJM in 1999 found that, all things being equal, physicians were **60% less likely** to refer Black women for cardiac catheterization than men and Whites. Hopefully, by being made aware of this unconscious bias, its effect can be mitigated and better care provided to all patients.

▶ **Objectives: Did you learn to …**
- Describe some health disparities based on race, culture, and ethnicity?
- Delineate the differences between the terms race, culture, and ethnicity?

▶ CASE 29.5

A 35-year-old comes to your office today to establish care with you. You see the first name of "Jennifer" is on the medical record. The patient is wearing a suit and tie and has a male style haircut. The gender listed on the medical record for this patient is female. Clearly the gender identity of this patient does not match the patient's gender designated at birth.

Question 29.5.1 How do you establish rapport with this patient and use correct terminology?

A) Ask the patient first thing, "Are you a man or a woman?"

B) Use the name Jennifer as well as female pronouns she/her/hers

C) Introduce yourself and your preferred pronouns, and ask the patient for their name and preferred pronouns

D) Say that you are glad they are here and that you have never had a patient "like them" before

E) Ask if he is from Iowa as you have heard Iowa is actually a pretty progressive state (or was until our conservative legislature overturned many of the gains made)

Answer 29.5.1 **The correct answer is "C."** Biological gender, gender identity, and gender expression are all different. Biological gender is defined by one's chromosomes, hormones, and reproductive organs. The assignment of gender is generally done at birth based on the appearance of external genitalia. Some newborns might be born with ambiguous genitalia but are assigned a sex at birth of either male or female. Gender identity is a person's innate, deeply felt psychological identification, which may or may not correspond to the sex assigned to them at birth. Gender expressions are the external characteristics and behaviors that are socially defined such as dress, grooming, mannerisms, and speech patterns. These can widely vary and are accepted as masculine, feminine, or neutral. Transgender is an umbrella term for people whose gender identity is incongruent from the sex assigned to them at birth. It is important to maintain respect for patients who identify as transgender in order to establish rapport and better care for the patient. Using preferred names and pronouns is extremely important in helping to establish respect. A good way to introduce yourself to a patient would be: "My name is Dr. X, my preferred pronouns are she/her/hers or he/him/his (or other); what are your name and preferred pronouns?"

HELPFUL TIP:
Transitioning is the process that some transgender people go through to begin living their affirmed gender identity. This may or may not include changing physical appearance and dress, initiating hormone therapy, and undergoing gender confirmation procedures and/or surgery. Treatment for transgender persons, including hormone therapy and surgery, has been deemed medically necessary to treat gender dysphoria. As with every community, there is a great deal of diversity within the transgender community, and each transgender person's transition is unique and may or may not include everything listed.

Jennifer indicates she actually prefers to go by female pronouns as she is of the female *biological sex*. However, she also prefers to identify and express herself as male *gender* at times. She returns to your office for an annual physical examination. She discloses on her intake form that she is in a long-term, monogamous relationship, but the sex of the partner is not asked on your intake form (which needs updating!) and thus isn't specified for you. She has regular periods and is not currently on birth control.

Question 29.5.2 Which of the following questions should you ask the patient:

A) "Are you using condoms with sexual activity?"

B) "What does your boyfriend/husband do for a living?"

C) "Would you like a pregnancy test today?"

D) "Are you sexually active with men, women, or both?"

E) You don't address the subject as you assume she is sexually active and already using protection to prevent pregnancy as she is in a stable relationship

Answer 29.5.2 **The correct answer is "D."** It can be very uninviting to patients when assumptions are made about the gender of the patient's sex partner(s). Knowing the patient's sexual identity (gay/lesbian, bisexual, heterosexual) as well as their past, current, and anticipated future sexual partner(s) and behavior is essential to providing comprehensive preventative screening and guidance. It is important to not assume the sexual identity or behavior of the patient, but rather ask a complete sexual health history prior to offering treatment or care to the patient.

▶ **Objectives: Did you learn to …**
- Describe the differences between biological sex, gender identity, and gender expression?
- Establish rapport by eliciting preferred pronouns?
- Obtain an appropriate sexual history without making assumptions regarding the patient's gender and sexual identities?

▶ **CASE 29.6**

You are on the board of your hospital's quality and safety committee and you have been asked to address the issue of a medication error. Ms. Jones, a 72-year-old patient with diabetes who was hospitalized for an acute myocardial infarction, died from what seems to be a sudden cardiac event. This was unexpected as she was recovering rather well. One of the nurses on the floor had told her supervisor that your partner, Dr. McTremble, had written an order for 6.0 U of insulin; but the new nurse, fresh out of nursing school, had misread this as 60 U of insulin and had proceeded to give the poor lady that amount, precipitating the hypoglycemic event that led to her death. The nurse is distressed as she thought she was only following orders. Around your office, Dr. McTremble's handwriting is a thing of legend: many pharmacists have had to call to double-check his prescriptions on more than one occasion. Time to move to electronic prescribing…

Question 29.6.1 Which of the following would have been an effective way to prevent the type of error that occurred?

A) The nurse should have called to confirm the dose of insulin before giving it

B) Writing out "units" rather than "U" and "6" instead of "6.0"

C) Use of computerized physician order entry
D) Having a clinical pharmacist as part of the team
E) All of the above

Answer 29.6.1 The correct answer is "E." It is estimated that between 44,000 and 98,000 deaths annually are attributable to medical errors, most of which are preventable. Although the numbers have been challenged, it is indisputable that medical errors continue to contribute to adverse outcomes in our patients. One of the most significant contributors to serious errors is mistakes in dosing and administering medication. One of the leading causes of medication errors is the use of potentially dangerous abbreviations and dose designations. The use of "U" as above has been reported in the literature to be problematic as it can easily be misread as a zero or a four, leading to up to 10-fold overdoses that can often have terrible consequences in patients using insulin. A decimal point may not be seen, leading to a factor 10 error (60 units of insulin being given rather than 6).

Question 29.6.2 Which of these would NOT be recommended as a way to prevent prescription errors (we will give you this one)?
A) Computerized order entry systems
B) A brief notation of the purpose for the prescription
C) Metric system for all therapies except those like insulin and vitamins that use standard units
D) Inclusion of age, and when appropriate, weight of the patient
E) A trailing zero after a decimal

Answer 29.6.2 The correct answer is "E." Nurses and pharmacists may not see the decimal point and thus give an order of magnitude higher dose of medication. All of the other options are recommended to help decrease medication errors and, thus, adverse patient events.

▶ **Objective: Did you learn to …**
· Recognize some causes of medication errors and ways to prevent them?

 QUICK QUIZ: HIPAA, HIPAA, HOORAY!

Which of these is prohibited by Health Insurance Portability and Accountability Act (HIPAA)?
A) Calling out patients' names in the waiting room
B) Leaving a message on a patient's answering machine or voicemail
C) Releasing health information to a specialist without patient authorization if that information is to be used for purposes of treatment, payment, or health operations
D) Faxing patient information
E) None of the above

The correct answer is "E." Since the HIPAA went into effect, many physicians have been confused as to what they can and cannot do under the HIPAA law. Providers can still call out patients' names in the waiting room ("A") as long as you do not go into particulars of their presenting complaint in front of other people (e.g., don't say to the whole waiting room, "Ms. Smith, I'm ready to check on your herpes infection"). You may leave a message on a patient's voicemail ("B") if the patient has authorized you to do so. You may fax information ("D") once you verify the fax number is correct—but you can only fax to persons the patient designates or consents to. If you fax health information to a wrong number, you are responsible and could be violating HIPAA. Finally, HIPAA gives physicians broad leeway in sharing information with other physicians, provided the information is used for treatment, payment, and healthcare operations ("C"). You must give a notice of your privacy practices to the patients and ask them to sign a form acknowledging receiving the notice or make a good-faith effort to get them to sign it.

Clinical Pearls

○ Always offer interpreter services to a patient if you do not speak their language. When using an interpreter, maintain eye contact with and address questions to the patient.

○ Do not overestimate the legal authority of the Health Insurance Portability and Accountability Act (HIPAA). Transmission of protected information is allowable for ongoing patient care.

○ Do not make assumptions about sexuality or gender. Simply ask. Same goes for race, ethnicity, etc.

○ Everyone possesses unconscious biases. Unconscious biases affect the care of patients. Simply recognizing these biases may mitigate their detrimental effects on patient care.

○ Gender identity and gender expression are affected by but are separate from sex assigned at birth. Ask transgender patients their preferred pronouns.

○ In addressing nonadherence, consider a patient's cultural background and enquire into how their cultural beliefs may conflict with those of traditional Western medicine.

BIBLIOGRAPHY

American Medical Association. *Cultural Competence Compendium: Section IV: Specific Populations Needs and Resources.* Chicago, IL: American Medical Association Press; 1999:153–178. Available at http://ww4.mgh.org/Physicians/Shared%20Documents/physicianCulturalCompendium.pdf. Accessed March 10, 2019.

Diaz VA Jr. Cultural factors in preventive care: Latinos. *Prim Care.* 2002;29(3):503–517.

Human Rights Campaign. Sexual Orientation and Gender Identity Definitions. Available at http://www.hrc.org/resources/entry/sexual-orientation-and-gender-identity-terminology-and-definitions. Accessed March 10, 2019.

Institute of Medicine Committee on Understanding and Eliminating Racial and Ethnic Disparities in Healthcare. Smedley BD, Stith AY, Nelson AR, eds. *Unequal Treatment:*

Confronting Racial and Ethnic Disparities in Health Care. Washington, DC: National Academies Press; 2003. Available at http://books.nap.edu/books/030908265X/html/. Accessed March 10, 2019.

National Center for Cultural Competence. Available at http://nccc.georgetown.edu. Accessed March 10, 2019.

National Coordinating Council on Medication Error Reporting and Prevention. Recommendations to enhance accuracy of prescription/medication order writing. Revised October 22, 2014. Available at http://www.nccmerp.org/recommendations-enhance-accuracy-prescription-writing. Accessed March 10, 2019.

Witt D, Brawer R, Plumb J. Cultural factors in preventive care: African-Americans. *Prim Care.* 2002;29(3):487–493.

Yarnall KS, Pollak KI, Østbye T, et al. Primary care: is there enough time for prevention? *Am J Public Health.* 2003;93(4):635–641.

Final Examination

30

Mark A. Graber, Jason K. Wilbur, and Brigit E. Ray

This is your final examination. See how you do. …

1) Which of the following IS NOT an *absolute* contraindication to cardiac exercise testing?
A) Unstable angina
B) Recent pulmonary embolism
C) Active pericarditis
D) Left bundle branch block

See question 2.2.2.

2) Which of the following is the preferred antiplatelet drug for treating chest pain in the emergency department?
A) Aspirin 81 mg PO
B) Aspirin 325 mg PO
C) Clopidogrel 75 mg PO
D) Clopidogrel 300 mg PO
E) Abciximab (ReoPro, a glycoprotein 2B/IIIA inhibitor)

See question 2.1.4.

3) This ECG, shown in Figure 30-1, represents a(n):
A) Inferior wall MI
B) Anterior wall MI
C) Inferolateral MI
D) Normal ECG
E) Pericarditis

See question 2.17.3.

4) The most appropriate initial treatment of this rhythm in a stable patient, shown in Figure 30-2, is:
A) Amiodarone
B) Adenosine
C) Diltiazem
D) Lidocaine

See question 2.3.5.

5) You admit a patient to the hospital after an episode of chest pain. The patient has a history of chronic kidney disease stage 4, type 2 diabetes mellitus, hypertension, hyperlipidemia, and obesity. At time of admission, troponin is elevated at 0.06 (normal <0.03). The medical student rotating with you on her family medicine clerkship asks the significance of the elevated troponin. You tell her which of the following?
A) An elevated troponin is always indicative of cardiac ischemia/infarct
B) Troponin rises after creatine phosphokinase (CPK) and stays elevated for a longer period of time
C) Pulmonary embolism and renal failure are two causes of an elevated troponin
D) CPK is overall the most sensitive (but not specific) cardiac marker for cardiac ischemia

See question 2.1.2: Helpful Tip.

6) Which of the following is true in a patient with known coronary artery disease?
A) A coronary calcium score will help to risk stratify this patient
B) The LDL goal is 90 mg/dL or less
C) A high sensitivity CRP (hsCRP) will help to risk stratify this patient
D) There is no LDL goal. Just start a maximal dose of a statin at time zero; there is no need to titrate the statin up

See questions 2.22.3 and 2.22.6: Helpful Tip.

7) Which of the following IS NOT a contraindication to the use of tPA in MI?
A) Blood pressure of >180/110 mm Hg
B) Noncompressible vascular puncture (e.g., subclavian line)
C) Major surgery within 3 weeks
D) Menstrual bleeding

See question 2.1.10 and Table 2-1B.

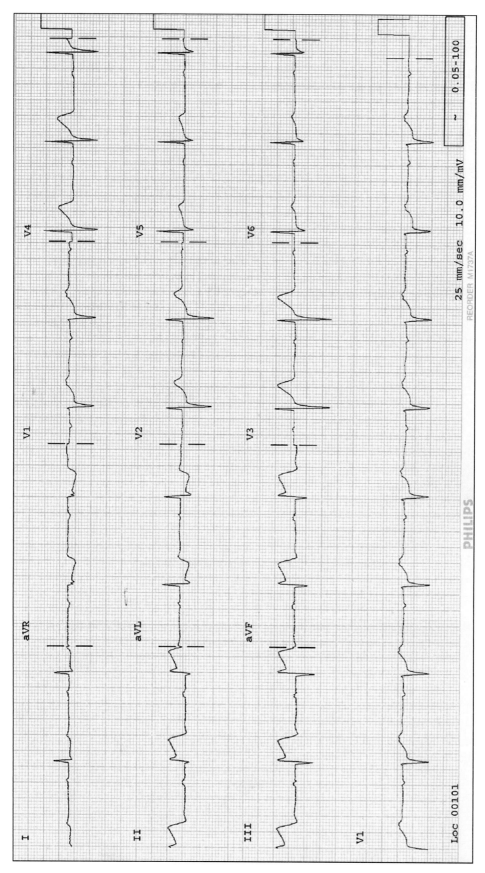

FIGURE 30-1.   Figure for Question 3.

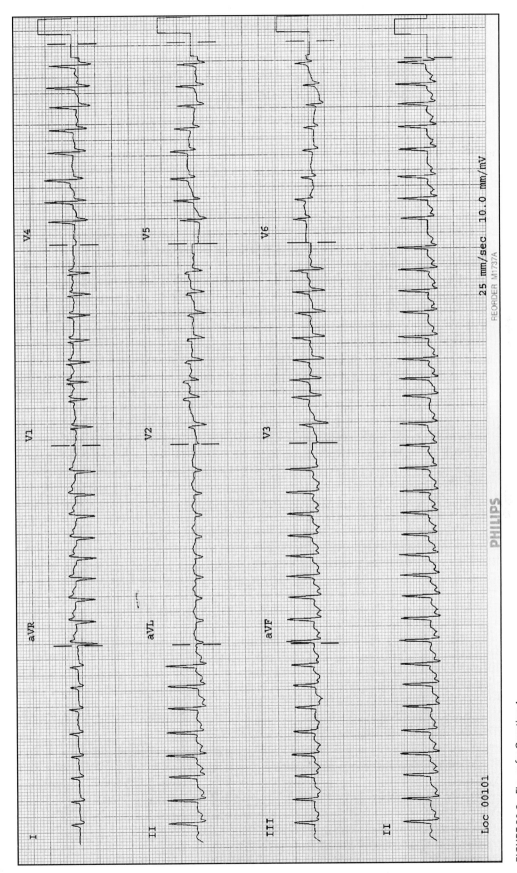

FIGURE 30-2. Figure for Question 4.

8) Which of the following IS NOT necessary for a class 1 indication for tPA in a patient with an acute myocardial infarction?

A) Greater than 1 mm ST elevation in 2 or more contiguous leads

B) Pain for less than 2 hours

C) Age <75

D) New complete left bundle branch block and typical history suggestive of MI

See question 2.1.10 and Table 2-1A.

9) Your patient has an elevation of his liver function tests (LFTs) after starting an HMG-CoA reductase inhibitor (i.e., statin). When would you consider stopping this patient's HMG-CoA reductase inhibitor?

A) Doubling of LFTs

B) Tripling of LFTs

C) Quadrupling of LFTs

D) Only when there is biopsy evidence of bridging fibrosis

See question 2.22.7.

10) Which medication(s) is (are) indicated in a patient with atrial fibrillation and a CHA2DS2-VASC score of 3?

A) Aspirin

B) Warfarin, rivaroxaban, dabigatran, or apixaban

C) Aspirin-dipyridamole (Aggrenox)

D) Clopidogrel

See question 2.4.1 and Table 2-6B.

11) Which of the following DOES NOT improve cardiovascular mortality in systolic heart failure (heart failure with reduced ejection fraction or HFrEF)?

A) Digoxin

B) Spironolactone

C) ACE inhibitors

D) Beta-blockers

See question 2.7.7.

12) Which statement is true regarding gastric lavage in a patient with a toxic ingestion?

A) Gastric lavage is of benefit even if it has been more than 1.5 hours, but less than 4 hours, since the ingestion

B) Gastric lavage should be done until the returned material is clear (maximum of 10 L)

C) Gastric lavage is associated with esophageal injury and aspiration

D) Gastric lavage is indicated for petroleum distillates within 1 hour of ingestion

See question 1.1.2.

13) Human papilloma virus (HPV) vaccine is indicated for all of the following EXCEPT:

A) All otherwise healthy 11- to 12-year-olds (boys and girls)

B) A 47-year-old female who has never been sexually active

C) An 18-year-old male with known HPV

D) Immunosuppressed 15-year-old female who is HIV positive

E) A 22-year-old female with cervical dysplasia

See question 14.5.3.

14) Topical tretinoin (Retin-A) is most effective in what kind of acne?

A) Cystic/nodular

B) Inflammatory papular

C) Pustular

D) Comedonal

See question 17.8.3: Helpful Tip.

15) In a study of drug A, 50% of patients in the treatment arm benefit versus 25% in the placebo group. What is the number needed to treat?

A) 2

B) 4

C) 6

D) 8

See question 28.3.1.

16) You are seeing a 27-year-old male in your clinic for evaluation of a rash which began about 2 days ago and is erythematous and macular with a pale center. He notes the rash itches. He denies any new lotions or creams. He has had recent cold-like symptoms including a sore throat. He has a past history only notable for chicken pox as a child. He is sexually active with several female partners. You diagnose him with erythema multiforme. He asks what could have trigged this. You counsel him that the *most* common cause of erythema multiforme is:

A) Herpes zoster

B) Streptococcal pharyngitis

C) Genital herpes

D) Rhus exposure ("poison ivy")

See Chapter 17 Quick Quiz: Erythema Multiforme.

17) "Sensitivity" is best defined as:

A) True positive rate/(true positive rate + false negative rate)

B) True positive rate/(prevalence of disease)

C) True positive rate/(true positive rate + true negative rate)

D) True positive rate/(true positive rate + false positive rate)

See Case 28.6.

18) Which of the following is true regarding isotretinoin (Accutane)?
A) Women should be on one form of birth control before using this drug
B) Pregnancy should be avoided for 3 months after discontinuation of this drug
C) Monthly pregnancy tests should be done on all women of reproductive age
D) Isotretinoin may increase the HDL

See question 17.8.4: Helpful Tip.

19) In general, what will happen with an innocent flow murmur during a Valsalva maneuver?
A) It gets louder
B) It gets softer
C) It is unchanged in volume
D) The sound becomes more harsh
E) It disappears entirely

See question 14.3.1.

20) What blood level of morphine is the most appropriate when treating pain from a terminal cause?
A) 1 µg/dL
B) 5 µg/dL
C) 10 µg/dL
D) Blood levels are irrelevant in determining the appropriate dose of morphine

See question 27.2.4: Helpful Tip.

21) Which of the following is NOT seen with an anticholinergic overdose?
A) Dry, flushed skin
B) Miosis
C) Confusion
D) Low-grade fever

See Chapter 1 Quick Quiz: Toxidromes and Table 1-1.

22) Which of the following IS NOT a cause of an elevated anion gap acidosis?
A) Methanol and other ingestions (e.g., salicylate)
B) Diabetic ketoacidosis
C) Uremia
D) GI bicarbonate loss

See question 1.4.3 and Table 1-3.

23) Reperfusion of extremities in hypothermia can cause all of the following EXCEPT:
A) Acidosis
B) Hypokalemia
C) Paradoxical central temperature drop
D) Arrhythmia

See question 1.12.3.

24) What is the appropriate course of action after treating a child with croup with inhaled epinephrine?
A) Admission for observation
B) Admission if room air oxygen saturation is less than or equal to 95%
C) Observation for 12 hours followed by discharge if stable
D) Observation for 2 hours followed by discharge if stable

See question 1.24.5.

25) Which of the following is NOT included in the "Coma Cocktail" for the unconscious patient?
A) Glucose
B) Thiamine
C) Naloxone (Narcan)
D) Flumazenil (Romazicon)

See question 1.20.1.

26) Which of the following is indicated in the child with croup (laryngotracheobronchitis) presenting to the emergency department?
A) Amoxicillin
B) Azithromycin
C) Dexamethasone
D) Oral theophylline

See question 1.24.4.

27) You are evaluating a 22-year-old woman in the ED who presents with left-sided pelvic pain. She is sexually active with men and does a poor job of remembering her oral contraceptive; condom use is only sporadic. Her last menses was 6 weeks prior. You are concerned about a possible ectopic pregnancy. Which of the following is true?
A) A negative pregnancy test effectively rules out ectopic pregnancy
B) Absence of an adnexal mass effectively rules out ectopic pregnancy
C) Every woman of reproductive age with a uterus in the ED with abdominal pain is pregnant until proven otherwise
D) The hCG should double every 5 days early in a normal pregnancy. Any less than this is indicative of an ectopic pregnancy

See questions 1.19.1 and 1.19.4.

28) Which of the following is the *one best drug* indicated for dyspnea in the terminally ill patient?
A) Buccal scopolamine
B) Lorazepam or other benzodiazepine
C) Morphine or other opiate
D) Nebulized lidocaine
E) Albuterol via inhaler

See question 27.1.6.

29) What is the one best drug to reduce headache and confusion secondary to CNS tumor with surrounding edema?
A) Acetaminophen
B) Dexamethasone
C) Morphine
D) Sumatriptan

Chapter 27 Quick Quiz: More than a little headache.

30) You are called by an anxious mother about her 3-year-old daughter who accidentally ingested lemon-lime smelling household cleaner at her grandparent's house thinking it was soda. Mom has been instructed by her parents, who were born in the late 1950s, that she should give ipecac to induce vomiting of the substance. You counsel her that ipecac:
A) Should not be used
B) Can be used if the ingestion may cause mental status changes
C) Is effective if used within 30 minutes of an ingestion
D) Is available over the counter in American pharmacies

See questions 1.1.1 and 1.22.5.

31) How frequently should methadone be dosed when used for pain control in the terminally ill?
A) Once daily
B) Every 8 to 12 hours
C) Every 4 to 6 hours
D) Methadone should not be used for pain management in the terminally ill

See question 27.2.6: Helpful Tip.

32) A 46-year-old male presents to clinic for evaluation of left shoulder pain. He has been taking over-the-counter ibuprofen 600 mg every 8 hours for the last 4 weeks. He is wondering if there are any possible long-term side effects of taking this medication. Most notably, he is concerned, as his wife has told him that ibuprofen can "tear up the gut." You tell him that NSAIDs, such as ibuprofen, can cause ulceration in:
A) The stomach
B) The duodenum
C) The colon
D) All of the above

See question 7.4.5: Helpful Tip.

33) What is true about the treatment of gastroesophageal reflux disease (GERD)?
A) Treatment of *Helicobacter pylori* is effective in curing GERD
B) Treatment should always start with a proton pump inhibitor
C) Surgical options (e.g., fundoplication) are often suboptimal with patients still requiring medication
D) Esomeprazole is vastly superior to omeprazole

See questions 7.1.3 and 7.1.4.

34) Which of the following is true regarding Barrett esophagus?
A) All patients with GERD should have an endoscopy to stage their disease vis-à-vis Barrett esophagus
B) Barrett esophagus is a change from the normal columnar epithelium to squamous epithelium
C) Barrett esophagus is present in >50% of patients with GERD
D) Barrett esophagus can regress with adequate treatment of GERD

See questions 7.1.2 and 7.1.5.

35) Which of the following lesions is considered premalignant on colonoscopy?
A) Inflammatory polyps
B) Hyperplastic polyps
C) Tubular adenoma/adenomatous polyps
D) Hamartomatous polyps

See question 7.5.4: Helpful Tip.

36) Which of the following histories in a patient with GERD is most concerning for serious underlying disease?
A) Food bolus impaction on two separate occasions
B) Dysphagia to solids followed in several months with dysphagia to liquids
C) Reflux of undigested food at night
D) Halitosis

See question 7.1.1.

37) Which of the following is NOT an appropriate test of cure for *H. pylori*?
A) Stool antigen test done 1 month after finishing treatment
B) Serum antibody test done 3 months after finishing treatment
C) CLO test done 1 month after finishing treatment
D) Breath urea test done 1 month after finishing treatment

See question 7.4.5.

38) Which of the following is true about a gastric feeding tube in the demented elderly?
A) It increases the patient's quality of life
B) It reduces the risk of pneumonia
C) It reduces mortality
D) It does nothing to improve quality of life but can cause complications

See question 21.5.14.

39) Which of the following is NOT a component of CREST syndrome?
A) **C**alcinosis
B) **R**enal failure
C) **E**sophageal dysmotility
D) **S**clerodactyly
E) **T**elangiectasia

See question 11.10.4.

40) Which of these drugs is indicated for control of an *acute* flare of Crohn disease?
A) Any 5-ASA moiety
B) Oral prednisone
C) Sulfasalazine
D) Thalidomide
E) Metronidazole

See questions 7.6.4 and 7.6.5.

41) Which of the following is a contraindication to use of sulfasalazine in Crohn disease?
A) Aspirin allergy
B) Heme-positive stools
C) Fever
D) Platelet count <100,000

See question 7.6.6.

42) Which of the following is the best screening test for hepatitis C virus (HCV)?
A) Quantitative HCV PCR
B) Hepatitis C antibody
C) Recombinant Immunoblot Assay (RIBA)
D) Qualitative HCV PCR

See question 7.10.1.

43) Which of the following is the most specific test for gluten enteropathy (nontropical sprue)?
A) Antiendomysial IgA antibody
B) Tissue transglutaminase antibody
C) Antigliadin antibody
D) Hydrogen breath test

See question 7.8.4.

44) *C. difficile* colitis has been linked to all of the following EXCEPT:
A) Hospitalization
B) Use of fluoroquinolones
C) Use of PPIs
D) Use of H_2 blockers
E) Use of metronidazole

See question 8.2.3: Helpful Tip.

45) You are seeing a 25-year-old female who works at a day care where there was a recent *Giardia* outbreak. She has been experiencing diarrhea, malaise, and nausea. You are concerned she may have contracted *Giardia*. Which of the following is recommended for treating *Giardia*?
A) Metronidazole
B) Vancomycin
C) Ciprofloxacin
D) Azithromycin
E) Mebendazole

See question 7.8.2: Helpful Tip.

46) You recently diagnosed a 30-year-old female with celiac disease. She is wondering what foods she should avoid. Which of the following foods DOES NOT contain gluten?
A) Wheat
B) Rye
C) Sticky (glutinous) Rice
D) Barley

See question 7.8.6.

47) Which of the following tests is the most sensitive for the diagnosis of bacterial overgrowth syndrome (of the GI tract)?
A) Urea breath test
B) D-Xylose breath test
C) Hydrogen breath test
D) CLO test

See question 7.8.3.

48) Treatment of hepatitis C with interferon is indicated as primary therapy for which of these patients?
A) Genotype 1
B) Genotype 2
C) Genotype 3
D) Interferon is no longer recommended as a primary therapy

See question 7.10.6.

49) Routine prenatal screening in the first trimester includes all of the following EXCEPT:
A) Blood type and antibody screen
B) Hepatitis B surface antigen
C) HIV antibody
D) MSAFP (maternal serum alpha-fetoprotein)
E) Rubella antibody

See question 15.1.7: Helpful Tips.

50) A 22-year-old G2 P2 female is ready to leave the hospital on postpartum day 2 after a normal spontaneous delivery, but she develops lower abdominal pain and fever. She denies urinary symptoms. She reports constipation and moderate lochia. Her temperature is 38.8°C. She had prolonged rupture of membranes and prolonged labor, and the placenta was removed manually. The most appropriate course of action now is:
A) Discharge with acetaminophen for fever and follow-up in 2 days
B) Discharge with amoxicillin and follow-up in 2 days

C) She likely has endometritis. Keep the patient in the hospital and obtain cultures for gonorrhea and chlamydia. Start oral penicillin

D) She likely has endometritis. Keep the patient in the hospital and start IV gentamicin and clindamycin

E) Manual exploration of the uterus for retained placenta

See question 15.2.9.

51) A 21-year-old G0 female presents for a physical examination and her first Pap smear. She has recently become sexual activity and has one lifetime partner. The results of the Pap smear show low-grade squamous intraepithelial lesion (LSIL). In accordance with guidelines, you recommend:

A) Immediate colposcopy

B) Immediate referral for excisional procedure

C) Return in 12 months for Pap smear

D) Do HPV on current sample and if negative, return in 3 years for Pap smear

E) Return in 6 months for colposcopy and Pap smear

See question 15.12.8: Helpful Tip.

52) A 48-year-old female presents with menopausal symptoms. She has had a total hysterectomy but her ovaries are intact. She would like to know the benefits and risks of taking estrogen-only hormone replacement therapy (HRT). You tell her that estrogen-only HRT is associated with:

A) Decreased risk of myocardial infarction

B) Decreased risk of ovarian cancer

C) Increased risk of colon cancer

D) Increased risk of osteoporosis

E) Increased risk of stroke

See question 15.14.3.

53) A 25-year-old G5P4 female at 28 weeks of gestation presents to labor and delivery with abdominal pain. The pain is sharp or tearing and located in her lower abdomen. She has not had any contractions. She just began to have a little vaginal spotting before she came in. Her pregnancy has been complicated by tobacco use and hypertension. What is the most likely diagnosis?

A) Cervical cancer

B) Normal labor

C) Placenta previa

D) Placental abruption

E) Uterine rupture

See question 15.2.1: Helpful Tip.

54) The USPSTF recommends screening for osteoporosis in:

A) All adults aged 65 and older

B) All men aged 75 and older

C) All women aged 65 and older

D) All women at onset of menopause

E) Women who smoke at age 50 and older

See question 21.2.3.

55) A 79-year-old male presents with his wife who complains that he has been more forgetful over the past month. The patient agrees and complains of forgetting where he put things, where the car is parked, and names of acquaintances. Also, he is more irritable and angers easily. He has trouble sleeping, and he has lost 5 lbs. He is healthy and takes no medications. He has poor eye contact, a blunted affect, and poor concentration. Neurologic exam is intact. His vitals and physical examination are otherwise normal. He can recall three items and draw a clock with no difficulty. The most likely cause of his symptoms is:

A) Delirium due to metastatic carcinoma

B) Delirium due to underlying systemic infection

C) Delirium due to Alzheimer disease

D) Dementia due to stroke

E) Depression

See question 21.5.2.

56) You are considering treating a 65-year-old male with supplemental testosterone due to low serum testosterone levels associated with fatigue, muscle weakness, and mild depression. After initiating testosterone, it is most important to check which of the following?

A) Creatinine

B) Hemoglobin

C) Potassium

D) Sodium

See question 16.7.3.

57) Delirium in the hospitalized elderly patient can be prevented by implementing all of the following interventions upon admission EXCEPT:

A) Assuring patient has access to usual aides (hearing aids, glasses, etc.)

B) Early mobilization

C) Lorazepam 1 mg QHS

D) Noise reduction at night

E) Orientation stimuli

See questions 21.3.4 and 21.3.5.

58) A 75-year-old male with mild dementia, atrial fibrillation (not on anticoagulation), osteoarthritis, and depression presents after sustaining a fall in his home 1 week ago. His son states, "He is a little banged up but otherwise fine." Your routine evaluation should include all of the following EXCEPT:

A) Asking about potential neglect and abuse

B) CT scan of the brain

C) Medication review

D) Neurological examination

E) Observation of the patient ambulating

See questions 21.4.1 and 21.4.2.

59) A 75-year-old female fell and injured her hip. She did not fracture it but has significant pain. She has a remote history of peptic ulcer disease. She takes lisinopril for hypertension and phenytoin for a seizure disorder. Which analgesic medication will be safest to initiate in this patient for her moderate pain?

A) Aspirin

B) Meperidine

C) Acetaminophen

D) Piroxicam

E) Fentanyl transdermal patch

See question 21.6.2.

60) An 80-year-old female nursing home resident with dementia recently started refusing medication and slapping at the staff when they try to bathe her. The nurse at the care center calls to request "something for her agitation." As the safest and most effective intervention, you recommend:

A) A behavior log to track when the agitation occurs and what might be causing it

B) Haloperidol 1 mg IV prior to bathing and medication administration

C) Haloperidol 1 mg PO BID

D) Restraints with bathing

E) Alprazolam 1 mg PO TID

See question 21.6.9.

61) The most appropriate next step for a 60-year-old male with a PSA level 12.5 ng/mL (normal range <4.0) is:

A) One month of a fluoroquinolone followed by repeat rectal examination and PSA

B) Referral for prostate biopsy

C) Repeat PSA in 6 to 12 months

D) Transrectal ultrasound of the prostate

E) Treatment of benign prostatic hyperplasia with terazosin

See question 16.8.3.

62) A 33-year-old male with depression had been taking paroxetine 60 mg daily for a year for depression. Due to sexual problems, he decided to try another medication, and his doctor prescribed bupropion. He stopped the paroxetine one day and started bupropion the next. He comes in 5 days later feeling dizzy, nauseated, and fatigued. He complains of myalgias, feelings of "electric shocks," and insomnia. These symptoms are most likely due to:

A) Adverse effects of bupropion

B) Hyperthyroidism

C) Major depression

D) Serotonin syndrome

E) Discontinuation of paroxetine

See question 23.9.1 and Table 23-1.

63) Concussion is defined as:

A) A disturbance in brain function caused by trauma

B) A traumatic event resulting in the loss of consciousness

C) A neurologic symptom that does not resolve within the first 24 hours of a traumatic injury

D) Absolutely any trauma involving the head and/or neck

See question 14.8.1: Helpful Tip.

64) A 17-year-old female runner with secondary amenorrhea should be further evaluated with all of the following EXCEPT:

A) Assessing calcium intake

B) MRI of the pituitary

C) Screening for eating disorders

D) Urine beta-hCG

See questions 14.2.2 and 14.2.4.

65) Gynecomastia in an adolescent male occurs as a response to which of the following mechanisms?

A) Excessive dehydroepiandrosterone

B) Excessive estrogen compared with testosterone

C) Excessive growth hormone

D) Excessive progesterone compared with testosterone

E) Rapidly developing obesity

See question 16.5.2.

66) Treatment of a patient in diabetic ketoacidosis (DKA) includes all of the following EXCEPT:

A) Aggressive volume replacement

B) Frequent glucose monitoring

C) Insulin

D) Potassium

E) Sodium bicarbonate

See questions 10.9.1 and 10.9.4.

67) A 30-year-old male presents with difficulty obtaining an erection sufficient for penetration. He has acid reflux and takes cimetidine. He reports a good relationship with his wife and denies depression. He does not smoke and rarely drinks alcohol. The most appropriate intervention at this time is:

A) To order a testosterone level

B) To perform cardiac stress testing

C) To refer him to a urologist

D) To replace cimetidine with omeprazole

E) To send him to a psychologist

See question 16.10.3.

68) Of the following, the *most* frequent side effect of metformin is:
A) Diarrhea
B) Hypoglycemia
C) Lactic acidosis
D) Renal failure
E) Weight loss

See question 10.10.7.

69) A 40-year-old male presents with generalized weakness for 1 month. He has lost some weight, perhaps 10 lb. He briefly lost consciousness yesterday while getting out of bed. He denies depression, drug or alcohol use, and any significant medical history. He is hypotensive but not tachycardic. He has orthostatic hypotension as well. Lab tests reveal mild anemia, low sodium, elevated potassium, and normal TSH, BUN, creatinine, and glucose. He is surprisingly tan for being a Caucasian farmer in the winter. (Did he just return from Cancun? No. He's not traveled. Good question.) To confirm your presumptive diagnosis, you order (which is the *best* test):
A) 24-hour urine catecholamines
B) Free T4 and T3
C) Cosyntropin stimulation test
D) Serum cortisol and adrenocorticotropic hormone (ACTH)
E) Serum testosterone

See question 10.8.2: Helpful Tips.

70) A 62-year-old female presents to the emergency department with a sudden "hole" in her right visual field developing today. She also has a right temporal headache present for the last 2 weeks, shoulder and neck pain for a month, and weight loss of 5 lbs. She is slightly hypertensive and has a prominent tender vessel at the right side of her head. Her CBC is normal but the ESR is 85 mm/hr. What is the most appropriate course of action?
A) Administer IV methylprednisolone and admit for further evaluation
B) Admit for cardiac monitoring and rule out myocardial infarction
C) Discharge to home with oral antibiotics
D) Discharge to home with referral to an ophthalmologist in the next week
E) Perform a CT scan of the brain and discharge to home if normal

See question 11.2.7.

71) You find a new and suspicious skin lesion in a patient who has had a liver transplant for hepatitis C and is on immunosuppressive therapy. You plan to perform a biopsy. If the skin lesion turns out to be malignant, it will most likely be:
A) Basal cell carcinoma
B) Distant metastasis from liver cancer
C) Melanoma
D) Squamous cell carcinoma
E) Kaposi sarcoma

See question 17.3.2.

72) The fractional excretion of sodium (FENa) is useful for determining:
A) If the patient has true hyponatremia
B) Whether the patient has oliguric or anuric renal failure
C) Whether the renal failure is due to acute tubular necrosis or another cause
D) Whether the renal failure is due to intrinsic renal disease or a prerenal cause
E) If the patient has pseudohyponatremia

See question 5.6.3.

73) The *major* Jones criteria for rheumatic fever include all of the following EXCEPT:
A) Carditis
B) Fever
C) Polyarthritis
D) Subcutaneous nodules
E) Sydenham chorea

See Chapter 11 Quick Quiz: An Ill Child.

74) A 29-year-old female daycare teacher presents with a severely pruritic rash that started at her wrists and has progressed to the web spaces of her fingers, under her arms, around her waist, and around her nipples. On examination, she has multiple excoriations and few small, erythematous papules. The most appropriate next step is:
A) Biopsy of normal-appearing skin
B) Biopsy of one of the papules
C) Empiric treatment with topical clotrimazole
D) Empiric treatment with topical lindane 1%
E) Empiric treatment with topical permethrin 5%

See questions 8.6.1 and 8.6.2.

75) A 60-year-old female with diabetic nephropathy is hospitalized with chest pain, and a cardiac catheterization is planned. Which one of the following is the best option to reduce her risk of contrast-induced nephropathy?
A) Administer ketorolac and IV saline
B) Administer mannitol and IV saline
C) Administer IV saline alone
D) Administer *N*-acetylcysteine

See question 5.1.7.

76) A 58-year-old man with hypertension, diabetes, heart failure, and chronic kidney disease (stage 4, GFR ~25 mL/min/1.73 m^2) presents for follow-up. His current medications are insulin, aspirin, metoprolol, and lisinopril. His blood pressure is 142/86 mm Hg and *he has significant dependent*

edema. **His labs reveal serum potassium of 5.3 mEq/L. To achieve his blood pressure to goal (<130/80) while avoiding adverse events, the best initial step is:**
A) Discontinue lisinopril
B) Furosemide 20 mg PO daily
C) Hydrochlorothiazide 12.5 mg PO daily
D) Increase lisinopril
E) Losartan 25 mg PO daily

See questions 5.1.10 and 5.6.6.

77) Which of the following is most likely to cause hypokalemia?
A) Excessive use of "lite" salt
B) Hypoaldosteronism
C) Hypomagnesemia
D) Overdose of propranolol
E) Renal tubular acidosis type 4

See question 5.5.2.

78) A patient presents with thickened, yellowish, dystrophic toenails. What is the most appropriate next step?
A) Recommend that the patient return for toenail removal
B) Send nail scrapings for KOH stain and/or fungal culture
C) Start treatment with a topical antifungal
D) Start treatment with an oral antifungal
E) Start treatment with an IV antifungal

See question 17.3.4.

79) All of the following are consistent with a diagnosis of syndrome of inappropriate antidiuretic hormone secretion (SIADH) EXCEPT:
A) High urine osmolality
B) Low plasma osmolality
C) Low urine sodium
D) Normal adrenal function
E) Normal thyroid function

See questions 5.7.2 and 5.7.3.

80) A 21-year-old male is brought in the emergency department by his girlfriend after he overdosed on aspirin. He took "a bottle, maybe 100 pills or so," but he denies other ingestions. He complains only of nausea. He becomes more somnolent during the evaluation. He is slightly tachycardic and febrile with a normal blood pressure. His blood gas shows: pH 7.38, PaCO$_2$ 20 mm Hg, PaO$_2$ 98 mm Hg, HCO$_3$ 15 mEq/L. His creatinine, CBC, and electrolytes are normal, except for low potassium. What is the best description of this patient's blood gas?
A) Metabolic acidosis and metabolic alkalosis
B) Metabolic acidosis and respiratory alkalosis
C) Metabolic alkalosis and respiratory acidosis
D) Pure metabolic acidosis
E) Normal blood gas (no acidosis or alkalosis)

Chapter 5 Quick Quiz: Acid-Base Disorder.

81) A 19-year-old college student presents to the emergency department with fever, headache, myalgias, and confusion. She has had a splenectomy but is otherwise healthy. The examination is notable for somnolence, fever, and nuchal rigidity. Due to her inability to follow directions, the neurological examination is difficult to complete, but it appears to be non-focal. There are several other seriously ill patients in the ED to triage. Which of the following interventions should not wait an hour and must be done now?
A) Administer ceftriaxone, vancomycin, and dexamethasone
B) Consult a neurosurgeon
C) Perform lumbar puncture
D) Obtain blood cultures
E) Order CT of the brain

See questions 8.3.1: Helpful Tip and 8.3.3.

82) You perform joint aspiration on a patient with a painful, swollen knee. Microscopic examination of the fluid shows rhomboid-shaped, positively birefringent crystals. Which one of the following is the most likely to alleviate the patient's acute symptoms?
A) Acetaminophen daily
B) Allopurinol daily
C) Ceftriaxone IM
D) Corticosteroid injection into the knee
E) Topical anti-inflammatory cream

See question 11.5.2.

83) A 23-year-old male with HIV stopped taking all of his medications 3 months ago due to cost. He was feeling fine until 3 weeks ago when he developed a cough. He now has daily fevers around 101°F, a non-productive cough, dyspnea on exertion, fatigue, chills, and tightness in his chest with inspiration. His examination is notable for fever, diaphoresis, bilateral crackles with inspiration, and mild tachypnea. Chest x-ray shows diffuse bilateral interstitial infiltrates. Which of the following is the most likely causative agent for this pulmonary infection?
A) Adenovirus
B) *Cryptococcus neoformans*
C) *Mycobacterium tuberculosis*
D) *Pneumocystis jiroveci* (PCP)
E) *Toxoplasma gondii*

See questions 9.1.9 and 9.1.10.

84) Which of the following is not useful in the treatment of hepatic encephalopathy?
A) Oral lactulose
B) Polyethylene glycol (Golytely)
C) Oral rifaximin
D) Lactulose enemas for acute encephalopathy

See question 7.13.2.

85) An otherwise-healthy 70-year-old female is admitted and started on ceftriaxone and azithromycin for pneumonia. On hospital day 3, her serum creatinine is found to have tripled from admission. She is mildly nauseated and has an erythematous, macular rash on her trunk and arms. Her CBC shows that her white cell count has declined from admission, but she now has a prominent eosinophilia. Urinalysis shows 1 + protein, and urine sediment shows white cell casts and eosinophils. The most appropriate next step is:
A) Add metronidazole to her antibiotic regimen
B) Bolus with IV 0.9% saline
C) Consult a nephrologist for possible renal biopsy
D) Discontinue ceftriaxone and consider an alternative antibiotic
E) Start furosemide to improve urine output

See question 5.13.3: Helpful Tip.

86) Each of the following patients is found to have asymptomatic bacteriuria. Who should be treated with a course of antibiotics?
A) An 88-year-old female nursing home resident
B) A 20-year-old pregnant patient
C) A 75-year-old male with an indwelling Foley catheter for obstructive BPH
D) All of the above

See questions 8.4.1 and 8.4.2: Helpful Tip.

87) In a patient with ascites, which of the following will cause a low serum-ascites albumin gradient (SAAG)?
A) Carcinomatous peritonitis
B) Portal hypertension
C) Budd–Chiari syndrome
D) Cirrhosis

See question 7.12.4: Helpful Tip.

88) A patient comes to the emergency department after sustaining a needle stick. She is a nurse who had just finished drawing blood for culture on a patient with AIDS, and somehow she stuck herself through her glove. She bled a little. She washed the area copiously. What is the most appropriate next step?
A) Prescribe antiretrovirals for 4 weeks
B) Prescribe single-dose antiretroviral prophylaxis
C) Reassure the patient as her risk of contracting HIV is negligible
D) Test her for HIV and treat based on the results

See question 9.3.2: Helpful Tip.

89) About half of patients with portal hypertension have esophageal varices, and one-third of these will experience a gastrointestinal bleed. Patients with varices may benefit from preventative therapy aimed at reducing bleeding risk. Which of the following IS useful in the prevention of variceal bleeding in patients with portal hypertension due to alcoholic cirrhosis?
A) Pentoxifylline (Trental)
B) Nadolol
C) Vitamin K
D) Cilostazol (Pletal)

See question 7.13.5.

90) Which of the following is generally true in alcohol-related liver disease?
A) AST is two times greater than ALT
B) ALT is two times greater than AST
C) Both ALT and AST are elevated to the same degree
D) The GGT is specific for liver disease and higher than either the ALT or AST

See question 7.15.2: Helpful Tip.

91) Appropriate antibiotic treatment of diverticulitis includes all of the following EXCEPT:
A) Ciprofloxacin + metronidazole
B) Amoxicillin clavulanate
C) Trimethoprim/sulfamethoxazole + metronidazole
D) Clindamycin + metronidazole

See question 7.17.3: Helpful Tip.

92) Which of the following is true about the treatment of pancreatitis?
A) Antibiotics should be used in most cases of pancreatitis
B) Oral feedings is the preferred method of nutrition if tolerated
C) Pseudocysts must be drained for pancreatitis to resolve
D) The Ransom criteria can be used at the time of admission to accurately predict mortality

See questions 7.15.8 to 7.15.12 as well as Helpful Tips.

93) Which of the following does NOT promote gastric emptying in gastroparesis?
A) Erythromycin
B) Metoclopramide
C) Amoxicillin
D) Cisapride

See question 7.16.2.

94) Of the following, the most common cause of acute pancreatitis in the United States is:
A) Hypertriglyceridemia
B) Biliary Tract Disease
C) Thiazide diuretics
D) Viruses

See question 7.15.7.

95) All of the following are causes of non-alcoholic fatty liver disease EXCEPT:
A) Statin use
B) Hypothyroidism
C) Diabetes
D) Obesity

See question 7.14.3.

96) The most common cause of the development of drug resistance in HIV is:
A) Failure to include zidovudine in the treatment regimen
B) Failure to initiate treatment until the patient has a known AIDS defining illness
C) Poor compliance with medications
D) Failure to include a protease inhibitor in the treatment regimen

See question 9.1.3.

97) At what CD4$^+$ level should one initiate prophylactic treatment of *Pneumocystis jiroveci* (previously *Pneumocystis carinii*)?
A) CD4$^+$ ≤50 cells/mm^3
B) CD4$^+$ ≤75 cells/mm^3
C) CD4$^+$ ≤100 cells/mm^3
D) CD4$^+$ ≤200 cells/mm^3

See question 9.1.4.

98) Which of the following recommendations regarding Pap smear screening in an HIV positive woman is true?
A) Start screening with a PAP smear 1 year after onset of sexual activity regardless of age
B) It is CD4$^+$ dependent. If the CD4$^+$ count is normal and the patient has two normal Pap smears at 1-year intervals, you can continue to do yearly PAP smears
C) It is CD4$^+$ dependent. If the patient has a CD4$^+$ count <200 cells/mm^3, screening should be done every 6 months regardless of whether or not the patient has had negative Pap smears
D) Pap smears can be suspended in HIV-positive patients since they will likely die from HIV before they die from cervical cancer

See question 9.2.14.

99) Which of the following statements best reflects the current thinking about treating influenza?
A) Rimantadine and amantadine are the most effective drugs for influenza B
B) Treatment with oseltamivir (Tamiflu) is highly effective, thus negating the need for influenza vaccine
C) Oseltamivir must be started within 48 hours of symptom onset to be of any benefit
D) There is no resistance of influenza A to oseltamivir

See question 8.1.3.

100) Assuming each of these patients has a negative chest x-ray, which of the following patients needs isoniazid treatment?
A) A patient with no risk factors who has a PPD reaction of 5 mm
B) A patient with recent exposure to TB and a PPD reaction of 5 mm
C) A healthcare worker with a PPD reaction of 5 mm
D) A patient with a PPD reaction of 10 mm 1 year after treatment for latent TB

See questions 8.4.4, Table 8-4, and 8.4.5.

101) The recommended *empirical* antibiotic treatment of meningitis in an immunocompetent adult age 40 is:
A) Ceftriaxone
B) Ceftriaxone + vancomycin
C) Ceftriaxone + ciprofloxacin
D) Ceftriaxone + TMP/SMX

See question 8.3.1 and Table 8-3.

102) The most common bacterial organism causing meningitis in adults is:
A) *Pneumococcus*
B) *Meningococcus*
C) *Haemophilus*
D) *Listeria*

See questions 8.3.1, 8.3.2, and Table 8-3.

103) All of the following can be used for malaria prophylaxis EXCEPT:
A) Doxycycline
B) Mefloquine
C) Azithromycin
D) Atovaquone/proguanil (Malarone)

See question 8.8.4.

104) Which of the following is true regarding the diagnosis of urolithiasis?
A) Over 95% of patients will have blood in their urine at the time of diagnosis
B) Urolithiasis may be difficult to differentiate from aortic dissection at the initial time of presentation
C) Hematuria will reliably differentiate urolithiasis from aortic dissection
D) A negative "FAST" ultrasound scan is considered the standard and if negative, rules out urolithiasis

See question 5.3.5: Helpful Tip.

105) Which of the following profiles are you likely to see in a patient with a pre-renal cause of elevated creatinine?
A) Urine sodium <20 mEq/L, fractional excretion of sodium <1%
B) Urine sodium <20 mEq/L, fractional excretion of sodium >2%

C) Urine sodium >40 mEq/L, fractional excretion of sodium <1%

D) Urine sodium >40 mEq/L, fractional excretion of sodium >2%

See questions 5.6.3 and 5.13.1.

106) Aldosterone resistance (such as occurs with diabetic nephropathy) or hypoaldosteronism will present with which of the following?

A) Hypokalemia

B) Hyperkalemia

C) Hyperphosphatemia

D) Hypophosphatemia

See question 5.1.9.

107) Which of the following regimens IS NOT recommended for treatment of a simple cystitis in an otherwise healthy, non-pregnant adult female?

A) Amoxicillin 500 mg PO TID for 3 days

B) Fosfomycin 3 grams once

C) Nitrofurantoin macrocrystals 100 mg PO BID for 5 days

D) TMP/SMX 1 PO BID for 3 days

See Chapter 5 Quick Quiz: Dysuria.

108) Which of the following drugs is LEAST LIKELY to reduce the progression of proteinuria?

A) Enalapril

B) Losartan

C) Verapamil

D) Nifedipine

See question 10.10.5.

109) The definition of nephrotic syndrome requires all of the following EXCEPT:

A) Hypoalbuminemia

B) Urine albumin excretion >3 g per day

C) Edema

D) Renal biopsy showing appropriate changes

See question 5.4.5.

110) Which of the following patients should have a carotid endarterectomy based on all current U.S. guidelines?

A) A 60-year-old female with a unilateral *symptomatic* 70% carotid plaque

B) A 60-year-old male or female with an *asymptomatic* 69% carotid plaque

C) Patient of either gender with bilateral 50% carotid plaque, *symptomatic* or *asymptomatic*

D) None of the above meet current qualification criterion

See Chapter 18 Quick Quiz: Carotid Artery Disease: When to Cut?

111) If cost were NOT an issue, which of the following drugs/ drug combinations would be the ideal regimen for the secondary prevention of stroke?

A) Aspirin + clopidogrel

B) Aspirin + dipyridamole

C) Aspirin alone

D) Clopidogrel alone

E) Warfarin

See question 18.1.5.

112) Which one of the following entities presents with reflexes preserved?

A) Guillain–Barré

B) Amyotrophic lateral sclerosis

C) Charcot–Marie–Tooth disease

D) Diabetic neuropathy

See question 18.6.4: Helpful Tip.

113) Which one of the following agents is most effective for controlling the pain of peripheral neuropathy?

A) Tricyclic antidepressant (TCA)

B) Gabapentin

C) Oxycodone or other narcotic

D) Carbamazepine or other traditional antiepileptic

See question 18.3.6: Helpful Tip.

114) Which of the following drugs IS NOT associated with rebound headaches?

A) Acetaminophen

B) Dihydroergotamine (DHE)

C) Nortriptyline

D) Sumatriptan

See question 18.4.6.

115) The risk of developing a seizure disorder after a single febrile seizure is:

A) 1% to 5%; the same as the rest of the population

B) 6% to 10%; slightly higher than the general population

C) 11% to 15%; significantly higher than the general population

D) Unknown

See question 18.14.4.

116) You determine that a 77-year-old female has Parkinson disease that is interfering with her daily life. The best drug or drug combination to alleviate her symptoms and improve her function is:

A) A COMT inhibitor (e.g., Entacapone)

B) A dopamine agonist (e.g., Requip)

C) Levodopa/carbidopa (e.g., Sinemet)

D) Apomorphine

See question 18.10.6.

117) The PRESENCE of a RAPD (relative afferent pupillary defect) can be indicative of:
A) Cataracts
B) Large retinal detachment
C) Bleed into the anterior chamber
D) Severe refractive error

See Chapter 19 glossary and question 19.2.1.

118) Which of the following patients has an indication for cataract surgery?
A) Vision 20/100 bilaterally in a patient who has no visual complaints or functional impairment
B) Vision 20/20 OD and 20/200 OS in a patient who can see well enough to do everything she desires
C) Vision 20/30 OD and 20/30 OS in a patient who is bothered by her inability to quilt
D) Vision unknown in a patient who can carry out all ADLs to her own satisfaction

See question 19.14.3.

119) All of the following intraocular muscles are innervated by cranial nerve III EXCEPT:
A) Inferior oblique
B) Inferior rectus
C) Lateral rectus
D) Medial rectus
E) Superior rectus

See question 19.15.1.

120) Skinnier, "politically correct" Santas are in vogue this year (bearing gifts of celery, no doubt). Your patient is in a tizzy: he has played Santa for years without the need for pillows. He wants to keep up his tradition as St. Nick. What can you tell him about weight reduction surgery?
A) "Sorry, even though you may lose weight, it will not help your overall health."
B) "You must have a BMI >40 kg/m² before qualifying for bariatric surgery regardless of other underlying weight-related conditions."
C) "You must have a BMI of 35-39 kg/m² AND significant reversible disease (e.g., hypertension, diabetes) to qualify for bariatric surgery."
D) "The reindeer union says it's members won't work if Santa's weight is under 300 lb—they need to keep 8 reindeer working the sleigh at all times."

See question 22.5.1.

121) A 70-year-old male patient complains of severe unilateral visual loss. He has no other symptoms. Here is a picture of his fundus (Fig. 30-3) that you took with your smartphone jerry-rigged to a direct ophthalmoscope. His diagnosis is:
A) Acute glaucoma
B) Acute venous disruption
C) Acute arterial occlusion
D) Diabetic retinopathy

See question 19.12.1.

122) What is the general course of rheumatoid arthritis during pregnancy?
A) Worsening during pregnancy
B) Worsening during pregnancy but only if methotrexate is used
C) It may remit during pregnancy and methotrexate is contraindicated
D) Morning sickness is worse in those with rheumatoid arthritis
E) Pregnancy has no effect on rheumatoid arthritis and vice versa

See question 11.1.8.

123) A diagnosis of rheumatoid arthritis can be made after symptoms have been present for at least:
A) 15 minutes
B) 2 weeks
C) 6 weeks
D) Duration of symptoms is no longer a criterion for diagnosing rheumatoid arthritis

See question 11.1.2: Helpful Tip.

124) You make a diagnosis of rheumatoid arthritis based on laboratory and clinical criteria. The best time to begin disease-modifying antirheumatic drugs (DMARDs) is:
A) At the time of diagnosis
B) After failure of 2 NSAIDs
C) After the failure of prednisone
D) When complications of rheumatoid arthritis occur
E) After waiting 6 months to see a rheumatologist

See question 11.1.3: Helpful Tip.

125) You are seeing a 57-year-old male in your practice who is complaining of bi-temporal headache. He checked the web and decided that he has giant cell (temporal) arteritis. The only problem is that his ESR is only 30 mm/hr. The CRP is not much more edifying. You appropriately respond to him:
A) "You may still have temporal arteritis since 15% or more will have normal ESR and CRP."
B) "You seem to be displaying drug seeking behavior since you came in to the ED with the same complaint 1 month ago."
C) "You may still have temporal arteritis, but we need to perform a temporal bone biopsy."
D) "You may still have temporal arteritis, but we will need to submit your head to the state lab for formal testing … You don't mind … do you?"

See question 11.2.2.

126) When treating gout, which one of these drugs for gout will be *ineffective* in those with renal insufficiency?
A) Allopurinol
B) Probenecid
C) Prednisone
D) Colchicine
E) Indomethacin

See question 11.4.6.

127) Regarding therapy for giant cell arteritis, which of the following statements best describes the appropriate relationship of aspirin, prednisone, and giant cell arteritis?
A) ASA (81 mg/day) can be used as adjunctive therapy for those on prednisone
B) ASA (325 mg/day) can be used as adjunctive therapy for those on prednisone
C) High-dose ASA (650 mg/day) can be used in those who do not tolerate prednisone
D) ASA has no role in the treatment of giant cell arteritis

See question 11.2.3.

128) The one best, first-line drug treatment of osteoarthritis pain is:
A) Acetaminophen
B) Celecoxib (Celebrex)
C) Ibuprofen
D) Naproxen
E) Morphine

See Chapter 12: General Note, at the start of the chapter.

129) Of the following options, the best initial pharmacologic therapy for fibromyalgia pain is:
A) Duloxetine
B) Ibuprofen
C) Nortriptyline
D) Tramadol

See questions 11.8.2 and 11.8.3: Helpful Tip.

130) Which of the following should NOT go into the calculus of what antibiotic to use for a patient with community acquired pneumonia?
A) Appearance of infiltrate on chest x-ray (lobar vs. "atypical")
B) Comorbid medical conditions
C) Likelihood of resistant organisms (based on prior cultures)
D) Patient age
E) Medication allergies

See question 3.12.1: Helpful Tip, 3.12.2, and 3.12.3.

131) Regarding depot medroxyprogesterone (Depo-Provera), which of the following is true?
A) Depo-Provera can cause bone mineral loss. However, recent data suggest that bone remineralization is possible after stopping
B) It is associated with an increase in breast cancer
C) More than 2 years of Depo-Provera is never indicated because of weight gain and other metabolic effects
D) It is a frequent cause of depression

See question 15.1.1: Helpful Tip.

132) Bleeding in a non-pregnant, amenorrheic patient in response to a "progesterone challenge" (e.g., medroxyprogesterone given for 10 days and then stopped) indicates that the patient has sufficient endogenous:
A) Follicle stimulating hormone (FSH)
B) Luteinizing hormone (LH)
C) Progesterone
D) Estrogen

See Chapter 15 Quick Quiz: Amenorrhea.

133) You get the following results on a vaginal wet prep: pH 5 and a positive "whiff" test. Wouldn't you know it, the rest of the results got lost. With the information available, the most likely diagnosis is:
A) Vulvovaginal candidiasis
B) Bacterial vaginosis
C) Vaginal trichomoniasis
D) Physiologic vaginal discharge

See Chapter 15: Table 15-13.

134) When is screening for Group B *Streptococcus* (GBS) in the pregnant female recommended?
A) Between 30 and 32 weeks of gestation
B) Between 32 and 34 weeks of gestation
C) Between 35 and 37 weeks of gestation
D) Intrapartum only

See question 15.1.8.

135) Which of the following is the most appropriate treatment of chronic menorrhagia in a 42-year-old female hypertensive smoker?
A) Low androgenic progesterone oral contraceptive
B) Levonorgestrel-containing IUD (e.g., Mirena, Liletta, Kyleena, or Skyla)
C) Copper IUD (Paraguard)
D) Low estrogen oral contraceptive

See questions 15.8.2: Helpful Tip and 15.9.4.

136) You are called to see a partner's patient who is G3P2 at 32 weeks gestation and is having regular contractions. After monitoring and an examination, you suspect that she is in labor. The SINGLE most important step, and the first step to take, at this point is:
A) Administration of corticosteroids to hasten fetal lung maturation
B) Administration of a tocolytic such as terbutaline
C) Insertion of a cervical cerclage to delay delivery
D) Antibiotic therapy (ampicillin) from now until delivery

See questions 15.4.2 and 15.4.4.

137) This fetal tracing, shown in Figure 30-3, is:
A) Reassuring
B) Worrisome
C) An indication for immediate C-section
D) An indication for the addition of Pitocin

See Chapter 15: Table 15-4 and question 15.2.7.

138) Which of the following *must* be present to make the diagnosis of pelvic inflammatory disease?
A) Adnexal pain
B) Elevated WBC count
C) Elevated CRP
D) Temperature of >38°C

See question 15.13.2: Helpful Tip.

139) A NEGATIVE fetal fibronectin suggests that:
A) The fetal lungs are immature
B) There is little likelihood that the patient will deliver within the next 7 days
C) There is an amniotic fluid leak
D) Is not helpful. A positive fibronectin suggests imminent delivery

See question 15.4.1.

140) Which of the following is true about tocolytics for premature labor?
A) They are effective at stopping labor and can arrest labor for an average of 1 week
B) They have very few side effects and should be used routinely in premature labor
C) Their use is mostly to buy time for antenatal steroids to work for those pregnancies between 24 and 34 weeks
D) Terbutaline is the only FDA-approved tocolytic

See question 15.4.3: Helpful Tip.

141) As you start a patient on fluoxetine for depression, you counsel him about the adverse effects of this class of medications. All of the following are common adverse effects of SSRIs EXCEPT:
A) Anxiety
B) Diarrhea
C) Headaches
D) Hypersexuality
E) Insomnia

See question 23.1.8.

142) A 12-month-old female presents to the emergency department after 24 hours of vomiting, diarrhea, and fever. She is lethargic, tachycardic, and hypotensive with poor skin turgor. What is the most appropriate initial method of providing her fluids?
A) Half-normal saline, 20 mL/kg bolus
B) Half-normal saline with 5% dextrose, 10 mL/kg bolus
C) Normal saline, 100 mL/kg bolus
D) Normal saline, 20 mL/kg bolus

See question 13.3.3.

143) A 15-month-old male is brought to the clinic by his parents. Like everyone else at his home, he has had some rhinorrhea and diarrhea in the last week. However, 4 hours ago the patient developed episodes of inconsolable crying accompanied by lying in "the fetal position" for 15 to 20 minutes at a time. At first his parents were puzzled but not too worried, but these episodes have occurred six to seven times now and he has become more lethargic. Finally, he had a bloody bowel movement, so they decided to bring him in to the office. On examination, he is afebrile, lethargic but arousable, and well hydrated. His abdomen appears benign. What is your leading diagnosis?
A) Cholecystitis
B) Gastroenteritis
C) Intussusception
D) Volvulus

See question 13.4.1.

144) Which of the following screening tests is recommended universally for all children in the United States?
A) Eye examination at 3 to 5 years
B) Hearing testing at 1 or 2 days old
C) Hemoglobin at 12 months
D) Lead level at 12 months

See Chapter 13 Quick Quiz: Congenital Infections, Helpful Tip.

145) During a visit for a physical examination, you note that this 33-year-old female has checked "depression" on her health-screening questionnaire. You ask her more about this and find that she has felt that her mood has been depressed

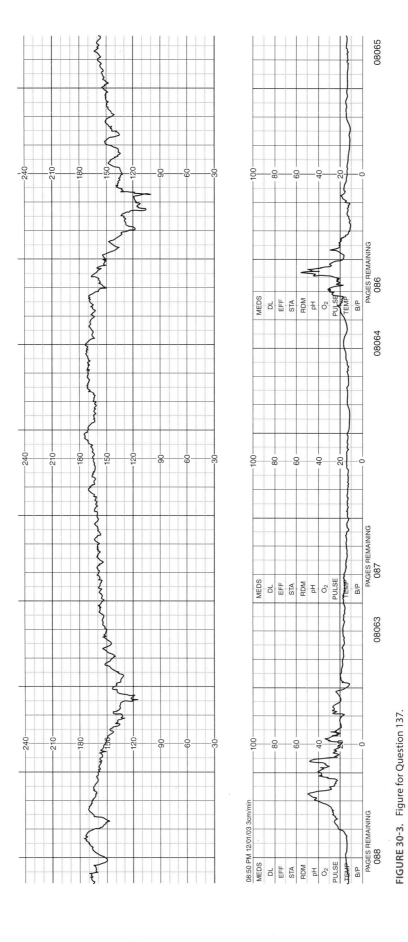

FIGURE 30-3. Figure for Question 137.

for 15 years or more. She generally feels fatigued and has low self-esteem, but she denies suicidal ideation and feelings of guilt and worthlessness. What diagnosis best characterizes her symptoms?

A) Avoidant personality disorder
B) Borderline personality disorder
C) Persistent depressive disorder
D) Major depressive disorder

See Chapter 23 Quick Quiz: Sad All the Time.

146) Which of the following symptoms would be LEAST likely to be due to a panic attack and therefore would prompt further investigation in a patient with known panic disorder?

A) Chest pain
B) Dyspnea
C) Palpitations
D) Syncope

See question 23.6.4.

147) A 23-year-old male presents with symptoms suggestive of panic attacks, an underlying anxiety disorder, and possibly panic disorder. You refer him for counseling services and recommend starting a medication. Which of the following drugs is LEAST effective for treating panic disorder?

A) Bupropion
B) Nortriptyline
C) Sertraline
D) Venlafaxine

See question 23.6.8.

148) All of the following are part of the CHA2DS2-VASC score EXCEPT:

A) Age
B) Sex/Gender
C) History of stroke, thromboembolic disease, etc.
D) Active cancer
E) Heart failure

See Chapter 2: Table 2-6A.

149) According to the USPSTF and CDC, hepatitis C screening is recommended for all of the following groups EXCEPT:

A) All individuals born between 1955 and 1975
B) Hemodialysis patients
C) Patients with a history of incarceration
D) Users of illicit injection drugs
E) Migrants from an endemic area (e.g., Southeast Asia)

See question 7.10.3: Helpful Tip.

150) Which of the following patients does NOT need a head CT scan per the PECARN rules?

A) A child with a GCS of 14 and no other symptoms or signs of intracranial injury
B) A 3-month-old with an occipital bruise after a fall of 3 ft
C) A 3-year-old with an occipital bruise and a fall of 3 ft
D) A 1-year-old child with a palpable skull fracture who is otherwise neurologically intact
E) A 1-year-old child with a scalp hematoma

See Chapter 1: Table 1-6.

151) Because _____ is the major unmeasured anion in the serum, the anion gap needs to be adjusted for the _____ level in the serum.

A) Albumin
B) Calcium
C) Phosphate
D) Total protein
E) Chloride

See question 1.4.2.

152) Your patient has just returned from Mexico where she sustained an ankle bite from a suspect dog. Rabies vaccine and immunoglobulin are not likely to be effective after:

A) 10 days
B) 20 days
C) 30 days
D) 90 days

See question 1.6.2.

153) Dislocation of which of the following joints is associated with the highest risk of arterial injury?

A) Wrist
B) Elbow
C) Shoulder
D) Knee
E) Ankle

See Chapter 1: Quick Quiz: Orthopedic Emergencies.

154) The Women's Health Initiative revealed which of the following statistically significant correlations?

A) Combined estrogen/progesterone therapy reduced breast cancer risk
B) Combined estrogen/progesterone therapy increased breast cancer risk
C) Estrogen monotherapy did not affect breast cancer risk
D) Estrogen monotherapy increased breast cancer risk

See question 15.14.3.

155) A 2-year-old child presents having missed his routine vaccines at 12 and 15 months. The patient should:

A) Restart all vaccines

B) Spread out the interval for his remaining vaccines to reduce the risk of side effects

C) Receive all of his missed doses of vaccines right now

D) Receive the vaccines due at age 12 months and continue on the "catch-up" schedule

See question 13.2.6: Helpful Tip.

156) A 12-month-old female infant presents for her routine well-child examination. She has some nasal congestion and her temperature is 100.4°C. She looks otherwise great. You should:

A) Administer her routine 12-month vaccines

B) Administer half her routine 12-month vaccines now and half in 2 weeks

C) Have her return for vaccines when she is afebrile for 24 hours

D) Never give her any more vaccines as she clearly has a febrile reaction just being close to them

See question 13.2.6.

157) A 20-year-old female with asthma presents to the ED wheezing and dyspneic. Within 5 minutes of a treatment with nebulized albuterol, her wheezing improves but she still feels dyspneic. The most appropriate next step is:

A) Prepare for imminent intubation

B) Administer IV magnesium

C) Administer IV ceftriaxone

D) Administer another dose of nebulized albuterol

E) Discharge her with a prescription for cough syrup

See question 1.14.4.

158) The diagnosis of chronic obstructive pulmonary disease is secured by:

A) Cough and sputum production in a smoker

B) Two or three of the following symptoms over the last 6 months: cough, dyspnea, sputum production

C) FEV_1/FVC ratio of <0.7

D) FEV_1 <70% predicted

E) $FVC > FEV_1$

See question 3.3.3 and Table 3-1.

159) A 16-year-old male with asthma and seasonal allergies presents for follow-up. His only asthma medication is an albuterol inhaler. In the past few months, he has needed the medication more and more, and is now using his albuterol inhaler one to two times per day. The most appropriate next step is to:

A) Add a low-dose inhaled corticosteroid (e.g., triamcinolone) twice daily

B) Add a long-acting bronchodilator (e.g., salmeterol) twice daily

C) Schedule his albuterol inhaler 4 times per day

D) Add a low-dose systemic steroid (e.g., prednisone) daily

E) Add a leukotriene inhibitor (e.g., montelukast) daily

See question 3.3.6 and Figure 3-1.

160) According to the USPSTF, the most appropriate modality and frequency for lung cancer screening is:

A) Posteroanterior and lateral chest radiographs annually

B) Low-dose CT of the chest annually

C) Low-dose CT of the chest every 3 years

D) Sputum cytology annually

E) None is recommended as the evidence is insufficient

See question 3.11.6.

161) A 30-year-old male is found unconscious, slumped in a chair outside the ED. You arouse him briefly with a sternal rub. He has pinpoint pupils and a respiratory rate of 8 per minute. The drug most likely to causing his current symptoms is:

A) Methamphetamine

B) Cocaine

C) Heroin

D) Ecstasy

E) Alcohol

See Chapter 1: Table 1-1.

162) You admit a 45-year-old male with cirrhosis for alcohol withdrawal. He meets criteria for complicated withdrawal. Which of the following medications will be safest and most effective at treating his withdrawal symptoms?

A) Chlordiazepoxide

B) Clonidine

C) Lorazepam

D) Metoprolol

See question 25.2.7.

163) You are admitting an 88-year-old male to a care facility with hospice due to declining overall health. In the last year, he has started to require total functional dependence in most activities of daily living. He has moderate-to-severe dementia, ischemic cardiomyopathy and heart failure with a left ventricular ejection fraction of 20%. When he was healthier, he had an implanted cardiac defibrillator (ICD) placed, which has fired once a year ago and caused him significant pain and distress. His daughter is his durable power of attorney and agrees with the patient that hospitalization, procedures, and CPR are not desired. He has made these same goals clear in past conversations with other care providers, documented in the medical record. When his daughter asks about his ICD, you recommend which of the following?

A) Deactivate the ICD

B) Change the settings so the ICD only fires for ventricular tachycardia

C) Surgically remove the ICD

D) Leave the ICD as it is

See questions 27.1.1 and 27.1.2.

164) A 58-year-old male tobacco connoisseur presents for increasing cough, dyspnea, and sputum production. He is afebrile. Oxygen saturation on ambient air is 88%. Lung examination demonstrates poor air movement and diffuse expiratory wheezing. His chest x-ray is consistent with COPD and shows no infiltrates. You decide to admit him. Which of the following drug regimens would be the best choice for this patient?

A) Nebulized albuterol every 4 hours as needed and IV methylprednisolone 125 mg daily

B) Tiotropium inhaler 1 puff daily, levofloxacin 500 mg PO daily, and nebulized albuterol every 4 hours as needed

C) Prednisone 50 mg PO daily, doxycycline 100 mg PO BID, and nebulized albuterol every 4 hours as needed

D) Morphine 5 to 10 mg IV every 2 hours to palliate his breathlessness

See question 3.4.1: Helpful Tip.

165) A 35-year-old male presents for follow-up, after an admission for pneumonia. Blood cultures grew *Streptococcus pneumoniae*. Over the past 10 years, he reports having several bouts of pneumonia and numerous sinus infections. Also, he has developed an autoimmune hemolytic anemia. What is the most useful test in making the diagnosis of an immune deficiency in this patient?

A) Complement levels

B) Immunoglobulin levels

C) CBC and differential

D) Bone marrow biopsy

E) Lymph node biopsy

See Chapter 4: Table 4-2.

166) You are evaluating a 70-year-old male for abdominal pain that you suspect may be due to mesenteric ischemia. You believe the best test would be a CT angiogram of his abdomen, but he has a contrast allergy. When you inquire about the allergy, he reports rash and shortness of breath. The most appropriate next step in the care of this patient is to:

A) Perform a non-contrast CT scan of the abdomen and pelvis

B) Perform a contrast-enhanced CT scan of the abdomen and pelvis and pre-treat the patient with prednisone and diphenhydramine

C) Perform a contrast-enhanced CT scan of the abdomen and pelvis and pre-treat with IV normal saline boluses and N-acetylcysteine

D) Consult a vascular surgeon or an interventional radiologist for an angiogram

E) Consult a surgeon for an exploratory laparotomy

See Chapter 4: Quick Quiz: Contrast Allergy.

167) A 12-year-old male presents with his mother for concerns about diplopia, which began two days ago. On examination, he has normal visual acuity when each eye is tested

individually, normal pupillary reflexes, and esotropia. What is the best next step to take in the care of this patient?

A) Reassurance that this is a normal, age-related change that will improve with time

B) Refer to an optometrist for corrective lenses

C) Refer to a physical therapy for "eye training"

D) Order an MRI of the brain

E) Order an EEG

See question 19.1.4: Helpful Tip.

168) A 3-year-old female returns for continued problems with hearing. Her parents are concerned about another ear infection. She has had three episodes of otitis media that you have treated over the last 6 months. Her hearing is diminished, per parents, and she indeed tests positive for hearing loss bilaterally. On examination, you note bulging tympanic membranes with clear, bubbly fluid in the middle ears, but no signs of inflammation. The intervention most likely to help this patient improve her hearing and prevent another infection is:

A) Eustachian tube exercises

B) Tympanostomy tubes

C) Prolonged antibiotics

D) Nasal steroids

E) Systemic decongestants

See question 20.1.9.

169) Which of the following findings is diagnostic of acute otitis media?

A) Child pulling at ears and fussing in the examination room

B) Child with fever and injected tympanic membrane on examination

C) Child with fever and an injected tympanic membrane that does not move when ear canal is insufflated

D) Child with history of acute otitis media whose tympanic membrane is clear but does not move when ear canal is insufflated

See questions 20.1.1 and 20.1.3.

170) A 72-year-old male presents with hearing loss. He has no other symptoms. He spent much of his life working in a machine shop after he was discharged from the army where he was assigned to an artillery unit. His real passion has been music: he continues to serve as a back-up vocalist and bass guitar player in a rock band. On examination, he has normal ears to inspection but high frequency hearing loss. Which of the following is the most likely diagnosis?

A) Presbycusis

B) Otosclerosis

C) Acoustic neuroma

D) Ménière disease

E) Otitis media with effusion

See question 20.4.2.

171) A 40-year-old obese female walks into the office requesting a refill on her oral contraceptives and asks to be seen for acute onset of shortness of breath. She reports that she just got back from a 3-week road trip when she developed dyspnea. She wonders if it could be related to her smoking. On examination, she is tachypneic and mildly tachycardic with an oxygen saturation of 92%. She has a tender, swollen lower leg on the left. Her lungs are clear to auscultation. The most appropriate next step in the care of this patient is to:

A) Order a d-dimer
B) Prescribe an albuterol inhaler
C) Order a contrast-enhanced chest CT scan
D) Prescribe a course of antibiotics
E) Order pulmonary function testing

See question 3.5.6.

172) A 65-year-old female presents for follow up after hospital discharge 8 days ago. She underwent laparoscopic cholecystectomy that was complicated by intra-abdominal hemorrhage and repeated surgical exploration. She was in the hospital for 10 days. Now, she complains of coughing fits that hurt her surgical wounds. She produces yellow sputum. She is currently febrile, tachypneic and tachycardic on examination. Chest x-ray shows a right middle lobe infiltrate. You decide to admit her and order the following antibiotic regimen:

A) Cefepime and vancomycin
B) Ceftriaxone and azithromycin
C) Linezolid
D) Clindamycin and metronidazole
E) Doxycycline

See question 3.12.5: Helpful Tip on HCAP.

173) A 60-year-old male presents to discuss lung cancer screening via low-dose CT scan. He has smoked 1 pack-per-day of cigarettes for 40 years. Consistent with USPSTF recommendations, you advise him to undergo annual screening with CT until he has quit smoking for:

A) 1 year
B) 5 years
C) 15 years
D) The rest of his life. There is no end time identified for former smokers

See question 3.11.6.

174) Which of the following medications is/are associated with urticaria?

A) Aspirin
B) Lisinopril
C) Morphine
D) All of the above
E) None of the above

See question 17.10.5: Helpful Tip.

175) A 45-year-old female with type 2 diabetes presents for follow-up. On examination, she has two brownish-red patches with yellowish areas through the center on her lower legs. The center of the rash appears shiny and has telangiectasia. When asked, she states the rash has been present for at least a year and is mildly tender if touched. It is not pruritic. Of the following, what is the most likely diagnosis?

A) Acanthosis nigricans
B) Atopic dermatitis
C) Cellulitis
D) Contact dermatitis
E) Necrobiosis lipoidica

See question 17.11.1.

176) All of the following are components of the "female athlete triad" EXCEPT:

A) Low energy availability with or without disordered eating
B) Recurrent stress fractures
C) Menstrual dysfunction
D) Altered bone mineral density

See question 14.2.2.

177) For adolescent athletes, what is the number one cause of sudden cardiac death?

A) Chest trauma (e.g., baseball hit to the chest)
B) Anomalous coronary artery
C) Hypertrophic cardiomyopathy
D) Patent foramen ovale

See Chapter 14 Quick Quiz: Adolescent Athletes.

178) A 29-year-old male presents with symptoms of fatigue, weight loss, palpitations, and anxiety. On examination, you note tachycardia, lid lag, fine tremor, and diffusely enlarged thyroid gland. Suspecting a hyperthyroid state, you order a TSH and free thyroxine (T4). The TSH is below the normal range but the free T4 is normal. What is the next step in the management of this patient?

A) Refer to an endocrinologist who can see him in 3 to 6 months
B) Check a calcium level
C) Check a thyrotropin-releasing hormone level
D) Check a free tri-iodothyronine (T3) level
E) Send for thyroid biopsy

See Chapter 10 Quick Quiz: Thyroid Tests.

179) Thyroid storm is diagnosed by:

A) History and physical examination findings
B) Elevated free T3 level
C) Free T4 level 10 times the upper limit of normal
D) TSH level immeasurably low
E) An endocrinologist, preferably a really old one with a long white beard

See question 10.2.6: Helpful Tip.

180) You are seeing a 75-year-old female with progressive memory impairment. In order to diagnose her with a neurocognitive disorder (dementia) according to DSM-V, she must demonstrate impairment in any one of the following EXCEPT:

A) Apraxia

B) Anosmia

C) Aphasia

D) Agnosia

E) Impairment in executive functioning

See questions 21.5.1 and 21.5.3.

181) Regarding the treatment of hepatitis C for genotype 1 patients, which of the following therapies has the highest cure rate?

A) Ledipasvir/sofosbuvir (Harvoni)

B) Ribavirin

C) Interferon alpha

D) Pegylated interferon alpha

E) Interferon alpha + ribavirin

See questions 7.10.6 and 7.10.7: Helpful Tip.

182) According to the 2018 ADA guideline, which of the following patients should be screened for diabetes mellitus EXCEPT?

A) A 25-year-old female whose mother is diabetic

B) A 40-year-old female whose BMI is 29 kg/m^2

C) A 40-year-old female with history of delivering a 9 lb 6 oz infant

D) A 25-year-old female who really, really likes soft drinks

See question 10.10.1: Helpful Tip.

183) You have diagnosed a 10-year-old child with immune thrombocytopenic purpura (ITP), and his platelet count is currently 10,000/μL. You are considering therapy to improve this patient's platelet count. All of the following are treatments for ITP EXCEPT:

A) Platelet transfusion

B) Corticosteroids

C) IVIG

D) Splenectomy

E) Rho(D) immunoglobulin (if he is Rh positive)

See question 6.2.2.

184) You are seeing a 45-year-old male with elevated liver transaminases. His serum bilirubin, alkaline phosphatase, and GGT are normal. He does not drink alcohol. In your evaluation of his liver disorder, you find that a liver ultrasound is unremarkable for anatomic abnormalities, serologic studies for hepatitis A, B, and C are negative for infection, and his ferritin level is 725 ng/mL (upper limit of normal 300 ng/mL). What is the preferred next step in diagnosing his disease?

A) Bone marrow biopsy

B) Liver biopsy

C) Hemochromatosis gene testing

D) Echocardiogram

E) Diagnostic and therapeutic trial of phlebotomy

See question 6.18.3: Helpful Tip.

185) Fournier gangrene is caused by infection with:

A) Virulent, flesh-eating viruses

B) Methicillin-resistant *Staphylococcus aureus*

C) Mixed aerobic and anaerobic bacteria

D) *Yersinia pestis*

See question 22.1.2.

186) Sepsis survival is improved by:

A) Early central line placement for hemodynamic monitoring

B) Early recognition with aggressive fluid resuscitation and antibiotic administration

C) Specific protocols guided by central venous pressures

D) Early intubation and ventilation

E) Early palliative care consultation

See question 22.1.5: Helpful Tip.

187) You are seeing a 30-year-old male in the ED. He has survived a motor vehicle collision in which the driver of the other car was killed. He has multiple traumatic injuries but is alert—in fact, he's screaming in pain. His blood pressure is 88/56 mm Hg. What is the best option for managing his pain?

A) A lollipop and reassurance that the trauma team is on the way

B) IV morphine

C) Oral morphine liquid

D) IV fentanyl

E) IV ketorolac

See question 22.2.1.

188) A 65-year-old female presents with 6 hours of abdominal pain. She also notes nausea but has not had emesis. She has not moved her bowels today. She has a history of abdominal surgeries, including hysterectomy, appendectomy, and cholecystectomy—all for benign reasons. Her vital signs are normal. Her abdomen is protuberant, tympanic to percussion, and mildly tender diffusely. Her bowel sounds are hypoactive. You suspect a partial small bowel obstruction due to adhesions. Your admission orders include all of the following EXCEPT:

A) IV fluids

B) Antiemetics

C) NPO status

D) NG tube to continuous suction

E) Analgesic medication

See question 22.4.3: Helpful Tip.

189) After weight loss surgery, patients are at risk of developing nutritional deficiencies. Which of the following deficiencies are patients NOT likely to experience?
A) Protein deficiency
B) Vitamin B1 (thiamine) deficiency
C) Vitamin B12 deficiency
D) Copper deficiency
E) Zinc deficiency

See question 22.5.4: Helpful Tip.

190) By definition, external hemorrhoids are located:
A) Proximal to the dentate line
B) Distal to the dentate line
C) Distal to the anal verge
D) In the gluteal cleft

See question 22.6.1.

191) A 55-year-old female presents with concern for a new mass she palpated in her left breast. She first noticed it a month ago and it has not changed. Your examination reveals a 2-cm firm mass in the upper outer quadrant of the left breast. The examination is otherwise normal. You find that a screening mammogram, done 6 months ago, was completely negative (BIRADS 1). The best next step in the management of this patient is:
A) Reassurance, as her mammogram was normal
B) Repeat a mammogram in 6 months
C) Have her return in 6 months for a follow-up breast examination
D) Refer for biopsy of the mass
E) All of the above are equally appropriate

See question 22.7.3.

192) A surgical colleague consults you on an 80-year-old female who broke her femur after falling. The patient underwent an uncomplicated open reduction and internal fixation. It is now postoperative day 4 and she has developed a fever of 39°C. Potential causes of postoperative fever in this patient include all of the following EXCEPT:
A) Atelectasis
B) Wound infection
C) Venous thrombosis
D) Pneumonia
E) Drug-induced fever

See Chapter 22: Table 22-3 and Question 22.8.3.

193) A patient with a history of heparin-induced thrombocytopenia and thrombosis syndrome CAN have:
A) Low–molecular-weight heparin for any reason
B) Bivalirudin and argatroban
C) Heparin or low–molecular-weight heparin for prevention of venous thromboembolism

D) No heparin products for the rest of his or her life

See question 22.8.9.

194) Which of the following tests has the highest sensitivity (i.e., misses the fewest) for appendicitis?
A) CBC
B) CRP
C) CT scan of the abdomen and pelvis
D) Ultrasound of the right lower quadrant
E) All of the above have equivalent sensitivity for appendicitis

See question 22.9.4.

195) A hysterical mother runs into the ED with her 2-year-old daughter in her arms, screaming, "She got scalded!" After a moment she is able to recount the story. The child was by the stove playing when she pulled on a pot handle and dumped hot water on herself. You find that the dorsum of her right hand and most of her dorsal right arm are covered in second- and third-degree burns. Using the "Rule of 9s," you estimate that she has burned:
A) 1% of her body surface area
B) 5% of her body surface area
C) 10% of her body surface area
D) None of the above. The "Rule of 9s" should not be used in children

See question 22.11.4: Helpful Tip.

196) A new test has been developed to detect pheochromocytoma (not really … just pretend). The test has a very high sensitivity but a very low specificity for pheochromocytoma. The prevalence of pheochromocytoma in the population is low. If this new test is applied to the general population, which of the following is likely to occur?
A) The specificity will increase
B) The sensitivity will increase
C) The positive predictive value will be low
D) The negative predictive value will be low

See Case 28.6: Helpful Tip.

197) You are seeing 23-year-old female for a routine physical examination. She tells you that she has a new male partner who has used injectable drugs in the past and has shared needles. His HIV status is not known. They do not always use condoms when sexually active. In addition to recommending consistent condom use, you also recommend pre-exposure prophylaxis (PrEP) with:
A) Tenofovir
B) Tenofovir/Emtricitabine (Truvada)
C) Efavirenz (Sustiva)
D) Tenofovir/Emtricitabine/Efavirenz (Atripla)
E) None of the above

See question 9.4.2.

198) A 5-year-old patient presents with "leg pain" that you determine is originating from the right hip joint. An x-ray demonstrates a density at the right femoral head. With your Spidey senses tingling, you order an MRI which shows osteonecrosis of the femoral head. The best next step in the care of this patient is:

A) Acetaminophen, rest, and physical therapy
B) Referral to orthopedic surgery for a hip replacement
C) Systemic steroids (e.g., prednisone)
D) Steroid injection of the hip joint

See question 12.2.3.

199) A 35-year-old male presents for foot pain one day after an injury. He was playing soccer when he twisted his right foot and ankle and fell. He has trouble bearing weight on the foot due to pain. You order an x-ray of his foot and ankle. The radiologist calls to tell you he has a Jones fracture. When you look at the x-ray, you expect to find a:

A) Proximal 5th metatarsal fracture (but distal to the tuberosity)
B) Distal 5th metatarsal fracture
C) Midshaft 5th metatarsal fracture
D) 5th metatarsophalangeal joint dislocation

See question 12.19.1.

200) You are watching a really bad grade B movie. Who do you think will win?

A) Mothra
B) King Ghidorah
C) Biollante (a bioengineered Godzilla including the genes of humans and roses)
D) Godzilla
E) Mechagodzilla

Never bet against Godzilla.

Number	Answer	Answer Location in the Chapter	Number	Answer	Answer Location in the Chapter
1	D	*See question 2.2.2*	58	B	*See questions 21.4.1 and 21.4.2*
2	B	*See question 2.1.4*	59	C	*See question 21.6.2*
3	A	*See question 2.17.3*	60	A	*See question 21.6.9*
4	C	*See question 2.3.5*	61	B	*See question 16.8.3*
5	C	*See question 2.1.2: Helpful Tip*	62	E	*See question 23.9.1 and Table 23-1*
6	D	*See questions 2.22.3 and 2.22.6: Helpful Tip*	63	A	*See question 14.8.1: Helpful Tip*
7	D	*See question 2.1.10 and Table 2-1B*	64	B	*See questions 14.2.2 and 14.2.4*
8	D	*See question 2.1.10 and Table 2-1A*	65	B	*See question 16.5.2*
9	B	*See question 2.22.7*	66	E	*See questions 10.9.1 and 10.9.4*
10	B	*See question 2.4.1 and Table 2-6B*	67	D	*See question 16.10.3*
11	A	*See question 2.7.7*	68	A	*See question 10.10.7*
12	C	*See question 1.1.2*	69	C	*See question 10.8.2: Helpful Tips*
13	B	*See question 14.5.3*	70	A	*See question 11.2.7*
14	D	*See question 17.8.3: Helpful Tip*	71	D	*See question 17.3.2*
15	B	*See question 28.3.1*	72	D	*See question 5.6.3*
16	C	*See Chapter 17 Quick Quiz: Erythema Multiforme*	73	B	*See Chapter 11 Quick Quiz: An Ill Child*
17	A	*See Case 28.6*	74	E	*See questions 8.6.1 and 8.6.2*
18	C	*See question 17.8.4: Helpful Tip*	75	C	*See question 5.1.7*
19	B	*See question 14.3.1*	76	B	*See questions 5.1.10 and 5.6.6*
20	D	*See question 27.2.4: Helpful Tip*	77	C	*See question 5.5.2*
21	B	*See Chapter 1 Quick Quiz: Toxidromes and Table 1-1*	78	B	*See question 17.3.4*
22	D	*See question 1.4.3 and Table 1-3*	79	C	*See questions 5.7.2 and 5.7.3*
23	B	*See question 1.12.3*	80	B	*Chapter 5 Quick Quiz: Acid-Base Disorder*
24	D	*See question 1.24.5*	81	A	*See questions 8.3.1:Helpful Tip and 8.3.3*
25	D	*See question 1.20.1*	82	D	*See question 11.5.2*
26	C	*See question 1.24.4*	83	D	*See questions 9.1.9 and 9.1.10*
27	C	*See questions 1.19.1 and 1.19.4*	84	B	*See question 7.13.2*
28	C	*See question 27.1.6*	85	D	*See question 5.13.3: Helpful Tip*
29	B	*Chapter 27 Quick Quiz: More than a little headache*	86	B	*See questions 8.4.1 and 8.4.2: Helpful Tip*
30	A	*See questions 1.1.1 and 1.22.5*	87	A	*See question 7.12.4: Helpful Tip*
31	B	*See question 27.2.6: Helpful Tip*	88	A	*See question 9.3.2: Helpful Tip*
32	D	*See question 7.4.5: Helpful Tip*	89	B	*See question 7.13.5*
33	C	*See questions 7.1.3 and 7.1.4*	90	A	*See question 7.15.2: Helpful Tip*
34	D	*See questions 7.1.2 and 7.1.5*	91	D	*See question 7.17.3: Helpful Tip*
35	C	*See question 7.5.4: Helpful Tip*	92	B	*See questions 7.15.8 to 7.15.12 as well as Helpful Tips*
36	B	*See question 7.1.1*	93	C	*See question 7.16.2*
37	B	*See question 7.4.5*	94	B	*See question 7.15.7*
38	D	*See question 21.5.14*	95	A	*See question 7.14.3*
39	B	*See question 11.10.4*	96	C	*See question 9.1.3*
40	B	*See questions 7.6.4 and 7.6.5*	97	D	*See question 9.1.4*
41	A	*See question 7.6.6*	98	A	*See question 9.2.14*
42	B	*See question 7.10.1*	99	C	*See question 8.1.3*
43	B	*See question 7.8.4*	100	B	*See questions 8.4.4, Table 8-4, and 8.4.5*
44	D	*See question 8.2.3: Helpful Tip*	101	B	*See question 8.3.1 and Table 8-3*
45	A	*See question 7.8.2: Helpful Tip*	102	A	*See questions 8.3.1, 8.3.2, and Table 8-3*
46	C	*See question 7.8.6*	103	C	*See question 8.8.4*
47	B	*See question 7.8.3*	104	B	*See question 5.3.5: Helpful Tip*
48	D	*See question 7.10.6*	105	A	*See questions 5.6.3 and 5.13.1*
49	D	*See question 15.1.7: Helpful Tips*	106	B	*See question 5.1.9*
50	D	*See question 15.2.9*	107	A	*See Chapter 5 Quick Quiz: Dysuria*
51	C	*See question 15.12.8: Helpful Tip*	108	D	*See question 10.10.5*
52	E	*See question 15.14.3*	109	D	*See question 5.4.5*
53	D	*See question 15.2.1: Helpful Tip*	110	A	*See Chapter 18 Quick Quiz: Carotid Artery Disease: When to Cut?*
54	C	*See question 21.2.3*	111	C	*See question 18.1.5*
55	E	*See question 21.5.2*	112	B	*See question 18.6.4: Helpful Tip*
56	B	*See question 16.7.3*	113	A	*See question 18.3.6: Helpful Tip*
57	C	*See questions 21.3.4 and 21.3.5*	114	C	*See question 18.4.6*
			115	A	*See question 18.14.4*

Number	Answer	Answer Location in the Chapter	Number	Answer	Answer Location in the Chapter
116	C	*See question 18.10.6*	168	B	*See question 20.1.9*
117	B	*See Chapter 19 glossary and question 19.2.1*	169	C	*See questions 20.1.1 and 20.1.3*
118	C	*See question 19.14.3*	170	A	*See question 20.4.2*
119	C	*See question 19.15.1*	171	C	*See question 3.5.6*
120	C	*See question 22.5.1*	172	B	*See question 3.12.5: Helpful Tip on HCAP*
121	C	*See question 19.12.1*	173	C	*See question 3.11.6*
122	C	*See question 11.1.8*	174	D	*See question 17.10.5: Helpful Tip*
123	D	*See question 11.1.2: Helpful Tip*	175	E	*See question 17.11.1*
124	A	*See question 11.1.3: Helpful Tip*	176	B	*See question 14.2.2*
125	A	*See question 11.2.2*	177	C	*See Chapter 14 Quick Quiz: Adolescent Athletes*
126	B	*See question 11.4.6*	178	D	*See Chapter 10 Quick Quiz: Thyroid Tests*
127	A	*See question 11.2.3*	179	A	*See question 10.2.6: Helpful Tip*
128	A	*See Chapter 12: General Note, at the start of the chapter*	180	B	*See questions 21.5.1 and 21.5.3*
129	C	*See questions 11.8.2 and 11.8.3: Helpful Tip*	181	A	*See questions 7.10.6 and 7.10.7: Helpful Tip*
130	A	*See question 3.12.1: Helpful Tip, 3.12.2, and 3.12.3*	182	D	*See question 10.10.1: Helpful Tip*
131	A	*See question 15.1.1: Helpful Tip*	183	A	*See question 6.2.2*
132	D	*See Chapter 15 Quick Quiz: Amenorrhea*	184	C	*See question 6.18.3: Helpful Tip*
133	B	*See Chapter 15: Table 15-13*	185	C	*See question 22.1.2*
134	C	*See question 15.1.8*	186	B	*See question 22.1.5: Helpful Tip*
135	B	*See questions 15.8.2: Helpful Tip and 15.9.4*	187	D	*See question 22.2.1*
136	A	*See questions 15.4.2 and 15.4.4*	188	D	*See question 22.4.3: Helpful Tip*
137	B	*See Chapter 15: Table 15-4 and question 15.2.7*	189	A	*See question 22.5.4: Helpful Tip*
138	A	*See question 15.13.2: Helpful Tip*	190	B	*See question 22.6.1*
139	B	*See question 15.4.1*	191	D	*See question 22.7.3*
140	C	*See question 15.4.3: Helpful Tip*	192	A	*See Chapter 22: Table 22-3 and Question 22.8.3*
141	D	*See question 23.1.8*	193	B	*See question 22.8.9*
142	D	*See question 13.3.3*	194	C	*See question 22.9.4*
143	C	*See question 13.4.1*	195	D	*See question 22.11.4: Helpful Tip*
144	A	*See Chapter 13 Quick Quiz: Congenital Infections, Helpful Tip*	196	C	*See Case 28.6: Helpful Tip*
145	C	*See Chapter 23 Quick Quiz: Sad All the Time*	197	B	*See question 9.4.2*
146	D	*See question 23.6.4*	198	A	*See question 12.2.3*
147	A	*See question 23.6.8*	199	A	*See question 12.19.1*
148	D	*See Chapter 2: Table 2-6A*	200	D	*Never bet against Godzilla*
149	A	*See question 7.10.3: Helpful Tip*			
150	C	*See Chapter 1: Table 1-6*			
151	A	*See question 1.4.2*			
152	D	*See question 1.6.2*			
153	D	*See Chapter 1: Quick Quiz: Orthopedic Emergencies*			
154	B	*See question 15.14.3*			
155	D	*See question 13.2.6: Helpful Tip*			
156	A	*See question 13.2.6*			
157	D	*See question 1.14.4*			
158	C	*See question 3.3.3 and Table 3-1*			
159	A	*See question 3.3.6 and Figure 3-1*			
160	B	*See question 3.11.6*			
161	C	*See Chapter 1: Table 1-1*			
162	C	*See question 25.2.7*			
163	A	*See questions 27.1.1 and 27.1.2*			
164	C	*See question 3.4.1: Helpful Tip*			
165	B	*See Chapter 4: Table 4-2*			
166	B	*See Chapter 4: Quick Quiz: Contrast Allergy*			
167	D	*See question 19.1.4: Helpful Tip*			

BIBLIOGRAPHY

Brunicardi F, Anderson DK, Biliar TR, Dunn DL, Hunter JG, Matthews JB, Pollock RE. eds. *Schwartz's Principles of Surgery.* 10th ed. New York, NY: McGraw-Hill; 2015.

Chaikof EL, Dalman RL, Eskandari MK, et al. The Society for Vascular Surgery practice guidelines on the care of patients with an abdominal aortic aneurysm. *J Vasc Surg.* 2018;67(1):2–77.

Hall JB, Schmidt GA, Kress JP, eds. *Principles of Critical Care.* 4th ed. New York, NY: McGraw-Hill; 2014.

Townsend CM, Beauchamp RD, Evers BM, Mattox KL. eds. *Sabiston Textbook of Surgery: The Biological Basis of Modern Surgical Practice.* 20th ed. Philadelphia, PA: Elsevier Saunders; 2017.

Index

Note: Page numbers followed by f and t indicate figures and tables, respectively.